DeJONG'S
THE NEUROLOGIC
EXAMINATION

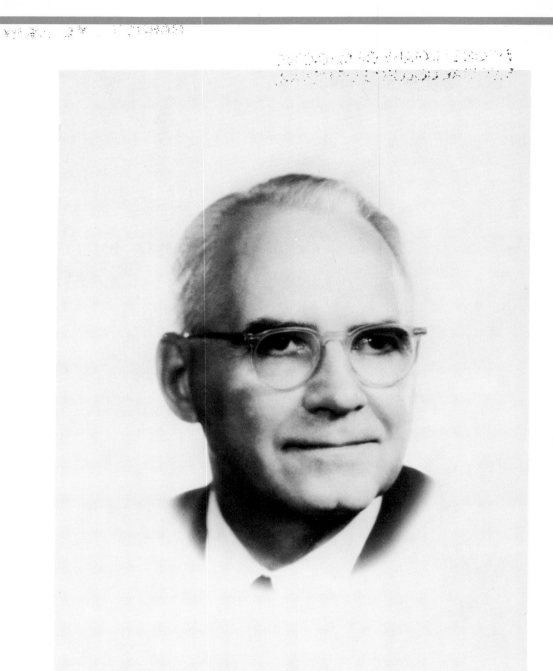

RUSSELL N. DeJONG, MD
1907–1990

DeJONG'S
THE NEUROLOGIC EXAMINATION

REVISED   BY

A.F. Haerer, MD

Professor of Neurology
University of Mississippi Medical Center
Chief of Neurology
United States Veterans Administration Hospital
Jackson, Mississippi

FIFTH EDITION

J.B. LIPPINCOTT COMPANY

PHILADELPHIA   NEW YORK   LONDON   HAGERSTOWN

Sponsoring Editor: Mary K. Smith
Assistant Editor: Anne Geyer
Project Editor: Lorraine D. Smith
Indexer: Anne Cope
Design Coordinator: Kathy Kelley–Luedtke
Interior Designer: Maria Karucinski
Cover Designer: Leslie Foster–Roesler
Production Manager: Helen Ewan
Production Coordinator: Nannette Winski
Compositor: Graphic Sciences Corporation
Printer/Binder: Arcata Graphics/Halliday

5th Edition

6 5 4 3 2 1

Library of Congress Cataloging in Publications Data

Haerer, Armin F., 1934-
    DeJong's The neurologic examination. — 5th. / rev. by
A.F. Haerer.
        p.   cm.
    Re. ed. of: The neurologic examination / Russell N. DeJong. 4th
ed. c1979.
    Includes bibliographical references and index.
    ISBN 0-397-51104-3
    1. Neurologic examination.   2. Nervous system—Diseases-
-Diagnosis.   I. DeJong, Russell N. Neurologic Examination.
II. Title.   III. Title: Neurologic examination.
    [DNLM: 1. Neurologic Examination.   WL 141 H136r]
    RC348.H28   1992
616.8'0475—dc20
DNLM/DLC
for Library of Congress   91-33731
                                                    CIP

The authors and publisher have exerted every effort to ensure
that drug selection and dosage set forth in this text are in
accord with current recommendations and practice at the time
of publication. However, in view of ongoing research, changes
in government regulations, and the constant flow of
information relating to drug therapy and drug reactions, the
reader is urged to check the package insert for each drug for
any change in indications and dosage and for added warnings
and precautions. This is particularly important when the
recommended agent is a new or infrequently employed drug.

PREFACE

Russell N. DeJong maintained a keen interest in neurology long after his retirement. As his vision and his health began to fail, he expressed a desire for a revision of his text, *DeJong's The Neurologic Examination*. The present edition attempts to comply with his wishes to continue to emphasize the importance of the neurologic history and examination in the assessment of patients.

The essentials of the neurologic examination have not changed with time. Dr. DeJong wanted the structure and the bulk of his text to remain unchanged as well. The chapter topics and sequences thus have remained as before. A new section has been added to Chapter 4, while significant deletions of obsolete material were made in the sections dealing with air contrast procedures and related topics. The text has been updated. Some new examination technics have been added. The later chapters, especially, reflect new knowledge and place the neurologic examination in the perspective of the 1990s, with the realization that the newer diagnostic tests and imaging studies have greatly influenced our patient evaluations. Some of the newer concepts of cerebrovascular disease, brain death, infections, and cerebrospinal fluid syndromes, among others, have been incorporated in the text where relevant to the examination phase of neurologic practice. No effort was made to include the vast new information on neurotransmitters, neurochemistry, neurogenetics, and neuroendocrinology in any detail in this discussion of the neurologic examination.

The overall size of this textbook has not changed. Many bibliographic items have been retained, some for their historic interest.

Drs. William Russell and S. H. Subramony kindly supplied the neuroimaging material for inclusion; Dr. Robert Currier gave continuing encouragement. Their help is appreciated.

Dr. DeJong died while this revision was in preparation. It is dedicated to his memory.

AFH, 1992

PREFACE TO THE FIRST EDITION

This volume is a textbook of the fundamentals of neurology and neurologic diagnosis. It has been designed to present, in some detail, the information necessary for a complete neurologic examination. More important, however, is the correlation of clinical neurology with its underlying anatomic and physiologic bases and, consequently, the explanation of neurologic disease by means of changes in nervous structure and function.

The approach to the subject in this textbook differs from that found in most standard texts. No attempt has been made to classify and describe the common neurologic entities or to give detailed accounts of their symptomatology, pathology, etiology, diagnosis, or therapy. Instead, these specific disease pictures are mentioned only as they are related to abnormalities of structure or function of the component portions of the nervous system, and the essentials of differential diagnosis are referred to only in the discussion of the effect of different disease processes upon a specific portion of the nervous system.

An adequate understanding of diseases of the nervous system requires a thorough knowledge of neuroanatomy and neurophysiology and of the effect of disease upon the normal structure and function. In no other field of medicine is there so close a parallel between morphology and physiology on the one hand and pathology and symptomatology on the other. The student of the nervous system must understand the basic laws pertaining to it before he can master the intrinsic aspects of nervous function. He must understand the normal anatomy and physiology in order to comprehend the changes that result from disease. He must understand both the normal and the pathologic in order to evaluate the signs and symptoms, interpret the disease process, and arrive at a diagnosis. Therefore, in dealing with the integral portions of the central and peripheral nervous systems, the anatomy and physiology are first presented and are related to the findings in the normal neurologic examination. Then changes in structure and function are outlined, and these are correlated with abnormalities in the examination. Reliable and standard methods of investigation are stressed, but experimental procedures are also described.

In general, the text follows the lectures on the neurologic examination that are given to junior and senior students in the University of Michigan Medical School. The various diagnostic procedures are described, their application and significance are explained, and abnormal findings are correlated with manifestations of disease. Certain portions of the examination, such as the interpretation of the visual fields, the investigation of vestibular function, and the examination of the autonomic nervous system, are discussed in some detail, even though these are usually performed by specialists in other fields. Their importance in neurologic diagnosis is so great, however, that it is advisable to stress them. The spinal puncture and the examination of the cerebrospinal fluid are included, since these usually constitute a part of the clinical evaluation, but other laboratory and auxiliary studies, such as psychometry, electroencephalography, and neuroroentgenology (including pneumoencephalography, ventriculography, myelography, and arteriography), which may also be essential to neurologic diagnosis, are mentioned only briefly. A complete description of these technics may be found in the many excellent monographs that are available.

It is the author's intent to make this work a practical guide to students and practitioners of medicine in the study of the essentials of the neurologic examination and the fundamentals of clinical neurology. It is designed to fill a need in the medical curriculum and to aid both the undergraduate and the graduate student to understand better the workings of the normal and the diseased nervous system and to correlate didactic lectures with the experience of the clinic. Furthermore, since the nervous system is the integrator and controller of all bodily functions and since knowledge of it is of importance and has implications in all fields of disease, the study of it cannot be separated from the study of other structures and functions with which it is in close relationship, nor can the study of the body as a whole, under either normal or pathologic conditions, be separated from that of the nervous system. Neither can one overlook the interdependence of the study of the nervous system and that of the mind. Consequently, this book should also be of value in general medical diagnosis and of benefit to internists, psychiatrists, and specialists in other fields.

One of the major difficulties that is encountered in any type of writing is the problem of determining how much material to include and how much to exclude. It is important to present all the relevant material that will contribute to the value and comprehensiveness of the work, and omit that which causes confusion, serves to complicate, and adds unnecessary details. There is a great volume of important past and current experimental work in neuroanatomy and neurophysiology, but only that which seems to have a definite clinical application has been included.

The bibliographic references are by no means exhaustive. A list of general references is given at the end of the book. Those at the conclusion of the various chapters or sections are incorporated to give appropriate credit for some of the newer theories and methods of examination, to cite collateral advances, and to mention the original contributions in controversial fields. Although these by no means cover the individual subjects, it is hoped that they may stimulate the reader. In general, only references in the English language have been listed.

I am deeply grateful for the helpful suggestions and criticisms of the many friends and colleagues who have assisted in the preparation of this book. I wish to express special appreciation to Dr. Elizabeth C. Crosby, who read many sections of the manuscript, advised me throughout the writing of the book, and gave me immeasurable assistance; to Dr. Lois A. Gillilan, who acted as assistant, secretary, and artist for a portion of the book; to Dr. Eugene S. McCartney, who read sections of the manuscript and gave much-needed help from an editorial standpoint; to Dr. Edmond L. Cooper, who read and criticized the portions dealing with neuroophthalmology; and to Miss Sue Biethan, who carefully checked all of the references. Individual credit is given to the authors and publishers who allowed me to reproduce illustrations from their books and articles, for which I wish to express my indebtedness at this time. Particular gratitude is due, however, to Miss Janet E. McLaughlin and Mrs. Elizabeth S. Eder, who made most of the original drawings herein contained; to Mr. Charles R. Burd and his assistants, Mrs. M. Rita Eriksen, Mrs. Eloise Duffy Bell, and Mr. Robert P. Logan, who took the original photographs that make an important part of the book; and to Mr. George J. Smith, who made the microphotographs. Dr. Robert Wartenberg was generous in lending not only illustrations from his articles, but also a large collection of valuable reprints of foreign articles. Finally, I wish to thank my secretaries, Mrs. Gertrude B. Null and Mrs. Virginia B. Gross, for their helpful assistance; to acknowledge the aid and cooperation given by my publisher; and to express my appreciation for the assistance rendered by my wife, without whose encouragement, patience, helpful editorial advice, and wise and critical judgment, the manuscript would never have reached completion.

R. N. DeJong
Ann Arbor, Michigan

CONTENTS

DeJONG'S
THE NEUROLOGIC
EXAMINATION

Part A

The Neurologic Examination: Overview, History, and Related Examinations

Chapter 1
INTRODUCTION

The importance of the neurologic examination in the diagnosis of diseases of the nervous system cannot be overemphasized. In no other branch of medicine is it possible to build up a clinical picture so exact with reference to localization and pathologic anatomy as in clinical neurology. To do this, however, one must have not only diagnostic acumen, but also a thorough knowledge of the underlying anatomy and physiology of the voluntary and involuntary (autonomic) nervous systems as well as the vascular supply to them, and of the changes in them that result from pathologic processes. This knowledge must be augmented by a comprehension of the ontogeny and phylogeny of the nervous system, neuropathology, psychology, psychiatry, psychopathology, pharmacology, and the effect of drugs on the normal and diseased nervous systems. Too frequently these subjects are studied individually in the medical curriculum and are separated from one another by long periods of time, but in the examination of the patient they must be synthesized and correlated. Current neurologic science also demands a knowledge of neuroradiology, the various imaging and blood flow procedures, electroencephalography, electromyography, biochemistry, microbiology, genetic principles, neuroendocrinology, neurotransmitters, immunology, epidemiology, and an understanding of the neuromuscular system as well as the nervous system.

The development of ever more sophisticated imaging studies of the nervous system along with many other sensitive laboratory technics has raised questions about the continued need and utility of the neurologic examination in the office or at the bedside. The neurologic examination will not become obsolete. It will not be replaced by mechanical evaluations; rather, a more precise and more directed neurologic examination will be needed in the future. The neurologic (and general) history and examination of the patient will continue to hold supreme importance in his evaluation. Laboratory technics will supplement the physician's observations and guide his reasoning. The neurologist will be the final judge of the significance of his own findings and those of special studies in every instance.

The nervous system is an essential part of the living organism, and neurologic diagnosis is a correlation of data in the study of the human nervous system in health and disease — a synthesis of all the details obtained from the history, examination, and ancillary studies. Nervous tissue, it has been said, makes up about 2% of the human body, yet it is supplied to all portions of the body. Should all the rest of the body tissues be dissolved away, there would remain an immense network of fibers, in addition to the brain, brain stem, and spinal cord. This network is the great receptor, effector, and correlating mechanism of the body. It acts in response to stimuli, acclimates the individual to his environment, and aids in defense against pathologic changes. In order to understand man, one must first understand the nervous system. Since the nervous system governs the mind and mental operations, one cannot study psychology without a knowledge of it.

Since the nervous system regulates and controls all the bodily functions, one cannot study disease of any organ or system of the body without a comprehension of neural function. Since the nervous system relates man to his environment and to others, one cannot study psychiatry or social pathology without first understanding nervous integration. We are not interested, however, in studying the nervous system alone nor primarily in disease, but in studying the person whose nervous system is diseased. We must insist that more important than the precise diagnosis of the case is its formulation in terms of the relationship of the individual to his disease and the relationship of the patient to his associates and his environment. If we bear this in mind, we can most effectively aid our patient, treat his illnesses, restore him to health, reestablish his personal equilibrium, and aid him to regain his place in society.

The problem of the neurologic diagnosis is often considered to be a difficult one by the physician who does not specialize in clinical neurology. Most parts of the nervous system are inaccessible to direct examination, and its intricate organization and integrated functions are difficult to comprehend on superficial observation. Many practitioners are of the opinion that all neurologic matters belong to the realm of the specialist, and, consequently, they make little attempt at the diagnosis of nervous disease. This impression is far from correct, for many neurologic disorders come within the everyday experience of most practitioners, who should know how to examine the nervous system, when additional studies might be helpful, and how to use the data collected. Furthermore, as will be stressed in Chapter 3, many systemic diseases may show evidence of nervous dysfunction as their first manifestations. Medical diagnosis cannot be made without some knowledge of neurologic diagnosis. There are certain rare conditions and diagnostic problems, it is true, that require long experience in the field of diseases of the nervous system for adequate appraisal, but the majority of the more common neurologic entities could and should be diagnosed and treated by the physician in general practice. It is hoped that this book will help the practitioner and the student to understand nervous function as a whole, and to appreciate the fact that not all neurologic questions are complex and esoteric, but that an understanding of certain fundamentals is necessary.

It should be emphasized, however, that there are certain complexities of nervous dysfunction that must be comprehended for critical evaluation of signs and symptoms. For instance, in pathologic neurophysiology one finds manifestations of destruction, release, irritation, and partial assumption of function by healthy tissues. Symptoms and signs of destruction result from a transient or permanent loss of function due to disease of a part; these are similar to the manifestations of disease that may be found in other systems of the body. If a nerve is injured, its continuity is interrupted and it no longer carries sensory and motor impulses or participates in trophic function and reflex action; as a consequence there is paralysis (loss of power), with anesthesia and areflexia in the distribution of the nerve. If an area in the cerebral cortex is destroyed, certain functions are lost, and paresis, hypesthesia, blindness, or intellectual loss may follow. The symptoms of release are somewhat more difficult to comprehend. Certain portions of the nervous system have a function of inhibition. When these areas are destroyed, there is an exaggeration of response owing to the loss of this inhibitory function and the release of intact centers from higher control. Such a phenomenon occurs to some extent in the presence of a lesion of the corticospinal system which is followed by increase in tone, increase in reflexes, and the presence of certain pathologic reflexes. These are positive rather than negative signs of disturbed function.

Positive signs are apparent in a different manner in the presence of **irritation,** or **excitation,** of a part of the nervous system. Here there is increased activity as a result of response to stimulation. The most characteristic examples of this are the pain and muscle spasm that follow disease of a peripheral nerve, and the so-called jacksonian convulsions in which signs of increased motor activity appear on one side of the body with irritation of the motor cortex.

In addition to these manifestations of destruction, release, and irritation, there may be **partial assumption of function by healthy tissues** to compensate for impairment or loss of function due to disease in another part. The destruction of one area may be followed by disruption of the nervous connections to neighboring or distant areas. There is, however, a certain amount of overlapping and duplication of function in the nervous system, and an intact center, nerve, or muscle may assume some of the physiologic activity of a diseased part. Furthermore, certain areas may be supplied with an overabundance of cells, so that a lesion in these sites, unless it is extensive, may be followed by a minimum of signs and symptoms. In parts of the nervous system, for instance, extensive lesions may be present without causing signs or symptoms, owing to a minimum of physiologic activity of the part, duplication of function, or compensatory activity elsewhere. For these many reasons neurologic diagnosis may present pitfalls.

The neurologic examination requires skill, intelligence, and patience. It requires accurate and trained observation, together with, in most instances, the help and cooperation of the patient. It must be carried out in an orderly manner if it is to be complete, and time and attention are necessary if the details are to be elicited. Each clinician eventually works out his own method, based on his personal experiences, but the student should make it an invariable rule to follow a fixed and systematic routine in every examination, at least until he is very familiar with the subject. Premature attempts to abbreviate the examination will result in costly errors of omission. A systematic approach is more essential in neurology than in any other field of medicine, for the multiplicity of signs and variations in interpretation may prove confusing. The specific order that is followed in the examination is not as important as the persistence with which one adheres to this order. The procedure herein outlined starts with the neurologic history and the physical and mental appraisals. In dealing with the neurologic examination *per se*, the sensory system is taken up first, because of the need for the patient's alertness in the sensory evaluation. Next the cranial nerves are investigated in sequence, followed by the motor system with all of its ramifications, including coordination, station, and gait. Since the reflexes depend upon the intergrity of both the motor and sensory functions, they are examined after the motor system. Then the autonomic nervous system, peripheral nerve and spinal cord localization, and cerebral localization are considered individually. Finally the investigation of special conditions (coma, hysteria, etc.) and the examination of the cerebrospinal fluid are undertaken.

It may, however, be necessary on occasion to vary the sequence of the tests or to modify them according to the state of the patient and the nature of his illness. Under certain circumstances, as in Parkinson's disease and chorea, it may be possible to make a diagnosis at a glance, but no neurologic examination — and this is especially true for the student — can be considered to be satisfactory unless it is complete. There should be no attempt to arrive at conclusions before the examination is finished. If the investigation is long and the patient's interest flags, or if he fails to understand the significance of and the need

for cooperating in diagnostic procedures whose purpose is not apparent or that seem to be unrelated to his presenting complaints, it may be well to explain the tests or their results to him, or to use other means to stimulate his interest and cooperation. On the other hand, if fatigue and lack of attention interfere with the results, it may be advisable to change the order of the examination or to complete it at a later date. Uniformity of procedure, however, greatly facilitates subsequent analysis of case records. The chief causes for incorrect diagnoses are insufficient examination, inaccurate observations, and, less commonly, false conclusions from correct and sufficient facts. More errors result from the omission of a part of the examination than from a misinterpretation of findings. It is important to bear in mind, however, that slight deviations from the normal may be as significant as more pronounced changes, and absence of certain signs may be as significant as their presence. On occasion clues may be obtained merely by watching the patient perform normal, routine, or "casual" actions, such as to dress or undress himself, tie his shoelaces, look about the room, or walk into the examining room. Abnormalities in carrying out these actions may point to disorders that might be missed in the more formal examination. The patient's attitude, facial expression, mode of reaction to questions, motor activity, and speech should all be noted.

Interpretation and judgment are also of extreme importance for evaluation and appraisal, and the ability to interpret neurologic signs can be gained only by carrying out repeated thorough and detailed examinations, and by keen and accurate observation. In the interpretation of a reflex, for instance, or in the appraisal of tone or of changes in sensation, differences of opinion may be evident. The only way in which the observer may become sure of his judgment is by experience, so that he may be certain of what is normal and of any variation from it. It must be borne in mind, however, that the personal equation may enter into any situation, and that conclusions may vary. The important factor is not a seemingly quantitative evaluation of the findings, but an interpretation or appraisal of the situation as a whole.

The use of a printed outline or form with a checklist for recording the essentials of both the history and the neurologic examination is advocated by some authorities and in some clinics. With such an outline various items can be underlined, circled, or checked as being either positive or negative, and numerical designations can be used to record such factors as the degree of activity of the reflexes or an approximate quantitation of motor strength. Such forms may serve as teaching exercises for the student or novice and as time-saving devices for the clinician, but they cannot replace a careful narrative description of the results of the examination. An outline of the major divisions of the neurologic examination is given in Chapter 4.

Neurologic diagnosis is a deductive process and is reached by a synthesis of all the details from the history, the examination, and laboratory studies. The physician must observe the findings, correlate and interpret them, and record them systematically. A conclusive diagnosis may have to await the results of laboratory tests or even therapeutic trials. On occasion, changes in the clinical state and either the development of new signs and symptoms or the disappearance of manifestations may alter the impression. Inexperienced physicians will need to learn when extended observation can help with neurologic diagnosis, as opposed to a flurry of laboratory tests.

The first step of the neurologic evaluation should be to determine whether an organic lesion of the nervous system exists; it may be a **focal lesion** with injury to all tissues within it regardless of their structures or functions, a **diffuse disease** with incomplete involvement in which some nerve cells and fibers suffer more than others, or a **systemic affection** in which only anatomically and functionally related systems of cells or fibers are involved. Secondly, an attempt should be made to localize the lesion with reference to the cell structures, nerve fibers, or tracts involved. The symptoms and signs may be primary ones, correlated directly with focal structural disease or local disorders of function, or secondary (indirect) manifestations, due to release from the inhibition that is normally exerted by the injured parts or the result of disordered reactions or disintegration of the physiologic mechanisms of the part injured. Then the nature and etiology of the lesion should be decided by interpreting symptoms and signs in terms of disordered function. When this information is available, a study can be made of the symptomatology of the disease process as a whole — the morbid phenomena, the pathologic anatomy and physiology. Finally, diagnosis having been made by distinguishing the pathologic process and differentiating it from similar processes, treatment, prognosis, and, in certain instances, epidemiology and prophylaxis may be determined. It does not matter whether the disease

process is secondary to disturbances of development, infection, toxic factors, trauma, neoplasia, vascular change, degeneration, or the aging process; in all, the essentials of diagnosis are the same.

No other branch of medicine lends itself so well to the correlation of signs and symptoms with diseased structure as does neurology, but it is only by means of a systematic examination and an accurate appraisal that one can elicit and properly interpret one's findings. Some individuals have a keen intuitive diagnostic sense and can reach correct conclusions by shorter routes, but in most instances the recognition of disease states can be accomplished only through a scientific discipline based on repeated practical examinations. Diagnosis alone, however, should not be considered the ultimate objective of the examination, but diagnostic investigations make up the first step toward treatment and toward attempts to help the patient.

Quantitative evaluation of neurologic abnormalities may be used for the accurate determination of a patient's clinical status, the study of the natural history of disease, and the measurement of response to either medical or surgical treatment. Such quantitative testing can be carried out for the appraisal of certain types of sensory and motor deficits, abnormal movements, reflex responses, and other functions and disturbances of function. It often, however, requires extensive instrumentation, and in the past has been carried out mainly for experimental purposes. There is a renewed interest in such testing, principally for the evaluation of response to various therapeutic regimens. References to such testing are given in chapters where they are applicable.

Ancillary diagnostic technics have, through the years, played important roles in neurologic diagnosis. The original electrodiagnostic technics of Duchenne, Erb, and others were introduced in the latter part of the nineteenth century. In this century neurologic diagnosis has been aided by the introduction of pneumoencephalography, ventriculography, myelography, electroencephalography, evoked potential studies, Doppler blood flow studies, angiography, electromyography, nerve conduction studies, radioisotope scanning, computed tomography, magnetic resonance imaging, blood flow studies by single photon emission computed tomography and inhalation methods, positron emission tomography, and others. There are excellent textbooks and research publications available dealing with each of these. Each is an individualized and specialized technic, usually carried out in a particular laboratory and by a person with specialized training. This book deals with the examination of the patient by the physician; therefore, it is felt that these other methods of examination are only of peripheral interest to it, and will be referred to but not described in detail. It is true that the methods for the electrical testing of nerves and muscles were described in the first three editions. However, owing to the specialization of these technics and the development of many additional ones they are now omitted and the reader is referred to textbooks dealing directly with them. Recent developments in internal medicine, immunology, epidemiology, genetics, and related fields, especially as they apply to metabolic processes affecting neural structures, will also be referred to in the book. Some of the newer laboratory procedures dealing with them will be mentioned, but no description of the technics will be given.

The new technics of imaging and the other laboratory studies alluded to above have indeed revolutionized the practice of neurology. However, their use must be integrated with the findings by history and neurologic examination.

The practice of "shot-gunning" the patient with laboratory tests is to be discouraged; it may even be dangerous at times. Such studies do not replace the examination. While often helpful and even essential, they may mislead the physician. By way of a few examples, it may be stated that imaging studies of the brain can be normal for variable times after the onset of an acute process; they may show incidental (or silent) lesions unrelated to the situation in question; they usually do not display the entire area of cerebral dysfunction; interictal electroencephalograms may be normal in epileptics; electromyographic changes may not manifest for 2 – 3 weeks after denervation; Doppler studies may insonate the wrong vessel; injection of contrast material for myelography may enter the subdural space instead of the subarachnoid area, and so forth.

BIBLIOGRAPHY

Ziegler DK. Is the neurologic examination becoming obsolete? Neurology 1985;35:559

Chapter 2

THE NEUROLOGIC HISTORY

A good clinical history often holds the key to diagnosis. This is true in the medical history, surgical history, and psychiatric history. It is especially true in the neurologic history, where a carefully obtained, properly analyzed, detailed account of the patient's symptoms, past and present, may lead to an accurate discernment of the nature and location of the disease process. A skillfully taken history, with a careful analysis of the chief complaints and of the course of the illness, will very frequently indicate the probable diagnosis, even before physical, neurologic, and laboratory examinations are carried out. In many instances the physician can learn more from what the patient says and how he says it than from any other avenue of inquiry. Every neurologic examination must be preceded by an accurate anamnesis if it is possible to obtain one. Many errors in diagnosis are due to incomplete or inaccurate histories. In certain disorders, some of which are common, the history is the only avenue available to arrive at a diagnosis, as the examination and laboratory studies are normal. Most persons with recurring headaches fall into this category, as do some with dizziness, sleep disorders, and episodic loss of consciousness.

The principal objective of the history is, of course, to acquire pertinent clinical data that will lead to a correct analysis of the patient's illness. Herein one elicits the **symptoms,** the subjective manifestations of disease as related by the patient, in contrast to the **signs,** the objective manifestations, which are revealed in the physical, the neurologic, and the laboratory examinations. Many dysfunctions of the nervous system are largely subjective without visible or outward signs of disease, and we can learn of their nature and course only by description. The information obtained in the history is not only essential to the diagnosis of the disease from which the patient is suffering, but is also valuable in the proper understanding of the patient as an individual and of his relationship to himself, to his disease, and to others. The elicited data become a permanent record which may be referred to from time to time during improvement or progression of the disease.

POINTS IN TAKING THE HISTORY

The taking of the history is no simple task. It may require greater skill and experience than are necessary to carry out a detailed examination. Time, diplomacy, kindness, patience, reserve, and a manner which conveys interest, understanding, and sympathy are all essential. The history is obtained most satisfactorily if the physician presents a friendly and courteous attitude, centers all his attention on the patient, appears anxious to help, words his questions tactfully, and asks them in a conversational tone. The mode of questioning may vary with the age and educational and cultural background of the patient. The physician should meet the patient on a common ground of language and vocabulary, and resort to the vernacular if necessary. The history is best taken in privacy, with the patient comfortable and at ease. An appearance of haste should be avoided. The method of questioning may vary from patient to patient, but the use of a regular order for recording the details is of value both in ensuring completeness and in facilitating future reference. One should never attempt, however, to elicit a history by following a stereotyped form or by repeating a memorized list of questions to each of which a specific answer is expected. No mechanical measures can take the place of a careful consideration of the patient's complaints. The reliability of the information obtained may depend largely upon the intuition of the physician and his ability to analyze and interpret the symptoms and to appraise the thoughts and personality of the patient. By following these precepts a favorable patient-physician relationship may be developed; the physician may acquire empathy for the patient and enter into his feelings or experiences, and rapport may be established, based on the confidence of the patient in the physician.

The history should be recorded clearly and concisely, in a logical, well-organized manner. It can never be sufficiently complete, and no symptom may be left unanalyzed. Each statement must be considered in its relationship to the whole. It is important, however, to stress the more significant manifestations, and to keep irrelevancies at a minimum; the essential factual material must be separated from the extraneous matter. Diagnosis involves the careful sifting of evidence, and the art of selecting and emphasizing the pertinent data may make it possible to arrive at a correct conclusion in a seemingly complicated case. It may be of value to record negative as well as positive statements, so that later examiners may know that the historian inquired into and did not overlook certain aspects of the disease.

The essentials of the history should be obtained from the patient himself, if at all possible. He must be encouraged to give a detailed account of his illness in his own words. The observer should intervene as little as possible, and only to exclude obviously irrelevant material, to obtain amplification on statements which seem vague or incomplete, or to lead the story into directions in which useful information may be obtained. Rarely, however, is the patient's narrative complete enough to be of value in diagnosis. It is the exceptional patient who recalls all the particulars of his illness and repeats them in an accurate, chronologic order without confusing symptoms and his interpretation of symptoms. Furthermore, if his mind is focused on a particular manifestation, he may fail to mention others of equal importance. Consequently, it is usually necessary to augment the patient's account by means of suitable questions, and often to do so

in great detail regarding specific factors, many of which he may not relate to his present condition, but the presence or absence of which may be of significance. The importance of an accurate and detailed record of events in cases involving compensation and medicolegal problems cannot be overemphasized. The patient should be allowed to use his own words, and any suggestion of symptoms or diagnoses should be avoided. The latter must be borne in mind especially in obtaining histories from overly suggestible and hypochondriacal patients. It may be necessary, however, to attempt to determine the precise meaning which the patient attaches to the words he employs, as ambiguity of language may make it difficult for the physician to interpret the exact significance of the symptoms described.

Special consideration may have to be used in taking the history of certain types of individuals. The timid, inarticulate, or worried patient may have to be helped by means of sympathetic questions or reassuring comments. The garrulous person may have to be stopped from losing himself in a mass of irrelevant detail. The evasive or undependable patient may have to be questioned more searchingly. The fearful, antagonistic, or paranoid patient may have to be questioned guardedly lest one arouse his fears or suspicions. The person with multiple or vague complaints may have to be held down to specificities. The elated patient may minimize or neglect his symptoms; the depressed or anxious patient may exaggerate them, and the excitable or hypochondriacal person may be overconcerned about them and describe them at length. Apprehension may impair logic. One must remember that the range of individual variations is wide, and this must be taken into account in appraising symptoms. What is pain to the sensitive, nervous, or exhausted patient may be but a minor discomfort to another. A blasé attitude, or seeming indifference may indicate a pathologic euphoria in one individual, but it may be a defense reaction in another. One person may take offense at questions which another would consider commonplace. Even in a single individual such factors as fatigue, pain, emotional conflicts, or diurnal fluctuations in mood or temperament may cause a wide range of variation in response to questions.

During the taking of the history the examiner has an unequaled opportunity to study the patient — his manner, attitude, behavior, and emotional reactions. The tone of voice, the bearing, the expression of the eyes, the swift play of facial muscles, the appearance of weeping or smiling, or the presence of pallor, blushing, sweating, patches of erythema on the neck, furrowing of the brows, drawing of the lips, clenching of the teeth, dilation of the pupils, or rigidity of the muscles may give information of great importance. Gesticulations, restlessness, delay, hesitancy, and the relation of demeanor and emotional responses to descriptions of symptoms or to details in the family or marital history should all be noted and recorded. These and his mode of response to the questions that are asked of him are of immeasurable value in the estimate of his character, personality, and emotional state. The manner of presenting his history may also give information with reference to the intelligence, powers of observation, attention, and memory of the patient. The examiner must, of course, be careful not to make a mental diagnosis of the patient's illness immediately upon meeting him, for some individuals are quick to sense and resent a physician's preconceived ideas about their symptoms. On the other hand, the patient's preconceived ideas should not alter the physician's interpretation of his symptoms, past or present.

The patient's story may not at all times be correct or complete. He may not possess full or detailed information regarding his illness; he may be misinterpreting his symptoms or giving someone else's interpretation of them; he may be wishfully altering or withholding information or may even be deliberately prevaricating for some purpose; he may be a phlegmatic, insensitive individual who does not comprehend the significance of his symptoms; he may be a garrulous person who cannot give a relevant or coherent story; he may have multiple or vague complaints which cannot be readily articulated. It may be necessary to ask for more historical details, or for confirmation of certain items on a later occasion. Infants, young children, comatose or confused patients obviously may be unable to give any history. Those who are in pain or distress, have difficulty with speech or expression, are of low intelligence, or are unable to speak the examiner's language may not be able to give a satisfactory history for themselves. Consequently, it may be necessary on many occasions to corroborate or supplement the history given by the patient with one given by an observer, relative, or friend, or even to obtain the entire history from someone else. Members of the family may also be able to give important information about changes in behavior, memory, hearing, vision, speech, or coordination of which the patient may not be aware. Under most

circumstances it is necessary to question both the patient and others in order to obtain a complete account of the illness. Data from earlier examinations and previous medical records should also be abstracted and added to the history.

The importance of the clinical history cannot be overemphasized. History taking is an art; it can be learned partly through reading and study, but it is completely acquired only through experience and repeated trials. The ability to elicit a satisfactory anamnesis is one of the prime requisites to neurologic diagnosis.

GENERAL OUTLINE OF THE HISTORY

The neurologic history, as is true of all clinical histories, usually starts with certain statistical data. These include the patient's name, sex, age, date and place of birth, residence, marital status, and handedness. Under certain circumstances it may be necessary to inquire about nationality, race, and religion.

Then one records the patient's major, or presenting, complaint. This is followed by a detailed description of the symptoms and course of the present illness, including a chronologic account of its development. The past medical history is then outlined. Herein are listed the following: a record of serious illnesses, operations, and injuries; known allergies or adverse reactions to drugs or treatments; a history of the birth and early development; a detailed account of symptoms referable to the various organs and systems of the body; the marital history; the occupational and educational history; a record of personal habits; and a personality inventory with history of adjustment to family, school, marriage, work, and community. The family history concludes the anamnesis.

THE PRESENTING COMPLAINT AND THE PRESENT ILLNESS

It is important to have the patient relate the presenting complaint or complaints in detail, because these are the symptoms for which help is being sought, and relief from them is the objective of treatment. The patient should give his complaints in his own words and as completely as possible. The examiner should record them as given and not in terms which he believes to be more descriptive scientifically. The physician, however, must clearly understand what the patient means by the terms that he uses; for instance, the expression "kidney trouble" may be used to indicate urinary incontinence, or "dizziness" to signify giddiness, unsteadiness, confusion, vertigo, and blackouts.

In obtaining the history of the present illness, each symptom is described and expanded. The historian should draw out the chronologic occurrence of each manifestation with the character, exact date and mode of onset, apparent precipitating or etiologic factors, duration, treatment, and progression or regression of each symptom. Statements are obtained regarding the stationary, remittent, intermittent, progressive, or regressive character of the illness, including circumstances which alleviate or increase the complaint, and seasonal, diurnal, and nocturnal variations. Trauma, for instance, and cerebrovascular accidents have an abrupt onset followed by general improvement which terminates in either complete recovery or stable incomplete resolution. Tumors and chronic progressive degenerative diseases have a gradual onset of symptoms. With certain neoplasms, however, hemorrhage may cause sudden onset or exacerbations. Multiple sclerosis is most often characterized by remissions and exacerbations, but with a progressive increase in the severity of symptoms; stationary, intermittent, and progressive varieties of multiple sclerosis are also encountered. Infections usually have a relatively sudden, but not precipitous, onset followed by gradual improvement, and either complete or incomplete recovery.

In many conditions symptoms may appear some time before striking physical signs of disease are evident, and before laboratory tests are useful in detecting disordered physiology. It is important to know when the patient last considered himself to be well, when he had to stop work, and when he was forced to take to his bed. A history of previous manifestations of the present symptoms, past evidences of disease which might in any way be related to the present disorder, and any physical illness, activity, trauma, emotional conflict, etc., which had any temporal relationship to the onset of symptoms or to remissions or exacerbations should be elicited, even though the physician may not believe an etiologic relationship exists. One must attempt to determine how disabling the illness is and what crystallized the patient's decision to undergo the examination just when he did. The social, environmental, and economic factors, including the patient's reaction to his illness and the reactions to his family and his employer,

may be of significance. Of equal importance is information regarding previous examinations and diagnoses and the patient's reaction to them, as well as his response to prior therapeutic regimens.

To illustrate the need for specific and detailed questioning, the convulsive disorder, one of the more common manifestations of disease seen in the neurologic clinic, may be taken as an example. The patient himself may feel that it is sufficient to state that he has "attacks," but inasmuch as convulsive seizures may be manifestations of such varying classes of nervous system and systemic diseases as inflammation, infections, toxemias, degenerations, neoplasms, and metabolic disorders, it is extremely important to question the patient in detail, and to question observers. The patient himself may be unconscious during the spell and may not be aware of its characteristics, he may withhold or alter information, or the relatives may withhold information from the patient.

In the first place, the presenting complaint may vary in individuals. One patient may say that he has "epilepsy," another may complain of "convulsions," another of "fits," "spells," "fainting attacks," "lapses," "seizures," or "falling spells." Some of these may be accurate so far as the patient knows, whereas others may be euphemisms to hide the true nature of the disorder.

Once the examiner has received the information that the patient is suffering from a convulsive disorder, he must obtain an adequate, detailed description of the manifestations of the individual attack in the order of occurrence. This is necessary for adequate diagnosis and interpretation, for differentiation between organic and hysterical attacks, for localization in the event of focal brain disease, and for information relative to possible therapeutic measures. First, one questions the patient regarding **precipitating factors** and the **aura,** or premonition of the attacks. "Have you any warning that an attack is imminent? If so, what are its nature and duration?" The aura may not be of localizing value. It may be described as a sensation of apprehension or anxiety, a queer feeling in the stomach, a pain in the stomach, a headache, or an increased frequency of small attacks. The aura, however, is often of localizing value, especially if it consists of auditory hallucinations or tinnitus, vertigo, visual illusions or hallucinations, an unusual odor or taste, or a recurring thought or memory. Of great localizing value are such manifestations as stuttering, aphasia, and numbness, tingling, or motor phenomena in one part of the body. In the presence of the latter one should elicit the area of onset, mode of extension, severity, and duration. In addition to asking the patient whether he himself is aware of such an approaching attack, he is asked whether observers can predict one, since they often become aware of an impending attack by noting flushing, pallor, sweating, staring, interruption of speech, confusion of thinking and speech, unusual sucking or swallowing movements, or sucking of the lips.

After information is obtained with reference to the aura, an adequate description of the attack itself is obtained. During the seizure the patient may be either flaccid or rigid, and either akinetic or hyperkinetic; movements may be either focal or generalized. Any localization of motor manifestations, either tonic or clonic, such as turning of the eyes, the head, the eyes and head, or the entire body to one side, either at the beginning or during the attack, may be of significance. The patient is asked whether he consistently falls to one side during attacks, or whether one arm, leg, hand, foot, or one side of the face moves before the other, and the nature of the movements and their duration and sequence. It is important to know whether the movements are bizarre and purposeless, or coordinated and purposeful, and directed toward persons or objects; fighting, kicking, and resistance to examination may suggest a nonorganic basis for the attacks, although such features may also be present in organic attacks. The automatisms of complex partial seizures are often seemingly purposeful. One should inquire whether there is amnesia or loss of consciousness during attacks, how deep the loss of consciousness is, whether it comes on gradually or suddenly, and how long it lasts. The presence of a cry at the onset of the attack or during it, flushing, cyanosis or pallor, incontinence of urine or feces, and frothing at the mouth may give relevant information, as may injury to the body during the attack, biting of the tongue, and chewing of the lips.

The postconvulsion manifestations are next investigated. The patient is asked whether he regains consciousness immediately and, if he does, how he feels, and whether he notices fatigue, sleepiness, confusion, or muscular soreness. He is asked whether there is weakness of any part of the body, such as the face, arm, or leg, and how long this weakness lasts; whether there is any unusual feeling in any part of the body, such as numbness, deadness, or tingling; whether there are nausea and vomiting or localized headache; whether speech is disturbed, and whether there

is partial or complete amnesia for the attack. If there is any difference in behavior after an attack, its nature and duration should be noted.

After an adequate description of the individual attack has been obtained, one inquires about the chronology of the disorder. It is important to know the age of the patient at the time of his first attack; the frequency of seizures and variations in their character; the relationship to rest, activity, sleep, emotional stress, irritability, presence of other people, and meals; the time of occurrence during the day or night and any relationship to the menstrual cycle. The birth history and the presence of convulsions immediately following birth or in infancy may be important, as may information about breath-holding attacks, dizzy or fainting spells, twitching of the muscles, brief periods of staring or confusion, temper tantrums, automatisms or episodic bizarre behavior, or recurring bouts of headache or abdominal pain. A detailed history should be obtained of any injury or illness preceding the onset of the attacks, especially trauma to the head, or a possible encephalitis or meningitis. The relationship to toxins and infections must always be borne in mind. Of importance, likewise, is information regarding previous diagnoses and the patient's reaction to them, and the response of the disorder to various therapeutic endeavors.

The convulsive attack is but one illustration of the diseases encountered in neurologic practice. An equally detailed description is obtained of every symptom and illness. In headaches, for instance, an accurate picture of the symptom may be of great help in diagnosis. A headache is a type of pain, and, consequently, is entirely subjective. One should determine whether the pain is localized or general, regional or diffuse, unilateral or bilateral, or bandlike. If it is localized, it is well to inquire whether it is frontal, occipital, temporal, or at the vertex, and whether there is localized tenderness. The character is also important—whether it is dull, aching, steady, throbbing, boring, burning, griping, sharp, lancinating, constricting, intermittent, continuous, or paroxysmal. One may have difficulty in evaluating its intensity, but may obtain indirect information by determining whether it is incapacitating and interferes with work or sleep, or can be endured, and whether it increases or lessens with activity or inactivity. The incidence, mode of onset, duration, frequency, periodicity of occurrence, time interval during the day or month, seasonal appearance, and the relationship to food, movement, exercise, position, coughing, mental effort, use of the eyes, emotional stress and strain, changes in mood, rest, and sleep are of importance, as are the mode of cessation and the response to special therapeutic or prophylactic measures. Finally, the presence of various associated phenomena such as nausea or vomiting, scotomas, diplopia, blurring vision, hemianopia, hyperacusis, hyperosmia, photophobia, tenderness, syncope, vertigo, aphasia, drowsiness, convulsions, or fever may be of diagnostic significance.

Similar information is obtained in every instance of pain or disturbance of sensation such as numbness, paresthesias, itching, tingling, or burning. One inquires about the location and distribution, including depth from the surface, radiation, extent of diffusion, and paths of reference; the mode of onset; the character; the severity; the relation to rest, position, motion, and sleep; the incidence, duration, and frequency or periodicity; aggravating factors; localized tenderness; muscle rigidity and spasm; associated symptoms, and finally, the method of alleviation.

In the narration of the present illness the patient may have disregarded certain data which have a distinct bearing on the present symptoms. Therefore, it is very important to record all pertinent facts, especially those dealing with disease of the nervous system. In addition to convulsions, headaches, pains, and paresthesias, the following should be stressed:

Motor Disturbances. If there is a history of paralysis, paresis, atrophy, or ataxia, one determines the time and mode of onset, location, severity, type, and progression or improvement. If there have been hyperkinetic manifestations, one ascertains their type or nature, location, onset, duration, amplitude, frequency, and exciting factors. Inquiry should also be made regarding weakness, fatigue, stiffness, and abnormalities of tone, clumsiness, stumbling, staggering, and disturbances of equilibrium. Response to attempted treatment should be noted.

Vertigo. Vertigo, giddiness, "dizziness," lightheadedness, and subjective and objective vertigo should be differentiated. If these are present, it is important to determine their nature, mode of onset, duration, frequency, severity, direction, and relationship to posture or change of position, and to inquire about the presence and laterality of associated symptoms such as staggering or falling. In organic vertigo there is usually a sense of rotation, either of the individual or of

the environment, and this may be accompanied by nausea, vomiting, deafness, tinnitus, perspiration, and prostration.

Visual Disturbances. Dimness or blurring of vision, scotomas, diplopia, transient blindness in one or both eyes, hemianopic defects in the visual fields, and formed or unformed visual hallucinations may be significant.

Auditory Disturbances. Tinnitus, deafness, and auditory hallucinations indicate cochlear nerve involvement; with abnormalitites of vestibular function there may be vertigo, unsteadiness, and disturbances of equilibrium.

Other Cranial Nerve Manifestations. These may include dysfunctions of smell, taste, salivation, and lacrimation; numbness or paralysis of the face; dysarthria; dysphagia for liquids or solids; and regurgitation.

Disturbances of Communication, Speech, or Expression. Abnormalities of speech, writing, and drawing, and of comprehension of spoken or written words or gestures should be noted.

Disturbances in Sleep Rhythm or State of Consciousness. A history of drowsiness, hypersomnia, attacks of uncontrollable sleep, insomnia, inversion of the sleep cycle, confusion, delirium, stupor, and coma may give diagnostic information.

Visceral Symptoms. Dysfunction of the autonomic nervous system may be indicated by changes in thirst, appetite, and elimination. Other important visceral symptoms include vomiting, which may or may not be projectile or accompanied by nausea; diarrhea and constipation; urinary symptoms including retention, frequency, urgency, dysuria, precipitancy, and incontinence; changes in potency or libido; sweating, flushing, and vasomotor disturbances.

Mental Symptoms. It is important to determine whether there is a history of delirium, confusion, personality change, memory difficulties, anxieties, nervous tension, alcoholism, abuse of street or prescription drugs, delinquency or misdemeanors, and "nervous breakdown."

If any of the aforementioned have been present, one should obtain exact data on the onset, nature, frequency, description, duration, progression or improvement, and degree of incapacity. It may be necessary to interrogate the patient in detail regarding symptoms and systems which apparently are not related to the present disorder. If there is a history of trauma to the head, one should inquire regarding loss of consciousness and its duration, confusion, disorientation, convulsions, amnesia (retrograde and anterograde), bleeding from the nose or ears, cerebrospinal fluid rhinorrhea, headaches, memory loss, and personality change. In all cases in which trauma plays a part the details of the accident must always be recorded, along with independent information from observers if it is possible to obtain it. One should get independent testimony in all instances in which industrial hazards or toxins or conduct disorders play a part and in those cases with possible forensic or medicolegal aspects.

THE PAST MEDICAL HISTORY

A history or an examination that is directed exclusively toward the central nervous system is incomplete. It may seem irrelevant at times to follow the history of the present illness with a detailed medical history. The nervous system, however, is but one part of the body, and neurologic manifestations or complications are frequently the first clinical evidence of serious systemic disease. In pernicious anemia and other blood dyscrasias, diabetes, syphilis, subacute bacterial endocarditis, hypertension, atherosclerosis, tuberculosis, acute infections, acquired immune deficiency syndrome, metabolic disorders, undulant fever, toxemias, and even in neoplasms in distant portions of the body, nervous system manifestations may be evident before one observes other signs or symptoms of the disease. Furthermore, the nervous system, through the central control of visceral function and through its autonomic division, is important in the regulation of heart rate, blood pressure, respiration, gastrointestinal function, and bladder control. Visceral dysfunction, either organic or psychogenic, may be of nervous system origin. For these and other reasons, the medical history should be detailed and complete.

First, the general health prior to the onset of the present illness is recorded, then a history of the past illnesses, operations, and accidents or injuries is obtained, with the date and nature of each, period of incapacitation, and sequelae. Information should be obtained about prior illnesses of all types and all hospitalizations, but often it is necessary to be somewhat skeptical in accepting previous diagnoses and to inquire instead about the symptoms and manifestations of the disease. In recording operations and injuries one should list the type of anesthetic used, the complications, the need for blood transfusions, and the end results. The patient is also questioned about his susceptibility to disease, his reactions to illnesses, operations, and injuries, and any known allergies or adverse reactions to drugs.

The history of the patient's birth and early development includes the following: the health of the mother during pregnancy, including vomiting, hypertension, eclampsia, and viral illnesses such as rubella; the possibility of Rh incompatibility of the parents; their age at the time of the patient's birth; the duration of gestation; any abnormalities of labor and delivery, such as prolonged labor, instrumental delivery, or precipitate birth; the type of anesthesia used for delivery; birth trauma; postnatal cyanosis, icterus, paralysis, or convulsions; birth weight; difficulty with respirations or with feeding after birth; health during infancy, with mode of feeding and gain of weight; age of weaning, dentition, holding head erect, sitting alone, standing, walking, talking, and development of toilet habits; the presence of delirium, "spasms," or convulsions with febrile states; handedness and possible shift of handedness; learning ability; mental characteristics, such as brightness and good nature, irritability, nervousness, peevishness, dullness, or timidity; habits and so-called neuropathic traits, such as enuresis, thumb sucking, somnambulism, nail biting, temper tantrums, night terrors, childhood fears, tics, and stammering. Not only is the somatic developmental history important, but one must also study the social development, including progress at school and a record of the adjustment of the individual to others and to his environment.

In relating his past illnesses the patient may list only the serious or outstanding ones, and may fail to mention individual symptoms that may be of diagnostic significance. As a consequence, detailed questioning is important in the diagnosis both of systemic and of psychophysiologic illnesses. Symptoms referable to the various *organs and systems* may be investigated by making inquiries about the following specific manifestations and details.

The Eyes. Visual difficulty, the wearing of glasses, the time of the last refraction, changes in vision following refraction, diplopia, blurring, transient blindness in one or both eyes, hemianopic defects, scotomas, pain, asthenopia, swelling, discharge, and inflammation.

The Ears. Hearing, tinnitus, deafness, pain, discharge, paracenteses, and vertigo.

The Nose. Head colds, discharge, allergic rhinitis, artrophic rhinitis, sinus disease, epistaxis, symptoms of obstruction, and olfaction.

The Mouth and Throat. Head colds, tonsillitis, sore throats, quinsy, difficulty in swallowing or talking, hoarseness, sore mouth or gums, the condition of the teeth, care of the teeth, roentgenographic examination of the teeth, and abnormalities of the tongue.

The Cardiorespiratory System. Colds, bronchitis, asthma, dyspnea, orthopnea, cough, sputum, hemoptysis, pleural pain, night sweats, cardiac pain or irregularity, tachycardia, palpitation, edema, history of blood pressure changes, and history of exposure to tuberculosis or inhalants.

The Gastrointestinal System. Habits of eating, changes in appetite or thirst, normal weight and changes in weight, nausea, vomiting, hematemesis, eructations, heartburn, pain and its location and character and relationship to meals, jaundice, flatulence, distention, bowel functions and habits, the use of cathartics, rectal incontinence with or without cathartics, character of stools, melena, hemorrhoids, fissures, and fistulas. A complete dietary history may give valuable information.

The Genitourinary System. Hematuria, pyuria, frequency, nocturia, enuresis, dysuria, urgency, precipitate micturition, incontinence, retention, and pain. An inquiry should also be made into the history of signs or symptoms of venereal diseases. A few frank questions should be asked of both sexes about childhood and adult sexual activity and adjustment, noting the mental attitude toward the sexual act and possible abnormalities of sexual function such as change in libido, impotence, frigidity, dyspareunia, nymphomania, autoerotic practices, and perversions. It is important to remember that some individuals will respond candidly and others will be offended by questioning on this subject, and the questions must be worded accordingly.

The Catamenial History. Age at the menarche and at the menopause and reactions thereto, the regularity of the menstrual cycle, recent changes in the menstrual cycle, the length of each period, amount of flow, dysmenorrhea, intermenstrual pain or bleeding, discharge, pruritus, and date of last period. If the patient has gone through the menopause, either physiologic or artificial, or if she is approaching it, one should inquire about hot flashes and other vasomotor and nervous symptoms.

The Orthopedic History. Injuries, growth disturbances, swelling of the joints, pain or redness, limitation of motion, and leg and back pains.

The Skin. Eruptions, urticaria, bruises, color changes, scaling, sweat disturbances and pruritus.

The Allergic History. Hay fever, allergic rhinitis, sneezing, urticaria, asthma, bronchitis, food intolerance, idiosyncracies to foods and drugs, previous sera and vaccines, pollen and dust sensitivities, and physical allergy.

The *marital* history should include the duration of marriage; the health of the partner and children; the number of times the patient has been married; the reasons for and circumstances leading to change in marital status; the number of children living and dead, with the cause of death; the number of miscarriages with their causes and the duration of pregnancy at the time of the termination, and abortions. Other important data deal with the adjustment to the marriage; the personality of the mate; conflicts, compatibility, fidelity, and objective of marriage; the use of, reason for, and type of contraceptive procedures.

The *occupational* history should give information about both present and past occupations, with special reference to contact with toxins, heavy metals, fumes, silica, unhygienic routines, and industrial hazards. Other significant factors include information on the duration, type, and nature of the employment; hours of labor; environment; physical and mental strain; work record, with history of promotions and data regarding future outlook. If there has been frequent change of employment or a poor work history with absenteeism and a dissatisfied attitude toward employment, the reasons should be elicited. If the patient is no longer working, one should determine when and why he stopped.

A *history of personal habits* is obtained, with special reference to the use of alcohol, tobacco, drugs, coffee, tea, etc., or the reasons for abstinence. Previous residences, especially in the tropics or in areas where certain diseases are endemic, may be of importance. One should also record a history of the routine of the day with information on the amount of and habits of sleep, regularity and habits of meals, diversions and avocations, exercise, energy output, and ease of fatigue.

A *personality inventory* of the patient is also included, especially in instances in which there have been changes in the individual's reactions as a result of the disease process. The mental characteristics during infancy and childhood about which one should have information have been mentioned, but the reactions, adjustment, and predominant emotional tendencies during puberty and adolescence and in adult life are equally important. One should determine whether the patient has been sensitive, shy, seclusive, shut-in, and given to daydreaming; sociable, gregarious, outgoing, friendly, and affectionate; submissive or aggressive; dependent or independent; good-natured and pleasant, with a ready sense of humor; moody, irritable, impulsive, suspicious, or jealous; rigid, stubborn, and obstinate; serious, persevering, and ambitious, or wavering, with ideas of inferiority. It is essential to learn how he has conformed to the mores and the social customs and legal restrictions. His attitude toward his body and his health are also pertinent — whether he is generally unconcerned about appearances or dress, or careful and meticulous; whether he is indifferent toward minor ills and pains, or is hypochondriacal in his attitude. One should ascertain whether he exhibits an excessive reaction to troubles and interests with wakefulness, anorexia, diarrhea, and exhaustion, and determine his attitude toward his present symptoms and his insight into and judgment regarding his illness.

The *social, economic, and adjustment* factors are of extreme importance: the patient's educational attainment and age at and reason for stopping school, with information about school records, repeated grades, truancy, and incorrigibility; the patient's place in the family — first child, last child, only child, etc.; his age at the time of the death of his parents, and his reaction to illness, separation, divorce, or death of relatives; the patient's employment and his reaction and adjustment to it; the financial and economic situation; the home situation — whether he lives in a house, apartment, tenement, rooming house, boarding house, or house trailer, or is a nomad; urban or rural residence; the number of rooms in the house and the number of people living in them; the presence of outsiders and in-laws in the home; separation or estrangement from parents or other relatives; likes and dislikes; hobbies and interests; social relationships; hopes and fears and goal ideal; capacity to enjoy life and profit by experience; crimes, misdemeanors, and prison sentences; special successes and difficulties. Forensic or medicolegal factors in the illness must always be borne in mind, especially if the symptoms are felt to be related to employment or injury. The possibility of later claims for compensation must be considered, even though the patient and his family may deny that any litigation is pending. If appropriate, a military history is elicited. Adjustment to military service and experiences, wounds and illnesses, promotions, and reasons for rejection or discharge should be stressed.

THE FAMILY HISTORY

Inasmuch as many neurologic conditions are of genetic or familial incidence, the family history should be obtained in detail. One records not only the age and cause of death of the parents and siblings, but also data with reference to their physical and mental health during life. More important than the fact that a parent died of pneumonia may be the knowledge that he died of pneumonia while in a hospital for treatment of mental diseases. One should determine the general health of the family and whether members of it are short- or long-lived. Information should be obtained regarding both the direct and collateral lines, and the possibility of consanguinity should be taken into consideration. In the neurologic history one is especially interested in inherited, familial, and congenital nervous and mental disorders and tendencies, including epilepsy, migraine, feeble-mindedness, organic or functional nervous or mental disorders, alcoholism, eccentricities, suicide, and criminal or other sociopathic tendencies. In certain neurologic disorders, such as Huntington's chorea, there is a single manner of inheritance which has been well documented; in others, such as the spinocerebellar ataxias and the myopathies, there are variable modes of inheritance; in others, such as the myotonias, individual members of the family may exhibit only certain aspects of the disease; in still others, such as certain of the inborn errors of metabolism, an inherited tendency is suspected but has not been proved. In some of the birth defects and chromosomal abnormalities, extrinsic factors may have altered the germ plasm or interfered with embryonic development. Recent developments in genetics stress the need for a careful and detailed family history. In addition to information about disorders related to the nervous system one should always include in the family history data about cancer, tuberculosis, diabetes, cardiovascular disease, hypertension, syphilis, acquired immune deficiency syndrome, and allergic disease. It is also important to obtain some history of the cultural and economic background of the family, with information regarding race, nativity, length of time in this country, religion, social and economic level, and the temperament and character of the parents and siblings.

Chapter 3
THE PHYSICAL EXAMINATION

The nervous system must be regarded as but one part of the body, and the clinical examination of it should be preceded, in every instance, by a physical examination and constitutional evaluation of the patient, and then by a mental appraisal. These are important preliminaries, and they must never be minimized or overlooked. An examination directed exclusively toward the functions of the nervous system is incomplete.

Neurology is closely linked to internal medicine. Serious nervous system manifestations and complications may not only accompany systemic disease, but may even be the first evidence of such disease. This may be true in the case of hematologic disorders, vascular disease, heart disease, diabetes, infections (including acquired immune deficiency syndrome), toxemias, neoplasms, metabolic disorders, and many other conditions. Furthermore, the patient with neurologic symptoms of either organic or psychogenic origin may also have symptoms referable to other organs and systems. These may result from central or autonomic nervous system effects on visceral function or they may be so-called psychophysiologic manifestations. All somatic complaints must be adequately appraised, and one cannot arrive at a diagnosis of disease of the nervous system without an adequate knowledge of the general physical status of the patient. The physical examination need not be so detailed or so painstaking as that made in an attempt to diagnose some obscure medical ailment, but it must be complete enough to bring to the fore any outstanding deviation, and no important physical sign should be overlooked. It is not within the scope of this book to dwell on the details of the physical examination and on physical diagnosis, but certain features will be stressed. The examination is most satisfactory and complete if an orderly routine is followed.

GENERAL OBSERVATIONS

The general appearance of the patient may yield important information. One looks for manifestations of acute or chronic illness, and special note should be made of signs of fever, pain, or distress; evidence of loss of weight, emaciation, or cachexia; the appearance of physical strength or weakness; the relative position of the trunk, head, and extremities; the posture and attitude in standing, walking, sitting, and lying; the general motor behavior, and any irregular or unusual attitudes, outstanding mannerisms, bizarre activities, restlessness, or increase or decrease in motor activity. The detailed examination of posture, gait, muscle tone, muscle atrophy, and hyperkinetic phenomena is discussed on Part D, "The Motor System," and the complete evaluation of the state of consciousness and the mental and emotional reactions in Chapter 4 and Chapter 54, but any outstanding motor manifestations and abnormalities in the behavior, attitude, and emotional reactions of the patient are noticed and recorded at the outset. One should make mention of the degree of cooperation, the appearance of apathy or lethargy and of fatigue, the presence of alertness or nervous tension, and the promptness or delay of responses.

The physique and habitus are taken into consideration, and the examiner observes the body build, the state of nutrition, the degree of development of the musculature, and the body contour. In the presence of obesity, the amount, texture, and distribution of the subcutaneous fat are significant. The aforementioned factors, together with the hair distribution and the extent of development of the primary and secondary sexual characteristics, are also pertinent in the appraisal of the degree of physical maturity in preadolescent, adolescent, and postadolescent subjects, and in the diagnosis of the endocrinopathies and disorders of the hypothalamus. Individual variations in the rate of physical development must, of course, be borne in mind, but observations of extremes and of wide deviations from the normal may be significant. This same individual variation must also be borne in mind in the evaluation of senility and the involutional processes. It is always well to note whether a patient looks his age or whether he appears to be older or younger than his stated age. Premature physical senility may connote early involution of the nervous system, although this is not necessarily the case. Premature graying of the hair may be familial in occurrence and of no clinical significance, but it is frequently observed in pernicious anemia and multiple sclerosis, and it may occur in hypothalamic and other disorders.

Note should be made of any outstanding abnormalities in development or structure such as gigantism, dwarfism, gross deformities, amputations, contractures, unusual conformations, or disproportion between parts of the body. Diseases of the nervous system are found in association with such skeletal and developmental anomalies as syndactyly, polydactyly, and arachnodactyly. Other developmental changes to be recorded include asymmetries; cranial abnormalities; deformities of the teeth, tongue, lips, palate, or uvula; abnormalities of the eyes or the ears; deformities of the face or jaw; disproportion of the extremities; genital anomalies; and spina bifida. The presence of gross tumor masses, signs of pregnancy, and injuries, scars, and bruises should also be mentioned.

Specific deformities constitute important criteria in the diagnosis of nervous system lesions. In spastic hemiparesis there is flexion of the upper extremity with flexion and adduction at the shoulder, flexion at the elbow and wrist, and flexion and adduction of the fingers; in the lower extremity there is extension at the hip, knee, and ankle, with an equinus deformity of the foot. In paraplegia in flexion there is a drawing up of both lower extremities. In Parkinson's disease and the related syndromes there is flexion of the neck, trunk, elbows, wrists, and knees, with stooping, rigidity, masking, slowness of movement, and tremors. A somewhat similar flexion of the neck and spine may be seen in ankylosing spondylitis and camptocormia. In the myopathies there may be lordosis, protrusion of the abdomen, a waddling gait, and hypertrophy of the calves. In amyotrophic lateral sclerosis and progressive spinal muscular atrophy there are atrophy of the muscles of the hands and shoulder girdle, deformities of the hands, and weakness of gait. In peripheral neuropathies involving the upper extremities there may be a wrist drop, or a claw or simian hand; somewhat similar deformities may be seen in Dupuytren's contractures or in deforming arthritis. A foot drop of the lower extremity may be a manifestation of poliomyelitis or of a peripheral neuritis; this should be differentiated from the equinus deformity of a spastic paresis, the cavus foot of Friedreich's ataxia, congenital clubfoot, and changes that may be due to trauma or arthritis. The deformities that result from changes in muscle power, tone, and volume are discussed in Part D, "The Motor System." As a part of the physical examination, however, one should appraise those deformities secondary to trauma, arthritic or periarthritic inflammations with consequent ankylosis, bursitis, or periostitis, muscular or tendinous strain or infiltration, disturbances of development, habitual postures, and occupational factors, and attempt to differentiate them from deformities of neurogenic origin.

THE FACIES

An evaluation of the facies, or of the facial expression, may aid in neurologic diagnosis. Gross abnormalities in the configuration of the face are found in such conditions as acromegaly, cretinism, myxedema, hyperthyroidism, and Down's syndrome. One may note outstanding manifestations, such as color changes, flushing, sweating, tears, pupillary dilation, tremors, muscular tension, or manifestations of anxiety, fear, or depression. The facies may suggest intelligence or stupidity, restlessness or lethargy, emotional lability or apathy, apprehension or resignation, depression or elation. The facial expression may be alert and mobile, attentive and pleasant, placid and cheerful, or it may be vacant, stolid, sulky, scowling, perplexed, distressed, distrusting, or fearful. In some neurologic disorders there are characteristic changes in facial expression or configuration. Among them are the fixed ("masked") face of parkinsonism, the immobile face with precipitate laughter and crying seen in pseudobulbar palsy, the grimacing of athetosis and dystonia, the ptosis and weakness of the facial muscles of myasthenia gravis, the localized atrophy and weakness of facial expression seen in some of the muscular atrophies and dystrophies, and the coarsening of facial features related to the use of some anticonvulsants.

THE PHYSICAL EXAMINATION

Although the details of the physical examination will not be presented, certain points will be stressed inasmuch as they may have particular significance in neurologic disease.

The *temperature, pulse, respiratory rate and rhythm,* and *blood pressure* are recorded, and it is also well to record the *height* and *weight,* especially if they are outside the normal range. These observations are followed by an examination by systems.

The Skin and Mucous Membranes. The appearance, consistency, texture, elasticity, tension, looseness or tightness, color, temperature, oiliness, and moisture or dryness of the skin are noted, as well as the color, moisture or dryness, and abnormalities of the mucous membranes. Aberrations of pigmentation, such as those seen in albinism, leukoderma, vitiligo, Addison's disease, pernicious anemia, argyria, icterus, carotenemia, and cyanosis, may be significant. The presence of redness or pallor, evidence of anemia or hyperemia, edema, eruptions, acne or furuncles, unusual markings, vasomotor changes, urticaria, dermatographia, scleroderma, ichthyotic change, striae, keloid formation, atrophy or hypertrophy, scars, needle marks or other evidence of intravenous substance abuse, bruises, trophic changes, such as indolent ulcers and decubiti, and tattoo marks should be noted. The degree of moisture or perspiration may be neurologically pertinent, and any localized or generalized increase or decrease in perspiration should be recorded.

Changes in the skin may be of diagnostic significance in the endocrinopathies, diseases of the hypothalamus, imbalance of the autonomic nervous system, and certain diseases of the cen-

tral and peripheral nervous systems. In encephalitis and parkinsonism the skin may be greasy and seborrheic. In herpes zoster there is a vesicular eruption in the distribution of the involved dorsal root ganglia. Hemangiomas of the spinal cord may be accompanied by skin nevi in the same metamere. Symmetrically placed, painless, recurring, poorly healing lesions of the skin of the extremities may be found in syringomyelia and in hereditary sensory neuropathy. In lesions of the peripheral nerves, tabes dorsalis, and transverse myelitis there may be trophic changes in the skin. In Raynaud's and Buerger's diseases there may be symmetric gangrene. In dermatomyositis there are erythema and skin rashes. In the neurocutaneous syndromes, or congenital ectodermatoses with associated nervous system involvement, cutaneous changes may accompany disease of the nervous system: in tuberous sclerosis (epiloia, Bourneville's disease), there are sebaceous adenomas suggesting acne rosacea (Fig. 3-1) together with localized areas of pigmentation and hyperplasia of the skin; in the peripheral type of von Recklinghausen's disease (multiple neurofibromatosis) there are café au lait spots, pigmentary changes, pedunculated polyps, and subcutaneous neurofibromas (Fig. 3-2); congenital nevi or port-wine marks, usually in the distribution of the trigeminal nerve, may accompany homolateral cortical cerebral

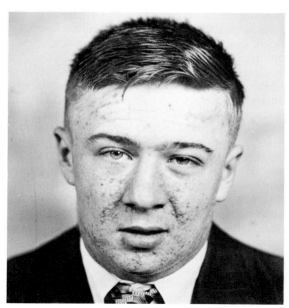

FIG. 3–1. A patient with tuberous sclerosis (Bourneville's disease) showing the characteristic distribution of sebaceous adenomas.

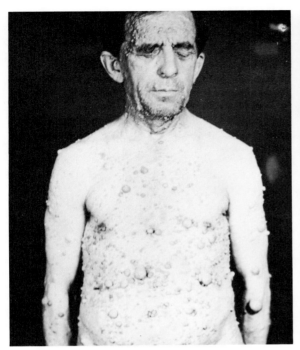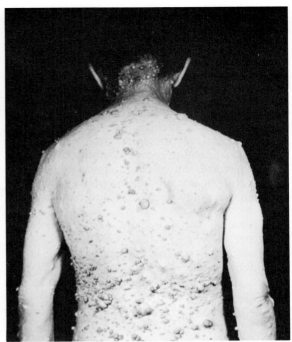

FIG. 3–2. A patient with neurofibromatosis (Recklinghausen's disease).

angiomas or telangiectases (encephalotrigeminal angiomatosis, or Sturge – Weber disease). Skin changes may also be of diagnostic consequence in the avitaminoses: in vitamin A deficiency there may be atrophy of the sweat and sebaceous glands and hyperkeratinization of the epithelium; in pellagra and niacin deficiencies the skin may be red and edematous, changing to a dull bronze or a deep brown; in thiamine deficiency there may be edema and trophic changes in the extremities; a deficiency in ascorbic acid may be accompanied by petechiae and ecchymoses.

The Hair and Nails. The texture, amount, distribution, color, and character of the hair, and baldness or premature graying are noted. Hair texture and distribution are important in the evaluation of the endocrinopathies and the degree of physical maturity. Hair loss may accompany peripheral neuritis or peripheral vascular disease. The nails should be examined, and attention is paid to their texture and smoothness; abnormalities such as fissuring, roughness, brittleness, cyanosis and splitting; and evidence of nail biting. Transverse discolorations (Mees' lines) may be seen in the nails with arsenic poisoning and certain debilitated states.

The Extremities. The appearance, temperature, moistness, and color of the extremities should be observed, and the character of the blood vessels determined by palpation. One looks for color change with change of position, pallor, redness, cyanosis, and edema. Any variation from the normal in the size or shape of the hands or fingers and the feet or toes, as well as deformities, joint changes, contractures, pain on motion, limitation of movement, localized tenderness, wasting, clubbed fingers, varicosities, and ulcerations may be significant. The consistency of the skin and muscles is noted, and it may be wise to measure the corresponding parts. The peripheral nerves, muscles, and tendons should be palpated, and tenderness, abnormalities of size and consistency, and signs of infiltration may be apparent.

The Eyes. The detailed examination of the eyes from the neurologic point of view, including ophthalmoscopy, is a part of the examination of the cranial nerves, discussed in Part C, "The Cranial Nerves." Structural changes in the eyes and their adnexa should, however, be included in the physical examination. One looks for abnormalities of the cornea, conjunctiva (including telangiectases), sclera, iris, lens, and eyelids. The width of the palpebral fissures, edema or discoloration of the eyeballs or lids, proptosis, chemosis, exophthalmos, lid lag, lacrimation, and the presence of a Kayser-Fleischer ring or arcus lipoides corneae (arcus senilis) should be noted.

The Ears and Nose. Significant findings in the examination of the ears include abnormalities in contour, stigmas, tophi, foreign bodies, impacted wax, and discharge. The size and shape of the nose, and the presence of deformities, discharge, edema, obstruction, deviation or destruction of the septum, and hypertrophy of the turbinates may give pertinent information.

The Mouth. In the inspection of the lips one notes the color, pallor or cyanosis, ulcerations, fissures, and herpetiform eruptions. The teeth should be examined for their appearance and condition, abnormalities in dentition, extractions, caries, and oral hygiene. The notched incisors described by Hutchinson are said to be pathognomonic of congenital syphilis. Significant changes in the gums include hypertrophy, pyorrhea, redness, bleeding, and a lead line. The color of the tongue is important, as well as fissuring, atrophy or hypertrophy of the papillae, coating or lack of coating, mucous patches, and scars. Abnormalities of the tongue, gums, or lips are diagnostic signs in various disease processes involving the nervous system. In pernicious anemia the tongue is smooth and translucent with atrophy of the fungiform and filiform papillae, and associated redness and lack of coating. In pellagra and niacin deficiency the tongue is smooth, and there are desquamation and atrophy of the papillae; in the acute stages it is scarlet red and swollen, but in chronic or mild deficiency states the papillae are mushroomed and the tongue is not so deeply red. In thiamine deficiency the tongue is smooth, shiny, atrophic, and reddened. In riboflavin deficiency the papillae are flattened, and the tongue may be purplish or magenta hue. Riboflavin deficiency may also result in cheilosis with fissuring of the lips at the angles of the mouth. Ascorbic acid deficiency may cause hypertrophy of the gums; a similar hypertrophy is often the result of exposure to hydantoins (Fig. 3-3).

The Throat. Abnormalities of the throat include redness, inflammation, exudation, hypertrophy of the tonsils, and edema of the palate and the pharyngeal wall. The character of the voice and any abnormality of the breath may be significant. A laryngeal examination should be

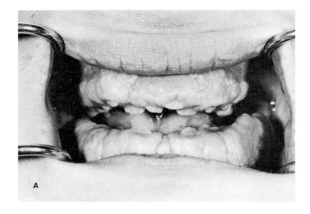

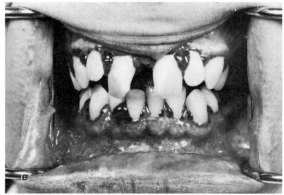

FIG. 3-3. Marked gingival hypertrophy following phenytoin therapy. **A.** Before surgical resection of hyperplastic tissue. **B.** After resection.

carried out if there are any suggestions of changes in structure or function.

The Respiratory System and Thorax. Special stress should be placed upon the examination of the respiratory and cardiovascular systems. In the examination of the former, the respiratory rate, rhythm, depth, and character of respirations are noted. Pain on breathing, dyspnea, orthopnea, or shortness of breath on slight activity may be significant. Abnormalities of respiration such as Cheyne–Stokes, Biot's, or Kussmaul's breathing may be seen in comatose states and other neurologic disorders. Either hyperpnea or periods of apnea may occur in increased intracranial pressure and in disturbances of the hypothalamus. The thorax is examined by inspection, auscultation, palpation, and percussion. The frequent association of cerebral complications with pulmonary disease, including cerebral metastases from lung abscesses and neoplasms, makes this portion of the investigation essential. In the examination of the thorax one should also inspect the breasts and search for lymphadenopathy in the axillas.

The Cardiovascular System.

The examination of the cardiovascular system is equally important because of the frequent occurrence of cerebral and other neurologic complications and manifestations with hypertension, atherosclerosis, acute and subacute bacterial endocarditis, valvuloplasty, mitral prolapse, and aortitis. The character of the peripheral blood vessels, especially the radial, brachial, and temporal arteries, and, under many circumstances, the dorsalis pedis and posterior tibial arteries, is significant. It must be stated, however, that peripheral or even retinal atherosclerosis may not always mean that cerebral atherosclerosis is present, nor is peripheral or retinal atherosclerosis necessarily present in individuals who have cerebral atherosclerosis. These do, however, occur together with enough frequency to be noteworthy. The blood pressure, both systolic and diastolic, is recorded for every patient, and it is well to determine the blood pressure in both arms, and with the patient upright, seated, and supine. The pulse rate and character are important, especially if increased intracranial pressure is suspected. The rate, rhythmicity, character, and tone of the heart sounds are recorded, as are murmurs, bruits, and other abnormal sounds.

The Abdomen and Genitalia.

In examining the abdomen one should observe the development and symmetry, and look for spasm, rigidity, tenderness, pain, abnormal masses, enlarged viscera, abnormal pulsations or respiratory movements, and the presence of fluid or hernias. Enlargement of the liver or the spleen is investigated by palpation and percussion, and palpability, motility, or displacement of the kidneys noted. The external genitalia are inspected for abnormalities of development, cryptorchidism, tumor masses, scars, ulcers, discharge, phimosis, varicocele and hydrocele, and evidence of inguinal lymphadenopathy. Often it is necessary to carry out rectal and pelvic examinations.

EXAMINATION OF THE HEAD, NECK, AND SPINE

A special examination of the head, neck, and spine should be a part of every physical examination in patients with nervous system disease.

The Head. By inspection one observes the posture, shape, symmetry, and size of the head, and any apparent abnormalities or irregularities such as deformities or developmental anomalies, hydrocephaly, macrocephaly, microcephaly, oxycephaly, asymmetries or abnormalities of contour, disproportion between the facial and the cerebral portions, acromegaly, tumefactions or tumor masses, enlarged frontal bosses, rachitic deformities, depressions, scars, and signs of recent trauma. It is informative to measure the skull, especially in infants. Exostoses may indicate an underlying meningioma; dilated veins, telangiectatic areas, or port-wine angiomas on the scalp or face may overlie a cerebral hemangioma, especially when such nevi are present in the distribution of the trigeminal nerve; scars of previous accidents, operations, or trephine openings may be significant. Next, by palpation, one searches for areas of tenderness, scars, deformities, old fractures, depressions, trephine openings, or residuals of craniotomies. The size or patency of the fontanelles is important in infants. Separation of the sutures is sometimes present in increased intracranial pressure in children, as is bulging of the fontanelles. If there is a postoperative skull defect, any bulging or tumefaction should be noted. Either tenderness or distention of certain extracranial arteries is of importance in the diagnosis of certain types of headache and of temporal arteritis. The tympanic percussion note should be observed. With tumors and subdural hematomas there may be a difference in the note on the two sides. The tympanitic percussion note found in hydrocephalus and increased intracranial pressure in infants and children is spoken of as **Macewen's sign,** or as the "**cracked pot**" resonance. Auscultation yields information. Percussion of the midfrontal area, accompanied by listening over various portions of both hemispheres with the stethoscope ("auscultatory percussion") often helps to identify unilateral cerebral masses by differences in the perceived sounds; a relative dullness is present over masses. Bruits are sometimes heard over angiomas, aneurysms, arteriovenous fistulas, and neoplasms that compress large arteries, and in the presence of atherosclerotic plaques that partially occlude cerebral or carotid arteries. They may also be present in the absence of disease. One should listen for them over temporal regions of the skull, the eyeballs, and the carotid arteries. A bruit heard over the eye in a patient with an arteriovenous aneurysm may disappear on carotid compression. Murmurs may be transmitted from the heart or large vessels; systolic murmurs heard over the entire cranium in children are not always of pathologic significance. Transillumination is often of value in the diagnosis of hydrocephalus and hydranencephaly.

The Neck. Adenopathy, thyroid masses or enlargement, deformities, tenderness and rigidity, tilting or other abnormalities of posture, asymmetries, changes in contour, and pain on movement are noted. Normally the neck can be flexed so that the chin can be placed upon the chest, and it can be rotated from side to side without difficulty. In meningeal irritation there may be nuchal rigidity, retraction of the head, and opisthotonos. Torticollis, or wryneck, is characterized by a retraction or turning of the head toward one side. The neck may also be tilted with some ocular palsies and its movement is restricted with cervical spondylosis. In the Klippel-Feil syndrome, syringomyelia, and platybasia the neck may be short and broad, movement is limited, and the hairline is often low. Gross abnormalities in the position of the head or neck in hysteria and rigidity with flexion deformities of the neck in cervical arthritis may simulate the changes of neurologic disease. The carotid arteries should be cautiously and lightly palpated bilaterally, one at a time, and any abnormality or inequality of them noted. Auscultation should also be carried out, and carotid bruits listened for.

The Spine. Inspection, palpation, and percussion are also used in the examination of the spine. Inspection may reveal the presence of abnormalities, deformities, or disturbances of posture or development. The motility (or limitation of movement) of the spinal muscles, active flexion and extension, lateral movement, asymmetries, kyphosis, lordosis, and scoliosis should be recorded. Palpation may aid in the diagnosis of structural abnormalities, and it is valuable in demonstrating arthropathies and localized tenderness and pain. One should also palpate the contiguous muscles and note their function and any apparent rigidity or spasm. Percussion of the individual spinous processes may further demonstrate the presence of localized pain or tenderness.

In Pott's disease and neoplasms of the spine there may be a marked kyphosis; in the muscular dystrophies, an increase in the lumbar lordosis; in poliomyelitis, syringomyelia, or Friedreich's ataxia, a scoliosis. In ankylosing spondylitis there may be deformities, pain, tenderness, and

rigidity. Localized rigidity with a slight list or scoliosis and absence of the normal lordosis are frequent symptoms of spinal irritation, sciatica, and ruptured intervertebral disks. Spinal rigidity and associated signs of meningeal irritation are described in Chapter 39 and manifestations of specific nerve root irritation in Chapters 44 and 45. Signs suggestive of spina bifida or meningocele, such as dimpling of the skin, unusual hair growths, or palpable abnormalities, should be taken into consideration. In all conditions in which bony abnormalities of the skull or spine are suspected, the physical examination is followed by radiologic examination or other imaging procedures.

The Extremities. The major aspects of the examination of the extremities are presented in Part D, "The Motor System." As part of the physical examination, however, special note should be made of obvious abnormalities of the extremities, such as absence of limbs or parts, limb deformities, contractures, edema, color changes, varicosities, and abnormal or absent arterial pulsations.

EXAMINATION OF PATIENTS WITH CEREBROVASCULAR DISEASE

Modification of the aforementioned methods of examination as well as certain special procedures are indicated in patients with symptoms suggesting the presence of atheromatous involvement, intermittent insufficiency, or partial or complete occlusion of either extracerebral or intracerebral circulation. These methods are as follows: Palpation of the carotid pulse may give important information about the patency of this artery or interruption of blood flow through it in certain cases. By careful palpation either low in the neck or just below the mandible, one may be able to distinguish between pulsations in the common and the internal carotid arteries; diminished, unequal, or absent pulsations may indicate either partial or complete obstruction. Some observers feel that palpation of the internal carotid artery by placing a finger in the anesthetized pharynx and against the posterolateral pharyngeal wall is more valuable than palpation in the neck. Auscultation may reveal the presence of bruits or murmurs over a partially occluded carotid artery; with complete occlusion of one artery, a bruit may be heard on the opposite side, but no bruit may be heard, or a bruit may even be present ipsilaterally. Bruits may be asymptomatic and in the elderly may resolve spontaneously. Either compression of the carotid artery or stimulation of the carotid sinus may also give important information, especially if they are monitored with electroencephalographic, electrocardiographic, and blood pressure recordings. Many physicians, however, are reluctant to use these technics because of fear of producing contralateral numbness or weakness, syncope, cardiac arrest, or seizures.

Other and more specialized technics may also be carried out. The time taken for intravenously injected fluorescein to appear in the retinal vessels may be compared on the two sides; there will be a delay on the side of a stenosed or occluded carotid artery. Abrupt tilting of a patient from a horizontal to an upright position may cause a sudden drop in the blood supply to the brain on the side where there is impairment of cerebral circulation; this may be accompanied by electroencephalographic changes and, at times, transient hemiparesis or syncope. Carotid as well as transcranial Doppler ultrasound technics help to identify obstructions and flow abnormalities of the large vessels noninvasively. Angiography may give the most specific and localizing information about the site, type, and extent of extracerebral and intracerebral vascular disease. In most instances indirect or retrograde angiography should be carried out to give information about the subclavian and innominate arteries and the origins of the carotid and vertebral arteries as well as the branches of these latter vessels. Digital arterial or venous subtraction technics of angiography may also be used. Measurement of carotid artery and cerebral blood flow may also be determined following the injection of radioisotopes. Included among these technics are single photon emission computed tomography, positron emission tomography, gas inhalation blood flow measurements, and others. Advanced magnetic resonance imaging may demonstrate flow abnormalities or blockages in some vessels. The technical aspects of these studies are discussed in texts devoted to them.

LABORATORY PROCEDURES

To complete the physical study of the patient, various laboratory examinations and related diagnostic procedures are carried out. Some of these are routine measures and should be done in every case; others are special tests which, under certain circumstances, may be essential to the diagnosis or to the complete evaluation of the patient; still others are procedures that are largely experimental but that in time may afford valuable diagnostic information.

The Urine. The routine urinalysis includes checking the color, specific gravity, and reaction; chemical tests for glucose, albumin, and acetone bodies; and microscopic examination for the presence of erythrocytes, casts, and microorganisms. Special studies may give additional information. Tests for excretion of bromides, barbiturates, phenothiazine or other drugs, or of lead, arsenic, mercury or other poisons may aid in the diagnosis of toxic states and coma; porphyrins may be found in the urine of patients with hematoporphyria; phenylpyruvic acid is found in phenylketonuria; other excessively excreted amino acids are found in a variety of aminoacidurias, metabolic disorders, and developmental disturbances; abnormalities of creatine and creatinine excretion as well as increased levels of certain enzymes are found in the myopathies; mixed aminoaciduria and increased urinary excretion of copper appear in Wilson's disease; myoglobin is present in the urine in many disorders including enzyme deficiencies such as McArdle's disease, acquired disorders characterized by muscle breakdown, exogenous toxins, alcohol, and drugs, metabolic derangements, and others; increased amounts of catecholamines and products of their metabolism are found in the urine of patients with pheochromocytoma; Bence Jones protein is found in cases of multiple myeloma; in diabetes insipidus the specific gravity of the urine and the measured fluid intake and urinary output are important; urea clearance and urine concentration tests may be essential to the diagnosis of renal disease; important abnormalities in electrolyte and nitrogen excretion may be found in patients with spinal cord and cerebral lesions as well as in those with systemic disease; in the myelopathies, bacteriologic studies, cultures, and chemical examinations of the urine are often indicated.

The Blood. An erythrocyte and leukocyte count of the blood, with a differential study and hemoglobin determination, should be carried out on every patient. Additional hematologic and associated studies may be indicated in patients with various blood dyscrasias, and in other instances it is necessary to study blood coagulation and clotting, determine blood groups, and investigate blood antibodies. An increased number of eosinophils is found in polyarteritis nodosa, trichinosis, and allergic conditions. Specific changes in the blood cells are found in disseminated lupus erythematosus, and a detailed study of the blood is essential to the diagnosis of malaria. A sternal puncture or bone marrow biopsy may give additional information in the blood dyscrasias and in multiple myeloma.

One of the serologic tests for syphilis should be done on most patients. An extensively used test is the VDRL (Venereal Disease Research Laboratory), a rapid, highly sensitive slide test employing cardiolipin antigen. When indicated, one of the tests for the detection of antibody to treponemes may be used, such as the *Treponema pallidum* immobilization (TPI), agglutination, complement fixation, or fluorescent treponemal antibody absorption (FTA-ABS) tests. An erythrocyte sedimentation rate gives information in certain infectious states and in giant cell arteritis. Blood cultures and agglutination tests are essential in the presence of infection.

Among the blood chemical studies included are the determination of the glucose content, blood urea nitrogen, uric acid, carbon dioxide combining power, pH, calcium, phosphorus, sodium, potassium, magnesium, bicarbonate, chloride, cholesterol, fatty acids, bilirubin, serum proteins and protein factors (including electrophoresis), blood ammonia, and various steroids. An abnormal content of many enzymes may be found in neurologic and neuromuscular disorders; these include ceruloplasmin, aldolase, and the phosphatases, transaminases, and dehydrogenases. The heavy metal, alcohol, prescription and other drug (and toxin) levels, including those of the various anticonvulsants, can be quantitatively identified in the blood. The rate of disappearance of Congo red from the blood gives information of importance in the diagnosis of amyloidosis. In certain cerebral disorders one finds elevated serum sodium, plasma chlorides, and blood nitrogenous bodies, with potassium depletion; this is associated with decreased urinary excretion of sodium and chlorides. In spinal cord lesions, on the other hand, there may be catabolism of body protein with urinary excretion of large amounts of nitrogenous bodies; spinal cord lesions may also have associated endocrine changes, with gynecomastia, testicular atrophy, and altered excretion of 17-ketosteroids.

Other Laboratory Procedures. Additional laboratory and diagnostic tests often add to the diagnosis. These include the following: radiologic procedures; cranial or spinal imaging with computed tomography or magnetic resonance; electroencephalography and at times prolonged monitoring with video recording; evoked potential studies of the visual, auditory, and somatosensory systems; electromyography and nerve conduction studies; complete investigation of the cerebrospinal fluid; radioisotope studies; metabolic and endocrine investigation; hepatic and renal function tests; chemical tests and spectrographic analysis of the skin, hair, and nails for the presence of heavy metals; determinations of osmolarity and osmolality of the blood and other body fluids, and arterial blood gas studies; microbiologic and immunologic investigation; skin testing in certain infections and in the diagnosis of allergic states; electrocardiography, and on occasion, electrocardiographic monitoring.

Expanding interest in cerebral chemistry, neurochemistry, neuropharmacology, and in endocrine changes in systemic and neurologic disease, has brought forth many additional laboratory procedures that are of value in diagnosis, but are not carried out routinely. Studies of cerebral blood flow, oxygen consumption, arteriovenous oxygen difference, and enzyme chemistry, for instance, give valuable information, but cannot be used regularly. This applies also to the chemical and other alterations in the blood, brain, spinal cord, and cerebrospinal fluid that have been found in experimental studies in multiple sclerosis, the convulsive disorders, the psychoses, and many other conditions. As scientific knowledge of the relationship between disorders of metabolism and disease of the nervous system expands, new methods of examination and diagnostic procedures increase in number. Research continues to add new methods and technics to the clinical diagnosis of the patient with disease of the nervous system.

Pathologic Examinations. These may include biopsy examinations of tumor masses or lymph nodes, especially in the diagnosis of malignant neoplasms and tumors of lymphoid tissues. In muscular diseases of various types, muscle biopsy examinations may give pertinent information. Nerve biopsy, too, has proved to give important diagnostic information. Pathologic examinations are also carried out for the diagnosis of inflammatory lesions, identification of parasites, and recognition of amyloid infiltration and other specific changes in muscle and nerve structure.

Rectal biopsy is of value in the diagnosis of amyloidosis and of the leukodystrophies and neurolipidoses. Cerebral biopsy has been employed for the purpose of distinguishing between various types of cerebral degeneration that can be differentiated only by histologic study, as well as in the diagnosis of neoplasms and herpes simplex encephalitis.

Technical details of the various diagnostic studies, as well as their specific descriptions, are beyond the scope of a text on the neurologic examination and are found in books devoted to them.

BIBLIOGRAPHY

Altman PL. Blood and Other Body Fluids. Washington DC, Federation of Societies for Experimental Biology, 1961

Austin JH. Metachromatic form of diffuse cerebral sclerosis. 2. Diagnosis during life by isolation of metachromatic lipids from urine. Neurology 1957;7:716

Evans OB. Manual of Child Neurology. New York, Churchill Livingstone, 1987

Goodgold J, Eberstein A. Electrodiagnosis of Neuromuscular Diseases. Baltimore, Williams & Wilkins, 1978

Guarino JR. Auscultatory percussion of the head. Br Med J 1982;284:1075

Henry JB (ed). Todd, Sanford, Davidsohn Clinical Diagnosis and Management by Laboratory Methods, 17th ed. Philadelphia, WB Saunders, 1984

Johnson EW (ed). Practical Electromyography, 2nd ed. Baltimore, Williams & Wilkins, 1988

Menkes JH, Richardson F, Verplanck S. Program for the detection of metabolic disease. Arch Neurol 1962;6:462

Schnitzlein HN, Murtagh FR. Imaging Anatomy of the Head and Spine. Baltimore, Urban & Schwarzenberg, 1985

Sutherland JM, Eadie MJ, Mann PR et al. Ancillary investigations in neurological diagnosis. Med J Aust 1967;2:542

Chapter 4
A. GENERAL OUTLINE OF THE NEUROLOGIC EXAMINATION
B. THE MENTAL STATUS EXAMINATION

A. GENERAL OUTLINE OF THE NEUROLOGIC EXAMINATION

The neurologic examination, as commonly applied, includes the major categories listed in Table 4-1 or minor modifications thereof. While it is customary or traditional in many institutions to record the neurologic examination in the general sequence outlined in Table 4-1, the examination itself does not need to be performed in such a sequence. For example, in the present text, the sensory examination follows the mental status examination and precedes the cranial nerve assessment. The neurologic examination must be fitted to each case and must be adapted for various settings. The order and completeness of the examination will vary; for example, only a rapid screening examination may be possible for unstable or severely ill persons until their condition stabilizes. The examination may have to be altered, and certain portions amplified or deleted, for persons in coma or for infants and children.

Physicians can evaluate certain neurologic functions in a variety of ways. For example, one certain test may be more useful to examine coordination and cerebellar function in one person, while a different test or set of tests may be needed in another individual to evaluate the same parameters, as the patient may not understand the first test or cannot carry it out for reasons unrelated to his coordination. Tests must be gauged to the patient's comprehension.

Careful observation of the patient as he enters and leaves the office may provide useful information. He may have a characteristic gait and station. His speech and voice may betray neurologic disturbances, as may his mannerisms, his ability to dress and undress, and even his handshake (which may reveal myotonia in affected individuals).

The neurologic examination must be detailed and painstaking. It may initially be more or less thorough depending upon the different circumstances of each case. The advent of modern imaging and other studies has produced a need for a more focused but not necessarily less thorough neurologic examination. Every physician develops his own sequence for the examination. If the patient is in discomfort or apprehensive, the examination may initially focus on the area or areas of his complaints, to be followed by a systematic evaluation of the entire nervous system.

A rapid "screening" or "mini" neurologic examination may initially be adequate for persons with minor or intermittent symptoms. One of a number of such possible abbreviated examinations is outlined in Table 4-2. The findings of such a screening examination will determine the emphasis of a more searching subsequent examination.

TABLE 4–1. *MAJOR SECTIONS OF THE NEUROLOGIC EXAMINATION*

Mentation
Cranial Nerves
Motor System
Sensory System
Reflexes
Cerebellar Function
Other Signs

TABLE 4–2. COMPONENTS OF A "SCREENING" INITIAL NEUROLOGIC EXAMINATION

> Not to replace traditional examination; abnormalities or specific symptoms should lead to more complete evaluations as listed for each section.
>
> 1. Mentation and communication during conversation with examiner
> 2. Cranial nerves II, III, IV, VI: Visual acuity, gross fields, funduscopic, pupillary reactions, extraocular movements
> 3. Cranial nerves VII, VIII, IX, X, XII: Facial musculature and expression, gross hearing, voice, inspection of tongue
> 4. Motor tone and strength, muscle bulk proximally and distally in all extremities; abnormal movements
> 5. Sensory: Pain or temperature medially and laterally in all extremities; vibration in ankles
> 6. Coordination: Rapid alternating movements of hands, finger-nose test, gait, station
> 7. Reflexes: Biceps, triceps, radial, quadriceps, achilles, plantar, clonus

B. THE MENTAL STATUS EXAMINATION

There are a number of reasons why a mental status evaluation is an extremely important part of the neurologic examination, or, indeed, of every physical examination. No appraisal of the neurologic status is complete without such an evaluation. We must know something about the patient's personality, intellectual status, and emotional reactions in order to understand him as an individual, to interpret his illness and the origin and progress of his symptoms, and to provide him with that type of care best suited to him. A good psychiatric history and a knowledge both of his premorbid personality and of the changes in his personality that the disease process has wrought are important in the appraisal of the patient and his adjustment in adolescent and adult life, in understanding why he reacts the way he does, and in comprehending why his illness has taken a specific course. The reliability of the history and of the responses to diagnostic procedures depends upon the patient's intelligence, memory, ability to express himself, emotional reactions, and state of consciousness.

The mental examination is also important in the differential diagnosis of neurologic disorders, and is often of aid in distinguishing between organic disease, psychotic states, hysteria, and malingering. Changes in the intellectual status and emotional reactions occur in many diseases of the nervous system — in toxic states, infections, neoplasms, vascular abnormalities, organic deliriums, posttraumatic syndromes, organic psychoses, and degenerative processes. In disease of the hypothalamus there may be changes in the emotions and the patient's reactions to them. Cortical lesions are often accompanied by abnormalities of memory, judgment, and intelligence, and it may be necessary to differentiate between a native defect of intelligence and intellectual deterioration. In diffuse disease of the cerebrum there may be marked psychic aberrations and disturbances of consciousness, with disorientation and abnormalities of thought content. In toxic encephalopathies, frontal lobe tumors, senile and presenile degenerations, and many other conditions there are pathognomonic mental syndromes. In psychophysiologic disorders there are changes in function of the autonomic nervous system. In other neurologic disorders, such as epilepsy, migraine, multiple sclerosis, and Parkinson's disease, specific personality types or features have been described, and the presence of such features may aid in diagnosis.

Neurology and psychiatry are interdependent, and a mental history and appraisal are important parts of a complete neurologic examination, just as a neurologic appraisal is essential to a complete psychiatric examination. Every neurologist must have an adequate knowledge of psychiatry and a comprehension of psychodynamics, and every psychiatrist must understand the fundamentals of neurology. Internal medicine is likewise dependent upon neurology and psychiatry, and both neurologic and psychiatric appraisals are essential in a complete physical examination and in the diagnosis of systemic disease.

The neurologic history may contribute important information to the mental appraisal of the patient. The developmental history, personality inventory, and social and economic review may give data regarding the patient's background, emotional reactions, personality pattern, and adjustment to his environment.

Furthermore, the careful observation of the patient during the narration of the history may aid in evaluating his emotional status, memory, intelligence, powers of observation, character, and personality.

It is not the purpose of this text to outline the procedure for the complete psychiatric examination, for such an examination is time-consuming and cannot be carried out on every neurologic patient. Certain manifestations must, however, be taken into consideration, and for this the following outline may be used.

STATE OF CONSCIOUSNESS

By the **state,** or **level, of consciousness** is meant the individual's awareness and the responsiveness of his mind to himself, to his environment, and to the impressions made by the senses. A patient may be conscious, alert, accessible, and attentive; drowsy or lethargic; apathetic with delayed responses; in a clouded or dreamy state; confused; delirious, semicomatose, stuporous, or comatose. In clouding of consciousness not only the reception of impressions but also their identification and interpretation are impaired, and responses are delayed. The detailed appraisal of sensorium, orientation, personal identification, and comprehension will be presented later in the mental examination. The diagnosis of the semicomatose and comatose patient is described in detail in Chapter 54.

APPEARANCE AND GENERAL BEHAVIOR

In observing the appearance, attitude, and general behavior of the patient, one includes not only the physical appearance of illness, pain, and tension (see "The Physical Examination," Ch. 3), but also his attitude, conduct, and reactions. One notices whether the patient looks strong, sick, or weak. He may be tidy, neat, clean, and of good appearance; slovenly, careless, dishevelled, and unkempt; cooperative and helpful; indifferent, irritable, hostile, resentful, and resistive; calm, quiet, reserved, adaptable, frank, social, friendly, and natural, free, and alert in his reactions; shy, anxious, perplexed, tense, agitated, fearful, suspicious, introspective, brooding, dull, strange, inhibited, negativistic, or withdrawn. One observes the patient's manner, speech, and posture, and looks for abnormalities of facial expression or motor activity, especially restlessness or stereotypy of movements, gestures and grimaces, bizarre mannerisms, and posturing. Eccentricities of dress and gait should be recorded.

One notes whether the patient shows interest in the interview and seems to be able to grasp the situation and to be in touch with his surroundings, or whether he is distractible, confused, absorbed, and preoccupied, with flagging of attention. It is valuable to observe the adaptability and manner of the patient both when he is and when he is not aware of being watched. The patient's attitude toward the physician and toward the examination is important, as are his insight into or his understanding of the general nature, cause, and implications of his illness, and his attitude toward his family and other patients. Finally, one takes into consideration the patient's ability to establish rapport with the physician, based upon the confidence of the patient in the physician. The physician's emotional reaction toward the patient, or his empathy, his ability to participate in the patient's feelings or ideas, may facilitate the establishment of rapport.

STREAM OF MENTAL ACTIVITY

The general stream of mental activity and character of the thinking processes are noted, both in the patient's spontaneous conversation and in his responses to questions and commands. The stream of thought should be clear, logical, relevant, and coherent. Any disorder of thought or abnormality in the tone, form, quantity, quality, rate, coherency, or spontaneity of speech or mental activity is significant — the overproductive, voluble, distractible, accelerated speech with flight of ideas that one sees in manic states; the hesitant, retarded, underproductive, inhibited speech, often with poverty of ideas, mutism, and negativism, that one sees in depressed states; the disordered, irrelevant, incoherent, rambling, circumstantial, repetitive, garrulous speech of organic cerebral deterioration; the sarcastic or bitter speech of the paranoid or sociopath; the concise, compulsive speech with careful choice of words seen in meticulous or obsessive – compulsive individuals; the evidence of evasion or fabrication seen in Korsakoff's psychosis or Ganser's syndrome; the inhibited, incoherent, hesitant speech with blocking that one sees in schizophrenic states. Such manifestations as verbigeration, neologisms, echolalia, palilalia, stereotypy, fragmentation, confabulation, clang associations, alliteration, rhyming, punning, and perseveration are pertinent. It is often valuable to obtain a tape or a stenogram, or detailed transcription of the patient's verbal productions, both spontaneous and in response to questioning. Other types of defects in speech, such as the dysarthrias and abnormalities of expression, will be discussed separately in Chapter 19 and Chapter 52.

Coincident with the stream of mental activity, one also observes the type and amount of **general motor activity** and any abnormalities of it — the restlessness, hyperkinesis, and overactivity that one sees in manic states and in delirium; the lack of initiative and spontaneity with diminished motor activity seen in depressed states and extrapyramidal syndromes; the bizarre mannerisms of schizophrenic states, and other gestures, eccentricities of movement, and abnormal motor manifestations. Both active and passive movements are noted, along with freedom and spontaneity of motor activity, apparent purposefulness of movements, response to commands, and outstanding abnormalities and paralyses.

EMOTIONAL STATE

The evaluation of the patient's emotional state is an extremely important aspect of the psychiatric appraisal, and one has to take into account both objective and subjective criteria. Somatic manifestations of the affective reactions, or mood, may be apparent in the physical examination — the occurrence of tears, pallor, flushing, tremor, muscular tension, tachycardia, hyperhidrosis, mydriasis, and other evidences of autonomic nervous system imbalance. The prevailing mood of the patient should be noted. He may present a normal emotional display and be calm, quiescent, and composed. On the other hand he may be cheerful, playful, silly, elated, euphoric, self-satisfied, boastful, grandiose, exalted, ecstatic, or excitable, as is seen in manic states; or bewildered, discouraged, despondent, despairing, and hopeless, as occurs in depressed states. In schizophrenia the patient may be cool, distant, aloof, disdainful, suspicious, defensive, perplexed, bewildered, silly, indifferent, withdrawn, apathetic, or dull. There may be emotional lability, irritability, or a striking variation in mood with or without apparent external causes. Diurnal or periodic fluctuations should be noted. One should determine not only the patient's current mood, but also his predominant emotional tendencies — whether he is social, friendly, and outgoing; has definite mood swings; is shy, seclusive, and withdrawn; or is by nature impulsive, irritable, and eccentric. If suicidal ideas are expressed or elicited, these should be recorded.

Especially important are the relationship between emotional expression and thought content, and the adequacy of emotional responses to the environmental situation. In schizophrenic states there is often an inappropriate emotional response or there are discrepancies between the patient's ideas and the accompanying mood, with an indifferent or smiling reaction in the presence of ideas which would normally call forth a depressive, anxious, or distressed response, or there may be unmotivated laughter or crying. In hysterical individuals there may be a martyrlike smile in describing severe pain, and the patient may appear to be passive and unconcerned in spite of what are said to be agonizing symptoms. Of course a tendency toward nonchalance or bravado or a defensive reaction in the presence of serious disease must be distinguished from true disharmony.

In certain organic diseases of the nervous system one may see variations in the personality and the affective responses. Patients with multiple sclerosis are frequently euphoric, with lack of insight and indifference, although they show emotional lability. They seem unconcerned over the seriousness of their disabilities and are generally hopeful, with an irrelevance between the prevailing mood and the amount of disability. In frontal lobe neoplasms there is often a silly, facetious behavior, with inappropriate joking and punning; there may be lack of inhibitions, with unrestrained behavior and alterations between dullness or apathy, and excitement. In the organic dementias there is emotional lability, and this is seen to an excessive degree in pseudobulbar palsies, where there often is precipitate crying or laughing which may appear to be unmotivated or may be brought on by a minimal stimulus.

CONTENT OF THOUGHT

In the review of the patient's mental trend and content of thought, his dominant attitudes and preoccupations are taken into consideration. Delusional ideas, obsessive trends, compulsive manifestations, hallucinatory phenomena, phobias, illusions, misinterpretations, fantasies, visions, feelings of familiarity (déjà vu), sensations of unreality or of depersonalization, grandiose or expansive ideas, and peculiar thoughts and experiences should be inquired about, not only in psychotic states but also in organic and functional diseases of the nervous system. Anxieties or fears, hypochondriacal mechanisms, somatic delusions, ideas of sin or unworthiness, feelings of self-accusation or self-depreciation, persecutory trends, ideas of unreality or nihilism, sensations of remote control or outside influence, suicidal trends, or other abnormalities of the content of thought may be present. A review of the patient's problems, his story in full, his reason for requesting his examination at the time he has chosen, his attitude toward his illness and toward the physician, his relationship to himself and others, his feelings toward the law, his thoughts in regard to his past conduct and his present situation, and his plans for the future are important. Special worries, recent deaths or disappointments, financial difficulties, or even small annoyances may be sources of concern. His aim in life and his goal ideal may give relevant information. Also, in this regard, information should be obtained relative to antisocial acts and tendencies, previous crimes and misdemeanors, and the general philosophic outlook of the patient.

Abnormalities of the content of thought are not as characteristic of organic as of functional nervous diseases, but hallucinations are encountered rather frequently in the former. Formed or unformed visual or auditory hallucinations may be encountered in focal brain disease. Visual, auditory, olfactory, or gustatory hallucinations may be experienced during the epileptic aura. Visual and auditory hallucinations may be symptoms of delirium, may be the result of use of hallucinogenic substances, and are seen in various toxic or withdrawal states. Olfactory and gustatory hallucinations are encountered in alcoholism, and tactile hallucinations in cocaine poisoning.

SENSORIUM AND INTELLECTUAL RESOURCES

Perhaps the most important part of the mental examination, from the organic neurologic point of view, is the review of the sensorium, mental grasp, and intellectual resources, including orientation, comprehension, insight, memory, judgment, reasoning power, general knowledge and information, and intellectual capacity. Inquiry into this field is essential in order to establish an estimate of the intellectual endowment and resources of the individual, both to appraise his innate abilities and to evaluate the changes that the disease process may have brought about. This is especially true in the organic cerebral disturbances, where a superficial review may reveal no apparent alterations, but a detailed examination may show evidence of severe changes in memory, judgment, reasoning power, and general knowledge. In a brief conversation the patient's stream of thought may appear to be logical and coherent, though slightly circumstantial; his responses seem adequate and his memory and judgment may appear to be within the normal range. On detailed questioning, however, gross defects in memory, judgment, comprehension, and intelligence may be demonstrated. One must be tactful in this portion of the examination, however, in order to avoid calling the patient's attention to these deficiencies. One must recall that in many conditions, especially instances of acute sensorial disturbance of toxic origin, there may be a fluctuation in the degree of impairment, oftentimes with a diurnal or nocturnal variation. Furthermore, in psychic retardation associated with depressions, in confusion, and in aphasic states there may be apparent disturbances of the sensorium and intellectual responses which must be evaluated with care.

Sensorium. The appraisal of the sensorium has in part been mentioned under the review of the state of consciousness. A more complete appraisal is carried out at this time, noting orientation, personal identification, attention, comprehension, and grasp of total situations. These may all be impaired in certain focal or diffuse cerebral conditions, namely in brain tumors, vascular and degenerative diseases, toxic and posttraumatic states, and encephalitis and other infections. Delirium and lowering of the state of consciousness may be characterized by clouding of the sensorium, loss of orientation and personal identification, flagging of attention, and lack of comprehension and insight.

Orientation. The patient should be tested for orientation with reference to time, place, and person. He is asked the time of day, the date, the day of the week, the month, the year, the season; the name of the city in which the examination is being carried out, the building, the type of building, the street; the identity of the examiner and of other physicians, nurses, patients, and relatives.

Personal Identification. In testing the personal identification one observes the patient's ability to give relevant data concerning his name, age, residence, the duration of his illness, the length of time he has been in the hospital, the date and place of birth, and to tell other historical facts about residence, employment, marriage, and family.

Attention. The patient's attention and his ability to maintain it and his interest and capacity to concentrate are worthy of observation. In pathologic states there may be distractibility, flagging or wandering of attention, abstraction, lowering of consciousness, confusion, lethargy, and negativism. In Bourdon's test for attention the patient is instructed to strike out or underline certain letters on a printed page, and his speed and accuracy are noted. In other methods of testing the examiner may recite a series of digits and ask the patient to tap his finger every time a specific one is repeated, or read a story and ask the patient to repeat it. In the tachistoscopic examination a group of objects or figures are shown to the patient for a fraction of a second, and he is then asked to recall them; this tests attention and also memory and speed of responses. There may be fluctuation in the attention threshold with flightiness and shifting of powers of observation; there may be absent-mindedness and loss af ability to concentrate. Apparent changes in attention may be associated with fatigue, a prolonged reaction time, or a slow, wandering stream of speech.

Comprehension. Comprehension is the ability of the individual to perceive, correctly interpret, and understand the meaning of visual, auditory, and other sensory stimuli, together with his interpretation and grasp of the total situation. Comprehension, perception, attention, reasoning power, and volitional functions are all complex factors, and they contribute to the other mental functions, such as memory, judgment, general knowledge, and intelligence, which are mentioned in following paragraphs. Loss of ability to appreciate or interpret certain specific types of sensory stimuli will be discussed in more detail in Chapter 52.

Insight. Comprehension and grasp of the total situation are revealed in a different manner in evaluating the patient's insight, or his understanding of and attitude toward the general nature, cause, and implications of his illness or problems. The patient should demonstrate, either spontaneously or in response to simple questions, this understanding, or lack of it. The most important practical aspects of insight are the ability to accept competent professional interpretation and advice regarding treatment, and the capability to plan for the future. One should determine whether the patient realizes that he is suffering from physical or mental symptoms, is aware of the presence of difficulties in memory and judgment, and appreciates that he needs treatment, or is indifferent to such symptoms and changes; whether he realizes that the difficulties are within himself, or ascribes them to external causes. If there is an apparent loss of insight, one should decide whether this is a true deficiency, an inappropriate emotional response such as facetiousness or euphoria which masks insight, or an attempt by the patient to hide his difficulties in order to save embarrassment to himself or his family.

Memory. The term memory is used as a generality to include various factors in the recall of past experiences. Memory is dependent on specific physiologic and psychologic processes which extend between the perception of a stimulus and its recall or reproduction. The perception itself is dependent upon, among other factors, attention, emotional state, and the content and strength of the stimulus. Recall and reproduction are evidence of the patient's ability to bring the engram to consciousness and to express it verbally. Clinically, a differentiation is made between remote memory, recent memory, and immediate recall. Some students of memory and its defects use the terms **long-term memory** (retrieval sometime after presentation, usually after hours, days, or years), **short-term memory** (retrieval after from several minutes to an hour), and **immediate memory** (retrieval immediately after presentation, within seconds or a few minutes). Usually, however, investigators use the terms immediate and short-term memory interchangeably, since the distinction between these and long-term memory is clearer than the difference between kinds of short-term memory. In this text the terms *remote memory, recent memory,* and *immediate recall* will be used.

Memory should first be tested by asking the patient a few general questions — whether he has noticed loss of memory, either recent or remote; whether he has had difficulty concentrating, been absent-minded, made mistakes in calculation, or made errors in his work. Significant defects in the patient's account of his illness, such as errors and discrepancies in dates and in the sequence of events, memory gaps and inconsistencies, and failure to remember important facts or symptoms, should be noted. If memory difficulty is present, one should determine whether this is due to an actual loss of memory or to failure to grasp the immediate total situation, and whether it is of recent onset or a manifestation of a native intellectual defect.

In testing *remote memory* one can obtain pertinent information from a review of the chronologic events in the life history — the date and place of birth; present age; places of residence with dates; age at the beginning and stopping of school; grade at which school was stopped; employment history, including wages earned and names of employers; date of marriage and age at the time of marriage; names, dates of birth, and ages of children; history of serious illnesses, with dates. Any discrepancies, such as between date of birth and age, or time of stopping school and age, should be noted. One also tests remote memory by noting the patient's ability to recite the alphabet, the Lord's prayer, or nursery rhymes or songs. General information, such as the names of the presidents of the United States in reverse order, dates of the presidents or of important wars, or other significant historical data or facts from the patient's own experiences may be relevant.

To test *recent memory* one may ask the patient his residence (with the street and number), the length of time he has been in the hospital, what he has done in the recent past, or what he has had for his recent meals. He may be asked when he came to the hospital, how he came and with whom, the names of the doctors and nurses, the events of the previous day or of a week ago. Historical data regarding the present illness may also give information in the realm of recent memory. The questions to determine both remote and recent memory may have to be modified to suit the particular situation, and in many instances the review of the patient's complaints, his present illness, and his general background will give the essential information. When testing remote and recent memory by asking the patient questions about his life history and recent experiences, it is assumed that the examiner has the necessary information available or can verify the patient's answers.

Registration, retention, and immediate recall may be tested in a variety of ways. The patient may be given a name, an address, a color, an object, or the time of day, and asked to recall this after 3 minutes, 5 minutes, or 1 hour. A commonly used test is carried out by asking the patient to remember three words. These are given to him early in the examination and he is asked to repeat them later in the interview. The test may be made more complex by using several short series of words, such as "old rocking chair" and "red delicious apple." In the digit span test the examiner recites a series of digits at the rate of one per second without rhythmic spacing,

and asks the patient to repeat them. An individual of normal intelligence and without memory impairment should be able to repeat seven or even eight digits forward, and should be able to return six digits in reverse order. A normal individual should also be able to repeat a sentence of several syllables without error. One that is commonly used is the Babcock sentence: "One thing a nation must have to become rich and great is a large secure supply of wood." Other tests for retention and immediate recall include giving the patient complicated commands that he is asked to carry out; reciting a series of words that the patient is asked to repeat; reading a short story and asking the patient to give the salient details; having the patient look at a group of objects placed on a table, and then name as many of them as possible from memory. He may be presented with a series of pairs of words, asked to fix them in his mind, and then respond with one of them every time the examiner mentions the other.

It must be borne in mind, in testing memory, that the ability to retain and recall are not isolated functions but are part of general cerebral function. In states of lethargy, fatigue, confusion, or lowering of the consciousness there may be impairment of memory; this is, of course, diagnostically significant, but an indication of a general rather than a specific defect. Lack of comprehension or attention will cause defects in memory, especially in registration, retention, and immediate recall, but also in remote memory. In the affective disorders there may be a memory defect, especially in depressed states; the difficulty is in part secondary to lowering of the emotional status and in part due to slowing of intellectual responses. Impairment of memory is one of the outstanding manifestations of intellectual deficiency, and one must be cautious in diagnosing a memory defect in mentally retarded persons.

Defects in memory are especially important in many types of disease of the nervous system. The variety of memory that is lost may have a special clinical significance. Registration, retention, and immediate recall, for instance, may be severely impaired in the organic dementias, while the remote memory may seemingly be intact, even remarkably keen. The patient may be able to recall without difficulty dates and events of the distant past, and yet he may have a gross disturbance of recent memory and of retention and immediate recall. A defect in registration is found in the acute organic reaction types, such as the toxic deliriums, but also in manic states and in hysteria; the difficulty is largely due to inattention. A defect in retention is characteristic of the organic cerebral disturbances in general, namely, the organic dementias and frontal lobe lesions. There may be a defect in recall in the various organic cerebral syndromes, including post-traumatic states, and the Korsakoff – Wernicke syndrome.

In amnesic states there may be a gap of memory or a loss of memory for a circumscribed period of time or for specific life situations without loss of orientation for the immediate environment. In posttraumatic syndromes and certain epileptic disorders there may be amnesia, both for the period of loss of consciousness and of an anterograde and/or retrograde type. In certain conditions, as in Korsakoff's psychosis, there is a tendency to minimize the difficulty by resorting to evasions or generalities or by filling in the gaps of memory by confabulation or the use of fabricated material. Similar confabulation may also be evident following cerebral trauma and in patients with subarachnoid hemorrhage. In Ganser's syndrome there is loss of orientation with evasion and consistently inaccurate replies to questions; this is usually of hysterical origin.

Judgment, Reasoning Power, and Abstract Thinking. An appraisal of judgment, reasoning power, and abstract thinking may be made during the process of taking the history and carrying out the mental tests. A history of indifference, change in personality, errors in judgment, loss of restraint, failure to observe the rules of social and ethical conduct, carelessness in habits of dress and personal hygiene, discrepancies in conduct, and sexual promiscuity may give relevant information. The attitude toward social, financial, domestic, and ethical problems is important. One may test judgment by asking the patient how he would conduct himself in certain social situations. Reasoning power is briefly appraised by asking the patient to define or differentiate abstract terms, such as to differentiate between a lie and a mistake, or between misery and poverty, and to detect absurdities. To test abstract thinking, he may be asked to interpret proverbs. One may inquire, for instance, about the meaning of "a rolling stone gathers no moss," or "a stitch in time saves nine." Needless to say, the interpretation should never be made by using the same words that appear in the proverb. Other tests of judgment and reasoning power are carried out in the psychometric examination.

General Knowledge and Information. It is often desirable to investigate the patient's ability to reproduce what he has learned at school, and to test his range of general information and his grasp of current events. The examination should, of course, be made with due regard to the nationality, place of birth, educational level, and general experiences of the individual. He may be asked simple questions in the fields of history, geography, and general science: names and political parties of the president, governor, and mayor; names and dates of recent presidents; dates of recent wars; important events taking place in the world; incidents from current newspapers; national holidays and why they are celebrated; names and population of the larger cities of the state or nation; names of the oceans, rivers, or Great Lakes; capitals of foreign countries; differences between a cable and a chain; metals that are attracted by a magnet; uses of electricity. Many other different questions may be asked if the occasion demands.

Language. During the taking of the history and the physical examination, the physician notes the patient's spontaneous speech and his answers to questions asked him. His comprehension or understanding of spoken words and sentences is also observed. He may be asked to repeat syllables, words, and phrases. He is then asked to spell simple and more complex words. Persons with low intelligence or intellectual decline may be able to spell their names forward but not backward.

Writing, Drawing, and Constructional Ability. The examiner should take notice of the patient's ability to write and the character of his handwriting. He is first asked to write his name and address, then to write a simple sentence, and finally to write a sentence that has been dictated to him. He is asked to draw simple forms such as a square, circle, or triangle, then more complex objects such as a three-dimensional cube, the face of a clock with the time of day, or something even more complex such as a flower or a tree. He is asked to draw from command first and then to copy an object drawn by the examiner.

Counting and Calculation. Ability to count and calculate may be evaluated by means of simple tests. The patient may be asked to count forward or backward; to count coins; to make change; to carry out simple addition, subtraction, multiplication, and division. He may be asked to subtract successive sevens from one hundred, and if he has difficulty with this, to subtract successive threes. He may be asked to solve simple problems: "If three apples can be bought for five cents, how many can be bought for a quarter?" "Given a three-pint vessel and a five-pint vessel, how can one measure out seven pints of water?" "If ribbon is fifteen cents a yard, how much would seven feet of ribbon cost?" "If one's salary is twenty dollars a day and one spends fourteen dollars a day, how long will it take to save three hundred dollars?" "If one is given fifty cents to spend and one buys individual items for ten, nine, and twelve cents, how much change would be left?" These simpler tests should be used on adults only if there is definite evidence of failure to pass the usual "adult level" examinations.

Reading and Writing. The patient's reading and his ability to recall what he has read, and his capacity to write spontaneously, from dictation, and by copying may also be reviewed. These faculties are investigated more completely in appraising the aphasic states (Ch. 52).

Intellectual Capacity. An appraisal of the patient's intellectual level, or capacity, may be an extremely important part of the neurologic examination. It may not only be of assistance in the diagnosis of the disease process, but it may also be of aid in judging the patient as a whole, in formulating some plan for therapy, and in determing the prognosis. A rough estimate of the patient's intelligence should be made in every case, but one must take into consideration, of course, his educational and professional level, his past experiences, and his opportunities for intellectual and social development. The vocabulary of the individual and his general choice of words should be noted. The intellectual level of the subject may be judged to a considerable extent by the results of the preceding parts of the examination — such as the appraisal of memory, judgment, general knowledge, and calculation. Some evaluation of the intelligence may be made on the basis of the school achievement record — the highest grade reached, the age at leaving school, and the number of grades failed. The patient who stopped school in the fifth grade at the age of 16 is obviously retarded unless, of course, he missed school because of illness or because of economic or geographic difficulties. One must also note the language factor

in judging intelligence, for an individual born in a foreign country or brought up in a foreign-speaking community in this country may have marked difficulty in responding to the testing. On the other hand, the failure to learn the English language may indicate either a subnormal intelligence or a poor adaptability. Halstead has postulated the concept of "biological intelligence" in contrast to psychometric intelligence; he believes that the latter, widely used in educational and clinical investigations, is a poor criterion of operational intelligence, and states that the results of a battery of special examinations give more accurate information regarding the biologically determined, adaptive behavior of the individual and of that aspect of intelligence which is necessary and usable in adjusting to the environment.

In many instances it is extremely valuable to have a quantitative measurement of the individual's intelligence rating. There are many psychometric tests which are helpful. These may be used to determine the various grades of mental deficiency; to differentiate between educational attainment, acquired knowledge, and native intelligence; to evaluate memory loss and intellectual deterioration; to give corroborative evidence of organic nervous system disease; to differentiate between mental deficiency, intellectual deterioration secondary to some pathologic process, hysterical amnesia, and certain psychotic states; to determine the patient's actual and potential abilities for rehabilitation. They require, however, special technics which fall in the realm of the clinical psychologist. Some of the better known tests are the Binet-Simon test as modified by Terman, Kuhlmann, and others, and the Wechsler adult intelligence scale.

In the Terman modification of the Stanford Simon – Binet test, intelligence can be determined from the mental age of 2 through the superior adult level, and printed blanks can be obtained for recording replies to oral questions. The intelligence quotient (I.Q.), an arbitrary statement of intellectual capacity, is obtained by dividing the mental age by the chronological age. The I.Q. of a normal or average adult should fall between 90 and 110. An I.Q. of 80 – 90 indicates a dull average intelligence, 70 – 80 is considered borderline. A score of 50 – 70 implies mild retardation, 30 – 50 moderate, and below 30, severe retardation. On the other hand, 110 – 120 indicates a superior intellectual level, 120 – 140, very superior, and 140 or more is termed "near genius." The Wechsler adult intelligence scale consists of verbal tests (information, comprehension, digit span, arithmetic, similarities, and vocabulary) and performance tests (picture arrangement, picture completion, block design, object assembly, and digit symbol) which are separately and completely standardized. In the very young the Kuhlmann modification of the Binet – Simon test or the Wechsler intelligence scale for children may be used, and in those of low intelligence, the Vineland social maturity scale. In certain instances group tests may be given, or abbreviated examinations such as the Kent emergency test. In examining patients who are unable to read or write one may make use of performance tests such as the Pintner – Paterson performance scale.

If it is not necessary or feasible to have a detailed psychometric examination carried out by a psychologist, the clinician evaluates the patient's intelligence by asking a few selected questions from the Binet–Simon or related tests. In this manner memory, calculation, general knowledge, reading, writing, and vocabulary are further tested, and abstract reasoning power, judgment, and comprehension are appraised. One may start with the 10-year level, if the patient is an adult, asking him to repeat 6 digits or a sentence of 22 syllables. He is given a short paragraph to read and is asked to repeat it. He is told to use 3 words, such as boy, ball, and river, or work, money, and men, in constructing a sentence. He is asked to draw designs from memory. His judgment and comprehension are tested by his response to such questions as: "What ought you to say when someone asks your opinion about a person you don't know very well?" "What ought you to do before undertaking something very important?" "Why should we judge a person more by his actions than by his words?" On the 12-year level he may be asked to repeat 5 digits backwards, and to define abstract words such as pity, revenge, charity, envy, justice. He should be able to give the similarities between such things as snake, cow, and sparrow; book, teacher, and newspaper; wool, cotton, and leather. His judgment is tested by his ability to interpret fables or proverbs and to detect absurdities. On the 14-year level he is asked to give three differences between a king and a president, and to state the time if the hands of the clock are reversed. He should be able to repeat 7 digits forward. On the average adult level he should be able to repeat 6 digits backward; to repeat a sentence of 28 syllables; to give the differences between abstract words such as laziness and idleness, evolution and revolution, poverty

and misery, character and reputation. In children and in older individuals with dementia or low native intelligence the questions asked will have to be from the lower levels of the scale. In infants and young children, a developmental quotient can be determined by comparison of the achieved motor and developmental milestones with those of the average child. Illustrations and details are found in pediatric and pediatric neurology texts.

A variety of abbreviated or screening mental status examinations, usually consisting of 10 – 12 questions have been described. Their advantages are brevity and consistency from patient to patient; their disadvantages are a lack of relative precision and depth.

The causes of mental deficiency are multiple and varied, including genetic and chromosomal disorders, maternal diseases, complications of labor and delivery, peri- or postnatal infections, deficiency states, trauma, toxins, cerebrovascular, environmental, and others.

THE MENTAL EXAMINATION IN ORGANIC CEREBRAL DISEASE

Changes in the mental status may occur in either focal or diffuse cerebral disease. There may be lowering or clouding of consciousness, abnormalities in the stream of mental activity and character of the thinking processes, variations in the affective responses and lability of emotions, hallucinatory phenomena and other abnormalities of the content of thought, confusion, disorientation, loss of attention, disorganization in visual perception, and a defect in sustained thinking and in organization of familiar material. The most characteristic changes, however, and those which can best be demonstrated objectively, are those in memory, reasoning power, planning, judgment, and intellectual capacity.

The deterioration of intellectual processes that occurs in cerebral diseases is characterized, early in its course, by loss of certain intellectual functions and preservation of others. Recent memory and retention and immediate recall are lost before remote memory is affected. Old mental habits and rote memory may be retained, while planning and reasoning are affected. Judgment and comprehension may be lost very early. A person's vocabulary tends to remain relatively constant throughout adult life, and even after the onset of cerebral disease the vocabulary may be used as an index of the original level of intellectual attainment.

Certain changes may be evident in the psychometric examination, which may show a "patchy" or "scattered" response with failures over a wide range. The Wechsler adult intelligence scale is helpful in determining the presence of intellectual deterioration, especially as distinguished from mental deficiency, in differentiating between psychoses with or without deterioration, and often in differentiating between organic and hysterical mental defects. Vocabulary, information, comprehension, and the ability to carry out object assembly and picture completion tests persist with age and in the presence of organic cerebral disease, whereas there is a loss of arithmetical reasoning, digit retention, appreciation of similarities, and relational thinking as shown in the digit symbol, picture arrangement, and block design tests.

The changes that have been mentioned previously are the most characteristic of diffuse brain dysfunction or of frontal lobe involvement; they are early manifestations of the cerebral dementias. Loss of memory and judgment may be present to such a degree that the patient is unable to carry on his business affairs and it may interfere with his social relations. The ability to perceive abstract relationships is lost before the simple, well-organized actions; the individual may be able to do ordinary things, but he is incapable of dealing with new problems, even though they may be within the scope or range usually handled by a person of his age and education. Tasks attempted are solved in a round-about manner; the most difficult to perform are those requiring the subject to break away from old mental habits and adapt to unfamiliar situations. Initiative and decision are lacking. The time and rate of reactions are lengthened; the patient fatigues rapidly. As the condition progresses there is lack of inhibitions, with facetiousness and unrestrained behavior. There may be marked emotional lability. The patient may fail to link immediate impressions with past experiences, and this leads to confusion and disorientation. The aforementioned changes may cause the patient to be suspicious of others, and even to have paranoid ideas. Impatience and irritability are common symptoms, and carelessness about personal appearance and dress are often evident. There may be a fluctuating level of awareness with periodic lowering of consciousness and confusion; this latter most often occurs at night.

In conditions in which the pathologic process is limited to the frontal lobes, irritability, confusion, and lack of restraint may be more pronounced. In frontal lobe tumors there is often indifference and apathy, or there may be facetiousness and *witzelsucht* (the telling of poor jokes and puns at which the patient himself is intensely amused). Toxic states, either due to exogenous toxins such as bromides, barbiturates, street drugs, or alcohol, or associated with febrile illnesses, may lead to hallucinatory experiences, principally in the visual and auditory spheres, along with confusion and disorientation. In trauma the period of loss of memory may be more extensive than the period of loss of consciousness, and the amnesia often extends in a retrograde direction. With improvement, however, there is a gradual lessening of the amnesic span.

The mental appraisal may constitute the most important part of the neurologic examination in the diagnosis of so-called brain-damaged children. Such children have variously been labeled as having an attention deficit disorder or minimal brain dysfunction in the milder forms; this may affect up to 10% of young children, mainly boys. Such patients often show variable degrees of distractibility, poor attention span, overactivity, aggressiveness, impulsivity, destructive behavior, negativism, failure to respond to reprimand or chastisement, and absence of fear. In addition to these readily apparent abnormalities, specific testing may show perceptual difficulties, disabilities of speech and reading, and poor motor coordination.

A detailed mental evaluation and psychologic examination, often with a battery of tests and the use of both objective and projective technics, may be not only helpful but also essential in neurologic diagnosis. Such procedures are important in both focal and diffuse cerebral disease, and they may provide essential data regarding the localization of the disease process as well as aiding in the diagnosis of the underlying disorder.

BIBLIOGRAPHY

Barbizet J. Psychophysiologic mechanisms in memory. In Vinken PJ, Brown GW (eds). Handbook of Clinical Neurology, Vol 3. Amsterdam, New Holland, 1969

Burgemeister BB. Psychological Techniques in Neurological Diagnosis. New York, Hoeber Medical Division, Harper & Row, 1962

Buschke H. Impairment of short term memory. Neurology 1965;15:913

Caird WK. Aging and short-term memory. J Gerontol 1966;21:295

Cheney CO. Outlines for Psychiatric Examinations. Utica, Utica State Hospital Press, 1934

DeJong RN, Haerer AF. Case taking and the neurologic examination. In Joynt RJ (ed). Clinical Neurology. Philadelphia, JB Lippincott, 1989

Drachman DA, Arbit J. Memory and hippocampal complex. Arch Neurol 1966;15:52

Garrett ES, Price AC, Deabler HL. Diagnostic testing for cortical brain impairment. Arch Neurol Psychiatry 1957;77:223

Goodenough FL. Mental Testing: Its History, Principles and Applications. New York, Rinehart & Co, 1949

Halstead WC. Brain and Intelligence: A Quantitative Study of the Frontal Lobes. Chicago, University of Chicago Press, 1947

Hecaen H. Cerebral localization of mental functions and their disorders. In Vinken PJ, Bruyn GW (eds). Handbook of Clinical Neurology, Vol 3. Amsterdam, North Holland, 1969

Hoedemaker ED, Murray MEM. Psychologic tests in the diagnosis of organic brain disease. Neurology 1952;2:144

Klein R, Mayer – Gross W. The Clinical Examination of Patients With Organic Cerebral Disease. Springfield, IL, Charles C Thomas, 1957

Kuhlmann F. Tests of Mental Development. Minneapolis, Educational Publications, 1939

Levin HS, Benton AC. Neuropsychologic assessment. In Joynt RJ (ed). Clinical Neurology. Philadelphia, JB Lippincott, 1989

McFie J. Psychological testing in clinical neurology. J Nerv Ment Dis 1960;131:383

Melton AW. Implications of short-term memory for a general theory of memory. J Verb Learn Verb Behav 1963;2:11

Pfeiffer E. A short portable mental status questionnaire for the assessment of organic brain defect in elderly patients. J Am Geriatr Soc 1975;23:433

Reitan RM. Investigation of the validity of Halstead's measures of biological intelligence. Arch Neurol Psychiatry 1955;73:28

Rowland LP (ed). Merritt's Textbook of Neurology, 8th ed. Philadelphia, Lea & Febiger, 1989

Spreen O, Benton AL. Comparative studies of some psychological tests for cerebral damage. J Nerv Ment Dis 1965;140:323

Strub RL, Black FW. The Mental Status Examination in Neurology. Philadelphia, FA Davis, 1977

Taylor EM. Psychological Aspects of Children With Cerebral Defects. Cambridge, Harvard University Press, 1959

Terman LM, Merrill MA. Measuring Intelligence: A Guide to the Administration of the New Revised Stanford – Binet Tests of Intelligence. Boston, Houghton Mifflin, 1937

Wechsler D. The Measurement and Appraisal of Adult Intelligence, 4th ed. Baltimore, Williams & Wilkins, 1958

Whitty CMW. The neurological basis of memory. In Williams D (ed). Modern Trends in Neurology, 3rd series. Washington DC: Butterworths, 1962

Young JZ. What can we know about memory? Br Med J 1970;1:645

Part B

The Sensory System

OVERVIEW

The sensory system places the individual in relationship with the environment. Every sensation depends upon impulses which are excited by adequate stimulation of receptors, or end-organs. These impulses are carried to the central nervous system by means of afferent or sensory nerves, and are then conveyed through fiber tracts to higher centers for conscious recognition, reflex action, or other consequences of sensory stimulation. The different types of sensation are classified in the following chapters. In this section, only general modalities of sensation are considered; special senses — smell, vision, taste, hearing, and vestibular sensation — will be discussed along with the cranial nerves which mediate them.

Receptors of various types are situated in the skin, subcutaneous tissues, muscles, tendons, periosteum, and visceral structures. Traditionally these receptors were considered to be specific for individual sensations, each responding only to certain stimuli. More recent observations have shown these receptors to be nonspecific: responding preferentially to a lower intensity of certain stimuli than to others, but capable of responding to most types of stimuli if they are sufficiently intense. The impulses are carried by individual types of nerve fibers to the dorsal (posterior) root ganglia which are situated just outside the cerebrospinal axis (*i.e.*, the spinal cord and brain stem), and then into the central nervous system. After one or more synapses, the impulses ascend specific fiber tracts and reach the central sensory areas of the brain. The type of sensation perceived varies with the types (size, diameter, myelination) of nerve fiber stimulated.

Abnormalities of sensation may be characterized by increase, perversion, impairment, or loss of feeling. Increase in sensation is usually manifested by pain — an unpleasant or disagreeable feeling that results from excessive stimulation of certain sense organs, fibers, or tracts. It may result from a stimulus that partially injures the sense organs, acting to make the patient aware of noxious stimuli and thus to protect him from them. The severity of pain depends upon a number of factors: the tissues affected; the duration, extent, and quality of the stimulus; the personality of the individual and his powers of discrimination. Pain is accompanied by an emotional state as well as by other physical reactions so that the entire pain experience is complex in nature. Often the patient's description of the symptom is the sole guide to its character and severity. Perversions of sensations take the form of paresthesias, dysesthesias, and phantom sensations. Some of these are associated with irritation of receptors, fibers, or tracts, whereas others are release phenomena (Ch. 1). Impairment and loss of feeling result from lessening of the acuity of the sense organs, decrease in the conductivity of the fibers or tracts, or dysfunction of higher centers with a consequent decrease in the powers of recognition or of perception.

The sensory examination is performed to discover whether areas of absent, decreased, exaggerated, perverted, or delayed sensation are present. The quality and type of sensation that is affected, the quantity and degree of involvement, and the localization of the change should be determined. There may be any of the following: loss, decrease, or increase of one or of all types of sensation; dissociation of sensation with loss of one type but not of others; loss in ability to recognize differences in degrees of sensation; misinterpretations (perversions) of sensation; areas of localized tenderness or hyperesthesia. More than one of these may occur simultaneously. The presence of trophic changes, especially painless ulcers and blisters, is also an indication for careful tests of sensation; these may be the first manifestations of a sensory disorder of which the patient is not aware.

Before starting the investigation, the examiner should determine whether the patient is aware of subjective changes in sensation or is experiencing spontaneous sensations of an abnormal type. The patient should be asked whether he notices pain, paresthesias, or loss of feeling; whether any part of the body feels numb, dead, hot, or cold; whether he has perceived sensations such as tingling, burning, itching, "pins and needles," pressure, distention, formication, or feelings of weight or constriction. If such symptoms are present, the examiner should attempt to determine their type and character, intensity, exact distribution, duration, and periodicity, as well as factors that accentuate, produce, and decrease them. Subjective pain sensations should be differentiated from tenderness, which results from touch or pressure. It should be recalled that pain and numbness may exist together, as they do in the thalamic syndrome and in peripheral neuritis. The patient's manner of describing the pain or sensory disturbance and the associated affective responses, the nature of the terms used, the localization, and the precipitating and relieving factors may aid in differentiating between organic and psychogenic disturbances. Psychogenic pains are often associated with inappropriate affect (either excessive emotion or indifference) and are vague in character or location, and reactions to them are not consistent with the degree of disability.

REQUISITES OF A SATISFACTORY SENSORY EXAMINATION

It is advisable, in most instances, to perform the investigation of the sensory system early in the course of the neurologic examination. It is most satisfactory if the subject is alert and his mind is keen. Fatigue causes faulty attention and slowing of the reaction time, and the findings are less reliable when the patient has become weary during the examination. Although a simple procedure, it must be painstaking and accompanied by critical evaluation. Its results depend largely upon subjective responses, and the full cooperation of the patient is necessary if conclusions are to be accurate. Not only the presence or absence of sensation, but slight differences and gradations should be recorded. Occasionally, objective manifestations, such as withdrawal of the part stimulated, wincing, blinking, and changes in countenance, may aid in the delineation of areas of sensory change. Pupillary dilation, acceleration of the pulse, and perspiration may accompany painful stimulation. Keenness of perception and interpretation of stimuli differ in individuals, in various parts of the body, and in the same individual under different circumstances.

It should be stressed at the outset that the results of the sensory examination may at times seem unreliable and confusing. The process may be a tedious one, and the findings difficult to appraise. Consequently, care must be used in drawing conclusions. It may be necessary to postpone the sensory investigation to a subsequent time if the patient has become fatigued, or to repeat the test on consecutive days if consistent and satisfactory results are to be obtained. In fact, the examination should always be repeated at least once to confirm the findings. This part of the neurologic appraisal, more than any other, requires patience and detailed observation for reliable interpretation.

There are other requisites for a reliable sensory examination. The patient must understand the procedure and be ready and willing to cooperate. Its purpose and method should be explained to him in simple terms, so that he comprehends what is expected. He should be able to understand and interpret the questions and commands of the examiner. Patients differ in intelligence and in powers of description. The findings are difficult to evaluate in individuals with low intellectual endowment, with language difficulties, or with a clouded sensorium, but it may be necessary to carry out the examination despite these obstacles. Furthermore, the confidence of the patient must be obtained, for a suspicious or a fearful patient never responds satisfactorily. At times sensations must be appraised in semi-stuporous, aphasic, or comatose individuals, when it may be possible to determine only whether or not the patient reacts to painful stimuli in various parts of the body. In young children it is often best to delay sensory testing until the end of the examination, particularly when even mildly uncomfortable, yet threatening, stimuli are applied. By so doing, cooperation is much more likely to be obtained during the rest of the examination. This may also hold true for some apprehensive adults.

During the examination the patient should be warm, comfortable, and at ease. Satisfactory results cannot be achieved if he is in pain, shivering, fearful, or confused, or distracted by sensations such as noise, hunger, or discomfort. If he is experiencing pain or discomfort, or if he has recently been given sedatives or narcotics, the examination should be postponed. The best results are obtained when the patient is lying comfortably in bed in a warm, quiet room. The areas under examination should be uncovered but it is best to expose the various parts of the body as little as possible. The patient's eyes should be closed or the areas under examination shielded to eliminate distractions and to avoid misinterpretation of stimuli. Symmetric areas of the body should be compared whenever possible.

The examiner must remember that the simpler the method of examination, the more satisfactory the conclusions will be. The subject should be asked to respond by telling the type of stimulus that he perceives, and its location. The examiner must be careful not to suggest responses. Sensory changes resulting from suggestion are notoriously frequent in emotionally labile individuals, but nonorganic changes can also be produced by suggestion in patients who have organic disease. If the patient notices no subjective changes in sensation, one can test the entire body rapidly, bearing in mind the major sensory nerve and segmental supply to the face, trunk, and extremities. If there are specific sensory symptoms (or motor symptoms such as atrophy, weakness, or ataxia), or if any areas of sensory abnormality are detected on the survey examination, sensory evaluation should be performed

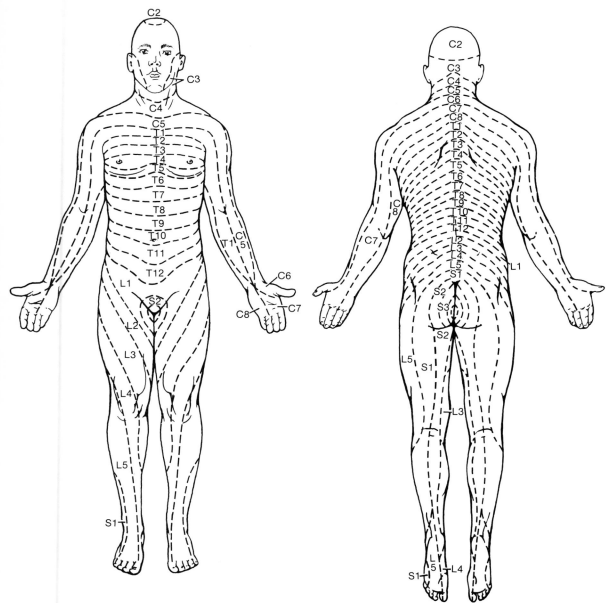

FIG. B–1. Sensory charts showing anterior and posterior aspects of the body.

in detail to determine the quality of sensation that is impaired and to delineate the areas of involvement. In persons with limited ability to cooperate or with short attention spans it may be desirable to examine the areas of sensory complaints first and then move to survey the rest of the body. The demonstrated changes can be drawn on the skin with a marker pencil and then recorded on a chart (Fig. B-1). Areas of change in the various modalities of sensation may be indicated on the chart by stippling, by the use of horizontal, vertical, or diagonal lines, or by the use of different colors. A code should be provided to give the meaning of the various symbols and colors. A note should also be made of the cooperation and insight of the patient as well as an estimate of the reliability of the examination. Well-executed sensory charts are helpful for comparison with the results of subsequent examinations in following the course of the patient's illness, as well as for comparison with the results of other examiners.

TYPES OF SENSATION

Sensations may be classified into various categories. Anatomists differentiate between somatic and visceral sensation, with general and special varieties of each. Most of those that can be tested clinically, however, fall into the general somatic group. The terms **epicritic** and **protopathic** sensibility were used by Head. By the former he meant the sensibility to stimuli that enables one to make fine discriminations of touch and temperature in order to bring about a clear appreciation of the nature of the contact and its localization. By the latter he meant the sensibility to strong stimulations of temperature and pain; this is coarser in degree and not well localized, and acts as a defensive agent against pathologic changes in the tissues. Others, including Edinger, Ariens Kappers, and Brock, have modified the terms used by Head, and have referred to **vital** and **gnostic** sensations. Included in the former group are such sensibilities as pain, temperature, and pressure, which are used in defense. The gnostic sensations are those of a discriminative or informative character, such as joint-position sense, vibration, touch, and two-point, weight, form, and texture discrimination.

These terms do have a place in clinical neurology, but a more practical classification is that of Sherrington, who listed **exteroceptive, proprioceptive,** and **interoceptive** sensations, basing his types on the location of the end organs and the types of stimuli that they mediate. It is this classification that will be used in the following chapters. To these is added the so-called **combined** sensations, or those which for their recognition require integrative cerebral functions.

The various sensations to be discussed are regarded as specific modalities with underlying anatomic and physiologic differences. Some investigators, however, question such specificity and express the belief that sensation should be regarded as a pattern or gestalt. They postulate that different cutaneous sensations arise because variable stimuli affect the same set of end-organs or conducting pathways in a different pattern, and not as a result of selective activation of specific receptors or fibers. They believe that the intensity and type of stimulus, threshold, discriminatory power, and possible "filtering" properties of cell groups in the sensory system may be important factors in the interpretation of stimuli. Most clinicians, however, believe that specificity, or at least preferential sensitivity, of both receptors and conducting pathways are important considerations in neurologic diagnosis.

BIBLIOGRAPHY

Adams RD, Victor M. Principles of Neurology, 4th ed. New York, McGraw – Hill, 1989

Adrian ED. The Basis of Sensation: The Action of the Sense Organs. London, Christopher's, 1928

Brodal A. Neurological Anatomy in Relation to Clinical Medicine, 3rd ed. New York, Oxford University Press, 1981

Head H. Studies in Neurology. London, Oxford University Press, 1920

Sherrington CS. The Integrative Action of the Nervous System. New York, Charles Sribner's Sons, 1906

Sinclair DC. Cutaneous sensation and the doctrine of specific energy. Brain 1955;78:584

Chapter 5
THE EXTEROCEPTIVE SENSATIONS

The exteroceptive sensations are those which originate in sense organs in the skin or mucous membranes in response to external agents and changes in the environment. They may also be designated the superficial or the cutaneous and mucosal varieties of sensation. There are three major types: pain, temperature (hot and cold), and tactile (light touch).

SUPERFICIAL PAIN SENSATION

Anatomy and Physiology

Impulses which carry superficial pain sensation arise in nociceptors, or free or branched endings, in the skin and mucous membranes. They travel along unmyelinated and thinly myelinated nerve fibers to the dorsal root ganglion, where the first cell body is situated. The impulses then traverse the lateral division of the dorsal root and enter the dorsolateral fasciculus of the spinal cord, or Lissauer's tract (Fig. 5-1). The axons synapse on the stellate cells (substantia gelatinosa of Rolando) or the funicular cells of the dorsal horn (nucleus proprius cornu dorsalis), or on both, within one or two segments of their point of entry into the cord, and the neuraxes of the second order cross the midline of the cord anterior to the central canal and ascend in the lateral spinothalamic tract (Fig. 5-2). Within this tract, the fibers which transmit impulses from the lower portions of the body are lateral to those from higher regions (i.e., are nearer to the surface of the cord), and are dorsal to those from the upper portion of the body (Fig. 5-3). Thus, the fibers which conduct impulses from the sacral areas lie near the anterior columns in the lumbar region, but in the cervical region, where the lateral spinothalamic tract occupies much of the ventrolateral portion of the cord, they are lateral to the ventral aspect of the corticospinal tracts. Here the fibers which conduct impulses from the sacral areas and lower extremities have moved dorsolaterally; those conducting impulses from the arms are ventrolateral, and those conveying impulses from the cervical region are ventromedial.

The cranial nerves which carry superficial pain sensation have ganglia corresponding to the dorsal root ganglia and pathways corresponding to the lateral spinothalamic tract. These are discussed in detail in Part C, "The Cranial Nerves" for the trigeminal, glossopharyngeal, and vagus nerves.

The lateral spinothalamic tract is situated dorsolateral to the inferior olivary bodies in the medulla, near the periphery. In the pons it is lateral to the medial lemniscus and medial to the middle cerebellar peduncle. In the mesencephalon it assumes a position dorsal to the medial lemniscus and remains peripheral, just dorsolateral to the red nucleus. It passes near the colliculi and then, just medial to the brachium of the inferior colliculus, it enters the diencephalon. Pain impulses carried through the trigeminal nerve ascend in the ventral secondary ascending tract of the trigeminal nerve (Ch. 12, Fig. 12-2) which is situated in close proximity to the lateral spinothalamic tract. These two fasciculi terminate in the nuclei ventralis posterolateralis and posteromedialis of the thalamus.

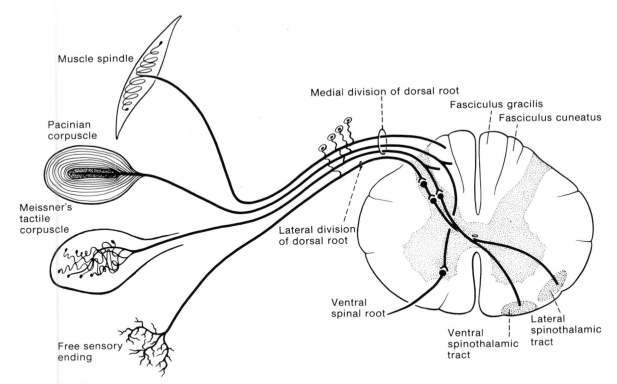

FIG. 5–1. Diagram of the spinal cord and dorsal root showing the peripheral sense organs and terminations of impulses from these organs within the spinal cord.

Here the fibers from the lower portion of the body are placed laterally and somewhat rostrally, those from the upper portion of the body are in an intermediate position, and those from the face are placed medially and caudally. Impulses are then transmitted to the most anterior portion of the parietal (somesthetic) cortex, on the posterior lip of the rolandic fissure, for conscious recognition. In the thalamoparietal radiations those fibers which carry sensation from the lower extremities are curved medially to the superior aspect of the surface of the medial longitudinal fissure; those from the upper portion of the body go to the midportion of the surface of the parietal lobe; those from the face terminate laterally on the inferior portion of the postcentral gyrus (Fig. 5-4).

End-organs serving pain perception are found in the skin and mucous membranes of the entire body. They are in close proximity on the tongue, lips, genitalia, fingertips, and in some of the fossae of the body, and they are farther apart on the upper arms, buttocks, and trunk. One fiber may innervate more than one end-organ; however, each end-organ may receive filaments from more than one nerve fiber. Itch and tickle sensations are closely allied to pain; they are probably perceived by the same nerve endings and are absent following procedures used for the relief of pain.

Two types of pain are described. **First,** or **fast, pain** is an initial discrete sharpness; it is bright and pricking in character. **Second pain** is slower and more diffuse; it is aching or burning in type and less accurately localized.

Fibers of the A group are the largest and they are the most susceptible to anoxia and pressure. The group is subdivided into A α, β, γ, and δ. The A α-fibers are the largest, about 16 μ in diameter, conducting impulses at greater than 50 m/sec; the smallest, or δ-fibers are 1 – 2 μ in diameter and carry fast pain impulses. The B group of small myelinated fibers (about 3 μ) are found in the autonomic nervous system. The unmyelinated C fibers conduct at rates of less than 1 m/sec, thus probably serving "second" or "slow" pain. The finely myelinated A δ-fibers conduct at about 15 m/sec and probably convey the fast pain perception. Centrally, the internuncial pool may reinforce the pain impulses.

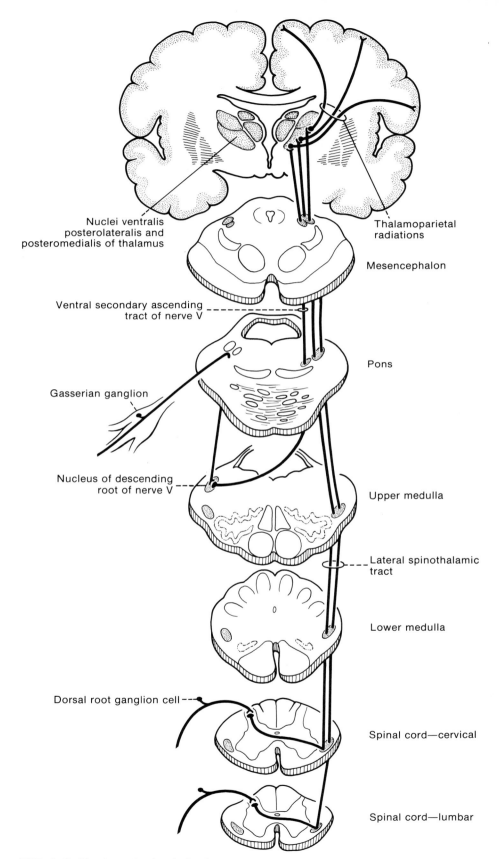

Nuclei ventralis
posterolateralis and
posteromedialis of thalamus

Thalamoparietal
radiations

Mesencephalon

Ventral secondary ascending
tract of nerve V

Pons

Gasserian ganglion

Nucleus of descending
root of nerve V

Upper medulla

Lateral spinothalamic
tract

Lower medulla

Dorsal root ganglion cell

Spinal cord—cervical

Spinal cord—lumbar

FIG. 5–2. The lateral spinothalamic tract.

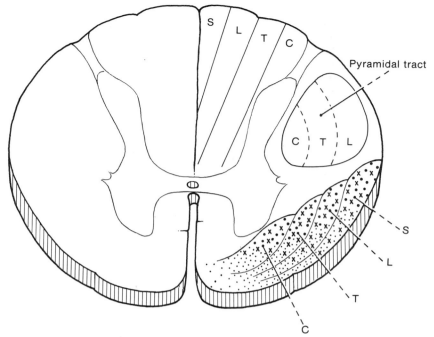

FIG. 5–3. Diagram of cross section of the cervical region of the spinal cord showing the arrangement of fibers in the spinothalamic and pyramidal tracts and dorsal columns. Heavy dots indicate fibers carrying temperature sensation, crosses indicate fibers carrying pain sensation, and fine dots indicate fibers carrying tactile impulses. **C, T, L,** and **S** indicate fibers from or destined for cervical, thoracic, lumbar, and sacral levels of the spinal cord.

The faster impulses may adjust the excitability of the synapses in preparation for the arrival of the later ones.

Within the lateral spinothalamic tract decussation takes place more promptly in the cervical and lumbar areas, which supply the extremities, than in the sacral and thoracic areas. Some impulses may ascend without decussation, and others by means of a series of short synapses, probably in the gray matter. The direct spinothalamic pathway, as described previously, is responsible for that type of pain which is felt immediately, is sharply localized, and lasts only as long as the stimulus, while a spinoreticulothalamic system is responsible for more diffuse, less well localized pain which has an appreciably slower conduction time to consciousness and which persists after withdrawal of the stimulus. These two pathways may travel together to the level of the inferior olive, then separate and join again in the thalamus.

Although the previously described central pathways and connections for pain perception are fairly well established, they are still being investigated by both anatomists and physiologists and there is still controversy about them.

Clinical Examination

Many methods of testing superficial pain sensation have been described. The simplest method, and one reliable as any, is to use a pin. The pin, however, should be a sharp one, so that with minimal pressure a brisk, distinct response of superficial pain may be elicited. A common safety pin (bent at right angles so that its clasp may serve as a handle) is often used. The pin or safety pin should be sterile and must be discarded after use on a single patient to avoid the risk of transmitting disease from accidental puncturing of the patient's skin.

Electrical and thermal stimulators are used experimentally in determining pain thresholds, but are not suitable for the routine sensory examination. Algesimeters and other apparatus for quantitative testing have been described and are sometimes recommended but actually these have little clinical application except for research work requiring reproducible segmental data. The experienced examiner learns to evaluate the intensity of the stimulus he applies, and to gauge the expected reaction to it. Dyck and associates have found that the clinical evaluation of superficial pain (and touch and temperature) sensation shows a reasonably good correlation with quantitative assessment.

It is best to examine the patient with his eyes closed. He should not be asked "Do you feel this?" or "Is this sharp?" Alternate stimulations should be made with the head and the point of the pin, and the patient instructed to reply "Sharp" or "Dull." He should also be asked about slight or relative differences in the intensity of the stimulus in different areas. This mode of examination, if carried out in a painstaking manner by an accurate observer, may be more satisfactory than one that involves the use of complicated instruments. Slight changes can sometimes be demonstrated in a cooperative patient by asking him to indicate the alterations in sensation when a nearly vertical pinpoint is stroked or drawn lightly over the skin. A sharp-pointed tailor's marking wheel aids in the rapid delineation of areas of major change. It must be sterilized after use on each patient. If the testing is done too rapidly, however, the area of subjective change may extend beyond a hypalgesic zone.

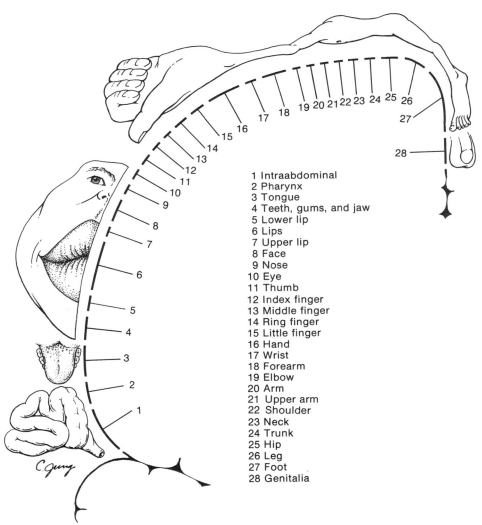

1 Intraabdominal
2 Pharynx
3 Tongue
4 Teeth, gums, and jaw
5 Lower lip
6 Lips
7 Upper lip
8 Face
9 Nose
10 Eye
11 Thumb
12 Index finger
13 Middle finger
14 Ring finger
15 Little finger
16 Hand
17 Wrist
18 Forearm
19 Elbow
20 Arm
21 Upper arm
22 Shoulder
23 Neck
24 Trunk
25 Hip
26 Leg
27 Foot
28 Genitalia

FIG. 5–4. Homunculus showing cortical sensory representation. (Modified from Penfield W, Rasmussen T: The Cerebral Cortex of Man. New York, Macmillan, 1950)

The latent time in the response to stimulation is eliminated and the delineation is most accurate if the examination is carried out by proceeding from areas of lesser sensitivity to those of greater sensitivity, rather than the reverse. That is, one should examine from areas of decreased sensation to those of normal sensation; if there is hyperalgesia, one should proceed from the normal to the hyperalgesic area. If the stimuli are applied in too close proximity and if they follow each other too quickly, there may be summation of impulses or, on the other hand, if conduction is delayed, the patient's response may refer to a previous stimulation. The terms **algesia** and **algesthesia** are used to indicate pain sensibility. In recording the response to pain stimulation, the terms **alganesthesia** and **analgesia** are used to designate areas insensitive to pain, **hypalgesia** for those having decreased sensitivity, and **hyperalgesia** for those showing increased sensitivity.

TEMPERATURE SENSATION

There are two types of temperature perception: hot and cold. Impulses which carry them arise in special sensory endings in the skin (corpuscles of Ruffini and end-bulbs of Krause) or in warm- and cold- sensitive spots. The latter are more superficial and numerous, although the relationship between the density of the temperature-sensitive spots varies in different parts of the body. None of these special sensory endings or spots are fully specific for warm or cold temperature stimuli, only relatively specific, and relative changes in temperature are more precisely appreciated than absolute temperature. Excess temperature, especially heat, stimulates free nerve endings, causing a sensation of pain. The conduction of temperature impulses from the endings in the skin to the parietal lobe is identical to that for superficial pain sensation. The impulses travel along unmyelinated or thinly myelinated fibers to the dorsal root ganglia, enter the fasciculus dorsolateralis through the lateral division of the dorsal root, synapse on the stellate or dorsal funicular cells or both within one or two segments of entry, decussate anterior to the central canal, and ascend in the lateral spinothalamic tract of the spinal cord. There is evidence that the paths for pain and temperature are distinct within the tract, the temperature fibers lying dorsally and medially, but the two are so closely associated, with so much overlapping, that spinal cord injuries will ordinarily affect both of them; dissociation of them may, however, occur with such lesions.

Temperature sensations may be tested by the use of test tubes containing cold water (or cracked ice) and hot water, or, better, by the use of cold or warm metal tubes or other metal objects, since glass is a poor conductor. As a screening test of cool perception, the tines of a tuning fork work well in a ventilated or air-conditioned room. A beam of light, which does not indent the skin and which stimulates a restricted area, is valuable in testing heat sensation. For quantitative evaluation one may use a thermophore, which is kept at a constant temperature by means of a rheostat, or an electric thermometer or thermopile. The patient is asked to respond by saying "Hot" or "Cold." For testing cold the stimuli should be 41° – 50° F (5° – 10° C), and for warmth, 104° – 113° F (40° – 45° C). Temperatures much lower or higher than these elicit responses of pain rather than of temperature.

It may be valuable in investigative work not only to determine whether the patient is able to recognize hot and cold sensation, and what the threshold for these sensations is, but also to test the ability to differentiate between slight variations in temperature, both in the normal and intermediate ranges and the more extreme degrees for hot and cold. A normal individual should be able to distinguish between stimuli differing from 2° – 5° in the middle ranges. Greater differences may be necessary in the extreme ranges. In the general examination, however, it is sufficient to determine whether the patient adequately differentiates hot and cold stimuli.

In almost every instance the absence of one variety of temperature sensation is accompanied by the absence of the other, but there may be occasional circumstances in which one is involved and the other remains partially intact; the cutaneous distribution of the absence of heat is usually larger than that of the absence of cold. Changes in temperature sensibility are recorded by the terms **thermanesthesia, thermhypesthesia,** and **thermhyperesthesia,** modified by the adjectives **hot** and **cold.** Sometimes, following cordotomy or lesions at high spinal cord levels, the patient perceives either cold or warm stimuli as warm; this is termed **isothermagnosia.**

TACTILE SENSATION

Anatomy and Physiology

Fibers which carry tactile, or light touch, sensation have their origin chiefly in specialized endings in the skin and mucous membranes.

Fibers which carry general tactile sensibility, or **thigmesthesia,** have their receptors mainly in the tactile disks of Merkel and around the hair follicles. Impulses traverse myelinated nerves to the dorsal root ganglia, and the axons enter the spinal cord through the medial divisions of the dorsal root and bifurcate into ascending and descending fibers (Fig. 5-5). These communicate with collaterals and synapse within several segments of their point of entry, and the axons of the neurons of the next order cross to the opposite ventral spinothalamic tract for ascent to the thalamus and then to consciousness. Anatomists often claim the ventral spinothalamic tract to be simply part of the lateral spinothalamic pathway. Fibers which carry discriminatory and localized tactile sensibility, or **topesthesia,** have as their most specialized receptors the corpuscles of Meissner in the hairless portions of the skin. They also enter the dorsal root ganglia through myelinated fibers. The axons enter the spinal cord through the medial division of the dorsal root and enter the ipsilateral fasciculi cuneatus and gracilis of the dorsal funiculus and ascend uncrossed and without synapse to the nuclei cuneatus and gracilis in the lower medulla, where they synapse, decussate as arcuate fibers, and ascend to the thalamus through the medial lemniscus. Tactile impulses carried through the trigeminal nerve ascend in the dorsal secondary ascending tract of the nerve, which is in close proximity to the ventral spinothalamic tract, as well as the ventral secondary ascending tract (Ch. 12, Fig. 12-2).

The distribution of the tactile impulses within the nuclei of the thalamus and their radiation to the parietal cortex follow in general that for pain and temperature impulses. Within the thalamus the tactile centers are placed slightly caudal to those conveying pain, and in the parietal lobe they are posterior to centers for pain although there is much overlap. Those fibers which ascend through the ventral spinothalamic tract transmit light touch and light pressure sensations, without accurate localization. The impulses which ascend uncrossed and without synapse in the dorsal funiculus are concerned with highly discriminatory and accurately localized sensibility, including spatial and two-point discrimination. Because there is some overlap and duplication of function, and because of the multisynaptic pathways for general tactile sensation, tactile sensibility is the least likely to be completely abolished with lesions of the spinal cord, and disturbances of it may fail to give localizing information.

Sensations of roughness and scraping, although essentially tactile, are probably not simple sensations but a combination of sensory qualities regarded as a perception rather than a sensation. Itching has been thought to be more clearly related to pain. "Pins-and-needles" sensations are probably caused by irritation or interruption of those fibers or tracts that carry tactile sensation. The tingling that follows ischemia of a limb has been attributed to stimulation of the tactile fibers by asphyxia, whereas the prickling and burning following release of compression have been attributed to stimulation of pain fibers.

Clinical Examination

Various means are available for evaluating the tactile sensations. General tactile sensibility is tested by the use of a light stimulus such as a camel's hair brush, a wisp of cotton, a feather, a piece of tissue paper, or even a very light touch with a fingertip. Touch is tested along with pain by stimulating alternately (but not in an even rhythm) with the sharp and blunt portions of a pin. Stroking of the hairs is also a delicate means of testing this type of sensation. For detailed or experimental investigations Frey's hairs or an aesthesiometer in which the stimulating element is a thin nylon wire may be used, but for routine examination simple methods are adequate, and it is sufficient to determine whether the patient recognizes and roughly localizes light touch stimulations and differentiates intensities. The stimulus should be so light that no pressure on subcutaneous tissues is produced. Allowance must be made for thicker skin on the palms and soles and the especially sensitive skin in the fossae. The patient is asked to say "Now" or "Yes" when he feels the stimulus and to name or point to the area stimulated and state the nature of the stimulus.

Similar stimuli are used for evaluating discriminatory tactile sensation but this is best tested on the hairless, or glabrous, skin, since motion of the hairs must be avoided. It is also tested by noting the patient's ability to localize the stimuli accurately and by investigating two-point discrimination. Localization is most accurate on the palmar surfaces of the fingers, especially the thumb and index finger. Two-point discrimination is considered both a delicate tactile modality and a more complex sensation requiring cerebral interpretation; methods of testing it are described in Chapter 8.

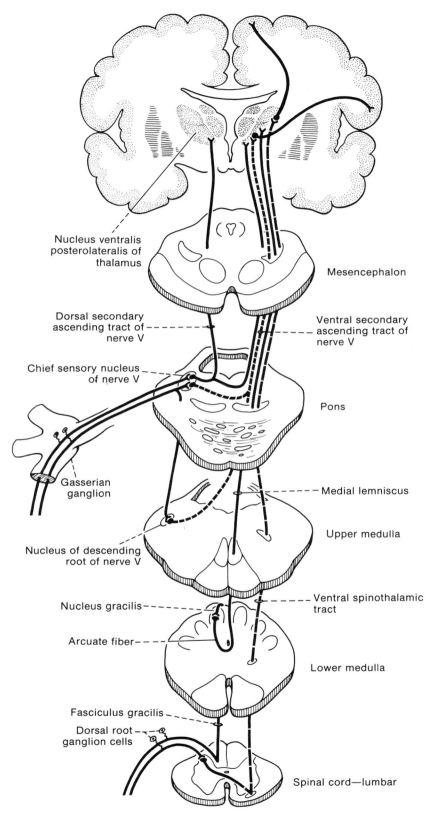

Nucleus ventralis
posterolateralis of
thalamus

Mesencephalon

Dorsal secondary
ascending tract of
nerve V

Ventral secondary
ascending tract of
nerve V

Chief sensory nucleus
of nerve V

Pons

Gasserian
ganglion

Medial lemniscus

Nucleus of descending
root of nerve V

Upper medulla

Nucleus gracilis

Ventral spinothalamic
tract

Arcuate fiber

Lower medulla

Fasciculus gracilis

Dorsal root
ganglion cells

Spinal cord—lumbar

FIG. 5–5. The tactile pathways.

The terms *anesthesia, hypesthesia,* and *hyperesthesia* are used to designate changes in tactile sensation, but, unfortunately, these terms also denote changes in all types of sensation. **Thigmanesthesia** denotes loss of light touch. Loss of sensation on stimulation to or movement of the hairs is known as **trichoanesthesia. Topoanesthesia** may be used to indicate loss of tactile localization. **Graphanesthesia** is the inability to recognize numbers or letters written on the skin; it is discussed with the cerebral sensory functions in Chapter 8. Pressure sensation, or touch-pressure, may be regarded as a distinct type of tactile sensation, involving more gross pressure from the skin. Most pressure impulses, however, arise from subcutaneous structures rather than from the skin, and pressure sense is herein considered to be a variety of proprioceptive rather than of exteroceptive sensation.

POINTS IN THE EVALUATION OF EXTEROCEPTIVE SENSATIONS

The subjective responses of the patient should be noted in testing all the exteroceptive sensations. **Paresthesias** are usually considered to be abnormal sensations that the patient experiences in the absence of specific stimulation; these include feelings of cold, warmth, numbness, tingling, burning, prickling, crawling, heaviness, compression, and itching. **Dysesthesias** are perverted interpretations of sensation, such as a burning or tingling feeling in response to tactile or painful stimulation. At times it is also of value to record the response to tickling, scraping, and roughness.

The examiner should carefully interpret and evaluate all changes in sensation reported by the patient. The following are some of the difficulties that may be encountered: The uncooperative patient may be indifferent to the sensory examination or may object to the use of painful stimuli. A child may be fearful of testing, and should be assured at the outset that the examination will be brief and not actually painful. The overly cooperative patient, on the other hand, may make too much of small differences and report changes that are not present. Some areas of the body, such as the antecubital fossae, the supraclavicular fossae, and the neck, are more sensitive than others, and apparent sensory changes in these regions may lead to false interpretation of the examination. The last of a series of identical stimuli may be interpreted as the strongest. Even though pain sensibility is absent,

a patient may still be able to identify a sharp stimulus with a pin. Occasionally in syringomyelia, with lost pain but preserved tactile sensibility, the patient may recognize the pin point in an analgesic area and give responses that appear to be confusing and inconsistent. In semistuporous and comatose individuals, pain may be tested by pricking or pinching the skin, but no accurate delineation of sensory change can be determined; comparison of the responses on the two sides of the body, however, provides valuable information.

One should observe not only the recognition and discrimination of pain, temperature, and tactile stimulation, but also accuracy in localization, which is important. The patient should be asked to name or point to the area stimulated. Responses on the two sides of the body should be compared. Slight gradations and differences in threshold should be recorded. In diseases such as tabes dorsalis a delayed response to painful or other types of stimulation is important for diagnosis.

To reemphasize, in testing all types of superficial sensation accurate results are best obtained by proceeding from the area of lesser sensation to that of greater sensation — that is, by going from the anesthetic to the normal zone, or from the normal to the hyperesthetic. There may be a definite line of demarcation between the areas of normal and abnormal sensation, a gradual change, or at times a zone of hyperesthesia between them.

Locating the Site of Neurologic Lesions.
In delineating and recording alterations in superficial sensations, it is important to differentiate between changes due to lesions of the peripheral nerves, the nerve roots, the spinal cord, or higher centers of the brain.

In *peripheral nerve lesions* the areas of anesthesia, hypesthesia, or hyperesthesia correspond to the areas of sensory distribution of specific nerves (Fig. 5-6). All types of sensation, including the proprioceptive sensations, are altered within the distribution of the affected nerve or nerves. It is necessary to bear in mind, however, that individuals show variations in the areas supplied by the peripheral nerves, and in one patient the resulting change will differ from that in another, as shown in variations in the radial nerve supply (Fig. 5-7). It is also important to recall that there are areas of algesic overlap for pain and temperature sensations. The demonstrable area of loss of pain and temperature perception in a lesion of a specific nerve is usually

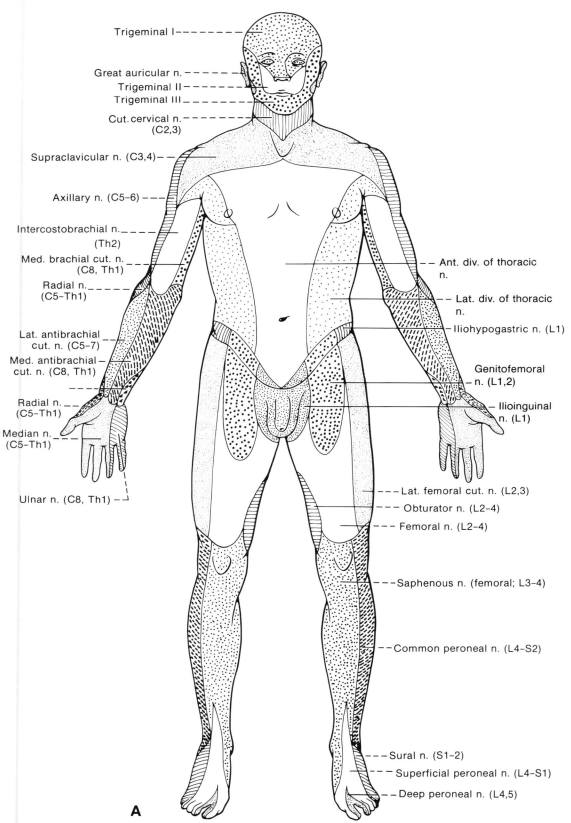

FIG. 5–6. The cutaneous distribution of the peripheral nerves. **A.** On the anterior aspect of the body. **B.** On the posterior aspect of the body *(continued)*.

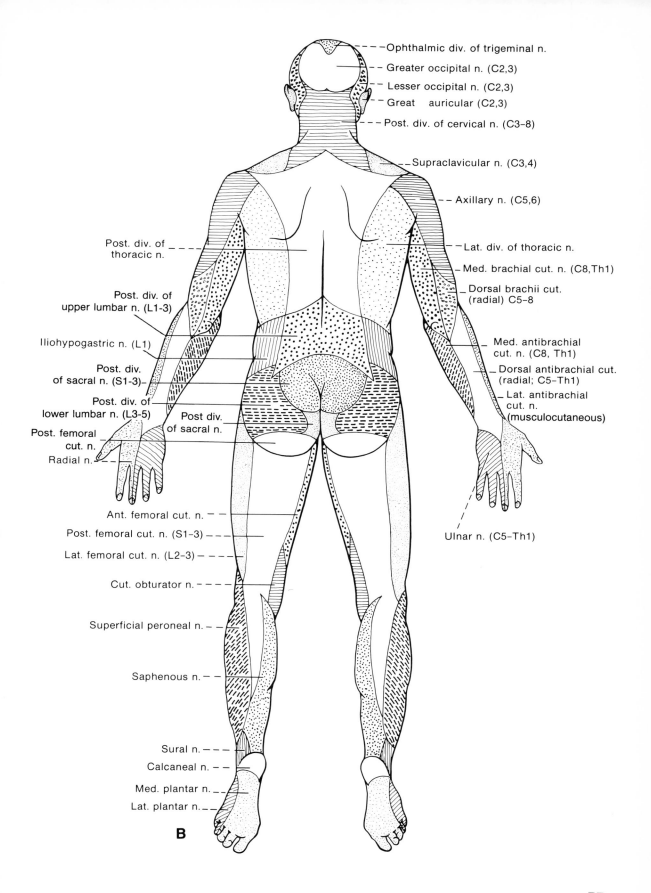

Ophthalmic div. of trigeminal n.

Greater occipital n. (C2,3)

Lesser occipital n. (C2,3)

Great auricular (C2,3)

Post. div. of cervical n. (C3-8)

Supraclavicular n. (C3,4)

Axillary n. (C5,6)

Lat. div. of thoracic n.

Med. brachial cut. n. (C8,Th1)

Dorsal brachii cut. (radial) C5-8

Med. antibrachial cut. n. (C8, Th1)

Dorsal antibrachial cut. (radial; C5-Th1)

Lat. antibrachial cut. n. (musculocutaneous)

Ulnar n. (C5-Th1)

Post. div. of thoracic n.

Post. div. of upper lumbar n. (L1-3)

Iliohypogastric n. (L1)

Post. div. of sacral n. (S1-3)

Post. div. of lower lumbar n. (L3-5)

Post. femoral cut. n.

Radial n.

Post div. of sacral n.

Ant. femoral cut. n.

Post. femoral cut. n. (S1-3)

Lat. femoral cut. n. (L2-3)

Cut. obturator n.

Superficial peroneal n.

Saphenous n.

Sural n.

Calcaneal n.

Med. plantar n.

Lat. plantar n.

B

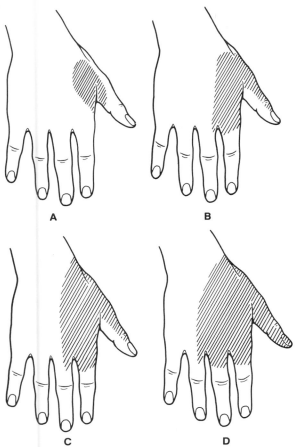

A   B

C   D

FIG. 5–7. Variations in the cutaneous distribution of the radial nerve. **A.** Frequent distribution. **B.** Typical distribution. **C.** Frequent distribution. **D.** Anesthesia beyond the usual limit. (Modified from Tinel J: Nerve Wounds. Rothwell F (trans). New York, William Wood & Co, 1917)

smaller than the distribution of the anatomically described cutaneous supply of the nerve. Consequently, with careful testing, one can identify an area of slight hypalgesia, with loss of ability to distinguish a slight difference in pain and thermal stimuli; then there is an area of marked hypalgesia and hypesthesia, within which, however, the patient may identify ordinary tactile stimuli; and finally an area of complete anesthesia and analgesia (Fig. 5-8). Occasionally there is spread of sensory loss beyond the field of an injured nerve. Those nerves supplying the face and body have a certain amount of "crossing" at the midline, more on the body than on the face. Therefore, an organic anesthesia usually ends before the midline is reached. The sensory and

other neurologic alterations associated with lesions of specific nerves are described in Part G, "Diagnosis and Localization of Disorders of the Peripheral Nerves, Nerve Roots, and Spinal Cord."

It is generally conceded that there is a definite relationship between nerve fiber diameter, sensory modality, rate of conduction of impulses, refractory period, and vulnerability to various types of injury. The greater the diameter of the fibers, the faster the speed of conduction. Cocaine, which blocks the conduction of the smaller fibers first, causes loss of sensation in the order of slow pain, cold, warmth, fast pain, touch, and position. Pressure, which blocks the conduction of the larger fibers first, causes loss of sensation in the order of position, vibration, pressure, touch, fast pain, cold, warmth, and slow pain. Aberrations of the skin sensibility casued by mechanical, thermal, radiant, or chemical insults are probably due to the liberation in the skin of some substance that reduces the threshold for stimulation of the pain endings.

In *lesions confined to the nerve roots*, areas of anesthesia or hypesthesia may be detected which are limited to the segmental distribution of these roots. All types of sensation are affected. Instead of sensory loss there may be hyperesthesia and radicular, or girdle, pains in the same distribution. The skin areas innervated by specific segments of the cord or their roots or dorsal root ganglia are called **dermatomes.** The distribution of these has been studied by Head, who based his observations on herpetic lesions and traumatic involvement of the spinal cord and the cauda equina, and later by Sherrington and Foerster, who performed isolated posterior root sections and noted the remaining, or unaltered, sensibility after certain roots were sectioned. Foerster also determined the distribution of the dermatomes by making use of antidromic responses (reverse conduction of impulses) and noting the vasodilation that followed stimulation of the cut end of a dorsal root.

There has been some variation in the results. The dermatome innervation of the extremities is extremely complex, in part due to the migration of the limb buds during embryonic development. As a result, the fourth and fifth cervical dermatomes approximate the first and second thoracic on the upper chest, and the first and second lumbar are close to the sacral dermatomes on the inner aspect of the thigh near the genitalia. According to both Head and Foerster there is an overlap of sensory supply by the nerve roots that is so widespread that it may not be possible to map out an area of sensory loss with a lesion involving only one nerve root, and it may be necessary to have involvement of two or more radicular zones in order to demonstrate an area of anesthesia or analgesia (Fig. 5-9). Head and Foerster delineated the sensory representation of only certain nerve roots in the distal portions of the extremities. Keegan, in a later study of a large series of cases of herniated intervertebral disks with the blocking of single nerve roots, has modified the dermatome representation in the extremities. He found little or no overlap, and was able to delineate strips of hypalgesia which extend to the most distal portions of the extremities (Fig. 5-10). The distribution of sensory roots also differs depending on whether a given root, e.g., C-6, is **not** functioning or is the only remaining root in an area of **non**functioning ones.

On occasion it may be necessary to differentiate between peripheral nerve and radicular lesions on the one hand and the more complex type of involvement that is found in lesions of the cervical, brachial, lumbar, or sacral plexuses on the other hand. A lesion of the upper trunk or the posterior cord of the brachial plexus, for instance, will result in changes in sensation which differ from those found in segmental or radicular involvement and from those arising from peripheral nerve lesions.

In *lesions of the brain stem and spinal cord,* or the *cerebrospinal axis,* the sensory changes are similar to those occurring with nerve root lesions. That is, they have segmental or dermatome distribution (see Figs. 5-10 A, B, C). The examiner can localize with fair accuracy the level

of involvement if he recalls the following: the first cervical segment has no supply to the skin; the interaural or vortex – meatal line forms the border between the areas supplied by the trigeminal nerve and the second cervical segment; the fifth and sixth cervical segments supply the radial side of the arm, forearm, and hand; the eighth cervical and first thoracic, the ulnar side of the forearm and hand; the fourth thoracic, the nipple level; the tenth thoracic, the umbilicus; the twelfth thoracic and first lumbar, the groin; the first three lumbar, the anterior aspect of the thigh; the fourth and fifth lumbar, the anterior and lateral aspects of the leg; the first and second sacral, the little toe, most of the sole of the foot, and the posterior aspect of the thigh and leg; the fourth and fifth sacral segments, the perineal region. In a spinal cord lesion there may be anesthesia of the body below the uppermost level of the lesion as a result of involvement of the ascending pathways. There may be hyperesthesia at the dermatome level of the lesion. There may be a zone of gradual transition. The level for pain and temperature sensations is most specific, and it may be difficult to delineate definite changes in tactile sensation. Furthermore, since the pain fibers from the lower portions of the body are lateral, pressure on the cord from one side may affect only the external fibers, and the resulting loss in pain sensation may be significantly below the level of the lesion.

It is also important to recall that the segments of the spinal cord and the spinous processes of the vertebrae are not on corresponding levels. In the upper cervical region the spinal cord level is about one segment higher than that of the corre-

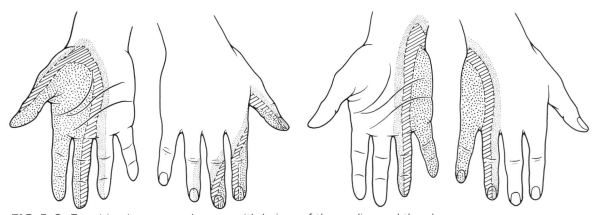

FIG. 5–8. Transition in sensory changes with lesions of the median and the ulnar nerve. The smallest area is completely anesthetic, the next area has decreased sensation, and the surrounding area has only slight decrease in sensation. (Modified from Tinel J: Nerve Wounds. Rothwell F (trans). New York, William Wood & Co, 1917)

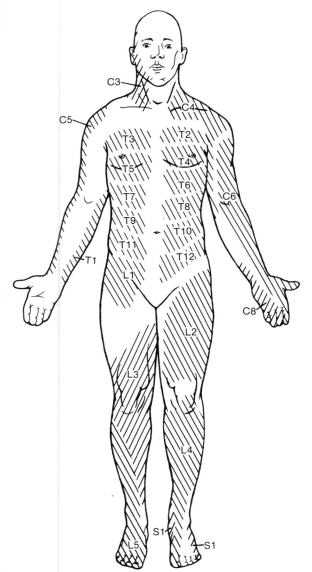

FIG. 5–9. *Segmental innervation of the body.*

The anatomic differentiation between the conduction of pain and temperature impulses on the one hand, and the conduction of tactile impulses on the other, is valuable in the diagnosis of neurologic disorders and in certain types of therapy. In syringomyelia, for instance, where the primary pathologic change is situated in the vicinity of the central canal of the spinal cord, the decussating pain and temperature fibers are interrupted. The earliest clinical manifestation may be a dissociation of sensation, with loss of pain and temperature modalities in the areas of the body supplied by the involved segments, whereas tactile sensation may not be affected. If the medial portions of the lateral spinothalamic tract are later involved, there may be interference with the conduction of pain and temperature sensations from other parts of the body. Occasionally, deep pain sensation is lost, with otherwise normal sensory perception. In hemisection of the spinal cord of the Brown–Séquard variety, pain and temperature sensations are lost on the opposite side of the body below the level of the lesion, whereas tactile sensation shows little if any evidence of change; usually a corticospinal paralysis and loss of proprioceptive sensations occur on the side of the lesion, often with anesthesia in the distribution of the involved segments on that side. With transverse lesions of the spinal cord all types of sensation are lost below the level of the lesion, the level for pain and temperature being the most distinct and well demarcated; the level is within one or two segments of the site of the lesion, owing to the immediate decussation of the fibers. There may be radicular pain in the distribution of the involved segments.

Perception Threshold Versus Reaction Threshold. In evaluating responses one must recall that not all portions of the body are equally sensitive, and that there are individual variations in the sensory reaction threshold. There is an irregular distribution of receptors in the skin, and the proximity of the sensory endings differs widely in various areas. The tip of the tongue, lips, genitalia, and fingertips are the most sensitive areas; the upper arms, buttocks, and trunk are much less sensitive. Calluses over the fingers, the palms, or the feet may impair sensory acuity.

Sensations are subjective phenomena, and individuals differ in powers of discrimination, sensory acuity, and reaction to pain. It is important to differentiate between a sensation and an individual's reaction to the sensation. Several inves-

sponding spinous process; in the lower cervical and thoracic regions there is a difference of about two segments, while in the lumbar region there is a difference of almost three segments. The spinal cord ends between the bodies of the first and second lumbar vertebrae in adults (Fig. 5-11). Furthermore, in lesions of the cerebrospinal axis there is often a dissociation of sensation, with loss, for instance, of pain and temperature sensations but little or no impairment of touch, owing to involvement of certain sensory pathways but the sparing of others.

tigators have demonstrated that the actual pain *perception* threshold is relatively uniform and stable and is independent of age, race, sex, experience, training, emotional state, or fatigue, but the pain *reaction* threshold may vary with any one of these.

The same individual may show variations in his reactions to pain from time to time as a result of fatigue, discomfort, alterations in the state of health, or emotional or physical factors. The actual pain threshold may be raised by distraction, concentration, suggestion, damage to the nervous system, local anesthesia, or the use of analgesic agents, and it may be lowered by alterations in the nervous system or inflammations of the skin. The threshold may be altered according to the site of the stimulus, type of stimulus, or strength of stimulus, irritability of the nerves, or the number of nerves involved. It can be modified by various physical and thermic factors, including changes in the end-organs, conducting pathways, and perception centers. There are probably no significant differences in the pain perception thresholds of normal and emotionally disturbed individuals, but there may be a significant lowering of the pain reaction threshold in the latter; they feel pain no sooner than others, but react sooner with a wince or withdrawal. The individual reaction to pain may be tested by the **Libman maneuver,** in which the examiner compares the patient's response to pain from pressure against the tip of the mastoid with that from pressure against the styloid process, and by similar tests. In all individuals, however, except those rare persons with congenital indifference to pain, overstimulation of a peripheral nerve results in the perception of pain.

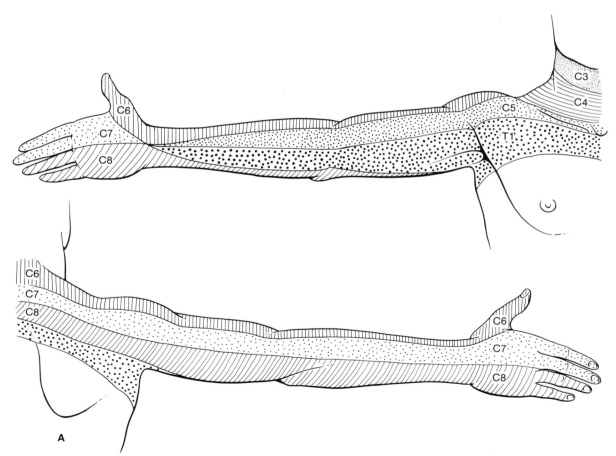

FIG. 5–10. The segmental innervation. **A.** The upper extremity. **B.** The lower extremity. **C.** The anterior and posterior aspects of the entire body. (Modified from Keegan JJ, Garrett FD: Anat Rec 102: 409–437, 1943) *(Figure continued on following pages)*

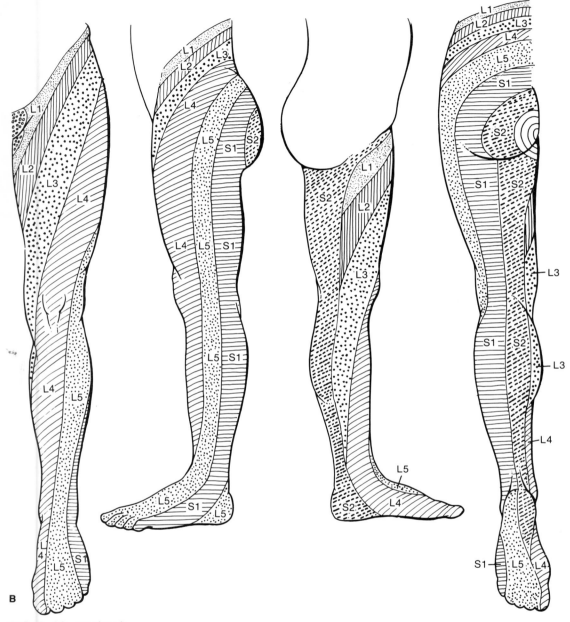

FIG. 5–10. (continued)

Sensibility Changes in Hysteria. In hysteria (conversion reaction), changes in sensory perception are found which do not correspond to organic nerve distribution and which may be influenced by suggestion. (The term **hysteria** is used herein for that condition in which there are sensory, motor, and other changes that are not of organic origin, and it does not necessarily have the complete psychiatric connotation of the clinical conversion neurosis.) In hysteria there may be anesthesia extending exactly to the midline or even beyond it; other changes which do not correspond to a peripheral nerve, root, or segmental supply, such as the so-called glove-and-stocking types of anesthesia, also are often indicative of hysterical change. There may be absolute loss of

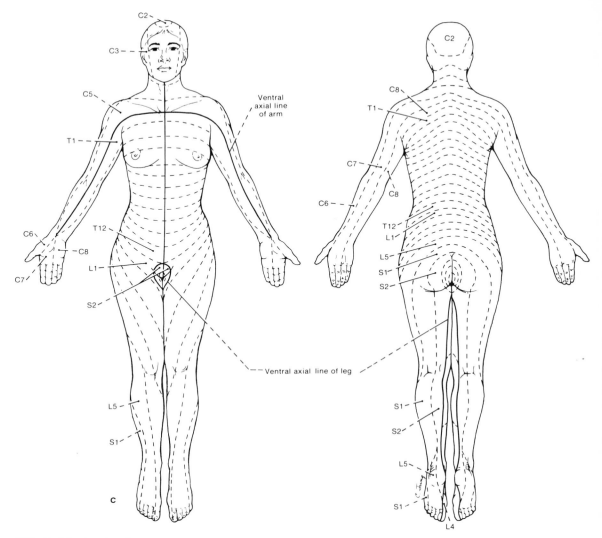

FIG. 5–10. (continued)

all cutaneous sensations. The borders of the anesthetic area are sharply defined, but they may vary from examination to examination. It may be noted, however, that in spite of marked anesthesia, these individuals can identify objects by touch and can perform skilled movements and fine acts for which cutaneous sensations are indispensable, and may retain postural sensation even though all other sensations are lost. There may be a midline change for the sense of vibration over the bony areas, such as the skull or sternum, anatomically impossible because of the continuity of the bone stimulated. Hysterical changes and malingering can often be demonstrated by asking the patient to say "Yes" when

he is stimulated and "No" when he is not stimulated; he will often say "No" every time the pseudoanesthetic area is touched.

All so-called hysterical sensory changes should be carefully investigated, but it must be remembered that apprehensive patients are often very suggestible, and that a skilled examiner can easily suggest glove-and-stocking and midline changes to many individuals if he so wishes. The presence of organic anesthesia may be demonstrated by the use of the dermometer and the determination of electrical skin resistance. There is a diminished galvanic skin response and an increase in skin resistance if the nerve pathways are interrupted. It has been said

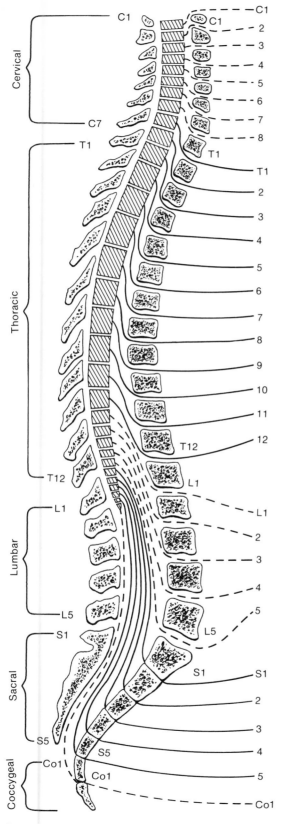

that hysterical individuals often have "hystero-genic" areas of hyperesthesia, especially in the inframammary region, over the ovaries, and over certain joints. Additional methods of examination in hysteria are described in Chapter 55.

Relief of Intractable Pain. In **cordotomy**, a therapeutic procedure for the relief of intractable pain, the ascending lateral spinothalamic pathway is sectioned with resulting contralateral anesthesia, usually from a level one to two segments below the level of the operation. Inasmuch as fibers which carry impulses from the upper portion of the body are medial and ventral to those from below, the level of relief depends upon the depth and anterior extent of the section. To obtain a high level of analgesia it is necessary to start at the attachment of the dentate ligament and carry the incision anteriorly and medially to a point just central to the emergence of the anterior roots. Occasionally a bilateral cordotomy is necessary for the relief of unilateral pain.

The lateral spinothalamic tract is also near the periphery in the medulla and in the mesencephalon, and it has been sectioned at these sites. It is sectioned in the medulla for the relief of high cervical pain. Here the incision is made at the level of the lower third of the inferior olivary nucleus, just caudal to the lowest filaments of the vagus nerve and the lower end of the fourth ventricle. The descending root of the trigeminal nerve is also sectioned at this site, and analgesia is produced on the ipsilateral side. In the mesencephalon it is possible to section both the spinothalamic tract and the ventral secondary ascending tract of the trigeminal nerve at the level of the posterior margin of the superior colliculus (anterior quadrigeminal body), across the brachium or the inferior colliculus to the base of the superior colliculus.

Pain in the distribution of a specific nerve or nerve root may be abolished by section of the nerve or root or by injection of local anesthetics, alcohol, or phenol into the affected nerve, root, or dorsal root ganglion or into the subarachnoid space. Posterior cordotomy has been performed for the relief of pain of a phantom limb. Peripheral nerve stimulations by such means as implants, transcutaneous nerve stimulation, and dorsal column stimulation have also been used

FIG. 5–11. The relationship of the spinal cord segments and spinal nerves to the vertebral bodies and spinous processes.

in the treatment of intractable pain, with variable success. Cerebral procedures for the relief of intractable pain will be discussed in Chapter 8.

Special Varieties of Sensory Changes. In the neuritides or in conditions where there is irritation of or pressure on the nerve roots, hyperesthesia may be present instead of anesthesia, together with demonstrable tenderness of the involved nerves. The ulnar, the radial, or the common peroneal nerves may often be palpated under the skin, and pressure on them may cause pain. Occasionally, as in the hypertrophic neuritis of Dejerine and Sottas and in leprosy, the hyperplasia of the nerves is palpable under the skin. In the neuritides there may also be pain on brisk passive stretching of the affected nerves.

There is increased susceptibility to ischemia in the presence of peripheral nerve and dorsal root lesions, and even in spinal and cerebral lesions, and constriction of a limb will accentuate both subjective and objective sensory changes; this can be used to evaluate both improvement and deterioration of nerve status. On the other hand, pressure and ischemia also cause paresthesias in the distribution of normal nerves, probably the result of impairment of conduction of some fibers and irritation of others. In conditions such as trigeminal neuralgia there is irritability of one or more branches of the nerves with resulting "trigger" or "dolorogenic" zones on the face. Hyperesthesia may precede the development of vesicles in herpes zoster. Hyperesthesia of the hands and the feet, in spite of demonstrable hypesthesia, is a frequent finding in patients with peripheral neuritis. This is especially true of the soles of the feet, which may be almost anesthetic to testing, yet extremely sensitive to all types of stimuli.

Spontaneous, or central, pain occurs most frequently with lesions of the thalamus. Similar pain, however, has also been described with cortical lesions, brain stem involvement (thrombosis of the posterior inferior cerebellar artery), and affections (usually post-traumatic) of the spinal cord. Either stimulation or section of the spinothalamic tract may cause a brief, intense, burning pain on the opposite side of the body, and neoplasms of the spinal cord may also cause contralateral pain. **Phantom,** or **spectral, sensations** are spontaneous sensations referred to insensitive areas; these may occur with lesions of the spinal cord or cauda equina. A **phantom limb,** on the other hand, is a sensation of the continued presence of an absent portion of the body, or of pain, paresthesias, or movement in it.

The terms **allachesthesia, allesthesia,** and **synesthesia** are used when the sensation of touch is experienced at a site remote from the point of stimulation; **allochiria** means the referring of a sensation to the opposite side of the body. Sensation in an affected area may be dulled when it and a normal area, usually the corresponding one on the opposite side of the body, are stimulated simultaneously; this denotes a cutaneous sensory **extinction,** or **suppression,** in the involved area, even though sensation may appear to be normal at the affected site if it is the only area stimulated. Occasionally a painful stimulus of high intensity in an analgesic area may cause perception of pain in adjacent regions on the same or opposite side of the body, owing to spread of excitatory processes within the segments of the cerebrospinal axis. After a cordotomy the patient may perceive pain on the normal side when the analgesic side is intensely stimulated.

Among the special varieties of sensory changes that may be found in the extremities are the following: **Causalgia** is a neuritis characterized by a disagreeable, burning type of pain, often accompanied by trophic changes, and most frequently seen in lesions of the median and sciatic nerves; **acroparesthesia** is a disease characterized by tingling, numbness, burning, and pain of the extremities, chiefly of the tips of the fingers and toes, often accompanied by cyanosis; **meralgia paresthetica** is a painful paresthesia in the area of distribution of the lateral femoral cutaneous nerve; **digitalgia paresthetica** is an isolated neuritis of the dorsal digital nerve of one of the fingers; **gonyalgia paresthetica** is a sensory neuritis of the infrapatellar branch of the saphenous nerve; **cheiralgia paresthetica** is an affection of the superficial branch of the radial nerve.

BIBLIOGRAPHY

Biemond A. The conduction of pain above the level of the thalamus opticus. Arch Neurol Psychiatry 1956;75:231

Bishop GH. The relation between nerve fiber size and sensory modality. J Nerv Ment Dis 1959;128:89

Bloedel JR, McCreery DR. Organization of peripheral and central pain pathways. Surg Neurol 1975;4:65

Bowsher D. Termination of the central pain pathway in man: The conscious appreciation of pain. Brain 1957; 80:606

Brodal A. Neurological Anatomy in Relation to Clinical Medicine, 3rd ed. New York, Oxford University Press, 1981

Casey KL. The neurophysiologic basis of pain. Postgrad Med 1973;53:58

Dyck PJ, O'Brien PC, Bushek W et al. Clinical vs. quantitative evaluation of cutaneous sensation. Arch Neurol 1976;33:659

Dyck PJ, Zimmerman IR, O'Brien PC et al. Introduction of automated systems to evaluate touch-pressure, vibration, and thermal cutaneous sensation in man. Ann Neurol 1978;4:502

Foerster O. The dermatomes in man. Brain 1933;56:1

Head H. Studies in Neurology. London, Oxford University Press, 1920

Kahn EA, Rand RW. On the anatomy of anterolateral cordotomy. J Neurosurg 1952;9:611

Keegan JJ, Garrett FD. The segmental distribution of the cutaneous nerves in the limbs of man. Anat Rec 1943;102:409

Lewis T. Pain. New York, Macmillan 1942.

Libman E. Observations on sensitiveness to pain. Trans Assoc Am Physicians 1926;41:305

Magee KR, Schneider RC. Syringomyelia. JAMA 1967; 200:135

Noordenbos W. Pain. Amsterdam, Elsevier, 1959

Noseworthy JH, Murray TJ, Lee SHA. Risks of the neurologist's pin. N Engl J Med 1979;301:1288

Notermans SLH. Measurement of the pain threshold determined by electrical stimulation and its clinical application. Neurology 1966;16:1071

Ogilvie WH, Thompson WAR (eds). Pain and Its Problems. London, Eyre & Spottiswoode, 1950

Schilling RF, Musser MJ. Pain reaction thresholds in psychoneurotic patients. Am J Med Sci 1948;215:195

Schwartz HG, O'Leary JL. Section of the spinothalamic tract in the medulla with observations on the pathway for pain. Surgery 1941;9:183

Sherman IC, Arieff AJ. Dissociation between pain and temperature in spinal cord lesions. J Nerv Ment Dis 1948;108:285

Sherrington CS. The Integrative Action of the Nervous System. New York, Charles Scribner's Sons, 1906

Spiller WG, Martin E. The treatment of persistent pain of organic origin in the lower part of the body by division of the anterolateral column of the spinal cord. JAMA 1912;58:1489

Szentágothai J, Kiss T. Projection of dermatomes on the substantia gelatinosa. Arch Neurol Psychiatry 1949;62:734

White JC, Sweet WH. Pain: Its Mechanisms and Neurosurgical Control. Springfield, IL, Charles C Thomas, 1955

Woolf HG, Wolf S. Pain, 2nd ed. Springfield, IL, Charles C Thomas, 1958

Young JH. The revision of the dermatomes. Aust NZ J Surg 1949;18:171

Chapter 6
THE PROPRIOCEPTIVE SENSATIONS

The proprioceptive sensations arise from the deeper tissues of the body, principally from the muscles, ligaments, bones, tendons, and joints. **Kinesthesia** is the sense by which muscular motion, weight, and position are perceived. **Bathyesthesia** is deep sensibility, or that from the parts of the body which are below the surface, such as the muscles and the joints. **Myesthesia** is muscle sensation, or the sensibility of impressions coming from the muscles. The aforementioned terms are sometimes used as synonyms for proprioceptive sensation, but the latter is somewhat more inclusive and specific varieties of it will be described.

The proprioceptive sensations which can be tested clinically are those of motion and position, vibration, and pressure; considered with the proprioceptive sensations, but somewhat different in nature, is deep pain.

ANATOMY

Traditionally, most impulses carrying proprioceptive sensation have been felt to ascend in the posterior columns of the spinal cord (dorsal funiculi). In recent years this concept has been challenged. The function of the dorsal columns is much more complex than had been believed. They are important in transferring peripheral inputs to the motor cortex necessary to plan, initiate, program, and monitor tasks requiring manipulative digital movements or intricate and precise sequences of phasic motor behavior (Davidoff). When the dorsal columns are com-

promised, any kind of discrimination is disturbed, as are knowledge of motion and position of the hands, along with ataxia and clumsiness. Nevertheless, the "clinical" viewpoint ascribing proprioceptive functions to the dorsal columns remains useful.

The peripheral sense organs most precisely dealing with proprioceptive information are situated in the muscles, tendons, and joints, the important ones being the neuromuscular and neurotendinous spindles, together with the pacinian and possibly the Golgi-Mazzoni corpuscles. These respond to pressure, tension, stretching of the muscle fibers, and related stimuli. The impulses travel along heavily myelinated fibers of the A type. The first cell body is situated in the dorsal root ganglion. The impulses traverse the medial division of the dorsal root (see Fig. 5-1, previous chapter), then going without a synapse into the ipsilateral fasciculi gracilis and cuneatus, within which they ascend to the nuclei gracilis and cuneatus in the lower medulla, where a synapse occurs. Following a decussation of the internal arcuate fibers, the impulses ascend in the medial lemniscus to the thalamus (Fig. 6-1).

Within the posterior columns the fibers carrying the impulses from the lower portions of the body are medial to those from the upper portions, and are pressed farther medially as additional incoming fibers enter the tracts. The fasciculus gracilis (column of Goll) transmits impulses from the sacral, lumbar, and lower thoracic nerves; it is medial to the fasciculus cuneatus (column of Burdach), which conveys impulses from the upper thoracic and cervical regions (see Fig. 5-3).

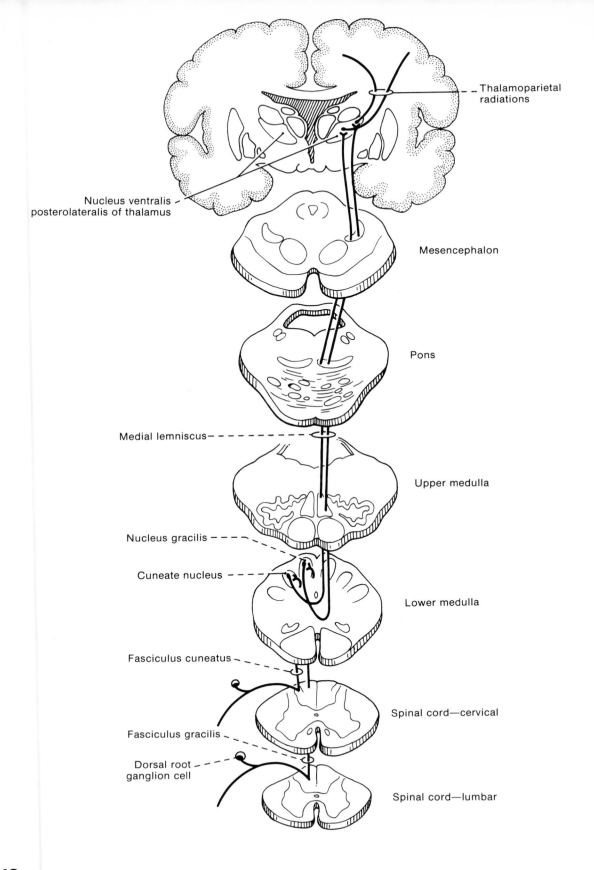

Thalamoparietal
radiations

Nucleus ventralis
posterolateralis of thalamus

Mesencephalon

Pons

Medial lemniscus

Upper medulla

Nucleus gracilis

Cuneate nucleus

Lower medulla

Fasciculus cuneatus

Spinal cord—cervical

Fasciculus gracilis

Dorsal root
ganglion cell

Spinal cord—lumbar

Within the medulla the medial lemniscus is a broad band of fibers situated along the median raphe; the fibers from the nucleus gracilis lie in the ventral position, and those from the nucleus cuneatus lie dorsally. In the pons the tract shifts to a ventromedian position, assuming the form of a flat band; the fibers from the nucleus gracilis are in the lateral position, and those from cuneatus, medial. In the mesencephalon the tract is in an oblique position; here the fibers from the nucleus gracilis lie dorsolaterally.

In the nucleus ventralis posterolateralis of the thalamus the posterior column terminations are caudal to those for pain and general touch, but the distribution is the same as for pain and touch; those from the upper portion of the body (cuneatus) are medial, and those from the lower portion of the body (gracilis) are in the lateral position. The thalamoparietal radiations then go through the posterior limb of the internal capsule, and the impulses are distributed on the cortex; those from the lower portions of the body pass medially; those from the upper areas pass laterally. Proprioceptive impulses for the posterior column pathway terminate in the parietal lobe posterior to those which convey touch.

Proprioceptive impulses from the head and neck enter the central nervous system with the cranial nerves. Many terminate on the mesencephalic root of the trigeminal nerve; others accompany motor nerves from the muscles they supply. Impulses probably reach the thalamus through the medial lemniscus.

SENSES OF MOTION AND POSITION

The sense of motion, also known as the kinetic sense, or the sensation of active or passive movement, consists of an awareness of motion in the various parts of the body. The sense of position, or of posture, consists of an awareness of the position of the body or its parts in space. **Arthresthesia** is used to designate the perception of joint movement and position, and **statognosis** to indicate the awareness of posture.

The sensations of motion and position are often tested together. They may be demonstrated by passively moving the digits to note the following: the patient's appreciation of movement and recognition of the direction, force, and range of movement; the minimum angle through which the digits have to be moved before he is aware of passive movement; his ability to judge the position of the digits in space. The appreciation of movement depends upon impulses arising as a result of motion of the joint and of lengthening and shortening the muscles. The normal individual should be able to appreciate movement of 1° or 2° at the interphalangeal joints. Quantitative devices for measuring joint movement are available. In minimal involvement there is first loss of the sense of position of the digits, then of motion; as the pathologic process becomes more extensive, loss of such recognition for an entire extremity develops, or even, at times, for the entire body. In the foot these sensations are lost in the small toes before they disappear in the great toe; in the hand involvement of the small finger may precede involvement of the ring, middle, or index finger, or thumb. There is some rise in the threshold for movement perception with age.

In testing, the completely relaxed digits should be grasped laterally with as little pressure as possible, and passively moved (Fig. 6-2). The examiner's fingers should be applied parallel to the plane of movement to eliminate variations in pressure. The digit being tested should be separated from adjoining ones so that no clues from contact are provided. The patient should be instructed not to attempt active movement of the digit, which may help to judge its position. If the senses of motion and position are lost in the digits, one should examine larger portions of the body, such as the leg and the forearm.

Reduction in the ability to perceive the direction in which the skin is passively moved may indicate impairment of position sense superficial to the joint. Such impairment usually is associated with joint-sense deficit as well. This is evaluated by the **pinch-press test.** The patient is asked to tell if the examiner is lightly pinching the skin or pressing it. Neither stimulus should be sufficiently intense so that either superficial or deep pain stimuli are induced.

Sensations of motion and position may also be tested by placing the fingers of one of the patient's hands in a certain position while his eyes are closed, then asking him to describe the position or to imitate it with the other hand. The foot may be passively moved while the eyes are closed, and the patient asked to point to his great toe or his heel. The patient may be asked to hold his hands outstretched; with loss of position sense one hand may waver or droop. One of the outstretched hands may be passively raised or lowered while the patient's eyes are closed, and the patient is asked to place the other extremity at the same level. One of the hands may be passively moved while the eyes are closed, and the patient asked to grasp the thumb or forefinger of

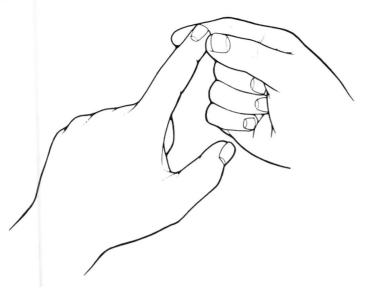

FIG. 6–2. *Method of testing position sense; done similarly with toe.*

that hand with the opposite hand. These latter tests, however, do not denote the side of involvement when a unilateral lesion is present.

Certain tests for ataxia, such as the finger-to-nose test and the heel-to-knee-to-toe test (see "Nonequilibratory Coordination," Ch. 30), are methods for examining the senses of motion and position if they are executed while the eyes are closed, assuming the tests are normal when the eyes are open. The senses of motion and position are also examined by observation of the station and gait. A patient with significantly disturbed sensations of movement and of position in the lower extremities is not aware of the position of his feet or of the posture of his body. A patient with tabes dorsalis, for instance, can assume a stable, erect posture when standing with his eyes open, but when his eyes are closed he tends to sway and fall; he can walk fairly well when his eyes are open, but when his eyes are closed he throws out his feet, staggers, and may fall (sensory ataxia). The **Romberg sign** is positive when the patient is able to stand with his feet together while his eyes are open, but sways or falls when they are closed; it is one of the earliest signs of posterior column disease. Sensations of motion and position contribute to the recognition of shape, size, and weight. Their absence may be manifested not only by recognizable changes in sensory acuity, but also by a difficulty in coordination known as **sensory ataxia** and by **stereo-anesthesia,** a difficulty in recognizing an object's shape, size, and weight by touch. The methods available for evaluating the senses of motion and position are all relatively

crude, however, and there may be definite impairment that is not adequately brought out by the testing procedures.

SENSE OF VIBRATION (PALLESTHESIA)

Pallesthesia is the ability to perceive the presence of vibration when an oscillating tuning fork is placed over certain bony prominences. A tuning fork of 128 Hz (C^0), with weighted ends, is most frequently used, although some authorities express the belief that a fork of 256 Hz (C^1) may detect finer changes in the vibratory threshold. Sensation is tested on the great toe, the medial and lateral malleoli of the ankle, the tibia, anterior superior iliac spine, sacrum, spinous processes of the vertebrae, sternum, clavicle, styloid processes of the radius and ulna, and the finger joints. It is also possible to test vibration perceived from the skin, or perceived from the bones and relayed via the skin and subcutaneous tissues; this may be tested on the pads of the fingertips. Not only the intensity of the stimulus which the patient perceives at the various sites, but also its duration, is noted. It is emphasized, however, that both intensity and duration depend to a great extent upon the force with which the fork is struck and the interval between the time it is set in motion and the time of application.

All observations are relative. There are some studies concerning the duration during which the normal individual perceives vibration at various sites of the body, but there are too many varying factors to make these statements reliable. Quantitative tests for vibration have been described in which an electrically stimulated oscillating rod or vibrating applicator (pallesthesiometer, clinical vibrometer, electronic biothesiometer) is used; this may vary in amplitude of vibration or in intensity but generally not in frequency, and thus the threshold of perception of vibratory sensibility can be determined. It is usually possible, however, for an adequate assessment to be made by using the tuning fork alone.

For clinical testing the tuning fork is placed in vibration and held on the great toe or over the lateral or medial malleolus until the patient no longer feels it vibrate in these places. The examiner then notes whether the vibration can still be felt at the wrist or over the sternum or clavicle, or, better still, compares the patient's perception of vibration with his own. Many examiners consider vibration sense to be "normal" when the patient perceives maximum vibration; a much more important criterion, however, is the ability to feel the fork when it has almost stopped vibrating, and relative differences are significant. The threshold for vibratory perception is normally somewhat higher in the lower than in the upper extremities. Loss of vibratory perception is referred to as **pallanesthesia**.

The receptors for vibratory stimuli are probably situated in the skin, subcutaneous tissues, muscles, periosteum, and other deeper structures of the body. Impulses are relayed with the proprioceptive tactile sensations through the large, fast-conducting, and the medium-sized myelinated nerve fibers, and traditionally ascend the spinal cord with other proprioceptive impulses in the dorsal columns. Many authorities express the belief that vibratory sensation is either a variety of deep cutaneous sensibility or a functional combination or elaboration of the primary senses of touch, rapidly alternating deep pressure, and position, rather than a specific proprioceptive entity, and dependent upon both cutaneous and deep afferent fibers. Bone may act largely as a resonator. For clinical diagnosis, it can be considered a specific type of sensation, however, changes in which are of definite diagnostic value. Netsky suggests, based on the pathologic study of a group of cases of syringomyelia, that vibratory sensation may be carried by the medial portions of the lateral columns of the spinal cord, rather than the posterior columns, while Calne and Pallis believe that it is carried in both the posterior and lateral col-umns. These concepts would explain the dissociation that is occasionally encountered between changes in motion and position senses and in vibration sense.

In patients with diseases of the posterior columns the sense of vibration is lost in the lower extremities much earlier than in the upper. Thus, the finding of a normal vibratory threshold in the distal lower extremities can usually obviate the need for detailed testing proximally or in the upper extremities, unless there are specific symptoms pointing to disease in these areas. A moderate decrease in vibratory perception in the lower extremities or a difference between the lower and the upper extremities may be clinically significant. It is important to remember, however, that with advancing age there is a progressive loss in the ability to recognize vibratory sense, and the sensation may be entirely absent in elderly individuals. The perceptions of motion, position, and vibration do not always parallel one another, and in some clinical conditions one is affected much more and much earlier than another. Occasionally, in localized spinal cord lesions, a "level" of vibration sense may be found on testing over the spinous processes. This variety of sensation may also be impaired or lost in lesions of the dorsal root ganglia, nerve roots, and peripheral nerves. Such sensory alterations may assist in the localization of a ruptured intervertebral disk. In certain peripheral neuropathies, especially those associated with pernicious anemia and diabetes mellitus, there may be marked loss of vibration sense in the distal portions of the extremities; there is also impairment in hypothyroidism.

PRESSURE SENSATION

Pressure or touch-pressure sensation is closely related to tactile sense, but involves the perception of pressure from the subcutaneous structures rather than light touch from the skin. It is also closely related to position sense and is mediated via the posterior columns. The more specific peripheral sense organs include the pacinian, or lamellar, and Golgi – Mazzoni corpuscles, which are found in the deeper layers of the skin, connective tissue, subcutaneous tissues, tendon sheaths, muscle aponeuroses, intramuscular septa, and periosteum, and near the tendons and joints. Pressure sense is tested by firm touch upon the skin with a finger or a blunt object, and by pressure on the subcutaneous structures, such as the muscle masses, the tendons, and the nerves themselves, either by the use of a blunt object or by squeezing between the fingers, and one tests both the appreciation and the localization of pressure. For quantitative testing the Head pressure aesthesiometer may be used, or the piesimeter, an instrument in which the differentiation in focal pressure is measured in grams. The term **piesesthesia** means pressure sensibility, and **baresthesia** is sometimes used to signify the sensibility for pressure or weight; this must be differentiated from **barognosis,** the appreciation, recognition, and differentiation of weight, which is described under the cerebral sensory functions. When strong pressure is applied over the muscle masses, tendons, and nerves, one tests deep pain sensibility.

DEEP PAIN SENSE, OR PRESSURE PAIN

The recognition of pain in the deeper tissues of the body is a proprioceptive sense in that the sense organs stimulated and the origin of the impulse are below the cutaneous level. It is more diffuse and less well localized than superficial pain. The neurons which carry deep pain do not follow the pathway of the other proprioceptive sensations, however, but ascend in the lateral spinothalamic tract with those which carry superficial pain. Deep pain is tested by squeezing the muscles or tendons, by pressure on those nerves which lie close to the surface, or by pressure on the testicles or the eyeballs. Deep pain sense is lost early in tabes, but here its loss is due not to involvement of the dorsal funiculi but to the presence of pathologic change in the dorsal root ganglia. Before the loss of deep pain there is a **delayed pain** reaction, for both superficial and deep pain, in which response to a painful stimulation is retarded.

Several maneuvers evaluate deep pain. **Abadie's sign** is the loss of pressure pain sense in the Achilles tendon, **Biernacki's sign** is the absence of pain on pressure on the ulnar nerve, and **Pitres' sign** is loss of pain on pressure on the testes; these are found in tabes dorsalis and other disorders affecting pain pathways. Increased sensibility and marked tenderness in the muscle masses, tendons, and nerves are present in the peripheral neuropathies, and occasionally there is palpable abnormality of the nerves. Muscle tenderness may also be present in myositis. Tenderness should not be considered an increased acuity for deep pain. **Tinel's sign** is a tingling sensation in the distal end of an extremity on pressure over the site of a divided nerve; it points to beginning regeneration of the nerve.

In addition to the above proprioceptive sensations, which are tested in every complete neurologic examination, there are other proprioceptive impulses and pathways which are important from both clinical and neurophysiological points of view. Afferent impulses are carried to the cerebellum through the dorsal and ventral spinocerebellar pathways (see "Anatomy and Physiology," Ch. 24). Impulses are carried to the brain stem through the spinotectal and spinoolivary tracts. There are impulses which function in exciting and inhibiting reflexes, in stretch excitation, and in postural and righting reflexes (see Part E, "The Reflexes"). Some of the above impulses arise in proprioceptors, others in less well defined end-organs. There are no methods for examining these as specific sensory modalities, however, and they may be described as afferent but nonsensory elements. Vestibular sensibility, or balance sense, is a proprioceptive sensation which arises in part from stimulation of the muscles, joints, and tendons, and is carried through pathways in the spinal cord. The principal sensory organs of the vestibular apparatus, however, are the semicircular canals, and vestibular sense may be regarded as one of the special senses, mediated through the cranial nerves (see "The Vestibular Nerve," Ch. 14).

BIBLIOGRAPHY

Brodal A. Neurological Anatomy in Relation to Clinical Medicine, 3rd ed. New York, Oxford University Press, 1981.

Calne DB, Pallis CA. Vibratory sense: A critical review. Brain 1966;89:723

Collens WS, Zilinski JD, Boas LC. Clinical vibrometer: An apparatus to measure vibratory sense quantitatively. Am J Med 1946;1: 636

Davidoff RA. The dorsal columns. Neurology 1989;39:1377

Fox JC Jr, Klemperer WW. Vibratory sensibility: A quantitative study of its thresholds in nervous disorders. Arch Neurol Psychiatry 1942;48:622

Goff GD, Rosner BS, Detre T et al. Vibration perception in normal man and medical patients. J Neurol Neurosurg Psychiatry 1965;28:503

Gordan DS. Pedal goniometer to assess ankle proprioception. Arch Phys Med Rehab 1988;69:461

Herrick CJ. The proprioceptive nervous system. J Nerv Ment Dis 1947;106:335

Kaplan FS, Nixon JE, Reitz M et al. Age-related changes in proprioception and sensation of joint position. Acta Orthopaed Scand 1985;56:72

Keighley G. An instrument for measurement of vibration sense in man. Milbank Mem Fund Q 1946;24:36

Nathan PW, Smith MC, Cook AW. Sensory effects in man of lesions of the posterior columns and of some other afferent pathways. Brain 1986;109:1003

Netzky MG. Syringomyelia: A clinicopathologic study. Arch Neurol Psychiatry 1953;70:741

Pearson CGH. Effect of age on vibratory sensibility. Arch Neurol Psychiatry 1928;20:482

Plumb CS, Meigs JW. Human vibration perception. I. Vibration perception at different ages (normal ranges). Arch Gen Psychiatry 1961;4:611

Schwartzman RJ, Bogdonoff MD. Proprioception and vibration sensibility discrimination in the absence of the posterior columns. Arch Neurol 1969;20:349

Steiness I. Vibratory perception in normal subjects. Acta Med Scand 1957;158:315

Yoss RE. Studies of the spinal cord: Part 3. Pathways for deep pain within the spinal cord and brain. Neurology 1953;3:163

Chapter 7
THE INTEROCEPTIVE, OR VISCERAL, SENSATIONS

The interoceptive sensations are the general visceral sensations, arising from the internal organs. The special visceral sensations such as smell and taste will be discussed individually in Part C, "The Cranial Nerves." The interoceptive sensations are important clinically, and the patient may, in the history, give information about pain, spasm, or distention of the viscera — a feeling of fullness in the stomach after a meal, gastric discomfort, spasm of the intestine, a pressure sensation in the chest, a sensation of fullness in the bladder or rectum, a desire for micturition, a sense of engorgement from the genitalia, or pain in the internal organs.

Visceral pain is often vaguely localized or diffuse, but is described by the patient as deepseated. Certain of the viscera are sensitive to direct stimulation; others are not. Pain endings are found in the parietal pleura over the thoracic wall and the diaphragm, although probably none are present in the visceral pleura on the lungs. The pericardium is probably insensitive to pain, but the vessels of the heart are extremely sensitive. The parietal peritoneum is sensitive, especially to distention, but the visceral peritoneum is probably not sensitive. Direct stimulation of the hollow viscera causes little or no pain, but spasm, inflammation, trauma, pressure, distention, or tension on them may produce severe pain if the stimulus is adequate, possibly the result of involvement of the surrounding tissues.

Afferent visceral fibers are found in the seventh, ninth, and tenth cranial nerves and in the thoracolumbar and sacral autonomic nerves. Their cell bodies are found in the cerebrospinal (dorsal root and associated cranial) ganglia, like the afferent fibers which accompany the somatic nerves, and impulses enter the central nervous system by way of the posterior roots and ascend to the higher centers through pathways close to those which carry somatic impulses. Although these fibers may be identified within the individual autonomic nerves, after reaching the dorsal root ganglia they are difficult or impossible to distinguish from fibers which carry the somatic afferent impulses. Controversy persists regarding the existence of any anatomic or physiologic differentiation between visceral and somatic afferent nerves. The distinction between the two may be entirely on the basis of peripheral distribution rather than associated with fundamental morphologic or functional variation. Authorities differ as to whether or not afferent axons are actually present in the autonomic nervous system. The so-called visceral afferent fibers may be indistinguishable from somatic afferent fibers, although they travel with the efferent fibers of the autonomic nervous system.

The afferent fibers that have been demonstrated in the autonomic nerves may function in visceral reflex action without conveying sensations to consciousness, or the autonomic nervous system may act as an accessory conduction system for painful and other impulses. The afferent impulses from the viscera may reach consciousness by a variety of routes. Some travel in somatic nerves and some with efferent autonomic nerves, while others travel near to nerves that are in close proximity to the blood vessels but later join the autonomic nerves. Some synapse in the dorsal horn, and the neuraxis of the neuron of the next order crosses to the opposite spinothalamic tract, where the fibers that carry visceral pain lie medial to those that carry superficial pain and temperature sensations. Many ascend for a greater distance in the white matter of the dorsolateral funiculus before a synapse, however, and some ascend by long intersegmental fibers in the white matter at the border of the dorsal horn, and reach the hypothalamus and thalamus without decussation. Still others may ascend in the ipsilateral spinothalamic tract. As a consequence, localization of visceral pain is not precise, and the threshold may be high. It has been said that the gyrus rectus rather than the parietal cortex may be the end station for visceral afferent sensation.

Visceral pain may on occasion be relieved by sympathectomy or sympathetic ganglionectomy, by means of which afferent neurons that run with the autonomic fibers are sectioned, but other factors may also contribute to the therapeutic results. The relief of the pain of angina pectoris by injection or section of the middle and inferior cervical and upper thoracic sympathetic ganglia may be effected not only by interruption of afferent fibers, but also by interruption of efferent pathways with consequent vasodilation, chemical alteration, and decrease in spasm. The mitigation of pain in Raynaud's disease by interruption of autonomic pathways is largely due to vasodilation and increased oxygenation of tissues. The relief of the pain of causalgia by sympathetic block may not be due to interruption of pain fibers in the autonomic nerves but to decrease in vasospasm and interruption of the efferent autonomic discharges from the hypothalamus, which may be causing direct irritation of the somatic afferent fibers.

Visceral pain on the aforementioned and other bases is also relieved by posterior root section and by section of the lateral spinothalamic tracts. However, because the visceral afferent fibers lie medial in the latter tracts, a cordotomy for the relief of visceral pain must be carried out with a deeper incision than one for the relief of somatic pain. Furthermore, because the afferent impulses from the viscera ascend for a greater distance before decussation, it is necessary to perform a cordotomy at a higher level to control visceral pain than to control pain from somatic structures. Also, because pain impulses from the viscera may be carried in both crossed and uncrossed pathways, a cordotomy done to control visceral pain may have to be bilateral. The pain of causalgia may also be relieved by posterior cordotomy and section of the long intersegmental fibers near the dorsal horn. It is stressed, however, that the mechanisms by which the autonomic nervous system effects conscious perception of pain are very complex and the technics mentioned previously are frequently unsuccessful in alleviating discomfort, particularly in disorders such as causalgia.

In addition to the pain experienced in the viscus itself, which may be vaguely localized and diffuse, but is deep-seated, there may be an associated somatic pain of reflex origin, known as **referred pain.** This is referred to the skin and subcutaneous tissues, and the area in which it is felt may be hyperalgesic to stimulation. It has been stated that this referred pain is experienced in the area of cutaneous distribution of the spinal nerves which corresponds to the level of the spinal cord segments that supply the viscus. Many years ago Head delineated the zones of pain and hyperalgesia which are found in disease of the various viscera. These are rather poorly localized; however, they vary widely, and the pain is frequently referred to distant areas. Referred pain may arise in the dermatome or skin segment directly over the involved organ, as a result of corresponding segmental innervation, or the pain may be quite distant, as a result of shifting of the viscus during embryonic development. Appendiceal pain is felt directly over the appendix; the pain of angina pectoris may radiate down the left arm, whereas renal pain is referred to the groin and diaphragmatic pain is referred to the shoulder or neck. The phrenic nerve, for instance, which is supplied by fibers from the third, fourth, and fifth cervical nerves, is motor to the diaphragm and is also sensory to it and to the contiguous structures, the extrapleural and extraperitoneal connective tissues in the vicinity of the gallbladder and liver. As a consequence, in irritation of the gallbladder, liver, or central portion of the diaphragm, there may be pain and hyperesthesia not only in the viscus involved, but also on the side of the neck and shoulder in the cutaneous distribution of the third, fourth, and fifth cervical nerves, or in the area supplied by the posterior roots of those nerves whose anterior roots supply the diaphragm. Some other hyperalgesic skin zones involved in referred visceral pain include mid-thoracic levels for stomach, duodenum, pancreas, liver, and spleen; upper thoracic levels for the heart; upper and mid-thoracic levels for the lungs; and low thoracic and upper lumbar levels for the kidney. With some exceptions, the referred pain appears on the same side of the body in which the diseased organ is located.

Referred pain has been said to be produced by the viscerocutaneous reflex (or the peritoneocutaneous reflex if the stimulus results from involvement of the peritoneum rather than the viscus itself) and to be brought about by central spread of the excitatory effects of noxious stimulation. At times there may also be tenderness and spasm of the musculature in the same area; this is a manifestation of the visceromotor, or peritoneomotor, reflex. It may be, however, that the pain and spasm, rather than being true reflex phenomena, are associated with a central mechanism in the internuncial pool. Both somatic and visceral afferent neurons may carry impulses which converge in and affect a common pool of secondary neurons. Sinclair, Weddell, and Feindel explain referred pain on the basis of branching of the axons which carry pain sensibility, one limb going to the site of irritation, the other to the site to which pain is referred; antidromic impulses are sent from the trigger point to the area of reference. Infiltration of this latter area with local anesthetic may relieve the pain, although residual discomfort may persist; this procedure may give indirect evidence which contributes to the neurologic examination and diagnosis.

Abnormal impulses arising from the viscera as a result of spasm or tension are usually due to pressure, inflammation, or trauma. They may be carried through special visceral fibers, or they may be mediated through somatic fibers, secondary to involvement of somatic tissues by the pressure, inflammation, or trauma.

Visceral sensations, regardless of their importance in clinical medicine, cannot be adequately evaluated by the procedures used in the routine neurologic examination. They are poorly localized and, due to their origin within the body, clinical methods for testing them are not available. Some of the sensations tested may be mediated by somatic nerves. There are, however, indirect procedures which may give some information. The use of atropine, for instance, to decrease intestinal spasm or bronchospasm, or of neostigmine to decrease distention, may afford a clue to the underlying mechanism. There are also tests for sensation in specific viscera, such as the appreciation of sensations of distention, pain, heat, and cold in the bladder during the process of cystometric examination; this subject will be considered more at length in Part F, "The Autonomic Nervous System."

BIBLIOGRAPHY

Freeman LW, Shumacker HB Jr, Radigan LR. A functional study of afferent fibers in peripheral sympathetic nerves. Surgery 1950;28:274

Head H. Studies in Neurology. London, Oxford University Press, 1920

Hinsey JC. The anatomical relations of the sympathetic system to visceral sensation. Assoc Res Nerv Dis Proc 1935;15:105

Livingston WK. Pain Mechanisms: A Physiologic Interpretation of Causalgia and Its Related States. New York, Macmillan, 1943

Pollock LJ, Davis L. Visceral and referred pain. Assoc Res Nerv Dis Proc 1935;15:210

Sinclair DC, Weddell G, Feindel WH. Referred pain and associated phenomena. Brain 1948;71:184

White JC. Conduction of pain in man: Observations on its afferent pathways within the spinal cord and visceral nerves. Arch Neurol Psychiatry 1954;71:1

Chapter 8
INTERPRETATION OF SENSORY DISTURBANCES

A. CEREBRAL SENSORY FUNCTIONS

The term **combined sensation** has been used to describe those varieties of sensation for the recognition of which more than one of the previously discussed senses is used. They are not mere combinations of sensation, however, and in most instances a cortical component is necessary for the final perception. This cortical component is a function of the parietal lobes, which act to analyze and synthesize the individual varieties of sensation; to correlate, integrate, and elaborate the impulses; to interpret the stimuli; and to call out memories to aid in discrimination and recognition. The resulting manifestations are perceptual and discriminative functions rather than the simple appreciation of the stimulation of primary sensory nerve endings. The more important combined sensory functions will be described.

Stereognosis is a faculty of perceiving and understanding the form and nature of objects by touch, and of identifying and recognizing them. When this ability is lost, the patient has **astereognosis**, or **tactile agnosia.** Astereognosis can be diagnosed only if cutaneous and proprioceptive sensations are present, for if these are significantly impaired, the primary impulses cannot reach consciousness for interpretation. Various qualities or steps may be noted in the recognition of objects. First, the size is perceived. Then the appreciation of shape in two dimensions is noted, then form in three dimensions, and finally there is identification of the object. Size perception may be tested by the use of objects of the same shape but of different sizes.

Shape perception may be tested by the use of objects of simple shapes, such as a circle, a square, or a triangle, cut out of stiff paper or plastic. Form perception is examined by the use of solid geometric objects, such as a cube, pyramid, or plastic or wooden balls. Finally, recognition is evaluated by placing simple objects such as a key, button, comb, pencil, or safety pin in the hand of the blind-folded patient and asking him to identify them. For more delicate testing the patient may be asked to differentiate coins, to identify letters carved out of wood or fiberboard, or to count the number of dots on dominoes. Stereognostic sensation, obviously, can be tested only in the hands. If weakness of the hands is present, the examiner must manipulate the object as it lies in the patient's fingers. When diminution of stereognostic sensation is evident, a delay in identification, or decrease in the normal exploring movements as the patient manipulates the unknown object, can be observed.

Recognition of texture may be regarded as a special variety of stereognosis in which the patient is asked to recognize similarities and differences, but it can probably be considered a specific type of combined sensation. It is tested by asking the subject to differentiate between cotton, silk, and wool, or between wood, glass, and metal.

Barognosis is the recognition of weight, or the ability to differentiate between weights. It is tested by the use of objects of similar size but of different weights, such as a series of plastic or wooden balls, or blocks loaded with different weights, which are appraised by holding them in the hand, either unsupported or resting on a table, but preferably the former. The senses of motion and position should be intact. Loss of ability to differentiate weight is known as **baragnosis.**

Topesthesia, or **topognosia,** is the ability to localize a tactile sensation. Its loss is known as **topoanesthesia,** or **topagnosia.** Localization is impossible if there is cutaneous anesthesia, but the loss of the sense of localization with an intact exteroceptive sensibility usually signifies the presence of a lesion affecting the parietal lobe.

Graphesthesia is a term used to designate the ability to recognize letters or numbers written on the skin. Letters or numbers 1 mm in height may be written on the finger pads, and up to 4 mm in height on the forearm and legs. A pencil or a dull pin is used to write the letters, and the patient is asked to identify them. Easily identifiable, dissimilar numbers should be used, e.g., 3 and 4 rather than 3 and 8. Loss of this sensation is known as **graphanesthesia.** The ability to identify letters written on the skin is interfered with in peripheral nerve and spinal cord lesions, and impairment of this ability may be a manifestation of slight involvement of cutaneous sensibility. Graphesthesia may be a finely discriminative variety of cutaneous sensation, but its loss in the presence of intact peripheral sensation implies the presence of a cortical lesion. This is particularly true when the loss is unilateral.

Two-point, or **spatial, discrimination** is the ability to differentiate cutaneous stimulation by one blunt point from stimulation by two points. A compass or a calibrated two-point esthesiometer is used, and the patient is stimulated randomly by a single point and by two points. Bending a paperclip to different distances between its two points is less quantitative but readily available for quick evaluation of differences between the two sides of the body. The patient's eyes should be closed during the test. It is best to start with the two points relatively far apart, and single and double points should be varied unpredictably; the points are approximated until the patient begins to make errors. One notes the minimum distance between two points that can be felt separately. The distance varies considerably in different parts of the body. Two points can be differentiated from one at a distance of 1 mm on the tip of the tongue, at 2 – 4 mm on the fingertips, at 4 – 6 mm on the dorsum of the fingers, at 8 – 12 mm on the palm, and at 20 – 30 mm on the dorsum of the hand. Greater distances are necessary for differentiation on the forearm, upper arm, torso, thigh, and leg. The

findings on the two sides of the body must always be compared.

Two-point discrimination is a highly discriminatory tactile sensibility, carried mainly through the posterior columns (dorsal funiculi). Loss of two-point discrimination with preservation of other discriminatory tactile and proprioceptive sensation may be the most subtle sign of a lesion of the opposite parietal lobe.

Recognition of electrical stimulation has been classified by some neurologists as a variety of combined sensation, but probably should not be so considered. Faradic stimulation probably affects mainly the tactile endings; galvanic current influences the temperature end-bulbs, and if sufficiently intense may stimulate the pain organs. Static electricity and electrical sparks may also affect the pain endings. The use of electricity in the sensory examination probably has little value.

Sensory extinction or **inattention** is the loss of ability to perceive sensation on one side of the body when identical areas on the two sides are stimulated simultaneously. Blunt points, cotton, or touch with the fingertip can be used as stimuli. One may also test the patient's ability to recognize double simultaneous stimulation of different segments of the body, on either the same or opposite sides, or to distinguish two cutaneous stimuli separated by a brief time interval.

Autotopagnosia, or **somatotopagnosia,** is the loss of power to identify or orient the body or the relation of its individual parts — a defect in the body scheme. The patient may have complete loss of personal identification of one limb or of one half of the body. He may drop his hand from the table onto his lap and believe that some other object has fallen, or he may feel an arm next to his body and not be aware that it is his own. Lack of awareness of one half of the body is referred to as **agnosia of the body half.**

In the syndrome of **finger agnosia** of Gerstmann there is an inability to recognize, name, and select individual fingers when looking at the hands. This may apply to both the patient's and the examiner's fingers. Accompanying this, in the full-blown syndrome, is loss of awareness of the position and identity of the parts of the body, with disorientation for right and left, agraphia, and acalculia.

Anosognosia is defined as the ignorance of the existence of disease and has been used specifically to imply the imperception of hemiplegia, or a feeling of depersonalization toward or loss of perception of paralyzed parts of the body, either due to anesthesia of the paralyzed parts or to amnesia for them. The patient may believe that he is able to use his paretic extremities in a normal manner. Anosognosia is most often found in lesions of the right parietal lobe.

The aforementioned are all complicated varieties of disturbances of cerebral sensory function, indicating involvement of parietal areas or their connections. Inasmuch, however, as they are actually types of agnosia, their characteristics and significance in localization are discussed in more detail in Chapter 52.

The *parietal cortex* receives, correlates, synthesizes, and elaborates the primary sensory impulses (Ch. 49). It is not concerned with the cruder sensations, such as recognition of pain and temperature, which are subserved by the thalamus (to be described later in this chapter). It is important in the discrimination of the finer or more critical grades of sensation, such as the recognition of intensity, the appreciation of similarities and differences, and the evaluation of the gnostic, or perceiving and recognizing, aspects of sensation. It is also important in localization, in the recognition of spatial relationships and postural sense, in the appreciation of passive movement, and in the recognition of differences in form and weight and of two-dimensional qualities. These elements of sensation are more than simple perceptions, and for their recognition it is necessary to integrate the various stimuli into concrete concepts as well as to call forth engrams. They are diminished or absent in lesions of the anterior portion of the middle third of the postcentral gyrus of the parietal lobe. The loss of each of these varieties of combined sensation may be considered a variety of **agnosia,** or the loss of the power to recognize the import of sensory stimuli.

Occasionally loss of ability to recognize the size and shape of objects is encountered with lesions of the cervical portion of the spinal cord and even of the posterior nerve roots and brachial plexus. Autotopagnosia also has been observed with lesions in these sites. In such instances, however, there is severe involvement of proprioceptive as well as of cutaneous sensation. The term **stereoanesthesia** is occasionally used when the difficulty results from infracerebral lesions, and the term **astereognosis** is reserved for disturbances that follow interference with cortical synthesis.

Lesions of the parietal cortex are not associated with anesthesia or complete loss of sensation. There may be diminution in the appreciation of the various modalities, with a raising of the threshold on the opposite side of the body, but both exteroceptive and proprioceptive sensations are perceived. Sensation is often disturbed more in the upper than in the lower extremity, trunk, or face. The distal parts of the extremities are affected more than the proximal portions, with a gradual transition to more normal perception as the shoulder and hip are approached. Perception becomes normal before the midline is reached on both face and trunk.

The threshold for pain stimuli is raised very little in parietal lesions, although a prick may feel less sharp than on the normal side; with deeper lesions the threshold is more definitely raised. The qualitative elements of heat and cold are present, but there is loss of discrimination for slight variations in temperature, especially in the intermediate ranges. Light touch perception is little disturbed, but tactile discrimination and localization may be profoundly affected. There often is severe impairment of postural sense; this results in sensory ataxia and athetoidlike movements. Vibratory sensation is only rarely affected. Astereognosis, baragnosis, graphanesthesia, and impairment of two-point discrimination may all be present. The period required for sensory adaptation is prolonged, and occasionally allachesthesia is experienced. Disorders of the body image such as autotopagnosia, anosognosia, and Gerstmann's syndrome occur with localized involvement.

Lesions between the thalamus and the cortex, especially those affecting the posterior limb of the internal capsule, cause more severe and extensive sensory loss than isolated cortical lesions. In this area the fibers are crowded closely together.

Detailed examinations of sensory perception and critical evaluation may be necessary to diagnose lesions of the parietal lobe. Both small and large objects may have to be used in testing for astereognosis; sometimes a delay in answering when objects are placed in the affected hand, with no delay when the other side is examined, may be a clue to minimal involvement. A similar detailed investigation of tactile localization and discrimination may be essential. Sensory inattention, or extinction, is often an early and important diagnostic finding in parietal lobe lesions. With involvement of one parietal area, the stimulus on the opposite side of the body will not be perceived, even though sensation on that side may be normal with routine testing. Critchley considers this to be the result of lack of attention to or local disregard of the affected body parts, whereas Bender believes that stimulation of the normal parietal lobe suppresses interpretation of impulses by the affected one, producing extinction. Bilateral simultaneous testing for stereognostic sense (placing identical objects in the patient's hands) may yield valuable information. The ability to distinguish two cutaneous stimuli separated by a brief time interval is also impaired with parietal lobe lesions. Double simultaneous stimulation above and below the presumed level of a spinal cord lesion in which there is relative but not absolute sensory loss may aid in demonstrating the level of the lesion. If the upper stimulus only is perceived, the lower is moved more rostrally until the intensity of both is equal; this may indicate the segmental level of the lesion. Bilateral or homolateral simultaneous stimulation of two different segments of the body (heterologous areas) shows that even in normal subjects one stimulus "dominates" the other, at least for the initial tests. In young children, patients with organic disease of the brain, and the aged this phenomenon is demonstrable still more frequently, and it appears that in general the more rostral area is the dominant one; when face and hand are stimulated, there is extinction of the hand percept (the **face-hand test**).

Sensory impulses that enter consciousness for interpretation by the parietal cortex must first pass through the *thalamus* and then be redistributed. The thalamus is thought to be the end-station in the quantitative interpretation of pain, heat, cold, and heavy contact, and is a receptive center wherein sensory impulses produce a crude, uncritical form of consciousness. A lesion in or near the thalamus may cause loss of various sensations, owing to interruption of the impulses on which they depend. A severe and extensive lesion may cause gross impairment of all forms of sensation on the opposite side of the body, probably as a result of damage to the nucleus ventralis posterolateralis (body) and posteromedialis (face). Marked loss of appreciation of heavy contact, posture, passive movement, and deep pressure perception occurs, and the thresholds for light touch, pain, and temperature sensations are raised.

In the **thalamic syndrome** of Dejerine and Roussy, which occasionally accompanies a cerebral hemorrhage or thrombosis, there is a characteristic group of symptoms, the result either of damage which predominates in the nucleus ventralis posterolateralis or of an interruption of the pathways from the thalamus to the cerebral cortex. The responsible lesion need not be limited to the thalamus. There is blunting, or raising of the threshold, of all forms of sensation on the opposite side of the body, without true anesthesia. All stimuli, however, when effective, excite unpleasant sensations, and any stimulus, even the lightest, may evoke a disagreeable, often burning, type of pain response. Slight hot and cold stimuli, and also light cutaneous sensations, excite marked discomfort. The overreaction is termed **hyperpathia,** and the diminution of all varieties of superficial and deep sensibility, accompanied by subjective intractable pain in the hypesthetic regions, is called **anesthesia dolorosa.** In addition to sensory changes, a hemiparesis or hemiplegia and a hemianopia usually occur and, less frequently, hemiataxia, choreoathetosis, and unmotivated emotional responses. Occasionally, pleasurable stimulation, such as that produced when a warm hand is applied to the skin on the affected side, may be markedly accentuated. This thalamic overreaction is due either to irritation of the thalamus or to release of thalamic function from normal cortical control by damage to higher centers. Every stimulus acting on the thalamus produces an excessive effect on the abnormal half of the body, especially as far as the affective element — the pleasant or unpleasant character in its appreciation — is concerned.

B. LOCALIZATION OF SENSORY DISORDERS

Diminution or loss of sensation may occur in the presence of lesions at various levels of the nervous system, as may abnormal sensations, such as pain or paresthesia.

Either diminution or perversion of sensation occurs in the presence of lesions involving the *end-organs*, or sensory receptors, such as the pain endings and Meissner's corpuscles. These are microscopic structures, and pathologic changes in them are difficult to evaluate. Quantitative studies of Meissner's corpuscles, however, have shown that they decrease in number with advancing age, and that their cholinesterase activity is decreased in the distribution of underfunctioning peripheral nerves. The pain that is perceived with irritation of the skin, traumatic denudements, and burns, as well as pruritus, paresthesias, and dysesthesias, may result from irritation of these distal structures or the nerve filaments to them, and decreased sensation in callosities and scars may result from involvement of the end-organs and smaller filaments. Infiltration of an area with a local anesthetic or freezing with ethyl chloride will cause anesthesia.

In lesions of the *peripheral nerves* there usually is a loss or diminution in all types of sensation in the distribution of the nerve or nerves affected. The areas of skin supplied by various nerves are shown in Chapter 43, "Peripheral Nerve Disorders." In peripheral neuritis, vibration is often the first modality to be found to be defective, but in severe cases all exteroceptive, proprioceptive, and combined modalities are impaired. An irritative lesion of a peripheral nerve may also cause abnormal sensation in the form of paresthesias or of pain that is either constant or lancinating in character. The nerves themselves may be hyperalgesic and sensitive, or tender to pressure, and there may be pain on brisk stretching of the affected nerves and increased susceptibility to ischemia. There sometimes is hyperalgesia in the cutaneous distribution of the nerves, even though the sensory threshold is raised. The unmyelinated fibers may be most affected, so the threshold for slow or aching pain is depressed, while the myelinated fibers may suffer less damage, and the threshold for fast or piercing pain is raised. In polyneuritis the distribution of sensory loss is variable, usually involving predominantly the distal segments. There may be what appears to be a glove and stocking distribution of altered sensation, but the margins of this area are poorly demarcated, and usually there is a peripheral blunting of sensation with no sharp border between the normal and hypesthetic areas.

The sensory examination is important in the diagnosis of peripheral nerve injuries and in the evaluation of progress in nerve regeneration. Pain in the distribution of a single nerve or group of nerves can be relieved by section of the nerves involved or injection with local anesthetic agents, alcohol, or phenol. Section or injection of a nerve peripheral to the dorsal root ganglion, however, may be followed by regeneration and return of pain.

Disease of the *dorsal root ganglia* (or corresponding ganglia of the cranial nerves) is also associated with sensory changes. In herpes zoster there is severe, lancinating pain in the distribution of the affected ganglia. In the now rare tabes dorsalis there is loss of deep pain, a delayed response to superficial painful stimulation, and, sometimes, impairment of superficial pain sensation. Transient, spontaneous "lightning" pains may develop. In hereditary sensory neuropathy the pathologic lesions are in the dorsal root ganglia; there is severe distal loss of all sensory modalities, along with trophic changes in the extremities.

The *nerve root* is in reality a part of the peripheral nerve, since it constitutes a part of the same neuron. Radicular lesions also are accompanied by diminution or loss of sensation, and by either pain or paresthesias, but the distribution is segmental in type. Irritation of the nerve roots causes pain in a radicular, sometimes girdle, distribution (i.e., encircling the body). The pain may be either constant or intermittent, but it is often of a sharp, stabbing, lancinating character. It is increased by movement, coughing, or straining. There may be either hypalgesia or hyperalgesia. Owing to algesic overlap, sensory changes may be difficult to demonstrate if but one root is involved.

Pain of a radicular distribution is sometimes relieved by injection or section of the root. If the nerve root is sectioned between the cerebrospinal axis and the ganglion, as in the rhizotomy or retrogasserian neurectomy done for the relief of pain in trigeminal neuralgia, no regeneration of the nerve occurs. Spinal anesthesia, caudal analgesia, or subarachnoid injection of alcohol or phenol also can relieve such pain by interrupting the conductivity of the nerve root.

With lesions of the *spinal cord* and *brain stem*, impairment of one or more modalities of sensation, or perversions of sensation in the form of either pain or paresthesias, may develop. The area of sensory diminution or loss, and the paresthesias as well, may involve the entire body below the level of the lesion, whereas the pain is usually segmental and involves only the dermatomes supplied by centers at the level of the lesion. The sensory loss is usually dissociated, with impairment of certain modalities and sparing of others. Despite a raised threshold for pain stimuli, there may be an overreaction to rapidly repeated stimulation.

When lesions of the spinal cord are present, involvement of pain, temperature, discriminatory, and proprioceptive sensations occurs. With brain stem lesions there may be ipsilateral sensory loss on the face and contralateral changes on the body. Lesions high in the cervical spinal cord and in the medulla may impair kinesthetic sensation in the upper extremities more than in the lower. As a result of the disturbance of proprioceptive sensations and a raised threshold for cutaneous senses there may be stereoanesthesia, which is difficult to differentiate from astereognosis. Extinction and even autotopagnosia may be present with such lesions. "Central" pain is occasionally experienced in patients with pontine, medullary, and spinal cord involvement. **Lhermitte's sign,** which consists of sudden electric-like or painful sensations spreading down the body or into the back or extremities on flexion of the neck, may be present with either local lesions of the cervical cord, or multiple sclerosis or other degenerative processes; the phenomenon may be secondary to disease of the posterior columns. It has also been reported following head injury; in such instances it may be the result of subdural or subarachnoid adhesions.

The pattern of sensory return with recovering spinal lesions is variable; the impairment may recede downward in a segmental manner; the return may start in the sacral distribution and ascend, or there may be a gradual recovery of function over the entire affected area. Pressure sensation returns first and its recovery is usually the most complete, followed, in turn, by tactile, pain, cold, and heat sensibilities. Intractable pain may be relieved by section of the ascending pathways in the spinal cord, medulla, pons, or mesencephalon.

Lesions of the *thalamus* are followed by diminution of various sensory modalities on the opposite side of the body without loss of sensation. They may be associated with abnormalities of sensation, such as paresthesias and hyperesthesias, or painful hyperpathias (Part H, "Diagnosis and Localization of Intracranial Disease"). Pain of central origin is most often associated with thalamic lesions, although it may occasionally be caused by stimulation of ascending pathways in the cerebrospinal axis or lesions of the cortex. When associated with cerebral lesions it probably is not a "spontaneous" pain, but rather an overreaction to stimuli capable of exciting affective reactions and sensations.

Involvement of the *sensory radiations* in the internal capsule causes variable and sometimes extensive diminution of all types of sensation on the opposite side of the body. The changes are similar to those which follow a thalamic lesion, and it may be difficult to differentiate between the two. Pain, however, is rarely experienced.

Lesions of the *parietal cortex* cause disturbances in the discriminatory sensations. There may be astereognosis, baragnosis, and sensory inattention or extinction, as well as autotopagnosia and anosognosia. Anesthesia is rare, but there is a raising of the threshold for both exteroceptive and proprioceptive sensations of the opposite side of the body (Part H, "Diagnosis

and Localization of Intracranial Disease"). Irritative lesions rarely cause pain, but they frequently cause paresthesias on the opposite side of the body. These paresthesias are especially important clinically when they assume the manifestations of a sensory aura preceding a jacksonian convulsion or constitute a focal sensory seizure.

The pains of causalgia and of phantom limb, which to a certain extent appear to be due to a hypersensitive receptive mechanism at the cortical level, have been relieved by interruption of the centripetal sensory pathways leading to consciousness; this has been achieved by removal of the cortical sensory representation of the part (gyrectomy or topectomy). Abnormalities of sensation in the form of anesthesias, paresthesias, or pain may be present in the absence of organic etiology and may be of psychogenic origin. In addition to the use of measures mentioned previously, such as nerve and nerve root block and section, anterolateral cordotomy, and tractotomy, other means have also been used for the relief of intractable pain or the patient's reaction to it; these include prefrontal lobotomy (severing the corticothalamic connections), cingulumotomy, and either stereotaxic surgery or the use of implanted electrodes to stimulate the nucleus ventralis posteromedialis and posterolateralis of the thalamus. The internal capsule and other structures have also been stimulated for such purposes. Apparently the patient's awareness of or concern over pain is lessened, even though there may be little or no change in the pain threshold.

Universal insensitivity or indifference to pain is a rare condition that is usually congenital. A few cases have been reported in which the absence of pain sensation was a part of a congenital sensory neuropathy or was associated with the absence of organized nerve endings or of Lissauer's tract and small dorsal root axons, but in others detailed investigations have shown no abnormality. In these latter cases the sensory defect may result from some anatomic, physiologic, or chemical abnormality in the cerebral integration of pathways concerned with pain appreciation, or it may represent a form of sensory agnosia.

It must be remembered that the perception of sensation and motor activity are interdependent, and that severe motor disabilities may follow impairment of sensory functions. This is particularly evident when lesions of the parietal cortex are present, but motor disabilities may also follow section of the posterior nerve roots or peripheral nerves and may accompany disorders affecting the posterior columns of the spinal cord or the afferent sensory pathways. On the other hand, motor dysfunction may affect sensory discrimination. It has been shown, for example, that when equal weights are placed in a patient's hands, he may underestimate the weight on the side on which there is a cerebellar dysfunction and overestimate it on the side of extrapyramidal dysfunction.

BIBLIOGRAPHY (SECTION A)

Babinski JFF. Anosognoise. Rev Neurol 1918;34:365

Bender MB. Disorders in Perception: With Particular Reference to the Phenomena of Extinction and Displacement. Springfield, IL, Charles C Thomas, 1952

Bender MB, Fink M. Green M. Patterns of perception on simultaneous tests of face and hand. Arch Neurol Psychiatry 1951;66:355

Brodal A. Neurological Anatomy in Relation to Clinical Medicine,. 3rd ed. New York, Oxford University Press, 1981

Cohn RA. Physiological study of rostral dominance in simultaneously applied ipsilateral somatosensory stimuli. Mt Sinai J Med 1974;41:76

Critchley M. The Parietal Lobes. London, Edward Arnold & Co, 1953

Dejerine J, Roussy G. Le syndrome thalamique. Rev Neurol 1906;14:521

French LA, Johnson DR. Examination of the sensory system in patients after hemispherectomy. Neurology 1955;5:390

Gardner WJ, Karnosh LJ, McClure CC Jr. Function following hemispherectomy for tumour and for infantile hemiplegia. Brain 1955;78:487

Gerstmann J. Fingeragnosie: Eine umschriebene Störung der Orientierung am eigenen Körper. Wien Klin Wochenschr 1924;37:1010

Halpern L. Astereognosis not of cortical origin. J Neurol Sci 1968;7:245

Head H. Sensory disturbances from cerebral lesions. Brain 1911;34:102

Henson RA. On thalamic dysaesthesiae and their suppression by bilateral stimulation. Brain 1949;72:576

Holmes G. Disorders of sensation produced by cortical lesions. Brain 1927;50:413

Hosobuchi Y, Adams JE, Rutkin B. Chronic thalamic and internal capsule stimulation for the control of central pain. Surg Neurol 1975;4:41

Mullan S. The transmission and central projections of pain. Med Clin North Am 1968;552:15

Riddoch G. The clinical features of central pain. Lancet 1938;1:1093

Riley HA. Discussion of Weinstein EA, Wechsler IS. Dermoid tumor in the foramen magnum with astereognosis and dissociated sensory loss. Arch Neurol Psychiatry 1940;44:162

Roland PE. Tactile discrimination after localized hemispheric lesions in man. Arch Neurol 1976;33:543

Sandifer PH. Anosognosis and disorders of body scheme. Brain 1946;69:122

Shapiro MF, Feldman DS. Double simultaneous stimulation phenomena in spinal cord disease. Neurology 1952;2:509

Walker AE. Anatomic basis of the thalamic syndrome. Arch Neurol Psychiatry 1938;39:1104

Woolsey CN. Patterns of sensory representation in the cerebral cortex. Fed Proc 1947;6:437

BIBLIOGRAPHY (SECTION B)

Bolton CF, Winkelmann RK, Dyck PJ. A quantitative study of Meissner's corpuscles in man. Neurology 1966;16:1

Boshes B, Brown M, Crouch RL. Sensory return in partial and recovery spinal lesions. Neurology 1952;2:81

Bourlond A, Winkelmann RK. Study of cutaneous innervation in congenital anesthesia. Arch Neurol 1966;14:223

Dickens WH, Winkelmann RK, Mulder DW. Cholinesterase demonstration of dermal nerve endings in patients with impaired sensation. Neurology 1963;13:91

Falconer MA. Relief of intractable pain by frontal lobotomy. Assoc Res Nerv Ment Dis Proc 1948;27:706

Foltz EL, White LE Jr. Pain "relief" by frontal cingulumotomy. J Neurosurg 1962;19:89

Kemp C. Electrical stimulation of the nervous system for the control of pain. Surg Neurol 1975;4:164

Magee KR. Congenital indifference to pain. Arch Neurol 1963;9:635

Mark VH, Ervin FR, Hackett TP. Clinical aspects of stereotactile thalamotomy in the human. I. The treatment of chronic severe pain. Arch Neurol 1960;3:351

Miles J, Hayward M, Mumford J et al. Pain relief by implanted electrical stimulators. Lancet 1974;1:777

Shealy CN, Maurer D. Transcutaneous nerve stimulation for control of pain. Surg Neurol 1974;2:45

Swanson AG, Buchan GC, Alvord EC Jr. Absence of Lissauer's tract and small dorsal root axons in familial universal insensitivity to pain. Trans Am Neurol Assoc 1963;88:99

Winkelmann RK, Lambert EH, Hayles RB. Congenital absence of pain. Arch Dermatol 1962;85:325

Part C
THE CRANIAL NERVES

INTRODUCTION

The examination of cranial nerve function is an exceedingly important part of the neurologic examination, and it should be performed carefully. The interpretation of the status of the individual nerves is valuable not only in the localization of disease processes within the central nervous system, but also in the diagnosis of systemic disease. An affection disturbing one or more of the cranial nerves may have significance in the localization of an intracranial lesion; it may indicate the presence of increased intracranial pressure; it may suggest the presence of some diffuse process such as meningitis, vascular disease, toxemia, diabetes, sarcoidosis, or generalized infection; or it may occur when there is a primary pathologic process at some distant site.

Cranial nerve function can be examined most thoroughly and most satisfactorily if each nerve is studied individually and if they are examined in consecutive order. In order to comprehend the significance of the signs and symptoms that may result from dysfunction of these structures, it is important to understand their anatomic relationships and functions. In this text the study of the cranial nerves is presented in the following order: first the anatomy and physiology of each is reviewed, then the procedure of the routine examination is outlined, and then some of the disease syndromes in which they may be involved are described.

Disorders affecting the cranial nerves may be divided into those which involve the peripheral nerve processes or trunks (**infra-nuclear lesions**), those which affect the nuclear center (**nuclear lesions**), and those which involve the central connections (**supra-nuclear lesions**). There are cerebral, or cortical, areas that govern the function of the various motor nerves and wherein the sensory impulses terminate for recognition or interpretation. The peripheral nerves extend from the nuclei to the ultimate distribution of their fibers, and often a part of their course lies within the brain tissue. Although a peripheral nerve may be involved independently of its nucleus, injury to the nucleus is always followed by a degeneration of the nerve. Owing to the proximity of many of the nuclei, especially those in the brain stem, and their proximity to other structures, it is rare to have a single nucleus affected without other involvement. The majority of the cranial nerves, the third through the twelfth, are similar in structure and function to the spinal nerves, and react similarly in disease processes. The first two nerves, the olfactory and the optic, however, have significant anatomic differences which will be described.

Chapter 9
THE OLFACTORY NERVE

ANATOMY AND PHYSIOLOGY

The peripheral neurons of the olfactory, or first cranial, nerves are bipolar sensory cells, the distal portions of which consist of ciliated processes which penetrate the mucous membrane in the olfactory region of the upper portion of the nasal cavity. These filaments are found on both the lateral and septal surfaces of the nasal mucosa in a relatively small area on the medial wall of the superior nasal concha, the upper part of the septum, and the roof of the nose. They are situated so high in the nasal cavity that by far the greater part of the inspired air which passes through the nostrils fails to reach the olfactory epithelium. Forceful inspiration, or sniffing, may be necessary to create sufficient current to have the air reach the olfactory endings. The central processes, or neuraxes, of these nerves are collected into approximately 20 branches on each side. These, the true olfactory nerves, penetrate the cribriform plate of the ethmoid bone as unmyelinated fibers and synapse in the olfactory bulbs (Fig. 9-1). As these nerves pass through the cribriform plate, each receives tubular sheaths from the dura and the pia mater, the former being continuous with the periosteum of the nose, the latter adjacent to the neurilemma of the nerve. The communication between the nasal and the intracranial cavities may be a portal of entry of infection to the meninges and the brain.

Within the olfactory bulbs the neuraxes of the incoming fibers synapse with the dendrites of the mitral and tufted cells in the olfactory glomeruli. The neuraxes of the neurons of the next order, mainly the mitral cells, course posteriorly through the olfactory tract in the tuberculum olfactorium and the olfactory trigone where they divide into the medial and the lateral olfactory striae, or roots. Some fibers decussate in the anterior commissure to join the fibers from the opposite side, and some go to the olfactory trigone and tuberculum olfactorium within the anterior perforated substance. The fibers of the medial olfactory stria terminate on the medial surface of the cerebral hemisphere in the parolfactory area, subcallosal gyrus, and inferior part of the cingulate gyrus. The lateral olfactory stria courses obliquely along the anterior perforated space and under the temporal lobe and terminates in the uncus, anterior portion of the hippocampal gyrus, and amygdaloid nucleus (Fig. 9-2). The hippocampal gyrus sends impulses to the hippocampus. The hippocampi and amygdaloid nuclei on the two sides are intimately related through the anterior commissure, and these structures in turn send projection fibers to the anterior hypothalamic nuclei, mammillary bodies, tuber cinereum, and habenular nucleus, and then to the anterior nuclear group of the thalamus, interpeduncular nucleus, dorsal tegmental nucleus, striatum, cingulate gyrus and mesencephalic reticular formation. Communications with the superior and inferior salivatory nuclei are important in reflex salivation. The olfactory bulbs and tracts are sometimes called the olfactory nerves, but the true nerves are the unmyelinated filaments, whereas the bulbs and tracts are in reality a part of the rhinencephalon of the brain. The olfactory tracts lie in the olfactory sulcus on the orbital surface of the frontal

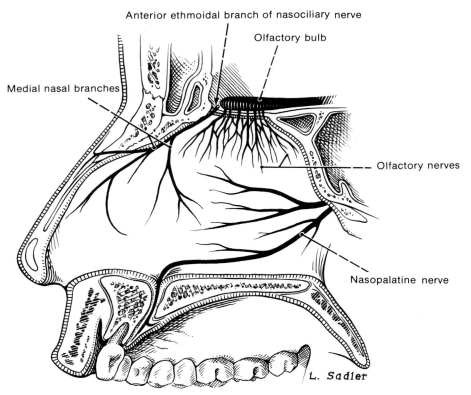

Anterior ethmoidal branch of nasociliary nerve

Olfactory bulb

Medial nasal branches

Olfactory nerves

Nasopalatine nerve

L. Sadler

FIG. 9–1. The distribution of the olfactory nerves within the nose.

lobes of the brain, and this proximity to the inferior surface of the frontal poles is an anatomic relationship that must always be borne in mind (Fig. 9-3).

Olfaction is phylogenetically one of the oldest types of sensation. In lower mammals in which the other sensory systems are only partially developed, olfaction is extremely important and the olfactory cortex constitutes a large part of the cerebral hemispheres. In higher primates and in man it is less essential, and authorities disagree as to just which structures should be considered olfactory cortex. Yet there remains in the brain a complex structure that is of consequence, especially in its relationship with the hypothalamus and with brainstem nuclei. Our knowledge concerning its structure and physiology has been derived largely from comparative neuroanatomy and phylogenetic development. The correlation, however, between the olfactory system, hypothalamus, and autonomic centers is pertinent in the understanding of many visceral functions.

The olfactory nerve is a sensory nerve with but one function, that of smell. The quantitative and qualitative ability to perceive and identify various odors differs from person to person. Only volatile substances soluble in lipids or water are perceived as odors. Lesions of the olfactory nerve are characterized by the presence of either **anosmia (anosphrasia)**, loss of smell, or **hyposmia,** impairment of olfaction. In true anosmia there is loss of ability to perceive or recognize not only scents but also flavors, for a large portion of what is interpreted as taste is perceived through the olfactory system. As discussed in Chapter 13, salt, sour, sweet, and bitter are the only true tastes; flavor is a synthesis of sensations derived from the olfactory nerves, taste buds, and other sensory end-organs within the mouth and pharynx. A patient with involvement of the olfactory system may complain of loss of taste rather than of smell, because he cannot appreciate the flavors of food, but some anosmic persons can identify and enjoy the flavors of many foods. Patients with unilateral anosmia may not be aware of any disturbance of olfaction. There is said to be a diurnal cycle in olfactory acuity, which is increased before meals and decreased after meals; this may be important in the regulation of appetite and satiety.

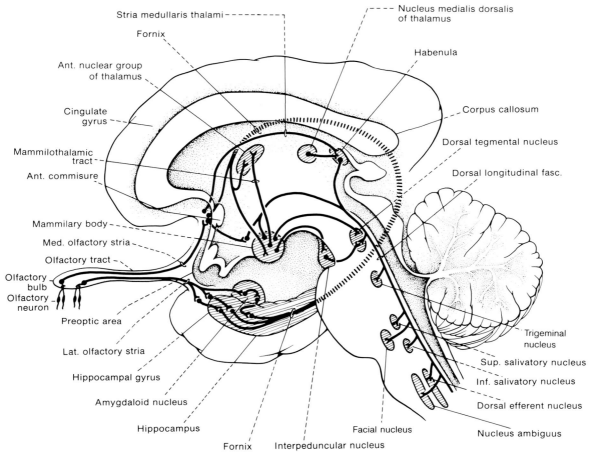

FIG. 9–2. The olfactory pathway and its central connections.

CLINICAL EXAMINATION

Smell is tested by the use of nonirritating volatile oils or liquids. Each nostril is examined separately while the other is occluded. With the patient's eyes closed, one nostril should be occluded and a vial of the test substance brought near the open one. The patient should be asked to inhale forcibly and then indicate whether he smells something and if so, to identify it. The process should be repeated for the other nostril to compare results between the two sides. Although more subjective, the perception of odor is probably more important than its identification. Such substances as oil of wintergreen, tar, oil of cloves, oil of roses, eucalyptus, oil of lavender, oil of cinnamon, oil of turpentine, vanilla, anise, almond water, and asafetida have been used for qualitative testing, but probably the most satisfactory test substances are freshly ground coffee, benzaldehyde (bitter almond oil), tar, and oil of lemon. Items such as toothpaste from the patient's bedside table may be used to carry out a rough qualitative test. One must avoid substances which, instead of stimulating the olfactory nerve, may stimulate gustatory end-organs or the peripheral endings of the trigeminal nerve in the nasal mucosa. Chloroform may stimulate gustatory as well as olfactory endings by imparting a sweet taste; pyridine may give a bitter taste. Peppermint, menthol, and camphor stimulate trigeminal endings and give a feeling of coolness; ammonia, strong solutions of acetic acid, alcohol, and formaldehyde also irritate the trigeminal endings.

Before evaluating loss or decrease of olfactory sensitivity, one must ascertain that the nasal passages are open. Intranasal conditions such as obstruction; allergic, atrophic, and hypertrophic rhinitis; mucoid changes; polyps; and sinusitis

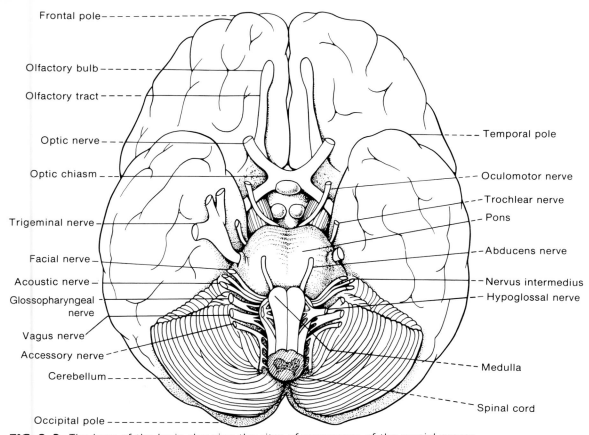

Frontal pole

Olfactory bulb

Olfactory tract

Optic nerve

Optic chiasm

Trigeminal nerve

Facial nerve

Acoustic nerve

Glossopharyngeal nerve

Vagus nerve

Accessory nerve

Cerebellum

Occipital pole

Temporal pole

Oculomotor nerve

Trochlear nerve

Pons

Abducens nerve

Nervus intermedius

Hypoglossal nerve

Medulla

Spinal cord

FIG. 9–3. The base of the brain showing the sites of emergence of the cranial nerves.

may seriously interfere with the sense of smell. One should observe the patient's ability to perceive, identify, and name the test substance. The results on the two sides should always be determined and compared, and any differences noted. In infants and hysterical patients, flaring of the alae nasi in response to strong odors may indicate that the sense of smell is intact. Perception of the presence of the odorous substances indicates the continuity of the peripheral nerve and its pathways; identification of the odor reveals intact cortical function as well. Since there is bilateral innervation, a lesion central to the decussation of the olfactory pathways never causes loss of smell, and a lesion of the olfactory cortex does not produce anosmia. The appreciation of the presence of a smell, even without recognition, is sufficient evidence to rule out anosmia.

The above method of testing olfactory sensation is dependent entirely upon the statements of the individual under examination, and is entirely qualitative. Various attempts have been made to devise instruments for the quantitative measurement of the sense of smell, but they are complicated and of little importance clinically.

DISORDERS OF OLFACTORY FUNCTION

The olfactory nerves themselves are rarely the seat of disease, but they are frequently involved in association with disease or injury of the surrounding structures. Loss of smell may occur in a variety of conditions. It may be either congenital or acquired. Anosmia, often accompanied by either perversions or loss of taste, may be a symptom of pernicious anemia. Trauma to the head with fractures of the cribriform plate of the ethmoid bone and hemorrhage at the base of the frontal lobes may cause loss of smell by tearing, crushing, or pressing on the olfactory filaments; this usually is permanent. Infectious processes involving the meninges at the base of the frontal lobes often cause anosmia, which frequently is a sequel of epidemic meningitis. Impairment of smell occurs in association with frontal lobe abscesses and osteomyelitis of the frontal or ethmoid regions. A number of toxic substances, including lead and calcium, cause anosmia. Anosmia is common with hydrocephalus. Some decrease in olfactory acuity may accompany aging. Overstimulation of the sense of smell may cause a temporary rise in the olfactory threshold to a particular odor, or it may cause permanent loss, as may excessive smoking, ingestion of amphetamine, or the prolonged use of cocaine.

Partial anosmia may occur with lesions of the trigeminal nerve as a result of trophic changes in the nasal mucosa. A decrease or loss of the sense of smell has also been reported to occur with viral infections, including viral hepatitis, in syphilis, in hypogonadism, and in gonadal dysgenesis, an idiopathic syndrome in which there are also disturbances of the sense of taste. Decreased sense of smell has also been reported in association with abnormalities in zinc metabolism. Disease of the anterior cerebral artery near its origin in the circle of Willis may produce homolateral loss of smell. Anosmia sometimes occurs, along with other anesthesias, in hysteria; usually in this condition taste is not affected. Hysterical loss of smell may be diagnosed by using irritating substances which stimulate the trigeminal endings, such as ammonia or acetic acid, as well as the volatile oils; in organic anosmia the former will be recognized but not the latter, whereas in hysteria neither will be recognized.

Loss of smell is frequently an early and important sign in the diagnosis and localization of intracranial neoplasms. This is especially true with meningiomas of the sphenoidal ridge and olfactory groove, gliomas of the frontal lobe, and parasellar lesions where there is pressure on the olfactory bulbs or tracts. The typical syndrome with sphenoidal ridge meningioma consists of unilateral optic atrophy or papilledema and exophthalmos, and ipsilateral anosmia. In meningiomas of the olfactory groove or cribriform plate area there is first unilateral anosmia, with retrobulbar neuritis or optic atrophy, progressing to bilateral anosmia. Frontal lobe tumors may also cause unilateral anosmia and optic atrophy, often in the form of the **Foster Kennedy syndrome:** anosmia and optic atrophy on the side of the tumor and papilledema on the opposite side. In parasellar and pituitary lesions bilateral anosmia may be an early manifestation.

Other disorders of smell, aside from hyposmia or anosmia, are occasionally encountered. **Hy-perosmia** is an increase in olfactory acuity. It occurs most frequently in hysteria, in certain psychotic states, and with certain types of substance abuse, but it may also be present, along with hyperacusis, in migraine, and it has been described in epidemic encephalitis and hyperemesis gravidarum, and as an accompaniment of the menstrual period. It is also reported to occur in cystic fibrosis, Addison's disease, and strychnine poisoning. **Parosmia,** or perversion of smell, and **cacosmia,** or the presence of disagreeable odors, also appear in psychic states and occasionally follow trauma to the head, especially to the uncus region. Olfactory hallucinations, which may be present in psychic states or as obsessional phenomena, are more frequently the result of an organic lesion. They indicate the presence of an irritative process in the central olfactory system, and thus are important in neurologic localization; they may occur with neoplasms or vascular lesions. In the so-called **uncinate fit** the seizure is preceded by an aura that consists of a disagreeable olfactory or gustatory hallucination, which may be accompanied, as the patient loses consciousness, by dilation of the nostrils, smacking of the lips, or chewing or tasting movements. Such attacks occur as the result of an irritative lesion in the uncinate gyrus, hippocampus, amygdala, medial portion of the temporal lobe, or neighboring structures. Olfactory stimulation has both arrested and activated such seizures. The uncinate fit, however, is not in itself a specific variety of seizure; rather, the olfactory hallucination is one manifestation (often the aura) of the complex partial or temporal lobe seizure, other elements of which may consist of memory disturbances, automatisms, auditory and visual phenomena, and psychic manifestations (Ch. 54). A neoplasm may or may not be responsible. There is never any evidence of objective loss of smell in these patients.

Disorders of olfactory function may thus be produced by lesions anywhere along the course of the peripheral nerve or its central pathways. Respiratory or inflammatory conditions may cause loss of smell due to obstruction of the nasal passages. Involvement of the nasal mucosa or of the cribriform plate area may be followed by a loss of smell as the result of destruction of the peripheral nerve fibers; infectious processes and toxic involvement may also affect the individual fibers. Intracranial lesions involving the olfactory bulb or tract may cause unilateral or bilateral loss of smell. Lesions of the olfactory radiations or of the olfactory cortex are never followed by loss of smell unless they are bilateral, owing to the decussation of the pathways, but they may produce lowering of olfactory acuity, or, occasionally, "smell agnosia." Irritative lesions in these areas may, however, cause perversions of smell and olfactory hallucinations.

BIBLIOGRAPHY

Adams RD, Victor M. Principles of Neurology, 4th ed. New York, McGraw – Hill, 1989

Adey WR. The sense of smell. In Field J, Magoun HW, Hall VE (eds). Handbook of Physiology. Washington, DC, American Physiological Society, 1959

Bedichek R. The Sense of Smell. Garden City, NY, Doubleday & Co, 1960

Brodal A. The hippocampus and the sense of smell: A review. Brain 1947;70:179

Caruso V, Hagan J, Manning H. Quantitative olfactometry in measurement of posttraumatic hyposmia. Arch Otolaryngol 1968;90:500

Elsberg CA, Levy I. The sense of smell. I. A new and simple method of quantitative olfactometry. Bull Neurol Inst NY 1935;4:5

Fordyce ID. Olfaction tests. Br J Ind Med 1961;18:213

Gorman W. Flavor, Taste and the Psychology of Smell. Springfield, IL, Charles C Thomas, 1964

Henkin RI. Studies on olfactory thresholds in normal man and in patients with adrenal cortical deficiency. J Clin Invest 1966;45:1631

Henkin RI. Abnormalities of taste and olfaction in patients with chromatin negative gonadal dysgenesis. J Clin Endocrinol 1967;27:1436

Henkin RI, Smith FR. Hyposmia in acute viral hepatitis. Lancet 1973;1:823.

Hussey HH. Taste and smell deviations: Importance of zinc. JAMA 1974;226:1669

Kristensen HK, Zilstorff – Pedersen K. Quantitative studies on the function of smell. Acta Otolaryngol 1953;43:537

Males JL, Townsend JL, Schneider RA. Hypogonadotropic hypogonadism with anosmia — Kallmann syndrome. Arch Intern Med 1973;131:501

Schneider RA. The sense of smell in man — its physiologic basis. N Engl J Med 1967;277:299

Seydell EM. Olfactory disturbances. JAMA 1932;99:627

Sumner D. On testing the sense of smell. Lancet 1962;2:895

Sumner D. Posttraumatic anosmia. Brain 1964;87:107

Chapter 10

THE OPTIC NERVE

ANATOMY AND PHYSIOLOGY

The optic nerve is not a peripheral nerve but is a fiber pathway that unites the retina with the brain. In common usage, however, it is referred to as the optic, or second cranial, nerve. The true peripheral optic nerves are situated in the cellular layers of the retina. The *receptors,* or end-organs through which visual impulses are mediated, are the rods and cones of the retina; these are stimulated by light impulses and synapse with the inner nuclear, or bipolar, layer, the cells of which in turn synapse with those of the ganglion cell layer (Fig. 10-1). The neuraxes of the ganglion cells make up the optic pathway referred to as the optic nerve.

The rods, which are more numerous than the cones, are scattered diffusely throughout the retina, but are absent in the macula. They react to low intensities of illumination and are concerned with peripheral vision, perception of movement, and night sight; they do not function in the perception of color. The cones are also scattered diffusely throughout the retina, although they are less numerous. The **macula (fovea centralis)**, the point of clearest vision at the center of the retina, is occupied entirely by cones, which are stimulated by light of a relatively high intensity and are concerned with discrimination of colors and fine details. The macula functions only in day vision. There are neither rods nor cones in the optic disk, or papilla, which constitutes the head of the optic nerve, and the disk itself therefore does not respond to visual stimuli. The consequent physio-

logic blind spot is described later in this chapter under "Scotomas."

The so-called *optic nerve,* which extends from the retina to the optic chiasm, is approximately 5 cm long. The major portion of its course, 3½ cm, is in the orbit, with 1½ cm in the optic foramen and within the skull. The approximately 1 million fibers of the optic nerve are usually unmyelinated in the retina and in the nerve head, but they become myelinated as they pass through the lamina cribrosa. The two optic nerves unite at the *optic chiasm,* which is situated superior to the sella turcica, usually over its posterior two thirds. The internal carotid arteries are lateral to the chiasm, the anterior cerebral and anterior communicating arteries are in front and above, and the third ventricle and hypothalamus are behind and above. The dural covering of the cerebrum is continuous over the optic nerve; at the bulb it fuses with Tenon's capsule, and at the optic foramen it is adherent to the periosteum. The pia and arachnoid also continue from the brain and envelop the optic nerve; at the termination of the nerve they fuse with the sclera where the nerve penetrates the sclera. The subdural and subarachnoid spaces around the optic nerve are continuous with those around the brain. The arachnoid, however, is very thin. The meningeal coverings of the optic nerve are sometimes referred to as the **vaginal sheaths.** The area between the dura and the pia is called the **intervaginal space;** it is divided by the arachnoid into a small subdural and a larger subarachnoid space.

The fibers which pass through the optic nerves primarily carry visual impulses, but they also

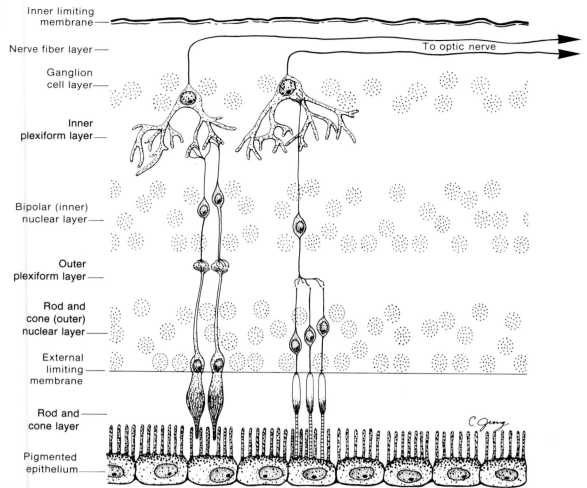

FIG. 10–1. The layers of the retina and their relationship to the optic nerve. (Modified from Ramon y Cajal S: Histologie du système nerveux de l'homme et des vertebres. Paris, A Maloine, 2 vols, 1909, 1911)

carry impulses which mediate accommodation and reflex responses to light and other stimuli. Throughout the extent of their entire course from the retina to the cerebral cortex, the fibers are grouped according to the retinal quadrants from which they arise. The fibers from the lateral (temporal) half of the retina are also situated in the temporal half of the nerve and pass through the chiasm without crossing; they continue to the ipsilateral reflex centers for pupillary reactions and to the ipsilateral visual areas (Fig. 10-2). The fibers from the medial (nasal) half of the retina go through the medial portion of the nerve; they decussate at the chiasm, and terminate on the contralateral centers. There are, however, intricacies in the chiasmal crossing. Some of the fibers

from the lower nasal retinal quadrant loop forward into the opposite optic nerve for a short distance before turning back again; consequently, a lesion of one optic nerve just anterior to the chiasm may cause a defect in the upper temporal field of the opposite eye. Also, some of the upper nasal fibers loop back briefly into the ipsilateral optic tract before decussation. In the chiasm the fibers from the upper retinal quadrants are dorsal and those from the lower quadrants are ventral.

Fibers from the macular portion of the retina (fovea centralis), which provide central vision, constitute the **papillomacular bundle.** In the peripheral portions of the optic nerve, near the eye, this is situated laterally and slightly

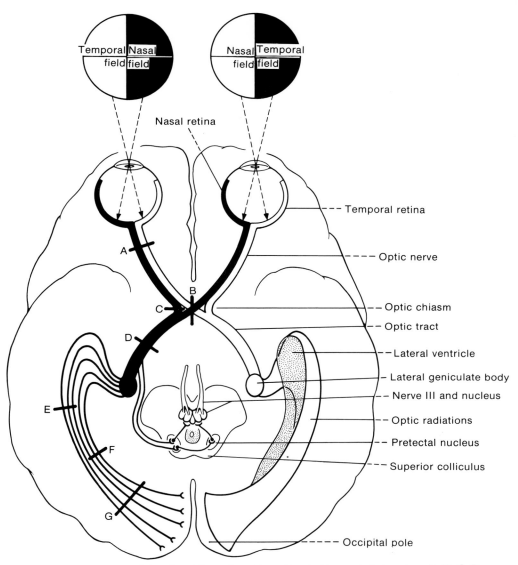

FIG. 10–2. The course of the visual fibers from the retina to the occipital cortex. **A, B, C, D, E, F,** and **G** show the sites of various lesions that may affect the fields of vision.

inferiorly separating the temporal fibers into dorsal and ventral quadrants. These in turn crowd and somewhat displace the nasal quadrants (Fig. 10-3). As the nerve approaches the chiasm this bundle approaches the center of the nerve, and the temporal fibers are lateral. The fibers from the medial half of the macula also decussate, whereas those from the lateral half do not. The fibers of the papillomacular bundle are the most vulnerable to toxins and pressure.

Posterior to the optic chiasm the fibers, part of which emanate from the temporal portion of the

ipsilateral retina, part from the nasal portion of the opposite retina, traverse the *optic tract,* and the majority of them terminate in the lateral geniculate body. The ratio of crossed to uncrossed fibers in the human optic tract is approximately 2:1, which roughly corresponds to the ratio of the area of the temporal field to that of the nasal field. There is a twisting of the fibers in the tract, and those from the macula gradually assume a dorsal and lateral position with a central wedge. The fibers from the upper retinal segments assume a medial and slightly dorsal

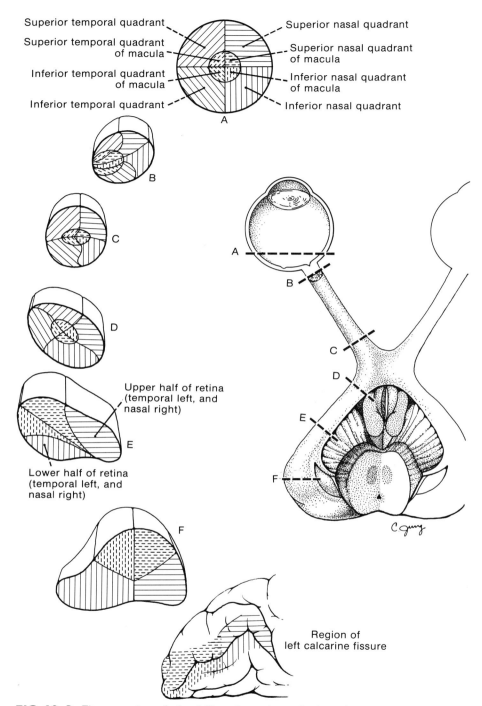

Superior temporal quadrant
Superior temporal quadrant of macula
Inferior temporal quadrant of macula
Inferior temporal quadrant

Superior nasal quadrant
Superior nasal quadrant of macula
Inferior nasal quadrant of macula
Inferior nasal quadrant

Upper half of retina (temporal left, and nasal right)

Lower half of retina (temporal left, and nasal right)

Region of left calcarine fissure

FIG. 10–3. The grouping of visual fibers from the retinal quadrants and macular area in the optic nerve, optic tract, lateral geniculate body, and occipital cortex.

position, and those from the inferior quadrants are ventral and somewhat lateral (Fig. 10-3).

Within the *lateral geniculate bodies* there is a definite localization corresponding to the various quadrants of the visual fields and the retinas. Fibers carrying impulses from the upper portion of the retina terminate on the ventromedial segment of the geniculate body; those from the lower portion of the retina terminate on the ventrolateral segment, and those from the macula occupy an intermediate position in the dorsal, middle, and somewhat caudal portion. Within the lateral geniculate bodies there is a stratification of fibers into six cellular layers, and those fibers from the ipsilateral temporal and contralateral nasal retina alternate. Some of the visual fibers pass over or through these structures and terminate in the pulvinar of the thalamus, but the significance of this connection has yet to be determined for vision or visual reflexes.

Neurons originating in the lateral geniculate bodies pass posteriorly as the *geniculocalcarine pathway,* or the *optic radiations,* and terminate on the striate cortex (area 17) of the occipital lobe (Fig. 10-4). In the anterior portions of the radiations the fibers carrying peripheral vision are placed medially, and then assume dorsal and ventral positions. The most dorsal, those from the upper retinal quadrants and the medial portion of the lateral geniculate nuclei, pass through the posterior limb of the internal capsule and the lower part of the parietal and occipital lobes and upper part of the temporal lobe, lateral to the posterior horn of the lateral ventricle, to terminate on the upper lip of the calcarine fissure (cuneus) and the medial surface of the occipital lobe. The most ventral, those from the lower retinal quadrants and the lateral portion of the geniculate nuclei, also pass through the posterior limb of the internal capsule, then through the temporal lobe, sweeping forward and lateralward above the inferior horn of the ventricle, and then laterally, down, and backward around the inferior horn in a loop (loop of Meyer and Archambault). They then course through the temporal and occipital lobes to terminate on the lower lip of the calcarine fissure (lingual gyrus). The fibers carrying macular vision come from the middle, dorsal, and caudal portions of the geniculate body; they are first lateralward, and then form the intermediate portion of the geniculocalcarine pathway, continuing to the posterior pole of the occipital lobe.

Fibers which carry visual impulses from the peripheral portions of the retina terminate on the anterior third or half of the visual cortex of the occipital lobe in concentric zones. Those from the fovea centralis, or macular area, terminate on the posterior portion of the occipital cortex. The macula has a wider cortical distribution than the peripheral portion of the retina, and it is represented in a wedge-shaped area, with its apex anterior, in the striate cortex. Some fibers carrying macular vision may cross to the opposite side through the splenium of the corpus callosum and end in the visual cortex on that side, although the concept of bilateral macular innervation has been disputed for many years. The temporal crescents that lie just outside the binocular visual field (see "The Visual Fields") are located in the most anterior portions of the visual cortex.

The *striate* or *calcarine cortex* (area 17 of Brodmann) is the sensory visual cortex. Its physiology is complex and has been the subject of intense investigation. The striate neurons are arranged in various patterns and respond to different visual stimuli. Surrounding the striate cortex are areas which function in visual associations. Area 18, the parastriate or parareceptive cortex, receives and interprets impulses from area 17. Area 19, the peristriate or perireceptive cortex, has connections with areas 17 and 18 and with the other portions of the cortex. It functions in more complex visual recognition, perception, revisualization, visual association, size and shape discrimination, color vision, and spatial orientation.

Optic Reflexes

Fibers carrying impulses which have to do with reflex responses to light and other optic reflexes pass through the optic chiasm in the same order as fibers which have to do with vision. They may travel in the medial part of the optic tract, and they leave the tract anterior to the lateral geniculate bodies. Those carrying light reflex impulses pass to the pretectal nucleus in the midbrain slightly above the level of the superior colliculi (anterior quadrigeminal bodies), where they synapse, and the neurons of the next order go to the Edinger-Westphal nuclei of the same and the contralateral sides, from which impulses are carried through the oculomotor nerve to the sphincter of the pupil. Those having to do with somatic visual reflexes, such as movement of the eyes and head in response to a visual stimulus, go to the superior colliculus; descending tectoo-

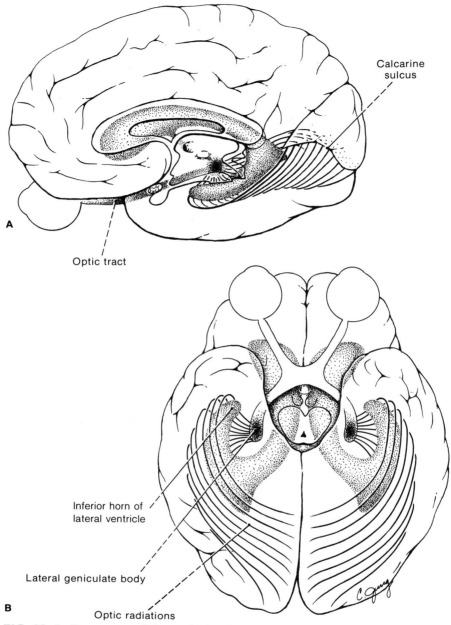

Calcarine
sulcus

A

Optic tract

Inferior horn of
lateral ventricle

Lateral geniculate body

B

Optic radiations

FIG. 10–4. The course of the geniculocalcarine fibers. **A.** Medial view. **B.** Inferior view.

culomotor fibers connect with appropriate areas in the nuclei of ocular nerves, and impulses going through tectospinal fibers innervate skeletal muscles for the response to a visual stimulus. For conscious modification of the visual reflex, impulses go from the lateral geniculate body to the visual cortex, and then to the superior

colliculus. Fibers also pass from areas 18 and 19 of the occipital cortex through the optic radiations to the superior colliculus. These subserve reflex reactions through connections with the eye muscle nuclei and other structures. The pathway is known as the **internal corticotectal tract.** Fibers which carry impulses having to do with visual-palpebral reflexes (such as blinking in response to light) go to the facial nuclei.

CLINICAL EXAMINATION; DISORDERS OF FUNCTION

The optic nerve is a sensory nerve and carries impulses which have to do with the special sense of vision, or sight. Rays of light pass through the cornea, crystalline lens, and vitreous and reach the rods and cones on the outer surface of the retina. From here, as described under "Anatomy and Physiology," impulses are carried to consciousness for recognition of light, form, and color. The other functions, such as the mediation of afferent impulses for light and visual reflexes, are tested with these reflexes. The major function of the optic nerve is tested by examination of the various modalities of the visual sense — namely, the quantity (acuity) of vision, the range (fields) of vision, and special components of vision, such as color vision and day and night vision. Finally, the optic nerve is the one cranial nerve that can be examined directly, and no neurologic, or indeed general, physical examination is complete without an inspection of the optic nerve and the retina by means of an ophthalmoscope.

The eyes are tested individually: when one is examining acuity, fields, and color vision it is important that the patient have one eye covered while the other is being tested. Before performing the functional examination of the optic nerve, one should look for local ocular changes such as cataract, conjunctival irritation, corneal scarring or opacity, iritis, uveitis, foreign bodies, or glaucoma. One should also record the presence of a prosthesis (so-called glass eye), of photophobia or abnormal intolerance to light, or of an **arcus senilis** (perhaps better termed **arcus lipoides corneae**). This last is a lipid infiltration in the corneoscleral junction. It is usually seen in elderly people, and is considered to be a part of the natural aging process. It is occasionally seen in younger persons, however, especially in black people, in whom its earlier development may be genetically determined. The presence of a unilateral arcus corneae with contralateral carotid disease has been reported. A Kayser – Fleischer ring is found in Wilson's disease (hepatolenticular degeneration); this is a zone of greenish-gold granular pigmentation on the posterior surface of the cornea near the limbus, often best seen with the slit lamp. It is the result of deposition of copper in the area. Cataracts may be pres-

ent in patients with myotonic dystrophy and certain rare hereditary conditions with disturbed lipid or amino acid metabolism, as well as in many other systemic and toxic disorders.

Visual Acuity

Visual acuity, or the resolving power of the eye for central or direct vision, is dependent upon the following functions: the **intensity threshold** (the sensitivity of the retina to light), the **minimum visible** (the smallest area that can be perceived), and the **minimum separable,** or **resolution threshold** (the ability to recognize the separateness of two closely approximated points or parallel lines). Visual acuity is tested for both distance and near vision. If glasses are worn, the examination is made with and without correction. In infants acuity can be tested only by noting pupillary reactions, blinking in response to bright light, and following movements. At the age of 4 months the acuity may be 20/400; it gradually increases, but does not reach a normal level until the age of 5 years.

Distance vision is examined by the use of the Snellen test charts. These consist of a series of letters of diminishing size that can normally be read at distances varying from 10 to 200 feet (Fig. 10-5). The letters are constructed so that each stroke of the letter subtends an angle of 1 min at the nodal point of the eye, and the whole character subtends an angle of 5 min at the usual distance from the eye. The charts are placed at a distance of 20 feet, or 6 meters, from the patient, since at that distance there is relaxation of accommodation and the light rays are nearly parallel. Normal vision is present when the subject is able to read at 20 feet, or 6 meters, the letters designed to be read at that distance, and the acuity is then recorded as 20/20 or 6/6. The eyes are tested separately, and one is covered during the examination. Any defect in vision is recorded fractionally. The figure 20, the distance from the test chart, is used as the numerator, and the distance at which the smallest type read by the patient should be seen by a person with normal vision constitutes the denominator. For example, if the patient is able to read at 20 feet only those letters which should be read at 40 feet, he has 20/40 vision. It must be borne in mind, however, that this does not mean that the patient has one half of normal vision, for the fraction is merely a record of his ability to read at 20 feet only those letters which are normally seen at 40 feet. It has been found, for instance,

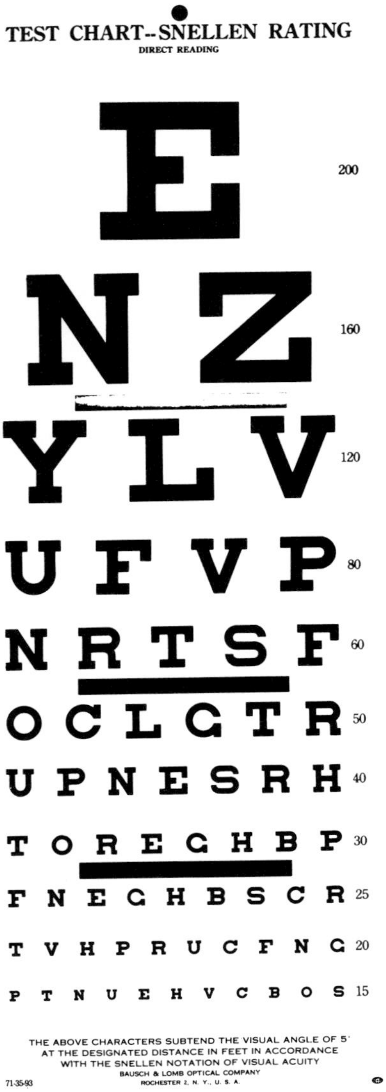

TEST CHART--SNELLEN RATING
DIRECT READING

E 200

N Z 160

Y L V 120

U F V P 80

N R T S F 60

O C L G T R 50

U P N E S R H 40

T O R E G H B P 30

F N E G H B S C R 25

T V H P R U C F N G 20

P T N U E H V C B O S 15

THE ABOVE CHARACTERS SUBTEND THE VISUAL ANGLE OF 5'
AT THE DESIGNATED DISTANCE IN FEET IN ACCORDANCE
WITH THE SNELLEN NOTATION OF VISUAL ACUITY
BAUSCH & LOMB OPTICAL COMPANY
71-35-93 ROCHESTER 2, N. Y., U. S. A.

FIG. 10–5. Snellen test chart.

that an individual with a Snellen notation for distance of 20/40 has only a 16.4% loss of vision, with an 83.6% maintenance of visual efficiency.

Near vision is tested by the use of ordinary printer's types, known as the Jaeger's test types. The finest is numbered 0, and successively higher numbers indicate coarser types (Fig. 10-6). Near vision is tested at the near point (14 in, or 35.5 cm).

Other test charts are available for use in examining distance vision and near vision in bed patients. For a rough approximation of vision the examiner may use ordinary print from a book or smaller print from a telephone directory, and compare the patient's vision with his own. Most physicians are aware of their own visual acuity, and if they have a defect, it is satisfactorily corrected by glasses. If the patient has a marked loss of acuity, the examiner should determine the distance at which he is able to count fingers, make out gross forms, discern moving objects, or tell light from dark. Testing for optokinetic nystagmus and visually evoked potentials may aid in evaluating the presence of vision in infants, comatose patients, hysterics, and malingerers.

It is important to remember that changes in visual acuity may result from either ocular disease or disease of the central nervous system, and that a large percentage of people have some error of refraction, such as myopia, hyperopia, or astigmatism, which may be present before the onset of more serious eye conditions or neurologic disease. This must be taken into consideration in noting visual acuity, as must corneal opacities and abnormalities of the media or retina. The **pinhole test** is useful in determining whether poor vision is due to a refractive error or to disease of the eyeball or to visual pathways. Vision which can be improved by looking through a pinhole can usually be improved by glasses. The test is made by requesting the patient to read the Snellen chart through a 1 mm pinhole in a disk that is held before one eye while the other eye is covered. Since the pinhole prevents peripheral rays of light from entering the eye and allows only the central rays to do so, defective vision due to refractive errors will be improved, but poor vision due to organic defects will not. Vision is recorded in the same manner as above, but with the letters "p.h." suffixed (e.g., 20/20 p.h.). Hysterical blindness or malingered defects may have to be appraised by special technics (Ch. 55). The term **amblyopia** is commonly used to designate defects of vision resulting from imperfect sensation of the retina without detectable organic lesions of the eye. Many varieties of amblyopia have been described, including amblyopia ex anopia (amblyopia from disuse) and alcoholic, toxic, traumatic, and uremic amblyopia. **Amaurosis** means blindness of any type, but in general usage means blindness without disease of the eye, or loss of vision secondary to disease of the optic nerve or brain.

Color Vision; Day and Night Vision

Color blindness (achromatopsia) is an inherited condition present mainly in men but transmitted by women. It occurs in about 3% – 4% of

J·o   BRILLIANT

If hope did not bring strength and encouragement when tr .ls and sorrows are sent, what a wretched miserable th'ng living would be. Who so strong and brave that they could endure the changes and burdens that sooner or later will inevitably come to all, if hope did not spring up in renewed vigor, with every add·   ·l Who can imagine the misery of - life if hope should veil her face and depart for ver?—Mrs Hen y Ward Beecher.

8 6 0 7 2

No. 1 Jaeger   DIAMOND

The bea·   ·l and good is with and around us; the evil and false is just as common,   have our choice a d can find whatever we look for, and see what the mind craves   · man who sees nothing in the e ▾   e tre da but dirt; nothing in the summer s sun but heat, nothing n the w nter's cold but d s worth, if he sees nothing in a tree but the fruit it bears, or its value for wood and timber, o· in the flower nothing but form, fragrance and color, will have a cold and stormy sunset.—C. L. Allen: "Nature a Series," in The Mayflower.

9 6 7 3

No. 4 Jaeger   AGATE

* * * Could the same unformed matter produce in one case a plant in a .other case a bird, in a third a man; and in each of these put bone, brain, blood and nerve in proper relations? Matter must be mind, or subject to a present working mind to do this. There must be a present intelligence directing e p·ocess laying the dead bricks, marble and wood in an intelligent order for a living temple.—H. W. Warren: "Recreations in Astronomy.'

3 8 2 0

                                                       TELEPHONE BOOK

Harper Jay L .8901 Buckingham.. . .. .FAircrest-6-8904
Lewis S Harold 28164 Landers......... ....CLifford 4-9661
Mason George W 8964 Windsor..... ....LIncoln 1-6096
Rollins Clyde N 40 Chase....... . ... WEather-9-8154
Simmons John C 2014 Cherry.... · WAshington-4-8456
Tilford F V 4891 Detroit... ....BLackhawk-3-0013

No. 7 Jaeger   BREVIER MOD.

When I read the names inscribed on the banners, they were those of men scattered far and wide about the world; some tossing upon distant seas; some under arms in d'stant lands—Washington Irving.

6 1 5 3 4

FIG. 10–6. Jaeger reading cards.

56 INCH TYPE—No. 4 Snellen, No. 11 Jaeger.   PICA.

There is a doctor in Mouse Alley who sets up f·r curing cataracts upon the credit of having, as his bill sets forth, lost an eye in the emperor s service. His patients come in upon this and he shows his muster roll, which confirms that he was in his imperial majesty's troops; and he puts out their eyes with great success.—Sir Richard Steele: "Quack Advertisements," in The Spectator.

72 INCH TYPE—No. 5 Snellen, No. 13 Jaeger.   GT. PRIMER.

The eye, it cannot choose but see;
   We cannot bid the ear be still;
Our bodies feel, where'er they be,
   Against, or with our will
              —Wordsworth.

108 INCH TYPE—No. 7 Snellen, No. 14 Jaeger.   2 LINE SMALL PICA.

"No action, whether foul
      or fair,
Is ever done, but leaves
      somewhere
A record." —Longfellow.

males and 0.3% of women. Disturbances of color vision, however, may also occur in disease of the choroid, optic nerve, visual pathways, etc., in which there is a disturbance of the visual sense. Loss of color vision may precede loss of general visual acuity or form perception. This is especially evident in the examination of the visual fields, and it has been noted that in diseases of the choroid the field for blue may be lost first, followed by loss for red, and then green, before form perception is lost. In field defects due to neurologic disease, red is usually lost first; this is sometimes referred to as red desaturation. Color blindness may be partial or total. There are various means for the testing of color vision. The patient may be asked to match or compare colors of skeins of yarn or, for more accurate testing, the pseudoisochromatic plates of Ishihara or of Hardy, Rand, and Rittler, or the Stilling test cards, may be used. Tests for color vision are important in the examination of certain industrial workers.

Day blindness, or **hemeralopia,** is a condition in which vision is poor in a bright light, but is better in dim lighting; it may be a fatigue syndrome and it is occasionally found in nutritional amblyopia, various conditions causing a central scotoma, and in beginning nuclear cataract formation; it may also be a side effect of trimethadione in the treatment of absence seizures. Bright lights may fatigue the retina in certain individuals, and since the pupil is contracted by illumination, only central vision is used; when the illumination is less bright, the pupil is dilated, and the individual is also able to use the periphery of the retina.

Night blindness (nyctalopia) is defective vision in feeble illumination or with the appearance of dusk, although vision may be normal when there is adequate illumination; this is often a symptom of pigmentary degeneration of the retina, but it is also observed in states of fatigue or exhaustion, chronic alcoholism, jaundice, Leber's disease, and debilitating diseases, and it is an early symptom of xerophthalmia. This last condition is the result of a deficiency of vitamin A, in which there is a poor adaptation to darkness and to changes in illumination.

The Visual Fields

The field of vision represents the limit of peripheral vision; it is the space within which an object can be seen while the eye remains fixed on some one point. As we fix the eye on an object, a sharp image falls upon the macula, the site of most distinct vision. Simultaneously, however, we are able to observe clearly, with the periphery of the retina, objects lying at some distance from that upon which the eye is fixed. Their images are not as distinct, however, and peripheral objects are more apparent if they are moving.

The examination of the visual fields is as important a part of the neurologic examination as the testing of visual acuity, and it may give more information in the localization of disease within the nervous system. In testing the fields the range of vision, the position, size, and shape of the physiologic blind spot, and abnormalities of either central or peripheral vision are determined. The normal visual field has a definite contour. A person is able to see laterally a distance of 90° – 100° from the fixation point, and medially only about 60°; he can see upward, at the center of vision, 50° – 60°, and downward 60° – 75°. The field of vision is wider in the inferior and lateral quadrants than in the superior and lateral quadrants (Fig. 10-7). There are individual variations in the field of vision, dependent to some extent upon the facial configuration, the shape of the orbital cavity, the position of the eye in the orbit, and the width of the palpebral fissure. An individual with a projecting brow or a highly bridged nose may have some resulting limitation in the extent of his vision, but such changes are inconsequential for clinical diagnosis in almost all instances. In binocular vision there is overlapping of the field of one eye by that of the other, with only a narrow crescentic, or sickle-shaped, area at the temporal aspect of the field which is seen by one eye only. This may extend from 60° – 90° on the horizontal meridian. In clinical testing, however, one is usually more concerned with the monocular than the binocular field.

Examining the visual fields requires cooperation of the patient. Results are most accurate in an individual who is alert and interested in the examination. The eye being examined should be fixed on an object, for any wandering of the eye impairs the evaluation. The illumination should be adequate and constant. Fatigue and weakness may lengthen the latent period between the patient's perception of the test object and his recognition of it or response to it, and may thus give a false impression of contraction of the fields. Close cooperation, good fixation, adequate illumination, and the absence of fatigue are essential for measurement of the blind spot and delineation of scotomas.

There are three standard methods of testing visual fields: the hand or confrontation method, the perimeter, and the campimeter or tangent screen. Methods of testing the visual fields by changing the rate of a flickering light and ob-

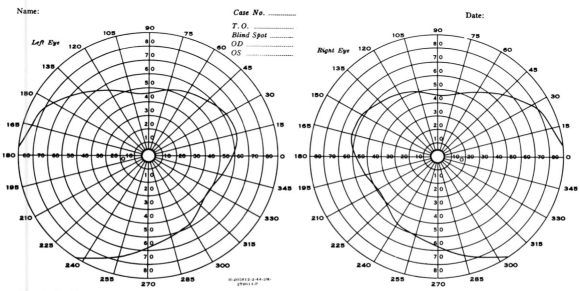

FIG. 10–7. The normal visual fields.

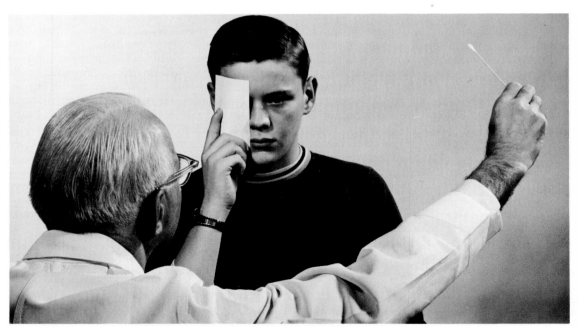

FIG. 10–8. Confrontation method of testing the visual fields.

serving when it is perceived as continuous (flicker fusion), by using ultraviolet light, and by visual evoked potentials are also available. There is also a rapid screening test by tachistoscopic presentation of simple, abstract patterns. These latter procedures, however, are used more for experimental and quantitative purposes than for clinical testing.

In the confrontation method the field under investigation is compared with the examiner's, which is used as a standard. The examiner stands, with one eyelid closed, in front of and 2 – 3 feet away from the patient, who also covers one eye and fixes the other on the examiner's nose. The opposite eyes are closed — i.e., if the examiner's left eye is closed, the patient closes his right eye. Each eye is tested individually. A pin with a white or colored head, a cotton-tipped applicator, a pencil, or a finger is used as a test object, and is brought into the field of vision through various meridians of vision (Fig. 10-8). The test object should be equidistant from the patient and the examiner. The patient is told to respond when he first notices motion, when he perceives whiteness or sees the object, when he can tell the color, and when he can distinguish the form of the object. The patient may also be asked to count fingers (either one or two) in the various quadrants of the visual field. After testing each eye, visual extinction, or inattention

(see "Visual Field Changes"), is evaluated by observing the patient's ability to see identical test objects, or movement of them, when they are presented simultaneously in the upper and lower temporal quadrants of vision of the two eyes.

By confrontation any gross defect in the field of vision may be detected, but minor changes and slight irregularities may be overlooked. The advantages of the confrontation method are that it is rapid, that it can be used at the bedside or in the home, and that it can be used on children, persons of low intellectual endowment or in states of lowered consciousness, and aphasic patients. However, it gives only approximate results and demonstrates only marked changes, and it is doubtful whether accurate delineation of the blind spot can be made.

At times major defects in the field of vision may be demonstrated in semistuporous or aphasic patients or the fields can be outlined in uncooperative patients, children, and malingerers by bringing in from the side some object that the patient would be interested in having such as a glass of water or a piece of candy, and noting how soon it is reached for. At the same time there is a turning of the eyes toward the object, an **optically elicited movement.** The presence of such movement indicates that the object is seen, and thus rules out gross field defects in malingerers. Turning of the head and eyes toward a diffuse light may be present in infants within a few days after birth. In testing aphasic patients and children one may move a flashlight with a small beam into the field of vision, and note when the patient blinks, or the examiner can bring his hand in rapidly from the side, as if to strike the patient, and notice whether he winces, draws his head back, or blinks. By this means the so-called **blink,** or **menace, reflex** is elicited.

The perimeter is an instrument by means of which one tests the field of vision through the arc of a circle. It is especially valuable for accurate delineation of the periphery of the field of vision. Many different types of perimeters and perimetric technics have been described. Flicker perimetry sometimes brings out visual field defects not evident with ordinary perimetry.

The patient is placed before the instrument and is asked to gaze at the fixation point. A test object is brought into the field of vision through multiple meridians. White test objects, varying in size from 1 – 5 mm, are usually sufficient, but for patients with diminished vision larger ones may be used. The places where the object is first seen are noted and recorded, and a line is drawn to join these points on the various radii and outline the field of vision. The smaller the test object, the smaller the visual field. The line representing the limits of the field for a given test object is called an **isopter.** Perimetric readings are expressed in fractions, with the numerator the size of the test object and the denominator the distance in millimeters. Thus 3/330 indicates that a 3 mm object was used at the ordinary perimetric distance of 330 mm. Defects in visual fields should be analyzed by plotting at least three isopters with targets of different sizes in order to gain an adequate understanding of the nature and extent of the field loss and to determine whether the defect has abrupt or sloping margins. If the size of a defect in the visual field is the same with all test objects used, it is said to have steep, or abrupt, margins. If, on the other hand, the defect becomes larger with decrease in the size of the test objects (isopters for smaller stimuli), its margins are said to be gradual, or sloping, in character.

Limits of the visual field vary according to the size and brightness of the test object, the intensity of illumination, the state of adaptation of the eye, and the cooperation of the patient. Colored test objects are sometimes used, because changes in the color fields precede gross field changes (**color desaturation**) and also because altered responses to color may aid in differentiating between lesions of the retina and of the connecting pathways. It is probable, however, that reported differences in color fields are not the result of differing receptor responses, but that the fields for all colors would be equal if size, light, intensity, and saturation of colors were equally perceptible. The perimetric examination is valuable because it gives a permanent record. The examination may be repeated periodically and the fields compared to observe changes accompanying progression or improvement in a lesion. It must be recalled, however, that a perimetric examination cannot be considered infallible: the cooperation of the patient and the competence of the perimetrist are important.

In the **tangent screen method,** a black screen, blackboard, or other flat surface is used instead of the arc of a circle, and the outlines of blind spots within the field of vision are charted as well as peripheral defects. The Bjerrum screen is a frequently used type of tangent screen (Fig. 10-9). Since the hemispheric field of vision is projected upon a flat tangential plane that is perpendicular to the line of fixation, only that portion of the field issuing from the central portion of the retina is studied, and usually only the central 30° of vision can be charted, but this area can be evaluated more accurately than with the perimeter. A test object of 1 – 3 mm is used, and the patient is seated 1 – 2 m from the screen. The reading may thus be expressed as 1/2000. A greater distance between the eyes and the screen furnishes a larger projection of any defect within the field of vision, and makes possible its earlier detection. The tangent screen is especially valuable in measuring the size of the physiologic blind spot and in demonstrating central defects. A more detailed method of testing central vision is possible with the stereocampimeter, by which each field is examined independently, but with binocular fixation; this is especially helpful in outlining central scotomas.

Devices are available for performing the visual field examination automatically, with computer generated randomly assigned visual stimuli of variable intensities to which the patient reacts by pressing a button when he sees them.

Visual Field Changes

Various changes in the visual fields may be demonstrated in neurologic disorders. Some of the more important of these are listed here.

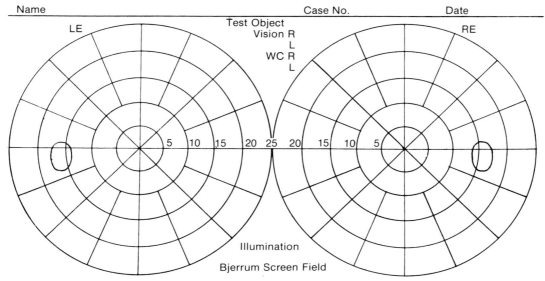

FIG. 10–9. The Bjerrum screen field.

Contraction. Contraction of the visual fields is characterized by a narrowing of the range of vision which may affect one or all parts of the periphery. Contraction may be regular or irregular, concentric or eccentric, temporal or nasal, and upper or lower. Regular, **concentric contraction** is most frequently seen. This is usually an early objective finding in optic atrophy, either primary or secondary, and is characterized by narrowing of the field of vision through all meridians. Concentric contraction of the visual fields also develops in degenerative diseases of the retina, especially in pigmentary degeneration. Narrowing of the fields due to fatigue, poor attention, or inadequate illumination must be excluded for proper diagnosis, as must "contraction" resulting from decreased visual acuity or delayed reaction time. Slight contraction of the field occurs when there is a significant refractive error.

A specific variety of contraction, the diagnosis of which is often important, is **tubular contraction**, a condition commonly regarded as a sign of hysteria (Fig. 10-10). Normally, the field of vision widens progressively as the test objects are held farther away from the eye, but in the hysterical individual this normal widening is not seen, and the entire width of the field is as great at 1 foot from the eye as it is at 2, 5, 10, or 15 feet. The tubular field is demonstrated either by testing the extent of the gross field at varying distances from a blackboard or screen, or by the use of test objects of different sizes at a constant

distance. Another type of contraction that is often difficult to evaluate is **spiral contraction,** in which there is a progressive narrowing of the field of vision during the process of testing it (Fig. 10-11). This is also said by some to be a sign of nonorganic disease, but it is probably more diagnostic of fatigue. Similar to the spiral field is the **star-shaped field,** in which there is an irregularity of outline. This may be seen in hysteria, fatigue, or poorly concentrated attention. Spiral and tubular fields and ring scotomas with a continual fluctuation of the visual threshold for different parts of the field and with concomitant phenomena of extinction have been described in patients with head injury.

Hemianopias. Loss of one half of the visual field is termed **hemianopia,** or **hemianopsia.** This may be either **homonymous** or **heteronymous. Homonymous hemianopia** is the loss of vision in the nasal half in one eye and the temporal half in the other eye. It is caused by lesions posterior to the optic chiasm, where there is interruption of the fibers from the temporal half of the ipsilateral retina and of the fibers from the nasal half of the opposite retina. With such lesions, vision is lost in the *nasal* field for the *ipsilateral* eye, and in the *temporal* field for the *opposite* eye, and inasmuch as the hemianopia is designated by the side of the field loss, a lesion posterior to the chiasm on one side always causes hemianopia on the opposite side (Fig. 10-12).

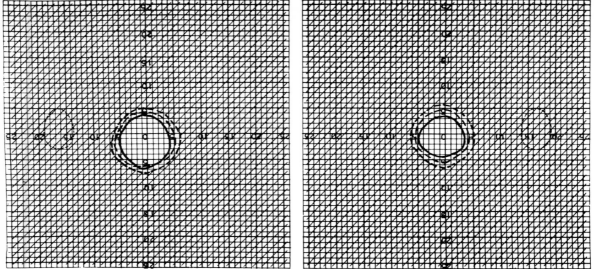

FIG. 10–10. Tubular contraction of the visual fields as shown on the tangent screen. The patient is tested at 1, 2, and 3 m from the screen.

If the lesion which causes a homonymous hemianopia is situated in the optic tracts anterior to the lateral geniculate body, the fibers subserving the light reflex are also involved, and there is a loss of the pupillary response when a pencil of light is focused on the involved half of the retina; this is termed **Wernicke's hemianopic phenomenon.** It has been suggested that even a small pencilled focus of light will usually diffuse through the cornea and eye structures so that Wernicke's hemianopic pupillary phenomenon, although a reasonable anatomic assumption, is not of clinical significance. The ipsilateral pupil may also be larger, and if optic atrophy is present, the phenomenon may be more marked in the ipsilateral eye. In tract lesions, furthermore, the hemianopia is usually **incongruous** — i.e., the field defects in the two eyes do not match exactly — as a result of the fibers from the corresponding retinal areas being unevenly mixed or intermingled in the tracts. There may also be incongruity in geniculate lesions owing to stratification of fibers.

If the lesion is posterior to the lateral geniculate body, within the optic radiations, the light reflex is not lost and the defect is usually congruous because fibers representing corresponding areas in the two retinas are closely associated. Wounds involving the intermediate portion of the radiations may cause a narrow, sector-shaped defect in the horizontal meridian, and with lesions of the anterior portion of the

visual cortex there may be sparing of the temporal crescent. In suprageniculate hemianopias there may be no subjective dimness of vision or darkness in the affected portions of the fields, and visual acuity may be normal.

Instead of a complete blindness in the hemianopic fields, other changes may be evident. A partial or irregular defect in one or both of the symmetric fields may be as significant as loss of the entire field. There may be relative rather than absolute loss of vision, or fluctuation of vision in the affected fields. There may be **extinction,** or suppression of vision toward one side without true loss of vision, or a failure to notice one object when a similar object is held simultaneously in the opposite field. This is also called **visual inattention.** Many investigators believe that in this phenomenon the stimuli originating in the normal field of vision suppress or obscure the image arising simultaneously in an affected field. Extinction may be present rather than hemianopia, or it may appear during the process of development of a hemianopia, and it should always be tested for. Of similar significance are the following: loss of visual discernment, or the inability to localize the object seen; impairment of the fusion threshold for intermittent light (as determined by flicker perimetry); and hemianopia for color, or hemiachromatopia.

It is often not possible to determine, from the field defect alone, the site of the lesion responsible for a homonymous defect. The most fre-

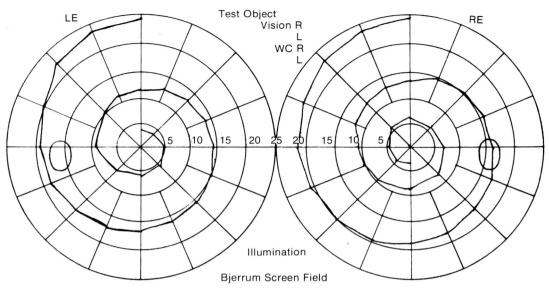

FIG. 10–11. *Spiral visual fields.*

quent location is in the occipital lobe, then the parietal and temporal lobes; optic tract and lateral geniculate lesions are infrequent. Lesions of the occipital lobe are most often of vascular origin. Parietal and temporal lobe lesions may be either vascular or neoplastic. A vascular lesion often has an abrupt onset and the resulting field defect has steep or abrupt margins. The field defects associated with neoplasms are often incomplete, gradual, and progressive in nature, and have gradual or sloping margins; occasionally they are incongruous.

An alteration or absence of optokinetic nystagmus toward the hemianopic side is found most often with parietal lobe involvement. With lesions near the tip of the occipital lobe, especially if in the dominant hemisphere, there may be **macular sparing,** or preservation of central

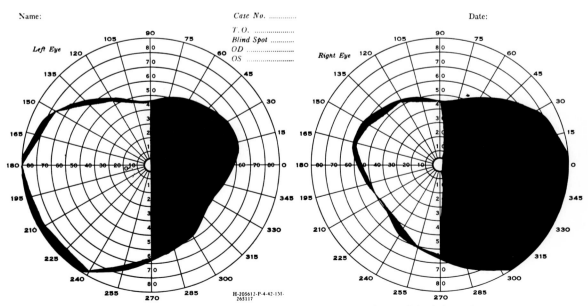

FIG. 10–12. *Right homonymous hemianopia in a patient with a neoplasm of the left occipital lobe.*

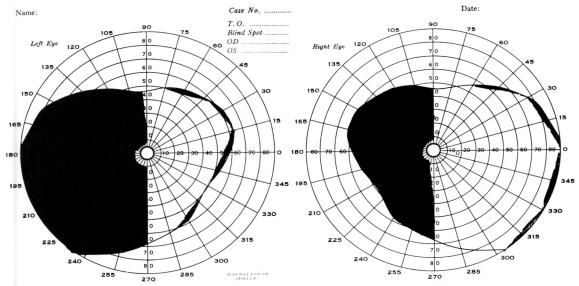

FIG. 10–13. Left homonymous hemianopia with macular sparing in a patient with a neoplasm of the right occipital pole.

vision in the otherwise blind half of the visual field (Fig. 10-13). Macular sparing was once explained on the basis of bilateral representation of the maculae in the occipital lobes, and it was believed that by means of either the radiation of fibers through both optic tracts or the crossing of fibers through the splenium of the corpus callosum the maculae were represented in the primary visual centers of both hemispheres; this has never been confirmed anatomically. The maculae do have wide distribution, however, both at the occipital pole and anteriorly in the depths of the calcarine fissure. The persistence of central vision with involvement of one occipital lobe can probably be explained by this extensive macular representation, or by incomplete destruction of the striate cortex by the lesion, overlapping of blood supply, or individual variations in the anatomic structure of the human brain. With occipital lesions a constant physiologic shift of fixation seems to occur. Therefore, macular sparing may be apparent rather than real, the change that appears in the visual fields being the result of instability of fixation and the establishment of an eccentric fixation point, both of which occur with loss of cortical integration and with interruption of corticotectal pathways. In the gradual onset of a hemianopia, macular vision is retained the longest, but it too may disappear.

Loss of one quadrant in the field of vision rather than an entire half may occur; this is termed **quadrantanopia,** or **quadrantic hemianopia** (Fig. 10-14). If the loss is in the lower quadrant, there has been involvement of the fibers that radiate through the parietal or upper temporal lobe and terminate on the upper lip of the calcarine fissure; an upper quadrantanopia signifies involvement of fibers that radiate through the remainder of the temporal lobe and around the lateral ventricle and terminate on the lower lip of the calcarine fissure.

A unilateral lesion limited to the posterior portion of the occipital lobe may cause a symmetric hemianopic scotoma. Calcarine, or cortical, blindness follows bilateral lesions. There may be bilateral homonymous hemianopias, owing to involvement of both optic tracts, radiations, or occipital lobes, or there may be bilateral central scotomas because of lesions of both occipital poles. Cortical blindness may be of vascular, traumatic, neoplastic, or degenerative origin, and occurs with injuries to the posterior parts of the brain; thrombosis of the basilar or of both posterior cerebral arteries; severe anoxia or blood loss; air embolism; hemolytic transfusion reactions; and at times demyelinating or degenerative disorders. Because the pupils may still react to light, cortical blindness is sometimes difficult to differentiate from hysterical blindness, although occasionally there is denial of loss of vision. Lesions of the more anterior portions of the occipital lobes may be accompanied by a disturbance in space perception and a loss of absolute localization of objects in the homonymous field without hemia-

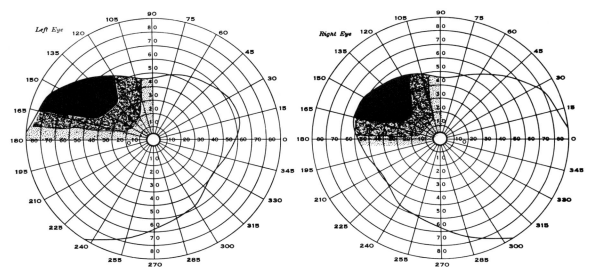

FIG. 10–14. Left superior quadrantanopia with sloping borders in a patient with a neoplasm of the right temporal lobe.

nopia, or by such defects as visual agnosia, or alexia (Ch. 53), loss of visual memory, denial of blindness, and loss of following and reflex movements of the eyes.

In **heteronymous hemianopia** either both nasal or both temporal fields are affected. The bitemporal variety is by far the more frequent, and is usually the result of involvement of the optic chiasm (Fig. 10-15), situated just above the sella turcica. The most common cause of bitemporal hemianopia is a pituitary adenoma, but it also results from other parasellar or suprasellar tumors or cysts such as meningiomas and craniopharyngiomas, as well as gliomas of the optic chiasm, aneurysms, trauma, and hydrocephalus. Interference with the decussating fibers

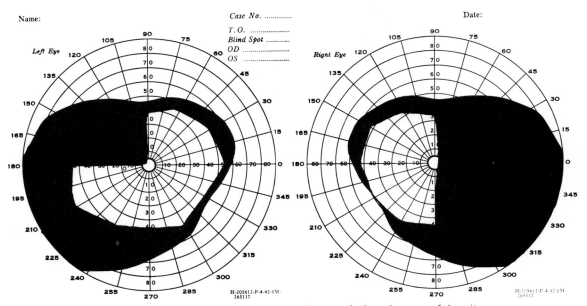

FIG. 10–15. Bitemporal hemianopia in a patient with a chromophobe adenoma of the pituitary gland. There is complete loss of vision in the right temporal field, and predominant involvement of the superior quadrant in the left temporal field.

which supply the nasal half of each retina, and carry vision from the temporal fields, is responsible for this field defect. It is unusual for the fields to be bilaterally symmetric. Because the fibers from the superior field of vision which travel in the ventral portion of the chiasm are usually first affected, the primary defect of vision appears in the superior quadrant. There may first be a superior temporal quadrantanopia in one eye, then a temporal field loss, followed by contraction or loss of the nasal field. One eye is usually involved before the other eye, and the visual loss develops more rapidly on that side. Occasionally there is blindness of one eye with a temporal field defect in the other, or the first manifestation may be a central scotoma. With successful treatment, recession with recovery of vision also takes place in sequence, in the reverse order to that of the advancing process.

A binasal hemianopia can occur with bilateral lesions which interrupt the continuity of the fibers from the temporal half of each retina without involving the crossing fibers. Binasal hemianopia is rare, although it is sometimes found when atherosclerosis or bilateral aneurysms of the internal carotid arteries are present, and it may be seen in demyelinating disorders. Unilateral nasal hemianopias are seen more frequently.

Altitudinal, or horizontal, hemianopias occur infrequently. They may be associated with a lesion of the sellar region, just below the optic chiasm, pressing on the ventral fibers and causing a superior field loss, or with internal hydrocephalus or a third ventricle lesion, pressing on the dorsal aspect of the chiasm and causing an inferior field loss. More often they may occur in the presence of bilateral lesions involving the occipital lobes.

Scotomas.   Scotomas are defects, or blind spots, of varying size, shape, and intensity within the field of vision. They are best demonstrated by the use of the tangent screen. In every field it should be possible to outline the **physiologic blind spot** (Mariotte's spot), a scotoma corresponding to the papilla, or nerve head, which contains no rods or cones and is therefore blind to all visual impressions. The physiologic blind spot is situated 15° lateral to and just below the center of fixation. It is elliptic in shape and averages 7° – 7½° in vertical diameter and 5° – 5½° in horizontal diameter, and extends 2° above and 5° below the horizontal meridian. If the blind spot is charted on the Bjerrum screen with the patient 1 m from the board, and tested with a 1 mm object,

the average measurements are from 9 – 12 cm in the horizontal diameter and from 15 – 18 cm in the vertical diameter. Testing at 2 m may give more accurate results. The blind spot is enlarged in papilledema and optic neuritis.

Pathologic scotomas, or blind spots, may be **relative,** or **indistinct,** in which the patient sees form but no color, or in which perception of objects is impaired but not destroyed; or they may be **absolute,** in which the patient sees neither form, color, nor light. Subjectively, scotomas may be positive, resulting from a lesion in or anterior to the retina or choroid, or negative, owing to a lesion of the optic nerve, tracts, or radiations. In **positive scotomas** the blind spots are seen by the patient as dark or blind areas; these are usually due to exudate or hemorrhage over the retina or changes in the media, and are not regarded as true scotomas. In **negative scotomas** the blind spots are not perceived by the patient until the visual fields are examined.

Scotomas are most frequently central, paracentral, annular, or peripheral in distribution. Scotomas secondary to lesions of the optic disk are usually cuneate (wedge-shaped), owing to involvement of one or more bundles of fibers.

A **central scotoma** is characterized by blindness that is limited to the area of the visual field which corresponds to the macula, or point of fixation, and it results from involvement of the macular area of the retina or involvement of the papillomacular bundle, which is especially susceptible to toxins and pressure (Fig. 10-16). A **paracentral scotoma** is one whose edge passes through the fixation point; it does not cause total loss of central vision. Enlargement of the physiologic blind spot is referred to as a **peripapillary scotoma.** A **cecocentral scotoma** involves both the macular area and the blind spot; it is usually accompanied by loss of all central vision, with preservation of a very small amount of peripheral vision, and frequently results from optic neuritis (Fig. 10-17). Peripheral scotomas may be present anywhere in the field of vision. In **annular,** or **ring, scotomas** there is a loss of vision surrounding the center of the visual field.

Ring scotomas may be present with pigmentary degeneration of the retina. In glaucoma there may be arcuate, cuneate, comma-shaped, or other partially ring-shaped scotomas. Gliomas of the optic nerve and drusen, or hyaline excrescences which may be either within or on the surface of the optic nerves, may cause scotomas, contraction of the visual fields, or sector defects. Although scotomas are most often the result of disease of the retinas or optic nerves, they may

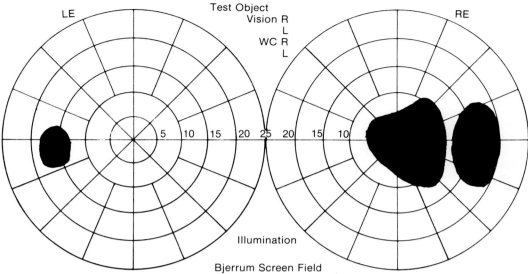

FIG. 10–16. *Screen fields of a patient with right-sided retrobulbar neuritis. There is a central scotoma together with enlargement of the physiologic blind spot.*

also be caused by cerebral lesions. Pressure on the intracranial portion of the ophthalmic artery may cause a blind spot within the field of vision, and localized lesions of the posterior portion of one or both occipital lobes may cause homonymous macular, paracentral quadrantic or hemianopic, or bilateral central scotomas. Central scotomas have been reported in hysteria; if present, they are usually bilateral.

All the scotomas noted previously can be demonstrated objectively, but there are also subjective scotomas which cannot be delineated in the field examination, such as the scintillating scotomas, or teichopsias, of migraine, and the muscae volantes ("flitting flies:" spots before the eyes) which many normal individuals experience. It should be remembered that scotomas of various types as well as field modifications of all varieties

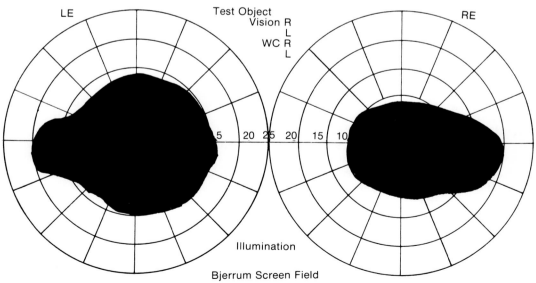

FIG. 10–17. *Screen fields of a patient with bilateral optic neuritis. There are bilateral cecocentral scotomas.*

occur in many ocular and intraocular conditions, such as retinitis, chorioretinitis, and glaucoma. These are not related directly to disease of the nervous system.

The Ophthalmoscopic Examination

The ophthalmoscopic examination is of extreme importance in the neurologic examination, and no evaluation of a patient is complete without it. This part of the examination is also significant in the diagnosis of many systemic diseases and in the differences between neurologic involvement, systemic disease, and various types of ocular morbidity.

Although the neurologist is most interested in the appearance of the optic disk, the entire fundus must be examined, and the lens and vitreous should also be appraised. Many varieties of ophthalmoscopes are available; nearly all are satisfactory when used by an experienced observer. It is only by practice that one learns to evaluate what one sees with the ophthalmoscope, and it is only by performing repeated examinations that one gains the ability to relax one's own accommodation, and thus more adequately visualize the fundus of the patient. Examining the fundi of many healthy persons helps to acquaint the beginner with the ranges and variations of normal appearance. Every ophthalmoscopist should be aware of his own error of refraction, so that he may correct it in studying the eyes of his patients by adjustment of the instrument.

The ophthalmoscopic part of the neurologic examination should be carried out without the use of mydriatics, if this is at all possible. The pupillary responses and their variations are an important part of the neurologic examination, and every attempt should be made to preserve them. In most instances, except when the pupil is miotic, as after administration of morphine-like substances (or drugs used to treat glaucoma, such as pilocarpine), it is possible to examine the optic nerve head, the macular area, the surrounding portions of the retina, and the blood vessels without dilating the pupil, especially if the patient is placed in a dark room for a short period before the examination is made. Sometimes, however, it is necessary to dilate the pupils, especially in examining the periphery of the fundus. This should be done only after the pupillary responses have been carefully noted. It is best to use mydriatics that do not cause cycloplegia (paralysis of accommodation) and whose action is of short duration.

The **retina,** which is transparent and assumes the color of the underlying choroid, varies from a pale orange-red in blond individuals to a deep red in brunets, and is even darker in those of very dark or black complexion. It is important to remember this variation in coloring, since one's interpretation of the coloring of the optic disk may be influenced by the contrast between the disk and the amount of pigment seen in the retina.

The **optic disk,** or **papilla,** represents the entrance of the optic nerve, and is situated just medial to and slightly above the center of the fundus. It is oval to elliptic in shape, and pale pink in color. The temporal half of the disk is slightly paler than the nasal half. The margins of the disk are usually sharply defined, and are slightly more distinct on the temporal aspect; at times they may be somewhat blurred nasally. Varying amounts of pigmentation are present in the retina near the temporal border of the disk, especially in dark-skinned persons, and at times there is a pigment ring which completely surrounds the disk. The white scleral and dark choroidal rings may sometimes be seen. The outer portions of the disk are elevated slightly above the center, or **physiologic cup,** and in the depressed central area is seen the cross-hatching of the lamina cribrosa, where the fibers of the optic nerve pass through the sclera (Fig. 10-18). Abnormalities of the contour or border of the disk may be caused by many physiologic or nonpathologic conditions: an excess of glial tissue may obscure the outline of the nerve head; myelination of some of the nerve fibers as they pass from the retina into the disk may give the latter an irregular, feathered outline; drusen may appear as shiny areas on the surface of the disk.

The central artery and vein emerge from the center of the disk and divide into superior and inferior divisions, whose nasal and temporal branches radiate out to supply the entire retina. The arteries are only 75 – 100 μ in diameter, but the 14-diameter magnification provided by the cornea and lens of the patient's eye makes these visible on the ophthalmoscopic examination. The arteries are smaller in caliber than the veins, in a ratio varying from 2:3 – 4:5. Their course is straighter, their color is lighter, and they show a bright reflex stripe along their surfaces. The veins are thicker, more tortuous, and of a deep reddish-purple color, and some terminate at the border of the disk.

The **macula lutea** is situated at the center of the fundus, about two disk diameters temporally to and slightly below the disk. It is an oval depression of the retina. Here the choroid is slightly darker or slightly granular, and this area is devoid of large blood vessels. There may be one or more bright spots corresponding to the position of the fovea centralis.

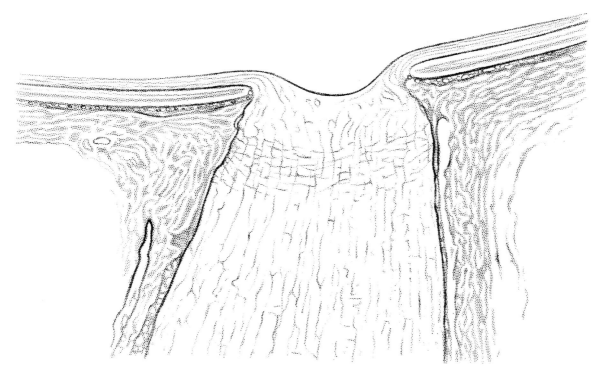

FIG. 10–18. Section of the optic nerve head showing the physiologic cup.

In the examination of the fundus, special attention must be paid to the optic disks and their color, size, and shape. The borders are inspected, as are the physiologic cup and lamina cribrosa. One should also observe the size, shape, and appearance of the vessels, and the appearance of the retina, choroid, and fovea centralis. Hemorrhages, exudates, aberrations in pigmentation, and other varieties should be noted and described.

There are many neurologic conditions in which important and characteristic abnormalities are apparent by ophthalmoscopy. Furthermore, the examination of the ocular fundus and the optic disk is a valuable part of the general medical examination and is often of distinct aid in the diagnosis of systemic disease.

Optic Nerve Disorders and Associated Findings

Optic Atrophy. When **primary optic atrophy** is present, the disk is paler than normal and somewhat smaller; it may be an opaque white or a blue-white color (Fig. 10-19). The disk margins stand out distinctly, the physiologic cup may be increased in depth and size, and the lamina

cribrosa is prominent and may extend to the margin of the disk. The capillaries which supply the disk are decreased in number and the larger vessels are diminished in caliber. Increased dark choroid pigment deposits about the margin of the disk may be present. Primary optic atrophy may develop in association with or as the result of many pathologic conditions. Some of the more

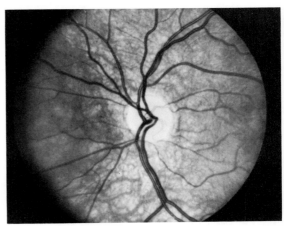

FIG. 10–19. Primary optic atrophy. (Courtesy of Richard A. Lewis)

important include retrobulbar neuritis, especially in association with multiple sclerosis, toxic amblyopia, deficiency states, diabetes, anemia, and Leber's disease (hereditary optic atrophy); central nervous system syphilis; pressure on the optic nerves due to pituitary tumors; craniopharyngiomas, suprasellar aneurysms and tumors, meningiomas, orbital tumors, gliomas of the optic nerve, Paget's disease (osteitis deformans), hydrocephalus, and oxycephalia; trauma, such as fractures or gun-shot wounds with severing of the nerve; interruption of the blood supply to the nerve (Fig. 10-20). In all of the aforementioned conditions there is primary damage to the nerve with resulting degeneration; sometimes the cause of optic atrophy is not determined. If there is marked recession of the disk, the term **cavernous** or **pseudoglaucomatous, optic atrophy** is sometimes used; this variety of atrophy is caused by interruption of the blood supply to the nerve, and occurs in vascular disease and pituitary tumors. In glaucoma there is both increase in the depth of the physiologic cup and atrophy of the optic nerve (Fig. 10-21). Glaucoma is a very common cause of optic atrophy.

In certain conditions, especially multiple sclerosis, there is apt to be increased pallor of the temporal portion of the disk. This may precede atrophy in multiple sclerosis, retrobulbar neuritis, and various toxic states. One cannot diagnose multiple sclerosis, however, on the basis of temporal pallor alone, for the pallor may be physiologic. The appearance of temporal pallor with visual loss, especially a central defect (due to involvement of the papillomacular bundle, which

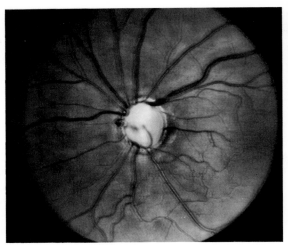

FIG. 10–21. Glaucomatous optic atrophy. (Courtesy of Richard A. Lewis)

runs through the temporal area of the disk), is significant. Leber's disease is a hereditary mitochondrial disease with loss of central vision, due to involvement of the papillomacular bundle, followed by atrophy of the optic nerve and retina.

In **secondary,** or **consecutive, optic atrophy,** which is most frequently a sequel of papilledema and optic neuritis, the appearance may be similar to that noted above, but there are usually residual signs of the previous condition. The disk is often a grayish-white color, and the margins are blurred and the lamina cribrosa may be hidden by connective tissue, glial proliferation, or residuals of previous exudation. Some authorities restrict the use of the term consecutive atrophy to that which follows disease of the retina or choroid rather than that which follows neuritis or edema.

Ischemic optic atrophy usually has an abrupt onset. Eye pain is mild and field defects are variable. It may develop after acute blood loss or in association with other disease processes such as diabetes mellitus, hypertension, or temporal (giant cell) arteritis.

It is often difficult to differentiate between primary and secondary optic atrophy, and the two may exist together. In both varieties there is loss of visual acuity, and concentric contraction of the visual fields which may be apparent before visible changes appear in the disk. In secondary atrophy, however, there may also be field changes which are the result of the previous inflammation or edema of the disk, or of the intracranial condition responsible for the disturbance of vision.

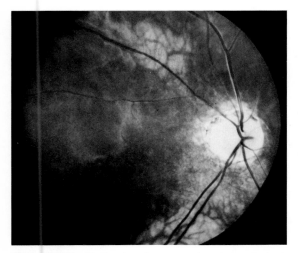

FIG. 10–20. Optic atrophy secondary to central retinal artery occlusion. (Courtesy of Richard A. Lewis)

Papilledema. Papilledema, or choked disk, is characterized by swelling of the nerve head, usually the result of increased intracranial pressure. The subdural and subarachnoid spaces of the brain are continuous along the course of the optic nerve, and increased pressure within the skull and subarachnoid space is conducted to the nerve. Papilledema is produced mechanically by increased cerebrospinal fluid (CSF) pressure in the vaginal sheath of the optic nerve, causing disturbed axoplasmic flow, swelling of the axons, and eventually vascular compression of the disk, with protrusion of the papilla into the globe of the eye (Fig. 10-22). The first visible change is hyperemia of the disk, with blurring of its margins, initially evident on the nasal, superior, and inferior borders; this is accompanied by a dilation of the veins and disappearance of venous pulsations (Fig. 10-23). Although the increase in intracranial pressure is the most important mechanism in the development of papilledema, swelling of the optic disk is also influenced (either hastened or retarded) by other factors, which include the intraocular tension, the pressure within the central retinal artery and vein, and systemic arterial and venous pressures, the condition of the capillary walls in the optic nerve, the composition of the blood, and the os-motic pressure of the vitreous body and the cerebrospinal fluid.

As the edema increases, the lamina cribrosa becomes obscured, the physiologic cup is obliterated, and the disk itself becomes reddened and elevated. The veins then become increasingly dilated and tortuous, the arteries are contracted, exudate forms over the disk and extends over the adjacent retina, and hemorrhages occur in the area surrounding the disk and into the retina (Fig. 10-24). The earlier hemorrhages are linear or flame-shaped and radiate out from the disk; these hemorrhages are present in the nerve-cell layer of the retina. Later, large hemorrhagic areas may be seen. Early in the process no interference with the blood supply through the central retinal artery is evident, but later this vessel may also be constricted.

The extent of elevation of the disk is recorded in diopters, and the reading is determined by noting the difference in the lens reading in diopters when focusing on the highest portion of the elevated disk and that, in turn, when focusing on an uninvolved portion of the retina. The use of a +2 lens to focus on the disk and a −1 lens to focus on the retina gives a difference of 3 diopters, or a papilledema of 3 diopters. Absence of spontaneous venous pulsations of the retinal

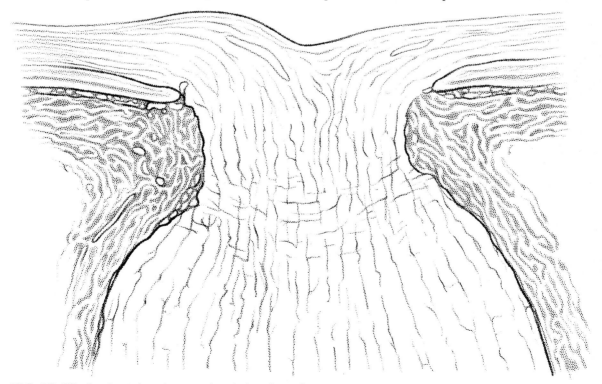

FIG. 10–22. *Section of optic nerve head showing edema.*

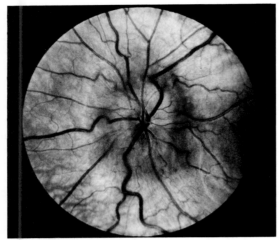

FIG. 10–23. Early papilledema. (Courtesy of Richard A. Lewis)

veins is one of the early signs of papilledema. In some 20% of normal persons, however, no pulsations can be seen in the absence of intracranial hypertension; if such is the case, it is often possible to bring out the pulsations by applying light pressure to the globe, thus raising the intraocular pressure above the venous pressure. In early stages of papilledema there may be no significant loss of visual acuity, and the only field changes may be an enlargement of the physiologic blind spot.

The presence of papilledema is usually an indication of elevation of the intracranial pressure. It is found most frequently in association with brain tumors, abscesses and other mass lesions, meningitis, encephalitis, posttraumatic states, subdural hematoma, subarachnoid hemorrhage, arachnoiditis, pseudotumor cerebri (benign or idiopathic intracranial hypertension), thrombosis of the dural sinuses, and hydrocephalus. Other pathologic states in which there may also be significant papilledema include the Guillain – Barré syndrome and other conditions in which there is a marked elevation of the protein content of the cerebrospinal fluid, profound anemia, leukemia, emphysema, hypertension, toxemia, plumbism, hypoparathyroidism, orbital tumors or pressure on the optic nerve in the orbit, decrease of the intraocular pressure, and various systemic and metabolic disorders causing alterations of the central nervous system. In the **Foster Kennedy syndrome,** which is usually the result of a neoplasm in the frontal lobe or in the region of the sphenoidal ridge, there is optic atrophy, usually with an associated central scotoma, on the side of the lesion, probably caused by direct pressure on the optic nerve, and papilledema in the opposite eye. Papilledema may fail to develop in spite of the presence of increased intracranial pressure if the optic nerves are atrophic, if the nerve heads are anomalous, as in severe myopia, or if the subarachnoid space around the optic nerves is sealed off from the intracranial subarachnoid space by the presence of adhesions.

It may be difficult, on occasion, to differentiate between papilledema and other conditions in which there is an apparent elevation of the papilla, such as optic neuritis, to be described below, and pseudopapilledema, which is seen in some hyperopic eyes. Here there is blurring of the disk margins, but the surface of the disk is not raised; there is no dilation of the veins, and no hyperemia or enlargement of the blind spot. High central branching of the retinal arteries may give an appearance of elevation of the disk margins. Papilledema must also be differentiated from neuroretinitis, which appears in hypertension and nephritis; from venous engorgement owing to neoplasms of the orbit, thrombosis of the central retinal vein, cavernous sinus thrombosis, arteriovenous aneurysm, and intrathoracic venous obstruction; and from drusen, or hyaline excrescences of the papilla, which may sometimes cause field defects and visual impairment. Photography of the fundus after the intravenous injection of fluorescein may aid in differentiating between early papilledema and so-called pseudopapilledema. In true papilledema there is increased capillary permea-

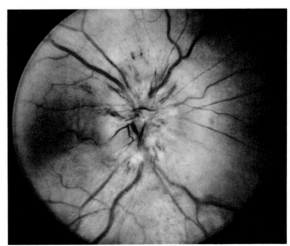

FIG. 10–24. Severe papilledema. (Courtesy of Richard A. Lewis)

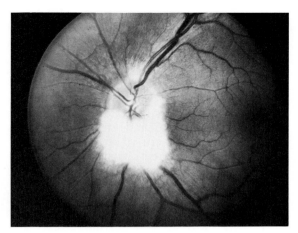

FIG. 10–25. Medullated nerve fibers. (Courtesy of Richard A. Lewis)

bility of the disk and the surrounding retina, and the fluorescein leaks into the extravascular tissues, where it remains for several hours. In pseudopapilledema due to hyperopia, medullated nerve fibers, drusen, and congenital anomalies, there is no such leakage (Figs. 10-25 and 10-26).

Optic Neuritis. Optic neuritis resembles papilledema and often is difficult to differentiate from it. Optic neuritis is an inflammation of the optic nerve, and while there may be elevation of the disk, the primary findings are congestion, infiltration, and exudation. The disk is a deep red or gray with red striations, the margins are blurred, the veins are dilated, and the arteries narrowed. There is extensive exudation over the disk, which often extends onto the retina, and there may be hemorrhages, choroidal changes, and pigment deposits. The retinal vessels are frequently hidden by exudate. The physiologic cup may be lost or the disk may be measurably elevated, but the actual edema is not in proportion to the other changes. In contrast to papilledema (where the onset is gradual, there may be little visual loss, and central vision is preserved until late), in optic neuritis there is a marked loss of visual acuity that is often abrupt — usually the best clue to the differential diagnosis — and there is a pronounced loss of the central field, often with a central scotoma and preservation of only a small amount of the peripheral field. Neuritis is usually associated with pain in and behind the eye, pain on movement of the eye, and tenderness to pressure, whereas papilledema is painless. Optic neuritis is often unila-

teral, and papilledema more frequently is bilateral. In papilledema the swelling, engorgement, and hemorrhages are more marked; in optic neuritis there rarely is marked elevation of the disk, but there is more exudation and retinal edema. Optic atrophy is frequently a sequel of optic neuritis.

Optic neuritis may be the first manifestation of neuromyelitis optica, or acute neuroencephalomyelopathy (see Fig. 10-17). The macular fibers and central vision seem to suffer the most, either because the center of the nerve is predominantly involved or because the papillomacular bundle is most susceptible to damage. The process may extend to involve the retina, causing a neuroretinitis. Optic neuritis may be a primary inflammatory condition of the optic nerve, in reality an encephalitis, or it may be secondary to infection elsewhere in the body. Both a perineuritis and an intraneural neuritis have been described. In the former the involvement is primarily in the sheath of the nerve, the result of extension of an inflammatory process from the meninges or orbit. Intraneural neuritis may be a primary infection or a part of neuromyelitis optica, or may be secondary to sinus disease (especially inflammation of the sphenoidal sinus) or to systemic infections such as measles, infectious mononucleosis, vaccinia, and various bacterial infections. Optic neuritis may also occur in multiple sclerosis, anemia, severe vitamin deficiency (especially of B_{12} and the B complex) or other malnutrition, or diabetes and other metabolic disorders, and may follow the ingestion of or exposure to certain toxins. Optic neuritis with

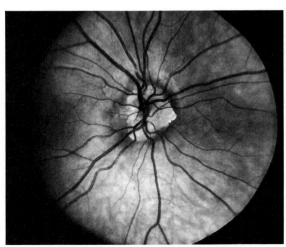

FIG. 10–26. Drusen of optic nerve head simulating papilledema. (Courtesy of Richard A. Lewis)

normal acuity has been reported but is rare; the preservation of vision has been explained by the sparing of the papillomacular bundle.

Retrobulbar Neuritis. In retrobulbar neuritis there is a marked loss of visual acuity, usually due to a defect in central vision, but no appreciable ophthalmoscopic change. It has been said that with retrobulbar neuritis, the patient "sees nothing" when he attempts to look out of his eye, and the examiner "sees nothing" (abnormal) when he looks into the eye. There is involvement of the optic nerve posterior to the globe, and especially of the papillomacular fibers, which are the most vulnerable to toxins and pressure. Although the appearance of the disk is usually normal, there may be either slight edema or temporal pallor. The condition is considered by many to be a clinical entity regardless of the ophthalmoscopic appearance of the disk, but it might be better to term it as a symptom complex. It may be similar to optic neuritis in etiology and pathophysiology, but the process is sufficiently posterior to the nerve head so that no changes are apparent on ophthalmoscopy. Computed tomography or magnetic resonance imaging of the orbit may show an enlarged optic nerve behind the globe in the orbit. The loss of acuity may vary from a 10% – 20% deficiency of vision to complete blindness. There may be central, peripheral, paracentral, or cecocentral scotomas. The process may either be self-limited or terminate in optic atrophy. Occasionally it occurs bilaterally.

Retrobulbar neuritis is seen most frequently in multiple sclerosis, but it may also occur in neuromyelitis optica, sinus disease, hereditary optic atrophy, allergic states, and hyperthyroidism; in certain of the conditions listed as causing optic neuritis (systemic infections, anemia, malnutrition, deficiency states, and diabetes); and following exposure to or ingestion of certain toxins, including lead, thallium, carbon disulfide, quinine, tryparsamide, and methyl alcohol. So-called tobacco – alcohol amblyopias are of deficiency origin. Pressure on the optic nerve by tumors and trauma may cause a syndrome resembling retrobulbar neuritis, as may certain vascular and circulatory disorders, such as temporal arteritis. In many instances the etiology of retrobulbar neuritis is not found, and the process resolves spontaneously. Statistical studies vary in incidence figures but in about 35% of such cases the patient later develops other manifestations of multiple sclerosis.

Vascular Disorders and Associated Findings

Ophthalmoscopic changes in the retinal arteries and veins may also have diagnostic importance. In retinal atherosclerosis, which may be part of cerebral or of generalized atherosclerosis, the arteries may be straight or tortuous. There is proliferation of the intima, and an endarteritis or periarteritis. The lumens of the vessels, especially the arteries, are narrowed, with widening of the reflex stripe and slight indentation of the veins at the arteriovenous crossings. As the process progresses, white lines seen along the borders of the arteries give an appearance of "silver-wire" arteries. Hemorrhages are frequently scattered along the blood vessels.

Obstruction of the central artery may cause sudden blindness. Within a few hours the entire fundus is pale and edematous, and the arteries are extremely thin and can be followed only a short distance from the disk. The veins are pale and may appear to be beaded, and there is a bright cherry-red spot at the fovea. Within a few days there may be degeneration of the retina, and within a few weeks atrophy of the nerve and of the retina. In thrombosis of the central vein there is marked distention of all the retinal veins, and the entire fundus may be covered with hemorrhages. The arteries are attenuated. The disk is blurred and may be elevated. Subhyaloid and vitreous hemorrhages are commonly encountered in patients with subarachnoid hemorrhage.

In hypertension retinal changes occur early and may be of prognostic significance. There is angiospasm, which progresses to angiosclerosis. The arteries are narrowed, the diameter ratio of arteries to veins is reduced, there is an increase in the reflex stripe, and there are localized areas of irregularity in the lumens of the arteries owing to spasm, in addition to arteriovenous compression, proliferation, and periarterial sheathing. As the process progresses the areas of spasm become more marked, with definite zones of constriction, straightening of the normal curves, and shortening of the arteries, so that the distal arteriolar segments are not seen. There may be hemorrhages and edema of the retina and the nerve head, which cause a diffuse angiospastic retinitis accompanied by exudation and elevation of the disk. Whitish deposits, or "cotton-wool" patches, form in the retina, edema develops in the macula, and a partial or complete star-shaped figure made up of white dots appears with the fovea as its center. Wagener and Keith have classified the retinal changes in hypertension and have expressed the belief that much information concerning the status of the patient, the differential diagnosis, and the prognosis, especially in cases of so-called malignant hypertension, can be derived from the retinal examination.

With cerebrovascular insufficiency of either the carotid or vertebrobasilar systems, visual symptoms may be prominent. Bilateral **amaurosis fugax,** or brief, recurrent attacks of binocular loss of vision and transient hemianopic defects may occur with insufficiency of the vertebrobasilar system. With atherosclerotic stenosis and insufficiency of either the common or internal carotid artery there may be attacks of transient, ipsilateral, monocular blindness (also called **amaurosis fugax**) due to temporal retinal ischemia, decrease in the central retinal artery pressure, or even occlusion of the central retinal artery. Occlusion of any of the arteries that supply the visual pathways or the cortex may cause permanent field defects. Atherosclerotic plaques at the bifurcation of the retinal arteries have been described in patients with carotid artery disease. In patients with so-called pulseless disease any of the above may be present and in addition, there may be multiple microaneurysms of the retinal arteries and dilated veins. Doppler ultrasound studies and angiography may help to delineate the status of the carotid circulation (see Ch. 3, "Examination of Patients with Cerebrovascular Disease").

Occlusion of the retinal vessels may also accompany carotid dissection, with transient or permanent visual loss on the ipsilateral side.

Ocular angiospasm, or angiospastic retinopathy, has also been described in association with other conditions. This and periphlebitis of the retinal vessels may be present in individuals with Buerger's and Raynaud's diseases or other types of peripheral vascular disease. Central angiospastic retinopathy has been described as a disease entity, probably of the autonomic nervous system. The attacks of spasm are accompanied by edema of the macula and by a marked disturbance of vision. The spasm may lead to ischemia and degeneration of the macular area. As the edema subsides, a mottled irregularity of pigmentation is noted in the region of the macula, frequently with discrete, punctate, yellowish spots around the fovea. The condition may progress to the development of a sharply outlined, punched-out hole in the macula. There may be a residual central scotoma. With temporal arteritis there may be visual defects due to ischemia of the optic nerve or retina. In patients with multiple sclerosis who have some visual impairment there may be increased blurring of vision immediately after exercise or with increased body temperature from any cause. Rucker has reported sheathing of the retinal veins with plaque formation and narrowing of the lumen in about 10% of patients with multiple sclerosis.

Other Retinal Disorders and Associated Findings

Congenital defects of the retina may occur especially in albinism. In Tay – Sachs disease and some related disturbances there is atrophy with lipid infiltration of the retinal ganglion cells, and the normal choroid at the macula stands out as a distinct red spot in contrast to the pale retina; there is also optic atrophy. In some late infantile and juvenile varieties of gangliosidosis there is a pigmentary degeneration of the retina, with deposits of black pigments in the periphery of the fundus and atrophy of the disk and retina. Pigmentary degeneration of the retina need not necessarily be associated with progressive intellectual deterioation, but it is often associated with other congenital anomalies such as deafness, mental deficiency, etc., and is part of the **Laurence – Moon – Biedl syndrome** which consists of retinitis pigmentosa, adiposogenital dystrophy, polydactyly, skull defects, and retardation (Fig. 10-27). Other degenerations of the

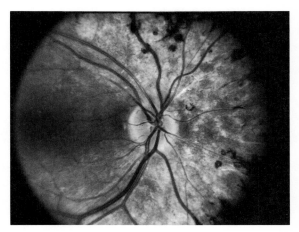

FIG. 10–27. Pigmentary degeneration of retina. (Courtesy of Richard A. Lewis)

retina include macular degeneration, colloidal changes, and fatty deposits. In tuberous sclerosis there may be retinal tumescences of glial or vascular origin that are called phakomas. In neurofibromatosis glial elevations may appear on the disk or retina. Choroiditis, especially in the macular area, is significant in the diagnosis of toxoplasmosis, often associated with human immunodeficiency virus syndrome.

Inflammatory changes are rarely limited to the retina, but are associated with disease of the choroid, **chorioretinitis,** or of the optic nerve, **neuroretinitis.** Syphilitic neuroretinitis and chorioretinitis are characterized by choroidal changes, pigment deposits, degenerative changes in the blood vessels, and areas of atrophy in the retina. In miliary tuberculosis retinal tubercles may appear. In exudative retinopathy (Coats' disease) there are areas of cicatricial tissue, the result of hemorrhages in the deep layers of the retina. Retinal vasculitis (Eales' disease) is a condition marked by recurrent hemorrhages into the retina and vitreous. In nephritis and diabetes there are characteristic changes that result in the so-called albuminuric and diabetic neuroretinitides, with tortuosity of the vessels, hyperemia and edema of the retina (especially in the macular area), microaneurysms, flame-shaped hemorrhages, exudation, redness of the disk with striation of its margins, and at times elevation of the disk. The changes are similar to those occurring in hypertensive retinopathy.

In anemia there may be pallor or even ischemia. Distention of the retinal vessels and cyanosis with hemorrhages are present in polycythemia and congenital heart disease. Dilation and tortuosity of the vessels, with numerous hemorrhages, are common in leukemia. In systemic vascular diseases there may be retinal changes, with distention of the vessels or embolic or thrombotic phenomena. Angiomatosis of the retina, von Hippel's disease, is frequently accompanied by a hemangioblastoma of the cerebellum (von Hippel–Lindau disease). There are, of course, numerous ocular and intraocular conditions, among the more important of which are glaucoma, separation of the retina, retinal and orbital tumors, and various congenital and traumatic eye conditions, all of which can be differentiated from neurologic disease largely by ophthalmoscopy.

SUBJECTIVE ANOMALIES OF VISION

In a complete discussion of the optic nerve one should also mention subjective anomalies of vision. Subjective scotomas, such as the scintillat-

ing scotomas of migraine, have already been referred to. In migraine there may also be photophobia, blurring of vision, and transient hemianopias that cannot be confirmed objectively. Simple visual hallucinations may arise from any portion of the visual pathway. They may be benign (phosphenes of advancing age, of ocular origin) or imply organic disease. Visual hallucinations and metamorphopsias (distortions of vision) occur in psychotic states and may constitute the aura of an epileptic attack, especially if the epileptogenic focus is in the visual cortex or temporal lobe. In lesions of the striate cortex the hallucinations are vague and unformed, but with involvement of the parastriate or peristriate cortex or temporal lobe there may be formed hallucinations or visual illusions. In the psychoses, toxic states, and delirium, formed visual hallucinations are common. Hallucinations of animals are often a part of delirium tremens or other withdrawal states. In epilepsy and in certain neurotic states there may be perversions of vision such as **macropsia** or **micropsia,** conditions in which objects seem larger or smaller than they really are. **Autoscopy,** the hallucination of seeing oneself, may be an epileptic phenomenon. Diplopia is caused by dysfunction of the ocular nerves, although monocular diplopia may occur. Its causes are usually retinal. **Aniseikonia** is a condition in which the ocular image of an object as seen by one eye differs in size and shape from that seen by the other; **metamorphopsia** is a distortion of objects seen. The visual aphasias and agnosias are discussed in "Aphasia, Agnosia, and Apraxia" (Ch. 52).

LOCALIZATION OF DISORDERS OF VISUAL FUNCTION

Disturbances of vision may result from disease processes in the eye, anywhere along the course of the optic nerve, at the optic chiasm, along the optic tract or radiations, or in the visual cortex. Disease of the retina may cause visual difficulty owing to involvement of the peripheral neurons, the rods and cones. In retinitis, chorioretinitis, vascular disease, hemorrhages, exudation, and separation of the retina there may be patchy or complete loss of vision in the involved eye, especially if the disease process is in the region of the macula.

Diseases of the optic nerve due to optic atrophy, degenerative conditions, optic or retrobulbar neuritis, infection, neoplasm, toxins, trauma, pressure, or vascular insufficiency may cause unilateral loss of vision progressing from a central scotoma or a partial field defect to complete blindness. If there is total loss of vision in one eye because of optic nerve disease, the direct light reflex is lost in this eye, but its consensual reflex is retained (see "Reflexes," under "The Pupils" in Ch. 11). If the lesion is immediately anterior to the chiasm, there may be a minimal defect in the opposite eye, especially in the upper temporal quadrant, as well as blindness of the eye involved.

A lesion at the optic chiasm may bring about a loss of acuity progressing to blindness. If the lesion is at the center of the chiasm, there is a bitemporal field defect, usually with loss of the upper quadrants before the lower quadrants; this may progress to optic atrophy. A lesion at one side of the chiasm causes a unilateral nasal hemianopic defect, while lesions at both sides of the chiasm produce bilateral nasal defects. Adenomas of the pituitary gland, craniopharyngiomas, meningiomas arising from the tuberculum sellae, and third ventricle tumors may cause defects in vision due to chiasmatic involvement. The visual changes may vary from unilateral or bilateral concentric contraction to sectoral, quadrantic, altitudinal, or hemianopic defects, or to complete blindness. Occasionally an homonymous hemianopia occurs with pituitary or parasellar lesions.

Involvement of the optic tract from the chiasm to the lateral geniculate body results in a contralateral hemianopic defect, with loss of the light reflex when a pencil of light is focused on the blind portion of the retina. Lesions of the geniculate body or of the optic radiations from the geniculate body to the cortex of the occipital lobe produce a hemianopic defect involving the contralateral fields, without loss of the light reflex when the light is focused on the blind portion of the retina. If the radiations through the temporal lobe, especially in their lower portion, are more affected, the upper quadrants of vision will be more involved, and if those subserving the upper portions of the retina are more affected, the lower quadrants of vision will be more involved. Lesions at these sites may be associated with intracranial neoplasms, abscesses, or granulomas, or may be caused by subdural hematomas or vascular involvement. The field defect appearing with tumors may be due either to direct involvement of the radiations or to interference with the blood supply. The anterior part of the optic tract is supplied by many branches from the arterial circle of Willis, and is not apt to be involved in vascular disease. The posterior part of the tract and the anterior part of

the radiations, especially the lower fibers, are supplied by the anterior choroidal artery. The middle cerebral artery supplies the middle portion of the radiations, and the middle cerebral and the calcarine branch of the posterior cerebral artery supply the posterior portion of the radiations. The geniculate bodies are supplied by the anterior choroidal artery and by the thalamogeniculate branches of the posterior cerebral. The striate cortex is supplied by the calcarine branch of the posterior cerebral and by other cortical branches of the posterior cerebral as well as cortical branches of the middle cerebral. Hemorrhage, thrombosis, embolism, spasm, or sclerosis of the arteries may cause visual changes.

Lesions of one occipital lobe will cause a contralateral hemianopic defect. If the involvement is localized to the cuneus or the upper lip of the calcarine fissure, there is a lower quadrantanopia, and if it is limited to the lingual gyrus or the lower lip of the calcarine fissure, there is an upper quadrantanopia. A lesion at the occipital pole will mainly affect central vision; focal lesions of the occipital lobes may produce localized loss of central vision. Occasionally sparing of the macula is seen in hemianopias associated with involvement of the posterior portion of the occipital lobe. Lesions slightly peripheral to the striate cortex may cause difficulty with fixation and with maintaining visual attention, loss of following and reflex ocular movements, loss of stereoscopic vision, impairment of visual memory and recall, difficulty in accurate discernment or localization of objects, disturbances in the spatial orientation of the visual image in the homonymous field, and loss of ability to discriminate with respect to size, shape, and color. There may be errors in the patient's ability to localize himself or stationary or moving objects in space, with a loss of visual perception of motion and of spatial relationships (**visual spatial agnosia**). **Simultagnosia** is the ability to perceive only one object at a time, or specific details but not a picture in its entirety. In the Charcot – Wilbrand syndrome there is loss of ability to recall visual images and to draw or construct from memory (Ch. 52). With bilateral lesions of the striate cortex there may be either marked loss of visual orientation or cortical blindness, often with anosognosia, or denial of blindness (**Anton's syndrome**). Lesions farther forward, in the region of the angular or supramarginal gyri, may cause other disturbances of visual perception, recognition, and comprehension. If they are in the dominant hemisphere they cause alexia (word blindness) or visual receptive aphasia. Such lesions may be neoplastic, vascular, or traumatic in origin. Stimulation or irritation of the calcarine cortex produces unformed visual hallucinations, such as flashes of light, in the corresponding field of vision, and irritation of the surrounding areas may cause formed visual hallucinations.

Psychogenic disturbances of vision may be of various types. There may be photophobia, blurring of vision, ocular fatigue, polyopia, monocular diplopia, tubular or spiral field defects, amblyopia, or blindness. **Asthenopia** is a weakness or fatigability of the visual organs. Field changes like those occurring in hysteria have been reported in patients with frontal lobe tumors.

BIBLIOGRAPHY

Adler FH. Physiology of the Eye: Clinical Application, 3rd ed. St. Louis, CV Mosby, 1959

Behrman S. Pathology of papilledema. Neurology 1964; 14:236

Bender MB, Rudolph SH, Stacy CB. The neurology of the visual and oculomotor systems. In Joynt RJ (ed). Clinical Neurology. Philadelphia, JB Lippincott, 1989

Berk MM. A critical evaluation of color perimetry. Arch Ophthalmol 1960;63:966

Breslin DJ, Gifford RW Jr, Fairbairn JF II et al. Prognostic importance of ophthalmoscopic findings in essential hypertension. JAMA 1966;195:335

Brickner RM, Franklin CR. Visible retinal arteriolar spasm in multiple sclerosis. Trans Am Neurol Assoc 1944;70:74

Brodal A. Neurological Anatomy in Relation to Clinical Medicine, 3rd ed. New York, Oxford University Press, 1981

Brodal A. The Cranial Nerves: Anatomy and Anatomico-clinical Correlations. Springfield, IL, Charles C Thomas, 1959

Cogan DG. Neurology of the Visual System. Springfield, IL, Charles C Thomas, 1966

Devinski O, Feldman E, Burrowes K et al. Autoscopic phenomena with seizures. Arch Neurol 1989;46:1080

Duke – Elder WS, Scott GJ. System of Ophthalmology: Neuro-ophthalmology. St. Louis, CV Mosby, 1971

Ellenberger C Jr. Modern perimetry in neuro-ophthalmic diagnosis. Arch Neurol 1974;30:193

Gans JA. The automation of visual fields. Trans Sect Ophthalmol Am Med Assoc 1962;34

Glaser JS. Neuro-ophthalmology. Hagerstown, Harper & Row, 1978

Glew WB. The pathogenesis of papilledema in intracranial disease: A review of some of the literature. Am J Med Sci 1960;239:221

Harrington DO. The Visual Fields: A Textbook and Atlas of Clinical Perimetry, 4th ed. St. Louis, CV Mosby, 1976

Hollenhorst RW. Neuro-ophthalmologic examination of children. Neurology 1956;6:739

Hollenhorst RW. Significance of bright plaques in the retinal arteries. JAMA 1961;178:23

Hoyt WF, Beeston D. The Ocular Fundus in Neurologic Disease. St. Louis, CV Mosby, 1966

Hoyt WF, Pont ME. Pseudopapilledema: Anomalous elevation of the optic disk. JAMA 1962;181:191

Hughes R. The Visual Fields. Oxford, Blackwell Scientific, 1954

Kahn EA, Cherry GR. The clinical importance of spontaneous retinal venous pulsations. Univ Mich Med Bull 1950;16:305

Kestenbaum A. Clinical Methods of Neuro-ophthalmologic Examination, 2nd ed. New York, Grune & Stratton, 1961

Larsen HW. Atlas of the Fundus of the Eye. Copenhagen, Munsgaard, 1964

Loder LL. Fundus and visual field changes accompanying lesions of the optic chiasm. Univ Mich Med Bull 1940;6:2

Macaraeg PVJ, Lasagna L, Snyder B. Arcus not so senilis. Ann Intern Med 1968;68:345

Miles PW. Testing visual fields by flicker fusion. Arch Neurol Psychiatry 1951;65:39

Miller NR. Walsh and Hoyt's Clinical Neuro-ophthalmology, 4th ed. Baltimore, Williams & Wilkins, 1988

Miller SJH, Sanders MD, Ffytche TJ. Fluorescein fundus photography in the detection of early papilledema and its differentiation from pseudo-papilledema. Lancet 1965; 2:651

Newman N, Kline LB, Leifer D et al. Ocular stroke and carotid artery dissection. Neurology 1989;39:1462

Petrohelos MA, Henderson JW. The ocular findings in intracranial tumors: A study of 358 cases. Am J Ophthalmol 1951;34:1387

Polyak SL. The Retina. Chicago, University of Chicago Press, 1941

Polyak SL. The Vertebrate Visual System. Chicago, University of Chicago Press, 1957

Reed H. The Essentials of Perimetry. London, Oxford University Press, 1960

Rucker CW. Sheathing of the retinal veins in multiple sclerosis. JAMA 1945;127:970

Smith JL (ed). The University of Miami Neuro-ophthalmology Symposium. Springfield, IL, Charles C Thomas, 1964

Smith JL, Susac JL. Unilateral arcus senilis: Sign of occlusive disease of the carotid artery. JAMA 1973;226:676

Traquair HM. An Introduction to Clinical Perimetry, 6th ed. London, Henry Kimpton, 1949

Uzman LL, Jakus MA. The Kayser – Fleischer ring: A histochemical and electron microscope study. Neurology 1957;7:341

Wagener HP, Keith NM. Diffuse arteriolar disease with hypertension and associated retinal lesions. Medicine 1939;18:317

Zuckerman J. Perimetry. Philadelphia, JB Lippincott, 1954

Since the oculomotor, trochlear, and abducens nerves all function in regulation of the eye movements, they are here referred to as the ocular nerves and are examined together. The cervical portion of the sympathetic (thoracolumbar) division of the autonomic nervous system functions with the third nerve in the innervation of the eyelid and of the pupil and, consequently, it also will be considered in the appraisal of the ocular nerves.

ANATOMY AND PHYSIOLOGY

The Oculomotor Nerve

The oculomotor, or third cranial, nerve nuclei of origin are in the mesencephalon, or midbrain. These nuclear centers are situated in the periaqueductal gray matter just anterior to the aqueduct of Sylvius, at the level of the superior colliculi (anterior quadrigeminal bodies). There are two, possibly more, separate nuclear groups (Fig. 11-1). The paired **lateral nuclei** are the largest, and are situated anterior and lateral to the others; their median portions are fused into an unpaired mass. These contain large cells, the neuraxes of which supply the superior rectus, inferior rectus, medial rectus, inferior oblique, and levator palpebrae superioris muscles. The cells supplying the inferior oblique and the medial and inferior rectus muscles are all in the ipsilateral oculomotor nucleus; the fibers to the superior rectus arise only contralaterally, while the levator palpebrae superioris receives fibers from both sides.

Convergence movements of the eyes are innervated by fibers originating in neurons for the medial rectus muscles. A so-called center for convergence ("Perlia's nucleus") has not been confirmed.

Posterior to the lateral nuclei, or somewhat between them at their rostral and dorsal extremities, are the **Edinger – Westphal** nuclei, which are made up of smaller cells and are a part of the craniosacral, or parasympathetic, division of the autonomic nervous system. There is a paired rostral portion and an unpaired medial and caudal portion that is sometimes called the **anteromedial nucleus.** Preganglionic fibers from these nuclei go to the ciliary ganglion. Postganglionic fibers related to cells in the rostral part of the nucleus supply the sphincter, or constrictor, of the pupil, and those related to the anteromedial nucleus supply the ciliary muscle and function in accommodation.

The fibers from these various nuclei course anteriorly through the mesencephalon, traversing the medial portion of the red nucleus, the substantia nigra, and the cerebral peduncle. They exit from the anterior surface of the midbrain. Shortly after leaving the brain stem these filaments are united to form the third nerve on each side. This nerve emerges just above the pons, between the superior cerebellar and the posterior cerebral arteries (see Fig. 9-3). It penetrates the dura just lateral and anterior to the posterior clinoid processes and enters the cavernous sinus, where it lies in the upper aspect, close to the lateral wall (Fig. 11-2). Here it is medial to the temporal lobe of the brain and lateral to the carotid artery. It enters the orbit through

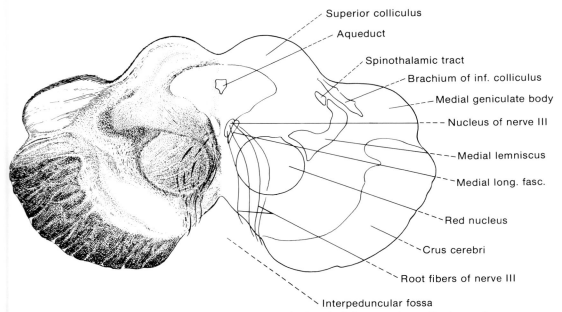

Superior colliculus

Aqueduct

Spinothalamic tract

Brachium of inf. colliculus

Medial geniculate body

Nucleus of nerve III

Medial lemniscus

Medial long. fasc.

Red nucleus

Crus cerebri

Root fibers of nerve III

Interpeduncular fossa

FIG. 11–1. *Section through the mesencephalon at the level of the superior colliculus and oculomotor nucleus.*

the superior orbital fissure, where it separates into superior and inferior divisions. The former supplies the levator palpebrae superioris and superior rectus muscles. The latter supplies the medial and inferior rectus and the inferior oblique muscles. It also sends a short root to the ciliary ganglion, from which postganglionic fibers go as the short ciliary nerves to supply the ciliary muscle and the sphincter pupillae (Fig. 11-3).

The superior, medial and inferior recti and the inferior oblique are extraocular muscles innervated by the oculomotor nerve. The superior rectus elevates the eyeball, especially if it is in abduction, and adducts it to a certain extent; it turns the eyeball upward and inward and rotates the adducted globe so that the upper end of the vertical axis is inward. The medial, or internal, rectus is an adductor of the eyeball. The inferior rectus depresses the eyeball, especially if it is in abduction, and adducts it to a certain extent; it turns the eyeball downward and inward and rotates the adducted globe so that the upper end of the vertical axis is outward. The inferior oblique elevates the eye, especially if it is in adduction, and abducts the eyeball; it turns the eye upward and outward and rotates the abducted globe so that the upper end of the vertical axis is outward (Fig. 11-4).

The levator palpebrae superioris supplies the striated musculature of the eyelid, which it ele-

vates. Not all of the striated musculature of the eyelid, however, is innervated by the levator; some is supplied by the orbicularis oculi, with which the fibers of the levator are closely intermingled. The sphincter pupillae causes constriction of the pupil. Contraction of the ciliary muscle causes relaxation of the ciliary zonule and decrease in the tension of the lens capsule, followed by an increase in the convexity of the lens to adjust the eye for near vision. This change in the shape of the lens is accompanied by convergence of the eye and constriction of the pupil.

A complete paralysis of the third nerve results in ptosis, or drooping of the upper eyelid, paralysis of medial and upward gaze, paresis of downward gaze, and dilation of the pupil (Fig. 11-5). A patient so afflicted is unable to raise his eyelid, and he is unable to turn the eyeball medially, directly downward, or laterally and upward. The eyeball is deviated laterally and somewhat downward; it can be moved still farther laterally owing to the function of the lateral rectus, and downward and laterally owing to the function of the superior oblique, but in no other directions. The completely dilated pupil does not react to light or in accommodation. The power to vary the curvature of the lens for near and distance vision is lost. It is stated that the third nerve may also send some fibers to the orbicu-

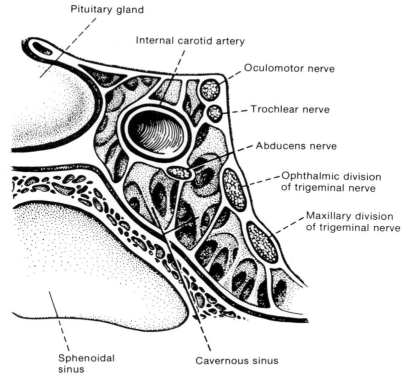

Pituitary gland

Internal carotid artery

Oculomotor nerve

Trochlear nerve

Abducens nerve

Ophthalmic division
of trigeminal nerve

Maxillary division
of trigeminal nerve

Sphenoidal
sinus

Cavernous sinus

FIG. 11–2. Oblique section through the cavernous sinus.

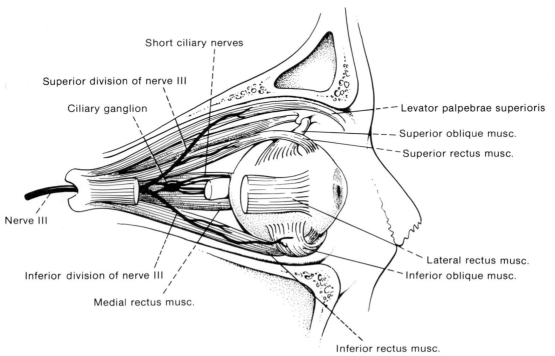

Short ciliary nerves

Superior division of nerve III

Ciliary ganglion

Levator palpebrae superioris

Superior oblique musc.

Superior rectus musc.

Nerve III

Inferior division of nerve III

Medial rectus musc.

Lateral rectus musc.

Inferior oblique musc.

Inferior rectus musc.

FIG. 11–3. The extraocular muscles and the third nerve in the orbit.

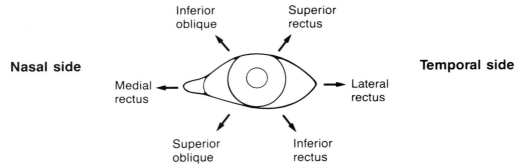

FIG. 11-4. Actions of the extraocular muscles on the left eye. Arrows denote the main directions of action for each muscle, resulting from a combination of movements of the globe in the three dimensions.

laris oculi, and as a result some weakness of this muscle may be seen in third nerve lesions.

A third nerve paralysis need not be complete: there may be paresis rather than paralysis of function, and only certain functions may be involved whereas others remain intact. If the lesion which causes dysfunction of the nerve is within the midbrain, where the nuclear centers and their neuraxes are still separated, or within the orbit after the nerve has redivided, only certain portions or functions may be involved. If, however, the lesion is along the course of the nerve between its emergence from the midbrain and its division within the orbit, there is apt to be

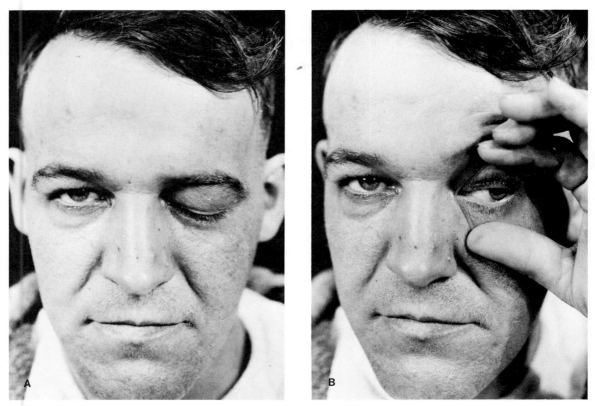

FIG. 11-5. Paralysis of the left oculomotor nerve in a patient with an aneurysm of the left internal carotid artery. **A.** Only ptosis can be seen. **B.** On elevating the eyelid it is seen that the pupil is dilated and the eyeball is deviated laterally.

paralysis of all functions. Paralysis of only the sphincter pupillae and ciliary muscle is called **internal ophthalmoplegia;** paralysis of only the extraocular muscles is called **external ophthalmoplegia;** paralysis of both is called **complete ophthalmoplegia.**

The Trochlear Nerve

The trochlear, or fourth cranial, nerve is the smallest of the cranial nerves. Its nuclei are situated just anterior to the aqueduct in the gray matter of the lower mesencephalon immediately above the pons (Fig. 11-6). They extend from the level of the lowest part of the anterior quadrigeminal bodies to the lower pole of the posterior quadrigeminal bodies and are immediately caudal to the lateral nucleus of the third nerve, but separated from it by a short distance. The fibers of the trochlear nerve curve posteriorly and caudally around the aqueduct and decussate in the anterior medullary velum. It is the only cranial nerve whose fibers emerge from the posterior aspect of the brain stem. The nerve then circles around the pons, the brachium conjunctivum, and the cerebral peduncle. It penetrates the dura just behind and lateral to the posterior clinoid processes, goes through the cavernous sinus, where it is lateral and inferior to the third nerve, and enters the orbit through the superior orbital fissure. It terminates on the superior oblique muscle on the side opposite to the nucleus of origin. This muscle depresses the eye, especially if it is in adduction, abducts the eyeball, and rotates the abducted globe so that the upper end of the vertical axis is inward. In paralysis of the fourth nerve these functions are lost. In a nuclear lesion of the fourth nerve, the contralateral superior oblique muscle is paralyzed, but in a lesion along the course of the nerve, after its decussation, the ipsilateral muscle is involved.

The Abducens Nerve

The abducens, or sixth cranial, nerve arises in the gray matter anterior to the fourth ventricle in the dorsal part of the tegmentum of the lower

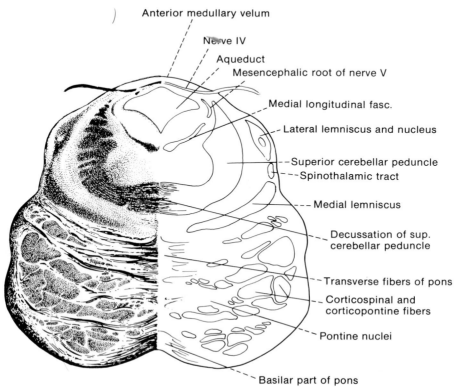

Anterior medullary velum

Nerve IV

Aqueduct

Mesencephalic root of nerve V

Medial longitudinal fasc.

Lateral lemniscus and nucleus

Superior cerebellar peduncle

Spinothalamic tract

Medial lemniscus

Decussation of sup. cerebellar peduncle

Transverse fibers of pons

Corticospinal and corticopontine fibers

Pontine nuclei

Basilar part of pons

FIG. 11–6. Section through the mesencephalon at the border of the pons, showing the trochlear nucleus and nerve.

pons (Fig. 11-7). The nucleus is situated just posterior to the nucleus of the facial nerve but within its looping fibers. The neuraxes of the sixth nerve leave the pons medially to those of the facial nerve (see Fig. 9-3). They emerge from the brain stem as a single nerve at the junction between the pons and the medulla, and as they emerge they cross the internal auditory artery (the posterior branch of the basilar artery). The sixth nerve has the longest intracranial course of all the cranial nerves. It passes anteriorly, lying between the pons and the anterior clivus; it finally pierces the dura at the dorsum sellae, where it lies between the posterior clinoid process and the apex of the petrous bone, in close relationship to the gasserian ganglion. In the cavernous sinus it is below and medial to the third nerve and lateral to the internal carotid artery. It also enters the orbit through the superior orbital fissure, and supplies a single muscle, the lateral, or external, rectus, which functions to abduct the eyeball, or deviate it laterally. When a lesion of the sixth nerve occurs, the eyeball is turned medially, and it cannot be moved laterally (Fig. 11-8). Because of its long intracranial course, this nerve is more frequently involved in disease processes than are the other cranial nerves, and an increase in intracranial pressure or exudate from inflammatory processes or hemorrhage may cause it to be pressed between the pons and the clivus and thus may interrupt its continuity. In such circumstances the sixth nerve involvement may be bilateral.

There are small groups of cells lying close to the motor cells of the abducens nucleus, which are sometimes termed the **parabducens nucleus,** and from which impulses are relayed through the medial longitudinal fasciculus to the oculomotor nucleus. The connection coordinates the contraction of the lateral rectus of one eye with the medial rectus of the other, so that both eyes move together in the same horizontal plane (**conjugate deviation**) toward the side of the contracting lateral rectus. The parabducens nucleus is also called the internuclear portion of the abducens nucleus.

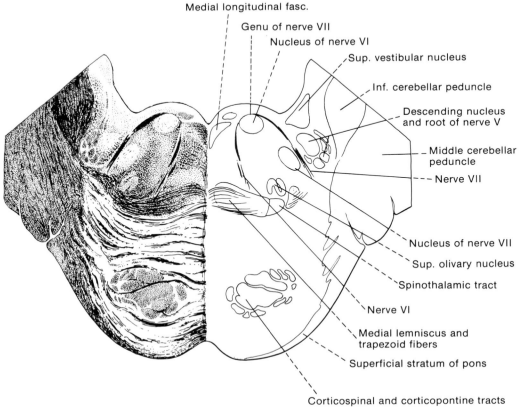

FIG. 11-7. *Section through the pons showing fibers of the abducens and facial nerves.*

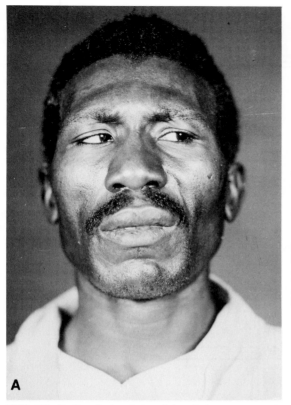 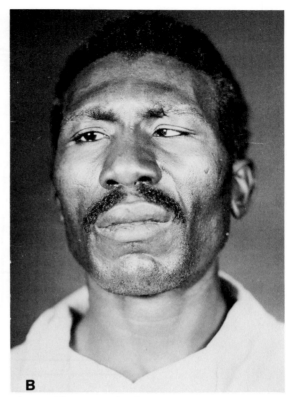

A   B

FIG. 11–8. Paralysis of the right abducens nerve in a patient with a posterior fossa neoplasm. **A.** Patient looking to left. **B.** Patient attempting to look in the direction of action of the paralyzed muscle.

The Medial Longitudinal Fasciculus

The oculomotor, trochlear, and abducens nuclei are situated one below the other in a more or less columnar arrangement in the brain stem. They are united for coordinated and conjugate action by the medial longitudinal fasciculus, which also connects them with the nuclei of the vestibular and cochlear portions of the eighth nerve, the trigeminal and facial nerves, the spinal accessory nerve, the hypoglossal nerve, the motor nuclei of the upper cervical nerves, the nucleus of the posterior commissure (nucleus of Darkshevich), and the nucleus of the medial longitudinal fasciculus (interstitial nucleus of Cajal), as well as with higher centers (Fig. 11-9). Owing to the function of this correlating mechanism, no isolated action of any eye muscle is ever possible, and movements of one eye are correlated with those of the other. Also, through the action of this fiber tract, head and even body movements are correlated with eye movements. Thus, in re-

sponse to visual, auditory, sensory, vestibular, and other stimuli, normal conjugate deviation of the eyes and the head occurs. This pathway has important functions in auditory-ocular reflexes, vestibular-ocular reflexes, and righting reflexes.

Sympathetic Innervation

The cervical portion of the sympathetic (thoracolumbar) division of the autonomic nervous system has its origin in the intermediolateral group of cells of the spinal cord extending from the eighth cervical or first thoracic segment through the upper four, five, or six thoracic segments. Those fibers which control oculopupillary action probably arise from the eighth cervical and the first and second thoracic segments (ciliospinal center). The preganglionic fibers go to the inferior, middle, and superior sympathetic ganglia in the neck. The postganglionic fibers follow the course of the internal ca-

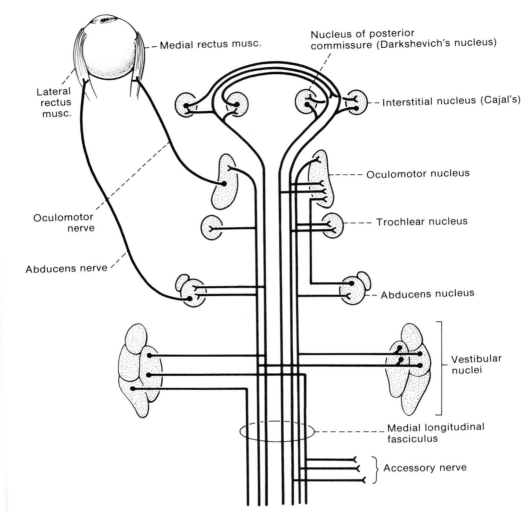

FIG. 11-9. *The medial longitudinal fasciculus.*

rotid artery into the head to the cavernous sympathetic plexus and then travel with the ophthalmic division of the fifth nerve into the orbit (Fig. 11-10). The sympathetic division supplies the sympathetic root of the ciliary ganglion, carried through the long ciliary nerves; fibers may pass without interruption through the ciliary ganglion into the short ciliary nerves. The cervical sympathetic nerves innervate the dilator of the pupil and also supply the tarsal muscles and the orbital muscle of Müller. The former are smooth muscle sheets in the upper and lower eyelids; the latter is a structure which, in the lower forms at least, keeps the globe of the eye forward in the orbit.

Paralysis of the cervical portion of the sympathetic division causes a **Horner's syndrome.**

This is characterized by miosis resulting from paralysis of the dilator of the pupil, a partial or pseudoptosis owing to paralysis of the upper tarsal muscle, enophthalmos owing to paralysis of the muscle of Müller, and often a slight elevation of the lower lid because of paralysis of the lower tarsal muscle (Fig. 11-11). In man the enophthalmos may be apparent rather than real. In addition, in a complete Horner's syndrome, there is ipsilateral dilation of the vessels of the face, head, neck, conjunctiva, and arm, with ipsilateral anhidrosis. There may be ocular hypotony with an acute Horner's syndrome, and heterochromia of the irises and atrophy of the side of the face if the defect dates from birth or is of long duration. Although there may be decreased sensitivity to atropine, this drug will usually di-

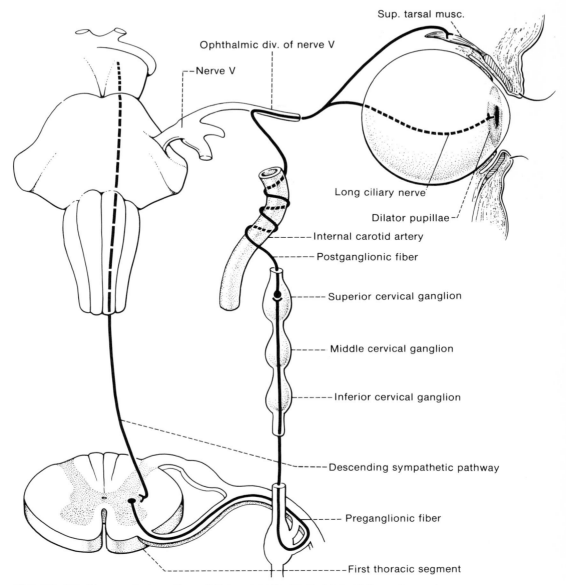

FIG. 11–10. *The cervical portion of the sympathetic division of the autonomic nervous system.*

late the pupil in Horner's syndrome, owing to its action in paralyzing the sphincter of the pupil, but cocaine, which stimulates the sympathetic endings, will not act as a mydriatic, and the ciliospinal reflex is lost. There may be hypersensitivity to epinephrine, especially if the lesion is a postganglionic one. Horner's syndrome may be the result of 1) the interruption of the descending ipsilateral sympathetic pathways in the brain stem or spinal cord; 2) lesions either in the cord at the level of the ciliospinal center or of the preganglionic fibers as or after they leave the cord; 3) injury to the cervical sympathetic ganglia; or 4) involvement of the postganglionic fibers.

Cortical Control

The principal cortical center for the regulation of the ocular nerves is situated in the posterior portion of the second and third frontal convolu-

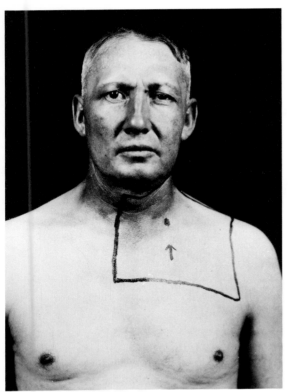

FIG. 11–11. Left Horner's syndrome in a patient with a pulmonary sulcus tumor.

tions, just anterior to the precentral fissure (area 8 of Brodmann) (Fig. 11-12). The impulses go through the corona radiata, internal capsule, and the cerebral peduncle, and then descend with the aberrant pyramidal fibers. They terminate in the centers for lateral gaze in the lower pons, which include the paramedian pontine reticular formation, the abducens nuclei (and parabducens), parts of the vestibular nuclei, and pathways connecting the ocular motor nuclei. There is almost complete decussation in the lower midbrain, and the cortical center of one hemisphere supplies the opposite ocular nuclei. This frontal center is concerned with volitional control of conjugate ocular movements, and stimulation of it causes a rapid deviation of the eyes to the opposite side, which may be accompanied by conjugate movement of the head. If the lower portion of this area is stimulated, the eyes are deviated upward as well as laterally, and if the upper portion is stimulated, the eyes are turned downward and laterally. Destruction or ablation of this area is followed by paralysis of conjugate gaze to the opposite side with turning of the eyes toward the involved side. This center may also have a regulatory effect over the levator palpebrae superioris, and when it is stimulated opening of the eyelids may accompany conjugate movements of the eyes.

The zone immediately surrounding the area striata, corresponding to areas 18 and 19 of Brodmann, especially the latter, is the cortical center for optically induced eye movements and optic fixation reflexes. Corticofugal fibers from this center pass through the optic radiations in the posterior limb of the internal capsule to the cerebral peduncle, and then follow the same course as those from the frontal lobes. Stimulation of this center also produces deviation of the eyes to the opposite side, but the movements are slower and less forceful; ablation is followed by loss of following movements and optic fixation reflexes, with retention of voluntary control. It is a reflex center rather than a volitional center, and is important in fixation and in maintaining visual attention. Stimulation of the dorsal part of area 19 or the ventral part of area 18 results in upward conjugate deviation of the eyes, and stimulation of the ventral part of area 19 or the dorsal part of area 18 causes downward conjugate movement. There are association pathways from the occipital to the frontal cortical areas, with radiation of some impulses to the frontal cortex before they descend into the brain stem. Still other centers for ocular movement have been described in the angular gyrus and temporal lobe (Ch. 49). Cortical areas for ocular deviation may also function in eye-centering, as may areas in the diencephalon, brain stem, and cerebellum. A center for lateral conjugate gaze is located near the abducens nucleus in the pons, whereas the vertical conjugate gaze center is felt to be in the pretectal midbrain tegmentum and the region of the posterior commissure. Convergence is controlled by neurons to the medial rectus muscles. The basal ganglia and the vestibular complex also play important parts in the regulation of ocular movements.

Cortical centers that control pupillary responses have also been described. Dilator impulses originating in the hypothalamus are conveyed to the frontal cortex, probably also to area 8, from which they descend to the ciliospinal center at the eighth cervical and upper thoracic segments of the spinal cord, where they synapse with the cells of the intermediolateral column. Stimulation of area 8 causes pupillary dilation. Pupilloconstrictor fibers may descend from the peristriate area to the Edinger–Westphal nucleus; stimulation of area 19 has

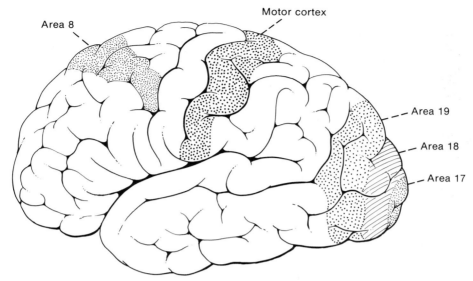

FIG. 11–12. Cortical centers related to vision and ocular movement.

been observed to produce pupillary constriction. The pupillodilator fibers and the afferent pathways that carry light reflex impulses from the retina are in close proximity in the midbrain.

CLINICAL EXAMINATION OF THE OCULAR NERVES AND THE CERVICAL SYMPATHETIC SYSTEM

In examining the functions of the oculomotor, trochlear, and abducens nerves, and the cervical sympathetic fibers to the intraocular structures, it is necessary to consider individually the pupils, the eyelids, the extraocular movements, and the position of the eyeball within the orbit.

The Pupils

The size, shape, equality, and position of the pupils, and their reflex responses, must be recorded. The pupils should be round, regular, centered in the iris, and equal, and should have specific reflex responses. Clinical observation is usually sufficient, and complicated procedures, such as pupillography, are used mainly for research.

Size. The size of the pupils varies greatly with the intensity of the surrounding illumination, but in lighting of average intensity they are usually 3 – 4 mm in diameter. The use of a small

ruler with holes varying from 1 – 9 mm in diameter aids in estimating their size (Fig. 11-13). The pupils are small and react poorly at birth and in early infancy. They are normally larger in young individuals, and some texts state that in moderate illumination the pupils of adolescents are about 4 mm in diameter and perfectly round. In middle age they are 3½ mm in diameter and regular, and in old age they are 3 mm or less in diameter and may be slightly irregular.

When the pupils are small (less than 2 mm in diameter) they are said to be **miotic.** They may be miotic in old age, atherosclerosis, syphilis, diabetes, and with levodopa therapy, and are sometimes so in hyperopia, occasionally in alcoholism, and frequently in drug intoxications, especially those associated with use of morphine or other opium derivatives. Miosis is also present in sleep, deep coma, increased intracranial pressure, and brain stem lesions with bilateral interruption of dilator fibers; the pupils may be pinpoint in size with acute pontine lesions. Miosis is present unilaterally with irritation of the third nerve or paralysis of the cervical portion of the sympathetic nervous system, and in association with corneal or intraocular foreign bodies. The pupils constrict slightly on expiration.

Dilation of the pupils (more than 5 mm in diameter) is called **mydriasis.** The pupils may be dilated in anxiety, fear, pain, hyperthyroidism, midbrain lesions, certain stages of coma and drug intoxication, cardiac arrest, and cerebral

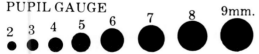

J. G. ROSENBAUM POCKET VISION SCREENER

95

874

2 8 4 3

	Point	Jaeger	distance equivalent
			$\frac{20}{800}$
			$\frac{20}{400}$
2 8 4 3	26	16	$\frac{20}{200}$
6 3 8 E Ш Ǝ X O O	14	10	$\frac{20}{100}$
8 7 4 5 Ǝ ṁ ш O X O	10	7	$\frac{20}{70}$
6 3 9 2 5 ṁ E Ǝ X O X	8	5	$\frac{20}{50}$
4 2 8 3 6 5 ш E ṁ o X o	6	3	$\frac{20}{40}$
3 7 4 2 5 8 Ǝ ш Ǝ x x o	5	2	$\frac{20}{30}$
9 3 7 8 2 6 ш ṁ E x o o	4	1	$\frac{20}{25}$
4 2 ṁ 7 3 9 E ш ṁ o o x	3	1+	$\frac{20}{20}$

Card is held in good light 14 inches from eye. Record vision for each eye separately with and without glasses. Presbyopic patients should read thru bifocal segment. Check myopes with glasses only.

PUPIL GAUGE

2   3   4   5   6   7   8   9mm.
● ● ● ● ● ● ● ●

FIG. 11–13. Reading card incorporating a gauge for estimating pupil size.

anoxia, after use of such drugs as atropine and belladonna, and sometimes in myopia. They also dilate with muscular activity, in response to loud noises, and in deep inspiration. Unilateral mydriasis accompanies paralysis of the third nerve, irritation of the cervical sympathetic nerves, and conditions in which there is a decrease in visual acuity or a reduction in the amount of light reaching the retina. On lateral movement of the eyes there may be slight dilation of the pupil of the abducting eye. Stimula-

tion of the hypothalamus or of the motor eye fields in the frontal lobe (see "Cortical Control") is followed by pupillary dilation. Persons with light irises have larger pupils than those with dark irises.

There is normally a certain amount of alternate fluctuation in the size of the pupil, designated as **pupillary unrest;** when this rhythmic contraction and dilation of the pupils is present to an excessive degree, it is called **hippus.** Hippus has been said to be associated with respiratory rhythm, but probably in most cases is an evidence of imbalance of the sympathetic and parasympathetic divisions of the autonomic nervous system. It may be present during recovery from a third nerve paralysis and during drowsiness. It is occasionally encountered in organic disease of the central nervous system but usually is of no significance in either diagnosis or localization.

Shape. The shape or outline of the pupil is also important in neurologic diagnosis. Normally the pupil is round and is regular in outline. Any irregularity, abnormality in shape, notching, or serration may be significant. Gross abnormalities in shape are usually the result of ocular disease such as iritis or eye surgery. There may be anterior synechiae (adhesions to the lens), a congenital coloboma (a gap in the iris), or defects owing to trauma or a previous iridectomy. A slight change in shape, however, such as an oval pupil, slight irregularity in outline, serration of the border, or slight notching, may be significant in the diagnosis of neurologic disease.

Equality. Equality of the pupils is also an important criterion. Comparison of the size of the two pupils may have more significance than the observation of size alone. Gross inequality of the pupils is called **anisocoria.** There may be a slight difference in the size of the pupils in 15% – 20% of normal individuals, on a congenital basis, but if this is at all marked it is noteworthy. A difference in the size of the pupils may also be caused by errors of refraction and unequal illumination. The physiologic basis of an inequality can often be established by demonstrating parallel reflex reactions of the two pupils to all stimuli and to drugs such as atropine.

A sympathetic paralysis on one side will, of course, cause a smaller pupil on that side, and sympathetic stimulation will cause mydriasis. A third nerve paralysis produces dilation, and stimulation of the oculomotor nerve, contraction. Unequal pupils may be caused by iritis. Alternating anisocoria has been observed with various nervous system diseases. The pupil of an amblyopic or blind eye is often larger, and acuity of vision should be noted in evaluating the size and equality of the pupils. The pupillodilator fibers are in close proximity to the tympanic plexus in the inner ear, and there may be ipsilateral constriction of the pupil in inner ear disease.

Unequal pupils or unilateral dilation and fixation of one pupil are frequently seen after cerebral vascular accidents or in association with severe head trauma. The presence of a dilated and fixed pupil in a comatose individual may give presumptive localization of a lesion in the ipsilateral cerebral hemisphere. If the dilation is marked and the pupil is fixed, one may assume direct pressure on the third nerve, probably the result of herniation of the hippocampal gyrus through the incisura of the tentorium cerebelli, causing pressure on the third nerve as it crosses the body of the sphenoid bone. On the other hand, involvement of the descending pupillodilator fibers from the frontal area as they pass through the internal capsule may cause miosis on the opposite side rather than an ipsilateral mydriasis. In hemianopia secondary to optic tract involvement the ipsilateral pupil may be dilated.

Position. The position of the pupil may also be significant. The pupil is usually situated in the center of the iris. Eccentric pupils, or ectopia of the pupils, may be the result of trauma or iritis and need not be pathognomonic of neurologic disease; the phenomenon, however, should be noted because it may give some clue to the underlying process. Some individuals have bilaterally eccentric pupils.

The Pupillary Reflexes

The evaluation of the pupillary reflexes is one of the most important parts of the neurologic examination. It is to preserve these reflexes that the use of a mydriatic is avoided if possible in carrying out the fundus examination. The principal reflex responses are those to light, those in accommodation and convergence, and those to pain, but others are also important.

The Light Reflex. The normal pupil reacts promptly when light is focused on the homolateral retina, and dilates when the light is withdrawn—the **direct light reflex.** The afferent

pathway is through the optic nerve to the pretectal nuclei, thence to the Edinger–Westphal nucleus, and the efferent fibers are carried by the oculomotor nerve through the ciliary ganglion. As a result of the semidecussation of fibers, both in the optic chiasm and en route to the Edinger–Westphal nuclei, the contralateral as well as the homolateral pupil responds — the **crossed,** or **consensual, light reflex.** Thus in a third nerve lesion the direct and consensual light reflexes are absent on the involved side, owing to paralysis of the sphincter of the pupil, but the consensual and the direct reflexes remain in the opposite eye. A blind eye does not respond directly to light, nor does its mate respond consensually, but a blind eye does respond consensually if its third nerve is intact and if the other eye and its optic nerve are not involved. In paralysis of the sympathetic pathway the light response is diminished.

Each eye should be tested individually for both the direct and the consensual reflexes, and it should be noted whether the responses are prompt, sluggish, or absent. For most accurate testing a distant source of light should be used; if a bright light is focused directly into the eye, the accommodation–convergence response as well as the light reflex is brought into action. The light reflex is best tested if the examiner stands beside and somewhat above the patient, who is asked to gaze at a lighted window or at some other distant source of light. The examiner then places his hands in front of the patient's eyes in such a way as to cut off the source of light, yet a sufficient distance to enable him to see the size of each pupil. The hands are withdrawn alternately, and the light is allowed to focus on the retina; as the hand is withdrawn on each side, the response of the homolateral pupil (direct reflex) and that of the contralateral pupil (consensual reflex) are noted.

The reaction to light is a relative phenomenon. If an eye is subjected to light of a certain intensity after having been adapted to less intense light, the pupil contracts. This same intensity of light, however, causes dilation of the pupil in an eye previously adapted to light of greater intensity. A reflex response to darkness has also been described, but it is difficult to state whether this is a true reflex or a tonic dilation due to relaxation of the sphincter on withdrawal of the light stimulus.

An **Argyll Robertson pupil** is one which does not react to light, though it does react to accommodation. The retina is sensitive to light, but the pupil is fixed. This condition is also spoken of as

reflex iridoplegia. It has been said that the Argyll Robertson pupil is pathognomonic of syphilis of the central nervous system, but it has also been observed in multiple sclerosis, encephalitis, Lyme disease, sarcoidosis, diabetes, alcoholic encephalopathy, and syringobulbia; with neoplasms of the posterior portion of the third ventricle or the pineal body, and lesions at the level of the superior colliculus; and in senile and vascular conditions. The true Argyll Robertson pupil is said to be less than 3 mm in diameter, and to show little variation in size. Both the direct and the consensual reflexes are absent. There is an active reaction in accommodation for near objects, and the convergence response may be increased and sustained. Dilation in response to pain is diminished, psychic and sensory responses are diminished or absent, the pupil dilates poorly in response to atropine, and there may be associated atrophy of the iris. The condition is usually bilateral, although the pupils are not necessarily equal. Less diagnostic than the Argyll Robertson pupil but also significant are pupils with a sluggish reaction to light, a reaction to light through a small excursion, a paradoxical reaction in which there is dilation rather than contraction, or a contraction followed immediately by dilation.

Various sites have been suggested for the lesion which causes the Argyll Robertson pupil, but it is quite obvious that such a lesion must involve both the afferent pathways carrying light reflex fibers from the retina and the autonomic connections. If a single lesion is responsible, it must occur at the point where these fiber tracts converge. Transmission of light impulses through the optic nerve must be intact. It is believed by most investigators that the phenomenon results from an inflammatory or a degenerative lesion in the periaqueductal region at the level of the anterior quadrigeminal bodies just ventral to the posterior commissure. At this area the light reflex fibers from the pretectal nuclei, which semidecussate to supply both Edinger–Westphal nuclei, run close to the sympathetic pupillodilator fibers. A lesion at this site interrupts both 1) the pathway from the retina which goes to the pretectal area and then to the Edinger–Westphal nucleus and through the third nerve to the iris, and 2) the adjacent pathway of the sympathetic pupillodilator fibers that descent from the hypothalamus and frontal cortex through the midbrain to the oculopupillary center in the upper thoracic spinal cord, and then through the cervical sympathetic chain to the iris. The syndrome may be the result of a sin-

gle lesion near the anterior quadrigeminal bodies, such as a tumor of the pineal gland, or there may be bilateral or more widespread lesions. Reliable observers differ, however, in their opinions on the site of the lesion that causes the Argyll Robertson pupil; it has been variously placed.

In **Adie's syndrome** there is also an impaired pupillary reaction to light and a better response in accommodation and convergence. The light reaction, however, is not absent: there is slow constriction on prolonged exposure to a bright light, especially if the patient has been in a dark room, with a gradual dilation after the stimulus has been withdrawn. The accommodation response is also slow and may be incomplete. The abnormality is unilateral in about 80% of cases, and the tonic, or myotonic, pupil is dilated in average light. The iris is not atrophic. The response to miotic and mydriatic drugs in the usual concentrations is normal. The Adie's pupil, however, constricts rapidly after a few drops of either 2.5% methacholine or 0.1% pilocarpine are instilled in the conjunctival sac, while the normal pupil fails to respond in this way. The lesion causing Adie's syndrome is in the ciliary ganglion and the postganglionic fibers. Progressive anhidrosis may also occur in persons with Adie's syndrome; this is evidence to suggest that it may be part of a widespread autonomic disturbance or neuropathy. The response to the abovementioned drugs suggests the presence of denervation hypersensitivity, secondary to a lesion in the ciliary ganglion or peripheral to it.

Adie's syndrome is usually a benign disorder, occurring most frequently in young women. Because the muscle stretch reflexes are often absent, is has been referred to as tonic pupils with absent tendon reflexes, and at one time was said to be easily confused with central nervous system syphilis. The above description, however, shows that the pupillary abnormality is quite different from the Argyll Robertson pupil. Furthermore, it is not the impaired response to light that brings the disorder to clinical attention, but the unilaterally dilated pupil, which sometimes seems to have an abrupt onset. It is not an uncommon cause of anisocoria. Tonic (Adie's) pupil has also been described as part of giant cell arteritis.

After an oculomotor ophthalmoplegia the pupil may contract on convergence but not in response to light; this may simulate the Argyll Robertson pupil. Under such circumstances, however, it may be observed that the pupil also contracts with other movements of the eyeball and with movements of the eyelid. Consequently, this abnormality of pupillary response, sometimes noted after a head injury complicated by a third nerve involvement, has no etiologic relationship to the classic reaction described by Argyll Robertson, but is, rather, a synkinetic reaction.

Wernicke's hemianopic phenomenon, in which light focused on one half of the retina causes a pupillary response while light focused on the other half does not, is present in hemianopias in which the interruption of the pathways is anterior to the departure of the fibers to the pretectal region (see "Hemianopias," Ch. 10).

In retrobulbar neuritis there may be a partial dilation of the pupil, which may react to light but not hold the reaction, or, paradoxically, may dilate slowly (the **Marcus Gunn pupillary sign**); the consensual reflex may be more prompt than the direct one. These changes can be brought about by rapid alternate stimulation of the eyes with a bright light (the **"swinging flashlight" test**). Several pupillary changes may occur with diabetes mellitus, including reduced pupillary size, decreased miosis in continuous light, and reduced pupillary unrest, all presumably related to autonomic neuropathy.

The Accommodation Reflex. The accommodation reflex, or the **accommodation – convergence synkinesis,** is elicited by having the patient shift his gaze to some near object after he has relaxed his accommodation by gazing into the distance. This is followed by a thickening of the lens, convergence of the eyes, and constriction of the pupils. There are two principal theories in regard to the mechanism of accommodation. The most generally accepted theory is that the ciliary muscle reduces or relaxes the tension of the zonular muscle, and this permits the elastic capsule of the lens to shape the lens and to increase its convexity in order to adjust the eyes for near vision. Others believe that the force of the ciliary muscle, acting through the zonule, tightens the zonule, and the vitreous forcefully molds a relatively plastic lens into the accommodated form. Convergence is produced by the action of both medial rectus muscles. The constriction of the pupils is called a reflex response, but many observers believe that the decrease in size of the pupils on accommodation and convergence is not a reflex in the ordinary sense of the term, but part of a synkinesis, or associated movement. The response depends upon the conduction of afferent impulses through the optic nerve and efferent impulses through the oculomotor nerve; afferent impulses may also be conducted through proprioceptive fibers from the extraocular muscles. It is generally believed, however, that there is also a cortical factor. The impulse probably reaches the occipital cortex by passing through the optic tract, lateral geniculate body, and optic radiations. It may then be carried directly to the midbrain through the internal corticotectal pathway, or it may pass by way of association fibers to the frontal cortex, and by way of descending pathways to the midbrain and the nuclear center of the oculomotor nerve. The contraction of the pupil accompanies accommodation even when convergence is prevented by prisms, and it accompanies convergence even when accommodation is prevented by atropine.

The constriction of the pupil in accommodation is occasionally lost in a postdiphtheritic paralysis of the ciliary mechanism, and in encephalitis. In both of these conditions there may also be a paralysis of convergence and some weakness of function of the medial rectus muscles. The pupil may continue to contract on accommodation in conditions where there is loss of convergence due to paralysis of the medial recti. There is no loss of pupillary response on accommodation in the Argyll Robertson pupil. It may be that there are two separate paths for pupillary contraction, and that the efferent pathway subserving the accommodation response differs from that for the light response. It has been said that the efferent pathway that has to do with pupillary constriction in the accommodation-convergence synkinesis goes through the third nerve to the episcleral ciliary ganglion and then to the ciliary body without passing through the ciliary ganglion.

The Pain Reflexes. The pupil may respond to a painful stimulus directed toward either a neighboring or a distant portion of the body. The **ciliospinal reflex** consists of a dilation of the pupils on painful stimulation of the skin of the neck on the ipsilateral side. In comatose states a similar response follows painful pressure on the cheek just below the orbit. The afferent impulses are relayed through the cervical (and trigeminal) nerves, and the efferent impulses through the cervical portion of the sympathetic division of the autonomic nervous system. The dilation is so minimal that it may be difficult to see in the normal individual, and it is best elicited in dim light, since in bright illumination the light reflex may interfere with the response. The reflex is absent with lesions of the cervical sympathetic fibers. The **oculosensory** or **oculopupillary reflex** consists of either constriction of the pupil or dilation followed by constriction in response to painful stimulation of the eye or its adnexa. It occurs in the presence of corneal or intraocular foreign bodies and in injuries to the eye or the side of the face. The afferent impulses are carried through the trigeminal nerve, and the efferent impulses through the oculomotor nerve. The so-called **paradoxical pupillary reaction of Byrne** consists of dilation of the pupil in response to pain in the lower portion of the body, usually in the opposite lower extremity or in the opposite sciatic nerve. This dilation, like the ciliospinal reflex, is doubtless a response to sympathetic stimulation.

The Orbicularis Reflex. Forceful closing of the eyes, closing of the eyes in sleep, and upward deviation of the eyeballs are followed by constriction of the pupils. The response is in all probability an associated movement. A variation of the orbicularis reflex is **Westphal's pupillary reaction,** which consists of pupillary contraction on attempts to close the eyes while the examiner holds them open.

The Cochlear or Cochleopupillary Reflex. Either a dilation or a constriction followed by dilation of the pupils occurs in response to a loud noise.

The Vestibular or Vestibulopupillary Reflex. This consists of either a dilation of the pupils in response to stimulation of the labyrinthine system, or a constriction during stimulation followed by dilation.

The Galvanic Reflex. Galvanic stimulation in the region of the temple causes constriction of the pupil. The mechanism is probably similar to that in the oculosensory reflex.

The Psychic Reflex. There is a dilation of the pupils in response to fear, anxiety, mental concentration, and sexual orgasm. It results from stimulation of the sympathetic division of the autonomic nervous system.

Effects of Drugs on the Pupil. The variation in size of the pupils in response to pharmacologic preparations may be designated the **drug responses.** These consist of dilation on either stimulation of the sympathetic division of the autonomic nervous system or paralysis of the parasympathetic division, and constriction on either paralysis of the sympathetic elements or stimulation of the parasympathetic. Atropine, homatropine, and scopolamine act as mydriatics by a paralyzing action on structures innervated by postganglionic cholinergic nerves; epinephrine, ephedrine, amphetamine, and cocaine dilate the pupil by stimulation of structures innervated by postganglionic adrenergic nerves. Pilocarpine, methacholine, and muscarine constrict the pupil by stimulation of structures innervated by postganglionic cholinergic nerves, and physostigmine (eserine) and neostigmine by inhibition of the action of cholinesterase. Ergot derivatives act as constrictors by blocking the action of postganglionic adrenergic nerves. Histamine may constrict the pupil by direct stimulation of the sphincter fibers. Nicotine has an irregular effect, depending upon whether the sympathetic or the parasympathetic endings are more stimulated. In man nicotine poisoning results in constriction followed by dilation. These responses are discussed further in Part F, "The Autonomic Nervous System." They may be used in the neurologic examination. Cocaine, for instance, will not dilate a miotic pupil if the miosis is secondary to sympathetic paralysis, but atropine will. Cocaine will cause further dilation of a mydriatic pupil if the mydriasis is due to paresis of the sphincter, but not if it is secondary to sympathetic stimulation. A myotonic pupil is abnormally sensitive to methacholine or pilocarpine.

The Eyelids

The function of the eyelids is examined by having the patient open and close his eyes, without and against resistance. The size of the palpebral fissures should be noted, as should associated contractions of the frontalis muscle. Paralysis of the levator palpebrae superioris causes **ptosis,** or drooping of the eyelid. This may be partial or complete. In lesions of the cervical sympathetic pathways there is pseudoptosis, owing to paralysis of the upper tarsal muscles: there is drooping of the lid to or below the margin of the pupil, but the patient can raise it completely by voluntary effort. There may also be slight elevation of the lower lid. In true ptosis, however, the striated, or voluntary, muscle is affected. If ptosis is complete, there is loss of ability to elevate the lid (Fig. 11-14); if partial, the lid is elevated only in part, and by voluntary effort. In evaluating ptosis and partial ptosis one notes the amount of iris or pupil covered by the lid. Slight weakness may become more apparent if the patient alternately elevates and depresses his lids through a

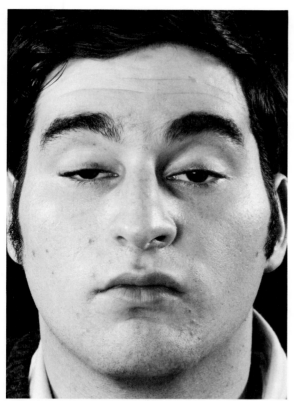

FIG. 11–14. Bilateral ptosis in a patient with myasthenia gravis.

small excursion. Partial ptosis may often be diagnosed by observing the contraction of the frontalis muscle when the patient attempts to open his eye on the involved side. If the examiner fixes the frontalis muscle with his finger, the patient may be unable to raise his eyelid. In ptosis of long standing there may be wrinkling in the forehead on the involved side, owing to constant contraction of the frontalis. In hysterical ptosis there is no associated overaction of the frontalis.

Any inequality of the palpebral fissures should be noted. The narrower fissure may denote a third-nerve or sympathetic involvement on one side, and the wider fissure may indicate a seventh-nerve (orbicularis oculi) paresis on the opposite side. A slight but perceptible difference in the width of the palpebral fissures occurs in 30% – 35% of normal individuals. In the absence of organic disease there is at times an appearance of ptosis in fatigue states. Bilateral partial ptosis of a benign nature may be familial or racial in origin. In myasthenia gravis there may be actual ptosis, either unilateral or bilateral, when the patient is fatigued, as well as

weakness of the orbicularis; these may almost disappear after either a period of rest or the administration of neostigmine or edrophonium (Fig. 11-15). Partial ptosis of congenital origin is present in the **Gunn phenomenon** (paradoxical lid retraction evoked by jaw movement) or **jaw-winking reflex;** the patient can raise the lid voluntarily and on upward gaze, but jaw movements are accompanied by exaggerated lid elevation (see "Other Trigeminal Nerve Disorders," in Ch. 12). In Parkinson's disease there is infrequent blinking and there may be some lid retraction. Lid lag, **Graefe's sign,** and increased width of the palpebral fissure (**Dalrymple's sign**) may be seen in hyperthyroidism (see below in section on exophthalmos). Loss of tone in the levator may cause a partial ptosis, but the eyelid can be elevated on upward gaze. With myotonia of the lids there may be difficulty in raising them immediately after forced closure; in myotonic lid lag the upper lids remain retracted briefly and then descend slowly on looking downward, immediately after a period of upward gaze. In myotonic dystrophy, partial bilateral ptosis may be present with the eyes in the normal position. In apraxia of lid opening the patient has difficulty in voluntarily initiating lid elevation although there is no paralysis of the levator.

Spasm of the eyelids may occur in psychogenic disorders, and a fine tremor of the lids (**Rosenbach's sign**) is seen in hyperthyroidism and hysteria. **Blepharospasm,** or spasmodic contraction of the orbicularis oculi and the levator, is common. It may have many etiologies. It may be psychogenic, a so-called habit spasm, which sometimes starts as a reflex response to pain in the eye or irritation of the cornea. On the other hand, it may be the result of hypersensitivity to light (photophobia), may be a post-encephalitic phenomenon, or may be a dystonia related to facial spasm or contracture (Meige syndrome).

The Ocular Movements

The eyes move in the service of vision. They bring objects of regard into the field of vision and then follow them if they move. Four basic types of movement have been described. **Saccades** are discrete, rapid movements from one object to another; the stimulus is either volitional or reflex. **Pursuit movements** are smooth following movements which maintain fixation. **Vergence movements** are accommodative or

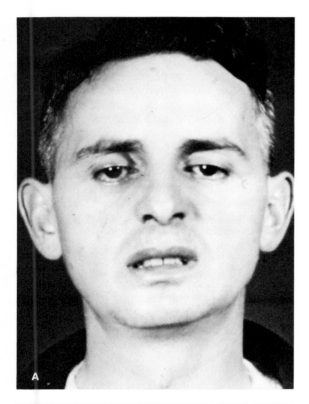

fusional. **Vestibulotonic movements** secure the relationship between the eyes and the environment during head and body movements. These various movements normally function harmoniously to secure and maintain vision.

The Visual Axes. The eyeball rotates in its socket around one or more of three primary axes that intersect each other at right angles near the center of the globe. One axis is vertical, and around it the lateral movements of abduction and adduction take place in the horizontal plane. A second is transverse, and is the axis of rotation for upward and downward movements. The third axis is in the anteroposterior plane, and torsion movements in the frontal plane take place around it. The eyes are said to be in their primary position, or position of rest, when their direction is maintained by the tone of the ocular muscles and gaze straight ahead and far away. The visual axes of the two eyes are then parallel. When the eyes view some definite object, they are turned by the contraction of the ocular muscles and are converged so that the visual axes meet at the observed object. An image of the object falls upon a corresponding point on each

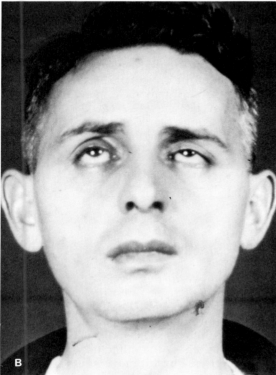

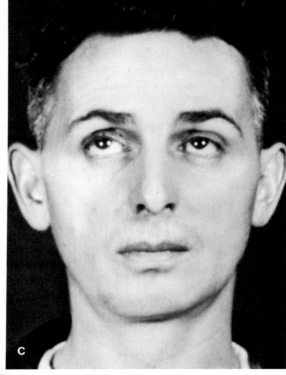

FIG. 11–15. Patient with myasthenia gravis. **A** and **B.** Ptosis and paresis of upward gaze. **C.** Absence of ptosis and normal upward gaze after administration of neostigmine.

macula. This movement of the eyes for acute observation is called **fixation.** The point where the visual axes meet is called the **fixation point.**

Conjugate Eye Movements. Normally the eye movements are **conjugate,** or **coordinated,** and there can be no isolated action of any ocular muscle. By means of the coordinating mechanism of the medial longitudinal fasciculus, various muscles of each eye contract and their antagonists relax in order to carry out any movement and, furthermore, the two eyes move together (Fig. 11-9).

Examination of the Ocular Movements

The ocular movements are tested by having the patient look in the six cardinal directions — laterally, medially, upward and laterally, upward and medially, downward and laterally, and downward and medially, as well as directly upward and downward, and then convergence is tested. Voluntary movements in response to a verbal command, and following movements using the examiner's finger, a flashlight, or a pointer for a guide, are first observed, and then reflex movements in which the patient fixes on a target and the head is passively moved from side to side and upward and downward are observed. Abnormalities of gaze may sometimes be brought out by having the patient perform a circular eye movement, following the slowly moving finger of the examiner. The range, speed, and smoothness of movement are noted, as well as the power to sustain lateral and vertical gaze. The **cover,** or **screening test** may aid in the demonstration of ocular muscle weakness. The eyes are focused on a light held at a reading distance, and they are alternately covered with a card. When an eye with a paretic muscle is covered, it will deviate away from the field of action of the affected muscle; when uncovered it will move back to the parallel position in order to focus on the light. When the sound eye is screened and the one with the paretic muscle is made to fix, the sound eye will deviate in a direction which is opposite to that of the paretic eye, and will return to the parallel position when uncovered.

The movements of individual muscles are first observed, and isolated pareses and paralyses noted; an attempt should be made to differentiate between nerve and muscle involvement. Then the conjugate movements are investigated for abnormalities of conjugate gaze and dissociation of movements. Certain reflex responses should be watched for, as well as the association between eye movements and contraction of the levator and frontalis muscles, and between eye and head movements. Finally, pathologic eye movements are evaluated. In examining infants, it should be borne in mind that binocular fixation is not established before the age of 6 months. By the age of 4 months, however, following movements and convergence can be tested. The cover test is especially helpful in evaluating ocular palsies in children. In both infants and comatose patients, reflex movements can be investigated, as described in the discussion of "Reflex Eye Movements." Eye movements may be recorded quantitatively by electrooculography.

Mechanisms of External Ophthalmoplegias

Paralysis of the individual ocular muscles produces a series of phenomena. Owing to loss of function of the individual muscle there is loss of certain movements of the eyeball. It must be remembered that there are no simple eye movements that are the result of the contraction of a single muscle, and that for any movement it is necessary to have not only the contraction of the prime movers, but also the relaxation of the antagonists. Consequently paresis or paralysis of one muscle is followed by secondary contraction of the antagonists. The pull of the nonaffected muscle or muscles results in primary deviation of the eyeball from parallelism with the normal eye, or noncorrespondence of the visual axes. This produces squint, or strabismus. If the patient attempts to fix his gaze on an object in the direction requiring the action of the affected muscle, and at the same time is prevented from seeing it with the normal eye, this eye will deviate too far in the required direction, owing to the increased effort resulting from the attempt to move the affected eye. As a result of the deviation there occurs an erroneous projection of the field of vision, always in the direction that the paralyzed muscle normally pulls the eye. Consequently there is a false image, with double vision, or **diplopia,** because the image of the object toward which the eyes are directed fails to fall on corresponding points of the two retinas. The false image is in the direction of the plane or planes of action of the paralyzed muscles. If the false image is on the same side as the eye which sees it, there is homonymous diplopia; if the image is on the opposite side, there is crossed diplopia. The farther the eyes are moved in the direction of the pull of the paralyzed muscle(s), the greater the separation of the images. Inasmuch as the face may be rotated and the head moved or tilted in the direction of action of a paralyzed muscle in an attempt to minimize the diplopia, there may be an abnormal posture, or attitude, of the head. Tilting of the head, however, occurs less frequently than the other manifestations. Vertigo and nausea may also be present.

Diplopia. Diplopia is usually preceded by blurring of vision. The patient's account of the two images seen in diplopia, especially if he is an intelligent observer, will give much information about the paretic muscles or nerves. If he sees double, he should be asked about the relationship of the two objects to each other — whether they are on the same horizontal plane, the same vertical plane, or separated both horizontally and vertically. He should be asked whether the diplopia is present at all times, or noted only when looking upward, downward, or to one side. It should be borne in mind that diplopia is not always the result of paralysis of ocular muscles; it may occur in conditions in which there is abnormality of the position of the eyeball, as in orbital inflammations or tumors. Monocular diplopia and polyopia often signify hysteria, but monocular diplopia may be present in ocular conditions such as cataracts, subluxation of the lens, and retinal detachment, and in cerebral lesions with dissociated visual projections of hemianopia of cortical origin. Slight monocular diplopia is said to be present in many eyes with normal vision, probably due to slight refractive differences in the lens substance; one image is much fainter than the other. **Aniseikonia,** a difference in the size and shape but not the position of objects seen with the two eyes is due to intraocular abnormality and not related to dysfunction of the ocular muscles.

A patient with diplopia may keep one eye closed to avoid seeing double, or may tilt his head to minimize the difficulty. In diplopia of long standing he may learn to suppress the vision of one eye. The diplopia is made more marked and the distance between the true and false images increases as the eyes are moved in the direction of the action of the paretic muscle. Diplopia is tested by holding a pencil or other object, or, best, a small light, in front of the pa-

tient; the relative position of the two perceived objects is noted when the eyes are at rest and when they are deviated in all directions of gaze. Then one eye is closed suddenly, and the patient is asked which object has disappeared. Minimal diplopia is increased and the images are more clearly differentiated if a colored glass (usually red) is placed before one eye and the patient asked to look at a small light held at a distance of 1 m. By moving the light into the various quadrants of vision, one can determine where the separation of images is the greatest. The relative positions of the two images may be recorded on a Lancaster chart (Fig. 11-16). A carefully made diplopia chart helps to identify the affected muscles; it also gives a permanent record of the degree of involvement, and thus aids in evaluating progression or improvement. Diplopia can also be tested by having the patient fix on an object with the paretic eye while the good eye is covered. Then the involved eye is also covered, and the patient is asked to point quickly at the object. If a muscle is paretic, he will point past the object in the direction of the apparent image when he looks in the direction of the pull of the paralyzed muscle.

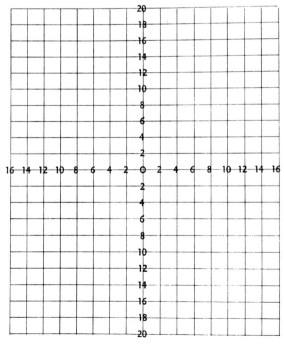

SUMMARY OF FINDINGS

FIG. 11–16. Diplopia chart.

Nuclear and Infranuclear Lesions

Isolated Paralyses (see also Fig. 11-4). An isolated paralysis of one or more of the extraocular muscles or nerves indicates the presence of either a nuclear or infranuclear lesion, that is, a lesion affecting the nucleus of the involved nerve, the course of the nerve from the nucleus to the muscles it supplies, or the muscle itself. In a paralysis of the superior rectus the eye is turned down and slightly outward. Upward movement is limited, especially when the eyeball is abducted. There is crossed diplopia on looking upward and laterally, and the secondary image is oblique; it is above and tilted away from the true image. The head may be deviated backward and rotated toward the affected side; the chin is elevated. In paralysis of the medial rectus the eyeball is turned laterally and cannot be deviated medially. Diplopia occurs on looking medially; it is horizontal and crossed, corresponding to the field of vision of the unaffected eye. The secondary object is vertical, and the face is turned toward the unaffected side. When the inferior rectus is involved the eyeball is deviated upward and slightly laterally, and cannot be moved downward when the eye is in abduction. Diplopia occurs on looking downward and laterally; it is crossed, and the false image is oblique, below the true image, but tilted toward it. The head may be tilted forward and toward the affected side; the chin is depressed. When the lateral rectus is paralyzed the globe is turned medially and cannot be abducted. Diplopia occurs on looking to the ipsilateral side, the two objects are on the same horizontal plane, and the false image is lateral, vertical, and homonymous. The face is turned toward the side of the involved muscle.

In paralysis of the inferior oblique the eyeball is deviated down and slightly medially, and cannot be moved upward when in abduction. Homonymous diplopia occurs on attempts to gaze upward and nasally, and the secondary image is oblique, above, and tilted away from the true image. The head is tilted backward and toward the shoulder of the affected side; the chin is elevated. With paralysis of the superior oblique there may be little deviation of the eyeball, but there is limitation of downward movement when the eye is adducted and there is no intorsion of the eye on looking downwards in abduction. Homonymous diplopia, with the secondary object oblique, occurs on looking downward and nasally; the secondary image is below

and lateral, and tilted toward the true image. The head may be deviated forward and toward the unaffected side, with the chin tilted toward the shoulder of the involved side.

In all the above, the position of the secondary object may vary, depending on whether the patient is fixing with his paretic or nonparetic eye. It is often difficult to differentiate isolated palsies of the cyclovertical muscles, except immediately after onset or when severe. Also, individual variations, incomplete or multiple involvement, and secondary contractures of opposing muscles may cause alterations in the position of the eyeballs or of the false image.

Nuclear and infranuclear involvement must be differentiated by noting associated signs and symptoms, or their absence. In a nuclear third nerve lesion there may be paralysis of individual extraocular muscles without palpebral involvement or associated internal ophthalmoplegia. Infranuclear affections usually result in a complete third nerve paralysis, unless the lesion is within the orbit, when isolated involvement may again occur. It is impossible to differentiate between nuclear and infranuclear fourth nerve abnormalities without considering other findings on the examination. A nuclear fourth nerve lesion causes a contralateral paralysis, whereas an infranuclear paralysis is ipsilateral. A nuclear sixth nerve involvement is usually differentiated from an infranuclear paralysis by the associated seventh nerve symptoms. Owing to the proximity of the nuclei of these nerves to the medial longitudinal fasciculus, nuclear lesions often result in complicated syndromes, and isolated nuclear palsies are rare, whereas infranuclear isolated palsies are common.

Strabismus. Isolated palsies should be differentiated from apparent palsies due to refractive errors, ocular or orbital disease, and muscular imbalance that causes strabismus, or squint. **Strabismus** is defined as deviation of one eye from its proper direction so that the visual axes of the two eyes cannot both be directed simultaneously at the same objective point. There is lack of parallelism of the ocular axes. The deviation may be divergent, convergent, upward, or downward, and may be unilateral or alternating. It may be latent, occurring only when the eye is occluded, or manifest, occurring when both eyes are open. It may be occasional, incipient, or constant. It may be concomitant, with the same amount of deviation regardless of the direction in which the eyes are looking, or noncon-comitant. Strabismus may be paralytic in disease of the ocular nerves, but in nonparalytic strabismus the involved eye can be moved throughout its complete range of movement, following the fixing eye with a constant error, even though it may diverge or converge at rest. In paralytic strabismus the defect is increased when the eyes are turned in the direction of the action of the paralyzed muscle. Since most strabismus is present from birth or early childhood, the patient learns to suppress one image, and usually develops amblyopia in the involved eye. **Heterotropia** is a generic term synonymous with strabismus, or squint, with a manifest deviation of the eyes. The term **esotropia** is used for convergent strabismus, or the turning inward of the visual axis of an eye; **exotropia** for divergent strabismus; and **hypertropia** for vertical strabismus with one visual axis elevated above the other.

Heterophoria is a generic term indicating a latent tendency to imperfect binocular balance rather than manifest involvement. **Hyperphoria** is a tendency for the visual axis of one eye to deviate above that of the other; **esophoria** is a tendency for the visual axes to deviate inward (latent convergent strabismus); and **exophoria** is the tendency to deviate outward (latent divergent strabismus). Esophoria may occur in individuals with hyperopia; exophoria, in those with myopia.

Supranuclear Lesions

Supranuclear involvement of ocular motion indicates the presence of a lesion either in the pathways connecting the various nuclei or in the higher centers. Disturbances of conjugate gaze may be found in association with midbrain, pontine, or cerebral lesions, resulting in paresis but rarely paralysis of conjugate gaze; there is a paresis of movement rather than a paralysis of muscles. The visual axes remain parallel, and there is neither strabismus nor diplopia.

Cerebral lesions may be either irritative or paralytic. Stimulation of the motor eye field in the frontal lobe (area 8) causes strong, rapid, involuntary conjugate deviation of the eyes to the opposite side, which may be accompanied by conjugate movement of the head and rotation of the trunk, usually of short duration. This occurs with irritation of either the cortex or the descending neuraxes, and may be part of a jacksonian convulsion. Destructive lesions of this cortical center or its descending fibers cause pa-

resis of gaze to the opposite side, usually not complete, with deviation of the eyes toward the side of the lesion. This deviation may be of considerable magnitude, and may be accompanied, for a short period of time, by conjugate movements of the head and rotation of the trunk to the same side; spontaneous recovery takes place within a few days or weeks. The head is turned in the same direction as the eyes, paralysis of associated muscles is symmetric, and there is usually paresis of the face and extremities on the side toward which there is paresis of gaze.

With destructive frontal lesions only voluntary motion is affected; the patient cannot turn his eyes laterally on command, but lateral following and reflex movements are intact. Vertical gaze may also be affected. Although the patient is unable to deviate his eyes, they will follow a test object that is moved slowly in the direction of paresis of gaze. They remain fixed on a stationary object when the head is passively rotated in the opposite direction (**optic fixation reflex**). Also, reflex movements in response to visual, vestibular, and acoustic stimuli and to turning movements of the head and body are retained or even exaggerated, as are the tonic neck reflexes. In **congenital ocular motor apraxia,** which occurs mainly in males, there is loss of voluntary horizontal eye movements, but random and involuntary movements are preserved; the quick phase of optokinetic nystagmus (see under "Induced Nystagmus") is absent in the horizontal plane. There are associated jerky head movements and reading difficulties. This syndrome is thought to result from a lesion of the cortical center for voluntary eye movements or of its connections with lower centers. Ocular motor apraxia may also be acquired, as part of the syndrome of ataxia telangiectasia, Gaucher's disease, and others.

In the **pseudoophthalmoplegia** described by Ford and Walsh there is loss of lateral or even vertical gaze, but the eyes move with passive rotation of the head; the phenomenon is brought on by optic fixation and labyrinthine reflexes, and may result from a lesion in the tectum.

Irritative and destructive lesions of the motor eye centers in the occipital lobe, and probably also in the temporal lobe and angular gyrus, cause similar conjugate deviation and paresis of conjugate gaze. With destructive lesions of the occipital centers (areas 18 and 19), however, voluntary movements may be little affected but there is impairment of following and reflex movements. Owing to associated involvement of the striate cortex or optic radiations, there may be difficulty with fixation and with maintaining visual attention, as well as field defects. Stereoscopic vision and visual memory may be lost. **Balint's syndrome** ("psychic" paralysis of optic fixation, optic ataxia, and alterations in visual attention) is said to be caused by bilateral parietooccipital lesions.

Pontine and midbrain lesions are usually paralytic rather than irritative. With irritative lesions affecting centers concerned with lateral gaze (the vestibular complex, the medial longitudinal fasciculus, secondary vestibular fibers destined for this tract, the parabducens nucleus, or the paramedian pontine reticular formation), there is ipsilateral deviation of the eyes. With destructive lesions of the structures there is paresis of gaze toward the side of the lesion, with contralateral deviation of the eyes that is of small magnitude but usually permanent; as with frontal lesions, voluntary motion is affected more than reflex and following movements. An abnormal position of the head is not a typical feature, but the head may be turned in the direction opposite to the ocular deviation. Paralysis of associated muscles may be asymmetric, and that of the face, if present, is collateral with the eye muscle paralysis, whereas paralysis of the extremities is on the opposite side; there may be additional nuclear palsies. Occasionally there is paralysis of conjugate gaze with retention of convergence.

A lesion at the level of the *superior colliculi* (anterior quadrigeminal bodies), the pretectal region, or the posterior commissure causes paralysis of conjugate upward gaze; the symptom complex is known as **Parinaud's syndrome,** and is found in tumors of the pineal gland or the posterior portion of the third ventricle, encephalitis, vascular lesions, multiple sclerosis, and other conditions (Fig. 11-17).

Lesions in the periaqueductal gray matter of the midbrain may cause impairment of convergence as may lesions of the fibers to the medial rectus muscles. Convergence loss may be seen in encephalitis, both acute and chronic, and in multiple sclerosis, trauma, vascular disease, and other conditions. Paralysis of convergence has also been reported with occipital and frontal lesions. A relative convergence insufficiency is seen in older individuals normally. Convergence spasm may be of functional or organic origin. Paralysis of divergence has also been described with lesions of the periaqueductal gray matter, and in brain tumors and extrapyramidal syndromes.

Partial loss of conjugate lateral movements and mixed gaze palsies are found with *inter-*

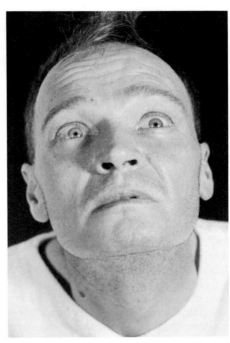

FIG. 11–17. *Paresis of upward gaze in a patient with a neoplasm of the posterior third ventricle.*

nuclear involvement. If there is a lesion of the medial longitudinal fasciculus that interrupts the impulses from the center for lateral gaze in the lower pons to the third nerve nucleus in the midbrain, there is paralysis of the medial recti on attempted conjugate lateral gaze. If the lesion is near the midbrain level (**anterior** or **superior internuclear ophthalmoplegia, Lhermitte's syndrome,** or **ophthalmoplegia internuclearis of Spiller**) there is paralysis of adduction of the contralateral eye on attempted lateral gaze to one side, and there is usually associated paresis of convergence. With a more caudal lesion (**posterior** or **inferior internuclear ophthalmoplegia**) there is paresis of abduction of the ipsilateral eye on attempted lateral gaze, which may be more marked than the paresis of adduction of the contralateral eye, and the latter may converge normally. In both of these syndromes the paretic muscles may respond to vestibular stimulation. Nystagmus usually is present, especially with posterior lesions, and is more marked in the abducting eye. It is most often horizontal, but may be rotatory or vertical. Some authorities dispute the existence of anterior versus posterior internuclear ophthalmoplegias. The internuclear ophthalmoplegias are often grouped together as the **syndrome of the medial longitudinal fas-**

ciculus. In the classic syndrome there is paralysis of adduction of the contralateral eye on attempted lateral gaze to one side, with normal convergence of that eye, together with variable paresis and monocular nystagmus of the abducting eye (dissociated, or "ataxic," nystagmus); there may be vertical nystagmus of both eyes on upward gaze. Convergence may be lost if the lesion is near the midbrain level. The syndrome is most often bilateral, and bilateral involvement is most often seen with multiple sclerosis. Unilateral involvement is more often the result of a vascular lesion. Either unilateral or bilateral internuclear ophthalmoplegias, however, may be present with vascular, neoplastic, inflammatory, or degenerative lesions of the brain stem or compression of the latter by neoplasms in the posterior fossa; under such circumstances there are usually symptoms and signs indicating involvement of neighboring centers and pathways.

Dissociation of eye movements is found in deep sleep and in coma, and it is often of serious prognostic significance in meningitis. In **skew deviation,** which is seen occasionally in cerebellar disease and posterior fossa lesions, the eye on the side of the lesion is turned downward and inward whereas the contralateral eye is deviated upward and outward. With *cerebellar lesions,* or involvement of cerebellar connections with other centers, disturbances of ocular fixation may result in ataxia or asynergy of extraocular movements. **Ocular dysmetria** is an overshooting of the eyes on attempted rapid fixation of gaze toward either side or on returning to the primary position; there may also be overshooting in following movements when the object of regard is suddenly stopped.

Under certain circumstances the smooth conjugate following movements of the eyes assume a jerky, irregular character and the eyes follow the moving visual object in a series of short steps, remain fixed for a moment, and then move again. They may overshoot the target or advance before it before coming to a jerky stop, and thus the movements resemble saccades. They may be brought out most effectively if the target is moved slowly across the visual field. They are seen most often in Parkinson's disease and postencephalitic parkinsonism, and are sometimes referred to as "cogwheel" movements. These movements are also seen in multiple sclerosis, post-traumatic states, and toxic or other cerebral disorders. The ocular movements during the first few months of life are also jerky. In the spinocerebellar ataxias both saccadic and pursuit movements are slow. In Huntington's chorea patients may be unable to move their eyes in rapid saccades, while smooth pursuit movements are preserved.

Reflex Eye Movements

Reflex movements of the eyes may be divided into two classes: movements that are carried out involuntarily but involve the mediation of consciousness, and true reflexes that are subserved by a subcortical mechanism.

The first group consists of the movements of fixation, **optically induced movements,** or the **visual,** or **psychooptical, reflexes.** These result from stimulation of the retina. When a light falls upon a peripheral portion of the retina the eye is moved reflexly in such a way that the image strikes the fovea, unless the intensity of the light is such that it causes closing of the eye. Both eyes respond in a coordinated manner, and the movement is a rapid one. There may be associated turning of the head. The afferent pathway travels through the optic tracts to the occipital cortex, whereas the efferent pathway goes to the midbrain and to the nuclei of the ocular nerves and other motor nuclei. Attention and conscious appreciation of the stimulus are probably necessary to the response. There may be a tendency for the eyes to remain directed on the object in central vision; this is sometimes termed the **optic fixation reflex.** With impairment of voluntary movement of the eyes, or with frontal lesions in which there is loss of cortical inhibition, this reflex may become exaggerated or dominant, and the patient may have difficulty in disengaging his vision from any point on which it is directed. Individuals with macular deficiencies or other severe ocular difficulties dating from birth may show, instead of fixation, gross, roving movements of the eyes ("ocular" nystagmus — see "Pathologic Nystagmus"). The **fusion reflex** determines the accurate directing of the eyes so that the images of the object toward which vision is directed fall on corresponding points of the two retinas. The **emergency light reflex** consists of pupillary constriction, closing of the eyes, lowering of the eyebrows, and sometimes even a bending of the head or an elevation of one arm in response to a sudden, strong visual stimulus. The afferent pathway goes through the optic tracts to the occipital cortex, and the efferent impulses go through the oculomotor, facial, accessory, and upper cervical nerves. It is a modification of the visual palpebral or blink reflex (see "Examination of the Reflexes," Ch. 13).

The second type of movements, true reflex movements, are produced by stimulation of the vestibular apparatus, otoliths, acoustic mechanism, or conjunctivae or cornea, and by changes in the position of the head or the body (postural reflexes, righting reflexes, and tonic neck reflexes). These latter are responses to proprioceptive impulses arising from the muscles of the neck or from the body as a whole, and in them eye movements are correlated with bodily responses and movements of the head and neck (Part E, "The Reflexes"). The **vestibulo-oculogyric reflex** (labyrinthine reflex) consists of either a lateral deviation of the eyeballs or nystagmus on stimulation of the labyrinthine apparatus or on sudden passive turning of the head (the **oculocephalic reflex** or **doll's head phenomenon**). The **auditory-oculogyric reflex** (a cochlear reflex) consists of a lateral deviation of the eyes in the direction of a sudden noise. In both of these responses the impulse travels through the constituent portion of the eighth nerve and its nuclei to the medial longitudinal fasciculus, and then to the nuclei of the ocular nerves. In states of lowered consciousness and coma it may be possible to test for the oculocephalic reflex even though voluntary motion is absent. It may also be tested in infants. The reflex is tested by holding the eyes open and passively but rapidly turning the head from side to side; if the eyes move in a direction opposite to that in which the head is moved, the reflex is intact. Absence of movement to one side suggests the presence of paresis of conjugate gaze to that side, and dissociation of response suggests the presence of brain stem involvement. The reflex is absent in near-terminal coma and severe brain stem disease.

The **corneo-oculogyric reflex** (a sensory reflex) consists of a contralateral or upward deviation of the eyes and a contraction of the orbicularis in response to irritation of the cornea. The afferent impulses are carried through the trigeminal nerve, and the efferent pathway is through the ocular and facial nerves. This response is related to the corneal reflex (see "Examination of the Reflexes," Ch. 12). The **oculogyric-auricular reflex** consists of a slight contraction of both auricles, greater on the opposite side, on lateral gaze toward one side. Proprioceptive impulses are carried through the oculomotor and abducens nerves, with the efferent pathway going through the facial nerve (see "Examination of the Reflexes," Ch. 13).

There are also associated movements between the ocular muscles, the levator palpebrae superioris, and the muscles of facial expression. Upward gaze is associated not only with elevation of the eyelid, but also with contraction of the frontalis. Elevation of the lid is associated with contraction of the frontalis. On contraction of the orbicularis oculi, with resultant closing of the eye, the eyeballs in most persons rotate upward; this occurs not only in voluntary closing of the eye, but also in sleep. This oculofacial associated movement is sometimes called the **palpebral-oculogyric reflex**. Proprioceptive impulses are carried through the facial nerve to the medial longitudinal fasciculus, and efferent impulses are relayed to the superior rectus muscles. The response is exaggerated in **Bell's phenomenon,** in which, in the presence of paralysis of the orbicularis, the eyeball rotates upward as the patient attempts to close his eye (see "Peripheral Facial Paralysis," Ch. 13). Associations between ocular and facial or head movements may also be observed in the vestibular, cochlear, sensory, and postural reflexes as well as in stimulation of the cortical or pontine centers, and there is absence of these movements in paralytic or destructive cerebral or brain stem lesions.

PATHOLOGIC EYE MOVEMENTS

Nystagmus

Nystagmus is a frequent manifestation in disease of the nervous system, and it is also observed in diseases of the eye and the inner ear. It may, however, be a normal phenomenon under certain circumstances or may be induced experimentally or as part of the clinical examination. There are many varieties of nystagmus, and in order to evaluate its significance in any individual instance, one must understand the underlying mechanisms and the mode of production of the phenomenon.

Nystagmus, or as it is rarely called, **talantropia,** may be defined as an involuntary oscillation or trembling of the eyeball. The term rhythmic is often included in the definition, but nonrhythmic varieties may be seen. Certain observers object to the inclusion of the adjective involuntary, as nystagmus of volitional origin has been described. Nystagmus is a coordinated movement, and usually both eyes move synchronously over a virtually equal range. Unilateral nystagmus, however, may occur, or there may be dissociation of movements or disproportion between the movements on the two sides. The motor response involves not only the contraction of certain muscles, but also the relaxation of their antagonists by reciprocal innervation, with alternating activity of agonists and antagonists.

Nystagmus may be described in various ways: by type, form, direction, rate, amplitude, duration, and intensity, and by relationship of the response to movements of the eyes, head, and body. It may be rhythmic or pendular in type. **Rhythmic** or **resilient nystagmus,** also known as **jerky, biphasic, directed,** or **spring nystagmus,** is characterized by alternate slow and quick ocular excursions, resulting in a jerky, unequal oscillation of the eyeballs. Usually there is a rapid movement in the direction of gaze (the **quick component,** or **rapid phase**) which is followed by a slower return movement away from the point of fixation (the **slow component** or **phase**). **Pendular** or **undulatory nystagmus** is characterized by more or less regular to-and-fro movements of approximately equal range and velocity toward each side of a central point.

Nystagmus may be horizontal, vertical, oblique, rotatory, or mixed in form, and to the right, left, upward, and downward in direction. In the rotatory variety the direction is recorded as clockwise or counterclockwise. Retraction nystagmus is occasionally seen; in this type of nystagmus the eyes appear to move back and forth in the orbits. Nystagmus may be slow, medium, or rapid in rate or velocity. If the movements are from 10 – 40/min, the nystagmus is slow; it is medium in rate if they are 40 – 100/min, and rapid if over 100/min. The oscillations may be fine, medium, or coarse in amplitude. The movements may be so gross that they cannot be overlooked, or so fine that they cannot be seen with the naked eye and are visualized only when the eye is examined with the ophthalmoscope or when strong convex lenses (Frenzel spectacles) are placed in front of the eyes. These not only magnify the nystagmus but also eliminate fixation. If the movements are of less than 5° or the excursions are less than 1 mm in amplitude, the nystagmus is fine; if they are over 15° or more than 3 mm in amplitude, the nystagmus is coarse; if they are between these, it is considered medium.

Nystagmus may be either abortive or sustained in duration. It is also classified by intensity. It is of first-degree intensity if present when the patient looks in the direction of the quick component; second-degree if present not only when looking in the direction of the quick component, but also while the eyes are in the neutral position; third-degree if present even when looking in the direction of the slow component.

Nystagmus may be either **congenital** or **acquired;** it may be **spontaneous** or **artificial (induced);** it may be present at rest, on fixation, or on deviation of the eyeballs. It may be **associated,** or **conjugate,** with the movements symmetric in the two eyes, or **dissociated,** with the movements of the two eyes unrelated. In **unilateral nystagmus** the movements take place in only one eye. In **disjunctive nystagmus,** which is rare, the movements are symmetrically opposite. A movement that appears to be simple to the naked eye may be irregular or complex when visualized through an ophthalmoscope or a lens. Nystagmus may vary from time to time in the same individual, depending upon the position of the body, head, and eyes, and other factors. It may be maintained or unimpaired in the presence of extensive ocular palsies. Rhythmic head movements may accompany it. Patients with nystagmus may notice blurring of vision and a sensation of movement at the onset of the manifestation, or they may notice a constant movement of the objects within the field of vision; this subjective manifestation, which is known as **oscillopsia,** is relatively rare.

Various methods have been described for the delineation and recording of nystagmus. A tambour may be placed against the closed eyelid, and a pneumatic tube used to transmit the movements of the eyeball to a kymograph. A photoelectric cell can record variations in an infrared beam focused on the eyeball. Videorecording may be used. The character and extent of the oscillations may be studied by means of the slit-lamp (biomicroscope). Electronystagmography, however, gives the most detailed information about the rate, amplitude, type, duration, and intensity of the nystagmus and, furthermore, provides a permanent record. Electrodes may be attached to the outer and inner canthi, the margins of the orbit, the anesthetized conjunctiva, or the ocular muscles, and the electrical potentials are recorded on an oscillograph or electroencephalograph. Both spontaneous and induced nystagmus may be studied, as well as other abnormalities of ocular movements.

There are many types of nystagmus and they appear to serve widely diverse purposes. The position of the eyes is influenced reflexly by impulses coming from the retinas, the ocular muscles, the labyrinths, and the cochlea, and by proprioceptive impulses initiated by movements of the head or the body. It is also influenced by impulses relayed from the cerebral cortex. Nystagmus may, in most instances, be considered a compensatory reaction of the eyeballs to defective or abnormal impulses from any of these sources. It may have many apparent purposes: to retain a specific field of vision, that is, to keep the eyes as long as possible in the same position in relation to the visual field; to increase incoming impulses; to aid in ocular fixation; to assist in orientation in space.

If the head moves or if the field of vision moves, the eyes move in the opposite direction in an attempt to remain fixed in the original field, to maintain as long as possible the same position relative to the visual field, or to preserve the image of the fixed object on the retina. Because of the limited excursion of the eyes, however, the original field cannot be held, and at their maximal deviation the eyes are jerked back to take up a new focus. If one labyrinth is stimulated, there is a slow movement of the eyes,

again in an attempt to retain the original field of vision (Fig. 11-18). The eyes, however, cannot be held in this position, and they are jerked back to take up a new focus in relation to the environment. If either of these movements persists, nystagmus results.

If, owing to poor macular vision, inadequate visual acuity, or inadequate illumination, the impulses focused on the macula are not sufficient to allow adequate perception, the eyes move from side to side in an attempt to increase or reinforce the incoming visual impulses, to find the sharpest image, or to achieve adequate fixation, with no relation to the movement of the head or of the field of vision. Here, also, a nystagmus results, but the movements toward each side are equal in amplitude and rate. If nystagmus is the result of movement of the field of vision or of at-

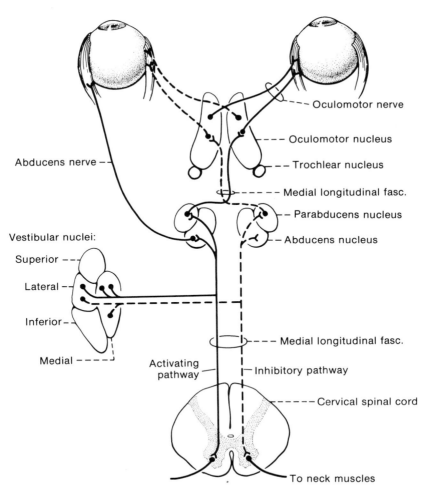

FIG. 11-18. Relationship of the vestibular system to the mechanism for conjugate lateral gaze.

tempts to increase vision, it is a reflex response to retinal stimulation and may be called an **oculocerebral reflex.** If it is the result of movement of the head or body or of irritation of the labyrinth, it is a reflex response to vestibular stimulation and may be called a **vestibulocerebral reflex.** Other mechanisms in the production of nystagmus will be described under the discussion of the specific varieties. Owing to the integrative action of the various components of the nervous system and their correlation with and interdependence upon each other, it is often impossible to separate visual, sensory (proprioceptive), vestibular, and other factors.

The slow phase of rhythmic nystagmus is said to be of peripheral or vestibular origin. The reflex arc involves the labyrinths, the vestibular nuclei, the medial longitudinal fasciculus, the nuclei of the extraocular muscles, and the ocular muscles themselves. There has been little agreement about the source of the rapid phase, which is often referred to as the cerebral or central component, but it probably is of brain stem origin. It has been found that all of the rapid discharges are mediated by the reticular formation. Nystagmus may disappear during anesthesia and return with return of consciousness. It may still be elicited after extirpation of the hemispheres, and even after section of the brain stem to the level of the nucleus of the oculomotor nerve. It has been demonstrated that the only portions of the central nervous system essential for the production of the slow and quick phases of nystagmus are the vestibular and oculomotor nuclei and the connections between them, although other regions and structures may exert a profound influence on the phenomenon. Clinicians, in referring to rhythmic nystagmus, usually name it from the direction of the rapid component, because this movement is more readily noticed and is more striking. The slow phase, however, represents the more active physiologic determinant, and in experimental literature it is used to indicate the direction of nystagmus.

In the appraisal of nystagmus, the eyes should be inspected in the resting position and on deviation in all directions, and with the patient both seated and recumbent. The direction, rate, amplitude, type, form, duration, and intensity of the nystagmus should be noted, and some of these features can be recorded graphically. One should also observe the relationship of the nystagmus to position or movement of the eyes, head, and body. It may change in direction or type or may even be brought on by change in position of the head or body. Nystagmoid jerks may be difficult to differentiate from clinical nystagmus. Some individuals have spontaneous rhythmic ocular movements during mental concentration while their eyes are gazing into the distance.

There is no generally accepted classification of nystagmus, and interpretation of the mechanism for and significance of different types vary widely. So-called physiologic varieties may appear in the presence of disease of the nervous system, and varieties usually considered to be pathologic are not always the result of a definite disease process. All types may be influenced by visual and vestibular stimuli, postural and tonic neck reflexes, the position of the head and eyes, and changes in the state of attention or alertness. The following classification includes the more commonly encountered and important categories; there may be mixed forms and irregular manifestations. The classification is first given in outline form, and the categories are then discussed individually.

I. Induced nystagmus
    A. Optokinetic or optomotor nystagmus
    B. Labyrinthine nystagmus

II. Pathologic nystagmus
    A. Nystagmus associated with disease of the eye or its adnexa
        1. Nystagmus of optic derivation
            a. "Ocular" nystagmus
            b. Occupational nystagmus
            c. Spasmus nutans
        2. Nystagmus of neuromuscular origin
            a. Paretic nystagmus
            b. Fatigue nystagmus
            c. Latent nystagmus
    B. Nystagmus associated with disease of the central nervous system
        1. Vestibular nystagmus
        2. Cerebellar nystagmus
        3. Nystagmus with lesions of the medial longitudinal fasciculus
        4. Other types of "central" nystagmus
    C. Miscellaneous varieties of nystagmus
        1. Toxic nystagmus
        2. Congenital or hereditary nystagmus
        3. Pathologic alterations of induced nystagmus
        4. Nystagmus due to involvement of the cervical portion of the spinal cord
        5. Positional nystagmus
        6. Hysterical nystagmus
        7. Voluntary nystagmus

Induced Nystagmus. Nystagmus may be produced clinically or experimentally by certain tests or methods of stimulation. The response is usually considered to be physiologic, and may be induced in normal individuals. Changes occur, however, in disease processes.

Optokinetic or Optomotor Nystagmus. When a person in a rapidly moving vehicle directs his eyes toward fixed objects, a jerky type of physiologic nystagmus appears. This is a conjugate or conjunctive response of the eyes to a succession of moving visual stimuli and has been known as **optic, railway,** or **elevator nystagmus.** When tested clinically it is called **optokinetic,** or **optomotor, nystagmus,** and is elicited by means of either an optokinetic drum or optokinetic tape (Fig. 11-19). The drum, painted with vertical black and white stripes, is rotated in front of the patient's eyes, or the tape, a series of 2-in. square red patches placed 2 in. apart on a white tape 1 yard long, is drawn across the patient's field of vision. The stimulus may be directed from the right or the left to elicit horizontal nystagmus, and from above or below to elicit vertical nystagmus. The slow phase is in the direction of movement of the drum or tape, with the quick return in the opposite direction. Thus the slow phase seems to indicate the pursuit of the moving object, with a quick return in an attempt at fixation on a new oncoming target. The nystagmus is fine, rapid, and rhythmic. The response is intensified if the subject looks in the direction of the quick phase. This phenomenon is a reflex response to retinal stimulation or to proprioceptive impulses from the eye muscles, and has been believed to be cortical in origin. It probably represents a cortical or an oculocerebral reflex, dependent on the continuity of the association pathways between the occipital and frontal cortices. There may be both active (cortical) and passive (subcortical) varieties. Optokinetic nystagmus is a physiologic response and its absence must be regarded as pathologic. The rotating drum test is used to demonstrate feigned or simulated blindness in a malingerer, to diagnose hysterical blindness, and to test for the presence of vision in an infant. In some disease states optokinetic nystagmus may be accompanied by vertigo, turning of the body, or irregular eye movements.

Labyrinthine Nystagmus. This is a physiologic response that follows the stimulation of the semicircular canals by rapid rotation of the body, spraying the external auditory canal with warm

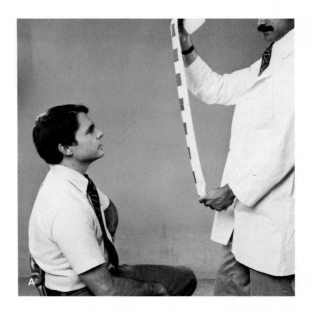

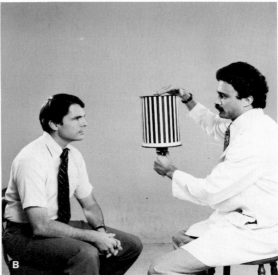

FIG. 11–19. Testing for optokinetic nystagmus. **A.** Using optokinetic tape. **B.** Using the rotating drum.

or cold water, galvanic stimulation, or pressure changes. It, too, is rhythmic in type. Its direction depends upon which semicircular canals are stimulated, and is thus dependent upon the position of the head during stimulation. The direction also varies with the type of stimulus used. The slow phase is said to be the resultant effect of the stimuli caused by the movement of the endolymph in the semicircular canals of the labyrinth. The head and eyes, and sometimes the body, are deviated in the direction of the endolymph current, and the slow phase of the ny-stagmus corresponds; the rapid phase is in the opposite direction. This variety of nystagmus is a reflex response to stimulation of the labyrinth, and thus is a vestibulocerebral reflex; pathologic variations may accompany disease processes. The details of the vestibular tests, and of the resulting nystagmus, are presented in Chapter 14.

Rhythmic nystagmus may be produced by loud auditory stimuli (**reflex acoustic nystagmus**) or by painful stimulation to the ear, face, or eye (**reflex sensory nystagmus**). These are rarely elicited and are of theoretical interest only.

Pathologic Nystagmus. This, in most instances, indicates the presence of some abnormal process in the eyes or the ocular muscles, or in the central connections concerned with ocular movement or bodily equilibrium. It is a **spontaneous nystagmus** and usually of clinical significance.

Nystagmus of Optic Derivation. Nystagmus may be associated with deficient vision, resulting either from impaired visual acuity or inadequate illumination and retinal fatigue. It is usually pendular rather than rhythmic in type, and the movements appear to result from an attempt to maintain fixation of vision in spite of deficient acuity or insufficient light. It may appear in early infancy or may be acquired; it is not congenital.

"Ocular" Nystagmus. This is of the pendular type and is usually coarse and slow, although sometimes rapid. It is characterized by to-and-fro movements, often of equal range and velocity, toward each side of a central point. The movements may be wide and aimless and of the so-called searching, wandering, or roving type. They may be highly irregular, and occasionally there is a rhythmic component. They are usually horizontal, sometimes vertical, and rarely rotatory. This variety of nystagmus occurs in persons who have had markedly deficient vision since birth, in persons whose vision has failed before fixation is learned or whose fixation is deficient, or in color-blind individuals or those with increased sensitivity to light. Thus it may be observed in persons with congenital cataracts, corneal scars owing to ophthalmia neonatorum or interstitial keratitis, congenital corneal leukomas, macular deficiencies, chorioretinitis, high errors of refraction (especially high-grade myopia), and albinism. It does not occur in persons

who are blind from birth. It develops shortly after birth, and probably begins when the infant first attempts fixation. As a result of poor vision or imperfect macular vision, a "searching" movement of the eye develops as the infant attempts to increase the incoming impulses, to find the sharpest image, or to achieve adequate fixation. The nystagmus is an adaptation to attain fixation in spite of defective vision. Sometimes there is an associated nodding of the head.

Ocular nystagmus probably does not develop in adults. When bilateral visual defects (especially loss of macular vision) are acquired late in life, there may be slow, seemingly aimless movements, which are not definitely pendular; these probably represent voluntary attempts at fixation rather than a true nystagmus. Unilateral nystagmus may occur in unilateral optic atrophy or other visual defects. An inconstant nystagmus is sometimes seen in homonymous hemianopic visual field defects, particularly when the patient is looking to the blind side. This is probably not entirely ocular in origin, as it usually is of the rhythmic type, and it may vary with position.

Occupational Nystagmus. Eyestrain caused by deficient illumination, repeated movements of the eyes, or retinal fatigue may cause nystagmus. This has been reported most frequently in miners, and is commonly referred to as **miner's nystagmus.** It develops after long exposure to poor illumination, especially after working in a stooped position with the eyes deviated upward, and is probably the result of insufficiency of binocular fusion. Only the rods are used for vision in imperfect light, and as there are no rods in the macula, there is inefficient macular vision in poor illumination; as a result, there is constant shifting of the axis of the eyes. Miner's nystagmus is usually pendular but occasionally rotatory. The movements are rapid and slow, constant or inconstant, and usually vertical in direction and increased in upward gaze; they may not be conjugate. There is defective fixation and there may be associated spasm of the levator palpebrae superioris. There often are associated symptoms of tremor, vertigo, and photophobia. Occupational nystagmus may develop in draftsmen, jewelers, train dispatchers, crane workers, painters, and others whose work necessitates movement of the eyes and strain on the ocular muscles or results in retinal fatigue. The movements may be either vertical or horizontal and show marked variation in rate; there may be associated blepharospasm, visual impairment, and ocular discomfort.

Spasmus Nutans. This condition is seen in babies from 6 months to 2 years of age. It consists of a rhythmic nodding or rotatory tremor of the head, tilting of the head, and a fine, rapid, pendular, or occasionally rhythmic, type of nystagmus. It is usually horizontal in direction, but it may be vertical. The movements may be unilateral or dissociated and may vary with the direction of gaze. Closing of the eyes may either reduce or increase the tremor, while forceful control of the tremor may increase the nystagmus. The condition has been ascribed to rickets, but it is known to occur in children who live in dark dwellings where no sunlight penetrates, regardless of the presence of rickets; at times it has no known cause. It may be of complex origin, both ocular and central; it is usually self-limited.

Nystagmus of Neuromuscular Origin. In a large percentage of normal persons a few fine, rapid nystagmoid movements are seen upon extreme deviation of the eyes. They are more marked on lateral gaze and are usually horizontal in direction. The rapid movement is in the direction of gaze, and the slow return represents the reflex contraction of the overstretched antagonists in an attempt to return the eyes to the central position. These movements are irregular and are usually transient; they may gradually disappear after five to ten jerks. This type of oscillation is referred to as **end-point nystagmus,** inasmuch as the movement is present only on extreme deviation of the eyes. These movements may also occur in normal persons when they attempt to fix their eyes on an object outside the field of vision without turning the head, or when they suddenly change the field of vision. The movements disappear when fixation has been established. The tendency toward the phenomenon is increased in fatigue states, paresis of the ocular muscles, and abnormal attempts at fixation, and is often seen in nervous individuals. Exaggerations occur as paretic, fatigue, or latent nystagmus.

Paretic Nystagmus. Paretic nystagmus is a rhythmic nystagmus that often occurs near the limit of the range of movement of a weak ocular muscle. When the subject is looking toward the paretic side, the weak agonist pulls the eyeball outward with a rapid jerk to avoid diplopia, and the antagonistic muscles slowly pull the eyeball back to the neutral position. There may be dissociation between the movements in the paretic and the normal eye. Paretic nystagmus may also occur with paresis of conjugate gaze.

Fatigue Nystagmus. This is similar to paretic nystagmus. It may follow excessive use of or increased fatigability of certain extraocular muscles, and may occur in general fatigue states and asthenia. It is usually observed only at extremes of lateral gaze and is usually abortive rather than sustained. It may occur when an individual attempts to hold his eyes in any extreme position for too long a period of time. In patients with myasthenia gravis one may observe nystagmus that may be of either the paretic or fatigue variety.

Latent Nystagmus. Latent nystagmus appears on covering one eye in subjects with poor visual acuity or without binocular vision, especially in those with unilateral amblyopia. The nystagmus is associated, and the rapid component is in the direction of the open eye. Latent nystagmus may be partially of ocular origin, inasmuch as it represents an attempt to aid vision, but the rhythmicity suggests that it is basically a neuromuscular phenomenon.

Nystagmus Associated With Disease of the Central Nervous System. Nystagmus is a frequent finding and is often of diagnostic import in association with diseases of the central nervous system. It may vary in form, rate, amplitude, and intensity. It may be spontaneous and present at rest, or it may occur only on fixation, at extremes of gaze, or on change of position of the head or body. It is of most significance if it is mixed or rotatory in form or if there is dissociation or disproportion of movements. Rhythmic head movements may accompany nystagmus or even be present in its place. Nystagmus of "central" origin is sometimes of localizing significance, but on most occasions it is not possible to identify the exact site or etiology of the lesion responsible for the nystagmus by clinical examination alone, even though its presence indicates that a pathologic process exists. Eye movements are influenced by the cortical centers in the frontal and occipital lobes, the corticofugal pathways from the centers, the basal ganglia and thalamus, the midbrain centers, the paramedian pontine reticular formation, the nuclei of the ocular nerves, the cerebellum, the vestibular mechanism, and the medial longitudinal fasciculus. Most pathologic nystagmus, however, appears to be associated with involvement of either the medial longitudinal fasciculus or the vestibular mechanism. Cortical irritation may cause conjugate jerking movements of the eyes, but this is not a true nystagmus, and it is probable that cerebral lesions do not cause nystagmus, although they may influence the type of directional preponderance of nystagmus that appears with disease in other parts of the nervous system.

Vestibular Nystagmus. This is a pathologic variation of induced labyrinthine nystagmus, and may be caused by either irritation or destruction of the semicircular canals, vestibular nerves, or vestibular nuclei. Afferent impulses pass from the labyrinths to the vestibular nuclei and then to the nuclei of the ocular muscles, and the efferent path is relayed to the individual muscles. The vestibular nuclei of the two sides are in tonic equilibrium, each nucleus tending to turn the head and eyes to the opposite side. A synergistic relationship between the cortical motor eye fields and the vestibular nuclei is necessary for conjugate movements. Stimulation of the labyrinths, of specific semicircular canals, or of the vestibular nerves or nuclei by a toxic process, pressure, edema, or inflammation produces essentially the same type of response as stimulation of these centers by rotation, heat or cold, or galvanic current, and the response depends upon the type of stimulus and the part of the vestibular system that is stimulated; the slow phase is usually to the opposite side. Destruction of one labyrinth or of one vestibular nerve results in a rhythmic, spontaneous nystagmus, the slow phase of which is toward the injured side, and there may be associated deviation of the eyes and head toward this side. The labyrinths are antagonistic, so that elimination of one acts as a stimulus to the other. The amplitude of the nystagmus is increased when the patient turns his eyes in the direction of the rapid phase or when fixation is eliminated by placing strong lenses in front of the eyes. Nystagmus that follows destruction of one labyrinth gradually diminishes and disappears if the other labyrinth is rendered functionless. It may last only 2 or 3 days and is usually gone in a week, as the loss of one labyrinth is compensated for by processes in the corresponding vestibular nuclei. Lesions of the lateral or medial vestibular nuclei produce a horizontal nystagmus, which may have a rotatory component. Lesions of the superior vestibular nuclei cause a vertical or oblique nystagmus. Vestibular nystagmus is usually accompanied by vertigo.

Hemorrhage into the labyrinth, suppuration of the labyrinth secondary to middle ear disease, increased or decreased pressure of the labyrinthine fluid, pressure on the inner ear, trauma to a vestibular nerve as a result of skull fracture, in-

tracranial hemorrhage, meningitis, involvement of a vestibular nerve by a neoplastic process such as a neurinoma of the cerebellopontine angle, or toxic or inflammatory involvement of the labyrinths or the vestibular nuclei may produce nystagmus that may be temporary or persistent. The nystagmus associated with toxic labyrinthitis may be due to stimulation of the vestibular end-organs by the toxic process, or it may be of the compressive variety, a result of increased pressure of the labyrinthine fluid in the semicircular canals. In Meniere's syndrome the nystagmus may be associated with increased secretion of endolymph or with a change in the acid-base or electrolyte balance. Caloric stimulation of the external auditory canal may differentiate between nystagmus due to irritation and that due to destruction of a labyrinth. With the former the nystagmus will be increased, whereas with the latter no reflex nystagmus will be elicited, and there will be no change in the nystagmus already present. In many disease processes, as in tumors of the cerebellopontine angle, multiple sclerosis, and lesions of the pons and medulla, vestibular nystagmus may be complicated by the existence of nystagmus resulting from involvement of the medial longitudinal fasciculus or other structures.

Cerebellar Nystagmus. This may be an ocular expression of cerebellar asynergia or ataxia, or a result of synergic disorders of fixation of cerebellar origin. It may also result from involvement of the cerebellar connections with the vestibular apparatus, the medial longitudinal fasciculus, or higher centers. The portions of the cerebellum most closely related to the vestibular complex are the flocculonodular lobe and the fastigial nuclei. The pyramis, however, and even the hemispheres, have some regulatory effect on vestibular function. With unilateral lesions of the cerebellum the eyes at rest may be deviated 10° – 30° toward the unaffected side. When the subject attempts to focus on an object directly in front of him the eyes wander slowly back to the resting position and are returned to the midline by means of quick jerks. When he looks toward either side, there are quick jerks toward the point of fixation with slow return movements to the resting point. The rapid movements are always in the direction of gaze, and the slow movements are toward the position of rest. The nystagmus is always more marked and the movements are slower and of greater amplitude when the patient looks toward the side of the lesion. It is said that cerebellar nystagmus is dependent upon fixation, in contrast to vestibular nystagmus, which is increased when fixation is eliminated by the use of strong lenses. In vestibular nystagmus the slow phase is toward the injured side, whereas in cerebellar nystagmus the slow phase depends upon the position of the eyes.

Nystagmus is a common sign in patients with cerebellar lesions of various etiologies, but owing to the multiplicity of connections between the cerebellum and other centers, it may be difficult to determine the exact site of the responsible lesion. Its presence usually indicates, however, that the vestibulocerebellar pathways are affected, and therefore most often suggests involvement of either the vermis region or the inferior cerebellar peduncle. The nystagmus with hemispheric lesions may be a pressure phenomenon or may represent an asynergia rather than a true nystagmus. Nystagmus is usually not present in parenchymatous cerebellar degenerations. With a tumor of the cerebellopontine angle the nystagmus is coarse on looking toward the side of the lesion, and fine and rapid on gaze to the opposite side.

Nystagmus With Lesions of the Medial Longitudinal Fasciculus.

Interruption of the impulses between the center for lateral gaze in the pons and the oculomotor nuclei (**internuclear ophthalmoplegia**) may cause dissociated lateral gaze palsies and dissociated nystagmus. In the **syndrome of the medial longitudinal fasciculus** there is usually paralysis of adduction of the contralateral eye on attempted gaze to one side, and a coarse monocular nystagmus of the abducting eye with the rapid movement in the direction of gaze. This is termed **dissociated,** or **ataxic, nystagmus;** there may also be vertical nystagmus. This syndrome, especially if bilateral, is often found in multiple sclerosis, but it may occur in vascular, neoplastic, and other lesions of the brain stem.

Other Types of "Central" Nystagmus.

It is often not possible to localize accurately the lesion responsible for nystagmus associated with various pathologic processes. Nystagmus of pathologic significance is produced mainly by lesions affecting structures in the region of the fourth ventricle, either its roof or floor, or by involvement of the brain stem, principally the zone between the oculomotor nuclei and the vestibular nuclei. Cerebral lesions probably do not cause spontaneous nystagmus, unless there is associated pressure on or involvement of other structures; they may, however, influence or alter

induced nystagmus and that produced by lesions elsewhere.

The presence of unequal movements in the two eyes, or of dissociated or disjunctive nystagmus, is usually indicative of interruption of impulses within the brain stem, but sometimes occurs with other lesions in the posterior fossa. Vertical nystagmus usually indicates involvement of the superior vestibular nuclei or their connections in the medial longitudinal fasciculus, but it may be present with peripheral labyrinthine lesions, intoxications, or even cerebellar disease. **Convergence nystagmus** (a rhythmic oscillation with slow abduction of the eyes followed by a quick adduction) occurs with anterior midbrain, posterior third ventricle, and periaqueductal lesions and is often seen with Parinaud's syndrome; the nystagmus may be precipitated by attempts at upward gaze. **Retraction nystagmus** (an oscillatory retraction of the eyeballs) is found with lesions in the region of the aqueduct, and also in Parinaud's syndrome; it may be brought out by testing for vertical optokinetic nystagmus with the stimulus directed downward.

"**Downbeat**" **nystagmus** has been described in association with brain stem lesions, acute meningoencephalitis and hypomagnesemia. "**Upbeat**" **nystagmus** is probably caused by lesions of the anterior vermis of the cerebellum. **Periodic alternating nystagmus** has also been described; its cause is uncertain. **See-saw nystagmus** is a vertical disjunctive variety in which one eye moves upward while the other moves down; there usually are associated torsional movements. Most cases have occurred in patients with tumors of the suprasellar region or anterior third ventricle or other lesions affecting the optic chiasm and causing a bitemporal hemianopia, although some investigators feel that a brain stem lesion can also cause this type of nystagmus.

The nystagmus of posterior fossa lesions is not necessarily the result of direct irritation or destruction of the aforementioned structures, but may be caused by pressure on them, edema, or interruption of the blood supply. The presence of associated signs and symptoms, such as cranial nerve palsies, conjugate gaze pareses, coordination difficulties, and sensory changes, may aid in the localization of the lesion. The nystagmus that occurs with conditions such as multiple sclerosis, Friedreich's ataxia, olivopontocerebellar atrophy, syringobulbia, encephalitis, and vascular, neoplastic, and degenerative diseases may be caused by lesions in various sites, and sometimes is the result of disseminated involvement.

Miscellaneous Varieties of Nystagmus.
Toxic nystagmus may be caused by the ingestion or injection of various drugs and toxins — barbiturates and related drugs, phenytoin, lead, nicotine, chloroform, quinine, alcohol. The movement is usually rhythmic, horizontal (but in severe cases vertical), rather coarse, and increased on lateral gaze, with the rapid component in the direction of gaze. The site of action of these drugs is not known, but they probably affect the vestibular connections and the brain stem; toxins associated with infectious states may affect the labyrinths. The nystagmus seen in patients with epilepsy is usually due to the anticonvulsant medication rather than a manifestation of the underlying disease process. The appearance of nystagmus in a patient receiving anticonvulsants does not call for withdrawal of the drug, but an increase in the nystagmus along with either vertigo or diplopia may be the first sign of intoxication; blood anticonvulsant levels usually settle the issue.

The intravenous administration of barbiturates or mephenesin or the injection of curare causes nystagmus to appear promptly. Coarse nystagmus on lateral gaze appears first, then nystagmus on vertical gaze, and finally nystagmus on direct forward gaze. Such administration of these drugs also causes inability to maintain gaze on voluntary deviation of the eyes, and abolishes optokinetic nystagmus. These drugs also alter induced and pathologic varieties of nystagmus. Small doses of barbiturates abolish optokinetic nystagmus and larger doses first increase and then abolish vestibular nystagmus. Barbiturates may also abolish the nystagmus on direct forward gaze in such conditions as multiple sclerosis and diseases of the brain stem; they may temporarily stop latent and some types of congenital nystagmus; they may alter the nystagmus of chronic alcoholics, and produce a fine shimmering variety. Meperidine may cause a downbeating nystagmus.

Congenital or Hereditary Nystagmus.
This variety, which dates from birth, must be differentiated from ocular nystagmus, which does not develop until fixation is attempted. It is not associated with grossly defective vision, and is usually rhythmic, rapid, and either horizontal or rotatory. It may vary in form and rate, however, and occasionally is vertical; it may be pendular at rest and rhythmic on lateral gaze, with

the rapid component in the direction of gaze. It is probably the result of hypoplasia or some other developmental anomaly of the central nervous system. Congenital nystagmus may be inherited as an autosomal dominant trait; it may be sex-linked, occurring only in males, or it may be irregularly dominant, occurring in both sexes. It may be associated with partial albinism.

Pathologic Alterations of Induced Nystagmus. Optokinetic nystagmus can be tested in states of lowered consciousness and caloric nystagmus in some stages of coma. Abnormalities of caloric response indicate interruption of brain stem pathways. The caloric responses are absent in near-terminal states of coma and severe brain stem disease. Optokinetic and labyrinthine nystagmus may be either altered or absent with lesions of various parts of the central nervous system. Contralateral optokinetic nystagmus is defective or diminished with deep cerebral lesions affecting the temporal, occipital, and parietal areas, especially the latter. This is true whether or not there is a hemianopic defect. With brain stem lesions there may be a dissociation of vertical responses or between vertical and horizontal responses, or a depression or unilateral defect of optokinetic nystagmus. On the other hand, with involvement of the posterior portion of the temporal lobe, there is a **directional preponderance** (i.e., increase in duration and intensity) of caloric or rotational nystagmus to the side of the lesion when tested with optic fixation maintained, but absence or reversal of this preponderance when optic fixation is abolished. These alterations of induced nystagmus in the presence of disease indicate that centers in various portions of the nervous system may either inhibit or exert directional control over these ocular movements.

Nystagmus Due to Involvement of the Cervical Portion of the Spinal Cord.
Lesions of the spinal cord, usually above the fourth cervical segment, may produce nystagmus. This is uncommon, but has been reported in syringomyelia, tumors, and other lesions. It may indicate involvement of the medial longitudinal fasciculus or of the spinovestibular pathways, or may be related to the tonic neck reflexes and their effect on ocular movement.

Positional Nystagmus. Nystagmus secondary to organic disease may be present only with alterations of the position of the head or body. One variety, which is usually transient, has been reported with posttraumatic vertigo and certain nonprogressive lesions of the nervous system; this has been termed **positional nystagmus of the benign, paroxysmal type,** and may be secondary to involvement of the utricle. Another variety, which persists as long as the critical head position is maintained, but may be accompanied by less severe vertigo, has been reported with metastatic involvement of the cerebellum and brain stem; this has been called **positional nystagmus of the central type.** Many of the other varieties of pathologic nystagmus may be altered or influenced by changes in the position of the head or body.

Hysterical Nystagmus. This has been described, but its actual existence is doubtful. The movements are said to be jerky and irregular, and occasionally accompanied by spasm of the orbicularis oculi and medial rectus muscles. If it does occur, it may be caused by inadequate neuromuscular control of the lateral eye movements and failure of alternate contraction of the agonists and antagonists on deviation of the eyes. It may be brought on by emotional strain, but it must be borne in mind that a true pathologic nystagmus may be increased by nervous tension, and nervous and fatigued individuals are especially apt to show nystagmoid movements or fixation nystagmus when they attempt to deviate their eyes and to fix them on some object.

Voluntary Nystagmus. Simulated nystagmus, or that of voluntary origin, has also been described. It is usually pendular and horizontal, and may be either unilateral or bilateral. The movements are extremely rapid; they are increased by fixation, convergence, and increasing the width of the palpebral fissures. The nystagmus disappears when the subject's attention is distracted or when vision is blurred by a convex lens placed in front of each eye. It is doubtful whether these voluntary movements of the eyeballs should be considered a variety of nystagmus.

Other Abnormal Movements

Oculogyric Crises. These consist of attacks of involuntary conjugate upward deviation of the eyeballs. Occasionally there is also some deviation to one side, or the eyes may be turned downward. The attacks may be transitory or last for hours, until the patient is able to get to sleep.

He may be able to turn the eyeballs downward for short periods of time, but be unable to keep them down. These phenomena are found in postencephalitic syndromes and as a side reaction from the use of phenothiazine and related drugs. The latter are the commonest cause of oculogyric crises at this time. There may be associated weakness of upward gaze between attacks, and jerkiness of ocular movements. Oculogyric crises from neuroleptic drugs may also be tardive or persistent. In absence seizures there may be brief spasms of upward gaze.

Spasmodic Lateral Deviation of the Eyes. Irritation of the cerebral centers controlling conjugate gaze may cause spasmodic lateral deviation of the eyes (Fig. 11-20). There may be associated turning of the head to the same side. This phenomenon is often seen in jacksonian convulsions, and it may be of localizing significance if it precedes generalized convulsions, although recent studies disagree on this point. A pseudospasm of conjugate gaze may be a feature of pontine lesions in which there is paralysis of gaze to the opposite side. Reflex deviation of the eyes in response to labyrinthine, cochlear, retinal, trigeminal, and postural stimulation has been mentioned previously.

Opsoclonus. The term **opsoclonus** has been given to rarely occurring coarse, irregular, nonrhythmic, "agitated" oscillations of the eyeballs in both horizontal and vertical planes. The movements, when present, may persist for long periods of time. They have been observed in encephalitis, cerebellar and brain stem disorders,

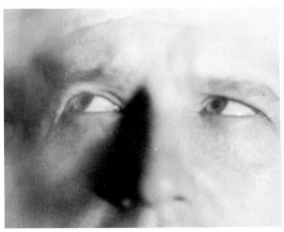

FIG. 11–20. Forced conjugate gaze to the right in a patient with a neoplasm of the left frontal lobe.

comatose states, metabolic encephalopathies and as part of paraneoplastic syndromes.

A description of other somewhat related and also rare abnormalities of ocular movement follows: Brief periods of **flutterlike** or **shimmering oscillations** are sometimes present with cerebellar lesions as well as on attempts to fix the eyes in a defective field of vision; they are also seen on occasion without disease in tense and nervous individuals. With some of the spinocerebellar degenerations there may be both flutterlike oscillations and dysmetria in pursuit movements. Brief bursts of rapid horizontal to-and-fro movements, called **lightning movements** or **ocular myoclonus,** may occur with midbrain or cerebellar lesions. Intermittent periods of coarse, synchronous, downward "bobbing" movements of the eyes (**ocular bobbing**) have been observed in coma and with pontine lesions. Ocular bobbing usually has grave significance, but may also be present in drug intoxications.

Rapid eye movements, which can be seen through the closed lids, occur periodically during sleep. During a normal night's sleep most individuals have four or five periods of what has been called paradoxical or activated sleep which takes up 20% – 25% of the sleeping time. The rapid eye movements (REM) are present during these periods (Ch. 54).

EXOPHTHALMOS AND ENOPHTHALMOS

Either exophthalmos or enophthalmos may occur in disease of the nervous system and may be of significance in neurologic diagnosis. Enophthalmos has already been referred to under the discussion of paralysis of the cervical portion of the sympathetic nervous system; it may also occur in intraorbital disease with loss of orbital tissue.

Exophthalmos may be bilateral, as it usually is in hyperthyroidism, but unilateral exophthalmos is more significant in the diagnosis of neurologic disease. It may be due to hypertonus of the smooth muscle of the orbit secondary to sympathetic overstimulation, but more frequently is a pressure manifestation. In the appraisal of exophthalmos one should note such phenomena as **Graefe's sign** (retarded descent of the eyelid during movement of the globe from the primary position to downgaze), lid lag (a static situation of the eyelid being higher than normal with the globe in downgaze), **Möbius'**

sign (insufficient convergence), **Dalrymple's sign** (increased width of the palpebral fissures), and **Stellwag's sign** (infrequent blinking). Malignant exophthalmos may occur spontaneously or following thyroidectomy; there may be associated ocular muscle palsies. Bilateral exophthalmos occasionally occurs in patients with increased intracranial pressure. Unilateral exophthalmos may be present in hyperthyroidism, but it is usually indicative of some localized intracranial or intraorbital disease. It may be seen in brain tumors, especially meningiomas of the sphenoidal ridge and olfactory groove. It may occur in association with a tumor or mucocele within the orbit, orbital cellulitis, deformities of the skull, or may be a sign of orbital pseudotumor. Pulsating exophthalmos may be caused by an intracranial aneurysm, angioma, or arteriovenous fistula; a pulsation may be felt or a bruit heard over the protruded eye. **Proptosis,** a marked forward displacement of the eyeball, is an exaggerated degree of exophthalmos. When it occurs in cavernous sinus thrombosis there is associated **chemosis,** or edema of the conjunctiva, together with edema of the eyelids and paralysis of the third, fourth, and sixth nerves. In determining slight degrees of exophthalmos and enophthalmos an exophthalmometer may be used.

DISORDERS OF THE OCULAR NERVES

Localization of Lesions of the Ocular Nerves

In appraising lesions of the nerves of ocular movement, one must differentiate between isolated involvement of a single nerve or of part of a nerve and involvement of these nerves in various combinations, and between infranuclear, nuclear, and supranuclear lesions. By noting in detail the manifestations of disordered function of these nerves, together with evidence of involvement of associated structures, one may be able to decide whether the pathologic lesion is in the cerebrum, midbrain, pons, medulla, or spinal cord; outside the brain or brain stem but within the skull; in the middle cranial fossa; or within the cavernous sinus or the orbit.

Paralysis of the *third nerve* may be either partial or complete. If the lesion is within the midbrain or within the orbit, the involvement is incomplete, but one along the course of the nerve may cause a complete paralysis. Among the more frequent causes of third nerve palsy are intracranial aneurysms, trauma, diabetes, neoplasms, compression of the nerve trunk by an atheromatous posterior cerebral artery, and compression by hippocampal herniation; since the pupilloconstrictor fibers are in the upper portion of the nerve, hippocampal herniation may affect only these, and there is pupillary dilation but no ptosis or ocular palsy. Incomplete palsies produce a variety of impaired movements; all may be weakened, or some may be defective and others paralyzed. One muscle only may be involved, or all except one. There may be paralysis of only the ciliary muscle, with resulting cycloplegia, or of the sphincter iridis, with resulting iridoplegia, or both may be involved. If the voluntary muscles are paralyzed, there may be either an external ophthalmoplegia or ptosis, or both. With faulty regeneration and misdirection of oculomotor fibers following third nerve paralysis certain synkinetic movements may appear: retraction of the upper lid, medial rotation of the eye, and constriction of the pupil take place on downward gaze (the **pseudo-Graefe syndrome**). If there is a residual partial ptosis, there may also be elevation of the lid on attempted medial and upward gaze, and the ptosis may increase with abduction.

An isolated *fourth nerve* paralysis is difficult to diagnose, since the ocular movements are only slightly disturbed and there is little deviation of the eyeball. The defect in function of the superior oblique may be hidden by the collateral action of the lateral and inferior recti. There is, however, a deviation of the face forward, downward, and toward the unaffected side, and the chin is tilted toward the shoulder of the involved side. The patient may complain of difficulty in descending stairs. In a nuclear palsy of the fourth nerve the defect is on the contralateral side, but in involvement of the nerve itself it is ipsilateral. An isolated fourth nerve paralysis most frequently follows trauma.

Isolated paralysis of the *sixth nerve* occurs more frequently than does that of the third or the fourth nerve, and bilateral sixth nerve paralysis may be present without localizing significance with increased intracranial pressure, diabetes, vascular disease, brain stem displacement, meningitis, and trauma to the skull.

Nuclear involvement of the ocular nerves may be the result of vascular lesions, such as hemorrhages or thromboses within the brain stem or vertebrobasilar artery insufficiency, or of inflammatory lesions, deficiency states, neoplasms, trauma, metabolic disorders, multiple sclerosis, syringobulbia, or other disorders of the midbrain and brain stem. Any or all of the nerves may be affected. Even though only one nerve may be paralyzed, there are usually associated manifestations that indicate extension of the process to involve the medial longitudinal fasciculus, the descending corticospinal pathways, the ascending sensory tracts, the cerebellar connections, or neighboring cranial nerve nuclei. Thus, nuclear third nerve lesions may be accompanied by involvement of the superior colliculus, red nucleus, substantia nigra, cerebral peduncles, medial longitudinal fasciculus, or ascending sensory pathways. In a nuclear lesion of the sixth nerve there is often involvement of other nuclei, such as that of the seventh nerve, or of other pathways, such as the medial longitudinal fasciculus.

Infranuclear lesions, resulting from involvement of the nerves after they have left the brain stem, may be caused by lesions within the skull, in the middle cranial fossa, in the cavernous sinus, in the superior orbital fissure, or in the orbit. Involvement within the skull may be produced by meningitis, basal hemorrhage, trauma to the skull, or concussion. Neuritic palsies may have the same etiologies as other polyneuritides—deficiency states, metabolic disorders, exposure to or ingestion of toxins, diphtheria and other infections, collagen disorders, amyloidosis, and others; they may be part of polyradiculoneuritis or the Guillain–Barré syndrome. Any or all of the nerves may be involved with lesions or fistulas within the cavernous sinus, lesions in the region of the superior orbital fissure, and with intracranial aneurysms, especially those involving the internal carotid artery or its branches. All may be involved, but in a different manner, in neoplasms, granulomas, or infections within the orbit. Pathologic changes within the muscles themselves, such as those associated with trichinosis, rheumatic infiltrations, myositis, fatty degeneration, and other strictly muscular disorders or disorders of the myoneural junction, may also produce disturbances of ocular movement.

Supranuclear lesions that cause disturbances of function of the ocular nerves may occur in the cerebral cortex, basal ganglia, internal capsule, midbrain, or brain stem. Neoplasms, vascular lesions, inflammations, trauma and degenerative changes of the cerebrum may affect the ocular nerves through involvement of either the cerebral centers which regulate their function or of the infracortical connections. Irritative lesions cause abnormalities of movement, whereas destructive lesions cause paresis of conjugate gaze and may also cause abnormalities in induced nystagmus. In disease of the extrapyramidal system there may be dyskinesias of ocular movement, such as the oculogyric crisis, along with slowness or jerkiness of movement. In progressive supranuclear palsy, there is often loss of conjugate downward gaze, whereas in Parkinson's disease conjugate upward gaze may be impaired.

Disorders Associated With Ocular Nerve Abnormalities

Abnormalities of the ocular nerves are especially important in the diagnosis of many diseases of the nervous system. In multiple sclerosis there may be nystagmus, ocular palsies with diplopia, ptosis, and pupillary abnormalities. Nystagmus is a very frequent finding; it is rhythmic, usually horizontal but occasionally rotatory or mixed, and relatively coarse. The presence of dissociated, or ataxic, nystagmus is significant. Inasmuch as multiple sclerosis may also be accompanied by retrobulbar neuritis, optic atrophy, scotomas, and changes in the retinal arteries and veins, the examination of the eyes is of extreme importance in its diagnosis.

In syphilis of the central nervous system the pupillary reflexes are especially important, but there may also be a third nerve paralysis, isolated palsies, ptosis, and other ocular manifestations. Most characteristically one finds Argyll Robertson pupils, but a sluggish or paradoxical pupillary response, anisocoria, or irregularity of the pupils may be significant. The manifestations may be caused by vascular, inflammatory, or degenerative changes associated with syphilitic involvement. Optic atrophy is also found in central nervous system syphilis, and cerebral involvement by gummas or thromboses may cause defects in the visual fields. Interstitial keratitis has been considered to be almost exclusively the result of congenital syphilis, but in **Cogan's syndrome** there is sudden onset of vertigo, tinnitus, and deafness accompanied by photophobia, blurred vision, and interstitial keratitis, which is nonsyphilitic; the etiology is uncertain, but it may either be of infectious origin or related to polyarteritis nodosa.

Congenital and developmental abnormalities may cause dysfunction of ocular motility and related phenomena. Strabismus and ocular imbalance, when present from birth, may be of muscular rather than neurologic origin. Ptosis may be congenital. A large percentage of pa-

tients with cerebral palsy of various types have strabismus, ocular palsies, or motor imbalance. There may be associated mental deficiency and epilepsy. All of these symptoms result from cortical or cerebral damage prior to, during, or immediately after delivery. Similar ocular signs, along with nystagmus, optic atrophy and other visual defects, may play an important part of the clinical picture in such inherited, developmental, and degenerative conditions as congenital hydrocephalus, craniostenosis, Down's syndrome, albinism, and the lipidoses.

Diplopia and ocular palsies are important in the diagnosis of acute encephalitis. **Polioencephalitis hemorrhagica superioris,** or **Wernicke's polioencephalitis,** is characterized by ocular palsies, nystagmus, ataxia, and disturbances of consciousness. It occurs mainly with chronic alcoholism, but also with hyperemesis gravidarum and other states of malnutrition, and is the result of thiamine deficiency. Diplopia, nystagmus, pupillary changes, and even complete ocular palsies are sometimes found in acute bulbar poliomyelitis. In polioencephalitis inferior and botulism the initial symptoms may be difficulty with convergence, followed by ptosis, dilated pupils, and paralysis of extraocular muscles. In postdiphtheritic paralysis there is loss of accommodation, often with associated weakness of convergence; blurring of vision for near objects is a common symptom.

In chronic progressive external ophthalmoplegia there is a gradually increasing weakness of the muscles of the eyelids and the extraocular muscles; the condition may be familial. It is often associated with progressive muscular alterations, rather than degeneration of nuclear centers, and is a myopathy or dystrophy of the ocular muscles; other evidence of muscular dystrophy may accompany or follow the ocular involvement. When progressive external ophthalmoplegia is associated with pigmentary degeneration of the retina and complete heart block, the term **Kearns – Sayre syndrome** is used. There is evidence that progressive external ophthalmoplegia may be a manifestation of more wide-spread mitochondrial disorders, many of which have been biochemically classified. In myotonic dystrophy there may be ptosis along with baldness and changes in the facial expression and voice; there is either myotonia of the lids or a myotonic lid lag.

The earliest symptoms of myasthenia gravis are often referable to the muscles supplied by the ocular nerves, and the patient may notice diplopia and ptosis that come on with activity and are relieved by rest. The amount of ptosis with ocular muscle weakness may fluctuate during a brief period of examination. There is often weakness of the frontalis and orbicularis oculi as well as of the levator. The weakness is often asymmetrical. The neostigmine or edrophonium tests may confirm the diagnosis. Ocular symptoms and signs similar to those of myasthenia may be found in the myasthenic syndrome of Eaton – Lambert.

In hyperthyroidism or excessive production of pituitary thyrotropic hormone there may be paralysis of extraocular muscles in addition to the exophthalmos and associated signs already mentioned (see "Exophthalmos and Enophthalmos"); hypothyroidism may cause edema of the eyelids that simulates ptosis. Diabetes mellitus is one of the more common causes of paralysis of the third and other ocular nerves; the pupil is often spared. However, in diabetes there may be an abnormality of the pupillary response of the Argyll Robertson type. Recurring cranial nerve palsies may be seen in sarcoidosis. Single or multiple cranial nerve palsies are also a feature of human immunodeficiency virus infections. Paralysis of the abducens nerve, and sometimes of the other ocular nerves, may be a complication or sequel of spinal anesthesia. Variable ophthalmoplegias have been reported with angioneurotic edema. Recurrent ocular palsies are seen in ophthalmoplegic migraine and in periodic paralysis of the familial type; both may result in permanent paralysis. There may be partial ptosis and miosis during the attacks of so-called cluster headaches. Cyclic oculomotor paralysis has been described.

In the syndrome of superior orbital fissuritis (**Tolosa Hunt syndrome**), acute episodes of painful ophthalmoplegia may occur which often respond promptly to steroids. Other syndromes of the superior orbital fissure may result from sphenoid sinusitis and skull fractures. The third nerve is affected and frequently the optic nerve as well. In Friedreich's ataxia, in other cerebellar familial ataxias, and cerebellar and labyrinthine lesions nystagmus is an important finding. In Gerlier's disease, or paralyzing vertigo, diplopia and ptosis are often present. Ocular torticollis may be associated with involvement of one or more of the ocular nerves, especially paralysis of the trochlear nerve. Ocular torticollis may date from birth or from the time of development of fusion; the deformity can usually be corrected voluntarily. In Parkinson's disease there may be saccadic or jerky ocular movements, sometimes referred to as "cogwheel" in type, and weakness of convergence or of upward gaze. There often is infrequent blinking and associated lid retraction, but repeated blinking movements may appear when threatening movements are made toward the eyes or when the bridge of the nose is tapped with a reflex hammer (**Myerson's sign**). These phenomena, together with oculogyric crises, blepharospasm, and abnormalities of the pupillary responses, occur more frequently in postencephalitic than in idiopathic parkinsonism. Abnormalities of ocular motility may also be present in Wilson's disease, progressive supranuclear palsy, and other extrapyramidal disorders.

In meningitis and trauma to the skull one finds various ocular palsies and pupillary changes. Ptosis, photophobia, and dissociation of ocular movements may also be present in meningitis. These same manifestations are seen in subarachnoid hemorrhage. Aneurysms of the internal carotid artery or of the circle of Willis may affect any or all of the ocular nerves. Such involvement in a patient who has had a subarachnoid hemorrhage usually indicates the presence of a localized aneurysmal dilation; supraclinoid carotid aneurysm is one of the most common causes of an isolated oculomotor paralysis. Thrombosis of the cavernous sinus, cavernous fistulas, and intraorbital neoplasms or infections may produce proptosis with ocular palsies. The typical syndrome of cavernous sinus thrombosis consists of ipsilateral proptosis, chemosis, edema of the eyelid and orbital tissues, paralysis of the third, fourth, and sixth nerves, and involvement of the upper divisions of the trigeminal nerve; papilledema is sometimes present.

Intracranial neoplasms, abscesses, granulomas, hematomas, hemorrhages, and thromboses may cause disturbances of function of the ocular nerves, and also of the optic nerves, which aid not only in diagnosis but also in localization. Significant findings include extraocular muscle palsies, disturbances of conjugate gaze, pupillary changes, and nystagmus. Also significant, as far as the second nerve is concerned, are papilledema, optic atrophy, and field defects. Increased intracranial pressure alone may cause either unilateral or bilateral abducens palsy. Such a sixth nerve palsy may be a false localizing sign not predictably ipsilateral to the mass lesion causing the pressure. The ipsilateral pupil may be dilated and fixed with expanding intracranial lesions, owing to compression by hippocampal herniation. A dilated unreactive pupil may also result from local irritation alone in children with bacterial meningitis. Hemorrhages, thromboses, and tumors of the brain stem are also important causes of ocular nerve dysfunction, as well as of transient blurring of vision, field defects, and conjugate gaze palsy. Brain stem hemorrhages and thromboses frequently cause marked miosis, owing to bilateral interruption of descending dilator pathways. Ocular palsies, nystagmus, and involvement of neighboring cranial nerves or ascending or descending pathways may aid in localization.

Many syndromes have been described in which there is involvement of the nerves of ocular movement and the cervical sympathetic pathways. Horner's syndrome has been mentioned under "Sympathetic Innervation." By evaluating the signs and symptoms of involvement of neighboring structures, it is often possible to localize, within the brain stem or spinal cord or along the sympathetic pathway, the responsible lesion. The syndrome may occur, for instance, in thrombosis of the posterior inferior cerebellar artery, with associated fifth and tenth nerve and spinothalamic involvement, or in **Raeder's paratrigeminal syndrome,** with associated motor and sensory changes in the trigeminal nerve. It has also been reported in association with thrombosis of the internal carotid artery.

Parinaud's syndrome, or paralysis of conjugate upward gaze, has also been mentioned; there may be, in association, fixed pupils or pupils which react in accommodation but not to light, and there often is paralysis of convergence. There may be convergence nystagmus or retraction nystagmus. This symptom complex is caused by lesions at the level of the anterior quadrigeminal bodies, and it is sometimes referred to as the **syndrome of the superior colliculus,** or the **pineal syndrome;** it is found in encephalitis and in tumors of the pineal gland, the posterior portion of the third ventricle, and the mesencephalon.

Gradenigo's syndrome consists of a lateral rectus palsy associated with pain, swelling, and tenderness behind the ipsilateral ear; it indicates inflammatory involvement of the petrous pyramid.

Benedict's syndrome, or the **tegmental syndrome of the midbrain,** is caused by a lesion of the midbrain involving the third nerve as it passes through the red nucleus. It is characterized by an ipsilateral oculomotor paralysis with contralateral ataxia, tremor, and hyperkinesis of the upper extremity. If the cerebral peduncle is also involved, there is a contralateral hemiparesis, and extension to the medial lemniscus

produces loss of proprioceptive sensation and diminished tactile sensation on the opposite side of the body. In **Claude's syndrome,** limited to the third nerve and red nucleus, there is an ipsilateral oculomotor paresis with contralateral ataxia and tremor. **Weber's syndrome,** or **superior alternating hemiplegia,** consists of an ipsilateral third nerve paralysis and a contralateral paresis of the lower face, tongue, and extremities. This is caused by involvement of the oculomotor nerve as it passes through the cerebral peduncle. In **Nothnagel's syndrome** there is a unilateral oculomotor paralysis combined with ipsilateral cerebellar ataxia, owing to involvement of the third nerve and the brachium conjunctivum. In the **syndrome of the mesencephalic gray matter** there are bilateral internal and external ophthalmoplegias, because of total bilateral oculomotor paralysis. The **syndrome of the interpeduncular space** consists of bilateral third nerve paralysis together with a spastic tetraparesis; there is involvement of the emerging fibers of both oculomotor nerves and of both cerebral peduncles.

Raymond's syndrome consists of an ipsilateral sixth nerve paralysis and a contralateral paresis of the extremities. More frequent is the **Millard – Gubler syndrome,** or **middle alternating hemiplegia.** In this there is an ipsilateral lateral rectus paralysis, probably because of nuclear involvement, with an ipsilateral facial paralysis, probably owing to involvement of the root fibers, and a contralateral spastic hemiplegia resulting from involvement of the corticospinal fibers.

Foville's syndrome is characterized by an ipsilateral facial paralysis owing to involvement of the root fibers, an ipsilateral paralysis of lateral gaze because of involvement of the center for lateral gaze or the medial longitudinal fasciculus, and a contralateral corticospinal hemiplegia. There is contralateral deviation of the eyes, and sometimes of the head as well. According to some authorities there is paresis of conjugate gaze and lateral rotation of the head contralateral to the lesion, with ipsilateral deviation, resulting from involvement of the aberrant oculogyric and cephalogyric pyramidal fibers.

In any of the last three syndromes there may be individual variations; involvement of the medial lemniscus causes loss of proprioceptive sensation and diminished tactile sensation on the opposite side of the body. The internuclear ophthalmoplegias and the syndrome of the medial longitudinal fasciculus have been described (see "Supranuclear Lesions").

The **Raymond – Céstan syndrome** has been described variously. Characteristically there is ipsilateral paralysis of conjugate gaze or contralateral ocular deviation because of involvement of the center for lateral gaze, or the medial longitudinal fasciculus, with contralateral hemiplegia and loss of proprioceptive and diminished tactile sensation, resulting from involvement of the corticospinal pathways and the medial lemniscus. In addition, there may be ipsilateral ataxia and dyssynergy as a result of involvement of the inferior cerebellar peduncle. Occasionally there is bilateral spastic paresis, with paralysis of lateral gaze in both directions and dissociation of eye movements, owing to involvement of both corticospinal pathways and both medial longitudinal fasciculi. The syndrome follows a hemorrhage or a thrombosis of the basilar artery or its pontine branches. Conditions in which the primary involvement is in the medulla (Ch. 18) may also influence eye movements.

In **Gerhardt's syndrome** there is a bilateral abducens palsy. **Möbius' syndrome** (see Fig. 13-7, Ch. 13) is characterized by paralysis or paresis of the ocular muscles, especially the abducens, together with paralysis or paresis of the facial muscles; pontomedullary necrotic foci and small calcifications have been found on imaging studies in patients with this syndrome. In **Duane's syndrome** there is widening of the palpebral fissure on abduction and narrowing on adduction of the affected eye. There is also limitation of lateral gaze, and there may be retraction and elevation of the globe on adduction. This has been explained on the basis of either aplasia of the abducens nerve with anomalous innervation of the lateral rectus by the oculomotor nerve or fibrosis of the lateral rectus and levator muscles. In the **syndrome of Foix,** found in cavernous sinus lesions and in periostitis, fractures, tumors, and aneurysms in the region of the superior orbital fissure, the third, fourth, and sixth nerves and the ophthalmic division of the trigeminal nerve are involved. The **syndrome of the tentorial notch,** or the **uncal syndrome,** occurs with herniation of the uncus and/or hippocampal gyrus through the incisura of the tentorium cerebelli, usually due to increased intracranial pressure or a mass lesion in the ipsilateral cerebral hemisphere. The first sign of this is a dilated pupil, which may not react to light, on the side of the compression. Later a complete third nerve paralysis appears, along with signs of lateral midbrain compression, causing a contralateral corticospinal paresis, progressive coma, and, finally, decerebrate rigidity. Compression of the posterior cerebral artery may cause a hemianopia. Occasionally there is a so-called central syndrome with Cheyne-Stokes respirations, constricted pupils, and bilateral corticospinal tract involvement. Pupillary dilation with passive neck flexion may indicate transient compression of the brain stem or its vascular supply, and thus may be a sign of impending uncal herniation.

Disturbances in function of the ocular nerves may also be on a *psychogenic basis.* Paresis of the ocular muscles or the levator rarely occurs, but there may be spasm of these muscles (Ch. 55). Spasm of convergence is most frequently encountered. Hysterical ptosis has been described; this is probably the result of spasm of the orbicularis (blepharospasm) rather than paresis of the levator. Diplopia, if present, may be monocular, or there may be polyopia. The existence of hysterical nystagmus is doubtful. In anxiety states and some psychoses the pupils may be large.

BIBLIOGRAPHY

Adams RD, Victor M. Principles of Neurology, 4th ed. New York, McGraw – Hill, 1989

Adie WJ. Tonic pupils and absent tendon reflexes: a benign disorder sui generis; Its complete and incomplete forms. Brain 1932;55:98

Adler FH. Physiology of the Eye: Clinical Applications, 2nd ed. St. Louis, CV Mosby, 1953

Anderson JR. Ocular Vertical Deviations and the Treatment of Nystagmus, 2nd ed. Philadelphia, JB Lippincott, 1959

Anderson NE, Budde – Steffen C, Rosenblum MK et al. Opsoclonus, myoclonus, ataxia, and encephalopathy in adults with cancer: A distinct paraneoplastic syndrome. Medicine 1988;67:100

Aschan G, Bergstedt M, Stahle J. Nystagmography. Acta Otolaryngol (suppl) 1956; 129:1

Bender MB (ed). The Oculomotor System. New York, Harper & Row, 1964

Bender MB, Rudolph SH, Stacy CB. The neurology of the visual and oculomotor systems. In Joynt RJ (ed). Clinical Neurology. Philadelphia, JB Lippincott, 1989

Büttner – Ennever JA, Akert K. Medial rectus subgroups of the oculomotor nucleus and their abducens internuclear input in the monkey. J Comp Neurol 1981;197:17

Büttner – Ennever JA, Büttner U, Cohen B et al. Vertical gaze paralysis and the rostral interstitial nucleus of the medial longitudinal fasciculus. Brain 1982;105:125

Cogan DG. Neurology of the Ocular Muscles, 2nd ed. Springfield, IL: Charles C Thomas, 1956

Crosby EC. Nystagmus as a sign of central nervous system involvement. Ann Otol Rhinol Laryngol 1953;62:1117

Currie J, Lessell S. Tonic pupil with giant cell arteritis. Br J Ophthalmol 1984;68:135

Dacso CC, Bortz DL. Significance of the Argyll – Robertson pupil in clinical medicine. Am J Med 1989;86:199

Dagi LR, Chrousos GA, Cogan DC. Spasm of the near reflex associated with organic disease. Am J Ophthalmol 1987;103:582

Daroff RB, Hoyt WF. Supranuclear disorders of ocular control system in man. In Bach-Y-Rita P, Collins CC (eds). The Control of Eye Movements. New York, Academic Press, 1970

Davson H (ed). The Eye: Muscular Mechanisms. New York, Academic Press, 1962

Duke – Elder WS, Scott GJ. System of Ophthalmology: Neuro-ophthalmology. St. Louis, CV Mosby, 1971

Dyken PR. Extraocular myotonia in families of dystrophic myotonics. Neurology 1966;16:738

Fisher CM. Ocular bobbing. Arch Neurol 1964; 11:543.

FitzGerald PM, Jankovic J. Tardive oculogyric crises. Neurology 1989;39:1434

Ford RF, Walsh FB. Tonic deviation of the eyes produced by movements of the head, with special reference to otolith reflexes. Arch Ophthalmol 1940;23:1274

Glaser JS. Neuro-ophthalmology. Hagerstown, Harper & Row, 1978

Goldstein JE, Cogan DG. Apraxia of lid opening. Arch Ophthalmol 1965;73:155

Gross – Tsur V, Har – Even Y, Gutman I et al. Oculomotor apraxia: The presenting sign of Gaucher disease. Pediatr Neurol 1989;5:128

Grove AS Jr. Evaluation of exophthalmos. N Engl J Med 1975;292:1005

Harvey JT, Anderson RL. Lid lag and lagophthalmos: A clarification of terminology. Ophthalmic Surg 1981;12:338

Hollenhorst RW. Neuro-ophthalmologic examination of children. Neurology 1956;6:739

Hoyt WF, Nachtigäler A. Anomalies of oculomotor nerves. Am J Ophthalmol 1965;60:433

Hreidarsson AB, Gundersen HJ. Reduced pupillary unrest. Autonomic nervous system abnormality in diabetes mellitus. Diabetes 1988;37:446

Kato I, Nakamura T, Watanabe J et al. Primary posterior upbeat nystagmus: Localizing value. Arch Neurol 1985; 42:819

Keane JR. Acute bilateral ophthalmoplegia: 60 cases. Neurology 1986;36:279

Kestenbaum A. Clinical Methods of Neuro-ophthalmologic Examination, 2nd ed. New York, Grune & Stratton, 1961

Kiloh LG, Nevin S. Progressive dystrophy of the external ocular muscles (ocular myopathy). Brain 1951;74:115

Lancaster WB. Physiology of disturbances of ocular motility. Arch Ophthalmol 1937;17:983

Langworthy OR. General principles of autonomic innervation. Arch Neurol Psychiatry 1943;50:590

Lowenstein O, Lowenfeld IE. Role of sympathetic and parasympathetic systems in reflex dilatation of the pupil: pupillographic studies. Arch Neurol Psychiatry 1950; 64:313

Lyle DJ. Neuro-ophthalmology, 2nd ed. Springfield, IL, Charles C Thomas, 1954

McGravey AR. A dilated unreactive pupil in acute bacterial meningitis: oculomotor nerve inflammation versus herniation. Pediatr Emerg Care 1989;5:187

Merritt HH, Moore M. The Argyll – Robertson pupil: An anatomic-physiologic explanation of the phenomenon, with a survey of its occurrence in neurosyphilis. Arch Neurol Psychiatry 1933;30:357

Miller NR. Walsh and Hoyt's Clinical Neuro-ophthalmology, 4th ed. Baltimore, Williams & Wilkins, 1988

Peter LC. The Extra-ocular Muscles, 3rd ed. Philadelphia, Lea & Febiger, 1941

Pola J, Robinson DA. An explanation of eye movements in internuclear ophthalmoplegia. Arch Neurol 1976;33:447

Robertson DA. On an interesting series of eye movements in a case of spinal disease, with remarks on the action of belladonna on the iris, etc. Edinb Med J 1869;14:696

Robertson DA. Four cases of spinal myosis; with remarks on the action of light on the pupil. Edinb Med J 1869;15:487

Smith JL. Optokinetic Nystagmus. Springfield, IL, Charles C Thomas, 1963

Smith JL (ed). The University of Miami Neuro-ophthalmology Symposium. Springfield, IL, Charles C Thomas, 1964

Smith JL. Cogan DG. Internuclear ophthalmoplegia: A review of 58 cases. Arch Ophthalmol 1959;61:687

Smith JL, Mark VH. See-saw nystagmus with suprasellar epidermoid tumor. Arch Ophthalmol 1959;62:280

Spiegel EA, Sommer I. Neurology of the Eye, Ear, Nose and Throat. New York, Grune & Stratton, 1944

Toglia JU. Electronystagmography. Springfield, IL, Charles C Thomas, 1976

Zinn KM. The Pupil. Springfield, IL, Charles C Thomas, 1973

Chapter 12
THE TRIGEMINAL NERVE

ANATOMY AND PHYSIOLOGY

The trigeminal, or fifth cranial, nerve is a mixed nerve, or one that carries both motor and sensory fibers. It is the largest of the cranial nerves, and, owing to connections with the third, fourth, sixth, seventh, ninth, and tenth cranial nerves and with the sympathetic nervous system, is one of the most complex. The nuclei of the trigeminal nerve are situated in the midportion of the pons (Fig. 12-1).

The Motor Portion

The motor nucleus of the trigeminal nerve is a prominent mass of large motor cells situated just anterior and medial to the outgoing fibers of the nerve in the lateral part of the reticular formation of the pons, near the floor of the fourth ventricle. The motor root, or portio minor, emerges from the lateral aspect of the pons in close association with, but anterior and medial to, the sensory root. It passes beneath the gasserian ganglion and leaves the skull through the foramen ovale. It joins the mandibular division immediately after leaving the skull, but soon separates from it to supply the muscles of mastication and associated muscles. The cerebral center which controls the motor functions of the trigeminal nerve is situated in the lower third of the posterior frontal convolution. Each cerebral center has bilateral connections with the motor nuclei. Impulses travel through the corona radiata, the internal capsule, and the cerebral peduncle to the pons, where many of them de-

cussate before supplying the motor nuclei. There is also extrapyramidal supranuclear innervation from the premotor cortex and the basal ganglia.

The principal function of the motor division of the trigeminal nerve is the innervation of the muscles of mastication, namely, the masseter, temporal, and internal and external pterygoid muscles. The masseter muscles elevate the mandible, and by means of their superficial fibers protrude it to a slight extent. The temporal muscles also elevate the mandible, and their posterior fibers serve to retract it; possibly the anterior fibers aid in protrusion. When the external pterygoid muscles act together they protrude and depress the mandible; when one acts alone it causes lateral movement to the opposite side. When the internal pterygoid muscles act together they elevate the mandible and assist the external pterygoids in protruding it; when one acts alone, it draws the mandible forward and causes deviation to the opposite side. Mastication consists of upward and downward movements of the jaw to open and close the mouth, together with forward, backward, and lateral motion. The masseters, temporals, and internal pterygoids elevate the mandible; the external pterygoids, assisted by the mylohyoids, digastrici, geniohyoids, and the other depressors of the hyoid bone, and also by gravity, depress the jaw; the internal and external pterygoids, assisted by the masseters and possibly the temporals, protrude the mandible; the temporals, assisted by the digastrici, retract the jaw, and the pterygoids produce side to side movement.

The trigeminal nerve also supplies the mylohyoid muscle and the superior belly of the

165

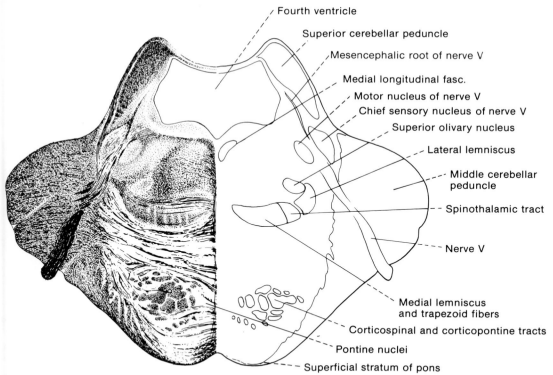

FIG. 12–1. Section through the pons at the level of the trigeminal nuclei.

digastricus. The former draws the hyoid bone upward and forward and raises the floor of the mouth, thus pressing the base of the tongue against the palate; if the hyoid bone is fixed, the mylohyoid tends to depress the mandible. The anterior belly of the digastricus raises and advances the hyoid bone if the jaw is fixed, or depresses and retracts the mandible if the hyoid bone is fixed by the antagonist muscles; if the mandible is fixed, it also assists the mylohyoid in drawing the base of the tongue upward and forward and pressing it against the palate during the first portion of the act of deglutition.

The tensor veli palatini and the tensor tympani are two smaller muscles which are also supplied by the trigeminal nerve but have less clinical significance. The former tenses the soft palate, draws it to one side, and raises it to a certain extent. This muscle aids in preventing food from passing from the oral to the nasal pharynx and also dilates the eustachian tube. The tensor tympani draws the manubrium of the malleus and the tympanic membrane medialward, thus tensing the tympanic membrane.

The Sensory Portion

The cells of origin of the sensory portion of the trigeminal nerve have their nuclei in the gasserian (semilunar) ganglion. The neuraxes which carry exteroceptive sensation terminate in the sensory nuclei in the pons and medulla.

The chief sensory nucleus, the pontine nucleus, is situated lateral and posterior to the motor nucleus in the lateral part of the reticular formation of the pons. It receives only tactile impulses, but receives both general and discriminatory and localized types of tactile sensibility. Only a small percentage of the trigeminal roots enter this nucleus. After a synapse here, the neuraxes which carry both discriminatory and general tactile sensations ascend to the thalamus near the medial lemniscus in the dorsal secondary ascending tract of the fifth nerve (Fig. 12-2). This is both crossed and uncrossed. Those neuraxes which carry general tactile sensation also descend and enter the ventral secondary ascending tract. Tactile impulses carried in the trigeminal pathway have central connections similar

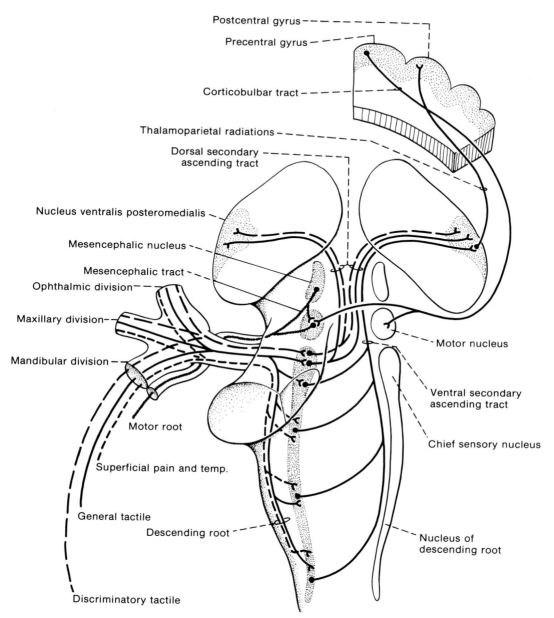

Postcentral gyrus

Precentral gyrus

Corticobulbar tract

Thalamoparietal radiations

Dorsal secondary
ascending tract

Nucleus ventralis posteromedialis

Mesencephalic nucleus

Mesencephalic tract

Ophthalmic division

Maxillary division

Mandibular division

Motor root

Superficial pain and temp.

General tactile

Descending root

Discriminatory tactile

Motor nucleus

Ventral secondary
ascending tract

Chief sensory nucleus

Nucleus of
descending root

FIG. 12–2. The trigeminal nerve and its connections.

to those from other parts of the body. In the nucleus ventralis posteromedialis of the lateral nuclear mass of the thalamus they terminate in a position medial to those conveying touch from the rest of the body, and on the parietal cortex they are below and lateral to those from the rest of the body.

The nucleus of the descending root, or spinal tract, of the trigeminal nerve extends downward

from the chief sensory nucleus, through the lower pons and medulla, and into the spinal cord, as far as the third or even fourth cervical segment. The descending root fuses with Lissauer's tract, and its adjoining nucleus fuses with the substantia gelatinosa rolandi. Pain, temperature, and general tactile impulses terminate on this tract and nucleus. The fibers from the maxillomandibular areas are in the dorsal part of this tract, and those from the ophthalmic area in the ventral part. The exteroceptive components of the facial, glossopharyngeal, and vagus nerves join the descending tract at their specific levels of entrance into the brain stem. The fibers descend for varying distances, depending upon the segmental distribution, but finally synapse, and neuraxes of the neurons of the next order cross and ascend to the thalamus in the ventral secondary ascending tract of the trigeminal nerve, or the trigeminothalamic tract. These terminate in the nucleus ventralis posteromedialis of the lateral nuclear mass of the thalamus, those carrying pain and temperature being somewhat rostral to those conveying touch. In the thalamus the trigeminal fibers are medial to those from the rest of the body, whereas on the parietal cortex they terminate laterally on the inferior portion of the postcentral gyrus.

A third sensory component, the mesencephalic root of the trigeminal nerve, runs with the motor root and then extends posteriorly and cephalad from the level of the motor nucleus into the mesencephalon. It carries proprioceptive impulses (including deep pain) from the muscles supplied by the trigeminal nerve and possibly also from muscles supplied by other cranial nerves.

The gasserian, or semilunar, ganglion (see Fig. 12-2) of the trigeminal nerve occupies a cavity (cavum meckelii) in the dura mater near the apex of the petrous portion of the temporal bone. Here it lies lateral to the internal carotid artery and the posterior part of the cavernous sinus. The ganglion cells are unipolar and the fibers bifurcate. The internal branches pass into the substance of the pons to terminate on the chief sensory and spinal nuclei, and the external branches pass outward as the sensory root (portio major) of the trigeminal nerve, which then forms its three constituent divisions.

The upper, or ophthalmic, division is the smallest of the three branches. It passes forward through the lateral wall of the cavernous sinus, where it lies beneath the third and fourth nerves and lateral to the sixth nerve, it enters the orbit through the superior orbital fissure, but just before leaving the cavernous sinus it gives off the tentorial and anastomotic branches and then divides into its lacrimal, frontal, and nasociliary branches.

The maxillary division passes through the lateral part of the wall of the cavernous sinus and leaves the skull through the foramen rotundum. Then it crosses the pterygopalatine fossa, enters the orbit through the inferior orbital fissure, traverses the infraorbital canal and groove, and reaches the face at the infraorbital foramen. Before leaving the skull the maxillary division gives off the middle, or recurrent, meningeal nerve which supplies the dura mater of the middle cranial fossa. The sensory root to the sphenopalatine ganglion and the zygomatic and posterior superior alveolar branches arise in the pterygopalatine fossa, and the middle and anterior superior branches, in the infraorbital canal. On the face, after leaving the infraorbital foramen, it divides into the terminal inferior palpebral, external and internal nasal, and superior labial branches.

The mandibular division, the largest of the branches, leaves the skull through the foramen ovale. The motor root of the trigeminal nerve, which lies in front of and medial to the sensory root, passes beneath the gasserian ganglion and also leaves the skull through the foramen ovale. Immediately after leaving the skull it joins the mandibular division to form a large trunk which directly divides into a small anterior, or chiefly motor, branch and a large posterior branch which is mainly sensory. Before dividing, the mandibular nerve gives off two branches. One is the spinous, or recurrent, branch which enters the skull through the foramen spinosum and supplies the dura mater, the greater wing of the sphenoid bone, and the lining membrane of the mastoid cells; the other is the nerve to the internal pterygoid muscle. The muscles supplied by the anterior portion have been listed; the sensory filaments of the anterior portion make up the buccinator nerve. The posterior portion of the mandibular nerve divides into three large branches. Two of these, the lingual and the auriculotemporal, are exclusively sensory, but the third, the inferior alveolar, also carries motor fibers to the mylohyoid muscle and the anterior belly of the digastricus.

The sensory portion of the trigeminal nerve carries exteroceptive sensations. The ophthalmic division supplies the skin of the forehead, temple, and scalp as far as the vertex; the upper eyelid; and the skin over the anterior and part of the lateral surface of the nose. It also supplies the eyeball; the upper conjunctiva; the cornea, ciliary body and iris; and the mucous membrane lining of the frontal sinus, parts of the sphenoid and ethmoid sinuses, and the upper part of the nasal cavity. It sends the sensory root to the ciliary ganglion, and branches to the lacrimal gland, the tentorium cerebelli, and the oculomotor, trochlear, and abducens nerves.

The maxillary division supplies the skin on the side and posterior half of the nose, the lower eyelid, upper cheek, anterior temporal region, and upper lip. It innervates the mucous membranes of the lower conjunctiva, maxillary sinus, parts of the sphenoid and ethmoid sinuses, lower nose, upper lip and cheek, oral part of the hard palate, soft palate except for its posterior border, uvula, and nasopharynx. In some individuals it supplies the tonsillar areas and the fauces, but these regions are also innervated by the ninth and tenth nerves. Its alveolar branches innervate the upper gingival areas, alveolar ridge, and teeth. The maxillary division also supplies the dura of the middle cranial fossa through the middle meningeal nerve, and sends the sensory root to the sphenopalatine ganglion where it communicates with the geniculate ganglion of the seventh nerve and with the sympathetic nervous system through the vidian and greater superficial and deep petrosal nerves.

The mandibular division supplies the skin of the side of the head, the posterior part of the cheek and temporal areas, the anterior portion of the pinna, the upper and outer walls of the external auditory canal, the anterior half of the tympanum, the lower lip and chin, the mucous membranes of the lower lip, the lower portion of the buccal surface, the tongue, and the floor of the mouth. The inferior alveolar nerve supplies the lower gingival area, lower alveolar ridge, and teeth. Its recurrent, or meningeal, branch innervates the dura of the middle and anterior cranial fossae, the greater wing of the sphenoid, and the mucous membrane lining of the mastoid cells. The mandibular division also supplies the temporomandibular joint and sends branches to the otic and submaxillary ganglia.

These three branches, or divisions, of the trigeminal nerve supply sensation to the entire side of the face except for the angle of the jaw, which is supplied by the second and third cervical nerves through the great auricular nerve. There is some midline crossing by the trigeminal nerve, but less than is found in the nerves supplying the trunk. Although the fifth nerve, through the lingual branch of the mandibular division, supplies the mucosa of the tongue, taste sensation to the anterior two-thirds of the tongue is a function of the seventh nerve, even though carried through the lingual nerve to the chorda tympani (Ch. 13).

With a lesion of the lingual nerve there will be loss of taste and of exteroceptive sensation on the anterior surface of the tongue. The various mucous membranes, including those of the pal-pebral conjunctiva, nose, and mouth, are supplied by pain, temperature, and tactile sensations. Only free sensory endings have been demonstrated in the cornea, but end-bulbs of Krause are also present at the corneal limbus. It is said that the cornea is sensitive only to pain stimuli, but light stimulation with cotton does cause an unpleasant sensation, and most observers believe that with careful testing tactile, pain, and temperature sensations can be differentiated on the cornea. Some corneal sensation and a diminished corneal reflex may persist after trigeminal tractotomy and medullary lesions; under these circumstances those impulses which descend in the spinal root are interrupted, whereas those tactile impulses going to the chief sensory nucleus remain intact.

The segmental distribution of the trigeminal nerve to the skin and mucous membranes of the face differs somewhat from the peripheral supply of the ophthalmic, maxillary, and mandibular divisions. Pain and temperature sensations, and to a lesser extent tactile sensations, were said by Dejerine to assume an "onion-skin" distribution (Fig. 12-3). The perioral area is supplied by those fibers whose neurons synapse and cross highest in the descending root of the nerve, whereas the fibers which descend for varying distances before they synapse and decussate supply a somewhat concentric distribution in gradually widening circles over the face and head, the most posterior and outermost segment, and that closest to the cervical sensory distribution, being innervated by those fibers which descend to the lowest portion of the spinal tract and nucleus. On the other hand, studies based on operative section of the spinal tract of the trigeminal nerve have suggested that the segmental representation in this tract may instead be in terms of, but inverse to, the peripheral divisions of the nerve, with the ophthalmic fibers descending to the most caudal part of the tract and the mandibular fibers terminating the most cephalad. This conclusion has been reached in part by the fact that section of the caudal part of the tract has caused analgesia which is limited to the territory of the ophthalmic division. The several viewpoints proposed by anatomists for the explanation of the cutaneous segmental distribution versus the peripheral distribution have been largely reconciled by Brodal.

Proprioceptive impulses from the muscles supplied by the trigeminal nerve are carried through the mandibular division and then to the mesencephalic root of the nerve. This conveys muscle sense, motion and position sensations,

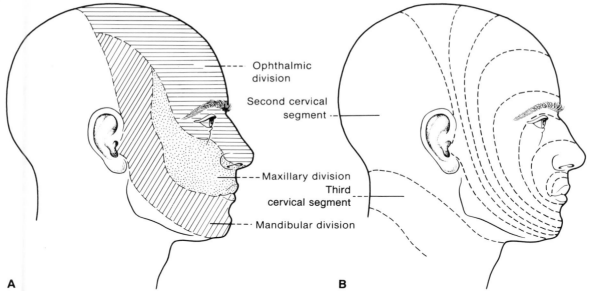

Ophthalmic
division

Second cervical
segment

Maxillary division

Third
cervical segment

Mandibular division

A

B

FIG. 12–3. Cutaneous distribution of the trigeminal nerve. **A.** Peripheral distribution. **B.** Segmental distribution.

and other kinesthetic impulses. The mesencephalic root of the trigeminal nerve may also carry proprioceptive impulses from the muscles supplied by the oculomotor, trochlear, abducens, facial, and other motor cranial nerves.

The divisions of the trigeminal nerve supply filaments to four ganglia in the head. The **ciliary ganglion,** situated in the posterior part of the orbit, receives its sensory innervation from the nasociliary branch of the ophthalmic division (the long root of the ciliary ganglion); it receives its motor (parasympathetic) supply from the Edinger-Westphal nucleus through the inferior division of the oculomotor nerve (the short root), and its sympathetic supply from the cavernous sympathetic plexus, running through the long ciliary nerves. Its branches, the short ciliary nerves, supply the ciliary muscle, sphincter and dilator of the pupil, and cornea. Involvement of these structures may follow a lesion of the ciliary ganglion.

The **sphenopalatine ganglion,** placed deep in the pterygopalatine fossa, receives its sensory innervation from the sphenopalatine branches of the maxillary division; it receives its motor (parasympathetic) supply from the facial nerve (nervus intermedius) through the greater superficial petrosal nerve, and its sympathetic supply from the internal carotid plexus through the deep petrosal nerve. These two latter nerves join to form the vidian nerve, or nerve of the ptery-

goid canal, before their entrance into the ganglion. The sphenopalatine ganglion sends ascending, or orbital, branches to the periosteum of the orbit and the mucous membrane of the posterior ethmoidal and sphenoidal sinuses; descending, or palatine, branches to the hard and soft palates, tonsils, and uvula; medial branches to the nasal mucosa; and posterior, or pharyngeal, branches to the mucous membrane of the nasopharynx. Fibers concerned with lacrimation pass along the zygomaticotemporal branch of the maxillary division to the lacrimal branch of the ophthalmic, and then to the lacrimal gland.

The **otic** ganglion, situated just below the foramen ovale in the infratemporal fossa, receives a motor and possibly a sensory branch from the mandibular division; motor (parasympathetic) and sensory branches from the glossopharyngeal nerve and to a lesser extent from the facial nerve, both through the lesser superficial petrosal nerve from the tympanic plexus; and sympathetic innervation from the plexus surrounding the middle meningeal artery. It may also communicate with the nerve of the pterygoid canal and the chorda tympani. It sends motor branches to the tensor tympani and tensor veli palatini muscles and secretory fibers to the parotid gland through the auriculotemporal nerve.

The **submaxillary ganglion,** situated on the medial side of the mandible between the lingual nerve and the submaxillary gland, receives its sensory supply from the lingual branch of the mandibular division, its motor (parasympathetic) supply from the superior salivatory nucleus of the facial nerve through the chorda tympani, and its sympathetic branch from the sympathetic plexus around the external maxillary artery. It sends secretory fibers to the submaxillary and sublingual glands and the mucous membrane of the mouth and tongue; those preganglionic fibers from the chorda tympani which supply the submaxillary gland pass through the ganglion to synapse on terminal ganglion cells in the hilus of the gland.

CLINICAL EXAMINATION

Examination of the Motor Functions

The principal motor functions of the trigeminal nerve are examined by testing the motor power of the muscles of mastication. In disturbance of function of the motor division of the nerve there is ipsilateral paresis or paralysis of the masticatory muscles. There is weakness or loss of power in raising, depressing, protruding, retracting, and deviating the mandible. The jaw is deflected toward the side of the involved nerve, and the patient is unable to deviate it toward the nonparalyzed side (Fig. 12-4). In bilateral paresis the jaw droops with gravity, and all muscle power is lost.

The function of the muscles of mastication may be tested by carrying out the following procedures: 1) The patient clenches his jaws while the examiner palpates the contraction of the masseter and temporal muscles on each side; if there is either weakness or paralysis on one side, there will be either impairment or absence of contraction on that side. 2) The patient opens his mouth; owing to the action of the pterygoids, especially the external pterygoids, which draw forward the condyle of the mandible and protrude the jaw, paralysis of the muscles of mastication will be evidenced by deviation of the jaw to the side of the paralyzed muscles. Deviation is appraised by noting the relation between the upper and lower incisor teeth when the jaw is opened and closed, not by the position of the lips. If the examiner places a ruler or pencil in a vertical position in front of the patient's nose, he may be able to tell whether there is deviation of the mandible. In paralysis of the facial nerve there may be an apparent deviation of the jaw because of weakness of the muscles of facial expression. 3) The patient moves his jaw from side

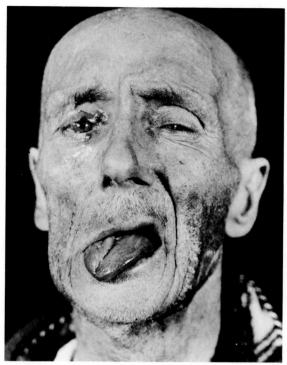

FIG. 12–4. *Infranuclear paralysis of the right trigeminal, facial, and hypoglossal nerves in a patient with metastatic carcinoma, showing deviation of the tongue and mandible to the right.*

to side against resistance; in paralysis of the fifth nerve on one side he is able to move the jaw to the paralyzed, not to the nonparalyzed side. 4) He protrudes and retracts the jaw, and any tendency toward deviation is noted. 5) He bites on a tongue depressor with his molar teeth, and the depth of the tooth marks is noted and compared on the two sides; if the examiner can pull out the tongue blade while the patient is biting on it, there is weakness of the muscles of mastication. 6) The jaw reflex is tested (see "Examination of the Reflexes"). 7) The tone, volume, and contour of the muscles of mastication are noted, and fasciculations sought for. If there is atrophy of these muscles, there are visible or palpable concavities above and below the zygoma.

Paresis or paralysis of the muscles of mastication is most marked in nuclear or infranuclear lesions, and in such it is followed by atrophy (Fig. 12-5). Because the motor nuclei of the trigeminal nerve have mainly bilateral supranuclear innervation, there is rarely any marked degree of paresis of the muscles of mastication in a unilateral cerebral, or upper motor neuron, lesion. There

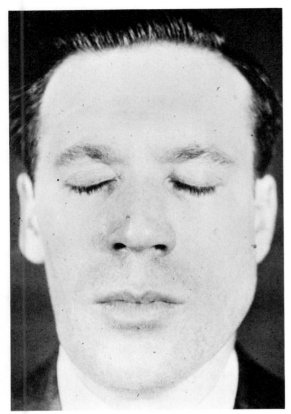

FIG. 12–5. Infranuclear paralysis of the right trigeminal nerve with atrophy of the muscles of mastication.

movement of the palate may be retained by the intact tensor. Paralysis of the tensor tympani is not apparent objectively, but the patient may complain of difficulty in hearing high tones and of dysacusis for high tones.

Examination of the Sensory Functions

In testing sensation in the distribution of the trigeminal nerve, both skin and mucous membranes are examined. The various exteroceptive modalities, namely, superficial pain, hot, cold, and light touch sensations, are examined individually in the same manner as elsewhere on the body (see Part B, "The Sensory System"), and changes in them are charted. The cornea, conjunctiva, nostrils, gums, tongue, and insides of the cheeks are also examined. With lesions of the sensory portion of the nerve there will be areas of altered or absent sensation. One should attempt to differentiate between changes of peripheral origin, that is, those resulting from lesions of one or more of the primary divisions of the nerve, and changes in the segmental distribution that result from lesions of the cerebrospinal axis (see Fig. 12-3). More important than finding of an onion-skin distribution with involvement of the descending root, however, is the dissociation of sensation with such a lesion: there may be loss of pain and temperature, but sparing of discriminatory and localized tactile sensations. In differentiating organic from hysterical anesthesias of the face, it is important to recall that there is less crossing at the midline on the face than there is elsewhere on the body, and that the skin over the angle of the jaw is not supplied by the fifth nerve, but by the second and third cervical nerves through the great auricular nerve. In trigeminal neuralgia and in certain neuritides there is an increased sensitivity at the emergence of the various sensory branches through their individual fascial sheaths and foramina, and stimulation of these "trigger" or "dolorogenic" zones may precipitate attacks of pain. Proprioceptive sensations carried by the trigeminal nerve cannot be adequately tested, but one can test for extinction and the ability to identify figures written on the skin.

may, however, be slight to moderate unilateral weakness of the masticatory muscles with deviation to the side of the paretic muscles, weakness of deflection to the opposite side, and exaggeration of the jaw reflex on the paretic side. The amount of involvement is dependent upon the extent of decussation. In bilateral supranuclear lesions there may be marked paresis.

The other muscles which are supplied by the fifth nerve cannot be adequately examined, but if possible their function should be evaluated. If there is paralysis of the mylohyoid and anterior belly of the digastricus, one may be able to note, on palpation, some flabbiness or flaccidity of the floor of the mouth. If there is paralysis of the tensor veli palatini, the uvula may be slightly tilted to the affected side, and the palatal arch on that side may appear broader and lower than normal. The levator veli palatini is more important than the tensor palatini, however, in elevation of the soft palate, and paresis of the tensor is masked if the muscles supplied by the tenth nerve are intact. In paralysis of the levator, some

Examination of the Reflexes

The trigeminal nerve participates in many reflex responses. Since it is the principal sensory nerve of the face, in most instances the afferent portion of the reflex arc is carried through the nerve, but in some of the responses it conveys the efferent portion of the arc as well.

The Jaw, Masseter, or Mandibular Reflex. To elicit the jaw (or jaw muscle) reflex the examiner places his index finger over the middle of the patient's chin, holding the mouth slightly opened and the jaw relaxed. He then taps his finger with the reflex hammer. The response is a contraction of the masseter and temporal muscles, causing a sudden closing of the mouth. The chin itself may be tapped, or the examiner may place a tongue depressor over the base of the tongue or the lower incisor teeth and tap the protruding end. All of the aforementioned call forth a bilateral response. A unilateral response may sometimes be elicited by tapping the angle of the jaw or by placing a tongue blade over the lower molar teeth and tapping the protruding end. The afferent impulses of this reflex are carried through the sensory portion of the trigeminal nerve, possibly through the mesencephalic root, and the efferent impulses through its motor portion; the reflex center is in the pons. The response is a rather minimal one, and usually is very slight and even absent in normal individuals. The jaw reflex is absent in nuclear and peripheral lesions of the trigeminal nerve, and is exaggerated with supranuclear lesions, or those affecting the corticobulbar pathways above the motor nucleus, especially if bilateral. It is sometimes possible to elicit jaw clonus.

In the **zygomatic reflex,** which may be considered a modification of the jaw reflex, percussion over the zygoma results in ipsilateral deviation of the mandible. Both the sensory and the motor portions of the reflex are carried by the fifth nerve. This response can be elicited only in the presence of supranuclear lesions.

The Head Retraction Reflex. With the head bent slightly forward, the upper lip is sharply tapped just below the nose. If the reflex is present, there is a quick, involuntary backward jerk of the head. This reflex is usually not elicited in normal individuals, but is obtained if there is exaggeration of the muscle stretch reflexes. It is present in bilateral supracervial lesions of the corticospinal tract. The sensory impulse is carried through the trigeminal nerve and the motor response through the upper cervical nerves to the retractor muscles of the neck. The reflex center is in the upper cervical portion of the spinal cord.

The Corneal Reflex. To elicit the corneal reflex, the examiner touches the cornea lightly with a wisp of cotton, a piece of string, or a hair; it is best to moisten the cotton to avoid irritating the cornea (Fig. 12-6). The patient should gaze in the opposite direction and the examiner should approach from the side to eliminate the blink, or visual–palpebral, reflex. Both the upper and lower portions of the cornea should be tested. In response to this stimulus there is a blinking, or closing of the ipsilateral eye, the **direct corneal reflex,** and also a closing of the opposite eye, the **consensual corneal reflex.** The afferent portion of the reflex arc is mediated by the ophthalmic division of the trigeminal nerve (in some persons the lower portion of the cornea is supplied by the maxillary division), whereas the efferent or motor response is a function of the facial nerve that conveys the impulse to the orbicularis oculi. The reflex center is in the pons. Electrical stimulation can quantitate the corneal reflex response.

In a unilateral trigeminal lesion, with resulting corneal anesthesia, stimulation fails to produce either the direct response on that side or the consensual response on the opposite, but stimulation on the opposite side elicits both responses. In a seventh nerve lesion with paralysis of the orbicularis oculi, the direct response is absent on that side, but the contralateral consensual reflex is maintained; when the opposite cornea is stimulated the direct response is present but the consensual reflex is absent. On occasion the bulbar conjunctiva, rather than the cornea, is stimula-

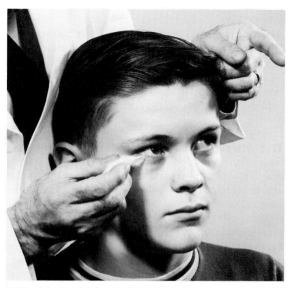

FIG. 12–6. *Method of eliciting the corneal reflex.*

ted — the conjunctival reflex; this may be absent in normal individuals, especially those with a high threshold for pain. It is much less significant than the corneal reflex.

Loss of the corneal reflex is an early sign of trigeminal nerve involvement, and indicates interruption of the sensory impulses carried through the ophthalmic division or its branches to the cornea or in the gasserian ganglion. With lesions of the nucleus of the descending root of the trigeminal nerve the reflex may be retained, but the response is diminished. It has been said that the corneal reflex also may be absent in hysteria, but loss of this reflex, especially if unilateral, indicates the presence of an organic lesion. The corneal reflexes are widely used as an index of the depth of anesthesia and of coma. The contralateral corneal reflex may be diminished or absent in patients with hemispheric cerebral disease, especially in those with lesions of the parietal lobe or internal capsule.

Modifications of the corneal reflex are as follows: the **oculosensory,** or **oculopupillary reflex** is characterized by a constriction of the pupil, or dilation followed by constriction, in response to a painful stimulus directed toward the eye or its adnexa. The afferent impulses are carried through the trigeminal nerve and the efferent impulses through the oculomotor nerve. The **corneo-oculogyric reflex** consists of a contralateral or an upward deviation of the eyes in response to stimulation of the conjunctiva or cornea. There is associated contraction of the orbicularis. Here the impulses are carried through the fifth, third, and seventh nerves. The **corneomandibular reflex** consists of contralateral deviation of the mandible, the result of ipsilateral contraction of the external pterygoid muscle, when one cornea is stimulated. Both the afferent and efferent portions of the reflex arc are carried through the trigeminal nerve. This response may be an associated movement rather than a true reflex; its presence indicates supranuclear interruption of the ipsilateral corticotrigeminal tract.

The Nasal, Sneeze, or Sternutatory Reflex. Stimulation of the nasal mucous membrane by tickling it with a hair or some similar object is followed by contraction of the nasopharyngeal and thoracic muscles with a violent expulsion of air from the nose and mouth. The afferent portion of the reflex arc is carried from the nasal mucous membrane through the trigeminal nerve, and the efferent impulses are carried through the trigeminal, facial, glossopharyngeal, and vagus nerves, and through the motor nerves of the cervical and thoracic portions of the spinal cord. There is also a visceral component relayed through the sympathetic nervous system. The reflex center is situated in the brain stem and in the upper portion of the spinal cord. The nasal mucosa may be stimulated not only mechanically, but also by the use of irritating inhalants such as pepper, acetic acid, ammonia, and formaldehyde. The effect of these upon the fifth nerve supply to the mucous membrane of the nose has been discussed in Chapter 9. Mechanical and gaseous stimuli and infections of the nasal mucosa, and even bright light in some persons, may evoke not only the sneeze reflex response, but also lacrimation, vasomotor reactions with increased secretion of mucus, and respiratory inhibition.

A modification of the above reflex is the **nasal reflex of Bechterew.** In this, tickling of the nasal mucosa causes contraction of the ipsilateral facial muscles. The afferent impulse is carried through the trigeminal nerve, and the efferent impulse through the facial nerve to the muscles of facial expression.

The **trigeminobrachial reflex,** found only in the presence of lesions involving both the corticospinal pathways and the sensory nuclei of the trigeminal nerve in the brain stem, consists of contralateral flexion and supination of the forearm following stimulation of an area in the distribution of one trigeminal nerve. The **trigeminocervical reflex** may be found in the presence of involvement of the corticobulbar pathways and the brain stem trigeminal nuclei; in this there is contralateral turning of the head following stimulation of an area in the distribution of one trigeminal nerve.

There are many other responses in which the afferent portion of the reflex arc is carried through the trigeminal nerve. These are described, however, under the discussions of the nerves that play the major role in the responses. The more important ones are the following: orbicularis oculi, trigeminofacial, nasomental, and lacrimal reflexes, Chapter 13; palatal, oculocardiac, and sucking reflexes, Chapter 15. Chvostek's sign is described in Chapters 13 and 39.

DISORDERS OF FUNCTION

Lesions of the trigeminal nerve may be manifested by any or all of the following: motor changes, either irritative or paretic in nature;

sensory alterations, consisting of diminution or loss of sensation, hyperesthesia, dysesthesias, or pain; abnormalities of the reflexes innervated by the trigeminal nerve; trophic or secretory changes.

Irritative Motor Phenomena. These may be either tonic or clonic in nature, and are usually the result of supranuclear lesions. An irritative focus in the precentral gyrus may produce a jacksonian convulsive seizure limited to the muscles of mastication; this is manifested by a clenching of the jaws with biting of the tongue or cheeks. In diseases of the extrapyramidal system there may be involvement of the masticatory muscles; a rhythmic tremor of the jaws is seen in Parkinson's disease, and arrhythmic movements in the choreas. Sometimes in basal ganglion disease there are yawning, gasping, "fish gaping,", and champing movements, the result of either irritative or release phenomena. In **trismus,** as seen in tetanus, and sometimes in encephalitis, rabies and tetany, there is irritability with marked spasm of the muscles of mastication: the teeth are tightly clenched, the muscles are hard and firm, and the patient is unable to open his jaws. Trismus may also occur in polymyositis and hysteria. Spasms of the muscles of mastication are also seen in strychnine poisoning, and chattering of the jaws occurs in chills and under emotional stress. Chewing movements and grinding of the teeth are sometimes present in psychoses, and chewing or tasting movements in complex partial seizures. Bruxism or chewing movements sufficiently severe to wear down the teeth may occur as a side reaction in patients receiving levodopa for parkinsonism. Chewing movements also occur as side effects of psychoactive drugs and as part of the orofacial dyskinesias.

Paretic Motor Phenomena. Owing to the fact that the motor nuclei of the trigeminal nerve have mainly bilateral cerebral innervation, there is rarely any marked degree of paresis of the muscles of mastication in a unilateral supranuclear lesion, although there may be slight weakness of the contralateral muscles with an exaggerated jaw reflex. There may be a transient deviation of the jaw to the paralyzed side in acute involvement. In bilateral supranuclear lesions, however, there often is marked paresis, and in bilateral cortical or internal capsule lesions, as in pseudobulbar palsy or amyotrophic

lateral sclerosis, there is striking weakness of the muscles of mastication with a grossly exaggerated jaw reflex. In supranuclear lesions no atrophy or fasciculations occur.

In lesions of the motor nucleus there is unilateral involvement, and if the lesion is a destructive one, the paresis is usually accompanied or followed by the development of atrophy and fasciculations in the involved muscles. The jaw reflex is absent. Irritative lesions of the motor nuclei may cause spasm of the muscles of mastication.

In infranuclear lesions there is unilateral paralysis with absence of the jaw reflex. The paralysis may be followed by atrophy of the involved muscles, but rarely by fasciculations. In both nuclear and infranuclear lesions the paralysis and atrophy of the muscles of mastication may be present to a marked degree (see Fig. 12-5). Lesions of the myoneural junction, as in myasthenia gravis, or of the muscles themselves (muscular dystrophies, inflammatory myopathies) also cause paralysis of the muscles of mastication.

Sensory Involvement. Sensory changes in the distribution of the trigeminal nerve are rarely the result of supranuclear lesions, although with involvement of the parietal lobe or sensory radiations there may be some raising of the sensory threshold of the contralateral face, especially for the discriminative elements, and with a thalamic lesion there may be hypesthesia with hyperpathia of the face.

Nuclear involvement is followed by loss of sensation in both skin and mucous membrane in the segmental distribution, and by loss of those reflexes in which the afferent arc is mediated by the trigeminal nerve. Lesions of the chief sensory nucleus result in diminished tactile sensation on the involved side of the face, and in lesions of the tract or nucleus of the descending root there is dissociation of sensation, with principally a disturbance of the pain and temperature modalities, and, possibly to a lesser extent, of tactile sense.

Involvement of the sensory portion of the trigeminal nerve after it leaves the pons is characterized by disturbance of all types of exteroceptive sensation. There may be loss or diminution of sensation, dysesthesias or paresthesias, or spontaneous pain. If the lesion is central to or at the gasserian ganglion, all three divisions are affected, but if it is peripheral to the ganglion, only isolated divisions are involved. In irritative lesions there is usually hyperesthesia of the peripheral branches at their points of exit from the skull, as at the supraorbital, infraorbital, mental, and alveolar foramina, and stimulation of these "trigger" zones may precipitate attacks of pain. If the painful lesion is a neuritis, there will be evidence of sensory change in the involved branches, together with reflex changes, such as absence of the corneal, sneeze, or palatal reflexes. If, however, it is a neuralgia, the routine examination will fail to show objective evidence of nerve involvement.

Trophic Phenomena. Trophic and sensory changes may also occur in disease of the trigeminal nerve. In lesions of the ophthalmic division there is anesthesia of the cornea, and this is sometimes followed by the development of corneal ulcerations and inflammation which may result in ophthalmia. This **neuroparalytic keratitis** may follow rhizotomy of the fifth nerve for the relief of tic douloureux. It is necessary to protect the eye very carefully whenever the cornea is anesthetic. Corneal ulcerations also occur in herpes ophthalmicus. In anesthesia of the nose there is inability to recognize such substances as ammonia and acetic acid; this is often accompanied by dryness of the nasal mucosa which may result in complete loss of smell. There may be trophic changes in the nasal mucosa and adjacent structures, sometimes with resulting erosion of the ala nasi. Caries of the jaw bone and loosening of the teeth may also be manifestations of a trophic disturbance.

Abnormalities in lacrimal, salivary, and mucous secretion, either a decrease or an increase in secretion, may be associated with lesions of the trigeminal nerve. This nerve, however, does not have secretory functions and does not normally produce these secretions. Lacrimation is a function of the facial nerve, and salivation and mucous production are functions of the facial and glossopharyngeal nerves and the sympathetic division of the autonomic nervous system. The fifth nerve, however, is intimately connected with these nerves through reflex centers and through the ganglia previously described. These various secretions may be reflex responses to stimuli mediated through the trigeminal nerve. Taste, too, which is not a function of the fifth nerve, is intimately connected with it and is carried through the lingual nerve to the chorda tympani. A Horner's syndrome (see "Sympathetic Innervation, Ch. 11), with characteristic eye findings and loss of sweating on the involved side of the face, may be seen with lesions of the fifth nerve, especially of the gasserian

ganglion. This, however, is the result of involvement of the sympathetic plexus which surrounds the carotid artery rather than of the nerve itself.

Localization of Fifth Nerve Lesions. Disorders of function of the trigeminal nerve may be the result of lesions at various sites in the central or peripheral nervous system. Some of the more frequent or important are as follows:

Supranuclear involvement of the trigeminal nerve is usually due to vascular lesions, neoplasms, degenerative changes, or inflammatory reactions affecting the cerebral center, internal capsule, basal ganglia, cerebral peduncle, or pons above the nuclear areas. The manifestations are predominantly motor in type, usually without profound paralysis unless there is bilateral involvement. There are no fasciculations or atrophy. The jaw reflex is exaggerated. There may be irritative motor phenomena in cortical or extrapyramidal lesions. In pseudobulbar palsy and amyotrophic lateral sclerosis there may be pronounced bilateral weakness. The former is usually the result of bilateral cerebral thromboses or hemorrhages, but is also found in association with cerebral neoplasms, encephalitis, or vascular, inflammatory, or neoplastic lesions involving the midbrain or pons above the motor nucleus. In thalamic lesions there may be anesthesia dolorosa of the contralateral trigeminal area.

Nuclear lesions may be of various types. Pontine neoplasms, inflammations, and degenerative and vascular lesions may affect either the motor or sensory nuclei or both. The motor weakness may be considerable and accompanied by atrophy and loss of the jaw reflex. In progressive degenerations, such as progressive bulbar palsy and syringobulbia, there are also fasciculations of the paretic muscles. Owing to the prolonged extension of the descending root and nucleus of the fifth nerve through the pons and medulla into the upper portion of the cervical cord, lesions far below the middle portion of the pons may cause sensory changes in the segmental distribution of the nerve. Multiple sclerosis, syringomyelia, polioencephalitis, and vascular lesions in the brain stem may affect the trigeminal nerve and may cause dissociation of sensation, absence of the corneal reflex, and pain in the distribution of the various divisions of the nerve, together with motor changes. Nuclear lesions are almost always accompanied by other symptoms referable to the pons or brain stem, such as involvement of other nuclei or centers, or interference with ascending or descending pathways. Inasmuch as the ascending lateral spinothalamic tract lies in close approximation to the tract of the descending root of the trigeminal, a lesion of one may involve the other, resulting in anesthesia of the ipsilateral side of the face and the contralateral side of the body. In thrombosis of the posterior inferior cerebellar artery and other medullary syndromes (Ch. 18) there are changes of fifth nerve function. The spasms which occur in toxic conditions and in tetany may result from nuclear involvement.

Infranuclear lesions also may involve the sensory filaments, the motor nerve, or both. In meningitis and in skull fractures, stab wounds, or other traumatic lesions, the trigeminal nerve may be injured just after its exit from the pons. Tumors of the cerebellopontine angle and other neoplasms or gummas involving the base of the skull or the meninges commonly affect the sensory branches with resulting pain, anesthesia, and loss of the corneal reflex. Various branches may be affected by lesions within the cavernous sinus, aneurysms of the circle of Willis or the internal carotid artery, infections of the petrous bone, orbital cellulitis or tumors, polyneuritis, or tumors or abscesses in the temporal lobe or middle cranial fossa. Branches of the trigeminal nerve are frequently involved in neoplasms of the nasopharynx and in metastatic malignancies (see Fig. 12-4). Branches of the nerve may also be affected by carotid artery dissection.

Neoplasms such as neurinomas of the fifth nerve usually occur at the gasserian ganglion but may involve the nerve itself. These cause not only pain and sensory changes, but loss of motor power as well, and owing to the proximity of the ganglion to the carotid artery and to its sympathetic plexus, there may be ptosis, miosis, and other evidence of a cervical sympathetic paralysis. The term **paratrigeminal** or **Raeder's syndrome** is used when a Horner's syndrome is present along with ipsilateral motor and sensory trigeminal nerve dysfunction; this is usually found with neoplasms of the gasserian ganglion or middle cranial fossa. Involvement of the muscles themselves or of the myoneural junction causes motor weakness without sensory changes. In myasthenia gravis the paresis may be so profound that the patient may have to use his hand to assist in closing his jaw when chewing.

Pain of Trigeminal Nerve Origin. Pains referred to the various branches of the trigeminal nerve occur frequently. They may be of re-

flex origin. A careful examination should always be made to determine a local cause. As a general rule, the radiation of pain is at first confined to one division, and search for the cause of the pain should always commence with a thorough investigation of those parts supplied by that division. When severe pain is present, however, there is radiation over the branches of the other main divisions. There may be associated spasm and contraction of muscles. Pain of this type may be associated with dental caries, alveolar disease, sinus involvement, glaucoma, and malignant disease within the sinuses. Neuritis of the trigeminal nerve is a result of the same processes which cause neuritis elsewhere in the body — infections, toxic processes, vitamin deficiencies, etc. It is usually predominantly sensory in nature. A specific type of neuritis may be associated with the industrial use of trichloroethylene, and a similar neuritis results if trichloroethylene is used in the treatment of tic douloureux. Stilbamidine isethionate, first used in the therapy of kala-azar and formerly for tic douloureux, also causes a neuritis confined largely to the distribution of the fifth nerve. Herpes zoster of the trigeminal nerve is an extremely painful condition, both in its acute stage and in the form of postherpetic neuralgia. Usually seen in elderly people, it most often affects branches of the ophthalmic division, and is known as **herpes ophthalmicus.** The pain and vesicles are distributed over the forehead, eyelid, and cornea, and the involvement of the latter may be followed by ulcerations and keratitis, resulting in corneal opacities and often in ophthalmia and blindness. There may be associated involvement of the motor division and the seventh and eighth cranial nerves and occasionally there are encephalitic manifestations or cerebrovascular insults.

Perhaps the most frequent lesion of the trigeminal nerve, if one excepts the limited reflex involvements associated with the diseases of the teeth or sinuses, is **trigeminal neuralgia,** or **tic douloureux** (Fothergill's neuralgia). This condition usually occurs in elderly people, and is characterized by sudden attacks of excruciating, lancinating pain of momentary duration in the distribution of one or more of the major divisions of the nerve. The attacks are usually brought on by stimulation of the trigger zones described previously, and accordingly the patient may refuse to eat, talk, wash his face, shave, or brush his teeth for fear of initiating an attack. Exposure to cold may also precipitate the pain. Objective examination shows no evidence of impairment of function of the nerve, and sensory tests, motor power, and reflexes are all normal. The symptoms may stop spontaneously for a period of time, but usually recur. The underlying etiology of and exact mechanism for this pain are still not known, but both central and peripheral pathophysiologic alterations have been suggested as possible explanations for the syndrome, including vascular pressure on the nerve outside the brain stem in the posterior fossa. In young persons tic douloureux may be a feature of multiple sclerosis, and the pain may even switch sides in this disorder.

Many alternate neurosurgical technics have been advanced for the treatment of trigeminal neuralgia, each of which gave varying degrees of relief. Decompression of the nerve, with separation of any pulsatile vessels from it in the posterior fossa has become a more common treatment in recent years, but there is still a place for the earlier ablative forms of surgery. Medical treatment in the form of carbamazepine and phenytoin gives relief in the majority of patients, and other drugs affecting transmission of nerve impulses have been used as adjunctive therapy. The use of these drugs has decreased the need for surgical therapy.

Pain similar to, if not identical with, tic douloureux is sometimes found in syringobulbia and tabes dorsalis. There are many atypical facial neuralgias that resemble tic douloureux but must be differentiated from it. **Sluder's syndrome,** or **neuralgia of the sphenopalatine ganglion,** is said to be characterized by pain in the orbital area, cheek, roof of the mouth, root of the nose, upper jaw, and teeth, and sometimes extending to the ear, occiput, neck, shoulder, and arm. The pain is said to be relieved by local anesthetic infiltration of the sphenopalatine ganglion, but the existence of such a symptom complex is questioned. So-called **vidian neuralgia** has a similar distribution, but pain in the ear is a more prominent symptom; this has been said to be due to irritation of the vidian nerve by infection in the sphenoid sinus. **Costen's syndrome** consists of unilateral pain in the face and head accompanied by pain in the ear, impaired hearing, tinnitus, and vertigo; this symptom complex results from distortion of and destructive changes in the temporomandibular joint, secondary to malocclusion. In **Eagle's syndrome** there is atypical facial pain, pharyngeal pain, and ear discomfort, presumably due to elongation of the styloid process of the temporal bone. Many of the atypical facial neuralgias may be reflex in origin, occasionally involving connections between the trigeminal nerve and other cranial afferent and cervical nerves, and others may be associated with autonomic nervous system disorders; often the pain is deep, boring, and agonizing, and is not relieved by section of the fifth nerve. Those of psychogenic origin are termed **psychalgias.** Migraine, especially of the hemicranial type, may simulate a neuralgia of the ophthalmic division of the fifth nerve, as may the so-called **cluster headache** (atypical migraine, Horton's headache, or histamine cephalgia). In neuritis of the fifth nerve resulting from various toxic, infectious, and deficiency factors there may be attacks of pain similar to those of the neuralgias, but there is residual pain between attacks, and a detailed examination should show impairment of sensation and loss of reflexes.

Other Trigeminal Nerve Disorders. The **Gunn phenomenon,** or **jaw-winking reflex,** occurs with partial ptosis of congenital origin; opening of the mouth and chewing and lateral movements of the jaw cause an exaggerated reflex elevation of the ptotic lid. This is probably a pathologic associated, or synkinetic, movement, and proprioceptive impulses from the pterygoid muscles are relayed to the oculomotor nucleus. The automatic closure of one eye on opening the mouth has been called the **inverted** or **reversed Gunn phenomenon,** or **Marin Amat's syndrome.** This has been explained as an associated movement involving the facial and masticatory muscles, but inasmuch as it is seen only in patients who have had a peripheral facial paralysis, it is probably an intrafacial associated movement.

The **auriculotemporal syndrome (Frey's syndrome)** consists of flushing, warmness, and excessive perspiration over the cheek and pinna on one side following the ingestion of highly seasoned food. It is usually a sequel of trauma or infection of the parotid gland, with injury to the regional nerves, and there may be associated trigeminal sensory changes. It is probable that in regeneration of the severed auriculotemporal nerve the secretory fibers to the parotid gland become misdirected to the sweat glands and the vasodilator endings, or there may be abnormal local irritability of cholinergic fibers. The symptoms have been relieved by interruption of the efferent arc by means of either alcohol injection or surgical section of the auriculotemporal nerve

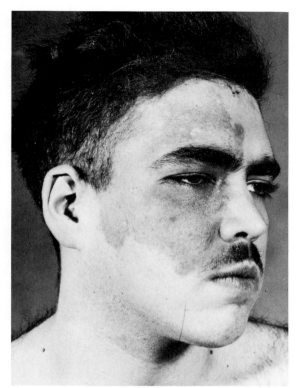

FIG. 12–7. A patient with encephalotrigeminal angiomatosis (Sturge–Weber syndrome).

or intracranial section of the glossopharyngeal nerve. In the so-called **encephalotrigeminal angiomatosis (Sturge – Weber syndrome,** or **Weber – Dimitri disease)** there are congenital nevi or angiomas over the side of the face in the trigeminal distribution with associated ipsilateral leptomeningeal angiomas and intracortical calcifications; there are also cerebral hemiatrophy with contralateral hemiparesis and focal convulsions (Fig. 12-7). Progressive facial hemiatrophy is described in Chapter 13.

BIBLIOGRAPHY

Accornero N, Berardelli A, Bini G et al. Corneal reflex elicited by electrical stimulation of the human cornea. Neurology 1980;30:782

Brodal A. Central course of afferent fibers for pain in facial, glossopharyngeal and vagus nerves: clinical observations. Arch Neurol Psychiatry 1947;57:292

Brodal A. Neurological Anatomy in Relation to Clinical Medicine, 3rd ed. New York, Oxford University Press, 1981

Cogan DG, Ginsburg J. Representation of corneal and conjunctival sensation in the central nervous system. Arch Ophthalmol 1952;47:273

Eagle WW. Elongated styloid process: Symptoms and treatment. Arch Otolaryngol 1958;64:127

Francis KR, Williams DP, Troost BT. Facial numbness and dysesthesia. New features of carotid artery dissection. Arch Neurol 1987;44:345.

Gunn RM. Congenital ptosis with peculiar associated movements of the affected lid. Trans Ophthalmol Soc UK 1883;3:283

Jaeger R. Permanent relief of the tic douloureux by gasserian injection of hot water. Arch Neurol Psychiatry 1957;77:1

Kerr FWL. The etiology of trigeminal neuralgia. Arch Neurol 1963;8:15

Magladery JW, Teasdall RD. Corneal reflexes: An electromyographic study in man. Arch Neurol 1961;5:269

Ross RT. Corneal reflexes in hemisphere disease. J Neurol Neurosurg Psychiatry 1972;35:877

Shelden HC, Pudenz RH, Freshwater DB et al. Compression rather than decompression for trigeminal neuralgia. J Neurosurg 1955;12:123

Singer PA, Chicarmane A, Festoff BW et al. Trismus. An unusual sign in polymyositis. Arch Neurol 1985;42:1116

Szentágothai J. Functional representation in the trigeminal nucleus. J Comp Neurol 1949;90:111

Szentágothai J, Kiss T. Projection of dermatomes on the substantia gelatinosa. Arch Neurol Psychiatry 1949;62:734

Taarnhøj P. Decompression of the trigeminal root and the posterior part of the ganglion as treatment in trigeminal neuralgia. J Neurosurg 1952;9:288

Walker AE. Anatomy, physiology, and surgical consideration of the spinal tract of the trigeminal nerve. J Neurophysiol 1939;2:234

Wartenberg R. Head retraction reflex. Am J Med Sci 1941;201:553

ANATOMY AND PHYSIOLOGY

The facial, or seventh cranial, nerve is predominantly a motor nerve, innervating the muscles of facial expression. In addition, however, it carries parasympathetic secretory fibers to the salivary and lacrimal glands and to the mucous membranes of the oral and nasal cavities, and it conveys various types of sensation, including exteroceptive sensation from the region of the eardrum, taste sensation from the anterior two-thirds of the tongue, general visceral sensation from the salivary glands and mucosa of the nose and pharynx, and proprioceptive sensation from the muscles it supplies. Anatomically the motor division of the nerve is separated from the portion which carries sensation and parasympathetic fibers; this latter part is frequently referred to as the **nervus intermedius,** or the **pars intermedia of Wrisberg.** Some authorities consider this a distinct nerve, although it is usually classed as part of the facial nerve.

The Motor Portion

The motor nucleus of the seventh nerve, the largest motor cranial nerve nucleus, lies deep in the reticular formation of the lowest part of the pons, medial to the nucleus of the descending root of the fifth nerve, anterior and lateral to the nucleus of the sixth nerve, and posterior to the superior olivary nucleus (see Fig. 11-7). Two groups of cells have been described. The dorsal group supplies the frontalis, upper facial, and zygomatic muscles and the upper half of the or-

bicularis oculi; the ventral group supplies the lower half of the orbicularis oculi, the lower face, and the platysma. The intrapontine root of the nerve arises from the dorsal surface of the nucleus and runs dorsomedially toward the floor of the fourth ventricle. It then passes upward, encircling the nucleus of the abducens nerve and producing an elevation, the facial colliculus, in the rhomboid fossa; this is the first genu of the facial nerve. The fibers then proceed forward, downward, and laterally through the pons, close to the facial nucleus, to emerge at the lateral aspect of the caudal border of the pons, between the pons and the medulla and between the inferior olivary body and the inferior cerebellar peduncle. Here the nerve lies in the cerebellopontine angle lateral to the exit of the sixth nerve and medial to the eighth. It enters the internal auditory meatus above the eighth nerve, with the pars intermedia between the acoustic and facial nerves. At the bottom of the meatus the nerve enters the facial canal, or fallopian aqueduct. It is at first directed lateralward, between the cochlea and vestibule, toward the medial wall of the tympanic cavity. It then turns suddenly backward, at its second genu, and arches downward behind the tympanic cavity to emerge from the stylomastoid foramen. After leaving the skull it runs forward in the substance of the parotid gland and divides behind the ramus of the mandible into its constituent parts (Fig. 13-1).

The cortical center of the muscles of facial expression is in the lower third of the precentral convolution. Impulses arising in the pyramidal and related cells are carried through the corona

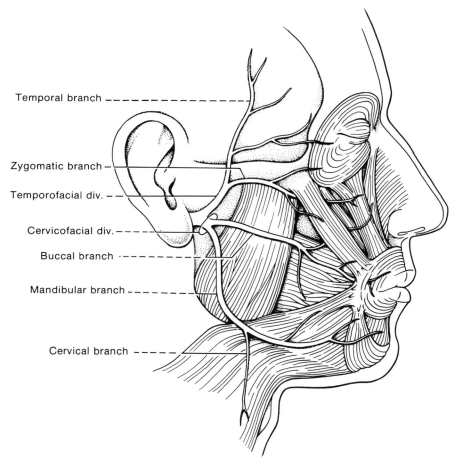

Temporal branch

Zygomatic branch

Temporofacial div.

Cervicofacial div.

Buccal branch

Mandibular branch

Cervical branch

FIG. 13–1. Branches and distribution of the facial nerve.

radiata, the genu of the internal capsule, and the medial portion of the cerebral peduncles, into the pons, where they decussate; the majority supply the facial nucleus on the opposite side. That portion of the nucleus which innervates the lower half to two-thirds of the face has predominantly crossed, unilateral supranuclear control, whereas the portion that supplies the upper third to half has bilateral control. There is some evidence that the muscles of the lower portion of the face receive more direct cortical innervation by way of the facial nucleus than do the muscles of the upper face and forehead. The facial nuclei also receive bilateral innervation from the extrapyramidal cortex and the basal ganglia, and possibly from the hypothalamus; this is concerned with the maintenance of tone in the facial muscles, and with automatic and emotional movements.

The motor branches of the facial nerve supply all the muscles of facial expression from the scalp and forehead through the platysma, including the extrinsic and intrinsic muscles of the ear. In addition they supply the stapedius, the posterior belly of the digastricus, and the stylohyoid muscles. The branch to the stapedius originates within the facial canal. At its exit from the stylomastoid foramen the facial nerve gives off the posterior auricular, digastric, and stylohyoid branches. The posterior auricular branch supplies the occipitalis, posterior auricular, and transverse and oblique auricular muscles. The digastric and stylohyoid branches supply respectively the posterior belly of the digastricus and the stylohyoid muscles.

Within the substance of the parotid gland the facial nerve divides into temporofacial and cervicofacial divisions at the so-called pes anserinus. The former divides into the temporal, zygomatic, mandibular, and cervical branches. The temporal branch innervates the frontalis and corrugator muscles, the upper part of the orbicularis oculi, the anterior and superior auricular muscles, and the intrinsic muscles on the lateral surface of the ear. The zygomatic branch is distributed to the lower and lateral part of the orbicularis oculi and some of the muscles of the nose and upper lip; it supplies in part the quadratus labii superioris, nasalis, caninus, risorius, and zygomaticus muscles. The buccal branches, which are larger than the zygomatic, also supply part of the orbicularis oculi, nasalis, caninus, risorius, and zygomaticus muscles, and in addition innervate the other muscles of the nose and upper lip, namely, the procerus, dilatores nares, orbicularis oris, and buccinator muscles. The mandibular branch supplies the muscles of the lower lip and chin, namely, the lower part of the orbicularis oris, the quadratus labii inferioris, mentalis, and triangularis. The cervical branch supplies the platysma.

The muscles of facial expression are responsible for all voluntary and involuntary movements of the face except those associated with movement of the jaws, and for all play of emotions upon the face. The frontalis raises the eyebrows and the skin over the root of the nose and draws the scalp forward, throwing the skin of the forehead into transverse wrinkles. The occipitalis draws the scalp backward. These two, with their aponeurotic connection, are called the epicranius, and acting together they cause movement of the entire scalp. The orbicularis oculi, or orbicularis palpebrarum, is the sphincter of the eyelids. The palpebral portion causes narrowing of the palpebral fissure and gentle closing of the lids. The orbital portion draws the skin of the forehead, temple, and cheek toward the medial angle of the orbit; it pulls down the eyebrow and draws up the skin of the cheek in order to close the eye firmly and give increased protection to the eyeball. The corrugator (corrugator supercilii) draws the eyebrow down and medially, producing vertical wrinkles in the forehead; it is the "frowning" muscle.

The muscles of the nose are as follows: The procerus (pyramidalis nasi) draws the medial angle of the eyebrows downward and produces transverse wrinkles over the bridge of the nose. The nasalis (compressor nares) depresses the cartilaginous portion of the nose and draws the ala toward the septum. The depressor septi draws the ala down and constricts the apertures of the nares. The dilatores nares posterior and anterior enlarge the apertures of the nares.

The orbicularis oris is the sphincter of the mouth; it closes the lips. By its superficial fibers it causes the lips to protrude, whereas with its deep fibers it draws them in and presses them against the teeth. The quadratus labii superioris elevates the upper lip and dilates the nostril, the caninus (levator anguli oris) muscle raises the angle of the mouth, and the zygomaticus draws the mouth backward and upward; all three of these aid in the formation of the nasolabial fold. The risorius retracts or draws out the angle of the mouth. The buccinator compresses the cheeks and keeps the food under pressure of the cheeks in chewing. The quadratus labii inferioris, or depressor labii inferioris, draws the lower lip downward and lateralward. The mentalis, or levator menti, raises and protrudes the lower lip and wrinkles the skin of the chin. The triangularis, or depressor anguli oris, depresses the angle of the mouth. The platysma draws down the lower lip and the angle of the mouth; it also depresses the lower jaw and raises and wrinkles the skin of the neck.

The extrinsic muscles of the ear are the posterior auricular, which retracts the pinna; the superior auricular, which elevates it; and the anterior auricular, which draws it upward and forward. The intrinsic muscles on the lateral surface of the ear, the helicis major, helicis minor, tragicus, and antitragicus, and those on the cranial surface of the ear, the transverse and oblique auriculars, are vestigial remnants and probably have little remaining function.

Additional muscles which are supplied by the facial nerve but are not muscles of facial expression are the stapedius, the posterior belly of the digastricus, and the stylohyoid. The former draws the head of the stapes backward and rotates it toward the posterior wall of the tympanic cavity; this increases the tension of the middle ear ossicles and of both the membrane which closes the fenestra ovalis and the tympanic membrane. The digastricus and stylohyoid act together to raise and draw backward the hyoid bone and thyroid cartilage. They also elevate and retract the base of the tongue, aid in swallowing, and prevent the return of food into the mouth in the second act of deglutition.

The Nervus Intermedius

The nervus intermedius, or sensory and parasympathetic root of the facial nerve, is lateral and inferior to the motor root (Fig. 13-2). Within the internal auditory meatus it lies between the motor root and the eighth nerve. The sensory

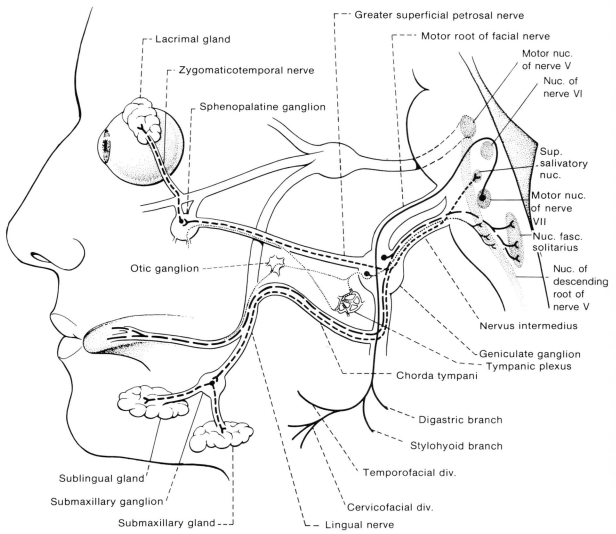

FIG. 13–2. *Course and branches of the facial nerve.*

cells are situated in the geniculate ganglion, at the bend of the facial nerve within the facial canal, and their neuraxes enter the pons with the motor root. The geniculate ganglion is continued distally as the chorda tympani which carries taste and general visceral afferent fibers as well as preganglionic parasympathetic fibers. The chorda tympani leaves the trunk of the facial nerve a short distance above the stylomastoid foramen. It goes forward and slightly upward in a minute canal in the posterior wall of the tympanic cavity and then enters and crosses the cavity. It passes to the base of the skull where it goes downward and forward to join the posterior border of the lingual nerve, a branch of the mandibular division of the trigeminal nerve.

The fibers which carry exteroceptive sensation have their cell bodies in the geniculate ganglion and terminate on the descending root and the nucleus of the descending root of the trigeminal nerve; their central connections are identical with those of the trigeminal nerve. It has been said that the pathway of the proprioceptive impulses is with the mesencephalic root of the fifth nerve, but the fibers which carry these impulses probably have their cells of origin in the geniculate ganglion, and terminate in the motor nucleus of the facial nerve. The fibers which carry gustatory and general visceral sensation terminate on the fasciculus solitarius and its nucleus. Secondary neurons pass from this structure to the superior and inferior salivatory nuclei, from which parasympathetic impulses go to the salivary glands. Other neurons pass to the reticular gray matter and descend in the ipsilateral and contralateral reticulospinal tracts to synapse with preganglionic sympathetic neurons on the intermediolateral column of the upper thoracic portion of the spinal cord. The neuraxes of these cells ascend to the superior cervical ganglia, and postganglionic fibers go to the salivary glands. Impulses which carry gustatory sensation to consciousness probably ascend with the contralateral medial lemniscus to the thalamus, and then, after a further synapse, terminate on the cortex in the lower part of the postcentral gyrus near the area for somatic sensibility of the tongue. Other impulses go to the hypothalamus for reflex stimulation of salivation. Smell and taste are functionally related, and the central connections dealing with gustatory sensation are correlated with those for olfactory sensation.

The *sensory distribution* of the facial nerve is not as definitely established as the motor supply, but it is generally accepted that the nerve carries mixed sensations. Exteroceptive sensations are conducted from part of the external auditory canal, tympanic membrane, and lateral surface of the pinna, and a small area behind the ear and over the mastoid process. There is a marked individual variation in this distribution. Taste sensation from the anterior two-thirds of the tongue is carried through the lingual nerve to the chorda tympani, and then to the geniculate ganglion. The seventh nerve may also carry taste sensation from the mucosa of the soft palate through the sphenopalatine ganglion. General visceral sensations are probably carried through the facial nerve from the lacrimal and salivary glands and the mucosa of the mouth and pharynx. Proprioceptive sensations may be mediated from all the muscles supplied by the nerve. The seventh nerve may also carry impulses of deep pain and deep pressure from the face.

The efferent preganglionic *parasympathetic fibers* that initiate salivary, lacrimal, and mucous secretion are also situated in the nervus intermedius. Those that stimulate salivary secretion arise in the superior salivatory nucleus in the pons. They pass through the nervus intermedius, geniculate ganglion, and chorda tympani, and terminate in the submaxillary gland (Langley's ganglion). Postganglionic fibers carry secretory and vasodilator impulses to the submaxillary glands and the mucous membrane of the mouth and tongue (see Fig. 13-2). These glands also receive a sympathetic supply from the thoracic autonomic division through the superior cervical ganglion and the carotid plexus. Stimulation of the parasympathetic fibers causes the formation of thin, watery saliva, and vasodilation, whereas stimulation of the sympathetics causes the formation of a scant supply of thick, turbid saliva, and vasoconstriction. Also, dry, acid, and sour foods induce a copious watery secretion, whereas moist foods cause the production of a scant, thick secretion. There is a central regulatory mechanism for salivary flow in the hypothalamus. Olfactory and gustatory impulses are received in the hypothalamus, and discharge paths go to the salivatory and sympathetic nuclei.

Impulses that stimulate lacrimation arise from a part of the superior salivatory nucleus or in a related nuclear mass which is sometimes called the lacrimal nucleus (see Fig. 13-2). Preganglionic fibers pass through the nervus intermedius and the geniculate ganglion into the greater superficial petrosal nerve. This goes forward through the hiatus of the facial canal and joins the deep petrosal nerve from the carotid sympathetic plexus to form the vidian nerve, or the nerve of the pterygoid canal. It supplies the motor, or parasympathetic, root of the sphenopalatine ganglion. Postganglionic fibers then travel in the zygomaticotemporal branch of the maxillary division to the lacrimal branch of the ophthalmic, and thus to the lacrimal gland. Stimulation of the trigeminal nerve in the eye or the nose produces tear secretion.

CLINICAL EXAMINATION

Examination of the Motor Functions

The examination of the motor functions of the facial nerve consists of an appraisal of the action of the muscles of facial expression. First the face is inspected, mobility of facial expression observed, and any asymmetry or abnormality of the muscles noted. A one-sided appearance while talking or smiling, inequality of the palpebral fissures, infrequent or asymmetric blinking, smoothness of the face and absence of normal wrinkling, or increased wrinkling may all give clues to facial nerve involvement. It should be noted whether the abnormality is more marked during emotional stress or during voluntary effort.

In making a detailed examination the patient is asked to contract the various muscles individually and in unison. He is asked to frown, wrinkle his forehead, raise his eyebrows, and corrugate his brow, to close his eyes, both singly and bilaterally, first lightly, then tightly, and then against resistance; to draw back the angles of his mouth, show his teeth, grimace, blow out his cheeks, purse his mouth, whistle, and retract the chin muscles. Retraction of the angles of the mouth is noted both on voluntary effort and on smiling, and voluntary and emotional responses of all muscles are compared. The patient may smile spontaneously after attempting to whistle. Function of the auricular muscles cannot be tested in most individuals, although some individuals can voluntarily contract the extrinsic muscles. The same is true of the occipitalis and scalp movements. Function of the platysma is tested by having the patient open his mouth against resistance or bite his teeth together firmly. The tone of the muscles of facial expression is noted, and atrophy and fasciculations are looked for. Abnormal movements such as tremors, spasms, tics, grimacing, and athetoid, myoclonic, and choreiform movements should be recorded, as should immobility, or masking, of the face. Special tests of motor function and confirmatory signs of facial paresis or paralysis, including the examination in stuporous patients, are discussed under disorders of function of the nerve. In infants, facial movements are observed during crying. Articulation of the labial sounds is discussed in Chapter 19.

The function of the stylohyoid muscle and the posterior belly of the digastricus cannot be adequately tested, but in paralysis of these there may be some weakness of deglutition with regurgitation of food. Weakness of the stapedius muscle is not apparent objectively, but the patient may complain of hyperacusis, especially for low tones.

Examination of the Reflexes

Certain reflexes should be elicited in the examination of the facial nerve. The corneal and nasal reflexes and their modifications are discussed in Chapter 12, the sucking reflex in Chapter 15, and the palmomental reflex in Chapter 35. The following responses are those in which the seventh nerve plays the major role, and which, therefore, may be considered tests for its function.

The Orbicularis Oculi Reflex. Percussion at the outer aspect of the supraorbital ridge, over the glabella, or around the margin of the orbit, or a sudden stretching of the orbicularis muscle, is followed by a reflex contraction of this muscle, with resulting closing of the eye. The response is usually bilateral. This reflex has been known by a number of names, such as the **supraorbital (McCarthy's),** the **glabellar,** and the **nasopalpebral reflex,** depending upon the site of application of the stimulus. It can sometimes be elicited by percussion of the forehead as far as the border of the hair, or by tapping the root of the nose. It is best tested by pulling back, between the thumb and index finger, a fold of skin on the temple lateral to the external canthus, and then applying a brisk tap to the thumb. There is an immediate contraction of the orbicularis, accompanied, to a similar degree, by a contralateral response. This is a muscle stretch reflex, and the corneal reflex may be considered its superficial counterpart. The afferent portion of the arc may be carried through both the facial nerve (as proprioceptive impulses) and the trigeminal nerve; the efferent impulses pass through the facial nerve, and the reflex center is in the pons. The strength of response varies in different individuals, but the reflex is diminished or absent in nuclear and peripheral lesions of the facial nerve, is absent in coma, and is preserved or exaggerated in supranuclear varieties of facial palsy and corticobulbar lesions above the nucleus of the seventh nerve. It is also exaggerated in extrapyramidal disease and the response may continue with repeated stimuli, particularly in parkinsonism, whereas in the normal individual it disappears after a few stimulations. This persistent response is sometimes referred to as **Myerson's sign;** it may disappear with medical therapy for Parkinson's disease.

The Palpebral Reflexes. Reflex contraction of the orbicularis oculi muscle and consequent closing of the eye may be a response to other stimuli. A reflex closing of the eyes in response to a sudden loud noise is known as the **auditory-palpebral, auro-** or **acousticopalpebral, cochleopalpebral,** or **cochleoorbicularis reflex.** The response usually is a bilateral one, more marked on the ipsilateral side. The sensory impulse is carried through the cochlear nerve, and the efferent portion of the reflex arc is mediated through the facial nerve. A reflex closing of the eyes in response to a strong light or a sudden visual stimulus is the **visuo-palpebral, visual-orbicularis, opticofacial, blink,** or **menace reflex.** In this response the afferent portion of the reflex arc is carried from the retina through the optic nerve to the visual cortex, and then to the facial nuclei. In a modification of this, the **emergency light reflex,** the closing of the eyes is accompanied by constriction of the pupils, lowering of the eyebrows, bending of the head, and, sometimes, elevation of the arm (see "Reflex Eye Movements," Ch. 11). Closing of the eyes in response to a painful stimulus to the face or in the region of the eye is known as the **trigeminofacial, trigeminopalpebral,** or **trigeminoorbicularis reflex;** the afferent portion of the reflex arc is carried through the trigeminal nerve. The trigeminofacial reflex may also be elicited by a sudden gust of air, or by cold or heat. The **palatopalpebral reflex** is a closing of the eyes in response to stimulation of the palate. The afferent impulse may be carried by the trigeminal, glossopharyngeal, or vagus nerves.

The Oculogyric-auricular Reflex. This consists of a retraction of the auricle and a curling back of the helix on lateral gaze in the extreme opposite direction, or a retraction of both auricles, more on the opposite side, on lateral gaze to one side. The afferent impulse is a proprioceptive one carried through the ocular nerves, and the efferent impulse is conveyed through the facial nerve to the auricular muscles.

The Palpebral-oculogyric Reflex. On contraction of the orbiculares and closing of the eyes, the eyeballs turn upward in the vast majority of healthy persons; this occurs not only with voluntary closing of the eyes, but also in sleep. It is actually an associated movement and not a reflex, but proprioceptive impulses are carried through the facial nerve to the medial longitudinal fasciculus, and efferent impulses are relayed through the oculomotor nerves to the superior rectus muscles. An exaggeration of this response is known as **Bell's phenomenon** and is seen in peripheral types of facial palsy (see "Peripheral Facial Paralysis"). The **orbicularis reflex,** a constriction of the pupils on either closing or upward deviation of the eyes, is discussed with the pupillary reflexes (Ch. 11).

The Orbicularis Oris Reflex. Percussion over the upper lip or the side of the nose is followed by a contraction of the ipsilateral quadratus labii superioris and cranius (levator anguli oris) muscles. If the mentalis (levator menti) muscles are also stimulated, there is, in addition, an elevation and protrusion of the lower lip and wrinkling of the skin of the chin. This reflex, which is also known as the **perioral, oral, buccal,** or **nasomental reflex,** is mediated through the trigeminal (sensory) and facial (motor)

nerves. It is not present to any degree in normal persons except during the first year of life, but is present and often exaggerated with corticobulbar lesions above the nucleus of the seventh nerve and also with disease of the extrapyramidal system. A slight or brief response to a single stimulus may not be significant. On the other hand, a strong stimulus in patients with upper motor neuron disease may evoke, in addition, either the jaw reflex when the lower lip is tapped or the head retraction reflex on stimulation of the upper lip. The reflex is difficult to test in edentulous patients.

When the response is increased, tapping of the upper or lower lip, or even sweeping a tongue blade briskly across the upper lip, is followed by contraction of both the upper and lower portions of the orbicularis and the muscles about the base of the nose, causing a puckering or protrusion of the lips known as the **snout reflex.** This is seen in bilateral supranuclear lesions and sometimes in diffuse cerebral degenerations associated with dementia, and is related to the sucking reflex (Ch. 15). The **palmomental reflex,** in which there is ipsilateral contraction of the mentalis and orbicularis oris muscles following stimulation of the thenar area of the hand, is described in Chapter 35.

Chvostek's Sign. This is a spasm or tetanic, cramplike contraction, of the ipsilateral facial muscles that appears on tapping over the exit of the facial nerve anterior to the ear. Degrees of response are discussed in Chapter 39. This is an important sign in tetany, but it is also observed in other conditions in which there is increased reflex irritability, such as dementia or upper motor neuron dysfunction. This may be either a trigeminofacial reflex, or a reflex involving only the facial nerve, the afferent impulse being proprioceptive and carried by this nerve. Electromyographic studies of latency time, however, indicate that the response is due to direct mechanical stimulation of the motor fibers in the nerve.

Examination of the Sensory Functions

The sensory functions of the seventh nerve are not easily tested. The exteroceptive sensations supply relatively inaccessible areas, namely, the external auditory canal and the tympanic membrane. These same areas also receive exteroceptive innervation from the trigeminal, glossopharyngeal, vagus, and great auricular (second and third cervical) nerves, with an overlap in distribution. As a result, no adequate examination can be made. General visceral, proprioceptive, and "deep" sensibilities cannot be evaluated. Consequently, the sensory examination of the seventh nerve is limited to the testing of taste, with a possible exception. Hitselberger and House express the belief that one of the earliest signs of the presence of an acoustic neurinoma is loss of exteroceptive sensation in the facial nerve. They recommend careful testing of sensation of the posterior aspect of the external auditory canal and tympanic membrane with a fine nylon wire or a wisp of cotton.

Gustatory sense, or *taste*, is closely associated with smell, and it is known that the flavor of many foods is a combination of both olfactory and gustatory sensation, together with somatic sensations experienced in the mouth, nasopharynx, and adjacent structures. Many anosmic patients complain that they have lost their sense of taste rather than of smell, because of inability to perceive the complex flavors of foods, but some persons with anosmia can recognize many food flavors and enjoy eating. There are, however, only four fundamental tastes: sweet, salty, sour, and bitter. Sweet taste is conveyed by many monosaccharides, disaccharides, synthetic sweeteners, and chloroform. Salty taste is most characteristically found in chlorides and bromides. Sour taste is conveyed by various acids. Bitter taste results from many alkaloids and glucosides. Some observers add alkaline and metallic tastes. The flavors of foods are probably blends of the above primary tastes, or combinations of them with olfactory sensations, tactile stimuli, and even visual stimuli. There is a difference, for various substances, in the latent period and in the threshold — man is most sensitive to bitter tastes, then to sour, sweet, and salty ones. The peripheral organs of taste are the taste buds embedded in the epithelium of the tongue, and to a lesser extent in the soft palate and epiglottis. Taste buds respond preferentially, but not solely, to one taste quality. It is said that sweet and salt are perceived best in the region of the vallate papillae and on the dorsum of the tip of the tongue, sour along the borders and the tip, and bitter at the back of the tongue and on the soft palate. Taste is also carried through the glossopharyngeal nerve and probably through the vagus nerve. These three nerves which convey taste act as one part of the afferent pathway for salivation.

Taste is tested with the four common flavors; solutions of sugar, sodium chloride, acetic acid, and quinine are most frequently used. It is important in testing taste to examine the anterior and posterior portions of each half of the tongue individually. In examining the functions of the facial nerve the examiner must be certain that the test substance is placed only on the anterior two-thirds of the tongue, without flowing to or communicating with the posterior third or the opposite half. Each time the patient speaks, he retracts his tongue into his mouth. This allows the saliva to flow over it, and possibly carries the test substance to the posterior third or the opposite half. For this reason, the tongue should be protruding during the entire test and the patient should not be allowed to speak during the examination. For an accurate test, the words "sweet," "salty," "sour," and "bitter" are first written on a piece of paper. The various test substances are then in turn placed upon the portion of the tongue that is being tested, and the subject is asked to point to the word that signifies the taste that he perceives. The test substances may be placed on the tongue either by using a cotton applicator that has been dipped in the solution or by using a pipette. Powdered test substances are sometimes employed, but their use is more difficult. The mouth should be rinsed with water between tests. Bitter substances should be tested last because they leave the most aftertaste.

Taste may also be tested by the use of a galvanic current, applying the naked copper electrode to the tongue. The anode is applied to the tongue and a current of 2 – 4 milliamperes is used. A galvanic current gives a sour, metallic taste. An electrogustometer, which regulates the galvanic taste stimulus with a potentiometer, can be used to determine taste thresholds and carry out quantitative testing.

Loss and diminution of taste are called respectively **ageusia** and **hypogeusia.** Perversions or abnormal perceptions of taste are **parageusias.** There is marked individual variation in taste. Complete ageusia is rare unless there is also loss of smell. Age, wasting diseases, certain drugs, coating of the tongue, and excessive smoking diminish the power of taste. If there is loss of taste one should first eliminate the possibility of disease of the tongue.

Examination of the Secretory Functions

The secretory fibers of the facial nerve can usually be evaluated by questioning the patient and by observation. Increased lacrimation is usually apparent, and a decrease in lacrimation may be determined from the history. The amount of tear secretion may be evaluated by hanging a strip of litmus or filter paper on each lower lid, and noting the amount of moistening on each side (**Schirmer's test**). In the so-called **lacrimal reflex** a secretion of tears, usually bilateral, is produced either by stimulating the cornea or by mechanical or chemical stimulation of the nasal mucosa (the **nasolacrimal reflex**). For the latter, irritating substances such as dilute solutions of ammonia or formaldehyde may be used.

Increased and decreased salivation are also apparent from the history. The secretory fibers to the submaxillary and sublingual glands may be examined, if the occasion arises, by placing highly flavored substances upon the tongue. The patient is then asked to elevate his tongue, and if there is no interference with secretory functions, a copious supply of saliva is seen to flow from the submaxillary duct. This may be called the **salivary reflex.** It is also possible to measure the submaxillary salivary flow through fine polyethylene tubes introduced into the submaxillary ducts. The patient is given a gustatory stimulus, such as a lemon drop, and the amount of flow from each side during a 5-min period is compared.

DISORDERS OF FUNCTION

Lesions of the facial nerve are most commonly evidenced by motor changes, either paresis or spasm, although there may also be changes in sensation and in the secretory functions.

Paretic Motor Phenomena

Paralysis of the facial nerve is of two general varieties. The peripheral type is the result of a lesion involving either the nucleus or the nerve peripheral to the nucleus; the central type follows supranuclear lesions.

Peripheral Facial Paralysis. In a peripheral facial paralysis, or **prosopoplegia,** there is flaccid paralysis of all the muscles of facial expression on the involved side, and the paralysis is usually complete. There is loss of function of the frontalis, corrugator, and orbicularis oculi muscles, and the nasal muscles, the muscles of the mouth, and the platysma, together with paralysis of the stylohyoid, the posterior belly of the digastricus, the auricular muscles, and, in some instances, the stapedius. The affected side of the face is smooth, there are no wrinkles on the forehead, the eyebrow droops, the eye is open, the inferior lid sags, the nose is flattened or deviated to the opposite side, and the angle of the mouth may be depressed (Fig. 13-3). The patient is unable to raise his eyebrow, wrinkle his forehead, frown, close his eye, laugh, smile, show his teeth, blow out his cheeks, whistle, purse his mouth, retract the angle of the mouth, or retract the chin muscles on the involved side. He talks and smiles with one side of the mouth, and the mouth is drawn to the sound side on attempted movement. The lips are narrower on the paretic than on the normal side. Food accumulates between the teeth and the paralyzed cheek. The cheek is flaccid and hollowed out; it puffs out in expiration, and the patient may bite his cheek or lip in chewing. He cannot drink liquids or retain them in the mouth, but is able to swallow. Saliva may drip from the paretic side of the mouth. The tongue may be protruded in the midline but is pushed to one side by the paretic angle of the mouth, so that there is an apparent deviation.

In a peripheral facial paralysis there is difficulty with articulation, especially in pronouncing the labials and the vowels which are produced by pursing the lips. The nasolabial fold is shallower than normal, or may be absent. The ala nasi is sunken and shows no movement on respiration. The platysma is seen to be weak when the patient depresses his chin against resistance. The palpebral fissure is wider than normal, owing to **lagophthalmos,** or inability to close the eye. In blinking the involved lid fails to close or lags behind the opposite one. When the patient attempts to close his eye on the involved side the eyeball turns upward until the cornea is hidden. This is known as **Bell's phenomenon,** and is a synkinesis of central origin in which the levator palpebrae superioris, the superior rectus, and the inferior oblique muscles participate. It is an exaggeration of the palpebral-oculogyric reflex. Owing to sagging of the lower lid there is epiphora, or an overflow of tears down the cheek; there may be increased lacrimation secondary to constant irritation of the cornea. The eye may be open at all times, even in sleep. If the patient had been able to move his scalp or ear voluntarily, he will have lost his power. Involvement of the scalp muscles and extrinsic muscles of the ear, however, can seldom be demonstrated. Paralysis of the stylohyoid muscle and the posterior belly of the digastricus is not easy to identify, but there may be some weakness of deglutition, and the base of the tongue may be depressed. When the stapedius is paralyzed there is hyperacusis, especially for the low tones, and these sound louder and higher.

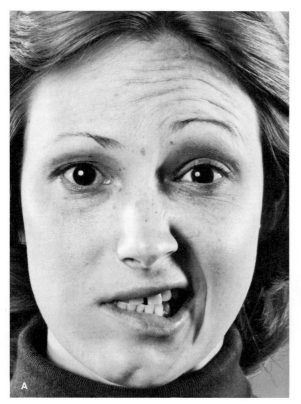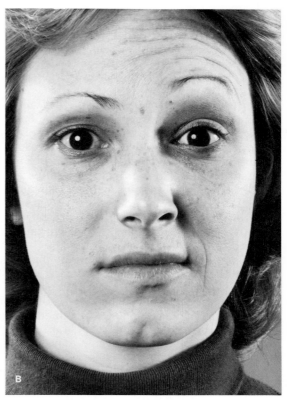

FIG. 13–3. A patient with a peripheral facial nerve palsy on the right. **A.** Patient is attempting to retract both angles of the mouth. **B.** Patient is attempting to elevate both eyebrows.

All of the above evidence of muscular weakness is present both on voluntary and involuntary contraction. The manifestations become especially marked when the patient talks or smiles, and on such occasions the asymmetry becomes much more obvious. The paralysis may result in atrophy of the muscles. The various reflexes that involve motor responses of the muscles supplied by the facial nerve are absent. The face may feel numb, but there is no objective evidence of reduction of cutaneous sensibility.

Certain confirmatory signs of facial paresis may be elicited when the peripheral paralysis is not a complete one. The patient, for instance, may be able to close his eye but is unable to close it against the resistance of the examiner's fingers. The examiner may find it easier to open the eye on the involved side against the patient's resistance than on the normal side. If the lids are passively opened and then allowed to close, the normal lid closes quickly but the closing is retarded and incomplete on the affected side. The patient should be asked to close each eye individually, and inability to close the eye on the involved side without simultaneously closing its mate may indicate a facial weakness or may be the only residual of a facial palsy. If the weakness is minimal, decreased or absent winking on the affected side may have diagnostic significance. In semicomatose or comatose patients the function of the facial nerve can be tested and the presence of a facial paralysis can be elicited by noting the response to painful pressure on the supraorbital ridge. With preserved facial nerve function, this is followed by a bilateral contraction of the facial muscles with closing of the eyes and retraction of the angles of the mouth. In paralysis of the facial nerve this response is obtained only on the normal side. The **levator sign** of Dutemps and Céstan is elicited by having the patient look down and then close his eyes slowly; when present, the upper lid on the paralyzed side moves upward slightly, being elevated by the levator palpebrae superioris because its function is no longer counteracted by the orbicularis. In **Negro's sign** the eyeball on the paralyzed side deviates outward and elevates more than the normal one when the patient raises his eyes; this is due to overaction of the superior rectus and inferior oblique. The **Bergara–Wartenberg sign** is the diminution or absence of palpable vibrations in the orbicularis oculi as the examiner attempts to open the closed eyelids against resistance; it is an early and sensitive sign of facial palsy, both peripheral and central. In the **platysma sign of Babinski** there is failure of the platysma to contract on the involved side when the mouth is opened. In facial paralysis the corneal reflexes, both direct and consensual, are absent on the involved side, a result of impairment of the motor portion of the reflex arc. The consensual reflex remains on the sound side when the cornea is touched on the involved side. The orbicularis oculi, nasomental, palmomental, and other facial reflexes are also absent on the involved side.

A minimal facial paresis on one side must be differentiated from a facial contracture on the opposite side; if the latter is present, the normal side appears to be the weaker. It must also be differentiated from developmental asymmetry and facial hemiatrophy. Unequal palpebral fissures resulting from ptosis on one side may suggest the presence of a facial weakness on the opposite side. Various special testing procedures are used in differentiating between peripheral and central types of facial palsy and in determining the prognosis of the former type. These include measurement of nerve conduction time in response to percutaneous electrical stimulation, nerve excitability tests, electromyography, and, on occasion, evaluation of lacrimal and salivary flow, and testing of the stapedius reflex.

There are different types of peripheral facial paralysis, depending upon the site of the lesion. The involvement may be nuclear, and within the pons, or infranuclear, anywhere along the course of the nerve. The different types may be identified and the site of pathologic change localized by noting the involvement of associated structures (see Fig. 13-2). These varieties are as follows:

1. Nuclear or infranuclear involvement within the pons: Lesions within the pons may affect either the nucleus of the facial nerve or its emerging root fibers. There is a complete peripheral facial nerve paralysis, often with evidence of disease of contiguous structures. There usually is preservation of sensation and secretory functions. In degenerative nuclear lesions such as progressive bulbar palsy and syringobulbia, fasciculations may appear in the muscles

supplied by the facial nerve. Owing to the proximity of the nucleus of the seventh nerve, and especially its root fibers, to the nucleus of the sixth nerve, pontine lesions frequently cause both an ipsilateral facial paralysis and an ipsilateral lateral rectus paralysis. In the **Millard–Gubler syndrome** a unilateral external rectus paralysis is accompanied by an ipsilateral facial paralysis, probably caused by a lesion of the root fibers, and a contralateral hemiplegia. In **Foville's syndrome** a facial paralysis resulting from involvement of root fibers accompanies an ipsilateral paralysis of conjugate gaze and a contralateral corticospinal hemiplegia (see "Disorders Associated with Ocular Nerve Abnormalities," Ch. 11).

2. Infranuclear involvement just peripheral to the pons or between the pons and the facial canal: The seventh nerve lies with the eighth nerve in the cerebellopontine angle and the internal auditory meatus. In lesions at these sites there may be involvement of the entire face, together with tinnitus, deafness, and vertigo. The nervus intermedius may be affected, with loss of taste on the anterior two-thirds of the tongue and diminution of salivary and lacrimal secretion. Lesions in the cerebellopontine angle commonly extend to the fifth nerve, cerebellar peduncles, and cerebellum, and cause ipsilateral pain or sensory changes, ipsilateral ataxia, and nystagmus.

3. Involvement within the facial canal between the internal auditory meatus and the geniculate ganglion: When lesions occur at this site, there commonly is a peripheral type of facial paralysis together with involvement of the nervus intermedius. Consequently ipsilateral loss of taste and diminution of lacrimal and salivary secretions accompany the palsy. There is often associated hyperacusis owing to paralysis of the nerve to the stapedius. The distance between the internal auditory meatus and the geniculate ganglion is very short, however, and lesions at this site are not common.

4. Involvement at the geniculate ganglion: A complete facial paralysis, hyperacusis, loss of taste, impairment of secretory functions, and pain in the region of the eardrum follow a lesion of the facial nerve at the geniculate ganglion. There may be a her-

petic eruption; the vesicles are present on the eardrum and in the external auditory meatus. This geniculate neuralgia, with herpes, is called **Hunt's syndrome.**

5. Involvement peripheral to the geniculate ganglion but central to the departure of the nerve to the stapedius: When a lesion occurs at this site, there is a peripheral facial paralysis accompanied by hyperacusis, loss of taste, and diminution of salivation. Lacrimation is not affected.

6. Involvement within the facial canal between the departure of the nerve to the stapedius and departure of the chorda tympani: Lesions here cause a peripheral type of facial paralysis, together with loss of taste on the anterior two-thirds of the tongue and diminution of salivary secretion. Neither hearing nor lacrimation is affected.

7. Involvement within the facial canal peripheral to departure of the chorda tympani: In lesions peripheral to the departure of the chorda tympani there is only a peripheral type of facial paralysis, with no accompanying changes.

8. Involvement in the parotid gland after emergence from the stylomastoid foramen: Lesions of the facial nerve after it has left the stylomastoid foramen may cause partial involvement, because only certain branches of the pes anserinus are affected, thereby paralyzing some but not all of the muscles of facial expression.

Facial Paralysis of Central Origin. In a central, or supranuclear, facial palsy there is paresis of the lower portion of the face, with relative sparing of the upper portion. The paresis is rarely complete and it is always contralateral to the pathologic lesion. As explained previously, under "Anatomy and Physiology," the nuclear center that controls the upper portion of the face has both contralateral and ipsilateral supranuclear connections, and direct innervation of this nuclear center may be less complete than for the center that supplies the lower portion of the face. The nuclear center that supplies the lower portion of the face has mainly or only contralateral supranuclear innervation. As a result, a cortical or subcortical lesion in one cerebral hemisphere will cause paralysis of the lower part of the face on the opposite side, but there is relative sparing

of the upper portion. It must be borne in mind that there is a great deal of individual variation in facial innervation, and the extent of involvement in a palsy of the central type may vary from the lower half to two-thirds of the face. There is usually a little weakness of the lower part of the orbicularis oculi, so that the palpebral fissure is wider on the involved side; there may also be some weakness of the upper portion of the orbicularis, although the frontalis and the corrugator are rarely or minimally involved. The inability to close the eye on the involved side without closing its mate may be the only defect of the upper face.

The levator sign and Negro's sign may be present in the central type as well as the peripheral type, and the patient may be unable to close his eye against resistance. The Bergara-Wartenberg sign and the platysma sign of Babinski are also present. Bell's phenomenon, however, is usually absent, the corneal reflex is usually present, and the orbicularis oculi reflex may be exaggerated. The lower portion of the face is smoother than normal, and the nasolabial fold is shallow. There is probably some bilateral innervation to the lower face as well as to the upper, and the paralysis of the lower face is never as marked in a central palsy as it is in a peripheral one. In a central palsy one rarely finds drooping of the angle of the mouth, blowing out of the cheek, difficulty in drinking liquids, and difficulty with the articulation of labials. There is some preservation of function, even in the involved muscles, and the central variety may be called a *paresis* of the lower face, whereas the peripheral variety is a *paralysis* of the entire face. The differentiation between the two is rarely a difficult one.

There are two principal varieties of central facial palsy, the volitional and the emotional types. In volitional palsy the involvement is most marked on voluntary contraction, and the paresis becomes apparent when the patient attempts to bare his teeth or retract the angle of his mouth. On involuntary contraction, such as spontaneous smiling, crying, or other expressions of emotion, there is preservation of function and there may be little or no evidence of paresis (Fig. 13-4). In fact, these automatic or involuntary movements may not only be preserved, but at times there is an exaggeration or dissociation of responses on smiling. This variety of paresis results from involvement of either the cortical center in the lower third of the precentral convolution that controls facial movements or the pathway between this center and

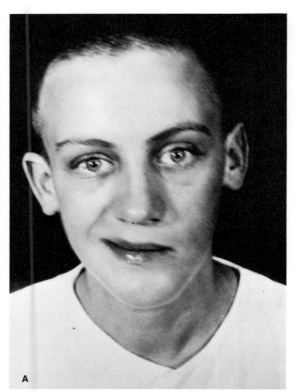 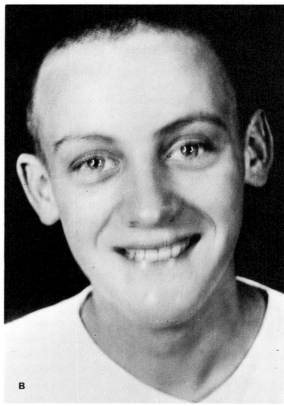

FIG. 13–4. Volitional type of facial paresis on the left associated with a neoplasm of the right frontal lobe. **A.** Patient attempting to retract the angle of the mouth. **B.** Patient smiling.

the motor nucleus of the facial nerve. The lesion thus may be either in the cortex or in the subcortical corticobulbar pathways as they go through the internal capsule, the cerebral peduncle, or the pons above the facial nucleus. Facial asymmetry has been described in epileptics with temporal lobe foci; the weaker side is usually contralateral to the temporal focus.

In the emotional or mimetic type of facial palsy, or amimia, the impairment is most marked on smiling and weeping, and the patient can voluntarily retract his mouth or blow out his cheeks without difficulty (Fig. 13-5). This type of palsy is considered to be the result of a deep-seated lesion, perhaps owing to extrapyramidal, basal ganglion, thalamic, or even hypothalamic, involvement. It has been described in lesions of the frontal lobe anterior to the precentral convolution and of the reticular portion of the pons just above the facial nucleus. The fibers carrying stimuli that produce an emotional response may go through pathways other than the direct corticobulbar tracts. Probably a close association exists between the centers or pathways controlling the emotional movements and those associated with respiration, and a smile may be accompanied by an arrest of respiration and laughter by a series of respiratory arrests and accelerations.

In many cases of central palsy there is both volitional and emotional involvement. In pseudobulbar palsy the paresis may be either voluntary or mimetic, but is usually predominantly the latter, and the involvement is bilateral. In addition there may be forced laughter and crying that are either unmotivated and spontaneous or precipitated by the slightest or most indifferent stimulus. This may be due to a short-circuiting from the ventral nucleus of the thalamus to the hypothalamus, or may be a result of failure of corticothalamic inhibition.

The *masked face* that is seen in Parkinson's disease and other related parkinsonian syndromes (Fig. 13-6) is sometimes classed as a third type of central facial paresis. Here there is no real pare-

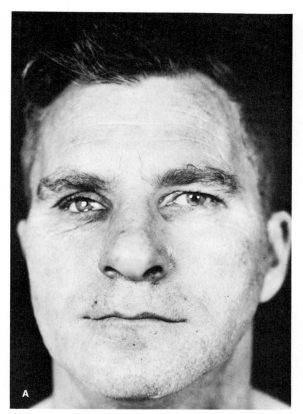 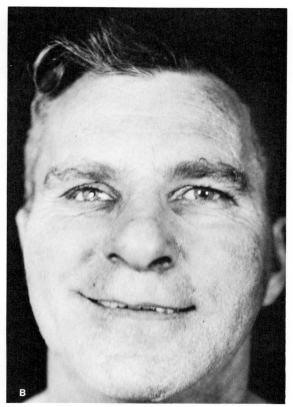

FIG. 13–5. Emotional type of facial paresis on the left following a cerebral infarction. **A.** Face at rest. **B.** Patient smiling.

sis, either of voluntary or emotional response, but the face is smoother than normal, the features are flattened, and the normal facial emotional responses are absent. There is a loss of associated movements, with infrequent blinking and smiling. The patient is able to smile, however, and when he does he frequently shows an exaggerated, frozen smile. In this variety there may also be forced or unmotivated laughing and crying. The masked face is also seen with degenerative and inflammatory diseases of the basal ganglia and extrapyramidal system and is often present in pseudobulbar palsy and progressive supranuclear palsy. Decreased facial expression may also be a feature of muscle disease, the so-called *myopathic facies.*

Conditions Characterized by Facial Nerve Paralysis. Paresis or paralysis of the facial nerve may result from a wide variety of lesions, and these lesions may be widely distributed throughout the central or peripheral nervous system. Neoplasms, vascular lesions, degenerative changes, and inflammations involving the motor cortex, the internal capsule, the cerebral peduncle, or the upper pons may cause one of the varieties of central palsy. Lesions of the lower pons or the cerebellopontine angle, lesions within the facial canal, or lesions affecting the nerve after exit may cause the peripheral variety. Pontine lesions are apt to be vascular in origin, but there may be involvement of the facial nuclei with neoplasms, polioencephalitis, multiple sclerosis, syringobulbia, and degenerative processes such as progressive bulbar palsy, in which there are also atrophy and fasciculations. Either unilateral or bilateral facial paralysis may be of congenital origin. When this is associated with paralysis of the extraocular muscles, especially the external rectus, it is known as **Möbius' syndrome,** or **congenital oculofacial paralysis** (Fig. 13-7; see also Ch. 12). There may also be paresis of the muscles of mastication and other muscles innervated by cranial nerves, and other developmental defects.

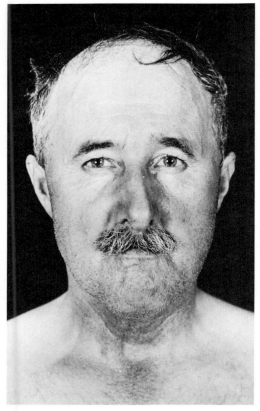

FIG. 13–6. The masked face of a patient with Parkinson's disease.

Just after its exit from the pons the facial nerve may be involved in meningitides and granulomas of various types, basal skull fractures, neoplastic changes, basilar aneurysms, extradural abscesses, or diseases of the base of the skull. The facial nerve is frequently affected in acoustic neurinomas and with other neoplasms such as meningiomas and chordomas in the cerebellopontine angle or at the base of the brain. It is involved early in chemodectomas, or tumors of the glomus jugulare, and the paralysis may be a progressive one. Tumors of the nerve itself are rare.

Within the facial canal many processes may affect the nerve. Inflammatory conditions at the geniculate ganglion, such as herpes zoster, may cause the Hunt syndrome, and it is very probable that many of the instances of spontaneous facial paralysis without herpes are due to a neurotropic virus infection. The facial nerve may be involved in various infectious processes, such as mumps, uveoparotid fever, scarlet fever, malaria, focal infections, and polyneuritis cranialis; in diabetic, alcoholic, and vitamin-deficiency neuritides; in vascular insufficiency; or by metastatic neoplasms and lymphomatous growths. Owing to the proximity of the facial canal to the middle ear and the mastoid process, the facial nerve is frequently involved in disease of the middle ear and its adnexa. Facial paralysis is seen as a complication of otitis media, petrositis, mastoiditis,

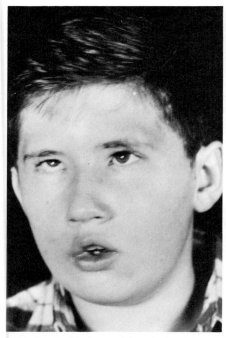
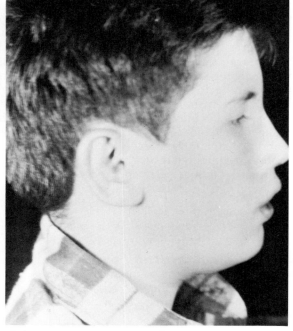

FIG. 13–7. Patient with aplasia of the right abducens and facial nuclei (Möbius' syndrome).

and suppuration of the temporal bone, and in association with a cholesteatoma; the ear should be examined in every case of peripheral facial paralysis, whether or not there are symptoms of ear disease. A facial paralysis may develop following a mastoidectomy if the nerve has been exposed during the operation or if the suppurative process has extended into the facial canal.

Paralysis of the peripheral branches of the nerve, after its emergence from the stylomastoid foramen, may result from disease or tumors of the parotid gland and from trauma to the face, especially that associated with cuts, slashes, or stab or gunshot wounds. Trauma at birth, especially a forceps delivery, may cause such an involvement. A neuritis of the great auricular nerve in the parotid gland has been said to cause facial palsy even though the seventh nerve is not directly affected. Paralysis of the terminal branches of the nerve is characteristic of leprosy; here there is involvement of individual muscles, often with extreme hypotonia and ectropion of the eye and mouth.

Bilateral peripheral facial paralysis is occasionally seen, especially in various types of peripheral neuritis, and facial diplegia may be one of the characteristic findings in the Guillain–Barré syndrome (Fig. 13-8). Facial diplegia has also been described in aneurysm of the basilar artery, and it may occur in polioencephalitis, and in myasthenia gravis and the myopathies.

The term **Bell's palsy** is often used as a synonym for the peripheral variety of facial paralysis, but the term should be used only if the paralysis is the result of a lesion peripheral to the geniculate ganglion, that is, one without neuralgia or herpes. This usually develops spontaneously, and the patient may not be aware of the paralysis until he sees his face in a mirror or notices difficulty in drinking or holding liquids in his mouth. Occasionally there is mild pain in the ear or some subjective numbness or stiffness of the face. Taste may or may not be affected. There is sometimes a history of exposure to cold or wind on the affected side or of a mild systemic infection prior to the onset of a paralysis, but the relationship of these to its etiology is not known. Most clinicians feel that either compression of the nerve by edema or periostitis of the facial canal, or ischemia of the nerve secondary to arteriolar spasm of the nutrient vessels, is responsible for most cases of idiopathic Bell's palsy. Either of these may cause a physiologic or an anatomic block of the nerve, and decompression of the facial nerve in its canal has been used in some instances to treat Bell's palsy. There is also evidence to suggest, however, that inflammatory

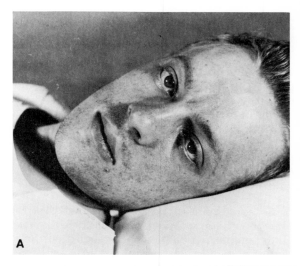

A

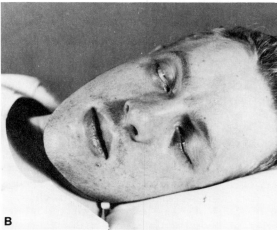

B

FIG. 13–8. Facial diplegia in a patient with Guillain–Barré syndrome. **A.** Face at rest. **B.** Patient attempting to close the eyes and retract the angles of the mouth.

involvement of the nerve (possibly viral, even in the absence of herpetic features) is responsible for a certain percentage of cases. The prognosis varies. In the majority of cases recovery is fairly prompt and complete. In a small group improvement is delayed; recovery may or may not be complete, or regeneration may be faulty, with the development of facial spasms. In a very small group there is little or no recovery. The prognosis for the speed and degree of recovery may at times be determined by electrodiagnostic testing. Bell's palsy is sometimes recurrent and may switch sides, for example, in multiple sclerosis. **Melkersson's syndrome** (or the **Melkersson – Rosenthal syndrome**) is characterized by recurring facial palsy, recurring facial edema, and a congenitally furrowed tongue (lingua plicata); it is sometimes familial and usually begins in childhood. It cause is unknown.

The muscles of facial expression may be involved in various other disease processes. In progressive bulbar palsy and amyotrophic lateral sclerosis there may be atrophy and fasciculations of the facial muscles; the atrophy is often difficult to recognize because the bulk of the facial musculature is small. In myasthenia gravis there often is marked weakness of the facial muscles, with a weak or "myasthenic" smile; the patient has difficulty in both closing and opening the eyes. In the myopathic facies, seen in the facioscapulohumeral type of muscular dystrophy of Landouzy and Dejerine, and in some other familial myopathies, the eyelids droop and cannot be tightly closed, and the lips cannot be pursed, but protrude and droop tonelessly, giving the *bouche de tapir*. On smiling the risorius pulls at the angle of the mouth, but because the zygomaticus is unable to elevate the lips, there results a transverse smile.

In **facial hemiatrophy,** or **progressive facial hemiatrophy,** there is either underdevelopment of congenital origin or a progressive atrophy of the muscles of mastication and facial expression and other muscles of one half of the face, together with trophic changes in the skin, subcutaneous fat, connective tissue, cartilage, and bone. Those in the skin include atrophy of the papillary layer with disappearance of subcutaneous fat and resulting scleroderma; trophic changes in the hair consist of loss of pigmentation and circumscribed alopecia. Occasionally instead of hemiatrophy there is hemihypertrophy. These processes probably have a central origin, and are due to a disturbance of development of the involved nuclei or their supranuclear centers, but the changes in the skin, subcutaneous tissues, bone, etc., may be associated with some disturbance of the autonomic nervous system. This, too, however, may have a central origin, and there may be involvement of the higher centers which leads to increased and unregulated activity of the lower centers.

Irritative Motor Phenomena

Irritation of the facial nerve causes abnormal motor manifestations rather than paralysis. Localized, or jacksonian, convulsive attacks occur with irritative lesions of the cortical center in the prerolandic convolution; tonic spasm or clonic movements of the contralateral facial muscles may be accompanied or followed by similar movements of the arm or leg or a conjugate turning of the head and eyes. Disease of the basal ganglia or extrapyramidal system can cause various hyperkinesias of the facial muscles — choreiform, athetoid, dystonic, grimacing, or myoclonic movements. Tremors of the face may accompany the masking of parkinsonism.

Irritation of the nucleus or of the nerve itself may cause contraction of the face, or spasm of the facial muscles. A facial spasm on one side with a corticospinal paralysis opposite is called **Brissaud's syndrome;** this occurs in the presence of irritation of the facial muscles, and is usually due to an inflammatory or neoplastic process. Irritation of the facial nerve anywhere along its course may cause spasm of the muscles it supplies. Reflex spasm may be a result of pain in the involved side of the face or irritation of the trigeminal nerve. Such spasm is sometimes seen with dental infections, tic douloureux, other painful affections of the face, and diseases of the parotid gland and mastoid. In Chvostek's sign (see "Examination of the Reflexes") there is marked hyperirritability of the facial nerves and muscles. In the risus sardonicus of tetanus there is increased activity of the muscles supplied by the facial nerve.

Abnormal associated, or synkinetic, movements resulting in facial spasms and even facial contracture may follow incomplete or faulty regeneration of the seventh nerve consequent to a peripheral type of palsy. It may first be noted that voluntary efforts to close the eye are accompanied by associated elevation of the corner of the mouth, contraction of the platysma, or wrinkling of the forehead; on baring the teeth there is an associated closing of the ipsilateral eye. These are **abnormal associated movements.** If the disorder progresses, the patient may exhibit a more or less rhythmic elevation of the corner of the mouth; on close inspection, however, it may be seen that this movement is synchronous with rhythmic blinking of the eye, and it may be noted that movements of the mouth, as in talking and smiling, are accompanied by narrowing of the palpebral fissure on the same side. These movements may progress to a stage of **facial spasm,** with repetitive, hyperkinetic, recurrent, spasmodic, clonic and occasionally tonic contractions of the muscles of the involved side of the face. The mouth twists to the affected side, the nasolabial fold deepens, the eye closes, and there is contraction of the frontalis muscle (Fig. 13-9). The spasm may involve the entire nerve or only certain branches; it may be propagated

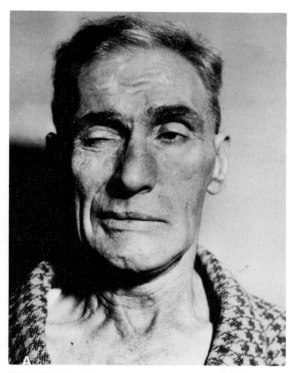

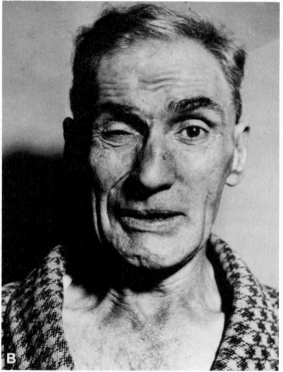

FIG. 13–9. Facial spasm following right peripheral facial paralysis. **A.** Patient attempting to close the eye. **B.** Patient attempting to retract the angle of the mouth.

from one branch to another. Instead of spasm, there may be a **facial contracture;** here one observes, instead of weakness of the involved side of the face, an apparent overactivity, with wrinkling of the forehead, narrowing of the palpebral fissure, drawing up or twisting of the angle of the mouth, and increased depth of the nasolabial fold. On casual inspection of a patient who has a facial contracture following a facial paralysis, one may gain the faulty impression that there is weakness on the opposite side instead. Careful testing, however, will show that the affected muscles are still somewhat paretic, even though in a state of contracture. It is generally believed that faulty regeneration or a misdirected outgrowth of regenerating fibers is responsible for the above phenomena: some fibers destined for the orbicularis oculi go to the orbicularis oris, and vice versa. Some observers do not accept this explanation, however, and express the belief that these are release phenomena resulting from either a central or a nuclear lesion.

Idiopathic or **cryptogenic hemifacial spasm** is a disorder that usually develops in middle-aged women. Twitching begins in the orbicularis oculi or the orbicularis oris followed soon by spread to all facial muscles on one side. It is strictly limited to the muscles supplied by the facial nerve. As the disorder spreads it may involve the auricular muscles even when the patient cannot move them voluntarily, and the platysma may also be affected. The cause is not known, but a redundant loop of the posterior inferior cerebellar artery touching the facial nerve may cause hemifacial spasm, and freeing the nerve from the pressure of this vessel may, in certain cases, relieve the symptoms. Hemifacial spasm has been described due to aneurysmal compression of the facial nerve. Pathophysiologically, ectopic excitation and ephaptic transmission have been shown to be part of hemifacial spasm.

Hemifacial spasms have on occasion been relieved either temporarily or permanently by neurolysis or decompression of the facial nerve. Section of the nerve will relieve the spasm but causes a permanent motor defect, while selective neurotomy of the most affected branches may afford relief without causing a significant motor deficit.

A true facial spasm, which is an organic condition, should be differentiated from the tic, or habit spasm, which is not organically initiated. In the latter there may be retraction of the angle of the mouth or contraction of the orbicularis oculi which may resemble that in the true spasm, but the movements are somewhat more bizarre and more purposeful, and other muscles besides those supplied by the facial nerve are brought into action. The eyebrow may be depressed instead of elevated. **Blepharospasm, or nictitating spasm,** at times relieved by injections of botulinum toxin A, is characterized by movements which involve principally the orbicularis oculi and frontalis muscles. This may start as a reflex response, associated with the presence of a foreign body in the eye, but may continue as a habit spasm. Bizarre grimacing movements of the face are also often habit spasms. Another type of reflex blepharospasm occurs in patients with organic disease and may appear following a cerebrovascular accident: voluntary opening of the eye is not impaired, but there is an exaggerated blink response to sensory and threatening stimuli. When this occurs the examiner may have difficulty in carrying out the ophthalmoscopic examination, because the stimulus of lifting the lid or focusing light in the eye causes an involuntary closing of the palpebral fissure. Blepharospasm may also be present in photophobia and in postencephalitic parkinsonism as well as other basal ganglion disorders.

Tremors of the face may be diagnostic of certain conditions. Perioral tremors are frequently seen in general paresis and alcoholism. Facial myokymia, or quivering of the muscles, occurs with lesions of the medulla near the facial nucleus, including multiple sclerosis, neoplasms, and Guillain–Barré syndrome. General facial tremors, especially of the eyelids, occur in psychogenic states. In Rosenbach's sign, seen in both hyperthyroidism and hysteria, there is a fine tremor of the closed eyelids. Fasciculations are present in progressive bulbar palsy and amyotrophic lateral sclerosis. There also may be choreiform, athetoid, and myoclonic movements of the face, which may or may not be accompanied by similar movement in other parts of the body. They sometimes consist of grimacing, perioral tremors, and pursing movements of the mouth — so-called **oral-facial dyskinesias.** If they follow the ingestion of phenothiazine and other psychoactive drugs, especially if they do not develop until these drugs have been used for some period of time, they are called **tardive dyskinesias.** Unfortunately, this term is also applied to similar movements of unknown etiology which do not follow drug ingestion. Similar oral-facial movements develop following levodopa administration and the use of dopamine agonist medications; usually they are dose related.

Sensory Involvement

Sensory phenomena are less frequently associated with lesions of the facial nerve than are motor phenomena, and are less easily diagnosed. Loss of exteroceptive, general visceral, and proprioceptive sensations may not be apparent to the patient and may not be elicited by the examination procedures.

In destructive lesions of the geniculate ganglion, or of the chorda tympani or the facial nerve central to its departure, there is loss of taste on the anterior two-thirds of the tongue on the involved side; in irritative lesions there is geniculate neuralgia, with paroxysmal bouts of pain, first deep in the ear, later radiating to the face. "Tic douloureux of the chorda tympani" has also been described. In lesions of the lingual nerve there is loss of taste together with loss of exteroceptive sensation on the involved side of the tongue, and there is usually subjective numbness.

Disturbances of taste and smell often occur together. Complete ageusia is rare unless there is also loss of smell. Ageusia or hypogeusia, often with associated anosmia or hyposmia, may occur with heavy smoking, viral infections, including viral hepatitis, and with hypogonadism, pseudohypoparathyroidism, diabetes, familial dysautonomia, and the use of some drugs such as thiouracil and penicillamine. In pernicious anemia there may be either perversions of taste or loss of taste for certain foods. Gonadal dysgenesis is an idiopathic syndrome in which there are also disturbances of smell and taste. Inability to taste phenylthiocarbamide is inherited as a mendelian recessive trait. Either transient or permanent ageusia may follow Bell's palsy or operations such as stapedectomy. A syndrome of idiopathic hypogeusia, with dysgeusia, hyposmia, and dysosmia, has been described. This seems to be associated with abnormalities of zinc metabolism. A deficiency of zinc is reported to cause a deficiency in the total number of taste buds and a disturbance of function in those that remain. Increased taste sensitivity occurs in patients with Addison's disease, pituitary deficiency, and cystic fibrosis. Distortions or alterations of taste may be the direct or indirect effects of malignancies.

In herpes zoster oticus, or the Hunt syndrome, there is, in addition to the peripheral facial paralysis and the sensory and secretory abnormalities described (loss of taste on the anterior two-thirds of the tongue, hyperacusis, and diminution of salivary and lacrimal secretion), pain behind and in the ear, and there are vesicles on the tympanum and in the external auditory canal, and also on the lateral surface of the pinna and in the cleft between the auricle and the mastoid process. Hunt has described two varieties of the syndrome — the otalgic form of geniculate neuralgia with pain in the ear, and the prosopalgic form with pain deep in the face, principally in the posterior orbital, palatal, and nasal regions. This latter variety is said to be the result of involvement of the sensory fibers which are carried through the greater superficial petrosal nerve to the sphenopalatine ganglion. Deep geniculate prosopalgia is usually accompanied by geniculate otalgia.

There is no loss of sensation in central lesions, but parageusias or gustatory hallucinations may be present. Hypergeusia and parageusias may be characteristic of certain psychoses and of hysterical states. Gustatory hallucinations may occur in tumors of or near the uncinate or hippocampal gyri or the parietal operculum, or as part of a seizure of the so-called complex partial or temporal lobe variety. Thus they are valuable in cerebral localization. There may be associated smacking of the lips and chewing movements before or during loss of consciousness in complex partial seizures. Frequently gustatory and olfactory hallucinations occur together. Elderly persons sometimes complain of either loss of taste or disagreeable tastes which may lead to anorexia.

Secretory Changes

Abnormalities of secretory function may be produced by lesions of the facial nerve. Peripheral involvement of the nervus intermedius, the greater superficial petrosal nerve, the chorda tympani, or the sphenopalatine or submaxillary ganglia may cause diminution or loss of lacrimal, salivary, or mucous secretion. There may also be vasomotor changes. Irritative lesions of the brain stem at the level of the superior salivatory nucleus may cause an increase in secretion, whereas destructive lesions may cause a decrease in flow. There is never absence of salivation, however, unless there are bilateral lesions. Changes in secretion may also be the result of central lesions, especially those involving the hypothalamus or the autonomic connections. Irritation of the rostral end of the hypothalamus produces an increase in salivation, whereas irri-

tative lesions of the posterior end or destructive lesions of the rostral regions cause a decrease in salivary flow with dry mouth and perversions of taste. Sialorrhea, and ptyalism are terms indicating an excess of saliva. Sialorrhea is sometimes present in Parkinson's disease. There is also ptyalism in the various types of bulbar palsy; this may be caused by excessive secretion of saliva or may be due to inability to swallow. Atropine and numerous other drugs often cause an unpleasantly dry mouth. In Sjögren's syndrome there is deficient secretion of the lacrimal, salivary, and mucosal glands, with resulting keratoconjunctivitis and dryness of the mouth and upper respiratory tract.

An increase or decrease in lacrimal or salivary secretion may occur on a psychogenic basis. Lacrimation, of course, is most frequently the result of a psychic stimulus. The secretion of saliva may be stimulated not only by the smell or taste of food but also by the thought or sight of food. Excitement may produce an increase of saliva; in nausea there is increased salivation. Depressed and anxious patients often complain of a decrease in salivation with dry mouth and perversions or loss of taste. An abnormal dryness of the mouth, of either central or peripheral origin, is referred to as **xerostomia.**

The syndrome of **crocodile tears** is an unusual residual of a peripheral facial palsy. It is a paradoxic gustatory–lacrimal reflex, and is characterized by the appearance of tears when strongly flavored foods are placed on the tongue. It is probably due to a faulty regeneration of the nerve fibers, in which filaments having to do with salivary secretion have grown along the pathway to the lacrimal gland. There may be abnormal local irritability of cholinergic fibers. The condition has been treated by section of the greater superficial petrosal nerve. In the chorda tympani syndrome there is unilateral swelling and flushing of the submental region after eating. The somewhat similar auriculotemporal syndrome is discussed in Chapter 12.

BIBLIOGRAPHY

Adams RD, Victor M. Principles of Neurology, 4th ed. New York, McGraw – Hill, 1989

Blatt IM. Bell's palsy: Diagnosis and prognosis of idiopathic paralysis by submaxillary salivary gland flow and chorda tympani nerve testing. Laryngoscope 1965;75:1081

Börnstein WS. Cortical representation of taste in man and monkey. I. Functional and anatomical relations of taste, olfaction, and somatic sensibility. Yale J Biol Med 1940;12:719

Börnstein WS. Cortical representation of taste in man and monkey. II. The localization of the cortical taste area in man and a method of measuring impairment of taste in man. Yale J Biol Med 1940;13:133

Boyer FC, Gardner WJ. Paroxysmal lacrimation (syndrome of crocodile tears) and its surgical treatment. Arch Neurol Psychiatry 1949;61:56

Brodal A. Neurological Anatomy in Relation to Clinical Medicine, 3rd ed. New York, Oxford University Press, 1981

Clark EC, Dodge HW Jr. Extraolfactory components of flavor. JAMA 1955;159:1721

Drachman DA. Bell's palsy: A neurological point of view. Arch Otolaryngol 1969;89:173

Editorial. Taste and smell deviations: Importance of zinc. JAMA 1974;228:1669

Fisher CM. Reflex blepharospasm. Neurology 1963;13:77

Gardner WJ, Sava CA. Hemifacial spasm — a reversible pathophysiologic state. J Neurosurg 1962;19:240

Gorman W. Flavor, Taste and the Psychology of Smell. Springfield, IL, Charles C Thomas, 1964

Henkin RI, Schechter PJ, Hoye R et al. Idiopathic hypogeusia with dysgeusia, hyposmia, and dysosmia: A new syndrome. JAMA 1971;217:434

Hitselberger WE, House WF. Acoustic neuroma diagnosis. Arch Otolaryngol 1966;83:218

Hunt JR. On herpetic inflammations of the geniculate ganglion: a new syndrome and its complications. J Nerv Ment Dis 1907;34:73

Jenny AB, Saper CB. Organization of the facial nucleus and corticofacial projection in the monkey: A reconsideration of the upper motor neuron facial palsy. Neurology 1987;37:930

Kugelberg E. The mechanism of Chvostek's sign. Arch Neurol Psychiatry 1951;65:511

Kugelberg E. Facial reflexes. Brain 1952;75:385

Mackenzie ICK. A simple method for testing taste. Lancet 1955;1:377

Maroon HC, Lunsford LD, Deeb Zl. Hemifacial spasm due to aneurysmal compression of the facial nerve. Arch Neurol 1978;35:545

Monrad – Krohn GH. On the dissociation of voluntary and emotional innervation in facial paresis of central origin. Brain 1924;47:22

Nielsen VK. Pathophysiology of hemifacial spasm. I. Ephaptic transmission and ectopic excitation. Neurology 1984;34:418

Pfaffman C. The sense of taste. In Field J, Magoun HW, Hall VE (eds). Handbook of Physiology, Vol 1. Washington, DC, American Physiological Society, 1959

Remillard GM, Andermann F, Rhi-Sausi A et al. Facial asymmetry in patients with temporal lobe epilepsy. Neurology 1977;27:109

Report of the therapeutics and technology assessment subcommittee of the American Academy of Neurology. Assessment: The clinical usefulness of botulinum toxin-A in treating neurologic disorders. Neurology 1990;40:1332

Shahani BT, Young RR. Human orbicularis reflexes. Neurology 1972;22:149

Stevens H. Melkersson's syndrome. Neurology 1965;15:263

Szentágothai J. The representation of facial and scalp muscles in the facial nucleus. J Comp Neurol 1948;88:207

Traverner D. Electrodiagnosis in Bell's palsy. Arch Otolaryngol 1965;81:470

Wartenberg R. Hemifacial Spasm: A Clinical and Pathophysiological Study. New York, Oxford University Press, 1952

Weil AA, Nosik WA. Electrophysiologic and clinical observations in hemifacial spasm. Neurology 1956;6:381

Weingrow SM. Facial reflexes. Arch Pediatr 1937;50:234

The eighth cranial, acoustic, or auditory, nerve is composed of two fiber systems which are blended into a single nerve trunk. These are the **cochlear nerve,** or the nerve of hearing, and the **vestibular nerve,** which subserves equilibration, coordination, and orientation in space. They originate in separate peripheral receptors and have distinct but also diffuse central connections. Although they are united along their course through the skull, they differ so greatly both in their anatomic relationships and their respective functions that they should be considered separately.

THE COCHLEAR NERVE

Anatomy and Physiology

The receptors, or end-organs, of the cochlear nerve are the hair cells, or auditory cells, in the organ of Corti, within the cochlea of the internal ear. Impulses travel to the bipolar cells of the spiral ganglia of the cochlea, from which the central fibers pass as the cochlear nerve, containing some 30,000 fibers. This nerve traverses the internal auditory meatus, where it is lateral and inferior to the facial nerve, it crosses the subarachnoid space between the pons and the medulla, entering the upper medulla at its junction with the pons. Its neuraxes pass around the restiform body to terminate on the dorsal and ventral cochlear nuclei at the dorsolateral and ventrolateral aspects of this body in the lower pons (Fig. 14-1). Within these primary nuclei, and all higher auditory relay centers, a fiber ar-

rangement reflecting the site of origin within the cochlea (tonotopic organization) is preserved. Fibers from the dorsal cochlear nucleus cross the floor of the fourth ventricle under the striae medullares (fibers of Piccolomini to the cerebellum), after which they pass ventrally into the pons, near the superior olivary nucleus, to terminate on the lateral lemniscus of the opposite side (Fig. 14-2). Some of the fibers from the ventral nucleus cross the pons as trapezoid fibers to the contralateral lateral lemniscus, and others communicate with the ipsilateral and contralateral olivary bodies, and through them with the nuclei of the third, fourth, and sixth cranial nerves. There are also communications with the nucleus of the trapezoid body and the nucleus of the lateral lemniscus. A few fibers from each cochlear nucleus, especially the dorsal, pass to the ipsilateral lateral lemniscus. Fibers from the lateral lemnisci ascend to the inferior colliculus (posterior quadrigeminal body) and the medial geniculate body. The former is an auditory reflex center, and the fibers from the latter, a station in the central auditory pathway, pass through the posterior limb of the internal capsule as auditory radiations to terminate on the cortex of the transverse temporal convolutions (Heschl's gyrus), especially the anterior part, and the adjacent portion of the superior temporal convolution.

The cochlear nerve has one function, that of hearing. Sound waves stimulate the special sensory receptors in the organ of Corti. The organ of Corti and the hair cells are induced to vibrate at the frequency of sound by tiny acoustically produced differences in pressure. The individual auditory fibers and their related hair cells are

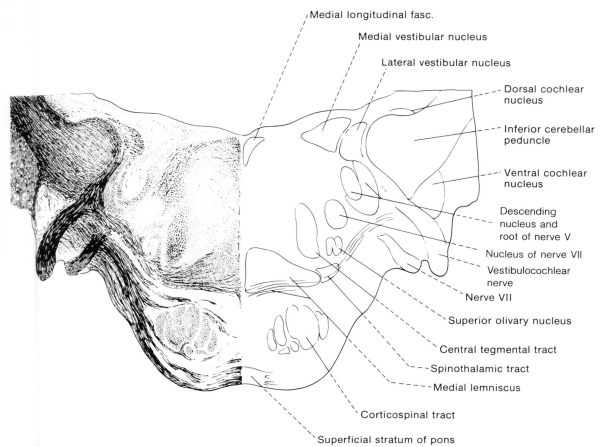

FIG. 14–1. Section through the junction of the pons and medulla at the level of the cochlear nuclei.

most sensitive to a particular frequency of vibration. Impulses are carried along the nerve to the cochlear nuclei, and then centrally to terminate on the auditory cortex in the temporal lobes of the same and the opposite sides. This work does not discuss in any detail the physics of sound or the physiology of sound conditions or recognition. Sound is a form of motion produced by some vibrating medium. A sound wave is a series or chain of alternate condensations and rarefactions in the surrounding air, by which the vibratory movements of the sounding body are conveyed to the tympanic membrane of the ear and then transmitted by the auditory ossicles to the inner ear. The **pitch,** or relative position of sound in the musical scale, depends upon the frequency or rapidity with which the vibrations follow one another. The pitch is raised as the number of vibrations per second is increased. The human ear normally appreciates and recog-

nizes tones of between 16 and 20,000 – 25,000 Hz (vibrations per second). The **intensity** with which a sound wave impresses the perceptive mechanism depends upon the amplitude of vibration. A physical law declares that the intensity of sound is proportional to the square of the amplitude. The **quality,** or **timbre,** is that property of sound by which one distinguishes between two tones of the same pitch or intensity. Sound is brought to the organ of hearing in two ways. It is conveyed by **air conduction** when the vibrating body is at some variable distance from the ear and the sound waves are transmitted through the medium of the surrounding air into the external auditory meatus and to the tympanic membrane. It is conveyed by **bone conduction** when the vibrating medium is in contact with the skull or the bones of the body, and waves are transmitted through the medium of the cranial bones.

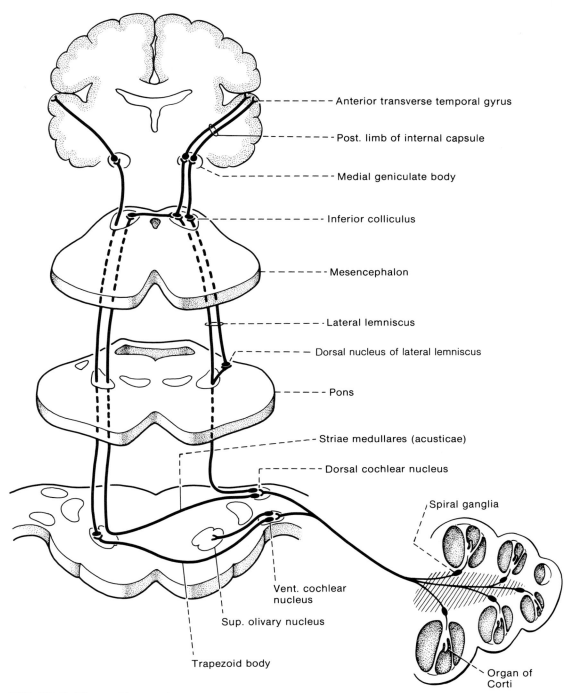

FIG. 14–2. The cochlear pathway.

Anterior transverse temporal gyrus

Post. limb of internal capsule

Medial geniculate body

Inferior colliculus

Mesencephalon

Lateral lemniscus

Dorsal nucleus of lateral lemniscus

Pons

Striae medullares (acusticae)

Dorsal cochlear nucleus

Spiral ganglia

Vent. cochlear nucleus

Sup. olivary nucleus

Organ of Corti

Trapezoid body

Clinical Examination

Hearing is evaluated in a variety of ways. Much information may be obtained by observation of the patient. Ability to understand soft and loud tones and low and high pitches is noted. Signs of deafness, such as a tendency to turn the head in listening, lip reading, speaking with a loud voice, or inability to hear high or low tones, may provide valuable information. If any history of difficulty in hearing is present or if hearing tests are to be made, the external auditory canal should be examined with the otoscope to eliminate the presence of wax, pus, blood, foreign bodies, and exudate, and to determine whether the tympanic membrane is intact. The mastoid region should be examined for swelling and tenderness.

In performing tests of hearing, the examiner may first note the distance from each ear at which the subject is able to hear either the whispered or the spoken voice. In carrying out the test one ear is kept closed, preferably with the moistened tip of the little finger, and the patient's head is turned so that he cannot see the examiner's lips. A whisper, if used, should be so light that the thyroid cartilage does not vibrate. This test, however, is not very accurate, since the intensity and pitch of the voice varies in individuals, and in the same individual from time to time. Certain tones are heard more loudly and at a greater distance than others. Sibilants, and the short vowels such as a, e, i, are heard at a greater distance than broad consonants such as l, m, n, and r, and such vowels as o and u. "Seventy-six" and "sixty-seven" can be heard at a greater distance than "ninety-nine" and "fifty-three." Monosyllables should be used rather than stock questions such as "How are you?" because hearing a single word of a group may enable the patient to understand the entire question. Words and numbers should be used alternately. The voice is inaccurate, but since it is more important to hear the human voice than any other sound, it may be more valuable from a practical point of view to test acuity for the spoken voice than to measure hearing accurately in terms of intensity or decibels. The voice test, if properly applied, can be useful and reliable.

Hearing may be tested by noting the patient's ability to perceive the noise made when the examiner rubs his thumb and index finger together in front of the external auditory meatus, but for more critical evaluation a ticking watch or clicking coins may be used. The source of sound is first held outside the range of hearing of one ear while the other one is closed; it is then brought toward the ear until the patient is first able to hear it. The distance from the ear is noted, and the examiner compares the patient's acuity of hearing with his own. Consistency is important in testing; the same watch or coins must be used for successive tests and patients. High-pitched sounds such as ticks, clicks, or finger rubs are not useful for testing persons with sensorineural deafness and in testing the elderly, many of whom have some high-frequency hearing loss. Some acuity for high tones is lost as early as the second decade, but usually is clinically most evident during or following the fifth decade. Politzer's acoumeter, an instrument which gives a loud clicking sound, may be used if the patient is unable to hear a watch or coins.

The use of a tuning fork also gives more specific information. The examiner may compare the patient's hearing with his own and note the patient's relative auditory acuity on each side. Air conduction is tested by placing the tuning fork in front of the external auditory meatus, and bone conduction by placing it on the mastoid process. Both the intensity, or quantity, of the sound and the duration are noted. In evaluating bone conduction, one must be certain that the patient *hears* the tuning fork rather than *feels* its vibration. In the **Schwabach test** a tuning fork of 128, 256, or 512 Hz (C^0, C^1, C^2) is used, and the patient's bone conduction is compared with that of the examiner. The duration of perception of tone is noted: the vibrating tuning fork is placed against the patient's mastoid process until he no longer hears it, and then is transferred to the examiner's mastoid process. The test can then be repeated for air conduction.

To perform the **Rinne test** the patient's air conduction and bone conduction are compared. The tuning fork is placed firmly against the mastoid process and the patient is asked to indicate when the sound is no longer heard; it is then placed in front of the external auditory meatus, and the time during which it is heard is noted. In the normal individual, or in the **positive Rinne,** the tuning fork is heard longer by air than by bone conduction. In conductive deafness, the **Rinne is negative;** air conduction is diminished and bone conduction is retained, and the fork is heard better when it is placed over the mastoid process. Often in deafness of this type bone conduction may even be exaggerated beyond the normal because occlusion of the external auditory meatus converts the cavity of the middle ear into a resonating chamber. In sensorineural deafness both bone and air conduction are diminished, but they retain their normal relationship and the Rinne is positive; if the deafness is severe, however, bone conduction may be absent.

The **Weber test** is carried out by placing a vibrating tuning fork over the forehead or the vertex of the skull. In the normal individual this is heard equally well in both ears, or it is not lateralized. If one ear is occluded, it is heard better or more loudly on that side. In conductive deafness the sound is usually lateralized to the involved side. In sensorineural deafness the fork is heard best in the uninvolved ear.

In testing loss of hearing throughout a wide range of pitch, a series of tuning forks varying from 64 to 2048 Hz (C^{-1} to C^4) may be used, but this is a complicated and often an unsatisfactory procedure.

For an accurate, quantitative test of hearing, the electronic audiometer is used and an audiogram is made. By means of this instrument, pure tones are produced as musical notes which vary in frequency of vibration, or pitch, and the intensity, or loudness, may be varied at any frequency. The vibrations are produced by means of electronic oscillators, and a set of headphones transforms the electrical energy of the audiometer into sound waves which are conveyed by air conduction through the external auditory meatus. For bone conduction a specially constructed receiver is provided. The normal range of hearing is said to be from 16 – 20,000 Hz, or some 10 – 11 octaves, although few adults beyond the fourth decade are able to hear above 16,000 Hz. With the audiometer, frequencies of 128 – 11,584 Hz, calibrated in octaves or half octaves, are tested. This includes the normal speech range, which is about 200 – 3,000 Hz. The ear is normally more sensitive to the middle of the pitch range where the practical hearing range is situated. Both air and bone conduction are tested, first without masking and then with one ear masked by producing a sound in it so that it cannot perceive the stimulus that is being directed to the opposite ear. The masking is done by an electronic noise generator, the intensity of which may be varied by calibrated steps. It may not be possible to eliminate the normal ear if it has 40 decibels more hearing than the ear being tested. Audiometric examinations should be carried out in soundproof rooms or with the use of rubber ear plugs if such rooms are not practicable.

Intensities of sound on the audiometer are measured in dynes/cm², and loss in ability to detect tones is charted in decibels. The degree of hearing loss throughout various ranges may thus be charted in a curve. The audiometer and the audiogram not only are important as aids in the detection and differentiation of acoustic deficiencies and in the recognition of obscure perceptive defects, but they also afford a permanent record that aids in evaluating alterations of a hearing defect and its response to treatment, and in the prescribing of hearing aids.

The audiometer has in general supplanted the watch, acoumeter, tuning fork, rods, bells, and whistles in the testing of hearing. It must be stated, however, that there are many varieties of audiometers, and that the instruments, or the interpretation of them, may not be without error. The making of an accurate audiogram takes patience and observation, and hastily made audiometric records are often valueless. In spite of the scientific accuracy of the instruments, the human element enters.

In testing large numbers of people, especially in the examination of school children, the "group audiometer" has been used. This is a player to which as many as 40 earpieces can be connected. Recordings of monosyllables or of numbers at different pitches are played, and the children are asked to write down those that they hear. Thus the number of mistakes or omissions shows the hearing defect.

Additional acoustic procedures are valuable in the differentiation of certain types of deafness. These are usually performed by the otologist or audiologist, and include the following: speech audiometry, including determination of the speech reception threshold and speech discrimination score; Fowler's binaural loudness balance test and determination of the loudness recruitment phenomenon; testing of auditory adaptation and fatigue and of tone decay; the use of various modifications of the Békésy continuous frequency automatic audiometer; determination of the short increment sensitivity index (SISI) and of the comfortable and uncomfortable loudness levels; appraisal of sound localization; electrophysiologic testing, including determination of the psychogalvanic skin response and brain stem auditory evoked responses. Special tests for psychogenic deafness are described in Chapter 55. Impedance measurements are also helpful in localizing abnormalities in the hearing chain. These include tympanometry to detect middle ear and ossicular chain disorders, and stapedius reflex measurements to detect lesions in the arc from the auditory nerve through the brain stem into the facial nerve.

It is again stressed that the ability to hear and understand the human voice is the most important functional aspect of audition. In certain types of deafness of clinical significance, the pure tone and even speech thresholds are normal, but there is a decrease of speech discrimination.

In the evaluation of hearing in the infant, in semicomatose individuals, in hysteria, and in malingering, certain reflex responses may be used. The **auditory-palpebral reflex** (auro- or acousticopalpebral, cochleopalpebral, or cochleoorbicularis reflex) consists of a slight blink, or contraction of the eyelids (more marked on the ipsilateral side) or even a reflex closing of the eyes in response to a loud, sudden noise. The **cochleopupillary reflex** is either a dilation of the pupils, or a contraction followed by dilation in response to a loud noise. The **auditory-oculogyric reflex** consists of a deviation of the eyes in the direction of a sound. The **general acoustic muscle reflex** is a general jerking of the body in response to a loud, sudden sound. Brain stem auditory evoked responses also provide reliable quantitative evaluations in persons who cannot cooperate with other hearing tests.

Disorders of Function

Disturbances in the function of the cochlear nerve and its connections are usually manifested by either diminution or loss of hearing (**hypacusis** or **anacusis**), with or without tinnitus. There may be such disturbances as hyperacusis, **paracusis** (perversion of hearing), auditory hallucinations, or auditory aphasia. **Hyperacusis,** or pathologic increase in auditory acuity, occurs with paralysis of the stapedius muscle (innervated by the facial nerve), but is also present in the aura of an epileptic attack, in migraine, and in certain psychiatric disorders and drug-induced states. **Dysacusis** is impairment of hearing that is not primarily a loss of auditory

sensitivity. **Diplacusis** is of two types. In the binaural type there is an apparent difference in the pitch or intensity of the same sound as heard in the two ears. The type in which a single sound is heard as two or as a group of sounds may be either monaural or binaural. Diplacusis is usually caused by disease of the inner ear, but disturbances elsewhere in the auditory pathway may also cause it.

There are two principal varieties of hearing loss: **sensorineural** (also known as **nerve** or **perceptive**) **deafness** due to disease of the cochlea, the cochlear nerve or its nuclei, or the central pathways concerned with hearing; and **conductive** (also known as **obstructive** or **transmission**) **deafness** due to interference with transmission of sound to the cochlea, usually the result of obstruction of the external auditory canal or disease of the middle ear.

In **sensorineural deafness** air and bone conduction are both diminished, but they may retain their normal relationship so that the Rinne is positive. The Schwabach response is shortened, and the Weber is referred to the side of the better ear. The hearing loss is especially marked for the higher tones as tested by the audiometer (Fig. 14-3) and the individual has most difficulty with sibilants, sharp consonants, and short vowels. He has especial difficulty with the letters s and t and the vowels e, a, and i, and will show loss of ability to recognize such words as *sister, fish, twenty, water,* and *date.* Occasionally the

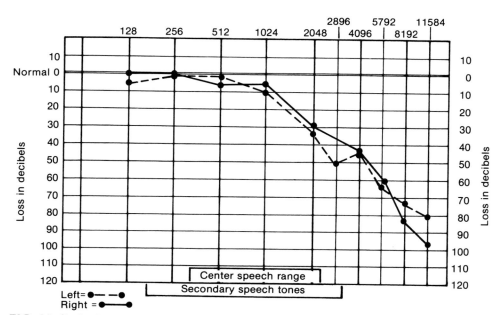

FIG. 14–3. Audiogram of a patient with sensorineural deafness.

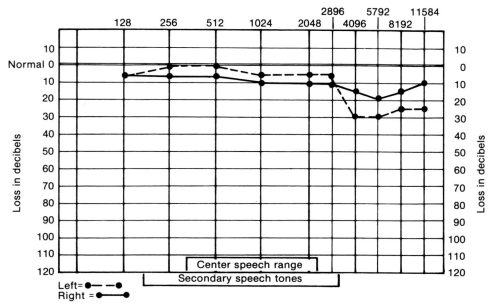

FIG. 14–4. Audiogram of a patient with early sensorineural hearing loss not affecting serviceable hearing.

audiogram will show loss of only certain ranges of speech, with "islands" in the chart (Fig. 14-4). In elderly individuals there is often a progressive loss of high tones, called **presbycusis,** that indicates an increasing sensorineural defect. This may not involve serviceable hearing at the out-

set, and may not be noticed by the patient until the loss reaches the 2148 Hz range (Fig. 14-5).

Special diagnostic testing may be used to differentiate sensorineural hearing loss due to disease of the cochlea or inner ear (**end-organ deafness**) from that secondary to involvement

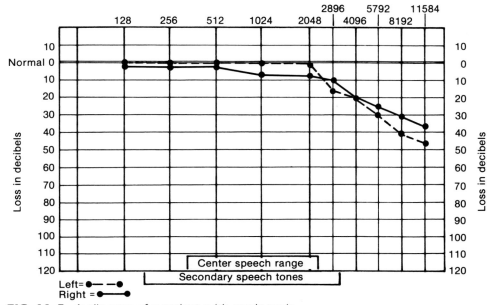

FIG. 14–5. Audiogram of a patient with presbycusis.

of the nerve itself or more central structures (**re-trocochlear deafness**). In the former the following may be found: loss of acuity for pure tones with parallel impairment of speech discrimination; recruitment of loudness, especially for tones of high frequency; near superposition of normal amplitudes of pulsed and steady-tone Békésy tracings (type II Békésy audiogram) (Fig. 14-6); a positive SISI; absence of significant tone decay; a lowered overload threshold but no threshold fatigue; diplacusis. With retrocochlear deafness the following are present: more loss of discrimination for speech than for pure tones; absence of or reverse recruitment; absent or minimal short increment sensitivity responses; more impairment in the ability to hear continuous rather than pulsed tones in Békésy recordings (Type III and IV Békésy audiograms); abnormal auditory adaptation by tone decay test; abnormal spread of masking; threshold fatigue. Brain stem auditory evoked potentials also aid in differentiating lesions at the end-organ from more centrally placed ones, depending on the presence, latency, form, and other characteristics of the evoked response peaks. Brain stem auditory evoked potentials are independent of consciousness. They are very sensitive in detecting acoustic nerve neoplasms, as are the imaging procedures, computed tomography and magnetic resonance.

In **conductive deafness** there is primarily a loss of air conduction, and bone conduction may be preserved or even exaggerated; consequently the Rinne is negative. The Schwabach response is shortened; the Weber is referred to the involved side. Low tones are lost, as are some of the broad or flat consonants and vowels such as m, n, l, r, o, and u, but, in general, speech discrimination is quite good and parallels the loss for pure tones. The hearing loss is frequently in the range of 128 – 1024 Hz, and in simple conductive defects there is rarely loss of more than

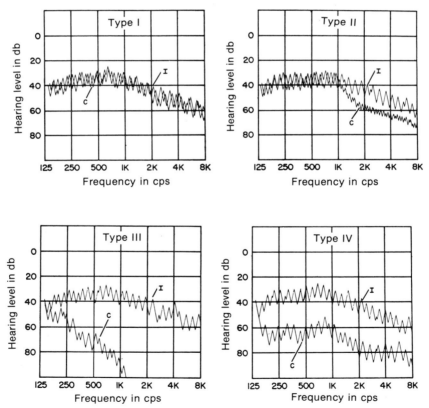

FIG. 14–6. The four types of Békésy audiograms. **C.** Hearing level for continuous tones; **I.** Hearing level for intermittent tones. **Type I** audiograms are found in normal persons and in association with disorders of the middle ear. **Type II** audiograms are obtained in patients with disorders of the cochlea. **Types III** and **IV** audiograms are obtained in persons with disorders of the eighth nerve.

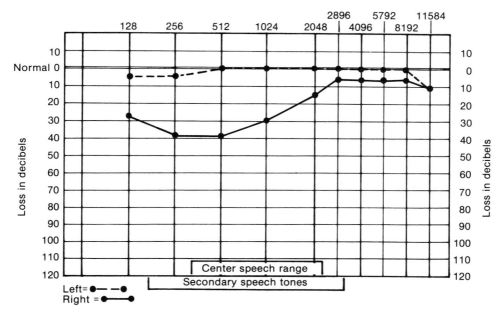

FIG. 14–7. Audiogram showing the hearing defect in patient with conductive deafness.

20 – 30 decibels in this range (Fig. 14-7). However, persons with conductive deafness tend to hear speech better in a noisy background than in a quiet setting. There is no recruitment, tone decay is within the normal range, and short increment sensitivity responses are absent or minimal. The pulsed and continuous tones are interwoven (type I Békésy audiogram).

Determining the type of deafness should always be attempted, but it is necessary to remember that there may be combined deafness with both nerve and middle ear involvement. If there is a loss of over 25 – 30 decibels, affecting both the higher and lower ranges, there is a mixed type of deafness with both conductive and sensorineural involvement (Fig. 14-8).

In deafness due to **otosclerosis** there is usually very gradual but progressive bilateral impairment of hearing. This condition is a hereditary one, and is characterized by replacement of the normal compact bone of the otic capsule by cancellous bone, causing deafness when there is obliteration of the oval window and immobilization of the stapes. Secondary metabolic degenerative changes may occur in the basal region of the cochlea with subsequent degeneration of associated cochlear nerve fibers. Early in the course of the disease there may be either a loss of low tones only or a mild impairment of hearing throughout the entire range with preserved bone conduction and a negative Rinne, suggesting a conductive hearing loss. With the development of secondary changes, however, there is increasing loss of higher tones as well, and evidence of an associated sensorineural type of deafness (Fig. 14-9). Otosclerosis is further characterized by severe and persistent tinnitus without vertigo and by **paracusis willisiana,** or the ability to hear better in the presence of loud noises. This differentiates the condition from sensorineural deafness, for most patients with involvement of the cochlea or cochlear nerve complain of profound inability to comprehend speech in the presence of noise.

Tinnitus aurium is characterized by the perception of abnormal sounds in the ear. It is a sensation of noise caused by the abnormal excitation of the auditory apparatus or its afferent pathways. It may vary in pitch and intensity, and may be continuous or intermittent. It is described in different instances as a singing, ringing, buzzing, blowing, whistling, humming, beating, pounding, ticking, swishing, or roaring sound. Tinnitus is commonly associated with deafness. It is most commonly seen in sensorineural hearing disorders, but may also be found in conductive deafness, and it is a fairly constant feature of otosclerosis. Tinnitus is often an early symptom of central nervous system disorders. Various factors may be responsible for the different types of tinnitus, and the mechanism underlying many types is not known. Stimulation or

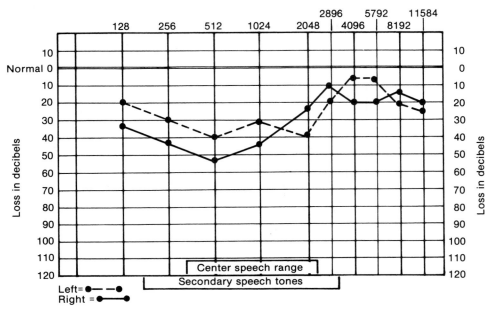

FIG. 14–8. Audiogram of a patient with mixed deafness.

irritation of the diseased nerve or central pathways may cause the symptoms, much as irritation of a peripheral nerve or afferent pathways causes paresthesias; total deafness could then be likened to the anesthesia that is produced by interruption of the continuity of the nerve.

Tinnitus due to external factors may be caused by wax or water in the external auditory canal or obstruction of the eustachian tube. It may be present in acute otitis media, and may persist after the infection has subsided. It is most commonly associated with irritation or disease of the

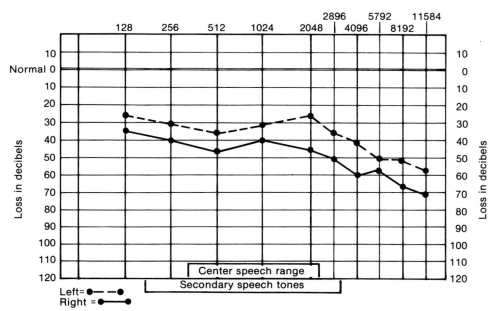

FIG. 14–9. Audiogram of a patient with advanced otosclerosis.

cochlea or the cochlear nerve and is found in circulatory disturbances of the internal ear or the central connections, as in anemia, atherosclerosis, or hypertension, and in toxic and inflammatory involvement of the cochlear nerve. Tinnitus is frequently found in presbycusis and in other types of sensorineural deafness. It may disappear by the time the deafness is complete, but may become apparent even before the deafness is noted, and increase after hearing is lost. Occasionally the symptom itself interferes with hearing. Tinnitus is often more noticeable at night when environmental noises are diminished, and may interfere with sleep. To the patient it may be more distressing than the accompanying deafness, and may cause marked depression in elderly individuals.

In the evaluation of tinnitus, an attempt should be made to determine its type and pitch, and to learn whether it seems to come from one or both ears, or to arise within the head without localization. The loudness of the tinnitus is not related to the type of hearing loss. True or intrinsic tinnitus should be differentiated from so-called extrinsic tinnitus, caused by extraneous noises. For example, a pulsating or intermittent tinnitus that is synchronous with the pulse may be present with hypertension or atherosclerosis, but is more often associated with angiomas or aneurysms of the internal carotid and vertebral arteries. It is in reality a bruit rather than a tinnitus, and is occasionally relieved by compression of the internal carotid artery. Muscle spasm, contraction of the tensor tympani, nasopharyngeal sounds, and temporomandibular joint clicking may also simulate tinnitus. Disease of the temporal cortex, principally that associated with atherosclerosis, hypertension, or decreased or increased cerebral blood flow, may cause the perception of abnormal sounds which, however, are more variable and complex than those perceived in a true tinnitus. Tinnitus may be psychogenic.

Loss of hearing may be the result of disease processes anywhere along the course of the auditory pathways. Conductive deafness may be caused by obstruction of the external auditory canal by foreign bodies; the presence of cerumen, water, blood, or exudate against the tympanic membrane; perforation of the tympanic membrane; disease of the middle ear; or disease of the nasopharynx with obstruction of the eustachian tube. Sensorineural deafness may be produced by disease of the cochlea, the cochlear nerve or nuclei, or the central auditory pathways. Sensory, or inner ear, deafness is caused by damage to the hair cells in the organ of Corti or the bipolar cells in the cochlea; this may follow acoustic trauma, may occur in Ménière's disease, and may result from certain infections and congenital abnormalities, such as the deafness resulting from rubella acquired by an infant from its mother during the first trimester of pregnancy. Retrocochlear deafness is that which follows lesions central to the inner ear. Cochlear nerve deafness is caused by degenerative and other pathologic alterations of the nerve itself; tumors of the nerve, injury associated with skull fracture, meningitis, syphilis, and various toxins or side effects of certain drugs cause this type of deafness. Nuclear lesions, either vascular, inflammatory, or neoplastic, occasionally cause impairment of hearing.

Presbycusis, the progressive decline in hearing acuity associated with aging, may have many causes. The sensory type results from atrophy of the organ of Corti and the nerve itself in the cochlea; the neural type is caused by loss of neurons in the auditory nerve and pathways; metabolic and mechanical etiologies have also been described.

Because supranuclear pathways are both crossed and uncrossed, unilateral lesions in the brain stem or temporal lobes are rarely followed by clinical loss of hearing, although detailed audiometric testing may show defects of the type found in sensorineural deafness, and brain stem auditory evoked potentials may show changes. Bilateral deafness may result, however, from midbrain lesions or from tumors of the posterior third ventricle or the aqueduct region with compression of either the medial geniculate bodies or the inferior colliculi.

Impairment of localization of sound has been described in the auditory field contralateral to a temporal lobe lesion. Bizarre types of tinnitus are found in some pontine lesions and cerebral lesions, and auditory hallucinations may occur in lesions of the temporal lobe. These frequently constitute epileptic auras. More bizarre hallucinations occur in psychotic states and drug-induced states.

Auditory receptive aphasia may be a manifestation of disease of the temporal lobe; it is characterized by inability to interpret or comprehend spoken words even though hearing is normal. In hysteria and other psychogenic disturbances there may be either partial or total and either unilateral or bilateral loss of hearing, with or without tinnitus.

THE VESTIBULAR NERVE

Anatomy and Physiology

The receptors of the vestibular nerve are situated in the neuroepithelium in the cristae of the ampullae of the semicircular canals and in the maculae of the utricle and saccule in the inner ear. Impulses are carried to the bipolar cells of the vestibular ganglion of Scarpa in the internal auditory meatus, from which central fibers pass as the vestibular nerve. This traverses the internal auditory meatus with the cochlear nerve and enters the medulla just below the pons (Fig. 14-10). Along their peripheral courses the two nerves are enclosed within a single sheath; the vestibular is larger. As they enter the brain stem the vestibular nerve is ventromedial to the restiform body and lies between it and the superior olivary body. The cochlear nerve is lateral and slightly caudal to the vestibular. Within the internal auditory meatus the facial nerve and

pars intermedia lie medial to and above the acoustic nerve. The peripheral fibers of the vestibular ganglia are composed of three branches: the superior branch arises from the sensory epithelium of the macula of the utricle and the ampullae of the superior (anterior vertical) and lateral (horizontal) semicircular canals; the fibers of the inferior branch arise from the macula of the saccule, and the fibers of the posterior branch arise from the ampulla of the posterior (posterior vertical) semicircular canal.

The majority of the vestibular fibers terminate on the four vestibular nuclei: the lateral, or Deiters', nucleus; the chief, dorsal, or medial nucleus, or nucleus of Schwalbe; the superior nucleus of Bechterew; and the inferior, spinal, or descending, nucleus (Fig. 14-10). Some of them, however, go without synapse into the cerebellum; these pass through the direct vestibulocerebellar pathway, which is one of the components of the inferior cerebellar peduncle. All four of the vestibular nuclei may send fibers into

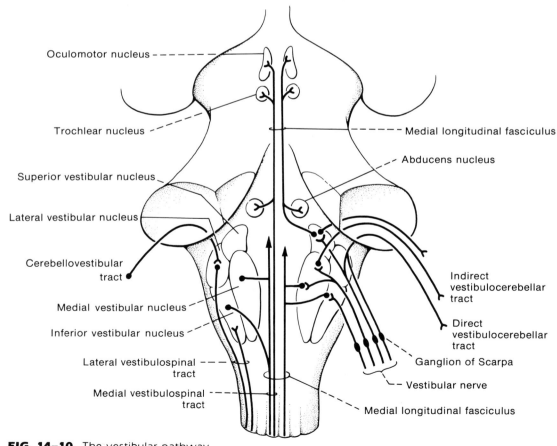

FIG. 14–10. The vestibular pathway.

the medial longitudinal fasciculus, but the vast majority of the ascending fibers arise from the superior and medial nuclei. This pathway, through connections with the nuclei of the oculomotor, abducens, and trochlear nerves, and the nuclei of the accessory and upper cervical nerves, is important in regulating movements of the eyes, head, and neck in response to stimulation of the semicircular canals. Impulses from the superior and medial nuclei go into the cerebellum as the indirect vestibulocerebellar pathway, whereas the latter nucleus receives cerebellovestibular fibers. Fibers from the lateral nucleus go down the spinal cord as the ipsilateral lateral, or direct, vestibulospinal pathway, which is important in the regulation of muscle tone and posture. Impulses from the medial vestibular nuclei descend to the cervical and upper thoracic spinal cord through the crossed medial vestibulospinal tract. The vestibular nuclei also have connections with the reticular gray matter of the brain stem and through this with the dorsal efferent nucleus of the vagus and with the spinal cord.

Ascending vestibular connections rostral to the mesencephalon have not been delineated with certainty. Thalamic cells with short response latencies to vestibular stimulation, suggesting a role in a primary projection pathway, have been found in the nucleus ventralis posterior inferior. Both experimental and clinical evidence documents some degree of vestibular involvement in all four cortical lobes. However, a primary vestibulocortical projection has been identified in animals posterior to the facial nerve zone in the somatosensory field of the parietal lobe. Such a parietal vestibular field may be involved in conscious perception of spatial orientation of the body. Vertigo, however, can be a symptom of temporal lobe irritation.

The labyrinth is composed of the semicircular canals and the utricle and saccule. The bony labyrinth comprises a series of osseous canals situated in the petrous portion of the temporal bone (Figs. 14-11 and 14-12). Within the bony canals are membranous tubes which contain endolymph and are separated from the osseous canals by perilymph (Fig. 14-13). There are three sets of semicircular canals, each at right angles to the other two. The lateral, or horizontal, canals are almost on the horizontal plane of the head, but are tilted 30° upward in their anterior arcs. The superior, or anterior vertical, canals are midway between the frontal and sagittal planes of the body, at an angle of 45° with the sagittal plane of the head and transverse to the long axis

of the petrous portion of the temporal bone. Their outermost portions are anterior, and the canals run inward and backward. The posterior, or posterior vertical, canals are also at an angle of 45° with the sagittal plane of the head and are parallel to the posterior surface of the temporal bone. Their outermost portions are posterior and the canals run inward and forward. The vertical canals are arranged in two diagonal pairs at right angles to the lateral canals and at right angles to each other. The posterior canal on one side is parallel to the superior canal on the opposite side. If the head is placed 30° forward, the lateral canals are horizontal and the vertical canals are vertical. Each semicircular canal has an ampulla, or dilated portion, which is twice the diameter of the rest of the canal. The ampullae lie at the anterior extremities of the horizontal canals and at the lateral extremities of the vertical canals. Within the ampullae are the cristae with the specialized epithelium, or hair cells, which are vestibular receptors. These are stimulated by movement of the endolymph. The sensory epithelium of the vertical canals is polarized so that displacement of endolymph away from the utricle is excitatory, whereas in the horizontal canal, the opposite is the case.

The semicircular canals are excited by movement in space and by changes in the direction and velocity of movement. They are influenced especially by rotatory motion of the head and rotatory acceleration. Stimulation of the canals gives evidence of the slightest alteration in the position of the body, and any change automatically calls for the appropriate motor response, a **kinetic labyrinthine reflex.** They are, thus, proprioceptive centers and regulate kinetic equilibrium. The semicircular canals and the vestibular apparatus are also important in the control of eye movements, ocular reflexes which follow changes in the position of the head and body, and ocular fixation. It is said that each canal has a major control over that pair of ocular muscles which moves the eyes in the plane of the canal. It is probable, however, that each labyrinth, directly or indirectly, has connections with all the ocular muscles of each eye through the medium of the medial longitudinal fasciculus, without a special relationship between canals and muscles.

Within the osseous vestibule are two membranous sacs, the **utricle** and **saccule.** Receptors similar to those in the semicircular canals are situated in these structures. The hair cells of the maculae are in contact with small calcareous masses, the **otoliths.** The otoliths of the utricles are known as the **lapilli,** and those of the sac-

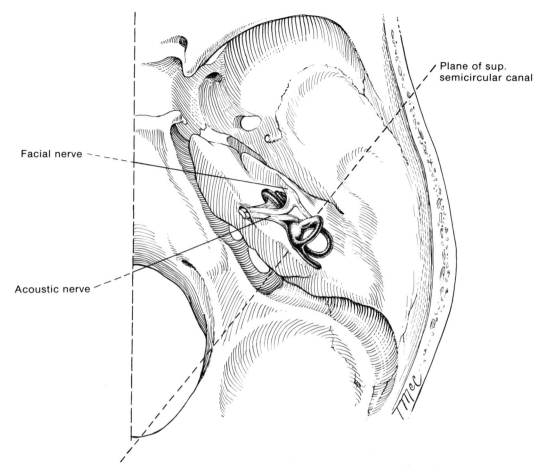

Facial nerve ---

Acoustic nerve ---

Plane of sup.
semicircular canal

FIG. 14–11. The right osseous labyrinth in the temporal bone viewed from above.

cules as the **sagittae.** The maculae of the utricle and saccule are stimulated by alterations of the position of the head and body in space, and by linear acceleration, gravity, and centrifugal force. The position of the otoliths with reference to the hair cells varies under the influence of gravity. The lapilli function synergistically, whereas the sagittae are opponents. When the head is erect, the two utricular maculae are approximately in a plane parallel to the ground, and the saccular maculae are perpendicular to them. The otolith mechanism, thus, conveys information concerning the position of the head and body in space, motion in a linear plane, and movement either with or against gravity. It exerts a tonic influence on the body musculature, reinforces muscle tone, and excites the muscular contractions necessary for the maintenance of equilibrium. It functions in static equilibrium, and is essential to the static, postural, tonic neck, and righting reflexes.

The vestibular apparatus, thus, has multiple and complex functions. Kinetic impulses which have their origin in the semicircular canals stimulate motor responses which involve compensatory movements and equilibrium. Impulses which arise from the otolith apparatus provide information about orientation in space and evoke reflexes which serve to maintain equilibrium in any posture. As a result of these functions and of its close relationship to the cerebellum, the vestibular complex plays an essential part in coordination, especially in the coordination of movements of the trunk and limbs in response to stimulation of the semicircular canals. The otolith mechanism, through the de-

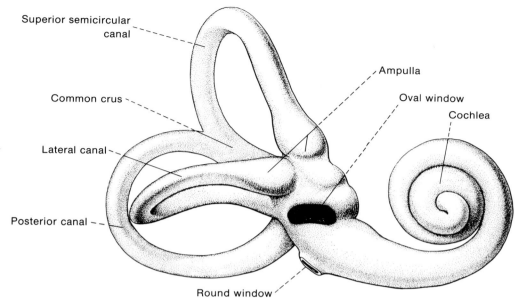

FIG. 14–12. The right osseous labyrinth, lateral view.

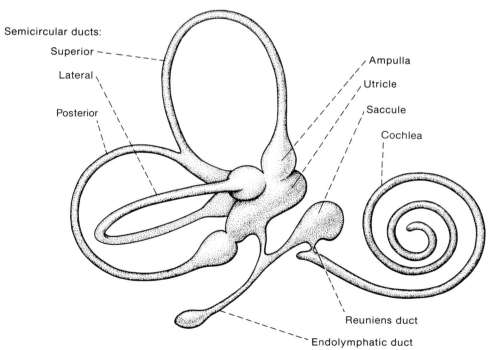

FIG. 14–13. The membranous labyrinth.

scending vestibulospinal pathways, is important in the regulation of muscle tone and is essential to postural and righting reflexes. Through the medial longitudinal fasciculus and the brain stem reticular formation and their connections with the ocular and cervical muscles, the vestibular apparatus is essential to ocular reflexes and fixation and to the conjugate movements of the head and eyes which enable the individual to keep his gaze on stationary objects while his head and body are in motion.

The most characteristic symptom in disease of the vestibular system is **vertigo,** usually described as dizziness by the patient. This is a sensation of movement, and is often accompanied by feelings of unsteadiness and loss of balance. True organic, or vestibular, vertigo is usually rotatory in type, and has been described as **objective** if external objects seem to be rotating around the individual, and as **subjective** if the individual himself seems to be rotating. All vertigo, however, is subjective, a sensation of a disturbed relationship with one's environment in some definite plane, often accompanied by a false sense of motion in that plane. Instead of subjective sensation of rotation, the patient may notice a feeling of vertical or horizontal movement, of a sense of tipping, of tilting, or of being pushed or pulled. Vertigo should be differentiated from giddiness or faintness, and from swimming, reeling, light-headed, or drunken sensations which may be interpreted as dizziness but are not true vertigo. In addition to vertigo there are often disturbances of equilibrium, manifested by unsteadiness and staggering. If the dysfunction is unilateral, the staggering is toward one side, and there is postural deviation, often accompanied by kinetic deviation, or past pointing. If the vertigo is severe, it may be accompanied by nausea, vomiting, diaphoresis, tachycardia, pallor, hypotension, and even shock and loss of consciousness. In most instances vestibular irritation or disease is accompanied by ocular deviation and nystagmus.

Clinical Examination

The clinical examination of the vestibular nerve should be preceded in every instance by a careful appraisal of the patient's symptoms. If the patient complains of dizziness, the examiner should attempt to determine whether there actually is vertigo rather than light-headedness or giddiness sometimes referred to as **pseudovertigo.** If vertigo is present, it is essential to know whether it is objective or subjective, episodic or constant, lateralized, and related to change of position. The presence of associated symptoms, such as nausea, vomiting, staggering, deviation of the eyes, disturbances of balance, prostration, tinnitus, hearing loss, or loss of consciousness, is important. The type, form, direction, rate, amplitude, duration, and intensity of spontaneous nystagmus should be noted, as well as abnormalities of coordination and of station and gait.

Certain tests of vestibular function and vestibular reflexes are closely related to the examination of other portions of the nervous system and are discussed elsewhere. Coordination *per se* is considered in detail in the examination of motor functions (Ch. 30); muscle tone is also discussed in the motor examination (Ch. 28); postural and righting reflexes are described in Part E, "The Reflexes;" ocular movements are considered in detail in Chapter 11. The **vestibulopupillary reflex** consists of either dilation of the pupil or constriction followed by dilation in response to stimulation of the labyrinthine system. The **vestibulo-oculogyric reflex** consists of movement of the eyeballs in response to vestibular stimulation. This is elicited by sudden passive movement of the head from side to side (the doll's head phenomenon) and also in performing the vestibular tests, which will be described in the following paragraphs. Usually only the lateral movements are investigated. These reflex movements may persist even after paralysis of voluntary movement. Certain **vestibulospinal reflexes** may be investigated by **Fukuda's stepping test.** The blindfolded subject is placed in the center of two concentric circles divided into angles of 30°, and is asked to mark time for 1 min. His rotation on his own axis and any movement forward, backward, or to the sides is noted; in normal individuals there is only minimal rotation and movement.

Tests for vestibular function essential to the neurologic appraisal are those which are carried out by stimulation of the semicircular canals or of vestibular nerve endings. The otolith organs are not available to direct testing by the clinician. The labyrinths, particularly the semicircular canals and/or the vestibular receptors, may be stimulated in three ways: by the use of the rotating chair, change in temperature (hot or cold), and galvanic stimulation. All of these are at times called Bárány tests.

In all of these tests the vestibular symptoms of vertigo, nausea, vomiting, and sometimes diaphoresis and prostration are reproduced, and the objective manifestations of deviation of the eyes, nystagmus, postural deviation, and past pointing are noted. It is believed that stimulation of the labyrinth by rotation or by the use of hot or cold water sets up a current of lymphokinesis in the endolymph within the semicircular canals, and that this, in turn, stimulates the vestibular nerves. Galvanic stimulation and pressure changes may act upon the vestibular nerve endings directly. It cannot be definitely stated whether the endolymph is static in the resting individual and is in motion only on stimulation of the labyrinth, or whether the fluid is bidirectional in the resting individual and becomes unidirectional by stimulation. Some authorities express the belief that there is no circulation in the fluid, but that pressure changes stimulate the cristae ampullaris. It is generally accepted, however, that the movement of the endolymph completely and consistently explains and accounts for the resulting phenomena.

The **nystagmus** which results from vestibular stimulation is rhythmic in type. Its direction depends upon the semicircular canals stimulated, and is thus dependent upon the position of the head during the examination. It is caused by stimuli initiated by movement of the endolymph; the slow phase is in the direction of the endolymph flow. The head and eyes, and sometimes the body, are deviated in the same direction. The vertigo is compensatory and is in the opposite direction, that is, in the direction of the rapid phase of the nystagmus. The excitation of a single semicircular canal produces nystagmus only in a plane parallel with the plane of that canal (**Flourens' law**), and the relationship between the direction of the flow of the endolymph and the direction of the nystagmus is a definite and constant one. Reversal of the flow of the endolymph causes a reversal in the direction of the nystagmus. Stimulation of more than one canal produces a more complex response and a more complex type of nystagmus. A horizontal semicircular canal is maximally stimulated by a movement of the endolymph within the canal toward its ampulla; a vertical canal is maximally stimulated by a movement of the endolymph away from its ampulla (**Ewald's first law**). Furthermore, maximal stimulation of a semicircular canal results in nystagmus with the rapid component toward the stimulated side, while minimal stimulation causes nystagmus with the rapid component toward the opposite side (**Ewald's second law**). The interval of time between the stimulation and the onset of the nystagmus should be noted, as well as the type, form, direction, duration, and intensity of the response. The amplitude of the nystagmus is increased on turning the eyes in the direction of the rapid phase. Placing strong convex lenses (Frenzel's spectacles) in front of the patient's eyes will aid in the observation of the nystagmus by magnifying it, and will be of further value by preventing the patient from fixing on any point or object. Electronystagmography, a recording of eye movements based on the corneal retinal potential, may aid in the evaluation of the responses and quantify wave forms, frequencies, and amplitudes.

Postural deviation is a tilting or reactive movement of the entire body in the direction of the flow of the endolymph. It is tested by having the patient stand with his feet together and noting persistent falling in any one direction. The patient may be asked to walk along a straight line or to walk tandem, placing one heel directly in front of the other foot, and any deviation is noted. **Past pointing,** or **kinetic deviation,** is a reactive movement of the extremities in the direction of the endolymph flow. It is tested by having the patient place his extended finger on that of the examiner; the patient closes his eyes and either lowers or raises his hand and then touches the examiner's finger again. Motion should take place at the shoulder joint. The degree of deviation to either side is noted. On repeated movements the amount of deviation may increase. Past pointing should be tested in both upper extremities. The nystagmus, postural deviation, and past pointing which follow vestibular stimulation must be differentiated from those signs of disease which may have been present before the tests were carried out. It is also valuable, in appraising the vestibular tests, to note the presence of such manifestations as subjective vertigo, nausea, vomiting, diaphoresis, and other symptoms. The patient may contribute information by comparing the vertigo which follows vestibular stimulation with vertiginous symptoms he may have had previously. Since the vestibular tests may be followed by unpleasant symptoms, it is best to carry them out after the neurologic examination has been completed.

The **Nylen-Bárány maneuver** for positional nystagmus and vertigo (often referred to as the **Hallpike maneuver**) is performed by seating the patient on the edge of an examining table and having him lie down abruptly with the head hanging for 45° backward and 45° to one side. The patient is observed for the development of nystagmus and symptoms of vertigo, and the onset, duration, and direction of the nystagmus are noted. The test is then repeated with the head toward the opposite side. The response is prompt and the vertigo of significant severity in patients with positional vertigo.

Rotation Tests. In the rotating-chair tests the patient is seated in the Bárány chair and rotated rapidly, about 10 times in 20 sec, and the movement is then abruptly stopped. The head is fixed by a head rest, and the eyes are closed to prevent the development of optokinetic nystagmus. On the completion of rotation the eyes are opened so that the nystagmus may be seen, and postural deviation and past pointing are tested. In the beginning of rotation, owing to inertia, the endolymph moves less rapidly than the body, and there is sensation of a brief movement in the direction opposite to that of the body. As a consequence, during rotation the eyes are drawn to the opposite side, and the slow phase of the nystagmus is opposite to the direction of rotation. This, however, is difficult to observe without the attachment of electronic recording devices on the rotating chair or the patient. Later the endolymph moves in the same direction as the body, and when the rotation ceases abruptly, the momentum of the labyrinthine fluid causes it to continue to flow in the direction of the recently completed movement of the body, even though the head is now stationary. This causes the **after-nystagmus,** which is what one observes clinically, and it is opposite in direction to the primary nystagmus. The slow phase of the nystagmus, deviation of the eyes, postural deviation, and past pointing are all correlated with endolymph displacement and are in the direction of the recently completed movement, whereas the vertigo is in the opposite direction.

In order to test the lateral (horizontal) canals, the head is tilted forward 30° so that these canals are on a horizontal plane. This plane is reached when a line drawn through the middle of the eye and the external auditory meatus is parallel to the floor. If the patient is rotated to the right, past pointing and postural deviation develop to the right, while vertigo develops to the left (Table 14-1). The after-nystagmus is characterized by a slow movement to the right with the quick phase to the left; it is horizontal in type. The opposite results are obtained by rotation to the left. The duration and intensity of the nystagmus and the degree of vertigo, nausea, and other symptoms depend upon the rapidity of rotation, the degree of sensitivity of the vestibular apparatus, and the duration of rotation. In the normal individual the nystagmus lasts 25 – 30 sec. This test involves the semicircu-

lar canals and vestibular apparatus on both sides, but the canal on the side toward which the subject is rotated is stimulated the most.

Rotatory and vertical nystagmus are produced by stimulation of the vertical canals, and diagonal or mixed nystagmus by stimulating more than one set of canals. The superior (anterior vertical) canals are placed in the plane of rotation and are stimulated by tilting the head either forward 90° – 120° so that the chin is against the chest, or backward 60°. The posterior (posterior vertical) canals are stimulated if the head is flexed 90° laterally toward the shoulder during rotation. The results which follow the stimulation of the vertical canals or of various combinations of the canals are sometimes confusing and are difficult to evaluate; they are summarized in Table 14-1. If the patient is rotated to the right with the head 90° – 120° forward there is rotatory nystagmus with the slow phase to the right, with postural deviation and past pointing to the right and vertigo to the left. If he is rotated to the right with the head extended backward 60°, there is rotatory nystagmus with the slow phase to the left, with vertigo to the right and deviation and past pointing to the left. If he is rotated to the right with the head bent 90° toward the right shoulder, there is vertical nystagmus with the slow phase upward, with a sensation of falling forward, past pointing upward, and, after the head is again erect, a tendency for the patient to fall backward. If he is rotated toward the right with the head 90° toward the left shoulder, there is vertical nystagmus with the slow phase downward, with vertigo backward, past pointing downward, and a tendency to fall forward after the head is erect. Nystagmus and deviation in the opposite directions are produced by rotation to the left. Mixed and diagonal types of nystagmus are elicited following rotation with the head in other positions, so that more than one set of canals is stimulated.

Caloric Tests. In the caloric, or thermal, tests the external auditory canal is douched with cold or hot water or air. A thermal stimulation of the auditory canal produces a change in the temperature of the endolymph. This sets up a convection current and causes the endolymph to circulate. Only those canals in the vertical plane are affected. Cold water causes the endolymph to flow from above downward, away from the ampulla, and toward the side stimulated, whereas hot water has the opposite effect. The advantage of the caloric test is that the vestibular apparatus on each side can be examined individually.

TABLE 14–1. VESTIBULAR TESTS

Rotation tests: Manifestations following rotation to the right (opposite results on rotation to the left)

Position of Head (patient seated)	Canals Stimulated	Nystagmus: Slow Phase (after-nystagmus)	Falling or Postural Deviation (after head is brought up)	Past Pointing (kinetic deviation)	Vertigo (hallucinated movement)
30° forward	Lateral	Horizontal to right	To right	To right	To left
90°–120° forward	Superior	Rotary to right	To right	To right	To left
60° backward	Superior	Rotary to left	To left	To left	To right
90° toward right shoulder	Posterior	Vertical upward	Backward	Upward	Forward
90° toward left shoulder	Posterior	Vertical downward	Forward	Downward	Backward

Caloric tests: Manifestations following douching of right ear with cold water (opposite results on douching with hot water; opposite results on douching left ear)

Position of Subject and Head	Canal Stimulated	Nystagmus: Slow Phase	Falling or Postural Deviation (after head is brought up)	Past Pointing (kinetic deviation)	Vertigo (hallucinated movement)
Lying down, head 30° forward	Lateral	Horizontal to right	To right	To right	To left
Seated, head 60° backward	Lateral	Horizontal to right	To right	To right	To left
Seated, head 90°–120° forward	Lateral	Horizontal to left	To left	To left	To right
Seated, head 30° forward	Superior	Rotary to right	To right	To right	To left

Before doing the caloric test the canal must be examined for the presence of cerumen or blood, and the tympanic membrane for perforations or other abnormalities. If the drum is perforated, air or an antiseptic solution should be used. If the drum is retracted, the response is accentuated. The patient's eyes should be fixed on a stationary object. In the original test water at 7° – 8° above or below normal body temperature was used, and either allowed to flow slowly into the canal through a rubber tube attached to a vessel suspended about 2 feet above the level of the ear, or injected gently from a large syringe. It may be necessary to instil 100 ml or more to elicit a response. The water may be allowed to run in the ear for 40 sec and this may be repeated if there is no response, or it may be injected until vertigo appears. In order to facilitate the test and to avoid the use of large amounts of water, many examiners use ice water (0° – 5° C); 5 ml are injected, and if there is no response the procedure is repeated with 10 ml. This may be repeated until there is a response. This method is less annoying to the patient, and less time-consuming. Warm water may be used first as a rough screening test; if similar responses are obtained bilaterally, the cold water stimulus can be omitted. When cold water is used, the past pointing and postural deviation develop toward the side of stimulation, and the slow phase of the nystagmus is in that direction. Hot water produces opposite effects. The nystagmus may be recorded graphically.

In order to stimulate the lateral canals and obtain horizontal nystagmus, the patient must either be lying down with his head tilted 30° forward, or seated with his head tilted 90° – 120° forward or 60° backward, so that the lateral canals are in a vertical plane. If the lateral canal of the right ear is stimulated with cold water when the patient is either lying down with his head 30° forward or seated with his head 60° backward, there is nystagmus with the slow phase to the right, with past pointing and postural deviation to the right and vertigo to the left (see Table 14-1). If the right ear is stimulated with cold water when the patient is seated with his head 90° – 120° forward, the vertigo is to the right, and the slow phase of the nystagmus, postural deviation, and past pointing are to the left. The nystagmus is horizontal on these occasions. The superior canals are stimulated and rotatory nystagmus is obtained when the patient is seated with his head tilted forward 30°, or when the patient is lying down with his head tilted forward 90° – 120° or backward 60°. If the right ear is stimulated with cold water when the patient is seated with his head forward 30°, there is rotatory nystagmus with the slow phase to the right, with postural deviation and past pointing to the right and vertigo to the left. The posterior canals are too far distant from the middle ear for stimulation in the test. If there is destruction of one labyrinth, or of the eighth nerve on that side, there is no response following caloric stimulation.

The **minimal ice water caloric test,** in which only a very small amount of water, but at a temperature of 1° – 3° C, is injected into the auditory canal, is a simple but sensitive test of vestibular function.

Galvanic Tests. The galvanic test is carried out with the patient standing upright with his feet together and his eyes closed. The cathode is placed in the patient's hand or over the sternum or back, and the anode over the mastoid prominence. Normally a current of 5 – 7 ma (milliamperes) causes nystagmus with the slow phase toward the side stimulated, and slight swaying and past pointing toward that side. The nerve endings in all the semicircular canals are stimulated directly, and the movement of the endolymph in the semicircular canals is not ordinarily affected; the nystagmus is of a mixed type, both horizontal and rotatory. If 1 – 2 ma evoke a response, there is a hyperirritability of the labyrinth, and if 10 – 15 ma are needed, there is impairment of function. Inasmuch as the galvanic stimulus may act directly on the vestibular nerve, there may be a response to the galvanic stimulation even though the labyrinth is destroyed and the caloric test is negative. Opposite results are obtained when the cathode is used as the stimulus.

Evaluation of Vestibular Function Tests. Of all the aforementioned tests, the caloric is the most practicable and the easiest to evaluate. The disadvantage of the rotation tests in neurologic diagnosis is that both labyrinths are stimulated simultaneously; however, rotation tests are sensitive measures of even minimal retained function of the labyrinths. Unilateral vestibular disease may be diagnosed more readily by the caloric and galvanic tests, which stimulate each side individually. The caloric test, which sets the endolymph in motion and thus stimulates the end-organ, is probably more valuable than the galvanic test, which may stimulate the nerve directly. Furthermore, specific canals are affected by caloric stimulation, whereas all the canals on one side are influenced by galvanic stimulation. In all instances the nystagmus, past pointing, etc. which may have existed prior to the test, must be differentiated from those which develop during the examination. Caloric, rotation, and galvanic stimulation may also be used to modify the stepping test; the patient's body rotates on its own axis in the direction of the slow phase of the nystagmus.

When the vestibular system is irritated, there is an exaggerated response to all of the aforementioned tests, and there are marked subjective symptoms in the form of vertigo, nausea, and vomiting. There is an individual variation in vestibular responses, which may be apparent clinically in the susceptibility of certain persons to motion sickness. With impaired vestibular function there is a diminished response on the affected side, especially in the caloric and galvanic tests. With destruction of the labyrinth or its connections or of the vestibular nerve on one side, there is absence of response to caloric or galvanic tests; there is no nystagmus, past pointing, postural deviation, or vertigo following stimulation of individual canals or of all canals on that side. Caloric testing can also be done in comatose patients; there is usually tonic conjugate deviation of the eyes without nystagmus toward the ear injected with cold water, but it may also be possible to bring out evidence of ocular muscle weakness, paresis of conjugate gaze, or abnormalities such as internuclear ophthalmoplegia.

With central lesions there may be a dissociation of responses, such as the presence of certain manifestations and the absence of others, lack of reaction to stimulation of certain semicircular canals but response of others, and perversion or inversion of reflex nystagmus. If there is interruption of connections with the medial longitudinal fasciculus on one side, stimulation of individual canals or of all canals on that side causes vertigo, past pointing, and postural deviation, but no nystagmus. With an intrapontine lesion there may be normal reactions from one set of canals and absence of response from others; there is especially apt to be absence of response to stimulation of the vertical canals. With a lesion of the inferior cerebellar peduncle on one side there is nystagmus following stimulation of the lateral canal on that side, but no vertigo, past pointing, or postural deviation. With a lesion of the middle cerebellar peduncle on one side there is nystagmus following stimulation of the superior canal on that side, but no vertigo, past pointing, or falling. With a unilateral cerebellar lesion there is nystagmus following stimu-

lation of all canals on that side, but no vertigo, past pointing, or falling. With a lesion of the midbrain there may be nystagmus following stimulation of all canals on both sides, but no vertigo, past pointing, or postural deviation. It must be emphasized, however, that one should not depend upon the vestibular tests alone for the localization of nervous system lesions. The other neurologic findings and the clinical history are essential to diagnosis, as are the findings on imaging studies.

Disorders of Function

As has been stated, vertigo is the most characteristic symptom of vestibular disease. Irritation or destruction of the labyrinths and increase or decrease in the pressure of the endolymph may cause vertigo, which may be accompanied by the objective signs of unsteadiness, staggering, incoordination, ocular deviation, and nystagmus, and by symptoms of nausea, vomiting, and prostration. Vestibular manifestations may be caused by disease of the labyrinths themselves, the vestibular nerve, the vestibular nuclei, or the supranuclear connections. Vertigo may also, however, be a symptom of general rather than focal disease, and in such cases it has no localizing value. The history is very important, and one should determine whether the patient experiences an actual sensation of rotation or movement, either of himself or of the environment; if such is present, one should inquire about its pattern, periodicity, direction, severity, and relationship to posture or change of position, as well as about associated ataxia, falling, deafness, and tinnitus.

Since the labyrinths are antagonistic to each other, the elimination of one acts as a stimulus to the other. If one labyrinth is destroyed there is nystagmus, usually with the slow phase toward the involved side, and there are associated deviations of the eyes, head, body, and extremities in the same direction. These manifestations do not persist, but are compensated for by processes within the corresponding vestibular nuclei and by visual and other nonlabyrinthine reflexes. It is often difficult to differentiate between manifestations associated with destruction and those secondary to irritation of the labyrinths or vestibular nerves, and between underactivity on one side and hyperactivity on the opposite side. In hyperirritability, however, the rapid phase of the nystagmus is usually toward the involved side, whereas in diminished irritability it is toward the opposite side. Hyperactivity and hypoactivity of the labyrinth may be caused by the same process. Shortly after the onset of a lesion there may be symptoms caused by irritation, whereas later those of destruction may predominate.

The labyrinths may be affected by inflammation, hemorrhage, edema, pressure changes, etc. Middle ear disease or mastoiditis with extension to the inner ear may cause a purulent or serous labyrinthitis, with vertigo and the attendant subjective and objective manifestations. The labyrinthitis may be either circumscribed or diffuse. Hemorrhage into the labyrinth may cause intense vertigo which may persist for a long time. Skull fractures through the labyrinth and labyrinthine fistulas may cause symptoms of vestibular dysfunction.

In motion sickness of various types, the vertigo and associated symptoms are probably the result of conflicting messages arriving simultaneously from two receptor systems, visual and labyrinthine (the semicircular canals and otolith organs). There is a marked individual variation in vestibular response, and such stimulation in especially susceptible individuals, such as those with hyperactive labyrinthine systems or sensitive vestibular mechanisms, causes vertigo, disturbances of equilibrium, drowsiness, vomiting, and pallor, perspiration, and other autonomic nervous system disturbances. Vision and psychic factors influence the symptoms. Nystagmus is often absent in motion sickness.

The term **Ménière's disease** has been used for both suppurative labyrinthitis and hemorrhage into the labyrinth, but currently it is applied to labyrinthine hydrops, which was once known as Ménière's syndrome. Ménière's disease is characterized by paroxysmal sudden attacks of labyrinthine vertigo, usually associated with unilateral tinnitus and deafness. The vertigo is often accompanied by nausea, vomiting, and unsteadiness, and may even result in prostration and loss of consciousness. At times the attacks are precipitated by change of position or sudden movements of the head. The patient is free from vertigo in between the attacks. The manifestations most frequently appear in middle age, and cochlear symptoms may precede those of labyrinthine involvement. The disease is usually unilateral, but occasionally becomes bilateral. When the cochlea is involved, hearing tests show an inner-ear or end-organ type of deafness, and the vestibular responses are usually decreased on the affected side.

There are many theories concerning the etiology of Ménière's disease. Most authorities express the belief that edema of the labyrinth with increased pressure of labyrinthine fluid (**labyrinthine** or **endolymphatic hydrops**) is responsible in most cases. Vasomotor changes (vasodilation or vasospasm), overproduction of endolymph, increase in the permeability of the capillaries with associated increase in intralabyrinthine pressure, disturbances of the autonomic nervous system, allergy, and changes in acid-base equilibrium with retention of sodium have all been listed as possible or contributory etiologies. Pathologically there are degenerative changes in the hair cells of the cochlea and the neuroepithelium of the semicircular canals. Individual cases seem to have been relieved by dehydration, restriction of sodium or increased intake of potassium, and the use of vasodilators and antihistamines or scopolamine. In severe cases the acoustic nerve or its vestibular portion has been sectioned as a therapeutic measure or destroyed with vestibulotoxic substances. Other approaches for relief of the symptoms by surgical and allied procedures include decompression of the labyrinth, fenestrated and surgical destruction of the membranous labyrinth, ultrasonic destruction or electrocoagulation of the labyrinth, stellectomy and dorsal sympathectomy, and section of the chorda tympani, the tympanic plexus, or both.

The terms **labyrinthitis** and **vestibular neuronitis** are used to signify disease processes in which the predominant symptom is vertigo, often with recurring attacks and usually without an associated cochlear disturbance. In the acute attacks there may be nausea and vomiting as well as nystagmus and kinetic and postural deviation. The vertigo is often brought on or increased by sudden movements or change in position of the head; it may be present only when the patient is in a certain position, as when recumbent, with positional nystagmus. There may be persisting dizziness between attacks. There may be either decreased or increased response to caloric testing on one or both sides; if the response is increased, the test may reproduce the symptoms. The syndrome may be associated with or follow some nonspecific infection, and occasionally occurs as so-called epidemic vertigo, but in most cases the etiology is not known and the condition is self-limited. The pathologic process may be in the labyrinth or in the vestibular nerve or nuclei. The symptoms may be due to stimulation of the vestibular end-organs by infection or by some endogenous toxin.

In addition to its peripheral origin, vertigo may also be of central, or even cortical, origin, or may be a symptom of disease elsewhere in the body, or of general disease. It is common in disease of the brain stem and cerebellum, and may occur with cerebral tumors and abscesses, increased intracranial pressure and intracranial aneurysms or other vascular disorders. Inasmuch as there may be associated symptoms of cochlear nerve dysfunction in such cases, these are discussed more in detail in the following paragraphs. Vertigo may be a prominent symptom in posttraumatic states, probably the result of focal injury to the vestibular pathways. In benign paroxysmal vertigo the symptom may be related to the position of the head or body, usually with rotatory nystagmus and vertigo when the patient assumes the supine position; the responsible lesion is felt to be in the posterior semicircular canals, due to dislocation of the otoliths from trauma or other causes. Ocular vertigo may be associated with imbalance of the extraocular muscles, ocular muscle palsies, and errors of refraction; vertigo experienced in high places may have a visual origin, but changes in atmospheric pressure may also be responsible. Systemic diseases such as atherosclerosis, hypertension, sudden fall in blood pressure, cardiac abnormalities, anemia, metabolic disturbances such as hypothyroidism and hypoglycemia, allergy, drug sensitivity, febrile states, and infections may cause vertigo. It may be difficult to differentiate between labyrinthine symptoms caused by peripheral lesions and those due to central nervous system changes or general or systemic disease. Those of peripheral origin, however, are usually episodic in character, aggravated by changes in posture, and accompanied by nystagmus. Vertigo of central origin is more apt to be continuous; it is less clearly defined and may not be accompanied by nystagmus, and there may be evidence of other central nervous system changes.

Dizziness is a common symptom in hysteria and the anxiety states. In these conditions, however, the patient rarely complains of true rotatory vertigo, but rather of giddiness or unsteadiness. The manifestations may be bizarre, and often are poorly described; there is no nystagmus; true postural deviation is rarely seen; and there are associated manifestations of the anxiety states.

LESIONS OF THE EIGHTH NERVE AND ITS CONNECTIONS

Although diseases of the peripheral apparatus, the cochlea and labyrinth, or diseases within the central nervous system may cause involvement of only one portion of the acoustic nerve or its connections, diseases of the nerve itself show evidence of impairment of function or irritation of both portions (Fig. 14-14). Both tinnitus and deafness may result from disturbance of cochlear function; while vertigo, abnormalities of equilibration, and nystagmus result from distur-

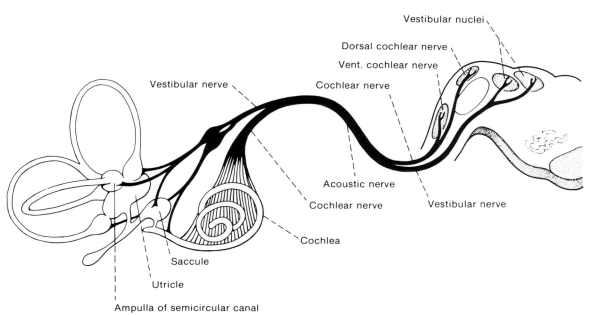

FIG. 14–14. The acoustic nerve and its connections.

bance of vestibular function. There may be symptoms of involvement of both branches in disease of the external, middle, or inner ear, with both vertigo and deafness. In obstruction of the external auditory canal by foreign bodies there is conductive deafness but there may also be vertigo. Otitis media, either acute or chronic, and either serous or suppurative, and obstruction of the eustachian tube, may cause symptoms referable to both branches. Mastoid disease, suppuration of the petrous apex, cholesteatomas, vascular lesions, angioneurotic edema, and trauma may cause both vestibular and cochlear symptoms. In otosclerosis there occasionally is vertigo as well as tinnitus and deafness.

The *end-organs* of both nerves within the cochlea and semicircular canals may be affected by various processes. Both are usually involved in Ménière's disease and in certain infections and congenital abnormalities, such as the syndrome resulting from rubella occurring early in pregnancy. Acoustic trauma, such as either blast injuries or repeated exposure to loud noises, as experienced in certain occupations or in the military, affects predominantly the cochlear endings. Streptomycin and its analogues frequently cause both vertigo and deafness. Streptomycin itself affects mainly the sensory epithelium of the semicircular canals and maculae, with secondary changes in the cochlea. If discontinued as soon as tinnitus is noted, serious deafness may be prevented; the effects are somewhat reversible, and the patient may learn to compensate for the labyrinthine dysfunction. Dihydrostreptomycin, kanamycin, and other aminoglycosides appear to have their major effect on the secretory epithelial structures of the inner ear, with secondary degenerative changes in the organ of Corti. Tinnitus and deafness follow. Occasionally deafness develops without the warning of tinnitus.

The *acoustic nerve itself* may be affected in many types of disease processes. It is frequently involved in basal skull fractures, and deafness and vestibular dysfunction may follow such a fracture or other types of cerebral or cranial trauma. Other disease of the base of the brain and its coverings, such as meningitis, granulomas, arachnoiditis, intracranial aneurysms, subarachnoid hemorrhage, and neoplasms, may involve the nerve, as may bone lesions such as Paget's disease and periostitis. Nerve deafness is one of the frequent sequelae of epidemic meningitis and it is one of the commoner stigmas of congenital syphilis, it also may result from intrauterine rubella infections. The eighth nerve is es-

pecially susceptible to various toxins, among which are quinine, lead, arsenic, alcohol, barbiturates, acetanilid, aminopyrine, hyoscine, chloroform, carbon monoxide, salicylates, cinchopen, and nicotine, as well as to endotoxic processes associated with disease of the gastrointestinal tract or uremia. It may be affected by either focal or systemic infections, and eighth nerve symptoms are common in any acute febrile illness. Progressive degeneration of the nerve may occur with increasing age or as a complication of central nervous system syphilis. A compilation of the many familial cochleovestibular atrophies appears in Adams and Victor. The nerve may also be affected in anemia, diabetes, gout, nephritis, leukemia, hypothyroidism, allergic states, avitaminosis, and myxedema and other hormonal imbalances.

Lesions of the *brain stem* may involve the nuclei or the central connections of either the cochlear or the vestibular nerve, but the latter are more commonly affected. The internal auditory artery supplies the entire inner ear, and the pontine branches of the basilar artery supply the nuclei of the eighth nerve. Intermittent insufficiency of the vertebrobasilar arterial system may cause recurring attacks of vertigo with or without hearing impairment and tinnitus. Thrombosis, aneurysms, angiomas, and other lesions of these or of other vessels of the pons or adjacent areas may cause both attacks of vertigo and deafness. Equilibrium is often affected; the nystagmus is often coarse and protracted and may be more marked toward one side or may be vertical in direction; there may be associated involvement of other cranial nerves or of the motor and sensory pathways that traverse the brain stem. Multiple sclerosis commonly causes vertigo and may cause either nerve deafness or "islands" of hearing loss; the damage may be in the nuclei or the ascending pathways. Other brain stem lesions that may cause similar symptoms include encephalitis and other inflammatory diseases, neoplasms, abscesses, granulomas including tuberculomas, tabes dorsalis and other forms of central nervous system syphilis, Friedreich's ataxia, syringobulbia, and platybasia or other congenital and developmental anomalies of the posterior fossa. Cerebellar lesions are often characterized by vertigo which may be the result of involvement of the vestibular pathways, but the symptom may also be associated with the ataxia and unsteadiness produced by the cerebellar dysfunction. Nystagmus, deviation, and past pointing are commonly encountered with cerebellar lesions. Patients with ataxia often complain of dizziness when referring to their sense of unsteadiness and lack of coordination.

Cerebral disturbances such as cerebral anemia, hyperemia, atherosclerotic or senile changes, concussion, and increased intracranial pressure may cause both vestibular and cochlear symptoms, as may cerebral neoplasms, abscesses, vascular accidents, and degenerative cerebral disease, especially if they involve the temporal lobes. Both tinnitus and vertigo may be present with migraine or as the aura of an epileptic attack. Vertigo and either unformed or formed auditory hallucinations may precede or accompany temporal lobe seizures. Vertigo is a common symptom in generalized cerebral disease, and may not have localizing value. Both tinnitus and vertigo have been produced by stimulation of the chorda tympani nerve. Both deafness and vertigo may be of psychogenic origin; the deafness is usually variable and inconsistent, whereas the vertigo may be vague and atypical.

There are a few neurologic syndromes in which involvement of the eighth nerve is especially significant. Perhaps the most important of these is the cerebellopontine angle neoplasm, usually a neurinoma or a neurofibroma, although occasionally a meningioma. The tumor arises on the eighth nerve within the internal auditory meatus, and its first symptoms are those of irritation or of loss of function of the nerve, namely, deafness and tinnitus, and later there are recurring attacks of vertigo. As the tumor grows in size there is involvement of the fifth nerve, with ipsilateral pain and anesthesia of the face and loss of the corneal reflex. Pressure on the cerebellum or its peduncles causes ataxia and coordination difficulties. There may be involvement of the seventh nerve with a peripheral facial palsy, and of the sixth, ninth, and tenth nerves. Later there are signs of increased intracranial pressure with headache, ocular manifestations, and occasional loss of consciousness. There are usually imaging signs of erosion of the internal auditory meatus or the presence of the mass itself in this location. On examination a sensorineural type of deafness is found, and the labyrinth on the involved side fails to respond to caloric or galvanic stimulation. Brain stem auditory evoked potentials are abnormal on the side of the lesion. There may, however, be atypical manifestations, with little impairment of hearing and unusual vestibular responses. Nystagmus is a common sign; it is coarse and slow on gaze toward the side of the lesion, and fine and rapid on gaze toward the

opposite side. Acoustic neurinomas may be part of generalized or localized neurofibromatosis (usually type II, especially if they are bilateral). Inflammatory lesions in the cerebellopontine angle may be difficult to differentiate clinically from neoplasms. In the former, however, motor symptoms predominate, whereas neoplasms affect sensory functions earlier and more severely.

Partial deafness may be an early symptom of a tumor of the glomus jugulare (chemodectoma); later there may be tinnitus, vertigo, and involvement of the facial, vagus, and other lower cranial nerves. On examination a vascular polyp may be found in the auditory canal or evidence of hemorrhage behind the tympanic membrane. **Bonnier's syndrome** consists of vertigo, nystagmus, and pallor, owing to involvement of Deiters' nucleus; these are often accompanied by hemiplegia, apprehension, tachycardia, and somnolence, and there may be evidence of associated involvement of the ninth, tenth, and third nerves. In **Lermoyez's syndrome** there are sudden attacks of dizziness which occur after increased deafness and are followed by improvement of hearing. In **Gerlier's disease,** or **paralyzing vertigo,** there are sudden transient attacks of vertigo accompanied by ptosis, paralysis of the arms and legs, pain in the back and neck, and muscular contractions. **Bruns' syndrome** consists of vertigo, vomiting, headache, and visual disturbances on change of position of the head; this is usually associated with a cysticercus infection of the fourth ventricle or with midline tumors of the cerebellum, and the symptoms are probably the result of disturbances of function of the vestibular pathways in the brain stem. When **deaf-mutism** is present, there is severe impairment of hearing from birth or from an early age, so that normal speech has not been acquired; there may or may not be impairment of vestibular function. There are many causes of deaf-mutism. Congenital deaf-mutism is usually inherited as a mendelian recessive trait, and may be due to aplasia of the cochlea, the labyrinth, or both. In **Cogan's syndrome** there are vestibular and auditory symptoms (vertigo, tinnitus, and deafness) along with a nonsyphilitic interstitial keratitis and some manifestations of systemic disease; this may be of infectious origin or a localized manifestation of polyarteritis nodosa.

BIBLIOGRAPHY

Adams RD, Victor M. Principles of Neurology, 4th ed. New York, McGraw – Hill, 1989

Alpers BJ. Vertigo and Dizziness. New York, Grune & Stratton, 1958

Atkinson M. Tinnitus aurium: Some considerations concerning its origin and treatment. Arch Otolaryngol 1947;45:68

Baloh RW. Neurotology. In Joynt RJ (ed). Clinical Neurology. Philadelphia, JB Lippincott, 1989

Baloh RW, Honrubia V. Jacobson K. Benign positional vertigo: Clinical and oculographic features in 240 cases. Neurology 1987;37:371

Bárány R. Physiologie und Pathologie (Funktionsprüfung) des Bogengang-Apparates beim Menschen: Klinische Studien. Leipzig, F Deuticke, 1907

Brodal A. Neurological Anatomy in Relation to Clinical Medicine, 3rd ed. New York, Oxford University Press, 1981

Brodal A, Pomeiano O, Walberg F. The Vestibular Nuclei and Their Connections. Springfield, IL, Charles C Thomas, 1962

Bunch CC. Clinical Audiometry. St Louis, CV Mosby, 1943

Carpenter MB. Central connections of the vestibular system. Arch Otolaryngol 1967;85:517

Cascino GD, Adams RD. Brainstem auditory hallucinosis. Neurology 1986;36:1042

Cawthorne TE. Examination of the vestibular system. Ann Otol Rhinol Laryngol 1965;77:727

Cawthorne TE, Fitzgerald G, Hallpike CS. Studies in human vestibular function. III. Observations on the clinical features of "Ménière's disease," with especial reference to the results of the caloric tests. Brain 1942;65:161

Davis H, Silverman SR (eds). Hearing and Deafness, 2nd ed. New York, Holt, Rinehart & Winston, 1960

DeWeese DD. Dizziness: An Evaluation and Classification. Springfield, IL, Charles C Thomas, 1954

Dix MR. Modern tests of vestibular function with special reference to their value in clinical practice. Br Med J 1969;3:317

Drachman DA, Hart CW. An approach to the dizzy patient. Neurology 1972;22:323

Favill J. The relationship of eye muscles to semicircular canal currents in rotationally induced nystagmus. Chicago, Privately printed, 1936

Fields WS, Alford BR. Neurological Aspects of Auditory and Vestibular Disorders. Springfield, IL, Charles C Thomas, 1964

Fischer JJ. The Labyrinth: Physiology and Functional Tests. New York, Grune & Stratton, 1956

Fukuda T. The stepping test. Acta Otolaryngol 1959;50:95

Glorig A (ed). Audiometry: Principles and Practices. Baltimore, Williams & Wilkins, 1965

Hawkins JE Jr. Biochemical aspects of ototoxicity. In Paparella MM (ed). Biochemical Mechanisms in Hearing and Deafness. Springfield, IL, Charles C Thomas, 1970

Jerger J. Audiological examination as an aid in diagnosis. Arch Otolaryngol 1967;82:552

Jerger J. Audiological findings in aging. Adv Otorhinolaryngol 1973;20:115

Jerger J. Modern Developments in Audiology. New York, Academic Press, 1973

Jeurs AL. Non-organic hearing problems. Laryngoscope 1966;76:714

Jongkees LEW. Vestibular physiology and tests. Arch Otolaryngol 1969;89:11

Kristensen HK, Zilstorff K. Modern diagnostic methods in otoneurology. Acta Otolaryngol (suppl) 1967;124:46

Lechtenberg R, Shulman A. The neurologic implications of tinnitus. Arch Neurol 1984;41:718

Naunton RF. The Vestibular System. New York, Academic Press, 1975

Nelson JR. The minimal ice water caloric test. Neurology 1969;19:577

Parker W, Decker RL, Richards NC. Auditory function and lesions of the pons. Arch Otolaryngol 1968;87:228

Pool JL, Pava AA. The Early Diagnosis and Treatment of Acoustic Nerve Tumors. Springfield, IL, Charles C Thomas, 1957

Rasmussen GL, Windle WF (eds). Neural Mechanisms of the Auditory and Vestibular Systems. Springfield, IL, Charles C Thomas, 1961

Spiegel EA, Sommer I. Neurology of the Eye, Ear, Nose and Throat. New York, Grune & Stratton, 1944

Stevens SS, Davis H. Hearing: Its Psychology and Physiology. New York, John Wiley & Sons, 1938

Uemura T, Suzuki JI, Hozawa J et al. Neuro-otological Examination. Baltimore, University Park Press, 1976

Von Békésy C. Experiments in Hearing. New York, McGraw–Hill, 1960

Wever EG, Lawrence M. Physiological Acoustics. Princeton, Princeton University Press, 1954

Wolfson RJ (ed). The Vestibular System and Its Diseases. Philadelphia, University of Pennsylvania Press, 1965

Chapter 15

THE GLOSSOPHARYNGEAL AND VAGUS NERVES

The glossopharyngeal and vagus, or ninth and tenth cranial, nerves are intimately associated with each other and are similar in function. Both have motor and autonomic branches with nuclei of origin in the medulla. Both conduct exteroceptive, general, and special visceral sensations to similar or identical fiber tracts in the brain stem. The two nerves leave the skull together and course through the neck in a similar manner, and in many instances they both supply the same structures. The two are frequently affected by the same disease processes. Often involvement of one may be difficult to differentiate from that of the other. For these reasons these two nerves are evaluated together.

THE GLOSSOPHARYNGEAL NERVE

Anatomy and Physiology

The glossopharyngeal nerve, as its name implies, is distributed principally to the tongue and pharynx. Its *motor fibers* originate in the cells of the nucleus ambiguus, which is situated in the reticular formation of the lateral part of the medulla, dorsal to the inferior olivary nucleus and ventromedial to the nucleus of the descending root of the trigeminal nerve (Fig. 15-1). The fibers first go posteriorly and medially toward the floor of the fourth ventricle, and then sweep laterally and somewhat forward, dividing to form multiple emergent root strands. The nucleus ambiguus, which extends from the level of entrance of the cochlear nerve at the upper border of the medulla to the level of the decussation of

the medial lemniscus, or even to the beginning of the corticospinal decussation, gives rise also to motor components of the vagus and accessory nerves.

The motor elements of the glossopharyngeal nerve go to the pharynx, but probably supply only the stylopharyngeus muscle. This muscle draws the posterior wall and the sides of the pharynx upward and lateralward, thus elevating the pharynx and increasing its transverse diameter. The stylopharyngeus also elevates the larynx in the act of swallowing and aids in closing the epiglottis. Although certain authorities have stated that the glossopharyngeal nerve also innervates the palatopharyngeus and palatoglossus muscles, and to a certain extent the superior constrictor of the pharynx, it is generally accepted that these latter muscles are supplied by the vagus nerve through the pharyngeal plexus, or possibly by the bulbar portion of the accessory nerve, fibers of which are distributed through the vagus. The cortical center which regulates the motor function of the ninth nerve is in the lower part of the precentral gyrus; the supranuclear innervation is bilateral, direct and indirect, and the motor path traverses the internal capsule, cerebral peduncle, and pons to the medulla.

Autonomic efferent fibers of the glossopharyngeal nerve have their origin in the portion of the dorsal efferent nucleus which is known as the inferior salivatory nucleus. The preganglionic fibers pass through Jacobson's nerve, the tympanic plexus, and the lesser superficial petrosal nerve to the otic ganglion, and the postganglionic fibers through the auriculotemporal branch

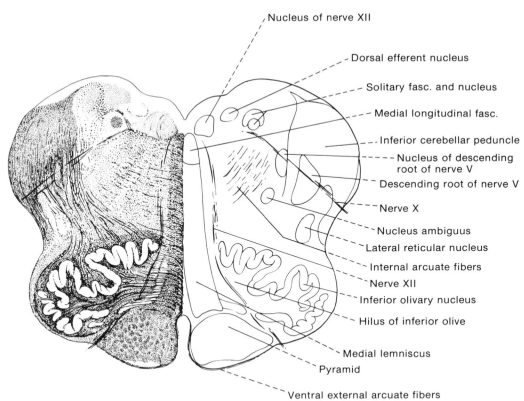

Nucleus of nerve XII

Dorsal efferent nucleus

Solitary fasc. and nucleus

Medial longitudinal fasc.

Inferior cerebellar peduncle

Nucleus of descending root of nerve V

Descending root of nerve V

Nerve X

Nucleus ambiguus

Lateral reticular nucleus

Internal arcuate fibers

Nerve XII

Inferior olivary nucleus

Hilus of inferior olive

Medial lemniscus

Pyramid

Ventral external arcuate fibers

FIG. 15–1. Section through the medulla at the level of the inferior olivary nucleus.

of the fifth nerve to the parotid gland. The glossopharyngeal nerve carries secretory and vasodilating impulses to the parotid gland. Salivation is also influenced by the sympathetic division of the autonomic nervous system, and is stimulated by gustatory and olfactory stimuli, by drugs such as pilocarpine, and by visual and emotional stimuli. The glossopharyngeal nerve, with the facial nerve, may supply impulses to the mucous membrane of the posterior and inferior portions of the pharynx and buccal cavity.

The *sensory branches* of the glossopharyngeal nerve have their nuclei in the petrous ganglion, situated in a depression in the lower portion of the petrous bone just below the jugular foramen, and in the superior, or jugular, ganglion, which is less constant and may be a part of the petrous ganglion. Fibers that carry exteroceptive sensation have peripheral pain, touch, and temperature endings in the posterior portions of the tympanic membrane and the external auditory canal. After passing through the petrous ganglion they terminate on the descending root of the trigeminal nerve and its nucleus within the medulla; their central connections are identical

with those of the other cranial nerves that carry exteroceptive sensation. Fibers that carry general visceral sensation from the mucous membrane of the pharyngeal wall, posterior and lateral portions of the soft palate, fauces, uvula, tonsils, tympanic cavity, mastoid cells, eustachian tube, posterior third of the tongue, and carotid body pass through the petrous ganglion, but terminate on the fasciculus solitarius and its nucleus. Fibers that carry the special visceral sensation, taste, have receptors in taste buds on the posterior third of the tongue and also terminate on the fasciculus solitarius and its nucleus.

Distribution and Branches. The glossopharyngeal nerve emerges from the medulla by means of three or four to six rootlets which are situated in the groove between the inferior olivary nucleus and the inferior cerebellar peduncle, below the emerging fibers of the seventh nerve and above and in line with those of the tenth (see Fig. 9-3). After leaving the medulla these rootlets unite to form the single nerve which leaves the skull through the jugular foramen with the tenth and eleventh nerves but within a separate sheath of the dura. It is lateral to and in front of these other nerves. At its exit from the skull the nerve passes forward between the internal jugular vein and internal carotid artery and descends in front of the latter vessel, but medial to the vein. It dips beneath the styloid process and follows the posterior border of the stylopharyngeus muscle with which it passes between the internal and external carotid arteries. It curves forward, forming an arch on the side of the neck, and reaches the lateral wall of the pharynx. It then disappears under the hyoglossus muscle, and divides into its constituent branches. The ninth nerve has intimate connections with the fifth, seventh, and tenth nerves and the cervical portion of the sympathetic division of the autonomic nervous system.

The branches of distribution of the glossopharyngeal nerve are the tympanic nerve and the carotid, pharyngeal, muscular, tonsillar, and lingual branches. The tympanic nerve, or Jacobson's nerve, arises from the petrous ganglion as the most important branch. It ascends to the tympanic cavity through a small canal on the under surface of the temporal bone, between the carotid canal and the jugular fossa. In the tympanic cavity it divides into branches which form the tympanic plexus. This plexus gives off the lesser superficial petrosal nerve and a branch to the greater superficial petrosal nerve; it receives sensory impulses from the mucous membrane lining of the tympanic cavity, the mastoid air cells, and the auditory canal. The lesser superficial petrosal nerve is a continuation of the tympanic nerve, supplemented by a filament from the geniculate ganglion of the facial nerve. It supplies motor (parasympathetic) and sensory roots to the otic ganglion, where there are further communications with the trigeminal and cervical sympathetic nerves. Postganglionic fibers pass in the auriculotemporal branch of the fifth nerve to the parotid gland. Carotid branches descend along the internal carotid artery to communicate with the pharyngeal branch of the vagus and the sympathetic nerves. They supply sensation to the carotid body and sinus for reflex control of respiration, heart rate, and blood pressure. Pharyngeal branches join those of the vagus and the sympathetic nerves to form the pharyngeal plexus, situated opposite the middle constrictor. Glossopharyngeal branches of this plexus supply the mucous surface of the pharynx and possibly some of its muscles. The muscular branch supplies the stylopharyngeus muscle. Tonsillar branches supply the tonsils, the soft palate, and the palatine

arches. The lingual branches are the terminal divisions. They supply the circumvallate papillae and mucous membrane of the base and posterior third of the tongue, the glossoepiglottic and pharyngo-epiglottic folds, the lingual surface of the epiglottis, and communicate with the lingual nerve.

Clinical Examination

The various functions of the ninth nerve are difficult to test, principally because the areas of distribution are also supplied by other, more important, nerves, and also because many of the structures it supplies are inaccessible.

Motor Function. The motor supply of the ninth nerve probably goes only to the stylopharyngeus muscle. If any dysfunction is evident at all, it will be a slight unilateral lowering of the palatal arch at rest, although the two sides elevate equally well on effort. The lateral wall of the pharynx may be neither elevated nor retracted. The "curtain movement" or *rideau* phenomenon, discussed with the vagus nerve in this chapter (see "The Pharynx," under "Examination of the Motor Functions") is probably associated with a lesion of the tenth rather than the ninth nerve.

Autonomic Function. The autonomic functions of the glossopharyngeal nerve can be evaluated by noting the function of the parotid gland. If highly seasoned foods are placed on the tongue, a copious flow of saliva may be seen to issue from Stensen's duct; this may be called the **salivary reflex.** Afferent impulses are carried through the glossopharyngeal nerve, and efferent impulses are conducted from the inferior salivatory nucleus to the parotid gland.

Sensory Function. The several sensory functions of the glossopharyngeal nerve are also difficult to test specifically. The areas to which branches of the glossopharyngeal nerve supply exteroceptive sensation are the posterior portion of the tympanic membrane and the posterior wall of the external auditory canal. These regions are also supplied by the fifth, seventh, and tenth cranial nerves. The glossopharyngeal nerve supplies the special visceral sensation, taste, to the posterior third of the tongue, and possibly with the vagus to the epiglottis, the region of the arytenoid cartilage, the hard and soft palates, the anterior pillars, and the posterior pharyngeal wall. This function may be tested in a similar manner to the testing of taste described in Chapter 13, but is examined more satisfactorily by the use of a galvanic current. However, such tests are not practical or necessary for ordinary neurologic diagnosis.

The function of the glossopharyngeal nerve that is most available to clinical testing is that concerned with general visceral sensation. Certain areas of this sensory supply, however, are inaccessible, but it is possible to test sensation in the region of the tonsils, fauces, opening of the eustachian tubes, lateral and posterior pharyngeal walls, posterior third of the dorsum of the tongue, and the lateral surfaces and a narrow rim along the inferior margin of the soft palate. With a lesion of the glossopharyngeal nerve these areas may be anesthetic, although owing to overlapping of supply in the throat by the tenth nerve and over the soft palate by the fifth, there may be a border of hypesthesia around the anesthetic zone. It has been found clinically, however, that in a large percentage of patients who have had a rhizotomy of the ninth nerve for glossopharyngeal neuralgia there is little or no objective sensory loss in the above distributions, and it is possible that the pharynx may derive a large part of its sensory innervation from the tenth nerve.

The Reflexes. The examination of the pharyngeal and palatal reflexes is an important part of the examination of the glossopharyngeal nerve. The **pharyngeal,** or **gag,** reflex is elicited by applying a stimulus, such as a tongue blade or an applicator, to the posterior pharyngeal wall, tonsillar regions, faucial pillars, or even the base of the tongue. The stimulus should be applied to each side of the pharynx. If the reflex is present, there will be elevation and constriction of the pharyngeal musculature, accompanied by retraction of the tongue. This reflex is used physiologically to initiate deglutition; its exaggeration may cause the vomiting reflex (see "The Vagus Reflex" later in this chapter). The afferent impulses of the reflex arc are primarily carried through the glossopharyngeal, the efferent elements primarily through the vagus nerve. The ninth may, however, contribute to the motor portion of the reflex arc, while the tenth may contribute to the sensory. The reflex center is in the medulla.

The **palatal** or **uvular** reflex is tested by stimulating the lateral and inferior surface of the uvula, or soft palate, with a tongue blade or a cotton applicator. Elevation of the soft palate and retraction of the uvula occur simultane-

ously. If the stimulus is directed toward one side of the soft palate, there is greater elevation on that side, together with ipsilateral deviation. The center for this reflex is also in the medulla. The motor portion of the reflex arc is carried through the vagus (and possibly the glossopharyngeal) nerve and the sensory component through the glossopharyngeal (and possibly the vagus) nerve. The trigeminal nerve, however, also supplies a part of the soft palate, and for this reason the palatal reflex may occasionally be retained in ninth nerve lesions. The palatal (uvular) reflex is less sensitive than the pharyngeal (gag) reflex. It may occasionally be absent normally.

These reflexes are absent if there is interruption of either the afferent or the efferent pathway. Occasionally their absence is without pathologic significance, but it usually indicates a lesion of the glossopharyngeal nerve, and the finding is most significant if it is unilateral. In some individuals the reflexes are markedly exaggerated, and when elicited, gagging and even retching and vomiting may occur. With pharyngeal anesthesia, regardless of its cause, no gagging results.

The **carotid sinus reflex,** which affects control of respiration, blood pressure, and heart rate, also receives its afferent supply from the glossopharyngeal nerve, but since this reflex is more closely related to vagal function, it is discussed with the vagus nerve later in this chapter, as are the cough and swallowing reflexes.

In summarizing the clinical examination of the glossopharyngeal nerve, it is repeated that the most important as well as the most readily available tests are the evaluation of sensation of the posterior pharyngeal wall and the soft palate, and the appraisal of the pharyngeal and palatal reflexes. Tests of the motor power of the stylopharyngeus muscle, the secretion of the parotid gland, exteroceptive sensations, and taste on the posterior third of the tongue are only rarely necessary for the proper interpretation of the neurologic examination.

Disorders of Function

Lesions of the glossopharyngeal nerve, especially isolated lesions, are not common. The nerve is small and is well protected. Isolated lesions of the ninth nerve are almost unknown and the nerve is usually involved only in association with the tenth, eleventh, twelfth, and other nerves. A lesion of the glossopharyngeal nerve may be followed by slight and transient difficulty in swallowing, especially of dry foods, due to paralysis of the stylopharyngeus muscle, but no disturbance of speech.

There is slight difficulty in retracting the lateral pharyngeal wall, and slight lowering of the palatal arch at rest may be noted. The tenth nerve is much more important than the ninth in both deglutition and articulation. Anesthesia in the distribution of the glossopharyngeal nerve rarely causes clinical symptoms, nor does loss of taste on the back of the tongue. Reflex swallowing and coughing may be lost in glossopharyngeal lesions because of the impairment of sensation and reflex salivation. The cough reflex elicited by stimulation of the tympanic membrane or the external auditory meatus may also be decreased.

Supranuclear lesions contribute to the syndrome of pseudobulbar palsy, but only if bilateral, and since the motor function of the ninth nerve is minimal, there is little or no clinical evidence of involvement of this nerve in pseudobulbar lesions. In nuclear lesions, such as progressive bulbar palsy, syringobulbia, multiple sclerosis, neoplasms, vascular lesions, granulomas, and botulism, there is usually associated involvement of the other medullary nerves, especially the tenth. Infranuclear lesions, such as gunshot or stab wounds in the neck, tumors, aneurysms of the carotid artery, skull fractures, and meningitis, also involve the tenth, eleventh, and other nerves. Tumors of the ninth nerve are rare, and usually also affect other nerves. Diseases of the middle ear, pharyngeal abscesses, extension of nasopharyngeal tumors, disseminated metastases from other neoplasms, and cervical adenopathy may cause disorders in the function of the nerve. Herpes zoster of the petrous ganglion has been described, but is rare. The otalgia which frequently accompanies throat disease is probably due in most instances to reflex involvement of the glossopharyngeal nerve. On the other hand, there is sometimes a disturbance of taste with increased salivation in diseases of the middle ear, owing to involvement of the tympanic plexus.

Perhaps the most important lesion of the ninth nerve is **glossopharyngeal neuralgia,** or "tic douloureux of the ninth nerve." In this condition the patient experiences attacks of severe lancinating pain originating in one side of the throat or tonsillar region and radiating along the course of the eustachian tube to the tympanic membrane, external auditory canal, and adjacent portion of the ear. As in trigeminal neuralgia, there may be trigger zones; they are usually in the pharyngeal wall, fauces, tonsillar regions, or base of the tongue. The pain may be brought on by talking, eating, swallowing, or coughing. The syndrome occasionally has been associated with cardiac arrest, syncope, or convulsions, because of stimulation of the carotid sinus reflex; associated hypersecretion of the parotid gland may also occur. The condition must be differentiated from neuralgia of the auriculotemporal or superior laryngeal nerves, and symptomatic pain secondary to irritation of the nerve by neoplasms or other diseases must always be considered before a diagnosis of glossopharyngeal neuralgia is made. Some authorities differentiate between glossopharyngeal neuralgia, in which the pain radiates from the throat to the ear, and Jacobson's neuralgia, in which the pain is limited to the ear and eustachian tube. The condition, if not responsive to medical measures similar to those effective for trigeminal neuralgia, is treated by intracranial section of the glossopharyngeal nerve, central to the petrous ganglion; this may be followed by little or no sensory deficit in the throat or loss of taste on the posterior portion of the tongue, in spite of complete relief of pain. As in trigeminal neuralgia, pain in the distribution of the glossopharyngeal nerve may also be relieved by intramedullary tractotomy (see "Pain of Trigeminal Nerve Origin," Ch. 12).

THE VAGUS NERVE

Anatomy and Physiology

The vagus nerve (the pneumogastric nerve in older terminology) is the longest and most widely distributed of the cranial nerves. The nuclei of origin of the vagus nerve are similar to and in many respects identical with those of the glossopharyngeal nerve, and the functions of the tenth parallel those of the ninth nerve.

The Motor Portion

The nuclei of the motor fibers of the tenth nerve are located in the vagal portion of the nucleus ambiguus (see Fig. 15-1). These fibers follow an almost identical course through the medulla with the motor fibers of the glossopharyngeal, and leave the skull through the jugular foramen. The cortical center which regulates the motor functions of the vagus nerve is in the lower part of the precentral gyrus; the supranuclear innervation is bilateral but predominantly crossed. The vagus nerve, or the vagus nerve together with the bulbar portion of the accessory, supplies all of the striated musculature of the soft palate, pharynx, and larynx with the exception of the tensor veli palatini and the stylopharyngeus. The tensor veli palatini, which renders the soft palate tense, is discussed in Chapter 12, and the stylopharyngeus, which raises and dilates the pharynx, in this chapter under the glossopharyngeal. It has been stated that the tensor veli palatini, musculus uvulae, palatoglossus, salpingopharyngeus, palatopharyngeus, and the superior and middle constrictors of the pharynx are supplied by the accessory nerve through the pharyngeal plexus, or that the palatopharyngeus, palatoglossus, and superior constrictor are supplied by the glossopharyngeal nerve. It is more probable, however, that these muscles are supplied by the vagus, or possibly by fibers of the bulbar portion of the accessory nerve which are distributed through the vagus.

The levator veli palatini raises the soft palate and pulls it backward; it blocks off the nasal passages in swallowing. The musculus uvulae, or azygos uvulae, shortens and bends the uvula backward and raises its tip; it helps to block off the nasal passages. The palatoglossus elevates the posterior part of the tongue and narrows the fauces in swallowing by approximating the anterior pillars; it also depresses the soft palate. The palatopharyngeus draws the pharynx and the thyroid cartilage upward and depresses the soft palate; it approximates the pharyngopalatine arches and closes the posterior nares and faucial orifice. The salpingopharyngeus, which blends with the palatopharyngeus, raises the upper and lateral portion of the pharynx. The superior, middle, and inferior constrictors of the pharynx flatten and contract the pharynx in swallowing. They play an important part in the final acts of deglutition by forcing the food into the esophagus and initiating the peristaltic waves that run through the digestive tract. Since the pharynx may be regarded as a resonator, and alterations of its form result in modifications of the voice, the constrictors of the pharynx are important in the production and modulation of speech.

All the intrinsic laryngeal muscles are supplied by the recurrent nerves, with the exception of the cricothyroid, which is innervated by the external branch of the superior laryngeal nerve. The arytenoid may receive some motor filaments from the internal branch of the superior laryngeal. The laryngeal muscles function to regulate the tension of the vocal cords and to open and close the glottis (abducting and adducting the vocal cords). The cricothyroids, posterior and lateral cricoarytenoids and thyroarytenoids are paired muscles. The cricothyroids are the chief tensors of the vocal cords; they stretch, or elongate, the cords by drawing up the arches of the cricoid cartilages and tilting back the upper borders of their laminae; they increase the distance between the vocal processes and the angle of the thyroid. The posterior cricoarytenoids are the chief abductors; they separate the vocal cords and consequently open the glottis by rotating the arytenoid cartilages outward. The lateral cricoarytenoids are the chief adductors; they close the glottis by rotating the arytenoid cartilages inward, so as to approximate the vocal processes. The thyroarytenoids draw the arytenoid cartilages forward toward the thyroid, and thus shorten and relax the vocal cords. The deeper portions of the thyroarytenoids (vocales) may also, if acting alone, modify the tension and elasticity of the vocal cords, and the external portions may act as adductors and narrow the rim of the glottis by rotating the arytenoid cartilages inward. The arytenoid, which is unpaired, approximates the arytenoid cartilages and closes the opening of the glottis, especially its posterior aspect. It is composed of oblique and transverse parts. The oblique arytenoid acts as the sphincter of the upper larynx, whereas the transverse arytenoid closes the posterior portion of the glottis. The extrinsic muscles of the larynx include those going to the hyoid bone, which is physiologically a part of the voice apparatus. These muscles are discussed with the infrahyoid muscles (see "Anatomy and Physiology," Ch. 17).

The Swallowing Mechanism. The process of deglutition is complicated. During the first stage the bolus of food is driven back into the fauces by the pressure of the tongue against the hard palate. At the same time the base of the tongue is retracted and the larynx is raised with the pharynx. During the second stage the entrance to the larynx is closed by the drawing of the arytenoid cartilages forward toward the epiglottis. After leaving the tongue, the bolus passes onto and glides along the posterior surface of the epiglottis for a certain distance. Then the palatoglossi contract behind the bolus and constrict the fauces. The palatine velum is slightly raised by the levator and is made tense by the tensor veli palatini. The palatopharyngei, by their contraction, pull the pharynx upward over the bolus; they nearly come together, and the small interval between them is filled by the uvula. By these means food is prevented from passing into the nasopharynx. The stylopharyngei draw the sides of the pharynx upward and laterally so as to increase its transverse diameter, and its anteroposterior diameter is increased as the tongue and larynx are carried forward in their ascent. The epiglottis is pushed back over the entrance to the larynx, which is closed. The bolus of food is then directed downward and backward into the pharynx. As soon as it is received there the elevator muscles relax, the pharynx descends, the constrictors contract on the bolus, and it is conveyed downward into the esophagus.

The Parasympathetic Portion

The parasympathetic, or visceromotor, constituents of the vagus nerve arise from the dorsal efferent nucleus, a long column of cells dorsolateral to the hypoglossal nucleus and extending from the upper pole of the inferior olivary body to the lowest portion of the medulla. In its upper portion it occupies the ala cinerea of the rhomboid fossa, and it extends into the closed part of the medulla along the lateral side of the central canal. The fibers go ventromedially and join those from the nucleus ambiguus, and leave the medulla as preganglionic fibers of the craniosacral portion of the autonomic nervous system. They terminate on ganglia close to the viscera which they supply and send postganglionic fibers directly to the muscular and glandular structures which they innervate. There may be bilateral cortical innervation, but central control is largely from the hypothalamus.

The parasympathetic functions of the vagus nerve are multiple and significant. The vagus is the largest and most important parasympathetic nerve in the body. It is essential to the regulation of heart action. It inhibits and depresses the activities of this organ by slowing the beat and weakening the contraction. It is also a vasoconstrictor of the coronary musculature. Vagus stimulation produces bradycardia, whereas vagus paralysis results in tachycardia. Vagus stimulation causes contraction of the smooth muscle of the trachea, bronchi, and bronchioles, with narrowing of the lumens of these structures, and it also stimulates the glands of the bronchial mucosa. Bronchial spasm may be relieved by the administration of a drug which inhibits vagus action. The vagus nerve supplies the alimentary tract from the pharynx through the esophagus, stomach, and small intestine; it also innervates the ascending and transverse colon,

and extends to the descending colon. In general it acts as a stimulant to alimentary function. It stimulates the secretion of gastric and pancreatic juices; it contracts the musculature of the gastrointestinal tract to render peristalsis more active; and it relaxes the sphincters of the upper alimentary tract. Through the lienal plexus the vagus stimulates the spleen; through the hepatic plexus it stimulates the liver and gallbladder; and through the celiac plexus it acts on the kidneys and adrenal bodies. It inhibits adrenal secretion. It must be remembered, however, that although the vagus nerve has a regulatory effect — motor, secretory, and inhibitory — on many important viscera, the vagus centers in the medulla that control these functions are themselves under the control of higher centers in the cortex and hypothalamus. Furthermore, the functions of the parasympathetic division of the autonomic nervous system connot be studied without including the study of the sympathetic division. The parasympathetic portion of the vagus nerve is considered in more detail in Part E, "The Autonomic Nervous System."

The Sensory Portion

The sensory branches of the vagus nerve have their nuclei in the jugular ganglion and ganglion nodosum. Fibers which carry exteroceptive sensation from the posterior portion of the external acoustic meatus, the adjacent part of the tympanic membrane, and a small area on the posterior aspect of the pinna have their first cell bodies in the jugular ganglion and terminate on the descending root of the trigeminal nerve and its nucleus. These fibers overlap with those from the seventh and ninth cranial nerves. A clinically demonstrable loss is rarely detected when they are affected. Fibers which carry pain sensation from the dura mater of the posterior cranial fossa and the transverse sinuses also go through the jugular ganglion to the trigeminal root, although it may be that some of these terminate on the fasciculus solitarius.

Fibers which carry gustatory sensation from the anterior and posterior surfaces of the epiglottis and the arytenoids, and with the glossopharyngeal nerve from the hard and soft palates, the anterior pillars, and the posterior pharyngeal wall, have their nuclei in the ganglion nodosum and terminate on the fasciculus solitarius and its nucleus. Fibers which carry general visceral sensation from the lower pharynx, the larynx, and probably from all the viscera to which the vagus nerve sends parasympathetic efferent impulses, pass through the ganglion nodosum and terminate on the fasciculus solitarius and its nucleus.

The jugular ganglion is situated in the upper part of the jugular foramen. It communicates by means of several delicate branches with the cranial portion of the accessory nerve, and also with the petrous ganglion of the glossopharyngeal nerve, the facial nerve, and the superior cervical sympathetic ganglion. The ganglion nodosum lies just beneath the jugular foramen. The internal branch of the accessory nerve passes through it to fuse with the vagus nerve, and this ganglion communicates with the hypoglossal nerve, the superior cervical sympathetic ganglion, and the loop between the first and second cervical nerves.

Distribution and Branches

The vagus nerve leaves the dorsolateral medulla in the dorsolateral sulcus between the inferior cerebellar peduncle and the inferior olivary body. There are eight or ten filaments in line with the ninth nerve above and the eleventh nerve below (see Fig. 9-3). These unite to form a single flattened trunk which courses outward beneath the flocculus of the cerebellum and leaves the skull through the jugular foramen with the ninth and eleventh nerves. It is behind the former and in the same dural compartment as the latter. The vagus nerve passes vertically down the neck within the carotid sheath. It lies between the internal jugular vein and the internal carotid artery as far as the upper border of the thyroid cartilage, and then between the internal jugular vein and the common carotid artery to the base of the neck. Branches leave the nerve in the jugular foramen to supply the meninges and the ear, and other branches leave just below to supply the pharynx and larynx, but the major portion of each vagus nerve goes into the thorax.

The branches of distribution of the vagus nerve are as follows: The meningeal and auricular branches arise from the jugular ganglion. The meningeal branch follows a recurrent course upward through the jugular foramen to supply the dura mater of the posterior fossa of the skull, especially in the vicinity of the transverse and occipital sinuses. The auricular branch, or nerve of Arnold, receives a filament from the petrous ganglion of the glossopharyngeal, passes behind the internal jugular vein, and enters the mastoid canaliculus. It then crosses the facial canal, passes between the mastoid process and the external auditory meatus, and divides into two branches. One communicates with the posterior auricular branch of the facial nerve; the other supplies exteroceptive sensation to the posterior part of the tympanic membrane and external acoustic meatus and the skin of the posterior part of the pinna. The pharyngeal and superior laryngeal branches arise from the ganglion nodosum. The pharyngeal branches pass across the internal carotid artery to the upper border of the middle constrictor of the pharynx where they divide into numerous filaments which join with branches of the glossopharyngeal and superior laryngeal nerves and sympathetic nerves to form the pharyngeal plexus. From this plexus the vagus sends motor nerves to all the muscles of the soft palate and the pharynx, with the exception of the stylopharyngeus and the tensor veli palatini, and sensory nerves are distributed to the mucous membrane of the pharynx. The superior laryngeal nerve passes medial to the external and internal carotid arteries and then divides into external and internal laryngeal branches. The external laryngeal branch is the smaller and descends to the larynx, beneath the sternothyroid, to innervate the cricothyroid muscle. It supplies branches to the pharyngeal plexus and the inferior constrictor of the pharynx and communicates with the superior cardiac nerve. The internal laryngeal branch passes between the middle and inferior constrictors of the pharynx, enters the larynx through the thyrohyoid membrane, and supplies filaments to the mucous membrane covering the pharyngeal and internal surfaces of the larynx as far as the vocal cord and branches to the mucous membranes of the epiglottis, the base of the tongue, and the aryepiglottic fold.

The superior cardiac branches arise from the vagus in the upper and lower parts of the neck. They communicate with the cardiac branches of the sympathetic division to form the cardiac plexus. The recurrent nerves are given off in the thorax and ascend to the larynx. That on the right arises in front of the subclavian artery, winds backward around it, and passes between the esophagus and the trachea and behind the common carotid artery and the thyroid gland. The left recurrent nerve arises on the left of the aortic arch, winds below the aorta, ascends to the side of the trachea, and follows a course similar to that of its fellow nerve. Both nerves pass under the lower border of the inferior constrictor of the pharynx and enter the larynx behind the articulation of the inferior cornu of the thyroid cartilage with the cricoid. They are distributed to all the muscles of the larynx except the cricothyroid; they communicate with the internal branch of the superior laryngeal nerve, and supply sensation to the mucous membrane of the lower part of the larynx and the trachea. The inferior cardiac branches arise on the right from the trunk of the vagus and from the recurrent, and on the left from the recurrent only, and end in the cardiac plexus.

Within the thorax, bronchial and pulmonary branches communicate with filaments from the sympathetic division to form the pulmonary plexuses; esophageal branches unite with each other and with filaments from the splanchnic nerves and thoracic sympathetic ganglia to form the esophageal plexus; and pericardial branches are given off by the vagus nerves and the pulmonary and esophageal plexuses. Within the abdomen branches of the two vagus complexes enter the gastric, lienal, celiac, and hepatic plexuses.

Clinical Examination

In spite of its great size, its many functions, and its importance in the regulation of essential visceral processes, the vagus nerve is tested with difficulty, and means for its examination are inadequate, particularly with regard to autonomic functioning. Although better evaluations of autonomic function would be useful not only to the neurologist but also to physicians concerned with thoracic and abdominal diseases, the evaluation of the motor functions of the nerve can provide great value to the neurologist.

Examination of the Motor Functions

The motor branches of the vagus nerve, which supply the soft palate, pharynx, and larynx, are easily available for clinical testing.

The Soft Palate. In the examination of the soft palate one observes the position of the soft palate and uvula at rest, and the position and movements during quiet breathing and on phonation. Asymmetry or absence of the uvula is usually related to prior tonsillectomy. Minor deviations of the uvula, regardless of cause, must be disregarded if symmetric elevation of the palatal muscles can be observed. The palatal reflex is tested, as described previously for the glossopharyngeal nerve. The character of the voice and the ability to swallow are appraised. Special attention should be paid to dysarthria and to dysphagia for liquids or solids.

Usually the uvula hangs in the midline and rises in the midline on phonation. In a unilateral vagus paralysis there is weakness of the soft palate, owing to disturbance of function of the levator veli palatini and musculus uvulae on the involved side. There is unilateral lowering with a flattening of the palatal arch, and the medial raphe is deviated to the normal side. On phonation the uvula is retracted to the nonparalyzed side (Fig. 15-2). The normally functioning tensor veli palatini, which is innervated by the trigeminal nerve, may prevent marked drooping of the palate. The palatal reflex is lost on the involved side, in this instance owing to interruption of the motor rather than the sensory pathways. There usually is little difficulty with articulation or deglutition, although in acute unilateral lesions there may be a nasal quality to the speech, dysphagia, more marked for liquids than solids, and some regurgitation of fluids into the nose when swallowing; these are usually transient.

When bilateral vagus nerve weakness develops the palate cannot be elevated on phonation although it may or may not droop to a significant

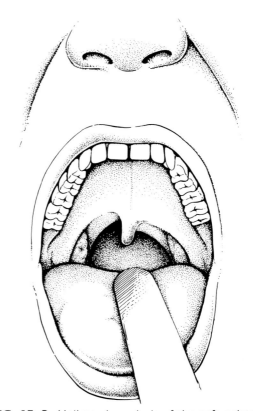

FIG. 15–2. Unilateral paralysis of the soft palate.

degree, owing to the action of the normally functioning tensors of the palate. The palatal reflex is absent bilaterally. The nasal cavity is not closed from the oral cavity, and on speaking air escapes from the latter into the former. The resonance mediated by the nasal cavity gives speech a characteristic nasal quality. There is especial difficulty with palatal and guttural sounds such as k, q, and ch. The sound b becomes m, d becomes n, and k becomes ng. The speech is similar to that of a patient with cleft palate. There may be severe dysphagia, especially for liquids, and fluids may be regurgitated into the nose on attempts to swallow.

The Pharynx. Functions and disorders of the pharynx are tested by observing the contraction of the pharyngeal muscles on phonation, by observing the elevation of the larynx on swallowing, by testing the pharyngeal reflex, and by noting the character of the patient's speech; he should also be given both liquids and solids to swallow, and any difficulty noted. If the superior constrictor of one side is not functioning, one may observe Vernet's *rideau* phenomenon, or a "curtain movement" of the pharyngeal wall toward the nonparalyzed side, on testing the pharyngeal reflex or at the beginning of phonation. Normally the larynx is elevated on swallowing; this is absent on one side in unilateral lesions of the vagus nerve, and on both in bilateral lesions.

In paresis of the pharynx, dysarthria may be present but this usually is minimal unless there is associated involvement of the soft palate or the larynx. Coughing may be impaired, and there may also be a decrease in the cough reflex. There may also be difficulty in swallowing, especially with solid foods. Dysphagia, however, is marked only in acute unilateral or in bilateral lesions.

The Larynx. In the examination of the larynx the character and quality of the voice, abnormalities of articulation, difficulty with respiration, and impairment of coughing are noted. A mirror examination of the larynx or a direct laryngoscopic examination should be carried out if there is hoarseness which is not readily explained by an acute inflammatory process or if there are any suggestions of vagus nerve involvement. Normally the vocal cords are abducted during inspiration and are adducted on phonation and coughing. In addition, there is reflex adduction on irritation of the larynx. In examining the larynx one notes the appearance and position of the vocal cords at rest, their movements during

phonation and inspiration, and their response on coughing and irritation. Sensation in the upper larynx may also be tested, a function of the internal branch of the superior laryngeal nerve. When paralysis of the laryngeal musculature is present, there may be difficulty in speaking, but occasionally there is almost complete involvement of the larynx on one side without an appreciable effect on the voice.

With paralysis of the cricothyroids, supplied by the superior laryngeal nerve, there is defective tension, with elongation of the vocal cord in phonation; high tones are lost, and the voice is deep and hoarse and fatigues easily. Inspiration is normal, and neither dyspnea nor stridor are present. In paralysis of the thyroarytenoid there is little difficulty with abduction, but adduction is slightly impaired. With bilateral thyroarytenoid paralysis the glottis has an oval instead of a linear appearance during phonation; the voice is hoarse, but there is neither dyspnea nor stridor. In paralysis of the arytenoid the glottis is closed only anteriorly, and the larynx shows a small triangular slit posteriorly during phonation; inspiration is normal.

In unilateral abductor palsy the involved cord lies close to the midline and cannot be abducted on inspiration. The voice may be hoarse, but in general phonation and coughing are little affected, since adduction is normal. Dyspnea is uncommon, for the normal cord is abducted in inspiration, but there may be some inspiratory stridor. With bilateral paralysis both cords lie close to the midline and cannot be abducted. The voice may be hoarse, but phonation is often slightly affected because both cords can still be adducted, and coughing is normal. There is severe dyspnea with inspiratory stridor, since the cords are drawn even closer on inspiration, but expiration is not affected.

With adductor palsy the cords are not adducted in phonation although they meet in the midline in coughing. Abduction is unimpaired and inspiration is normal. There is neither stridor nor dyspnea, and coughing is normal, but the voice is either lost or cannot be raised above a whisper. The loss of voice is usually sudden. The difficulty is almost always bilateral. Psychogenic or dystonic origin is often suspected. Unilateral adductor palsy is occasionally seen in trauma and in peripheral neuritides; there is paralysis of one lateral cricoarytenoid, with hoarseness and also *impairment* of *coughing*.

With total unilateral palsy both adduction and abduction are affected and the involved cord lies in the cadaveric position, motionless in midabduction. The voice is low-pitched and hoarse and there is difficulty in coughing, but phonation may not be much affected since the normal cord may cross the midline. There is little or no dyspnea, and inspiratory stridor is absent or is slightly present on deep inspiration. In bilateral palsy both cords are in the cadaveric position and phonation and coughing are lost. Marked dyspnea with stridor is present, especially on inspiration.

The most common type of laryngeal palsy is the result of a unilateral recurrent nerve lesion. Three stages have been described in a recurrent paralysis. The first manifestation is a lessened abduction of the involved side, resulting from isolated involvement of the posterior cricoarytenoid; next there is tension, or secondary contracture, of the adductors; and finally there is complete paralysis with the cord in the cadaveric position. The uninvolved cord crosses the midline on adduction. The voice may be coarse and husky, and there is loss of the ability to sing. Coughing may be ineffective, but little dyspnea or stridor is present. Aphonia, however, is not present, for the healthy side crosses the midline to meet the paralyzed cord. Owing to anatomic variability of the recurrent nerves, especially of their terminal divisions, the paralyses with lesions of these nerves may be complex and varied. With slight weakness of the vocal cords or pharynx, hoarseness and dysphagia may be apparent only when the head is turned to either side. With bilateral recurrent paralysis, stridor is present and the dyspnea may be so marked that tracheostomy is necessary. The absence of laryngeal movements in bilateral recurrent palsy is called **Gerhardt's sign.**

Examination of the Autonomic Functions

Although the vagus nerve is the most important parasympathetic nerve in the body, its autonomic functions are very difficult to test clinically. Certain functions, however, may be evaluated, and special attention should be paid to the cardiac and respiratory rates and rhythms in every neurologic examination. Because the pulse may be slowed with medullary compression, the rate must be followed closely in all patients with increased intracranial pressure.

Since the vagus nerve is the inhibitor of the heart, paralysis of it causes tachycardia, whereas stimulation causes bradycardia. It is apparent, however, that abnormalities of cardiac rate may result from many other causes. The heart rate and, to a certain extent, the respiratory rate may be slowed slightly by pressure on the eyeball or by painful stimulation of the skin on the side of the neck. This is called the **oculocardiac reflex,** or **Aschner's ocular phenomenon.** The afferent portion of the reflex arc is carried through the trigeminal nerve and the efferent portion through the vagus nerve. The reflex is inconstant, unstandardized, and influenced by emotion. Usually the pulse is not slowed more than 5 – 8 beats/min, and it may be necessary to test the response with electrocardiographic monitoring to be certain of the results. The slowing may be accompanied by extrasystoles. The oculocardiac reflex is an index of vagal hyperirritability and is absent in vagus paralysis. It may be either exaggerated or diminished in hyperthyroidism, absent in tabes dorsalis and heart block, and abolished by the use of atropine. It is demonstrated to a significant degree only in such pathologic conditions as paroxysmal tachycardia, where the overactivity of the heart may on occasion be controlled by vagus stimulation.

Vagus paralysis may also cause depression, acceleration, or irregularities of the respiratory rate and alterations of gastrointestinal function. Detailed investigation of cardiac abnormalities, of pulmonary function and vital capacity, and of the gastrointestinal tract are usually not considered as parts of the neurologic examination. Some of the autonomic functions of the vagus nerve can be tested by pharmacologic means, and are discussed in Part F, "The Autonomic Nervous System." It is common knowledge, for example, that the bronchial spasms present in asthma may be relieved by atropine or related anticholinergic drugs and that cardiospasm or spasm of the intestine may also be relieved by similar drugs, whereas peristalsis may be stimulated by the use of cholinergic drugs, such as neostigmine and pyridostigmine.

Examination of the Sensory Functions

The sensory elements of the vagus nerve cannot be adequately tested. The exteroceptive branches supply the tympanic membrane, part of the external acoustic meatus, and part of the pinna. These areas are difficult to examine, and furthermore are also supplied by the fifth, seventh, and ninth cranial nerves. Sensation to the meninges cannot be tested. Taste in the region of the epiglottis is difficult to examine, and is of no known clinical significance. The general visceral afferent supply, too, is distributed to areas that are inaccessible for testing, except for the lower pharynx and larynx. The vagus nerve also carries some sensation from the tonsillar area and posterior pharyngeal wall; the ninth nerve is considered the more important in this respect, and while there is rarely anesthesia of the pharynx in isolated vagus lesions, preserved sensation after interruption of the ninth nerve indicates that the vagus also contributes to pharyngeal sensation.

Examination of the Reflexes

The vagus nerve plays a part in many autonomic, or visceral, reflexes, and loss of these reflexes may follow a lesion of the tenth nerve.

The Vomiting Reflex. The pharyngeal (gag) reflex has already been mentioned in connection with the ninth nerve. Exaggeration of it may cause the **retching, vomiting,** or **regurgitation reflex,** also carried through the ninth and tenth nerves. Excessive stimulation or hyperirritability may initiate reverse peristalsis in the esophagus and stomach, with forceful ejection of material from the stomach. The reflex center is in the region of the dorsal efferent nucleus; such a center has been described in the dorsolateral border of the lateral reticular formation of the medulla. The vomiting reflex may also be produced by stimulation of the wall of the lower pharynx, the esophagus, the stomach, the duodenum, or the lower gastrointestinal tract; in all these the sensory portion of the reflex arc is carried through the tenth nerve, probably to the fasciculus solitarius. From there the impulse is relayed to the dorsal efferent nucleus, and also down the spinal cord to innervate the diaphragm and the abdominal muscles, as well as sympathetic centers. The cardiac sphincter is inhibited by impulses mediated through the vagus nerve, and the pyloric sphincter is constricted by impulses which leave the spinal cord through the splanchnic nerves.

The Swallowing Reflex. Stimulation of the pharyngeal wall or back of the tongue initiates swallowing movements. The afferent impulses are carried through the fifth, ninth, and tenth nerves, and the efferent impulses through the ninth, tenth, and twelfth nerves. Food is moved into the esophagus by action of the tongue, palatine arches, soft palate, and pharynx. The presence of the bolus of food acts as a stimulus for the various stages of the process of deglutition.

The Cough Reflex. Stimulation of the mucous membrane of the pharynx, larynx, trachea, or bronchial tree, or stimulation of the tympanic membrane or external auditory canal elicits a cough response. The afferent portions of the reflex arc are carried by the glossopharyngeal and vagus nerves to the fasciculus solitarius, and the efferent impulses descend to the pharyngeal muscles, tongue, palate, and larynx, and to the diaphragm, chest, and abdominal muscles. The reflex response consists of a deep inspiration followed by forced expiration with the glottis momentarily closed by approximation of the vocal cords. There is spasm of the diaphragm and throat. The pressure of the abdominal muscles and the diaphragm continues until sufficient tension is exerted to open the vocal cords.

The Nasal, Sneeze, or Sternutatory Reflex. A violent expulsion of air through the nose and mouth occurs in response to stimulation of the nasal mucous membrane. The afferent impulse is carried through the fifth nerve and the efferent through the vagus and phrenic nerves with associated function of the fifth, seventh, ninth, and upper thoracic nerves, and the sympathetic pathways. The reflex center is in the brain stem and upper spinal cord. The reflex is similar to that in coughing, but there is also contraction of the faucial pillars with descent of the soft palate, so that the air is directed chiefly through the nose. The threshold of this reflex varies from person to person. Some individuals are especially sensitive to certain types of stimuli. Sneezing on exposure to bright light may be an inherited response in some families.

The Sucking Reflex. In the infant, stimulation of the lips is followed by the production of a series of sucking movements which involve the lips, tongue, and jaw. The afferent impulses are carried through the fifth and ninth nerves, and the efferent through the fifth, seventh, ninth, tenth, twelfth, and spinal nerves. The response is elicited by touching, stroking, or tapping the lips near the buccal angle. The baby will turn his head toward the stimulus, open his mouth, and make sucking movements with the lips and tongue. If an object, such as a nipple or finger, is placed at the mouth, it is grasped by the upper and lower lips, hard palate, tongue, and mandible. The pharynx is closed off from the nasal cavity and the mandible is depressed, causing a partial vacuum. Respirations are interrupted only during deglutition. This reflex is normally present at birth, but is lost after infancy. Like the snout reflex (see "Examination of the Reflexes," Ch. 13), it is present in some adults with supranuclear corticospinal tract involvement and some of those with diffuse brain disease associated with dementia; however, its presence is not diagnostic of any particular disorder. Testing for the orbicularis oris reflex may cause not only puckering or protrusion of the lips, but also sucking and even tasting, chewing, and swallowing movements. This exaggerated response is also known as the **Atz, mastication,** or **"wolfing" reflex.** When present, it may be elicited by lightly touching, stroking, or tapping the lips, stroking the tongue, or stimulating the palate. When grossly exaggerated, there may be automatic opening of the mouth and smacking and chewing movements even when an object is brought near the lips, a visual rather than tactile sucking response.

Hiccup or Singultus. This is a sudden reflex contraction of the diaphragm, causing a forceful inspiration. There is an associated laryngeal spasm with sudden arrest of the inspiration by closure of the glottis, which produces the peculiar inspiratory sound. The phenomenon usually results from some irritation of the stomach wall or the diaphragm or occasionally the pharynx. The phrenic nerves are the important pathways, but the vagus nerve may also play a part, through both its sensory and motor functions.

Yawning. Yawning is deep, prolonged inspiration, usually involuntary, through the open mouth; it is often accompanied by stretching movements of the neck and body. Under most circumstances it can be considered a complex respiratory reflex which occurs during sleepiness and fatigue, usually a response to chemical stimulation. It may serve to restore depleted oxygen in the blood. Yawning may be a symptom of encephalitis or brain stem or cerebral disorders; it may also be brought on by suggestion or boredom.

The Carotid Sinus Reflex. Stimulation of the carotid sinus or of the carotid body by digital pressure at the bifurcation of the common carotid artery (either unilateral or bilateral) causes reflex stimulation of the vagus nerve and of the cerebral centers governing autonomic functions. The afferent impulses are carried through the carotid branch of the glossopharyngeal nerve to the medulla, and efferent impulses are carried through the vagus and sympathetic nerves. Normally, pressure on or massage over the carotid sinus or body causes no change in autonomic functions, but in certain susceptible individuals, usually those with atherosclerosis or hypertension, such stimulation may cause slowing of the heart rate, a fall in blood pressure, a decrease in cardiac output, and peripheral vasodilation; this is the **hyperactive carotid sinus reflex.** In pathologic states, such stimulation may cause vertigo, pallor, loss of consciousness (**carotid sinus syncope**), and occasionally convulsions. However, in individuals with extensive atherosclerotic disease both of the carotid and vertebrobasilar arterial systems, pressure on one carotid artery may cause syncope and sometimes convulsions or contralateral hemiplegia secondary to cerebral ischemia. If either hyperactivity of this reflex or carotid artery stenosis is suspected, pressure over the sinus and artery should be carried out with extreme caution, and only unilateral stimulation should be used.

Three types of pathologic carotid sinus syndrome responses have been described: the vagal type, in which the predominant response is slowing of the heart rate; the depressor type, in which the fall in blood pressure is the principal manifestation; and the cerebral type, characterized by syncope or loss of consciousness. Receptors similar to those in the carotid sinus and body are found in the aortic sinus and body. Impulses aroused by stimulation of these latter structures are probably carried through the vagus nerve. Both the carotid and aortic receptors respond to chemical as well as mechanical stimuli, and are important in the regulation of both circulation and respiration. Carotid sinus syncope has been relieved by either denervation of the carotid body or intracranial section of the glossopharyngeal nerve. Currently, drugs are available allowing surgery to be avoided in most instances.

In *summarizing the examination* of the vagus nerve, it is again stressed that the motor functions are the most readily available for clinical testing. The soft palate is examined at rest and on phonation, and the palatal reflex is tested. The pharynx is examined during speaking and swallowing, and the pharyngeal reflex is elicited. Dysphagia and dysarthria are appraised. If there is any disturbance of speech, the larynx is examined either directly or indirectly. Of the autonomic functions, those most available for testing are the regulation of the heart and respiratory rates. The most important autonomic reflexes, as far as the examination is concerned, are the oculocardiac and carotid sinus reflexes, although the integrity of the vagus nerve is essential to many important visceral reflexes. The sensory functions are not significant in the clinical examination.

Disorders of Function

Total *paralysis* of one vagus nerve is followed by paresis of the soft palate, pharynx, and larynx on the affected side, together with certain sensory and autonomic changes. The paresis of the soft palate and pharynx are not marked but in acute lesions difficulty in swallowing both liquids and solids is present. The voice may be moderately impaired, with either a nasal quality or hoarseness. The only definite sensory change is an anesthesia of the larynx due to involvement of the superior laryngeal nerve. Rarely is it possible to demonstrate loss of sensation behind the pinna and in the external auditory canal. The palatal and pharyngeal (gag) reflexes are absent on the involved side. Autonomic reflexes which lead to vomiting, coughing, and sneezing are usually retained in unilateral lesions. Heart action may be increased and the oculocardiac reflex may be lost on the involved side, but usually there are no cardiac symptoms. Gastric disturbances are slight or, more often, absent.

Bilateral complete vagus paralysis is not compatible with life. It causes complete paralysis of the palate, pharynx, and larynx, with marked dysphagia and dysarthria; rapid, irregular heart action; slow, irregular, dyspneic breathing; loss of hunger and thirst; vomiting, abdominal pain, and dilation and atonia of the stomach and intestines.

Paralysis of any branch of the vagus nerve may occur. Involvement of the meningeal and auricular branches causes changes which are entirely sensory, usually asymptomatic. Paralysis of the pharyngeal branches produces difficulty in swallowing; the function of the superior and middle constrictors of the pharynx is especially affected, and there may be paralysis of the soft palate; palatal and pharyngeal reflexes are lost. Paralysis of the superior laryngeal nerve causes anesthesia of the larynx if the internal branch is involved, and paralysis of the cricothyroid if the external branch is involved. There may also be weakness of the inferior constrictor of the pharynx. Paralysis of the recurrent nerve, the most common type of vagus lesion, has been discussed under "The Larynx." Isolated involvement of the visceral branches with sparing of the others is unusual.

Irritation of the vagus nerve may be followed by slowing of the pulse, reflex coughing and vomiting, and hypertonus of the gastrointestinal tract. The bradycardia and projectile vomiting which occurs with increased intracranial pressure may be the result of vagal irritation. Various respiratory disturbances associated with vagus nerve involvement include Cheyne-Stokes, Biot's, and Kussmaul's breathing, respiratory tics, forced yawning, and other abnormalities of breathing. The hyperventilation syndrome that occurs in emotional disturbances, such as hysteria, produces symptoms based in large part on irritation of the vagus nerve; this may lead to changes in acid-base equilibrium with symptoms suggestive of tetany.

Spasm of the constrictors of the pharynx, also known as **pharyngismus** or **cricopharyngeal spasm,** may be associated with central nervous system disorders, such as rabies, or may be present secondary to local irritation. It is frequently of psychogenic origin, and is responsible for the so-called **globus hystericus** in which there is a feeling of constriction or of a foreign body in the throat. Spasms of the larynx also may be present in rabies and tetany. Laryngeal spasms may also follow irritation of the larynx and excessive use of the voice. In **laryngismus stridulus** in children there is the sudden development of laryngeal spasm with "crowing" respiration and cyanosis. This may occur either as an independent disease, especially in connection with rickets, or in laryngeal inflammations. A partial laryngeal spasm may result in stuttering, with explosive speech, or in ticlike or compulsive coughs. The "epileptic cry" at the onset of a tonic – clonic seizure is probably due to spasm of the larynx. In asthma and in acute allergic states such as anaphylactic shock there may be spasm not only of the larynx, but also of the bronchi and bronchioles. Spasm of the esophagus, cardia, pylorus, and intestinal tract may be caused by organic and nonorganic factors.

Rhythmic movements of the palate and associated muscles are sometimes seen. Although no proper term has been applied to this condition, it is usually referred to as **palatal myoclonus** or **palatal nystagmus.** The contractions may range from 50 – 240/min. Occasionally there are associated movements of the eyes, neck, and diaphragm. Sometimes the contractions are audible to the patient or to others. Occasionally the syndrome is congenital but more often it has a sudden onset in patients with a history of cerebrovascular disease. It probably results from a brain stem lesion with interruption of the connections between the inferior olivary body, the dentate nucleus, and the red nucleus (the triangle of Guillain and Mollaret).

In neuralgia of the superior laryngeal nerve there are lancinating pains which radiate from the larynx to the ear. This bears some resemblance to glossopharyngeal neuralgia, and the pain is brought on by talking or swallowing, but the trigger zone is usually in the region of either the pyriform sinus or the thyroid cartilage. Occasionally the pain radiates to the angle of the jaw before going to the ear. It is very rare. Similar pain may be present on a reflex basis. Pain from a sore throat may radiate to the ear owing to vagus stimulation, as it does in stimulation of the glossopharyngeal nerve. Laryngeal crises have been described in tabes. There may be hyperesthesia of the tragus in vagus irritation, and pressure on the external auditory meatus may cause coughing.

Vasovagal attacks (fainting spells or syncope) are characterized by palpitation, dyspnea, peripheral vasomotor constriction, faintness, and loss of consciousness. There may also be gastric and precordial distress, a slow pulse, and respiratory arrhythmia, and even brief convulsive movements. These are manifestations of imbalance of the autonomic nervous system. There is often associated intense anxiety, and fainting may be precipitated by emotional stimuli but also develops secondary to pain, shock, fright, or loss of blood. It may also be brought on by hyperventilation. Somewhat similar symptoms are present in the so-called diencephalic attacks which occur as part of complex partial seizures.

Vagus involvement may result from supranuclear, nuclear, or infranuclear lesions. *Supranuclear involvement* is significant mainly when it is bilateral. In pseudobulbar palsy the dysphagia and dysarthria are due in part to bilateral supranuclear vagus involvement. Irritative supranuclear lesions are rarely encountered. Extrapyramidal supranuclear involvement bilaterally may cause difficulty with swallowing and talking, and in postencephalitic states there may be tics and anomalies of respiratory rhythm. Laryngeal spasm with stridor may be present with Parkinson's disease or other extrapyramidal disorders.

Nuclear involvement may occur in **bulbar** poliomyelitis, the Guillain–Barré syndrome and related disorders, neoplasms, vascular lesions such as thromboses and hemorrhages, multiple sclerosis, diphtheria, developmental anomalies of the base of the skull, and many other conditions. In botulism there may be dysphonia, dysphagia, vomiting, dry mouth, and respiratory difficulties. If the nuclear lesion is a slowly progressive one, such as occurs in progressive bulbar palsy, the bulbar form of amyotrophic lateral sclerosis, syringomyelia, and some neoplasms, there may be fasciculations in the palatal, pharyngeal, and laryngeal muscles. If there is medullary compression at the foramen magnum due to trauma, increased intracranial pressure, or edema of the brain, there may be marked slowing of the heart and respiratory rates, projectile vomiting, and increased or decreased blood pressure. This syndrome, along with progressive bulbar and pseudobulbar palsies and other specific nuclear syndromes are described in Chapter 18.

Infranuclear involvement may follow lesions at the base of the brain, in the jugular foramen, or along the course of the vagus nerves. Extramedullary but intracranial involvement occurs in association with meningitis, basal hemorrhages, extramedullary tumors, intracranial aneurysms, and skull fractures. Lesions at the jugular foramen or in the retroparotid space may also involve the ninth, eleventh, twelfth, and cervical sympathetic nerves. Such lesions may be due to stab wounds, gunshot wounds, periostitis, thrombosis of the jugular bulb, and retroparotid abscesses. Either intracranially or extracranially the vagus may be involved in diabetes or in the toxic, deficiency, and other multiple neuritides that affect peripheral nerves in other parts of the body. Diphtheritic involvement of the tenth nerve is now rare; in this condition there is often paralysis of the soft palate with nasal speech and regurgitation of fluids. Individual branches of the vagus nerve may be involved by disease processes in the neck, upper mediastinum, thorax, and abdomen. Tumors occasionally affect the vagus nerve, but the diagnosis may be difficult. The vagus, along with the other lower cranial nerves, is often affected in tumors of the glomus jugulare or chemodectomas. Involvement of the esophageal musculature in myotonic dystrophy may cause difficulty in swallowing.

The recurrent nerve is the most frequently affected. This may be damaged by tumors in the neck, especially carcinoma of the thyroid, cervical adenopathy, metastatic lesions, Hodgkin's disease, lymphosarcoma, aortic aneurysms, mitral stenosis with enlargement of the left atrium, pericarditis, mediastinal and apical tumors, stab wounds in the neck, or accidental trauma during a thyroidectomy or other surgical procedure. The superior laryngeal and pharyngeal branches may be involved in trauma, or in neoplasms or abscesses in the neck.

Muscular weakness of the pharynx and larynx with dysphagia and dysarthria may be prominent symptoms in myasthenia gravis, the myasthenic syndrome, oculopharyngeal forms of muscular dystrophy, myotonic dystrophy, polymyositis, and other myopathies.

Psychogenic disturbances frequently affect the structures innervated by the vagus nerve. In globus hystericus (pharyngismus, esophagismus, or cricopharyngeal spasm) the patient may complain not only of constriction and a sense of a lump in the throat but also of dysphagia. In hysterical aphonia or dysphonia there may be paresis of the adductors of the larynx. Cardiospasm, pylorospasm, spastic constipation, and various forms of functional dyspepsia may in part be due to vagus involvement secondary to psychogenic problems. Respiratory tics and other anomalies of respiration may also result from psychogenic involvement, and irregularity in the heart rate, tachycardia, bradycardia, and palpitation may be a reflection of emotional influence on the cardiac system.

Vagotomy has been used in the treatment of gastric and duodenal ulcers. Either trunk of the nerve may be sectioned or selective gastric denervation may be performed. Relief of pain and healing of the ulcer occur, probably because of a reduction of gastric motility and decrease in the volume and acidity of gastric secretion, as well as other less tangible effects. Section of the vagus nerve has also been performed for the treatment of ulcerative colitis and regional enteritis and for the pain associated with the gastric crises of tabes dorsalis. The cough reflex has been interrupted and bronchial pain relieved by section of the vagus nerve below the origin of the recurrent nerves.

BIBLIOGRAPHY

Amols W, Merritt HH. Vomiting: Neural mechanisms and control by chlorpromazine. Neurology 1955;5:645

Brodal A. Central course of afferent fibers for pain in facial, glossopharyngeal and vagus nerves. Arch Neurol Psychiatry 1947;57:292

Brodal A. Neurological Anatomy in Relation to Clinical Medicine, 3rd ed. New York, Oxford University Press, 1981

Bulteau E. The aetiology of bilateral recurrent laryngeal nerve paralysis. Med J Aust 1973;2:776

Droulias C, Tzinas S, Harlaftis N et al. The superior laryngeal nerve. Am J Surg. 1976;42:635

Edwards H. Neurological disease of the pharynx and larynx. Practitioner 1973;211:729

Engel GL. On the existence of the cerebral type of carotid sinus syncope. Neurology 1959;9:565

Forrester JM. Sneezing on exposure to bright light as an inherited response. Hum Hered 1985;35:113

Gurdjian E, Webster JE, Hardy WG et al. Nonexistence of the so-called cerebral form of carotid sinus syncope. Neurology 1958;8:818

Misuria VK. Functional anatomy of tensor palatini and levator palatini muscles. Ann Otolaryngol 1976;102:265

Palmer ED. Disorders of the cricopharyngeus muscle: A review. Gastroenterology 1976;71:510

Chapter 16
THE SPINAL ACCESSORY NERVE

ANATOMY AND PHYSIOLOGY

The spinal accessory, or eleventh cranial, nerve is composed of two distinct parts. The **cranial part,** or the **accessory portion (ramus internus)**, is the smaller of the two, and is accessory to the vagus. It arises from the cells within the caudal prolongation of the nucleus ambiguus and the dorsal efferent nucleus, probably mainly from the former. Its fibers emerge from the medulla as four or five delicate rootlets below the roots of the vagus. The nerve goes laterally to the jugular foramen, where it becomes united with the spinal portion for a short distance and also communicates with the jugular ganglion of the vagus nerve. It leaves the skull through the jugular foramen, separate from the spinal portion, passes through the ganglion nodosum without interruption, and blends with the fibers of the vagus nerve (Fig. 16-1). It is distributed principally with the pharyngeal and superior laryngeal branches of the vagus. It has been suggested by some authorities that the levator veli palatini, musculus uvulae, palatoglossus, salpingopharyngeus, and superior and middle constrictors of the pharynx are supplied by the cranial portion of the accessory nerve, but it is probable that these are mainly supplied by the vagus nerve. A few fibers from the accessory nerve may also innervate the intrinsic muscles of the larynx with the recurrent nerve, and a few fibers which originate in the dorsal efferent nucleus may carry parasympathetic impulses and join the cardiac branches of the vagus nerve.

The major portion of the eleventh nerve is the **spinal portion (ramus externus)**. Its fibers arise from the motor cells of the accessory nuclei in the central cell group of the ventral horn of the spinal cord from the lower end of the medulla to the fifth or even the sixth cervical segment. Rootlets from these nuclei pass through the lateral funiculus of the cord and unite to form a single trunk which ascends within the dura between the dentate ligament and the posterior roots of the spinal nerves. This trunk enters the skull through the foramen magnum and is directed toward the jugular foramen, where it joins the cranial portion of the nerve for a short distance, and probably receives one or two filaments from it. It leaves the skull, as does the cranial portion, through the jugular foramen. It is within the same dural sheath as the vagus nerve, but separated from it by a fold of arachnoid. It descends in the neck behind or in front of the internal jugular vein and behind the digastricus and stylohyoid to the upper part of the sternocleidomastoid. It passes through this muscle and supplies filaments to it, and then courses obliquely across the posterior triangle of the neck to end in the deep surface of the trapezius. In the neck it unites with the second and third cervical nerves, and beneath the trapezius it forms a plexus with the third and fourth cervical nerves. The nuclei of the spinal portion of the accessory nerve communicate with the nuclei of the oculomotor, trochlear, abducens, and vestibular nerves through the medial longitudinal fasciculus.

The cerebral center which governs the action of the spinal accessory nerve is in the lower portion of the precentral gyrus. The supranuclear innervation is bilateral in part, but comes pri-

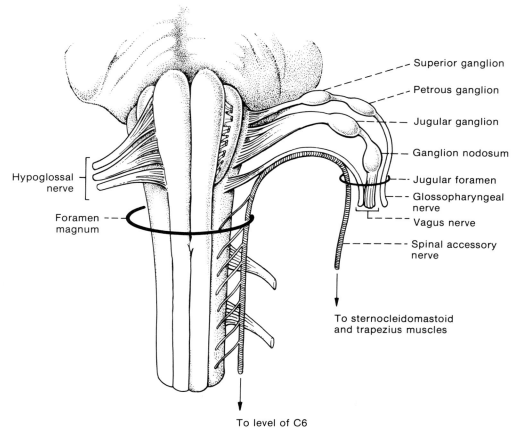

Superior ganglion

Petrous ganglion

Jugular ganglion

Ganglion nodosum

Jugular foramen

Glossopharyngeal nerve

Vagus nerve

Spinal accessory nerve

Hypoglossal nerve

Foramen magnum

To sternocleidomastoid and trapezius muscles

To level of C6

FIG. 16–1. Relationship of the cranial and spinal portions of the accessory nerve to the vagus and glossopharyngeal nerves.

marily from the contralateral hemisphere. The descending axons going to the two muscles supplied by the accessory nerve are separate in the brain stem, permitting dissociated involvements of the two muscles.

Essentially, the eleventh nerve is entirely motor in function, although it may contain some proprioceptive fibers. The accessory portion functions with the glossopharyngeal and vagus nerves, and cannot be distinguished from them. It in reality contributes to the function of the vagus nerve. The spinal portion of the nerve supplies two important muscles, the sternocleidomastoid and the upper portion of the trapezius. The innervation of the former muscle is via the eleventh nerve, although it may be supplied by a few fibers from the anterior divisions of the second and third cervical nerves. The amount of innervation to the trapezius differs in different individuals, but only the upper part is supplied by the accessory nerve; the lower part is innervated by the third and fourth cervical nerves.

The sternocleidomastoid muscles function with the other cervical muscles in flexing the head and in turning it from side to side. When the muscle on one side contracts, the head is drawn toward the ipsilateral shoulder and is rotated so that the occiput is pulled toward the side of the contracting muscle, while the face is deviated in the opposite direction, carried forward, and tilted upward. Acting together from their sternoclavicular attachments, the two muscles flex the cervical part of the vertebral column and bring the head forward and downward; they also rotate the head from side to side. When the head is fixed, the two muscles assist in elevating the thorax in forced inspiration.

The trapezius retracts the head and draws it to the corresponding side. It also elevates, retracts, and rotates the scapula, and assists in elevating the abducted arm above the horizontal. When the muscle on one side contracts while the shoulder is fixed, the head is drawn to that side. When the two muscles act together, the head is drawn backward and the face is deviated upward. When the head is fixed, the upper and middle fibers of the trapezius elevate, rotate, and retract the scapula and shorten the distance between the occiput and the acromion. The lower fibers depress the scapula and draw it toward the midline.

The sternocleidomastoid and trapezius muscles act together to rotate the head from side to side and to flex and extend the neck.

CLINICAL EXAMINATION

The functions of the cranial portion of the eleventh nerve are so closely allied to those of the vagus nerve that they cannot be distinguished from them clinically or examined separately. As a consequence, the examination of the spinal accessory nerve is limited to an evaluation of the functions of the sternocleidomastoid and trapezius muscles.

The function of the sternocleidomastoid is appraised by inspection and palpation as the patient rotates his head against resistance. The muscle usually stands out well, and its contours are distinct even at rest; its contractions can be seen and felt (Fig. 16-2). In unilateral paresis there may be little change in the position of the head in the resting state, and rotation and flexion can be carried out fairly well by the other cervical muscles, but a weakness of rotation can be observed if the examiner places his hand

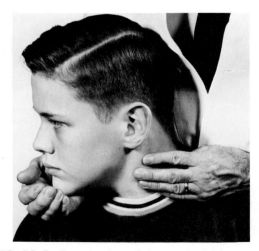

FIG. 16–2. Examination of the sternocleidomastoid muscle. When the patient turns his head to the right against resistance, the contracting muscle can be seen and palpated.

against one side of the patient's chin and the patient is asked to counteract this resistance. Even when the muscle is completely paralyzed the other cervical muscles allow some neck movement to the other side and only occasionally does the head turn so that the face deviates to the other side. If the chin is bent down against resistance there is further deviation of the face toward the paralyzed side, and contraction of the platysma may be observed. The paralyzed muscle is flat and does not contract, and it no longer stands out or becomes tense when attempts are made to turn the head toward the opposite shoulder or to flex the neck against resistance. Contracture of the contralateral, normally functioning, muscle may develop. The two sternocleidomastoid muscles can be examined simultaneously by having the patient flex his neck while the examiner exerts pressure on the forehead, or by having the patient turn the head from side to side. If both are paralyzed there is difficulty in anteroflexion of the neck, and the head assumes an extended position.

In addition to testing the motor power of the sternocleidomastoids, one should note their tone, volume, and contour. With a nuclear or infranuclear lesion there may be atrophy, and fasciculations may be seen with the former. The **sternocleidomastoid reflex** may be elicited by tapping the muscle at its clavicular origin. Usually there is a prompt contraction. The reflex is innervated by the accessory and upper cervical nerves and is lost in disease of these nerves. However, this reflex has little significance in neurologic diagnosis.

The function of the trapezius is tested by having the patient shrug and retract the shoulders against resistance. The movements may be observed and the contraction may be seen and palpated (Fig. 16-3). Muscle power should be compared on the two sides. In unilateral paralysis of the trapezius the patient cannot elevate and retract the shoulder, head tilting toward that side is weak, and it is difficult for him to elevate the arm above the horizontal level. There is a lowering of the arm on the affected side, and the fingertips touch the thigh at a lower level than on the normal side; if the palms are placed together with the arms extended anteriorly and slightly below the horizontal, the fingers on the affected side will extend beyond those of the normal side. There is a tendency for the upper portion of the scapula to fall laterally while its inferior angle is drawn inward, and there may be some "winging" of the scapula when the arm is extended anteriorly to the horizontal; this is

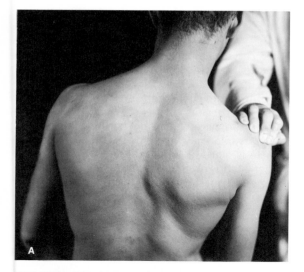

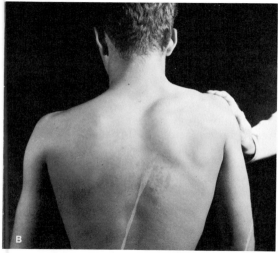

FIG. 16–3. Examination of the trapezius muscle. **A.** Examiner pressing shoulder down against patient's resistance. **B.** Patient attempting to elevate shoulder against examiner's resistance.

The two trapezius muscles can be examined simultaneously by having the patient extend his neck against resistance. When paralysis of both is present, there is weakness of extension of the neck and the head may tend to fall forward; the patient is unable to raise his chin, and the shoulders appear to be square or have a drooping, sagging appearance as a result of atrophy of both muscles. The relationship of the trapezius muscle to the movements of the shoulder girdle and the examination of the functions of its lower fibers are discussed under "The Shoulder Girdle" in Chapter 27.

When bilateral paralysis of the spinal accessory muscles is present, diminished ability to rotate the neck is present and the neck may tend to droop or even fall backward or forward, depending upon whether the sternocleidomastoids or the trapezei are more involved. Inasmuch as other cervical muscles, among which are the scaleni, splenii and obliqui capitis, recti capitis, and longi capitis and colli, are also of importance in rotation, deviation, flexion, and extension of the head and neck, a complete paralysis of the neck muscles does not develop with even bilateral lesions of the spinal accessory nerve.

DISORDERS OF FUNCTION

Paralysis or paresis of the muscles supplied by the spinal accessory nerve may be caused by supranuclear, nuclear, or infranuclear lesions.

much less marked, however, than the winging seen with a paralysis of the serratus anterior, which is most marked when the arm is extended to the horizontal (Ch. 27, Fig. 27-6). The outline of the neck is changed; there is a depression or drooping of the shoulder contour, and the levator scapulae becomes subcutaneous (Fig. 16-4). The paralyzed muscle becomes atrophic and fasciculations may be seen after several weeks. With unilateral paralysis of the trapezius, contracture of the normal muscle occasionally develops.

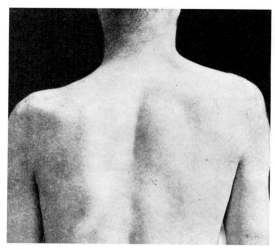

FIG. 16–4. Paralysis of the left trapezius muscle. There is a depression in the shoulder contour with downward and lateral displacement of the scapula.

Supranuclear involvement in the cerebrum and brain stem may cause only moderate loss of function since central regulation of the accessory nerve is in part bilateral. In hemiplegia there is usually no deviation of the head, but on testing there may be slight weakness of the sternocleidomastoid (or sometimes marked weakness in acute hemiplegia), with difficulty in turning the face to the side opposite the paralysis. There is often, however, moderate depression of the shoulder resulting from weakness of the trapezius on the affected side. Atrophy and fasciculations do not develop. Cerebral vascular accidents, degenerative disorders, neoplasms, and inflammatory conditions, among others, may cause a supranuclear palsy. More frequent than paralytic supranuclear lesions are irritative ones, which cause a turning of the head, and often of the head and eyes, in the direction opposite to the involved hemisphere. This turning of the head or head and eyes is seen in jacksonian epilepsy, and is often the first manifestation of the seizure. Dissociated weakness, of the trapezius on one side and the sternocleidomastoid on the other, may occur with lesions above the third nerve nuclei ipsilateral to the weak sternocleidomastoid. Extrapyramidal lesions (Ch. 22) may also involve the sternocleidomastoid and trapezius muscles, principally the former, with resulting rigidity, akinesis, or hyperkinesis. Deviation of the head is a frequent postencephalitic manifestation, and abnormal movements of the head and neck are seen in the several types of chorea, athetosis, dystonia musculorum deformans, and other dyskinesias.

Lesions of the brain stem above the accessory nuclei may cause dysfunction of the sternocleidomastoid and trapezius muscles either separately or together, depending on the area in the brain stem involved. The supranuclear (corticobulbar or extrapyramidal) pathways may be disrupted, as may be the medial longitudinal fasciculus. This tract (Ch. 11), which connects the nuclei of the third, fourth, sixth, and eleventh nerves with the cochlear, vestibular, and other centers, is important in controlling conjugate deviation of the head and eyes in response to auditory, vestibular, and other stimuli.

Nuclear involvement of the accessory nerve is not frequently encountered, but it may occur in association with such conditions as progressive bulbar palsy and the other forms of degenerative motor neuron disease, syringobulbia, and syringomyelia. In nuclear lesions there is not only paresis of the involved muscles, but also atrophy and fasciculations.

Infranuclear, or *peripheral, lesions,* either extramedullary but within the skull, in the jugular foramen, or in the neck, are the most common causes of impairment of function of the accessory nerve. Basal skull fractures, meningitis, or extramedullary neoplasms most commonly affect the nerve within the skull or at the foramen. Usually evidence of involvement of other structures, principally the vagus, glossopharyngeal, or hypoglossal nerves is present. Within the neck the accessory nerve may be affected by severe cervical adenitis, neoplasms, trauma, or abscesses. The nerve is occasionally injured in operations in the cervical area, or it may be surgically sacrificed for anastomosis into a nonfunctioning facial nerve. Among other causes of peripheral accessory nerve involvement are dislocations of the cervical spine, lesions in the mediastinum and at the pulmonary apices, and multiple neuritis. Injuries to the nerve in the posterior cervical triangle will impair only the supply to the trapezius. Muscular disorders which affect the sternocleidomastoid and trapezius muscles include the myopathies, myasthenia gravis, and myositis. Atrophy of both sternocleidomastoid muscles is a prominent feature of myotonic dystrophy (Fig. 16-5).

Torticollis

Hyperkinetic manifestations with tonic or clonic spasm of the muscles supplied by the accessory nerve are encountered more frequently than paralytic phenomena. The sternocleidomastoid muscles are most frequently involved, but the trapezius and the other muscles of the neck may also be affected. The muscular contractions cause a turning, or deviation, of the head or neck, known as **wryneck** or **torticollis.** The head and occiput are pulled to one side, and the face is turned toward the opposite side (Fig. 16-6). Abnormal function of inhibitory interneural networks between the trigeminal and accessory nerves has been implicated as a cause. The movements may be jerky, clonic, or spasmodic at first, and may be present only in attacks. They may present the manifestations of a tic. Later the difficulty becomes tonic, with constant deviation. The hyperkinesis usually starts in one sternocleidomastoid, but in far-developed cases there is some involvement on both sides and the other neck muscles are also affected. The trapezius may pull the head backward or the shoulder upward on the involved side, and the obliqui capitis, recti capitis, and splenii capitis may also

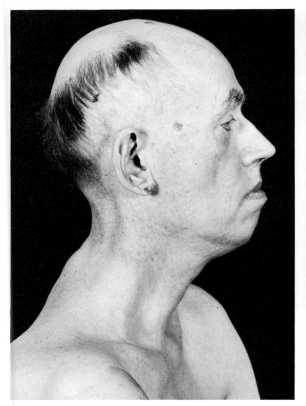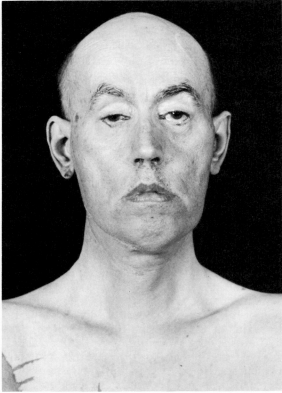

FIG. 16–5. A patient with myotonic dystrophy. There is atrophy of the sternocleido-mastoid muscles.

be implicated. The involved muscle or muscles may become tense and firm and may hypertrophy in the course of time because of the continued contraction.

In advanced torticollis, more or less stereotyped deviation of the head into an abnormal position develops. It varies from a slow twisting movement to a complete deviation with sustained muscular contractions. In spite of the tonic spasmodic turning of the head to one side, it can usually be deviated voluntarily to the midline or to the opposite side, especially if the patient is allowed to press some object against his chin. A minimal amount of manual assistance may aid in deviation of the head to the opposite side. The turning of the head in spasmodic torticollis is usually painless, but occasionally there is pain in the contractured muscles. Though the deviation of the head in torticollis is by far most often a lateral one, a backward (**retrocollis**) or a forward (**anterocollis**) deviation sometimes develops.

There are many causes and varieties of torticollis, and the syndrome should not be considered an entity. Congenital, structural, traumatic, and myogenic factors include birth injury, congenital atrophy or hypertrophy of one sternocleidomastoid muscle, congenital fusion of the cervical vertebrae, the Klippel–Feil syndrome, spina bifida, rickets, fracture or dislocation of the cervical spine, cervical arthritis, and trauma to the muscles. Symptomatic, or reflex, torticollis may be secondary to occipital neuralgia, vascular lesions, tumor or scar formation in the neck, neoplastic metastases to the cervical lymph nodes, or some infectious process such as cervical adenitis, caries of the cervical spine, lesions of the mediastinum or pulmonary apex, retropharyngeal or retrotonsillar abscesses, myositis, arthritis, or synovitis. Occupational torticollis may occur in cobblers and tailors. Torticollis has also been reported due to increased cerebrospinal fluid pressure, neurovascular compression by the posterior inferior cerebellar artery, and as a sequel to radiation therapy.

The more important varieties of torticollis, however, from a neurologic point of view, are those associated with disease, either organic or

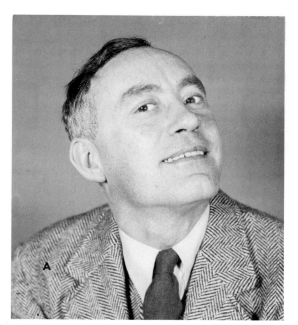 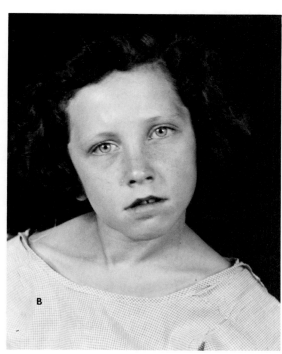

FIG. 16–6. *Spasmodic torticollis.* **A.** *Of psychogenic origin.* **B.** *Of congenital origin. In both cases there is contraction of the right sternocleidomastoid muscle with deviation of the chin toward the left shoulder.*

functional, of the nervous system. Paralytic torticollis may follow either a lower motor neuron or an upper motor neuron paresis. Ocular torticollis is associated with paresis of one or more of the extraocular muscles; there is no true contracture of the sternocleidomastoid muscle, the deformity can usually be corrected voluntarily, and there is no facial asymmetry. Neonatal torticollis occurs secondary to hemorrhage and its sequelae which may or may not be associated with other developmental anomalies, and occasionally is due to fibrous tumors of the sternocleidomastoid muscle. Aural or labyrinthine torticollis is secondary to involvement of the cochlear or the vestibular mechanisms, including the medial longitudinal fasciculus and the vestibulospinal pathways.

Disorders of the extrapyramidal system, especially of the basal ganglia, are probably the most frequent cause of neurologic torticollis. It develops during the course of encephalitis and in dystonia; it may be the only symptom, or there may be associated rigidity, deviation of the eyes, or athetoid movements. Torticollis can also result from the use of phenothiazine and other psychoactive drugs, and although other abnormal involuntary movements are usually present tor-

ticollis can occur as an isolated phenomenon. In some instances spasmodic torticollis may develop on a psychogenic basis, possibly as a conversion mechanism. It may start as a tic, nodding spasm, negation tremor, or compulsive turning of the head to one side, but later there is spasmodic or tonic deviation of the head.

The treatment of torticollis is difficult. Very few cases resolve spontaneously or respond to conservative therapy. Pharmacotherapy is often ineffective. Various approaches to surgical therapy have been made, including anterior cervical rhizotomy and subarachnoid spinal accessory neurectomy, sometimes followed by other neurectomies. Such measures have given some relief on occasion, but in other cases spasmodic movements have persisted in spite of extensive surgery. Selective thalamotomy has also been used, with questionable results. Suppression of the vestibular system by applying iontophoresis has also been advocated for relief of the syndrome, but failed to produce the expected results. Injection of the involved muscle or muscles with botulinum toxin may give temporary relief. Although some cases have been felt to be of psychogenic origin, psychotherapy, too, has failed to bring about relief of symptoms.

BIBLIOGRAPHY

Baquis GD, Rosman NP. Pressure-related torticollis: An unusual manifestation of pseudotumor cerebri. Pediatric Neurology 1989;5:111

Brodal A. Neurological Anatomy in Relation to Clinical Medicine, 3rd ed. New York, Oxford University Press, 1981

Cooper IS. Effect of thalamic lesions upon torticollis. New Engl J Med 1964;270:967

Gilbert GJ. Spasmodic torticollis effectively treated by medical measures. New Engl J Med 1971;284:896

Herz E, Glaser GH. Spasmodic torticollis. II: Clinical evaluation. Arch Neurol Psychiatry 1949;61:227

Landan I, Cullis PA. Torticollis following radiation therapy. Movement Disorders 1987;2:317

Pagni CA, Naddeo M, Faccani G. Spasmodic torticollis due to neurovascular compression of the 11th nerve. Case report. J Neurosurg 1985;63:789

Sorenson BF, Hamby WB. Spasmodic torticollis: Results in 71 surgically treated cases. JAMA 1965;194:706

Svien HJ, Cody DT. Treatment of spasmodic torticollis by suppression of labyrinthine activity: Report of a case. Mayo Clin Proc 1969;44:825

Chapter 17

THE HYPOGLOSSAL NERVE

ANATOMY AND PHYSIOLOGY

The hypoglossal, or twelfth cranial, nerve is a purely motor nerve, supplying the tongue, with its origin in the cells of the hypoglossal nuclei. These are upward extensions of the anterior column of the spinal cord, and consist of a long column of large, multipolar cells, similar to those in the anterior horns. The paired nuclei extend almost the entire length of the medulla; their upper portions are just underneath the floor of the fourth ventricle, close to the midline, under the medial aspect of the trigonum hypoglossi (Fig. 17-1), and the lower portions are situated in the gray matter on the ventrolateral aspect of the central canal. Numerous fibers connect the nuclei of the two sides. The nerve roots leave the ventral side of the nucleus and go forward and laterally through the reticular formation to emerge from the medulla in the ventrolateral sulcus between the pyramid and the inferior olivary body, medially to the ninth, tenth, and eleventh nerves (see Fig. 15-1).

The hypoglossal nerves leave the medulla in 10 – 15 rootlets on each side (see Fig. 9-3). These are collected into two bundles which perforate the dura mater separately, pass through the hypoglossal canal, and then unite. This united nerve descends through the neck to the level of the angle of the mandible, and it then passes forward to supply the extrinsic and intrinsic muscles of the tongue. In the upper portion of its course it is situated beneath the internal carotid artery and internal jugular vein, and is intimately connected with the vagus nerve. It then passes forward between the artery and vein,

loops around the occipital artery, and crosses the external carotid and lingual arteries. It goes forward above the hyoid bone, beneath the tendon of the digastricus, deep to the stylohyoid and to the mylohyoid and lateral to and above the hyoglossus, and breaks up into a number of fibers to supply the various muscles of the tongue.

The hypoglossal nerve communicates with the ganglion nodosum of the vagus nerve shortly after it leaves the skull, and it also gives a branch to the pharyngeal plexus. In the neck it communicates with the superior cervical ganglion of the sympathetic trunk and is joined by a filament from the first or first and second cervical nerves. Lower in the neck it communicates with the descending cervical branch from the second and third cervical nerves. At the base of the tongue it is in close communication with the lingual branch of the mandibular nerve.

The branches of the hypoglossal nerve are the meningeal, descending, thyrohyoid, and muscular. The meningeal branches send filaments to the dura mater in the posterior cranial fossa and to the diploë of the occipital bone; since the hypoglossal nerve is essentially motor, these branches are doubtless supplied by the first and second cervical nerves. The descending ramus leaves the hypoglossal nerve as it loops around the occipital artery and descends in front of or in the sheath of the carotid vessels. It gives a branch to the superior belly of the omohyoid and then joins the descending cervical communicating branch from the second and third cervical nerves to form the loop known as the **ansa hypoglossi** (Fig. 17-2), which supplies the inferior belly of the omohyoid and the sternohyoid

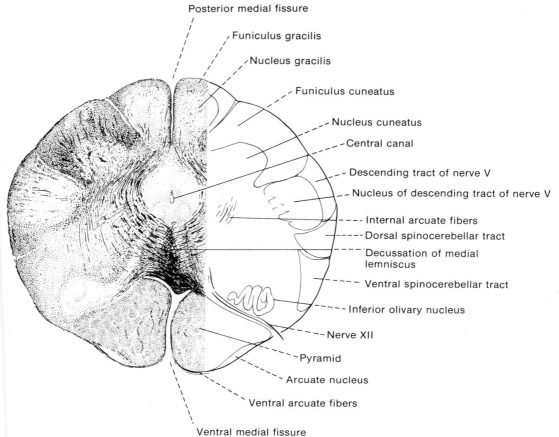

Posterior medial fissure

Funiculus gracilis

Nucleus gracilis

Funiculus cuneatus

Nucleus cuneatus

Central canal

Descending tract of nerve V

Nucleus of descending tract of nerve V

Internal arcuate fibers

Dorsal spinocerebellar tract

Decussation of medial lemniscus

Ventral spinocerebellar tract

Inferior olivary nucleus

Nerve XII

Pyramid

Arcuate nucleus

Ventral arcuate fibers

Ventral medial fissure

FIG. 17–1. *Section through the medulla at the level of the decussation of the medial lemniscus.*

and sternothyroid muscles and may communicate with the phrenic and cardiac nerves. The thyrohyoid branch arises near the posterior border of the hyoglossus and supplies the thyrohyoid muscle. The descending and thyrohyoid branches may carry hypoglossal fibers to a limited extent, but they are innervated mainly by the cervical plexus.

The muscular, or lingual, branches constitute the real distribution of the hypoglossal nerve. They supply the genioglossus, styloglossus, hyoglossus, and chondroglossus muscles, the intrinsic muscles of the tongue, and possibly the geniohyoid.

The cerebral center for the regulation of tongue movements is situated in the lower portion of the precentral gyrus near and within the sylvian fissure. The supranuclear fibers pass through the genu of the internal capsule and the middle of the cerebral peduncle. Supranuclear control to the genioglossus muscle is primarily

crossed, while the supply to the other muscles is bilateral, although some authorities feel the entire supranuclear pathway is crossed.

The hypoglossal nerve controls the movements of the tongue. It supplies all of the extrinsic muscles of the tongue except the palatoglossus, the intrinsic muscles, and possibly the geniohyoid muscle. The extrinsic muscles pass from the skull or the hyoid bone to the tongue, and all are in pairs and are symmetrical; the intrinsic muscles arise and end within the tongue.

The extrinsic muscles of the tongue and their functions are as follows: The genioglossi, by means of their posterior fibers, draw the root of the tongue forward and thus protrude the apex. The anterior fibers draw the tongue back into the mouth and tend to depress and retract the organ. The two work together to draw the tongue downward and make its superior surface concave from side to side. The posterior fibers of the genioglossus on one side push the tongue to-

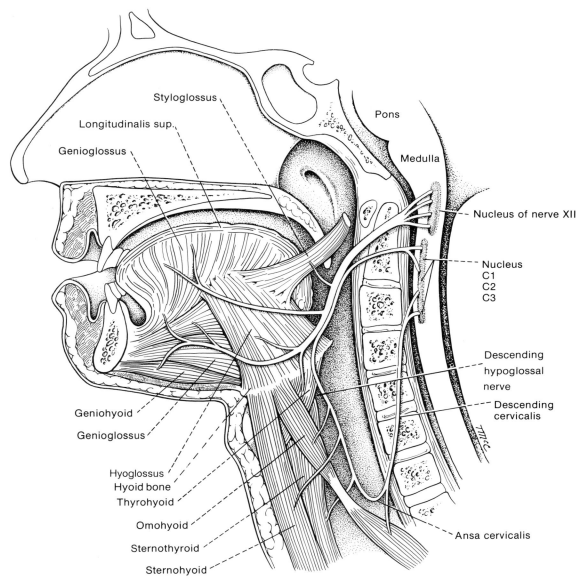

FIG. 17–2. Ansa hypoglossi and muscles supplied by the hypoglossal nerve.

ward the opposite side. The hyoglossi retract the tongue and depress the sides; they make the superior surface convex. The chondroglossus is sometimes described as a part of the hyoglossus, and is a depressor and retractor. The styloglossi draw the tongue upward and backward; they retract the organ and elevate the root. They also elevate the sides, and thus aid in the production of transverse concavity of the dorsum. The palatoglossus, which aids in drawing the root of the tongue upward, may also be classified as one of the extrinsic muscles of the tongue. It is more

closely associated in location and function, however, with the muscles of the soft palate. It is innervated by the vagus nerve.

The intrinsic muscles of the tongue are the superior and inferior longitudinales, the transversus, and the verticalis. They are mainly concerned with altering the shape of the tongue; they cause it to become shortened, narrowed, or curved in different directions. Both longitudinales shorten the tongue; the superior longitudinalis also turns the tip and sides to make the dorsum concave, whereas the inferior longitudinalis pulls the tip down and makes the dorsum convex. The transversus narrows and elongates the tongue, and the verticalis flattens and broadens it.

The suprahyoid muscles also influence the movement of the tongue by bringing about the movement of the hyoid bone. The geniohyoid raises and advances the hyoid bone and the base of the tongue during deglutition; it depresses the mandible when the hyoid bone is fixed. Some anatomists state that this muscle is supplied by the hypoglossal nerve, but other authorities express the belief that its innervation is derived mainly from the first and second cervical segments of the spinal cord through the cervical plexus, although the fibers are carried through the hypoglossal nerve. The other suprahyoid muscles, which function with the geniohyoid in raising the hyoid bone and the base of the tongue and in depressing the jaw when the hyoid is fixed, are the mylohyoid and the anterior belly of the digastricus, which have been discussed with the trigeminal nerve, and the stylohyoid and the posterior belly of the digastricus, which have been discussed with the facial nerve.

The infrahyoid group of muscles exert no specific action on the tongue, but through their innervation they are related to the hypoglossal nerve. The sternohyoid depresses the hyoid bone and the larynx after these structures have been drawn up by the pharynx in the act of deglutition. The sternothyroid acts as a depressor of the thyroid cartilage of the larynx. The omohyoid depresses the hyoid bone, which it carries backward and to one side; it also contracts and renders tense the cervical fascia. The thyrohyoid elevates the thyroid cartilage when the hyoid bone ascends; it draws the thyroid cartilage up and behind the hyoid bone. These muscles are innervated by the first three cervical nerves through the descending and thyrohyoid branches of the hypoglossal and the ansa hypoglossi. They may receive some innervation from the hypoglossal nerve as well.

CLINICAL EXAMINATION

The clinical examination of the functions of the hypoglossal nerves consists of an evaluation of the movements of the tongue. Motor power is tested; the position of the tongue on protrusion and at rest, and the strength and rapidity of movement in all directions, are noted; weakness,

paralysis, atrophy, and abnormal movements are observed.

The position of the tongue when at rest in the mouth is first noted, and the patient is then asked to protrude it, to move it in and out, from side to side, upward and downward, both slowly and rapidly, and to press the tip against each cheek while the strength of this pressure is tested with the finger placed on the outside of the cheek. A more precise method of testing involves asking the patient to protrude his tongue, placing a tongue blade against the side of it, and then asking the patient to press against it firmly; the procedure is then repeated on the opposite side. He may also be asked to curl the tongue upward and downward over the lips, and to elevate the lateral margins.

When unilateral paralysis or paresis of the tongue is present it deviates toward the involved side on protrusion (Fig. 17-3) owing to the action of the normal genioglossus, which produces a stronger movement than do the other tongue

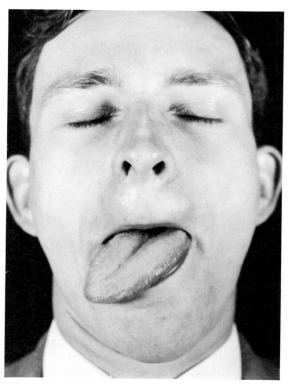

FIG. 17–3. Infranuclear paralysis of muscles supplied by the hypoglossal nerve: Unilateral atrophy and deviation of the tongue following a lesion of the right hypoglossal nerve.

muscles. It protrudes the apex of the tongue by drawing the root of the organ forward and pushing the distal portion outward and toward the paretic side. As the tongue lies in the mouth at rest it may deviate or curl slightly toward the healthy side, owing to the unopposed action of the styloglossus, which draws the organ upward and backward. There is a diminution or loss of the ability to deviate the protruded tongue toward the nonparetic side and of the ability to push it against the cheek on the sound side, but the patient is able to push it against the cheek on the paralyzed side. Lateral movements of the tip of the nonprotruded tongue toward the sound side may be preserved, as they are controlled by the intrinsic tongue muscles. The tongue may be unable to remove food from between the teeth and the cheeks on either side.

If the paralysis is not accompanied by atrophy, the tongue may appear to bulge slightly and to be higher and somewhat more voluminous on the paralyzed side, but when atrophy supervenes the paralyzed side becomes smaller and the tongue may become curved toward the paralyzed side, giving a sickle-shaped deformity. In bilateral paralysis of the tongue the patient may be able to protrude the organ only slightly or not at all. If paralysis of the facial muscles or of the muscles of mastication is also present, it may be difficult to evaluate deviation of the tongue. The paretic angle of the mouth may have to be retracted by the examiner, so that the relationship of the tongue to the central incisors can be compared. With either weakness or coordination difficulties, rapid movements may be impaired. The presence of unilateral atrophy may be confirmed by palpation of the tongue. In myotonia, sharp percussion of the tongue may cause the formation of a dimple which disappears slowly.

When atrophy is present, there is a loss of muscle substance, first apparent at the borders or at the tip (Fig. 17-4). The tongue is wrinkled, furrowed, and obviously wasted, and the epithelium and mucous membrane on the affected side are thrown into folds. The protruded tongue may curve toward the atrophic side. Atrophy may be accompanied by fasciculations, which at times may give the appearance of a wriggling mass of worms. The fine, rapid tremors seen in general paresis and toxic states may be difficult to differentiate from fasciculations when the tongue is protruded, but the tremors usually disappear when the tongue is lying at rest in the mouth, whereas fasciculations persist.

Coarse tremors of the tongue are present in parkinsonian states. All tremors may be brought

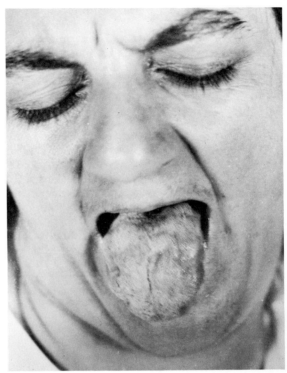

FIG. 17–4. Nuclear paralysis of muscles supplied by the hypoglossal nerve: Atrophy and fasciculations of the tongue in a patient with amyotrophic lateral sclerosis.

out or accentuated by protrusion of the tongue or by talking. Other hyperkinesias of the tongue are observed in various diseases of the motor system. In chorea there may be irregular, jerky movements of the tongue, and often the patient is unable to keep his tongue protruded. Athetoid and dystonic movements, habit spasms, and tics may involve the tongue; lingual spasm has been described in tetanus and in emotional disturbances. Oral–facial dyskinesias, usually involving the tongue, occur in patients suffering from side effects of phenothiazines and other psychotropic drugs. Dyskinesias that are similar in appearance may also occur during the use of levodopa and dopamine agonists in the treatment of parkinsonism.

Morphologic changes in the tongue may be of diagnostic significance. Ankyloglossia, or tongue-tie, may simulate paresis. Macroglossia is seen in cretinism and Down's syndrome. There may be hypertrophy of the tongue in conditions such as parkinsonism and other dyskinesias where there is constant protrusion. The presence of coating or lack of coating, fissuring, redness, scars, mucous patches, and atrophy or hypertrophy of the papillae may give some clue in the diagnosis of physical disease. The term **atrophic glossitis** is used to designate changes that occur in the tongue in certain deficiency states. In these, however, the atrophy involves only the papillae, and there is no neurogenic atrophy of the musculature. The tongue of pernicious anemia is smooth and translucent, with atrophy of the fungiform and filiform papillae; in some stages of the disease the tongue is pale and in other stages red, but in all there is a lack of coating. In thiamine deficiency the tongue is smooth, shiny, atrophic, and reddened. In pellagra and niacin deficiency the tongue is smooth, and there is atrophy with desquamation of the papillae; in acute stages it is scarlet red and swollen, but in chronic or mild deficiency stages the papillae are mushroomed and the organ is not so deeply red. Fusion and atrophy of the papillae and fissuring may produce the so-called geographic, or scrotal, tongue. In riboflavin deficiency the papillae are flattened and the tongue may be a purplish or magenta hue.

DISORDERS OF FUNCTION

Lesions of the hypoglossal nerve or its central connections cause paresis or paralysis of the tongue. A unilateral paralysis may cause few symptoms; speech and swallowing are little affected. In bilateral paralysis the tongue cannot be extended or moved laterally; the first stage of deglutition is impaired, and there is difficulty with articulation, especially in pronouncing the linguals. With bilateral nuclear or infranuclear lesions swallowing may be difficult and speech indistinct; there may be respiratory difficulty, as the tongue tends to slip back into the throat. There are no sensory changes with lesions of the hypoglossal nerve. Glossodynia, or burning of the tongue, is often accompanied by parageusias, or abnormalities of taste, and by repeated movements of the tongue against the teeth; these symptoms are not related to lesions of the hypoglossal nerve, but may be secondary to atherosclerosis, psychogenic disorders, and other conditions.

Paralysis of the tongue, or glossoplegia, may be due to a supranuclear, a nuclear, or an infranuclear lesion. In supranuclear involvement there is paresis, with deviation but no atrophy. The impairment of power is rarely complete. Since the genioglossus, the principal protractor of the tongue, has mainly crossed supranuclear

innervation, the tongue protrudes toward the paralyzed side, but to the side opposite the cerebral lesion. In nuclear and infranuclear lesions there is atrophy of the involved side in addition to paralysis and deviation. The protrusion is toward the paralyzed side, which is also the side of the lesion. If the nuclear lesion is a progressive one, such as progressive bulbar palsy, amyotrophic lateral sclerosis, or syringobulbia, there are also fasciculations.

Supranuclear paralysis of the tongue may follow lesions of the cerebral cortex, the internal capsule, the cerebral peduncle, or the pons. The paresis is usually the result of a destructive lesion of the cortex or the corticobulbar pathway. If the lesion is an irritative one, there may be involuntary protrusion of the tongue to the opposite side; this may be seen in jacksonian convulsions. In dystonia, athetosis, oral–facial dyskinesias, and chorea there may be abnormal movements, and in other extrapyramidal disorders there may be slowing of tongue movements, with thickness of speech and difficult protrusion. In pseudobulbar palsy there is bilateral paralysis; the tongue may be small and the patient may be unable to protrude it beyond the teeth. Patients with aphasia may have apraxia of tongue movements, and often are unable to protrude the organ on command.

Nuclear lesions may be of the progressive varieties described previously, or may be due to neoplasms, vascular lesions, polioencephalitis, multiple sclerosis, syphilis, abscesses, granulomas, or botulism. In progressive bulbar palsy and amyotrophic lateral sclerosis the atrophy may be so severe that the tongue cannot be protruded, and it is seen lying on the floor of the mouth, exhibiting extensive fasciculations. In nuclear lesions there may be evidence of involvement of contiguous structures, such as the ascending sensory or descending motor pathways. In hypoglossal alternating hemiplegia (Ch. 18) there is a nuclear paralysis of the tongue on the side of the lesion, and a contralateral spastic hemiplegia.

Infranuclear lesions may be extramedullary but within the skull, within the hypoglossal canal, or in the neck. Basal skull fractures, subarachnoid hemorrhage with exudation and organization, meningitis of various types, granulomas, extramedullary neoplasms or abscesses, basilar impression (platybasia), compression of the medulla into the foramen magnum by increased intracranial pressure, or dislocation of the upper cervical vertebrae may affect the nerve before it leaves the skull. After the exit of the nerve from the hypoglossal canal or within the neck it may be injured by trauma of various types (examples include stab or gunshot wounds), carotid aneurysms, infections in the retroparotid or retropharyngeal spaces, tumors of the neck, tumors of the base of the tongue, salivary gland tumors, or operations on the neck, mouth, or tongue. Primary tumors of the twelfth nerve have been reported. When the hypoglossal nerve is involved with the ninth, tenth, and eleventh, and occasionally with the cervical sympathetic nerves in lesions in the retroparotid space, the Collet–Sicard or Villaret syndromes are seen (see "Syndromes of Intramedullary or Extramedullary Involvement," Ch. 18). Isolated neuropathies may cause weakness of the tongue, and it may be involved unilaterally or bilaterally in the Guillain–Barré syndrome and related polyneuropathies.

Weakness of the tongue may be a symptom of myasthenia gravis; usually there is no atrophy. The tongue may be protruded a few times, but soon fatigues. The localized contraction following percussion in myotonia has been described previously. The tongue may be weak in the various myopathies as well. In psychogenic paralysis of the tongue the patient may appear unable to deflect it to the paralyzed side, but instead protrudes it to the nonparalyzed side.

Hyperkinetic manifestations of the tongue have already been mentioned. Tremors, fasciculations, and choreiform and athetoid movements may be manifestations of supranuclear, nuclear, or psychogenic disturbances. Forced deviation of the tongue may be a part of a jacksonian seizure. Tics, lingual spasm, lisping, stammering, and other speech abnormalities may be present. **Aphthongia** is the name given to a form of spasm occurring in speakers and similar in nature to writer's cramp. Either tonic or clonic spasm of the tongue may be seen in hysteria, as a result of reflex irritation, or in tetanus or rabies.

BIBLIOGRAPHY

Brodal A. Neurological Anatomy in Relation to Clinical Medicine, 3rd ed. New York, Oxford University Press, 1981

Riggs JE. Distinguishing between extrinsic and intrinsic tongue muscle weakness in unilateral hypoglossal palsy. Neurology 1984;34:1367

Chapter 18

MEDULLARY AND RELATED SYNDROMES

The medulla, or medulla oblongata, may be considered either the caudalmost portion of the brain stem or an upward projection of the spinal cord. The caudal portion of the posterior cerebral vesicle of the embryo is called the myelencephalon. This term implies functions of both spinal cord and brain, or transition from spinal cord to brain. The medulla and the lower part of the fourth ventricle develop from the myelencephalon.

The medulla extends from the bulbopontine sulcus and the striae medullaris acousticae, above, to the lowermost roots of the hypoglossal nerve and the lowest plane of the pyramidal decussation, just rostral to the highest rootlet of the first cervical nerve. The structure is 24 – 30 mm in length. The medulla contains the motor nuclei of the glossopharyngeal, vagus, cranial portion of the accessory, and hypoglossal nerves; the parasympathetic nuclei of the glossopharyngeal and vagus nerves; and the nuclei of termination of the sensory components of the glossopharyngeal and vagus nerves. Some of the vestibular nuclei are in the medulla, and the cochlear nuclei are situated at the junction between the medulla and the pons. It also contains the nuclei of gracilis and cuneatus, inferior olivary bodies and accessory olives, reticular formation, inferior cerebellar peduncles, arcuate fibers, and sensory and pyramidal decussations. Structures which pass through the medulla are the pyramidal (corticobulbar and corticospinal) pathways, lateral and ventral spinothalamic tracts, medial lemniscus, descending tract and nucleus of the trigeminal nerve, medial longitudinal fasciculus, fasciculus solitarius, ascending spinocerebellar

and spinovestibular and descending vestibulospinal pathways, descending sympathetic pathways, and other fibers of passage.

The functions of the medulla are vital and numerous. The presence of the nuclei of the ninth, tenth, and twelfth nerves renders it an important center in the control of the reflex action of the pharynx, larynx, and tongue, and thus of articulation and deglutition. It receives taste and visceral sensations and is concerned with many visceral reflexes such as coughing, swallowing, sneezing, salivation, sucking, and vomiting, and with various secretory responses. It contains the medial longitudinal fasciculus, which is important in the regulation of head and neck movements and of coordinated movements of the head and eyes. It is a center for cochlear and vestibular responses and a relay station for the nerves concerned with them. It is a region of passage for long ascending and descending pathways which relate it to lower and higher centers. The reticular formation plays an important part in the facilitation and suppression of motor activity, in the regulation of tone and conduction of sensation, in postural and other reflex activity, and in the control of consciousness and of visceral and autonomic functions. In addition, through the dorsal efferent nucleus and the vagus nerve, the medulla aids in regulation of respiratory, cardiovascular, digestive, and the other metabolic processes of the body.

Symptoms and Signs of Medullary Lesions. Owing to the small size and compact form of the medulla, a focal lesion may affect structures having widely varying functions, and this may lead to varied and pronounced symptoms and signs. Such lesions may involve the nuclear centers and cause specific and multiple cranial nerve palsies. They may damage the fiber tracts and produce motor and sensory changes in the face and body. They may affect the vital functions and bring about bradycardia, hypotension, abnormalities of respiration, and disturbances of gastrointestinal function. Usually, owing to the proximity of the relationships, a very small lesion of the medulla involves combinations of the above and causes neurologic syndromes which include cranial nerve palsies, sensory changes, corticospinal tract and cerebellar dysfunction, and oftentimes disturbances of respiration, circulation, and digestion. Since the corticospinal and some sensory pathways decussate in the medulla, unilateral lesions may produce ipsilateral paralysis of individual cranial nerves, together with contralateral motor and sensory changes of the body and limbs. The signs referable to the ipsilateral cranial nerve dysfunction indicate the level of the lesion. Involvement of the ninth, tenth, and twelfth nerves may cause dysphagia, dysarthria, and nasal regurgitation of liquids. In unilateral lesions complete paralysis of deglutition or of articulation is not present, but in extensive or bilateral lesions severe impairment of these functions is present.

Involvement of the fibers of passage may result in monoplegia, hemiplegia, alternating hemiplegia, or sensory dissociation. Because of the proximity of the two corticospinal pathways, there may be a paraplegia or a decerebrate type of rigidity. Involvement of the dorsal efferent nuclei or of both vagus nerves or pressure on the medullary centers may lead to profound disturbances of cardiac function, blood pressure, and respiratory action, and convulsions and/or coma and death may result. If death does not take place at once, there may be some recovery, but the residual paralysis of deglutition may lead to an eventual pneumonia.

Lesions of the medulla or of the medullary nerves may be acute, subacute, or chronic in course, and vary in etiology and in site of pathologic change. Intramedullary lesions involve the cranial nerve nuclei and fibers of passage directly; extramedullary lesions within the posterior fossa affect the roots of the cranial nerves and also may cause pressure manifestations; supranuclear lesions interrupt the continuity of the corticobulbar pathways; extrinsic lesions, that is, those outside the skull or within the neck, involve the peripheral course of the bulbar nerves in various combinations.

Specific syndromes of the midbrain and pons are not dealt with in this chapter, but those in which there is also medullary involvement are described. The midbrain, which is the seat of the nuclei of origin of the oculomotor and trochlear nerves, also contains the red nucleus, substantia nigra, cerebral peduncles, superior cerebellar peduncles, the geniculate and quadrigeminal bodies in part, and ascending and descending pathways. The syndromes involving specific cranial nerves are discussed with those nerves, and disturbances of motor function associated with lesions of the red nucleus and substantia nigra or their connections are described in Part D, "The Motor System." The cranial nerve nuclei from the trigeminal through a part of the acoustic are situated within the pons. The pons also contains, in addition to the long ascending and descending pathways, the pontine nuclei and the brachium pontis (middle cerebellar peduncle). Syndromes characterized by cranial nerve involvement are described with those nerves. Owing, however, to the proximity of the pons to the medulla, and to the fact that the two structures may be supplied by the same blood vessels, pontine involvement may occur in medullary lesions, and it may be difficult or impossible to differentiate the two. Many pontine lesions, such as those which produce alternating hemiplegia and hemianesthesias, cause syndromes that are very similar to medullary syndromes, and in many vascular lesions there may be involvement of both structures. Those pontine syndromes which occur with medullary ones and those of specific vascular origin are considered in this chapter.

Causes of Medullary Disorders. Neoplasms may be either intramedullary (gliomas or ependymomas) or extramedullary (neurofibromas, meningiomas, hemangiomas, metastatic or other tumors). The symptoms and signs vary, but the course is progressive; occasionally increase of intracranial pressure appears late, particularly in brain stem gliomas, and there sometimes is a paucity of neurologic signs in spite of the size of the tumor. Extrinsic metastases and neoplasms that spread by direct extension from the nasopharynx and neighboring sites may cause widespread cranial nerve involvement and bone erosion with signs of medullary compression. Tuberculomas, sarcoidosis, and other granulomas may cause symptoms similar to those present with neoplasms. Vascular lesions, such as those secondary to hemorrhage, thrombosis, or embolism are intramedullary in site and usually acute in onset. Aneurysms of the basilar or vertebral arteries or their branches, and hemangiomas, however, may cause extramedullary compression and cranial nerve involvement. Arteriovenous malformations may cause intramedullary or extramedullary involvements, depending on their extent and location. Extravasation of blood about the base of the brain from either subarachnoid or intracerebral hemorrhage may affect the cranial nerves as they leave the skull. Hemorrhages into the midbrain, pons, and medulla may cause hyperthermia, respiratory difficulties, coma, and finally death in patients with brain tumors, subarachnoid hemorrhage, cerebral hemorrhage, trauma, or other conditions with an acute increase in intracranial pressure. The venous drainage from the medulla goes caudally into the venous plexus surrounding the spinal cord, and that from the pons and midbrain goes cephalad into the middle cranial fossa; consequently compression at either the foramen magnum or the tentorium may cause bleeding into the brain stem.

Other causes of intramedullary involvement include bulbar polioencephalitis accompanying poliomyelitis, multiple sclerosis, syringobulbia or syringomyelia, progressive bulbar palsy, congenital abnormalities and disturbances of development, and many other infectious, toxic, and degenerative processes. Extramedullary syndromes may be caused by trauma, basal skull fractures, abnormalities of skeletal development, acute and chronic meningeal inflammations, and a sudden increase of intracranial pressure, causing herniation of the medulla into the foramen magnum. Extrinsic lesions include, in addition to neoplastic invasion, trauma, tuberculosis, other granulomas, and aneurysms. Some of the aforementioned will be discussed in detail in the following paragraphs.

VASCULAR LESIONS

Vascular lesions of the medulla (and/or pons) may be either intermittent in course or abrupt in onset. The medulla receives its blood supply from the vertebral arteries; the pons, from the basilar (Fig. 18-1). These arteries, however, also supply the cerebral peduncles and the major portion of the cerebellum, and the terminal posterior cerebral branches of the basilar artery supply the occipital lobes, part of the temporal lobes, the hypothalamus, and the posterior portions of the thalamus and internal capsule (Ch. 51). When embolization of the vertebral and/or basilar arteries or their branches occurs, or atherosclerotic narrowing develops in these vessels or in the subclavian arteries from which the vertebral arteries arise, **transient ischemic attacks** often occur. These are characterized by temporary dysfunction of the nuclear centers, ascending and descending pathways, and other structures supplied by them. These take the form of brief episodes, usually less than 30 minutes, of unilateral or bilateral weakness of the limbs, fleeting dimness or loss of vision or visual field defects, diplopia or paresis of conjugate gaze, nystagmus, nausea and vomiting, vertigo, ataxia, deafness or tinnitus, subjective or objective sensory changes involving either the trigeminal distribution or the extremities, dysphagia, dysarthria, drowsiness, mental confusion, headaches, or sudden attacks of loss of tone and occasionally of consciousness (drop attacks).

Ischemic attacks (and permanent occlusions) may also be the result of trauma, arthritic narrowing, neck manipulations, and other mechanical factors influencing the flow through the proximal portions of the vertebral vessels. Basilar-vertebral transient ischemic attacks occasionally are part of the subclavian steal syndrome with reversed flow in the posterior circulation. Recurring ischemic episodes may cause increasingly severe deficits, and permanent occlusion of the branches of these vessels may cause the syndromes to be described. Extensive involvement of the major vessels may lead to sudden death due to circulatory or respiratory involvement. However, there is wide individual variation in the vascular supply of the brain stem, and as a result the symptom complex that follows either occlusion or hemorrhage of these vessels may differ considerably in individual cases. Furthermore, medullary infarcts are often multiple.

The *anterior spinal artery* is formed by the union of branches from each vertebral artery; the site of union may vary. It supplies the pyramids, medial lemniscus, and emerging hypoglossal fibers. Thrombosis of this artery is usually followed by either an **alternating hypoglossal hemiplegia,** or an **alternating hypoglossal hemianesthetic hemiplegia.** In the former, also known as **crossed hypoglossal paralysis,** or the **syndrome of the pyramid and the hypoglossal nerve,** there is an ipsilateral flaccid paralysis of the tongue due to involvement of the hypoglossal nucleus or the emerging root fibers of the hypoglossal nerve, with a contralateral corticospinal paresis of the arm and leg, a result of involvement of the corticospinal

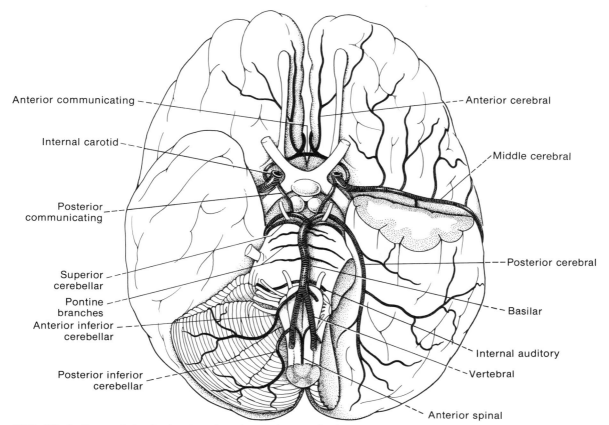

FIG. 18–1. Base of the brain showing the major cerebral arteries and some of their branches.

tract before decussation. In the latter, also known as the **syndrome of the pyramid, the medial lemniscus, and the hypoglossal nerve,** a contralateral loss of proprioceptive and discriminative tactile sensibility is also present, resulting from extension of the lesion to involve the medial lemniscus. The spinothalamic tract is spared in most instances; therefore, there is no loss of pain and temperature sensations. Lesions that cross the midline to affect both corticospinal tracts or both medial lemnisci may be involved in either syndrome. In **bilateral anterior spinal thrombosis,** in which the circulation is cut off on both sides, or in thrombotic instances in which only one anterior spinal artery exists, double hemiplegia and hemianesthesia (for discrimination, tactile, and proprioceptive sensations), with a bilateral or alternating paralysis of the tongue, usually more marked on one side, may occur. Both the paralysis and the sensory change spare the face. Lesions of the anterior spinal artery do not always involve the hypoglossal nerve. They

may affect the medial longitudinal fasciculus and cause nystagmus. They may affect adjacent structures to cause a disturbance of bladder and bowel function. All of the aforementioned are sometimes referred to as **Dejerine's anterior bulbar syndrome** (Fig. 18-2).

In **hemiplegia cruciata, crossed hemiplegia,** or the **syndrome of the decussation,** there is a lesion at the level of the decussation of the pyramids, with a contralateral spastic paresis of the lower extremity due to involvement of the corticospinal fibers to the leg which have not yet decussated, and an ipsilateral spastic paresis of the upper extremity attributable to damage to those fibers to the arm which have already crossed. Ipsilateral flaccid paresis, atrophy of the sternocleidomastoid and trapezius muscles, and occasionally ipsilateral paralysis of the tongue may be evident. The crossed hemiplegia may result from anterior spinal artery involvement or from trauma. A more extensive lesion or one just above the decussation may produce a spastic tetraplegia.

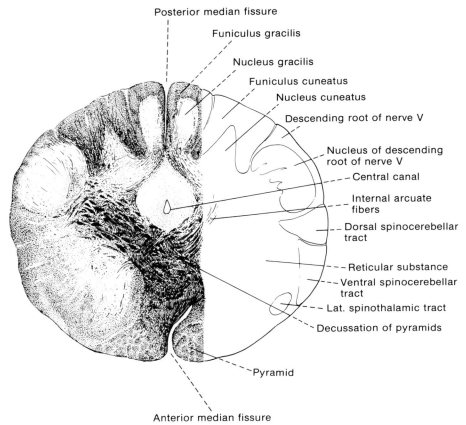

Posterior median fissure
Funiculus gracilis
Nucleus gracilis
Funiculus cuneatus
Nucleus cuneatus
Descending root of nerve V
Nucleus of descending root of nerve V
Central canal
Internal arcuate fibers
Dorsal spinocerebellar tract
Reticular substance
Ventral spinocerebellar tract
Lat. spinothalamic tract
Decussation of pyramids
Pyramid
Anterior median fissure

FIG. 18–2. *Cross section of the medulla at the level of the decussation of the corticospinal tracts.*

Occlusions of the posterior inferior, the anterior inferior, and the superior cerebellar arteries or their branches may produce a variety of abnormalities, some more typical of a particular vessel, or fitting into a named syndrome, others not so. Significant variations exist in the distributions of these vessels from person to person. Thus, while it is desirable to attempt to ascribe a symptom complex to a lesion of a certain vessel in the brain stem, a listing of the several neurologic deficits will be more precise in localization than would be the assignment to a vascular territory. Improving imaging technics will also define the extent of a lesion more precisely in the future.

The *posterior inferior cerebellar artery*, usually a branch of the vertebral artery, comes off just below the union of the two vertebrals to form the basilar artery; occasionally it is a branch of the basilar artery. It supplies the inferior cerebellar peduncle (restiform body), the dorsolateral tegmentum of the medulla, and the inferior surface of the vermis and adjacent cerebellar cortex. Thrombosis of this artery, also called the **lateral medullary** or **Wallenberg's syndrome,** is the most frequently encountered medullary syndrome (Fig. 18-3). The nucleus ambiguus and the emerging fibers of the ninth and tenth nerves, the descending tract and nucleus of the trigeminal nerve, the descending sympathetic pathways, the restiform body and the afferent spinocerebellar tracts, and the lateral spinothalamic tract are usually affected. The resulting manifestations include ipsilateral paralysis of the soft palate, pharynx, and larynx with dysphagia and dysphonia; ipsilateral anesthesia of the face for pain and temperature sensation with loss of the corneal reflex; ipsilateral Horner's syndrome, and ipsilateral cerebellar asynergy and hypotonus. Contralateral loss of pain and temperature sensations on the limbs and trunk is present. Sixth, seventh, and eighth nerve involvements on the side of the lesion are occasionally evident. The vestibular nuclei and

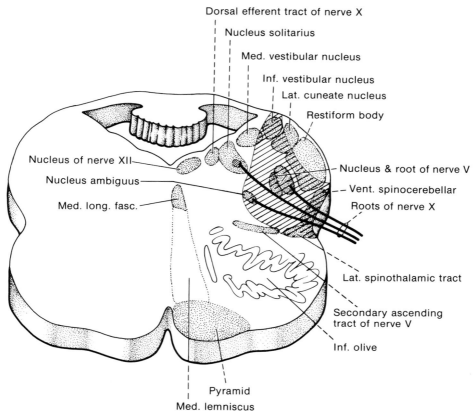

Dorsal efferent tract of nerve X
Nucleus solitarius
Med. vestibular nucleus
Inf. vestibular nucleus
Lat. cuneate nucleus
Restiform body

Nucleus of nerve XII
Nucleus ambiguus
Med. long. fasc.

Nucleus & root of nerve V
Vent. spinocerebellar
Roots of nerve X

Lat. spinothalamic tract

Secondary ascending
tract of nerve V

Inf. olive

Pyramid
Med. lemniscus

FIG. 18–3. Cross section of the medulla illustrating the site of the lesion following thrombosis of the posterior inferior cerebellar artery.

olivary connections may be affected. Headache or pain in the back of the neck may occur at the time of the occlusion; vertigo, nausea, vomiting, nystagmus, conjugate deviation of the eyes, and singultus are frequent manifestations. The patient may be unable to talk and swallow at the onset. Survival is the rule; a certain amount of improvement occurs. The ability to swallow and talk returns, although residual hoarseness and persistent ataxia and sensory changes may remain. This syndrome also often results from occlusion of the vertebral rather than of the posterior inferior cerebellar artery. It has also been described secondary to aneurysms, hematomas, arteriovenous malformations, and metastatic neoplasms.

The *anterior inferior cerebellar artery* supplies the lateral tegmentum of the upper medulla and lower pons, the restiform body, lower portion of the middle cerebellar peduncle (brachium pontis), flocculus, and inferior surface of the cerebellar hemisphere. This vessel is usually a branch of the basilar artery, but is the most

variable of the arteries supplying the medulla and cerebellum. Thrombosis of this artery usually causes, ipsilaterally, cerebellar asynergy, loss of pain and temperature sensation and diminished light touch sensation on the face; Horner's syndrome usually causes deafness, and a peripheral type of facial palsy. Contralaterally, incomplete loss of pain and temperature sensations on the limbs and body may occur. Postoperative thrombosis of this artery may follow excision of a cerebellopontine angle tumor.

The *superior cerebellar artery* supplies the lateral part of the tegmentum of the pons and midbrain, upper portion of the brachium pontis, brachium conjunctivum (superior cerebellar peduncle), superior surface of the cerebellum, and cerebellar nuclei. In thrombosis of this artery (not a medullary syndrome), ipsilateral cerebellar asynergy with hypotonus and involuntary movements develop, often choreiform or choreoathetoid in type, and an ipsilateral Horner's syndrome may be present. Contralaterally there is loss of pain and temperature sensations on the face and body owing to involvement of the spinothalamic tract and the ventral secondary ascending tract of the trigeminal nerve. Occasionally a central type of facial palsy and partial deafness may be detected.

Lesions of the *vertebral artery* may be either partial or complete. Various syndromes compatible with life have been described which are secondary to vertebral artery thrombosis.

The rare **medial medullary syndrome** may be due to a small branch occlusion of the vertebral artery. Ipsilateral involvement of the hypoglossal nerve is accompanied by contralateral hemiparesis and loss of proprioceptive and discriminatory tactile functions on the contralateral side. The **syndrome of Avellis** may follow thrombosis of the vertebral artery, and is characterized by involvement of the spinothalamic tract and of the nucleus ambiguus, usually with associated involvement of the bulbar nucleus of the accessory nerve. Occasionally involvement of the medial lemniscus and the tract of the solitary fasciculus may be present. Ipsilateral paralysis of the soft palate, pharynx, and larynx, with contralateral loss of pain and temperature sensations on the trunk and extremities is evident. There may also be loss of proprioceptive sensibility and diminution of discriminatory tactile sensation on the opposite side of the body, and ipsilateral anesthesia of the pharynx and larynx and loss of taste. An ipsilateral Horner's syndrome and a contralateral corticospinal tract paralysis may be detected in this syndrome.

The **syndrome of Céstan – Chenais** is caused by occlusion of the vertebral artery below the point of origin of the posterior inferior cerebellar artery. The syndrome may be caused by more than one lesion. Lesions of the nucleus ambiguus, restiform body, and descending sympathetic pathways cause paralysis of the soft palate, pharynx, and larynx, with cerebellar asynergy and Horner's syndrome on the side of the lesion, while involvement of the corticospinal tract and the medial lemniscus produces hemiplegia with loss of proprioceptive sensibility and diminution of discriminatory tactile sensation on the opposite side of the body. This differs from posterior inferior cerebellar thrombosis principally in the presence of corticospinal tract signs and medial lemniscus involvement and the absence of changes in pain and temperature sensations. Occasionally, however, the symptoms in the syndrome of Céstan–Chenais may be extensive and variable. Nuclei of the eleventh and twelfth nerves may be involved, with ipsilateral paralysis of the sternocleidomas-

toid and trapezius muscles and of the tongue; there may be involvement of the descending root of the trigeminal nerve, resulting in ipsilateral loss of pain and temperature sensations on the face; and there may be spinothalamic involvement, with loss of pain and temperature sensations on the opposite side of the body.

The **syndrome of Babinski – Nageotte** is in many respects similar to that of Céstan – Chenais, but it is believed to be caused by multiple or scattered lesions, chiefly in the distribution of the vertebral artery. There is usually involvement of the nucleus ambiguus, solitary fasciculus, descending root of the trigeminal nerve, restiform body, sympathetic pathways, corticospinal tract, and medial lemniscus, and often of the hypoglossal nucleus as well. There is ipsilateral paralysis of the soft palate, pharynx, larynx, and sometimes of the tongue, with loss of taste on the posterior third of the tongue, loss of pain and temperature sensations on the face, cerebellar asynergy, and Horner's syndrome, together with contralateral spastic hemiplegia, loss of proprioceptive sensibility, and diminution of tactile sensation. Contralateral loss of pain and temperature sensations on the trunk and limbs results if the lateral spinothalamic tract is involved. Some authorities claim that the Céstan–Chenais syndrome differs from that of Babinski-Nageotte in that tenth nerve involvement is present in the former but not in the latter. Variations may be found in the descriptions of these syndromes; again, description of deficits is more useful than assignment to a given eponymic syndrome.

Occlusion of the *basilar artery* may have a gradual onset or a somewhat fluctuating course, with some prodromata, but often the symptoms appear precipitously, and death may occur within a short period of time. Bilateral cranial nerve and long tract abnormalities develop. With total occlusion there is either a hemiplegia on one side and a partial hemiplegia on the other, or a quadriplegia; this is accompanied by bilateral involvement of the supranuclear fibers to the bulbar nuclei and of the ascending sensory pathways as well. Pseudobulbar palsy with severe dysphagia and dysarthria result, together with disturbance of both deep and superficial sensations on the body, extremities, and sometimes the face. The pupils are usually miotic. Decerebrate rigidity, either profound coma or akinetic mutism, and respiratory and circulatory difficulties usually result. The symptoms of basilar artery hemorrhage are similar but warning symptoms are less apt to occur. Hemorrhages into and edema of the brain stem may also occur following intracranial surgery or cerebral trauma or with sudden increase of intracranial pressure, subarachnoid hemorrhage, and rapidly expanding supratentorial mass lesions. Death is the usual result of complete basilar artery occlusion.

Thrombosis of the medial pontine branches of the basilar artery may cause involvement of the nuclei of the sixth and seventh nerves or their emerging fibers, the medial longitudinal fasciculus, the corticospinal tract, and the medial lemniscus, with ipsilateral facial paralysis and paralysis of lateral rectus movement or of conjugate lateral gaze, contralateral hemiplegia, loss of proprioceptive sensibility, and diminution of tactile sensation. Lateral pontine branches of the basilar artery supply the middle cerebellar peduncle, superior olivary body, facial nucleus, vestibular and cochlear nuclei, and in part the motor and sensory nuclei of the trigeminal nerve, medial longitudinal fasciculus, and spinothalamic tract. Thrombosis of these branches causes ipsilateral cerebellar asynergy with symptoms referable to the fifth, seventh, and eighth cranial nerves, often with contralateral loss of pain and temperature sensations on the trunk and limbs. There may also be contralateral hemiplegia and loss of discriminative tactile and proprioceptive sensations.

When thrombosis of the upper pontine branches of the basilar artery occurs, a contralateral corticospinal hemiplegia including the face and tongue develops. There is also contralateral loss of pain, temperature, and proprioceptive sensations and diminished tactile sensation on the face, trunk, and extremities, resulting from involvement of the corticospinal tract, the medial lemniscus, the spinothalamic tract, and the ventral and dorsal secondary ascending tracts of the trigeminal nerve. Thrombosis of the *internal auditory artery* produces ipsilateral deafness and loss of vestibular function.

SYNDROMES OF INTRAMEDULLARY OR EXTRAMEDULLARY INVOLVEMENT

Many other specific syndromes are characterized by involvement of the medullary nerves and pathways in various combinations. They result from either intramedullary or extramedullary lesions, and may be of vascular origin, or found in association with syringobulbia, multiple sclerosis, polioencephalitis, trauma, neoplasms, or other lesions. They are associated with the names of the individual observers who described them, but the descriptions in the literature vary widely, and in many instances there is a difference of opinion regarding the specific characteristics of each syndrome. The **syndrome of Jackson,** or **vago-accessory-hypoglossal paralysis,** is caused by a nuclear or radicular lesion of the tenth (nucleus ambiguus), eleventh, and twelfth nerves on one side; there is ipsilateral flaccid paralysis of the soft palate, pharynx, and larynx, with flaccid weakness and atrophy of the sternocleidomastoid and trapezius (partial) muscles, and of the tongue. The **syndrome of Schmidt,** or the **vago-accessory syndrome,** is caused by a lesion of the nucleus ambiguus and of the bulbar and spinal nuclei of the eleventh nerve and/or their radicular fibers; there is ipsilateral paralysis of the soft palate, pharynx, and larynx, with flaccid weakness and atrophy of the sternocleidomastoid and trapezius (partial) muscles. Inasmuch as the sternocleidomastoid and trapezius muscles are involved in both the syndrome of Jackson and the syndrome of Schmidt, it is unlikely that a nuclear lesion in the lower third of the medulla is responsible. Both are probably caused by extramedullary lesions which involve the fibers before they leave the skull. The **syndrome of Tapia,** or **vago-hypoglossal palsy,** is characterized by ipsilateral paralysis of the soft palate, pharynx, and larynx, and paralysis and atrophy of the tongue. This results from a tegmental lesion in the lower third of the medulla involving the ambiguus and hypoglossal nuclei, but since the soft palate and pharynx are spared, the syndrome of Tapia may also result from an extramedullary lesion with involvement of the hypoglossal and vagus nerves high in the neck. The syndrome of Avellis, characterized by involvement of the nucleus ambiguus and the bulbar nucleus of the accessory nerve, together with the spinothalamic tract and the medial lemniscus, has been described previously under "Vascular Lesions."

The **syndrome of Vernet** is caused by a lesion at the jugular foramen, and is characterized by ipsilateral paralysis of the ninth, tenth, and eleventh nerves. It is usually of traumatic origin and may follow a basilar skull fracture, however, vascular and neoplastic lesions, thrombosis of the jugular bulb, aneurysms of the internal carotid artery, and granulomas may also be etiologic factors. The **syndrome of Villaret** is the result of a lesion in the retropharyngeal space. Ipsilateral paralysis of the ninth, tenth, eleventh, and twelfth nerves and of the cervical sympathetic fibers (producing Horner's syndrome) is detected. The **syndrome of Collet and Sicard** is similar to that of Villaret, with the exception of the Horner's syndrome. The syndromes of Villaret and Collet – Sicard may be difficult to differentiate. With tumors of the glomus jugulare (chemodectomas), involvement of the ninth, tenth, and eleventh nerves at the jugular foramen may be evident, as well as evidence of seventh and eighth nerve dysfunction. **Garcin's syndrome** consists of paralysis of all the cranial nerves (or of only the third through the tenth nerves), usually on one side but occasionally on both, which is most often the result of involvement by metastatic neoplasm, but may also be caused by invasion by a neoplasm of the nasopharynx or retropharyngeal space or by granuloma or infection.

CHRONIC MEDULLARY SYNDROMES

Chronic medullary syndromes occur more frequently than either the acute and subacute or the localized varieties. The two principal types, progressive bulbar palsy and pseudobulbar palsy, bear some resemblance to each other but are important to differentiate in clinical diagnosis. In both the outstanding symptoms are dysphagia and dysarthria, and both run a chronic course.

Progressive, or **true, bulbar palsy** is a relentlessly progressing degenerative disease of the motor neurons which involves the nuclei within the medulla and sometimes those within the pons and midbrain. It is closely related to progressive spinal muscular atrophy, in which the process is limited to the anterior horn cells of the spinal cord, and amyotrophic lateral sclerosis, in which there is involvement of the bulbar nuclei, the anterior horn cells, and the pyramidal cells within the motor cortex. Progressive bulbar palsy is usually a disease of late adult life; most frequently the onset is in the sixth and seventh decades, although younger individuals may be affected. The degenerative process in the motor nuclei causes atrophy of the muscles supplied by the specific nerves, and this atrophy is accompanied by fasciculations and progressive paralysis. Inasmuch as the centers which supply the tongue, pharyngeal musculature, palate, and sometimes the lips are predominantly involved, the condition is often referred to as glossopalatolabial, glossolabiolaryngeal, or glossopharyngolabial paralysis.

The disease usually starts in the nucleus of the twelfth nerve and ascends. Among the first manifestations may be atrophy, fasciculations,

and paralysis of the tongue. These symptoms are bilateral from the onset; in the beginning there may be fatigability of the tongue, but in far-advanced cases the patient may be unable to protrude his tongue or to push food back into his mouth. The lingual involvement is followed or accompanied by dysphagia, usually for both liquids and solids, and by dysarthria. Regurgitation of fluids is an outstanding symptom, and it may lead to choking and aspiration. The defect in articulation is of the bulbar type, and is the result of involvement of the soft palate, the larynx, and the tongue. It is best described as a "thick" speech with a definite nasal factor — the speech observed in edema of the throat or when the mouth is filled with soft food. At the outset the most pronounced difficulty is in the pronunciation of the linguals and palatals, but later the labials, too, are affected. In far advanced cases speech is reduced to unmodified laryngeal noises that are quite unintelligible. There is often marked drooling of saliva. Sometimes atrophy and fasciculations may be seen in the palate and pharynx as well as in the tongue, and the condition may ascend to the facial nucleus and even the muscles of mastication. Occasionally the sternocleidomastoid and trapezius muscles are affected, and there may be autonomic involvement with tachycardia. The palatal and pharyngeal reflexes disappear early. There are no sensory changes, and no corticospinal tract manifestations unless amyotrophic lateral sclerosis develops. The condition is a progressive one, and there is no known cure. Death is usually caused by aspiration pneumonia. Progressive bulbar palsy may be associated with progressive spinal muscular atrophy, or it may be the first manifestation of amyotrophic lateral sclerosis. It is occasionally familial.

Progressive bulbar palsy is also a manifestation, often the terminal aspect, of Werdnig – Hoffmann paralysis, or progressive muscular atrophy of infancy and early childhood. Progressive bulbar paralysis of childhood, which may show a clinical course similar to that of the adult type, is known as Fazio – Londe's disease (Ch. 21). Congenital flaccid bulbar palsy may be related to either Möbius' syndrome or the congenital myopathies.

In **pseudobulbar (supranuclear) palsy** difficulties with articulation, mastication, and deglutition which resemble those of progressive bulbar palsy are present, but the underlying mechanism is entirely different. Pseudobulbar palsy is caused by bilateral lesions which interrupt the pathways of the suprasegmental fibers (corticobulbar tracts) to the bulbar nuclei. The pathologic process is supranuclear, but the symptoms are referred to the medulla. Since the bulbar nuclei are to some extent bilaterally innervated, or receive impulses from both the ipsilateral and the contralateral motor cortices, a unilateral supranuclear lesion rarely causes difficulty in talking, eating, or swallowing. Bilateral lesions, however, do cause severe problems. The most common causes of pseudobulbar palsy are repeated bilateral cerebral vascular lesions caused by multiple hemorrhages, thromboses, or emboli. The syndrome may also occur in encephalitis, multiple sclerosis, multiple or diffuse neoplasms, trauma, cerebral anoxia, or other disease processes that interrupt the corticobulbar pathways on both sides. The lesions may be at the cortex or in the corona radiata, internal capsule, basal ganglia, or cerebral peduncle, or in the pons or medulla above the nuclear centers. They are situated most frequently, however, in the internal capsule. Usually a history is elicited of a vascular lesion that caused paralysis or paresis of one side of the body, followed by improvement. At the time of the original attack a history of slight and transient impairment of speech, chewing, or swallowing is obtained. A later vascular lesion on the opposite side, involving the remaining supranuclear fibers to the bulbar nuclei, causes the syndrome of pseudobulbar palsy. Speech is thick and slurred, but is more frequently explosive in type. There is difficulty in swallowing, with regurgitation, choking, holding of food in the mouth, and drooling. Although the dysarthria is marked, there is less tendency to choke than in progressive bulbar palsy, since palatal and pharyngeal reflexes are present. There is neither atrophy nor fasciculations of the tongue, but the patient may be unable to protrude the tongue beyond the lips because of the bilateral paralysis. The palate rises only slightly. Weakness and spasticity of the muscles of mastication, an exaggerated jaw reflex, and snout and sucking reflexes may be present, along with paresis of the muscles of facial expression and "masking" of the face. Corticospinal tract signs are present in most patients. Sensory changes may be present. Frequently, deficient emotional control with spontaneous, or unmotivated, laughter and crying is evident. The prognosis is no more favorable than in progressive bulbar palsy and the outcome is dependent upon the etiologic factor in the individual case. Aspiration pneumonia often terminates the illness in both disorders.

Two types of pseudobulbar palsy have been described, one due to scattered lesions which affect the corticobulbar fibers, and one due to involvement of the basal ganglia or the extrapyramidal pathways. In both there is disturbance of the tongue, pharynx, lips, cheeks, and muscles of mastication, with difficulties in articulation, phonation, mastication, and deglutition. On occasion respirations may be severely affected, and swallowing may evoke a cough reflex. Evidence of cerebral involvement may coexist, with aphasia, extensive motor and sensory changes, incontinence, and dementia. In striatal pseudobulbar palsy there are additional signs of basal ganglion involvement, with rigidity, hyperkinesias, and a parkinsonian attitude.

Progressive supranuclear palsy (the **Steele – Richardson – Olszewski syndrome**) is characterized by supranuclear ophthalmoplegia, especially paresis of downward gaze. As the disease progresses there is supranuclear paresis of other eye movements also, and then of the muscles of facial expression, articulation, and deglutition. There is often dystonia of the neck muscles, and the presence of facial masking and rigidity resembling those seen in Parkinson's disease. Progressive dementia is often part of the syndrome. Degenerative lesions are found in the brain stem, basal ganglia, and cerebellum.

In myasthenia gravis (asthenic bulbar paralysis) the dysarthria and dysphagia of the bulbar type resembles that of bulbar palsy. Weakness and fatigue of the facial, masticatory, and ocular muscles, the levator palpebrae superioris, and the general skeletal musculature are usually present. Ptosis, diplopia, difficulty in chewing, and general weakness are frequent symptoms. All of these manifestations are brought on by use of the affected muscles and are symptoms of abnormal fatigability; they are relieved by rest. Myasthenia gravis is not a true bulbar disease, but is rather a disease of the myoneural junction (Ch. 21). Signs and symptoms similar to those of myasthenia may occur with the myasthenic syndrome of Eaton and Lambert. Weakness resembling bulbar palsies may at times be part of the muscular dystrophies and other myopathies; the involvement is confined to the muscles themselves.

OTHER SYNDROMES AFFECTING THE MEDULLA

Diphtheritic palsy is manifested by a bulbar syndrome with involvement of the soft palate and pharynx, and sometimes of the tongue. There is nasal speech, with regurgitation of fluids owing to paresis of the soft palate, and sometimes there is difficulty in swallowing solids owing to weakness of the pharynx. If the laryngeal musculature is involved, hoarseness and even aphonia may be present. There often is associated paralysis of accommodation and of convergence. Furthermore, there frequently are manifestations of either a peripheral neuritis or an ascending myelitis, and of cardiac involvement. The pathogenesis of these changes is not entirely understood, but they are believed to be caused by the selective action of the diphtheritic toxin.

Botulism involves the bulbar centers, often along with some of the higher nuclear groups. After a short incubation, symptoms of dysarthria, dysphonia, and dysphagia develop, along with paresis of the tongue, palate, pharynx, and ocular movements. Photophobia, vertigo, blurred vision, diplopia, ptosis, vomiting, and generalized muscle weakness are other important symptoms.

In tetanus spasm of the pharynx may accompany trismus.

In rabies spasmodic contractions of the muscles occur spontaneously on attempts to swallow. Bulbar type weakness may be a part of the Guillain – Barré syndrome and related polyneuritic disorders.

Central pontine myelinolysis runs a fulminating course. It may start with diplopia, dysphagia, dysarthria, and other evidence of brain stem involvement, followed by quadriplegia and by mutism and extensor rigidity before its usually fatal termination. Cases have been reported in chronic alcoholics or in patients with severe malnutrition or chronic debilitating systemic or central nervous system diseases. Widespread, symmetric myelin loss within the central portion of the pons and occasionally of the adjacent midbrain and medulla is found pathologically. The lesion may at times be visible antemortem on magnetic resonance imaging. A deranged sodium metabolism is often observed with this syndrome, and overly rapid correction of hyponatremia, or, less often, hypernatremia, may be an etiologic factor.

The terms **locked-in syndrome, akinetic mutism,** and **coma vigil** are often used more or less synonymously. In this syndrome all motor functions are paralyzed except for ocular and eyelid movements. The patient is speechless and motionless and often makes little response to stimuli. He appears to be asleep, but can be aroused, and his eyes may follow moving objects and deviate in the direction of loud sounds. In some cases the patient may be aroused sufficiently so as to follow directions and respond to

questions requiring "yes" and "no" answers by opening and closing the eyes once or twice. This syndrome occurs with basilar artery thrombosis, traumatic, neoplastic, and other lesions of the upper brain stem, with pathologic changes affecting the descending corticobulbar and corticospinal pathways and the reticular formation at lower midbrain and upper pontine levels.

Pressure on the midbrain and brain stem secondary to supratentorial mass lesions can cause either the syndrome of the tentorial notch (uncal syndrome) with third nerve involvement and signs of lateral midbrain compression (see "Disorders Associated with Ocular Nerve Abnormalities," Ch. 11) or the so-called central syndrome with constricted pupils, Cheyne – Stokes respirations, bilateral corticospinal tract involvement, decorticate rigidity, and progressive impairment of diencephalic, midbrain, pontine, and medullary function.

In bulbar poliomyelitis there is paralysis of the throat, tongue, and respiratory muscles. In epidemic encephalitis there may be true bulbar or pseudobulbar involvement. Syringomyelia and syringobulbia may cause varying syndromes of medullary involvement, as may multiple sclerosis, tabes dorsalis, and bulbar neoplasms. Medullary manifestations are also seen in such conditions as Friedreich's ataxia, Marie's cerebellar ataxia, and olivopontocerebellar atrophy, but in these the cerebellar symptoms are more outstanding. So-called palatal myoclonus is discussed in Chapters 15 and 31.

The syndrome of the herniation of the medulla and the cerebellar tonsils into the foramen magnum may occur in association with increased intracranial pressure. It may take place precipitously following the removal of cerebrospinal fluid by the lumbar route in the presence of increased intracranial pressure, if the increased pressure is caused by posterior fossa tumors and abscesses, but also if caused by supratentorial brain tumors and other masses. Compression of the medulla produces impairment of vital functions, with profound bradycardia, slow or rapid respirations, a fall or marked rise in blood pressure, soaring temperature, convulsions, unconsciousness, and death. On postmortem examination a "pressure cone" may be seen on the medulla.

Developmental or congenital anomalies of the occipital bone, atlas, and axis frequently cause medullary involvement, with characteristic neurologic syndromes. The bony walls of the foramen magnum and upper portion of the vertebral canal have a close anatomic relationship with the medulla, upper cervical portion of the spinal cord, and cerebellum. The neurologic manifestations may be produced by mechanical compression of the medulla and spinal cord by the bony deformity; there may be associated malformations of the nervous system, or both factors may be important. The bony abnormalities consist of malformations of the occipital foramen, basilar impression or invagination (platybasia), malformation or occipitalization of the atlas, fusion of the atlas with the occiput, abnormal position of the axis in relation to the occiput and the atlas, absence of one or more of the cervical vertebrae and fusion of certain of the cervical vertebrae (the **Klippel – Feil syndrome**), and cervical spina bifida. The principal nervous system anomalies are the **Arnold – Chiari** deformity, with caudal displacement of the cerebellar tonsils and/or the inferior portion of the vermis and of the lower medulla and fourth ventricle into the spinal canal; maldevelopment and heterotopic changes in the brain stem and cerebellum; dysraphic conditions with incomplete closure of the medullary tube; syringobulbia; and meningocele.

The skeletal and nervous system developmental anomalies usually occur together. In severe cases with obstruction of ventricular outflow, hydrocephalus develops. The neurologic examination demonstrates both medullary and cerebellar signs, with palsies of the ninth through twelfth cranial nerves, involvement of the corticospinal tracts and sensory pathways, nystagmus, and signs of compression of the spinal cord at the foramen magnum; increased intracranial pressure may develop. Some of the neurologic signs of dysfunction are entirely developmental in origin; others may arise on a mechanical basis secondary to traction. In the **Dandy – Walker syndrome** there is dilation of the fourth ventricle and associated hydrocephalus. This arises following maldevelopment in fetal life and has been attributed to atresia of the foramina of Luschka and Magendie. Anomalies of the cerebellum are also present, and these, rather than atresia of the foramina, may be responsible for the syndrome.

BIBLIOGRAPHY

Adams RD. Occlusion of the anterior inferior cerebellar artery. Arch Neurol Psychiatry 1943;49:765

Adams RD, Victor M, Mancall EL. Central pontine myelinolysis. Arch Neurol Psychiatry 1959;81:154

Amarenco P, Hauw J-J. Cerebellar infarction in the territory of the anterior and inferior cerebellar artery. A clinicopathological study of 20 cases. Brain 1990;113:139

Aring CD. Supranuclear (pseudobulbar) palsy. Arch Intern Med 1965;115:198

Atkinson WJ. The anterior inferior cerebellar artery: Its variations, pontine distribution, and significance in the surgery of cerebello-pontine angle tumors. J Neurol Neurosurg Psychiatry 1949;12:137

Barnett HJM, Mohr JP, Stein BM et al. Stroke. Pathophysiology, Diagnosis, and Management. New York, Churchill Livingstone, 1986

Bell HS. Paralysis of both arms from injury of the upper portion of the pyramidal decussation: Cruciate paralysis. J Neurosurg 1970;33:376

Brown HW, Plum F. The neurologic basis of Cheyne – Stokes respiration. Am J Med 1961;30:489

Brown JR, Baker AB. Poliomyelitis. I. Bulbar poliomyelitis: A neurophysiological interpretation of clinicopathological findings. J Nerv Ment Dis 1949;109:54

Currier RD, Giles CL, DeJong RN. Some comments on Wallenberg's lateral medullary syndrome. Neurology 1961; 11:778

D'Agostino AN, Kernohan JW, Brown JR. The Dandy – Walker syndrome. J Neuropathol Exp Neurol 1963;22:450

Davison C. Syndrome of the anterior spinal artery of the medulla oblongata. Arch Neurol Psychiatry 1937;37:91

Davison C, Goodhart SP, Savitsky N. Syndrome of the superior cerebellar artery and its branches. Arch Neurol Psychiatry 1935;33:1143

Escourolle R, Hauw J-J, Der Agopian P et al. Les infarcts bulbaire: Etude des lésions vasculaire dans 26 observations. J Neurol Sci 1976;28:103

Ferbert A, Brückmann H, Drummen R. Clinical features of proven basilar artery occlusion. Stroke 1990;21:1135

Gillilan LA. The correlation of the blood supply to the human brain stem with clinical brain stem lesions. J Neuropathol Exp Neurol 1964;23:78

Hauw J-J, Der Agopian P, Trelles L et al. Les infarcts bulbaire: Etude systematique à la topographie lésionelle dans 49 cas. J Neurol Sci 1976;28:83

Kubik CS, Adams RD. Occlusion of the basilar artery: A clinical and pathological study. Brain 1946;69:73

List CF. Neurologic syndromes accompanying developmental anomalies of occipital bone, atlas, and axis. Arch Neurol Psychiatry 1941;45:577

Millikan CH, McDowell F, Easton JD. Stroke. Philadelphia, Lea & Febiger, 1987

Steele JC, Richardson JC, Olszewski J. Progressive supranuclear palsy: A heterogeneous degeneration involving the brain stem, basal ganglia and cerebellum with vertical gaze and supranuclear palsy, nuchal dystonia, and dementia. Arch Neurol 1964;10:333

Toole JF. Cerebrovascular Disorders, 3rd ed. New York, Raven Press, 1984

Tyler HR. Botulism. Arch Neurol 1963;9:652

Chapter 19
DISORDERS OF ARTICULATION

The terms *phonation, speech,* and *articulation* are often used synonymously. In correct usage, however, they must be distinguished. **Phonation** is the production of vocal sounds without word formation; it is entirely a function of the larynx. **Speech** is defined as the utterance of vocal sounds which convey ideas, or as the faculty of expressing thoughts aloud by means of words (articulate sounds which symbolize and communicate ideas). It is the entire process by which meanings are comprehended and expressed in words; it involves psychologic as well as physiologic factors, and is largely a function of the cerebral cortex. **Articulation,** on the other hand, is the enunciation of words and phrases, or the power of forming words by the larynx together with the pharynx, tongue, palate, teeth, and lips; it is a motor action whereby words, having been formulated, are audibly expressed. It is largely a function of the organs and muscles innervated by the medullary nerves.

Various types of abnormalities in sound production and word formulation may be produced by organic lesions of the nervous system. Disorders of function of the larynx may cause disorders of the volume, quality, or pitch of the voice, called dysphonia; complete loss of voice is aphonia. Lesions of the cerebral centers and connections which deal with word formulation and power of expression by speech, even though articulation may be adequate, cause **aphasia** or **dysphasia.** Involvement of the organs and muscles of articulation, the nerves to them, the nuclei of these nerves, or the central regulation of the nuclei (corticobulbar, extrapyramidal, or cerebellar) causes **dysarthria,** or the imperfect utterance of sounds or of words; verbal formulation is normal, phonation is preserved, but enunciation of words is faulty owing to difficulty in performing the coordinated muscular movements necessary for the production of the vowels and consonants which make up syllables and words. If the disorder is so marked that it causes total inability to articulate, because of a defect in the control of the peripheral speech musculature, there is **anarthria.** Many varieties of dysarthria have been described. In **pararthria** there is imperfect or disturbed utterance of speech in which single sounds or syllables cannot be pronounced in proper succession. **Bradyarthria,** or **bradylalia,** is slow or labored speech.

Dyslalia is a disturbance of utterance in which no organic neurologic defect is present, but there is either structural abnormality of the organs concerned with speech or a disorder of articulation without dysfunction of the articulatory mechanisms. **Mutism** results in an inability to speak or loss of the power of speech; usually the patient appears to make no attempt to speak or make sounds. **Alalia,** or mutism, is usually of psychogenic origin if present in a patient who appears to be conscious, but may occur in association with lesions of the cerebrum and brain stem.

In the present discussion only the motor components of word production are considered. The central control of speech and its disorders are discussed elsewhere (Ch. 52).

Anatomy and Physiology of Articulation. Sounds are produced by the expiration of a current of air from the lungs, through the trachea and upper air passages, and over the partition formed by the movable vocal cords. For true articulated speech, it is necessary that coordination exists between the diaphragm, intercostal muscles, lungs, air passages, larynx, pharynx, soft palate, tongue, lips, and facial and masticatory muscles. Respiratory movements determine the strength and rhythm of the voice. Variations in pitch are effected by alterations in the tension and length of the vocal cords and the rate and character of the vibrations transmitted to the column of air which passes between them. Modifications in sound are produced by changes in the size and shape of the glottis, pharynx, and mouth, and by changes in the position of the tongue, soft palate, and lips. The pharynx, nasopharynx, and mouth act as resonating chambers and further influence the timbre and character of the voice. Toneless speech may be possible in the absence of vocal cords, and whispered speech may be carried out in inspiration as well as in expiration.

Several cranial nerves are involved in articulation, and for an adequate appraisal of speech, the function of each must be evaluated. The trigeminal nerves control the muscles of mastication and thus open and close the mouth. The facial nerves control the functions of the muscles of facial expression, especially branches to the orbicularis oris and other smaller muscles about the mouth. The vagus nerves, assisted to a degree by the glossopharyngeal nerves, supply the soft palate, pharynx, and larynx, and the hypoglossal nerves regulate the functions of the tongue. Thus articulation may be considered one of the important bulbar functions. The upper cervical nerves, which have communications with the ninth, tenth, eleventh, and twelfth nerves and in part supply the infrahyoid and suprahyoid muscles, also contribute to normal speech, as do the cervical sympathetic nerves which in part supply the pharyngeal plexus, and the phrenic and intercostal nerves.

Types of Speech Sounds. In order to understand the production of disturbances in articulation, it is important to understand some of the more significant types of sound formation. Voiced sounds are produced when the glottis is narrowed so that the vocal cords approach each other or touch lightly. Voiceless sounds are made while the glottis is open for outgoing breath. Both types of sound may be modified by changes in the size, shape, and position of the passageways through which the air must pass after leaving the larynx. Vowels are largely of a laryngeal origin, but are modified by the resonance of the vocal cavities. Consonants may be either voiced or voiceless; they are formed chiefly by the origins of articulation and are characterized in enunciation by constriction or by closure at one or more points in the breath channel. This distinction between vowels and consonants, however, is not absolute. Fricative sounds (either voiced or voiceless) are characterized by a frictional rustling of the breath as it is emitted with the oral passage largely closed.

From the point of view of phonetics, speech sounds may be placed in various categories. From the anatomic point of view, however, it is more important to recognize the individual organs which are chiefly responsible for the various sounds. The **articulated labials** are consonants which are formed principally by the lips, they are b, p, m, and w. The **modified labials** are vowels which are altered by contraction of the lips, mainly through the action of the orbicularis oris; they are o and u, and to a lesser extent i, e, and a. **Dentolabials** are formed by placing the teeth against the lips; f and v belong to this group. The **linguals** are sounds which are formed with the aid of the tongue. T, d, l, r, n, and th are **tongue-point,** or **alveolar,** sounds and are formed by contact of the tip of the tongue with the upper alveolar ridge. S, z, sh, zh, ch, and j, are **dentals,** or **tongue-blade** or **palatoalveolar** sounds. The **velars,** or **tongue-back sounds (gutturals)**, are articulated between the back of the tongue and the velum, or soft palate; they are k, g, and ng. The **palatals** are formed when the dorsum of the tongue is approximated to the hard palate; they include the German ch and g, and the French gn. Certain vowel sounds such as i, a, and y are modified by the palate and the velum. Whispered sounds are entirely articulatory. Humming with the mouth open is solely phonation.

Normal articulation is dependent upon many factors. Not only is the proper neuromuscular control of the organs of articulation and phonation necessary, but also normal cerebral synthesis and correlation. A proper development of the tongue, larynx, and soft palate, and adequate hearing are essential to correct enunciation. A normal attention span and adequate intelligence are also important. In appraising speech one must take into consideration the cultural and emotional background of the individual. It must be remembered that normal variations in enunciation and articulation result from training as well as being associated with geographic areas. No two individuals possess the same speech patterns. This is true not only for pitch and timbre, but also for the quality, duration, and intensity of tones and sounds, and for the ability to pronounce certain words and syllables. Some individuals never acquire the ability to formulate certain sounds. Education and training both enter into speech, and the uneducated, the illiterate, and the mentally deficient may mispronounce letters and syllables even though their powers of articulation are normal. Those who learned to speak another language before learning English may never learn to enunciate certain English sounds. Within the United States, as well as in all other countries, there are marked regional variations or "accents," evident in the pronunciation of vowels and many of the consonants.

EXAMINATION OF ARTICULATION

To examine the articulatory process one first notes the patient's spontaneous speech in normal conversation. This may be accomplished while the history is being taken. Then the patient may be asked to read aloud some simple printed matter. The mode of expression, character of enunciation, rate of speech, resonance, and prosody (variations in pitch, rhythm, and stress of pronunciation) are noted. Any abnormalities of articulation such as tremulousness, stammering or stuttering, slurring or eliding of letters or words, scanning, explosive characteristics, and difficulties with specific sound formations should be noted.

For a detailed examination of articulation, the patient may be asked to repeat some of the so-called test phrases. These phrases have been selected to test principally the labials and linguals — such letters as l, r, b, p, t, and d— and as the patient repeats them, various aspects of dysarthria may become evident. These phrases are time-honored, perhaps above their actual value, and are to a certain extent colloquial, but many of them serve a need in testing articulation. The more commonly used are such phrases as "truly rural," "third riding artillery brigade," and "Methodist Episcopal," but such phrases and words as "liquid electricity," "voluntary retribution," and "irretrievable" are also useful. A more accurate evaluation of articulation can be made, however, by the use of weighted words, phrases, and sentences in which the significant consonants and vowels are placed in the initial, medial, and final positions. Ataxia and so-called

scanning speech are detected most effectively by having the patient repeat a fairly long sentence. Weakness and fatigability of articulation, as well as disturbances in rhythm and quality, may be made evident by having the patient count quickly and at an even rate to 30 or beyond. Disturbances of laryngeal function and of rhythm may also be elicited by having the patient attempt prolonged phonation with an "ah" or "ee" sound.

DISORDERS OF ARTICULATION

Abnormalities of articulation may be caused by many different pathologic conditions. Disturbances in the respiratory rhythm produce an interference with speech. Paresis of the respiratory muscles causes an enfeebled voice with abnormalities in regularity and rhythm. Laryngitis, neoplasms, or other abnormalities of the larynx may be responsible for severe impairment, but whispered speech may be possible in the presence of extensive disease of the larynx. In children, articulation disturbances may be developmental and often temporary. Local disturbances and craniofacial structural defects, congenital or acquired, such as cleft palate, harelip, ankyloglossia (tongue-tie), adenoids, edentulism, stomatitis, nasal obstruction, or perforated nasal septum may cause abnormalities in sound production. Speech is affected when there is interference with the symbolic formation of ideas, but articulation may be normal in spite of the presence of aphasia.

Neurologic disturbances of articulation or vocalization may be caused by primary muscle diseases affecting the tongue, larynx, and pharynx; disorders of the myoneural junction; disease of the lower motor neuron, involving either the motor nucleus or the peripheral nerves which supply the muscles of articulation; dysfunction of the cerebellum, the basal ganglia, or the upper motor neurons; difficulties in symbol formation or word expression; psychomotor disturbances; and abnormalities of rhythm in vocal expression or respiratory control.

Diseases of the *neuromuscular level* (those which involve the lower motor neuron, the myoneural junction, or the muscles) produce various alterations of articulation, dependent upon the specific nerves or muscles that are involved. With lesions of the hypoglossal nerve, nuclear or peripheral, or with specific disorders of the tongue such as ankyloglossia, especial difficulty in pronouncing the lingual sounds is evident, although there may be impairment of all enunciation. The speech is lisping in character and is clumsy and indistinct. When paralysis of the larynx is present, the voice may be hoarse, and the patient may not be able to speak above a whisper. Specific difficulty with vowel sounds is detected. A similar change in articulation occurs in laryngitis and in tumors of the larynx.

With unilateral laryngeal muscle weakness, or in paralysis of the recurrent laryngeal nerve, the voice is low-pitched and hoarse, but occasionally almost complete unilateral paralysis may be present without appreciable effect on phonation, owing to unimpaired adduction and crossing the midline by the normal vocal cord. With slight weakness of the vocal cords hoarseness may become evident by having the patient talk with his head turned to one side. In bilateral abductor paralysis speech is moderately affected, but in bilateral total paralysis it is lost. With paralysis of the cricothyroid, the voice is hoarse and deep and fatigues quickly. In adductor palsy the loss of speech is out of proportion to the involvement detected by laryngoscopy.

If the paralysis is limited to the pharynx, little impairment of articulation is detected, but when paralysis of the soft palate is evident there is marked dysfunction with resulting nasal speech, or **rhinolalia,** caused by undue patency of the posterior nares with a resultant inability to shut off the nasal cavity from the mouth. An abnormal resonance is added to all voice sounds. There is special difficulty with the velar sounds, but those formed by the lips and tongue are also weakened, for much of the air which should be used for their production escapes through the nose. The speech is similar to that encountered in a patient with a cleft palate. Characteristically, b becomes m, d becomes n, and k becomes ng. The dysarthria is more noticeable when the head is tipped forward; it is less evident when the patient is lying with his head back, for then the paralyzed soft palate falls back by its own weight and closes off the nasopharynx. Amyotrophic lateral sclerosis and myasthenia gravis are common causes of this type of speech difficulty.

When paralysis of the seventh nerve is present there may be difficulty in pronouncing the labials and the dentolabials. This defect is noticeable only in peripheral facial involvement: the central type of facial paralysis is usually too mild to cause interference with articulation. Occasionally in a Bell's palsy there may be a marked dysarthria because of inability to close the mouth, purse the lips, and distend the cheeks. Similar articulatory defects are found in myopathies involving the labial muscles, especially the facioscapulohumeral or oculopharyngeal types, and in harelip and wounds of the lips. Tremors of the lips, such as those of dementia paralytica and toxic states, may interfere with speech. There is little impairment of articulation in paralysis of the trigeminal nerves unless the involvement is bilateral, and in such instances there usually are other characteristics of bulbar speech. In trismus, as for example in tetanus, speech may be affected because the patient is unable to open his mouth. Lesions of the ninth and eleventh nerves usually have no effect on articulation.

Diseases of the lower motor neuron causing difficulties in articulation of the types just described may occur in neuritides of the cranial nerves or all other disorders of the cranial nerves discussed in previous chapters. They may also occur in neuromuscular disorders such as botulism, myasthenia gravis, and other disorders of the myoneural junction. In myasthenia gravis, prolonged speaking such as counting may cause progressive weakness of the voice with a decrease in volume and at times the development of a bulbar or nasal quality, which may even proceed to anarthria. An occasional myasthenic patient may have to close the jaw with the hand in order to enunciate. In progressive bulbar palsy the defect is the result of multiple paralysis of motor functions of cranial nerves which affect the tongue, pharynx, and larynx, soft palate, and, to a lesser extent, the facial muscles, lips, and muscles of mastication. Both articulation and phonation may be affected; speech is slow and hesitant with failure of correct enunciation, and all sounds and syllables may be distinct. The patient talks as though his mouth were filled with soft food, and the resulting change in articulation is often known a "hot-mush" or "hot-potato" speech. It is thick and slurred, often with a definite nasal quality. It may have a halting, drawling, monotonous character. The tongue lies in the mouth, more or less immobile; the palate rises very little, and swallowing is difficult. The impairment may progress to a stage in which speech is reduced to unmodified, unintelligible laryngeal noises. If the disease is so extensive that the patient is completely unable to talk, there is anarthria.

Supranuclear lesions, or involvement of the corticobulbar pathways, may cause disturbances of speech or of articulation. Unilateral cortical lesions do not usually affect speech unless they are in the dominant hemisphere and cause dysphasia, although occasionally some dysarthria accompanies dysphasia. Rarely, small lesions in the cortical motor system for articulation have resulted in severe dysarthria (aphemia) without aphasia. Both dysarthria and dysprosody, or a defect in rhythm, melody, and pitch, have been described with localized frontal lobe lesions; these may be due to a dyspraxia of speech. In acute hemiplegia there may be transient slurring or thickness of speech, dependent upon the degree of weakness of the face and tongue. Bilateral cortical lesions, however, or bilateral lesions of the corona radiata, internal capsule, cerebral peduncles, pons, or upper medulla (vascular, inflammatory, neoplastic, degenerative, etc.) may cause pseudobulbar palsy, with its characteristic dysarthria. There is a thick bulbar type of speech, similar to that in progressive bulbar palsy, but somewhat more explosive in nature; it rarely progresses to complete anarthria. The muscles which govern articulation are weak and spastic, the tongue may appear smaller than normal and is protruded with difficulty, and there may be spasticity of the muscles of mastication. In spastic diplegia, especially congenital spastic paraplegia, the speech may be slow and slurred, with poor enunciation, and there may be spasm of the pharyngeal muscles; owing to an abnormal breathing rhythm, there is poor correlation between breath control and voice production, and thus the speech is irregular and jerky.

Lesions of the *basal ganglia* affect articulation. When athetosis is present, the grimaces of the face and tongue interfere with speech. Irregular spasmodic contractions of the diaphragm and other respiratory muscles, together with spasm of the tongue and pharynx, may give the speech a curious jerky and groaning character. In addition there may be a pseudobulbar element with slurred, indistinct, spastic speech. When chorea is present, the violent movements of the face, tongue, and respiratory muscles may make the speech jerky, irregular, and hesitant; the patient is unable to maintain phonation. Occasionally there is loss of ability to speak.

In Parkinson's disease and the parkinsonian syndromes associated with encephalitis or treatment with phenothiazines or other psychotropic drugs, there is **bradylalia;** speech is feeble, slow, and slurred owing to muscular rigidity and immobility of the lips and tongue. There is dysprosody and the speech lacks inflections, accents, and modulation. The patient speaks in a monotone, and the words are slurred and run into one another. The voice becomes increasingly weak as the patient talks, and he may become unable to speak above a whisper; as the speech becomes more indistinct it may become inaudible or practically disappear. Tremor of the voice may be apparent; words may seem to be chopped off, and there may be sudden blocks and hesitations, or the speech may stop abruptly. There may be repetition of syllables or **palilalia.** Like the gait associated with Parkinson's disease, the speech may show festination, with a tendency to hurry toward the end of sentences or long words.

Palilalia may also be a feature of **Gilles de la Tourette's syndrome,** or the syndrome of multiple tics. Involuntary vocalizations, sometimes of expletives (**coprolalia**) may also occur intermittently.

With *cerebellar lesions* or temporary dysfunctions (toxic, etc.) there is a defect of coordination, or asynergy, of the speech, which is slow, slurred, irregular, labored, intermittent, and jerky. It is often explosive or staccato in character. Words are enunciated with irregular force and speed, with variations in loudness and pitch. Often the words or syllables are broken, causing a jerky, syllabic, sing-song cadence, the so-called **scanning** type of speech which resembles the scanning of poetry. It may be accompanied by grimaces and irregular respirations.

In patients with voice tremor, or tremor of phonation, there are rhythmic alterations in loudness and pitch; there may be associated tremor of the extremities or head or other signs of neurologic dysfunction. Organic voice tremor is often an inherited condition, a variant of the familial tremor which most commonly affects the hands.

Specific types of speech defects or anomalies of articulation may be observed in association with various organic diseases of the nervous system. The exact type of disorder in articulation varies in individual cases and depends upon the site of the predominant pathologic change.

In dementia paralytica there is a tremulous, slurring type of dysarthria; there are special difficulties with the linguals and labials. The defect is brought out when the patient repeats the various test phrases. He hesitates and repeats. Letters, syllables, and phrases are omitted, elided, or run together. The speech is slovenly, with ataxia, stumbling, and alliteration. Tremors of the lips, tongue, and face are increased when the patient is talking. Articulation may be made more difficult by the presence of aphasia and memory loss.

In multiple sclerosis the speech is characteristically scanning in type; there are explosive and staccato elements, with slowness, stumbling, halting, slurring, and ataxia of a cerebellar type. The spacing of the sounds with perceptible pauses between words and irregular accenting of the syllables give the sing-song or scanning character which has been described as pathognomonic of the disorder. In Friedreich's ataxia the ataxic, staccato, and explosive elements predominate. Speech is clumsy, often scanning in type, and the pitch may be suddenly changed in the middle of a sentence.

In alcoholic intoxication the speech is slurred and indistinct. There is difficulty with the labials and linguals and there may be tremulousness of the voice. Furthermore, the conversation is often characterized by a tendency toward garrulousness, and the patient may repeatedly utter words that can be pronounced and enunciated correctly, whereas the use of other words is avoided. This obviously results from loss of cerebral cortical control over thought and resultant word formulation and speech rather than from a primary articulatory disturbance. In delirium tremens the speech is tremulous and slurred. In various toxic states, including intoxications with barbiturates, phenothiazines, benzodiazepines, and bromides, speech is thick and slurred. Severe spasm of the muscles in tetanus may impair speech. A milder disorder of speech occurs in myxedema with a low-pitched, harsh and husky, slow and monotonous voice. Rarely, the inability to relax muscles causes slight impairment of speech in myotonia.

Spastic dysphonia is a disorder characterized by a striking abnormality of voice production. Excess excretory pressure against a tightly constricted laryngeal sphincter causes a choked quality of the voice. This varies during the course of a sentence. It is most marked in stressed vowels. Synkinetic facial and other body movements may occur. The dysphonia frequently is absent when the patient sighs or whispers. It has been suggested that the condition is related to writer's cramp and similar disorders. There is dispute over the extent of the role of psychic influences versus organic disease as the cause of the condition. Some authorities feel it is a focal dystonia. Spastic dysphonia often improves with unilateral section of the recurrent laryngeal nerve. Injection of botulinum toxin is also effective in some cases.

Dyslalia associated with damage to or structural abnormalities of the external speech organs or the articulatory apparatus may be caused by wounds of the lips, tongue, palate, or floor of the mouth; maxillofacial injuries; perforation of the palate; congenital harelip and cleft palate; abnormal shortness of the frenulum of the tongue; enlarged tonsils and adenoids; and dental malalignment. Secondary speech disturbances may also occur without abnormalities or specific dysfunction of the articulatory apparatus. They are seen in individuals with hearing defects, delayed physical development, mental retardation, and psychogenic disturbances. The nature and degree of speech disorders resulting from hearing loss depend largely upon the amount of loss and the individual's ability to cope with it; the disorder may vary from a mild abnormality of articulation to the indistinct and often unintelligible speech of deaf-mutism. A child with slow physical development or psychologic problems may retain childish speech until later years. In delayed puberty and in eunuchism the male voice retains the juvenile or feminine characteristics, while in the virile woman it may be low-pitched and coarse. In mild mental retardation, also, childish speech may be retained. In moderately retarded persons speech may be indistinct and difficult to understand; it is slow and labored, develops late, and the vocabulary is limited. Similar characteristics may be observed in cretinism and Down's syndrome. In the severely retarded speech is babbling and grunting in character, with a tendency toward echolalia.

Emotional and *psychogenic* factors influence articulation. In agitation the speech may be broken and tremulous. In nervous tension it may be high-pitched, uneven, and characterized by breathlessness. In hysterical dysphonia the speech defect may vary in type from time to time. It often is bizarre in character, and does not correspond to any organic impairment and function. Oftentimes there is an abrupt onset of the difficulty with sudden periods of remission. The speech may be rapid and jumbled (tachyphemia or tachylalia), or there may be stuttering, lalling, "baby talk," or mutism. In hysterical aphonia there is imperfect adduction or even paresis of adduction of the vocal cords; even though the speech difficulty is profound, there is no disturbance of coughing or of respiration. In habit spasms, Tourette's syndrome, and obsessive-compulsive states, there may be articulatory tics which are characterized by grunts, groans, or barking sounds. In lingual spasm there is marked difficulty with articulation. **Aphthongia** is a type of anarthria due to spasm of the speech muscles; it occurs in speakers and is similar in nature to writer's cramp, possibly a dystonia. The term **dysphemia** may be used for any type of speech disorder due to psychogenic factors.

In manic states, with psychomotor acceleration, there may be a rapid flow of words, often with an abrupt change of ideas from one subject to another. In depressed states there may be slowing of speech, sometimes with mutism. In schizophrenia there may be hesitancy with blocking, or there may be negativism with resulting mutism, or alalia. Palilalia, echolalia, and perseveration are often psychotic manifestations but can all occur with organic lesions. **Palilalia** is the pathologic repetition of syllables, words, or phrases. **Echolalia** is the meaningless repetition by a patient of the words addressed to him. **Perseveration** is the persistence of one reply or one idea in response to various questions; this may also be observed in certain aphasias. In certain psychotic states patients utter **neologisms,** or new words, usually meaningless, coined by the patient. Some aphasic patients, however, also do this. Alliterative sentences, repetition, and confusion are found in delirious and in psychotic states. **Idioglossia** is imperfect articulation with utterance of meaningless sounds; the individual may speak with a vocabulary of his own. Idioglossia may be observed in patients with partial deafness, aphasia, and congenital word deafness. The term **dyslogia** is used for disorders of speech, or impairment of reasoning power and speech, due to mental disease.

Stuttering is a variety of faltering or interrupted speech characterized by difficulty in enunciating syllables and joining them together. Speech is stumbling and hesitant in character, with habitual and spasmodic repetitions of consonants or syllables, alternating with pauses which interfere with communication. **Stammering** is also a faulty, spasmodic, interrupted speech; there are involuntary hesitations in which the subject is unable to produce the next expected sound. **Cluttering** is characterized by sudden irregular acceleration of speech with shifting of stress and syllable division. Stuttering and stammering are often considered to be synonyms although the term stuttering is more emphatic. Stammering often indicates embarrassment or hesitation. Stuttering indicates a more severe disturbance of articulation. In both the flow of speech is broken by pauses during which articulation is entirely arrested. There may be localized cramps, spasms, and ticlike contractions of the muscles essential to articulation, and these may be accompanied by grimaces, spasms and contractions of the muscles of the head and extremities, and spasm and incoordination of the respiratory muscles. The individual may be unable to pronounce certain consonants, with particular difficulty in using dentals and labials. Often the first syllable or consonant of a word is repeated many times. A failure of coordination between the laryngeal and oral mechanisms of speech and between voice production and respiratory rhythm is evident. There may be spasm of the articulatory apparatus and the individual may remain with his mouth open until the spasm relaxes, when the words rush out in an explosive manner until the breath is gone. He then takes another breath, and the process is repeated. The difficulty is markedly influenced by emotional excitement and by the presence of strangers. In spite of difficulty in speaking, the individual may be able to sing without hesitation.

Many theories have been offered regarding the etiology of stammering and stuttering (or **spasmophemia** as the two are sometimes called) and both organic and psychogenic factors are cited.

In **lalling,** or **lallation,** the utterance is childish or infantile in type; it is characterized by a lack of precision in pronouncing certain consonants, especially the letters r and l. A uvular is substituted for a lingual-palatal r, so that "broken reed" is pronounced "bwoken weed." The diphthong ow or other letters may be substituted for the letter l, or sometimes l may be substituted for r. T and d may be substituted for k, c, s, and g. In **lisping** the sibilants are imperfectly pronounced, and th is substituted for s; a similar defect in articulation may be associated with partial edentulism. Lalling may occur secondary to hearing defects, mental or physical retardation, or psychogenic disorders. If that is not the case, it and lisping are usually due to imperfect adjustment of the organs of articulation (as in children), persistent faulty habits of articulation, imitation of faulty patterns of articulation, poor speech training, habit, or affectation.

BIBLIOGRAPHY

Aronson AE. Psychogenic Voice Disorders. Philadelphia, WB Saunders, 1973

Bicknell JM, Greenhouse HA, Pesch RN. Spastic dysphonia. J Neurol Neurosurg Psychiatry 1968;31:158

Blitzer A, Brin MF, Fahn S et al. Clinical and laboratory characteristics of focal laryngeal dystonia: Study of 110 cases. Laryngoscope 1988;98:636

Brown JR, Simonson J. Organic voice tremor: a tremor of phonation. Neurology 1963;13:520

Darley FL, Aronson AE, Brown JR. Motor Speech Disorders. Philadelphia, WB Saunders, 1975

Darley FL, Brown JR, Goldstein NP. Dysarthria in multiple sclerosis. J Speech Res 1972;15:229

Espir MLE, Rose FC. The Basic Neurology of Speech, 2nd ed. Oxford, Blackwell Scientific Publications, 1976

Greene MC. The Voice and Its Disorders. Philadelphia, JB Lippincott, 1964

Kaplan HM. Anatomy and Physiology of Speech. New York, McGraw – Hill, 1960

Lass NJ, McReynolds LV, Northern JL et al. Handbook of Speech – Language Pathology and Audiology. Toronto, BC Decker, 1988

Schiff HB, Alexander MP, Naeser MA et al. Aphemia. Clinical – anatomic correlations. Arch Neurol 1983;40:720

Whitty CWM. Cortical dysarthria and dysprosody of speech. J Neurol Neurosurg Psychiatry 1964;27:507

PART D
The Motor System

Chapter 20
LEVELS OF MOTOR ACTIVITY

The examination of motor functions involves many factors and is often a complex process. It includes not only the determination of muscle power, but also an evaluation of muscle tone and bulk, a study of coordination and gait, and the observation of abnormalities of movement. Electromyography and the determination of nerve conduction velocities and repetitive nerve stimulations may be needed to obtain additional information about the status of the lower motor neuron, the peripheral nerve, the myoneural junction, and the muscle. All parts of the peripheral and central nervous systems participate in motor activity, and various functional components have to be evaluated individually.

By means of our motor system we move our bodies in space and the various parts of the body in relation to one another. We also maintain postures and attitudes in opposition to gravity and other external forces. All movements, except for those of the viscera and other structures supplied by the autonomic nervous system, are effected by contractions of striated muscles through the control of the nervous system.

The intricate organization of the motor system and its evolutionary development from the simple responses of unicellular organisms to the patterns of behavior of animals and man account for the complexity of motor function. From anatomic and functional standpoints it can be demonstrated that there are certain phylogenetic levels, or stages of development, which increase in intricacy as the phylogenetic scale ascends. In the lower vertebrates all motor activi-

ties are effected through subcortical centers, but with the greater development of the cerebral cortex in higher mammals, some of these functions are significantly altered. The older centers, however, retain their original functions, although they are modified by cortical control. They are not replaced, but are incorporated into an elaborate motor system, subordinate to the cortex. They continue to function as levels of motor activity. They all work together, however, and the efficiency of each depends upon its collaboration with the others. Certain diseases of the nervous system may involve, or predominantly involve, these individual levels; various segments or functional units may be affected while others are spared. In other clinical conditions, however, a complexity of motor phenomena may be encountered, and it may be difficult to separate the actions of different mechanisms which may be affected simultaneously. An understanding of the relationships between certain anatomic structures of the nervous system and their functional activity is necessary for adequate comprehension of disease of the motor system.

The various approaches to the understanding of the different aspects of motor disorders make a clear-cut analysis difficult. Overschematization of syndromes and rigidly ascribing certain symptoms to particular anatomic systems may interfere with knowledge. In order to understand the function of the motor system as a whole, however, and to evaluate the changes in motor activity that occur in disease, one is justi-

281

fied in analyzing first the morphology and function of the constituent parts of the changes in each that result from pathologic processes. Then one can synthesize and correlate their functions. This does not mean that any one part ever acts individually. Each does, however, have its own functions and its changes in disease processes, and an understanding of each part aids in comprehension of motor function as a whole. In this text the description of the individual components is followed by a discussion of the examination of the various motor functions.

THE LEVELS OF MOTOR FUNCTION

There are many varieties of movement; some of them are independent of consciousness, whereas others are directly under the influence of the will. Certain neurologists have referred to the various stages, or levels, of nervous function, and especially of motor function. Hughlings Jackson described the "hierarchy or evolution of the motor centres" and listed three levels of the central nervous system, each sensorimotor and each representing impressions and movements from all parts of the body. The first, or lowest, level consists of the anterior horn cells in the spinal cord and their homologues, the motor nuclei in the brain stem and the sensory input to them; it is that sensorimotor division of the nervous system through which pass nerves to and from every part of the body. It is the lowest level in the evolution of the central nervous system and, in its motor elements, represents the simplest movements of all of the parts of the body. His second, or middle, level was placed in the motor centers of the cerebral cortex, possibly including the basal ganglia. This level mediates more complex movements. He named as his highest motor centers those which have their origin in the prefrontal lobes of the brain — the motor division of the "organ of the mind." This description of the motor system was presented in the nineteenth century and marked one of the early attempts to differentiate various motor functions. It is now known that the motor system is much more complex and that these three divisions are far too limited to allow an understanding of movement.

Orton listed six phylogenetic levels, or stages of development, which are as follows: 1) the stage of direct muscular responses in which there are no nerve responses and the muscles react directly; 2) the asynaptic level in which the nerve filaments go from cell to cell and there is a spread of responses in all directions without polarity; 3) the ganglionated cord, or nerve trunk, level in which there is a pair of dorsally placed nerve trunks, one on each side of the midline; this is found first in Crustacea; 4) the spinal cord level in which there is a fully developed neural axis with nuclei and pathways; this is found in Amphioxus; 5) the midbrain level; 6) the cortical level.

Cobb stated that there are seven levels of motor integration: 1) the neuromuscular, or the final common path along which all impulses from above travel to reach expression in the muscles; 2) the spinal, which is characterized by relatively simple reflexes with little if any postural element; 3) the hindbrain, which involves the simple postural and standing reflexes; 4) the midbrain, which is characterized by more complex standing and righting reflexes; 5) the striatal, where locomotor reflexes and automatic movements originate; 6) the cortical motor, which functions to integrate skilled movements; 7) the cortical associative, which involves such mechanisms as initiative, memory, and symbolization. The cerebellum gives coordination to the first six levels. He refers to the first five as the "old motor system" which is important in man for all automatic locomotor responses. The "new motor system" is found only in the higher forms and reaches its most complete development in man. It works on and through the lower centers.

The evolutionary development of motor function from simple to complex movements is duplicated to a certain extent in the maturation of motor skills in man. At the time of birth simple spinal and brain stem reflexes have already been established, and more complex postural and righting reflexes appear during the first few weeks of life. Then, following the maturation of the cortex and commissural pathways, acts requiring associated sensory functions (grasping and groping) are possible. Still later volitional control of movement appears, and then the ability to perform skilled acts with a high degree of precision.

In order to carry out a discrete movement, the initiation of contraction of the prime mover must be accompanied by graded relaxation or contraction of the antagonists and synergists and by fixation of the more proximal muscles to free the distal ones for use. If the act is to be performed smoothly and accurately, there must be the ability for the movement to be stopped at a given degree of contraction, and either reversed or started again at a degree of contraction necessary to accomplish the desired purpose. Stereotyped and patterned movements, integrated at lower levels, can be used as part of the act. Postures must be assumed that can be modified or shifted easily and instantly for adjustment to the next movement. Throughout all this, the volitional elements and purposive aspects of the act are of paramount importance. Thus, all of the aforementioned levels of motor integration enter into precision of movement.

In the present analysis of the anatomy and physiology of the constituent portions of the motor system, the following useful levels will be discussed: 1) The simplest constituent part to be considered is the spinomuscular level, the motor impulses of which arise in the anterior horn cells of the spinal cord and the motor nuclei of the brain stem and go to the myoneural junctions and then to the individual muscles. Pathologic processes which are situated in the motor nuclei may be considered as diseases of the spinal level; those placed in the motor nerves, as diseases of the neural level; and those which originate at the myoneural junction and within the muscles, as diseases of the neuromuscular and muscular levels. 2) The extrapyramidal level has its nuclei of origin in the basal ganglia and their complex connections. 3) The corticospinal (pyramidal) level has its origin in the motor nuclei of the cerebral cortex. 4) The cerebellar level is the coordinating mechanism. 5) The psychomotor level has to do with memory, initiative, and conscious and unconscious control of motor activity; it corresponds to Jackson's highest level. Discussed with the extrapyramidal level, but considered more in detail with reflex activity, are the hindbrain and midbrain centers which give rise to the vestibulospinal and related pathways (Ch. 37). These are of importance in postural mechanisms and standing and righting reflexes.

It is not suggested that these so-called levels are individual motor systems, or that they in any way act individually or separately. Anatomists continue to have difficulty in even defining the constituents of some of these levels, e.g., the corticospinal or pyramidal versus the basal ganglion or extrapyramidal. These levels are components of the motor system as a whole; each, with its constituent cellular centers, is a part of the complex motor apparatus. Each contributes its share to control of the primary motor neuron on which, as the final common pathway, all efferent pathways converge. Disease of each is characterized by certain signs and symptoms. Many syndromes of motor involvement may, however, embrace more than one of these constituent levels of the motor system, and the newer knowledge of cerebral and motor functions shows an even closer relationship between the individual parts than was formerly suspected. Furthermore, it must always be remembered that all purposive movements are initiated and guided in their performance by a constant stream of afferent impulses that reach the cerebral cortex. Sensory and motor functions are interdependent in the performance of volitional movement, and it is not possible to consider the motor system apart from the sensory system. Impairment of sensation may affect all aspects of motion — volitional, reflex, postural, tonic, and phasic.

BIBLIOGRAPHY

Brodal A. Neurological Anatomy in Relation to Clinical Medicine, 3rd ed. New York, Oxford University Press, 1981

Cobb S. Foundations of Neuropsychiatry, 3rd ed. Baltimore, Williams & Wilkins, 1944

Jackson JH. A contribution to the comparative study of convulsions. In Taylor J (ed). Selected Writings of John Hughlings Jackson. London, Hodder & Stoughton, 1931

Orton ST. Neuropathology. Arch Neurol Psychiatry 1926; 15:763

Chapter 21
THE SPINOMUSCULAR LEVEL

ANATOMY AND PHYSIOLOGY

The structure and function of striated muscles depend upon their connections with the central nervous system. The spinomuscular level of motor integration has, as its primary units, the motor nuclei in the anterior horn cells of the spinal cord and their homologues, the motor nuclei in the midbrain, pons, and medulla. Impulses which originate in these cells are carried through their neuraxes, the peripheral motor nerves, to the motor end-plates of the muscles. Stimulation of the nuclear center causes contraction of the muscle which it supplies. Sherrington, in 1904, described the anterior horn cell, from the point of view of function, as the "final common pathway" through which all nervous impulses from higher centers must pass to reach the myoneural junction and influence striated muscle. The terms **lower motor neuron** and **primary motor neuron** are applied to this structural unit. Inasmuch as clinical symptoms may result from pathologic change in the motor unit, in its neuraxis, or peripheral to the motor unit, either at the neuromuscular junction or in the muscle itself, the spinomuscular level of motor activity is subdivided into spinal, neural, neuromuscular, and muscular components.

The primary functional unit of the spinal level, or of any motor level, is the reflex, or response to a stimulus (discussed further in Part E, "The Reflexes"). The essential unit of the reflex is a center of adjustment, together with the conductors necessary to connect this center with the appropriate receptor and effector apparatus. The receptor is the peripheral sensory ending; the primary conductor is the afferent nerve fiber; the center of adjustment is the motor unit with its associated synapses; the secondary conductor is the efferent nerve fiber, the neuraxis of the motor neuron; the effector is the muscle stimulated. There may be intermediate or interposed association and commissural neurons.

In the spinal level is found one of the most primitive reflex arcs. The impulse is carried from a receptor in the skin, subcutaneous tissue, tendon, or periosteum, through the dorsal root ganglion and into the dorsal horn of the spinal cord, where there is a synapse and the neuron of the second order, or the intercalated neuron, carries the impulse to the anterior horn cell (Fig. 21-1). On stimulation of this center of adjustment the motor impulse is relayed through its neuraxis, which goes by way of the ventral root of the spinal cord and the α-subgroup of the A fibers in the peripheral motor nerve to the motor end-plate of striated muscle, where it stimulates the muscle and causes it to contract. The arrival of the motor impulse at the nerve ending is associated with the liberation of acetylcholine, which causes depolarization of the muscle membrane at the neighboring end-plate. This, in turn, starts a wave of excitation with resulting contraction of the muscle fibers. There is immediate hydrolysis of the acetylcholine by cholinesterase, and the end-plate returns to its former state of polarization so that the next impulse can again cause depolarization and excitation. This normally takes place repeatedly and in rapid succession. Any interruption or break in this reflex arc causes loss of muscle response. Such loss may be caused by any pathologic process that involves the periph-

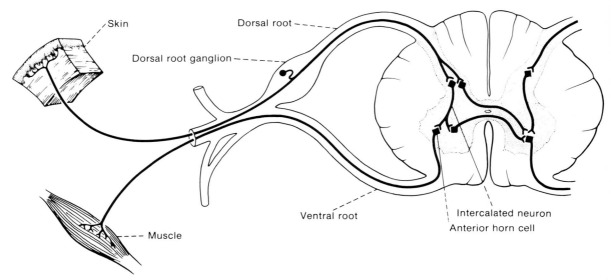

FIG. 21–1. Diagrammatic section through the spinal cord, showing the anterior horn cell and its afferent and efferent connections that make up the simple reflex arc.

eral sense organ, sensory nerve, or dorsal root ganglion; the spinal cord with damage to the synapse, intercalated neuron, or motor neuron; the efferent motor fiber; myoneural junction; or muscle. Disease of the motor neuron, its neuraxis, the myoneural junction, or the muscle causes not only loss of reflex response but also loss of motor function.

The α-motor neuron in the anterior horn of the spinal cord is the terminal neuron of the voluntary motor system. It supplies the main large muscle fibers, and its neuraxis goes directly to the motor end-plate, or neuromuscular junction. One α-motor neuron innervates from less than 50 to 200 or more individual fibers, the number varying in different muscles. (In muscles designed for discrete movement, such as the ocular muscles, the ratio of nerve to muscle fibers is much smaller.) This group of fibers constitutes a **fasciculus;** the anterior horn cell, its neuraxis, and the fasciculus it supplies make up a single **motor unit.** All variations in the force, range, and type of movement are determined by the number and size of motor units called into activity. The γ-motor neurons in the anterior horn area are smaller in diameter than the α-motor neurons and are efferent to small, specialized fibers in the muscle spindles, the **intrafusal** or **fusiform fibers.** These latter in turn act as receptor organs, and stimulation of them causes afferent impulses to be sent to the anterior horns to initiate contraction of the muscle by reflex action of the α-motor neurons, thus producing the muscle stretch reflex. Special interneurons within the dorsal and ventral horns of the spinal cord, including the Renshaw cells which have an inhibitory action on the motor neurons of the anterior horn region, also play a part in the reflex activity of the cord, which is connected by means of synapses with interposed association and commissural neurons and with the higher levels of the nervous system. All motor impulses, whether part of the spinomuscular reflex arc or a part of a higher, more complex arc, are relayed to the muscle through the neuraxes of the anterior horn cells, which are acted upon by the corticospinal, rubrospinal, tectospinal, olivospinal, vestibulospinal, reticulospinal, intersegmental, intrasegmental, and other reflex levels (Fig. 21-2). Through the combined function of these various elements, normal muscular control is made possible. The parts played by the fusiform (γ-efferent) system, which functions to regulate the sensitivity of muscle stretch receptors, and by the inhibitory interneurons, the Renshaw cells, are referred to here but not discussed in detail; these play an important part in the regulation of reflex activity and of tone and posture, but participate little if at all in voluntary motor function. Within the anterior horns there is a somatotopic arrangement of the motor neurons, those innervating the trunk and neck being medial to those of the extremities, and cells innervating distal extremity muscles being dorsal to those of the proximal muscles.

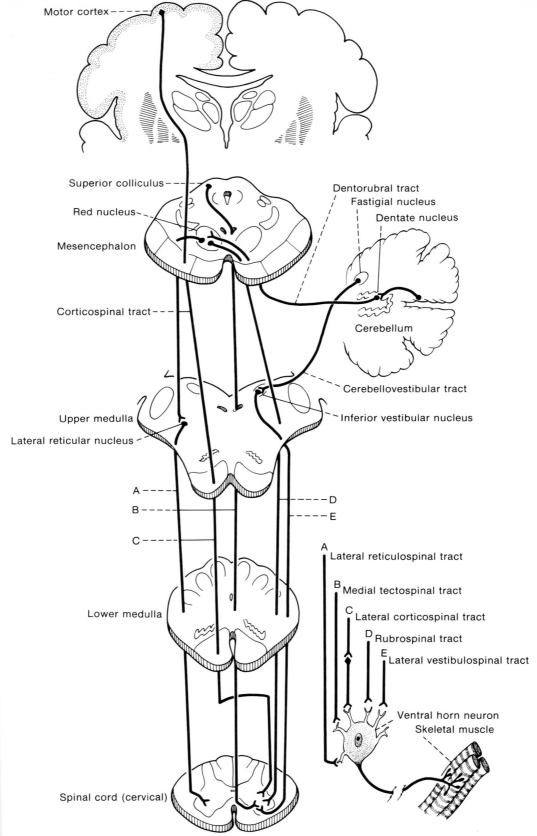

FIG. 21–2. The most important descending pathways that act upon the anterior horn cell of the spinal cord (final common pathway).

The arrangement of motor cells in the anterior horns was originally metameric: those of one segment innervated the muscles of the corresponding myotome. Owing, however, to complexities of development and the intermingling of the motor roots in the plexuses from which the peripheral nerves take origin, one nerve may contain fibers from several roots, and individual muscles may receive nerve impulses from more than one segment of the spinal cord. As a consequence, a disturbance of motor function which is caused by disease of the anterior horn cells may differ in distribution from one which is produced by injury of a peripheral nerve (Part G, "Diagnosis and Localization of Disorders of Peripheral Nerves, Nerve Roots, and Spinal Cord").

A physiologic classification of the various muscles which participate in any simple movement divides these into the following groups: the agonists, or **prime movers (protagonists)**, are the muscles which directly perform the desired movement; they are those whose contraction is essentially responsible for the muscular activity. The **antagonists,** or **moderators,** are those which oppose the agonists; the antagonists must be relaxed in order to have the agonists contract. The **synergists** assist the agonists and reduce unnecessary movement to a minimum; when the agonists have two or more actions and only one of them is required for a certain movement, the contraction of the synergists prevents the undesired action. The **muscles of fixation** bring about stability of the neighboring joints prior to movement in order to afford a firm base for muscular action; they place the parts of the body in a position appropriate for the movement. Thus the flexor carpi ulnaris is an agonist when it flexes and adducts the wrist, an antagonist when it resists passive extension at the wrist, a synergist when the fingers are extended with the wrist in flexion, and a fixator when it contracts to fix the pisiform bone for the action of the abductor digiti quinti. Any movement is dependent upon the combined action of all four groups — the ability of the agonists to contract while the antagonists relax, together with the associated function of the synergists and the fixators. Loss of function of any of these will impair the motor response.

The integrity of the various components of the motor unit may be assessed by electromyography and nerve conduction studies to supplement the clinical findings.

CLINICAL MANIFESTATIONS OF DISEASE OF THE SPINOMUSCULAR LEVEL

Certain specific clinical findings become manifest in disease of the anterior horn cell, its neuraxis (which includes the nerve root, plexus, and peripheral nerve), the myoneural junction, or the muscle itself (Table 21-1). In all, loss of

TABLE 21-1.   Changes in Motor Function

	Loss of Power	Tone	Atrophy	Fascicu-lations	Ataxia
Spinomuscular lesion					
a. Anterior horn cell	Focal	Flaccid	Present	Present	Absent
b. Nerve root, plexus, peripheral nerve	Focal or segmental	Flaccid	Present	Occasionally present	Absent
c. Neuromuscular junction	Diffuse	Usually normal	Usually absent	Absent	Absent
d. Muscle	Diffuse	Flaccid	Present but later than in a. and b.	Absent	Absent
Extrapyramidal lesion	None or mild	Rigid	Absent	Absent	Absent
Corticospinal tract lesion	Generalized Incomplete	Spastic	Absent	Absent	Absent
Cerebellar lesion	None; ataxia may simulate loss of power	Hypotonic (ataxic)	Absent	Absent	Present
Psychogenic disorder	Bizarre No true loss of power May simulate any type	Normal or variable Often increased	Absent	Absent	Absent (may simulate ataxia)

TABLE 21–1. Changes in Motor Function (Continued)

	Reflexes	Abnormal movements	Pathologic associated movements
Spinomuscular lesion			
a. Anterior horn cell	Decreased or absent	None except for fasciculations	Absent
b. Nerve root, plexus, peripheral nerve	Decreased or absent	None except for rare fasciculations	Absent
c. Neuromuscular junction	Usually normal	None	Absent
d. Muscle	Decreased	None	Absent
Extrapyramidal lesion	Muscle stretch reflexes normal or variable Superficial reflexes normal or slightly increased No corticospinal tract responses	Present	Absent
Corticospinal tract lesion	Muscle stretch reflexes hyperactive Superficial reflexes diminished to absent Corticospinal tract responses	None	Present
Cerebellar lesion	Muscle stretch reflexes diminished or pendular Superficial reflexes normal No corticospinal tract responses	May be present (intention tremor and ataxia)	Absent
Psychogenic disorder	Muscle stretch reflexes normal or increased (range) Superficial reflexes normal or increased No corticospinal tract responses	May be present	Absent

motor power is evident. The weakness is focal, or restricted, and is segmental, affecting only the muscles or muscle groups that are supplied by the involved cells or nerves. It is dependent upon and proportional to the number of motor neurons (cells or neuraxes) affected, but there is complete paralysis of the affected muscle fibers. There is a loss of ability to contract the affected muscles voluntarily and in response to stimulation, with weakness of all movements in which the affected muscles play a part. The paralysis is characterized by a loss of tone of the involved muscles; this is called **flaccidity,** or **hypotonicity** (Ch. 28). If the motor neurons are destroyed, all of the muscle fibers supplied by these undergo **atrophy,** or loss of volume (Ch. 29); owing to degeneration of specific fibers or fasciculi, this is focal and is proportional to the degree of fiber loss. With denervation atrophy some 70%–80% of the original muscle mass may be lost within 3 months. With diminution in size, an overgrowth of connective tissue replaces the degenerated fibers. Contractures with resulting deformities may be caused either by contraction of the antagonists whose action is no longer opposed by paralyzed muscles, or by atrophy

and fibrosis of affected muscles. Denervated muscle fibers undergo spontaneous contractions, known as **fibrillations;** these are too fine and rapid to be seen with the naked eye but can be demonstrated electromyographically. Fibrillations are contractions of bundles, or fibrillae, of muscle fibers which usually constitute a unit supplied by a single anterior horn cell (see under "Fasciculations," Ch. 31). Electromyography carried out after the lesion has been present for a sufficient period of time, usually 14–21 days, will show the presence of fibrillations and other signs of denervation. Biopsy and chemical examinations of the muscles will show the presence of histologic and biochemical alterations. Finally there will be a diminution or loss of muscle stretch reflexes in the areas involved (Ch. 33). No pathologic reflexes are found. Trophic changes in the skin, nails, hair, and bone and abnormal vasomotor phenomena may be present. There are no sensory changes if the lesion is restricted to the motor units.

Poliomyelitis may be considered as one of the more characteristic of the disease processes which involve particularly this level of the motor system. It is a disease of the spinal portion of the spinomuscular level. In this disorder, in which the predominant pathologic change is an acute inflammatory process in the anterior horn cells, there develops a flaccid paralysis, as previously described, with focal involvement of certain muscles or muscle groups which is complete for the area involved. This is accompanied sooner or later by atrophy; there is a loss of muscle stretch reflexes without pathologic reflexes. Electrical signs of denervation become apparent. Eventually fibrous change takes place in the involved muscles and at the unused joints, and contractures develop.

Progressive spinal muscular atrophy, both the adult type of Aran – Duchenne and the infantile type of Werdnig – Hoffmann, **progressive bulbar palsy,** and **amyotrophic lateral sclerosis** (Fig. 21-3) are related conditions, sometimes familial, in which the predominant pathologic change is a slow but progressive degeneration of the anterior horn cells and the motor nuclei within the brain stem and their neuraxes, with resulting progressive wasting of muscle tissue. Flaccid paralysis, atrophy, and areflexia are present, but the atrophy is the outstanding manifestation and it precedes the paralysis and areflexia. One of the most characteristic manifestations in this group of disorders is the presence of fasciculations in the affected muscles (Ch. 31). Another type of spinal atro-

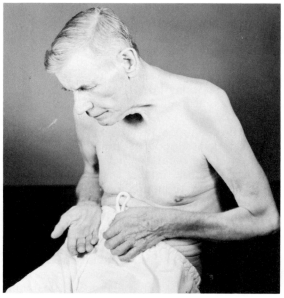

FIG. 21–3. A patient with amyotrophic lateral sclerosis, showing advanced atrophy of the muscles of the hands and shoulders.

phy, usually beginning in childhood, is the **Wohlfart – Kugelberg – Welander syndrome,** which is characterized by slow progression and involvement primarily of proximal rather than distal muscles. Other progressive degenerations of the anterior horn nuclei, such as may occur with syringomyelia and intramedullary neoplasms, also cause atrophy and fasciculations. All these diseases of the anterior horn cell and motor nerve may result ultimately in trophic changes and muscular contractions. **Peroneal muscular atrophy** (progressive neural muscular atrophy or Charcot – Marie – Tooth disease) causes similar changes; here, however, the pathologic alterations are mainly in the peripheral nerves and nerve roots (Fig. 21-4).

Radiculitis, with irritation or disease of the ventral nerve roots, and **peripheral neuritis,** discussed in Chapter 43, with involvement of the motor nerves, cause clinical manifestations that are similar in many respects to those in poliomyelitis. There is a lesion of the neural portion of the spinomuscular level: the disease process is in the neuraxis rather than in the nucleus, although there may be an ascending degeneration that eventually involves the nucleus as well. Owing to impairment of conduction of the motor impulse, there is a flaccid paralysis of certain groups of muscles, with atrophy, signs of denervation, and areflexia. The involvement is limited to those muscles supplied by the specific nerve roots or peripheral nerves affected. Often a radiculitis and usually a neuritis will involve afferent as well as efferent fibers, so sensory changes are often present, and there may be associated pain and hyperesthesia. In the absence of coexisting spinal cord tract involvement, it may be difficult to differentiate clinically between anterior root and anterior horn cell disease; in the absence of sensory changes it may be difficult to differentiate clinically between affections of the peripheral nerve, anterior root, and anterior horn cell. Nerve conduction studies can help to localize blocks in the conduction of impulses along the peripheral nerves. Electromyography and evoked potential studies can also help to differentiate the lesions at various levels of the motor unit.

The pathologic physiology is situated at the myoneural junction in **myasthenia gravis** and the myasthenic syndrome of Eaton – Lambert. In myasthenia gravis there is impairment of conduction of the motor impulse at the myoneural junction of striated muscles due to destruction of acetylcholine receptors. In the myasthenic syndrome there is inadequate release of quanta of

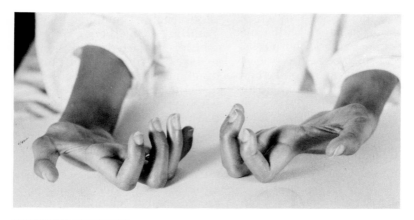

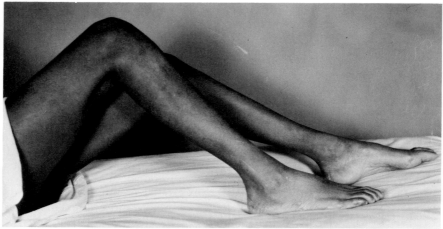

FIG. 21–4. A patient with Charcot–Marie–Tooth disease (peroneal muscular atrophy), showing wasting of distal muscles and contractures of the hands and feet.

acetylcholine at the motor end-plate. Both disorders are characterized by fatigability of muscles, which is followed by weakness and may result in pseudoparalysis or even true flaccid paralysis. Atrophy and areflexia are usually absent but may occur if muscles are severely affected. Tests of strength show increasing fatigability as maneuvers are repeated. Electrical tests also show muscle fatigue but repetitive nerve stimulation with electromyographic recording can usually differentiate myasthenia gravis from the myasthenic syndrome. Myasthenia gravis is temporarily relieved with anticholinesterase drugs, whereas guanidine may improve the symptoms of the myasthenic syndrome.

Familial periodic paralysis is a disease of the myoneural junction and muscle; there are recurring attacks of flaccid paralysis with areflexia. The symptoms come on abruptly and may last from a few hours to 3 or 4 days. There is a fall in

the potassium content of the blood during attacks, and the symptoms are often relieved by the administration of this ion. In certain cases, at least, the syndrome is related to intermittent aldosteronism. There is retention of sodium shortly preceding an attack, which brings about a drop in potassium at the time of the onset of symptoms; the paralysis may be prevented by decreasing sodium intake. Disturbances of carbohydrate and thiamine metabolism may be present. The periodic paralysis that occurs in association with hyperthyroidism is also characterized by hypokalemia. In addition, muscle weakness due to hypokalemia may occur secondary to either urinary (renal tubular necrosis) or gastrointestinal (severe or chronic diarrhea) loss of potassium, or due to chelation of potassium by certain chemicals.

A hyperkalemic variety of familial periodic paralysis has been described — so-called **hered-**

itary episodic adynamia of Gamstorp. The attacks develop during a period of rest after activity, and there is an increase in serum potassium during attacks; they may also be provoked by the administration of potassium. Myotonia is a symptom in some cases. A third, or normokalemic, type has been reported; this type is worsened by the administration of potassium and treated by the use of sodium. The muscle weakness of Addison's disease may be secondary to hyperkalemia, or there may be variations in muscle strength and muscular excitability resulting from alterations in body electrolytes, with a fall and a rise of intracellular and extracellular sodium and potassium as significant factors.

Other abnormalities of electrolytes and metabolism as well as the action of various drugs and toxins may cause paralysis and other evidence of motor dysfunction by their effect on the neuromuscular junction. Muscular activity is accompanied by an exchange of sodium and potassium across the cell membrane, and potassium can also excite muscular contraction by causing depolarization; consequently, abnormalities in both potassium and sodium metabolism may alter function. Increased aldosterone production causes retention of sodium with a resulting deficiency of potassium, which leads to a periodic muscular weakness as well as tetany. With calcium deficiency there is heightened sensitivity of the motor end-plate, causing a lowered threshold of muscle to both stimulation and acetylcholine. Magnesium in high concentrations causes neuromuscular depression, blocking contraction by a curarelike effect; a deficiency of magnesium results in weakness, tremors, and tetany. Curare and tubocurarine raise the threshold of the motor end-plate to acetylcholine and thus prevent depolarization by acetylcholine. Decamethonium and succinylcholine cause depolarization; after a brief initial stimulation a neuromuscular block occurs, and the muscle no longer responds. Organic phosphates cause paralysis both by central action and by irreversible inhibition of cholinesterase. Botulinum toxin causes paralysis of muscle by inadequate synthesis or release of acetylcholine. The bites of certain ticks, snakes, spiders, and marine organisms, and the toxin of some mushrooms also cause paralysis at the neuromuscular junction, but the exact mode of action is incompletely understood.

Descending the spinomuscular level, there are many diseases which primarily affect the muscle itself. They may be characterized by a flaccid weakness similar to that seen in disorders of the motor nucleus and its neuraxis, but there is no areflexia until after extensive atrophy has occurred. The most characteristic diseases of this group are the **myopathies,** which include pseudohypertrophic muscular dystrophy of Duchenne, the facioscapulohumeral type of Landouzy – Dejerine, scapulohumeral dystrophy, other less common familial dystrophies, distal myopathy of Gowers and Spiller, and the several varieties of congenital myopathy. In the myopathies the anterior horn cells and the nerve trunks remain intact, but degeneration of the muscle fibers, often with replacement by connective tissue and fat, causes loss of contractility without loss of excitability (Fig. 21-5). The pathophysiology of many of these disorders remains to be explained; because of heritable patterns, it is probable that a basic biochemical defect is present. Some forms of hereditary myopathy, notably Duchenne dystrophy, relate to specific chromosomal defects. Duchenne dystrophy is x-linked, with an absence of the protein, dystrophin. Amyotonia congenita, or Oppenheim's disease, is generally considered to be a type of myopathy, although changes have been reported in the motor nuclei of the spinal cord or in the motor cortex. Related to amyotonia congenita but definitely of myopathic origin are the syndromes of congenital hypoplasia of muscle, benign congenital hypotonia, and the congenital nonprogressive myopathies. Congenital aplasia or nondevelopment of muscles, focal or generalized, represents another form of myopathy. Several of the glycogen storage diseases have associated myopathies; for example, myophosphorylase deficiency (McArdle's disease) presents with cramps, pain, and weakness of muscles after exercise. Some of the mitochondrial disorders, such as the Kearns – Sayre syndrome and carnitine deficiency, also present as myopathies.

Motor changes of muscular origin may also be found in the various types of **myositis,** such as polymyositis, dermatomyositis, fibromyositis, trichinosis, polyarteritis nodosa, myositis ossificans, rheumatic myositis, vascular myosclerosis, ischemic myositis (Volkmann's contracture), thyrotoxic, carcinomatous, steroid and other medication-induced myopathies, and localized panatrophy, as well as in other types of muscular dysfunction. In these, all of which are muscular disorders, there is no involvement of the motor neuron or its neuraxis. There is a flaccid loss of power with focal involvement of certain muscles or groups of muscles. This may result in atrophy and areflexia. In myotonia and myotonic dystro-

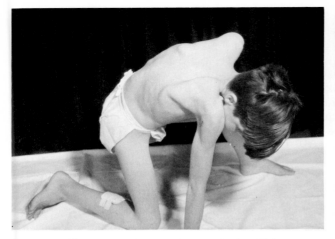

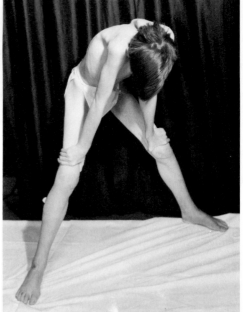

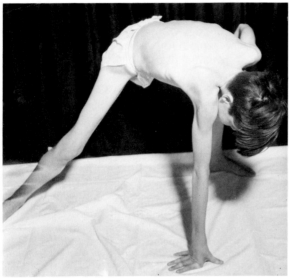

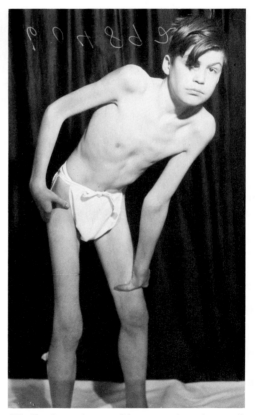

phy, as well as in paramyotonia and occasionally in myxedema, there is a delayed relaxation of muscles with a myotonic electrical response. In myotonic dystrophy there is muscular atrophy as well as myotonia. Electromyography, muscle biopsy, and enzyme studies are important procedures in the diagnosis of the myopathies, both primary and secondary, and in the differentiation of them from the muscle atrophies of neural and anterior horn cell origin.

Diseases of the sensory portion of the reflex arc, which include the sensory neuropathies and radiculopathies, are discussed in Chapters 43 and 44. It must be recalled that in such conditions there is areflexia and there may be decreased muscle tone, but if the anterior horn cell or its neuraxis is not involved there is no paralysis and no atrophy. Certain lesions of the afferent system, however, especially if they affect dorsal nerve roots, posterior columns, or the pa-

FIG. 21–5. A patient with muscular dystrophy, showing wasting of the musculature in the shoulders and thighs; weakness and atrophy of the glutei cause difficulty in assuming the erect position, and the patient "climbs up on his thighs" (Gowers' maneuver) in order to stand erect.

rietal cortex, may cause impairment of voluntary motor function and interference with purposeful movement.

BIBLIOGRAPHY

Adams RD, Victor M. Principles of Neurology, 4th ed. New York, McGraw – Hill, 1989

Adrian ED. General principles of nervous activity. Brain 1947;70:1

Brodal A. Neurological Anatomy in Relation to Clinical Medicine, 3rd ed. New York, Oxford University Press, 1981

Dale H. The physiological basis of neuromuscular disorders. Br Med J 1948;2:889

Dyck PJ, Thomas PK, Lambert EH et al. Peripheral Neuropathy, 2nd ed. Philadelphia, WB Saunders, 1984

Gamstorp I. Adynamia episodica hereditaria. Acta Paediatr Scand 1956;Suppl 45, 108:1

Johnson EW (ed). Practical Electromyography, 2nd ed. Baltimore, Williams & Wilkins, 1988

Kakulas BA, Adams RD. Diseases of Muscles, 4th ed. Philadelphia, Harper & Row, 1985

McArdle B. Myopathy due to a defect in muscle glycogen breakdown. Clin Sci 1951;10:13

Riker WF Jr. Some aspects of the pharmacology of neuromuscular function. Am J Med 1953;15:231

Rowland LP, ed. Merritt's Textbook of Neurology, 8th ed. Philadelphia, Lea & Febiger, 1989

Sherrington CS. The Integrative Action of the Nervous System. New York, Scribner's, 1906

Walton J (ed). Disorders of Voluntary Muscle, 5th ed. Edinburgh, Churchill Livingstone, 1988

Chapter 22
THE EXTRAPYRAMIDAL LEVEL

The extrapyramidal level is discussed before the pyramidal (or corticospinal/corticobulbar) level because it is phylogenetically more primitive. It has been referred to as the most highly developed portion of the "old motor system." The extrapyramidal system, however, should not be regarded as an anatomic or physiologic entity; it is, instead, a functional concept, and our understanding of it has been derived mainly from clinicopathologic data on diseases characterized by disturbances of tone, movement, and/or posture. While its major or best known centers are in the basal ganglia, other important areas described subsequently are functionally related, and it is closely allied with centers of motor integration in the brain stem, especially with the midbrain and vestibular components that are important in the regulation of tone, in primitive postural and righting reflexes, and in facilitation and inhibition of motor responses. It is also intimately connected with those portions of the cerebral cortex which have to do with motor control.

According to Fulton and Kennard, the term *extrapyramidal* should embrace all the nonpyramidal projection systems. Such a division of the projection systems is clearly useful since it allows separation of the voluntary corticospinal or pyramidal pathway from the other motor systems which have to do primarily with postural and other involuntary adjustments. The extrapyramidal system clinically is generally considered to comprise only the **motor** functions of the basal ganglia. However, anatomists disagree as to what should be properly included in the extrapyramidal system, and some decry the con-tinued use of the term. The concept of an extrapyramidal level, however, continues to be clinically useful. The extrapyramidal level is not an independent neural mechanism nor a single unitary system, but a group of complex neural organizations which, while not directly concerned with the production of voluntary movement, are closely integrated with other levels of the motor system for the control of muscular activity. Although the cerebellum would be included in this use of the term extrapyramidal, for practical clinical purposes cerebellar functions are usually considered separately because of the marked variance in clinical manifestations of lesions of the cerebellum and its pathways and those of the basal ganglia and their connections.

ANATOMY AND PHYSIOLOGY

The extrapyramidal phase of motor activity has also been referred to as the **basal ganglion, striatal, pallidal,** or **thalamopallidal level.** It cannot, however, be separated functionally from related centers in the brain stem or from important connections with the cerebral cortex. Phylogenetically and ontogenetically the basal ganglia comprise the oldest portion of the cerebrum. They reach a high state of development in birds.

The basal ganglia which contribute most extensively to the extrapyramidal system are the caudate and lenticular nuclei. These structures lie deep in the substance of the cerebral hemispheres between the lateral ventricle and the insula (Fig. 22-1). The caudate nucleus is a pear-shaped mass of gray matter. Its head is on the

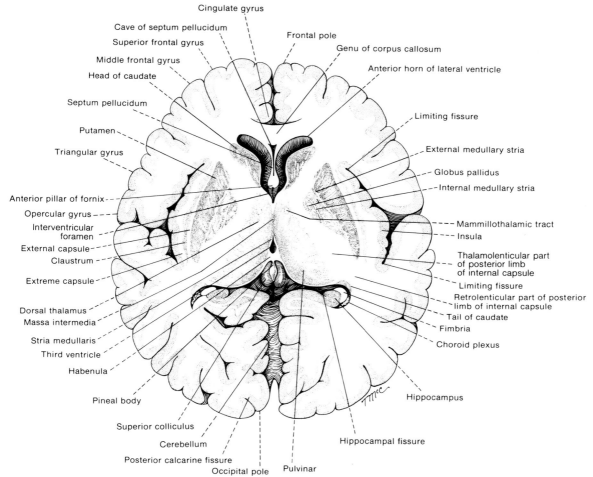

Cingulate gyrus
Cave of septum pellucidum
Superior frontal gyrus
Middle frontal gyrus
Head of caudate
Septum pellucidum
Putamen
Triangular gyrus
Anterior pillar of fornix
Opercular gyrus
Interventricular foramen
External capsule
Claustrum
Extreme capsule
Dorsal thalamus
Massa intermedia
Stria medullaris
Third ventricle
Habenula
Pineal body
Superior colliculus
Cerebellum
Posterior calcarine fissure
Occipital pole

Frontal pole
Genu of corpus callosum
Anterior horn of lateral ventricle
Limiting fissure
External medullary stria
Globus pallidus
Internal medullary stria
Mammillothalamic tract
Insula
Thalamolenticular part of posterior limb of internal capsule
Limiting fissure
Retrolenticular part of posterior limb of internal capsule
Tail of caudate
Fimbria
Choroid plexus
Hippocampus
Hippocampal fissure
Pulvinar

FIG. 22–1. *Drawing of the superior surface of an unstained horizontal section of the adult human brain, through the internal capsule, basal ganglia, and thalamus.*

lateral side of the anterior horn of the lateral ventricle, into which it bulges, and its tail runs backward in the floor of the ventricle and then downward and forward in the roof of the descending horn. The lenticular, or lentiform, nucleus, is composed of the putamen and globus pallidus. The former, which makes up the outer segment of the nucleus, is separated from the insula by a narrow zone of gray matter, the claustrum, and by the external capsule. The caudate nucleus is continuous with it, and histologically the two structures are identical; they contain a few large (Golgi type I) and many small (Golgi type II) ganglion cells. The globus pallidus is medial to the putamen and is separated from the thalamus and the caudate nucleus by the internal capsule. It is divided into a

lateral and medial zone, and contains only large ganglion cells.

The nomenclature of these nuclei varies. The caudate and putamen are frequently referred to as the striatum, in contrast to the globus pallidus, or pallidum. Sometimes all three are classed as parts of the striatum, and the caudate and putamen are called the neostriatum, whereas the globus pallidus is the archi- or paleostriatum. Two structures classed as basal ganglia on an anatomic basis, the claustrum and the amygdaloid nucleus, are not functionally related to these structures, and are usually not considered to be parts of the extrapyramidal system.

Other structures, however, are functionally and clinically related to the basal ganglia and must be considered parts of the extrapyramidal motor system. The subthalamic nucleus or corpus Luysii is a small, lens-shaped gray mass situated in the ventral thalamus just dorsal to the cerebral peduncle (Fig. 22-2). The red nucleus is located in the tegmentum of the midbrain at the level of the anterior quadrigeminal bodies. It contains both large and small cells. The substantia nigra is a gray mass that lies between the cerebral peduncle and the tegmentum of the midbrain, also at the level of the anterior quadrigeminal bodies. It is composed of two parts, the zona compacta that contains large melanin-bearing ganglion cells, and the zona reticulata that contains nonpigmented, spindle-shaped ganglion cells. The lateral and medial nuclear groups of the reticular formation are situated in the tegmentum of the midbrain, and other constituents of the reticular formation that either inhibit or facilitate motor responses are placed caudally in the brain stem.

The inferior olivary nucleus is located in the medulla. The dentate nucleus and possibly the other nuclei of the cerebellum, the zona incerta, the vestibular nuclei, the interpeduncular nucleus, the tegmental nuclei, the nucleus of the posterior commissure (Darkshevich's nucleus), the interstitial nucleus (Cajal's), and the gray matter of the quadrigeminal plate are intimately associated with the basal ganglia. All these are in close approximation to the thalamus, which is not only the sensory reception center for both the basal ganglia and the cortex but also receives fibers from and relays impulses to most of the aforementioned structures as well as the cerebral cortex.

The basal ganglia have rich connections with one another and with brain stem structures, as well as with certain areas of the cerebral cortex and with lower centers (Fig. 22-3). The caudate nucleus receives projections from the frontal

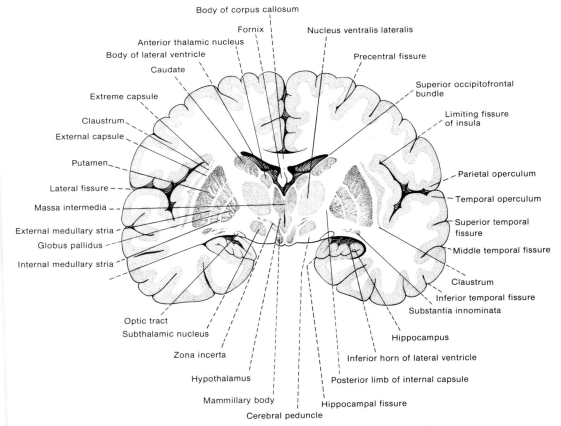

FIG. 22–2. Drawing of the posterior surface of an unstained coronal section of the adult human brain, through the posterior limb of the internal capsule, basal ganglia, and mammillary bodies.

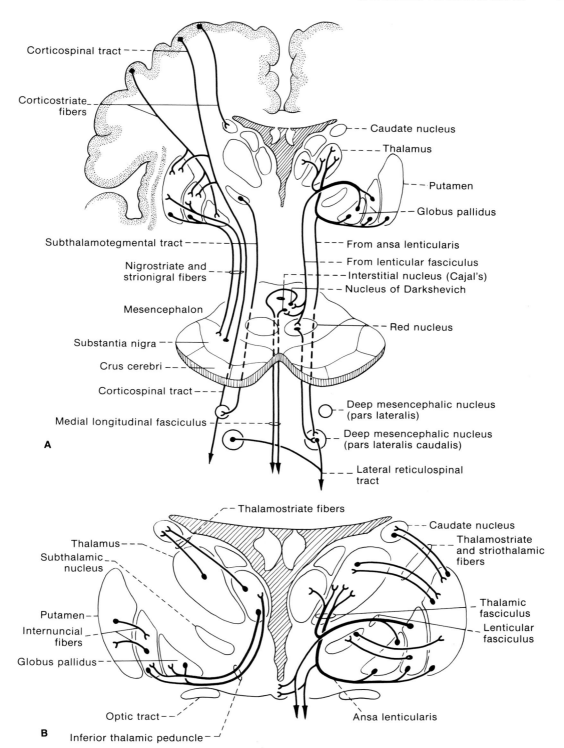

FIG. 22–3. A. Principal connections of the basal ganglia. The thalamocortical portions of the loops (cortex–basal ganglia–thalamus–cortex) are omitted. **B.** Detail giving connections between the basal ganglia and thalamus.

cortex, principally from Brodmann's areas 4s and 8, and possibly from area 4 through collaterals from the corticospinal neurons, and from areas 2, 6, and 9 (see Fig. 23-1). It also receives fibers from the nuclei medialis dorsalis and ventralis anterior of the thalamus (thalamostriate fibers) and from the putamen, and sends fibers to the thalamus (striothalamic fibers) and to the putamen and globus pallidus. The small cells of the caudate nucleus are receptor in function, and are believed to give rise to the internuncial fibers that make up short association pathways with the other basal ganglia and terminate in the putamen and globus pallidus. The large cells are efferent in function and send impulses to the globus pallidus and possibly also to the subthalamic nucleus, red nucleus, and substantia nigra.

The connections of the putamen are similar; it receives fibers from cortical areas 4 and 6 and from the thalamus, and has a large connection with the caudate. It also receives fibers from the subthalamic nucleus (subthalamic fasciculus of Forel) and from the substantia nigra (comb bundle). It communicates directly with the globus pallidus, although the large cells may project as do those of the caudate. Some fibers may enter the ansa lenticularis.

The globus pallidus receives impulses from the nuclei medialis dorsalis and ventralis anterior of the thalamus, through thalamostriate fibers and the inferior thalamic peduncle, and from area 6 of the cerebral cortex and possibly from area 4 through collaterals from the corticospinal neurons. Its principal afferent innervation, however, is from the caudate and putamen. There are internuncial fibers within the ganglion. Its efferent pathways are numerous and important. The lenticular fasciculus of Forel (H_2 bundle), which emerges from the dorsal surface of the globus pallidus, is distributed to the hypothalamus, the nucleus of the posterior commissure, the interstitial nucleus, the red nucleus, and the tegmentum dorsal and lateral to the rostral end of the red nucleus (deep mesencephalic nucleus, pars dorsalis and pars lateralis). The thalamic fasciculus (of Forel) carries fibers to the nucleus ventralis anterior of the thalamus and probably also conveys thalamopallidal fibers. The ansa lenticularis, which emerges from the ventral surface of the globus pallidus (and also putamen), carries fibers to the hypothalamus and to the reticular formation and tegmental nuclei (deep mesencephalic nucleus, pars ventralis, pars lateralis, and pars lateralis caudalis). The subthalamic fasciculus

(of Forel) conveys fibers to and from the subthalamic nucleus. The inferior thalamic peduncle carries efferent as well as afferent fibers. The globus pallidus also sends impulses to and receives them from the substantia nigra, and sends impulses to the inferior olivary nucleus. Those to this latter structure arise through synapses in the field of Forel and descend in the thalamoolivary tract; there are further synapses in the tegmental region.

The subthalamic nucleus receives impulses from the globus pallidus and probably the striatum and sends impulses to the globus pallidus and putamen through the subthalamic fasciculus of Forel, and to the thalamus. It communicates with the tegmentum of the midbrain (deep mesencephalic nucleus, pars lateralis) through the subthalamotegmental tract, and with the contralateral subthalamic nucleus through the supramammillary decussation of Forel. Connections with area 6 of the cerebral cortex have been described, and those with the red nucleus and substantia nigra have been hypothesized. The red nucleus receives impulses directly from area 4 of the frontal cortex as well as from the globus pallidus, the contralateral dentate nucleus, and possibly the caudate and putamen. Its large cells give rise to the rubrobulbar and rubrospinal tracts that cross in the decussation of Forel and descend; the latter course through the brain stem into the cervical portion of the spinal cord. The rubroreticular and rubroolivary fibers from the small celled portion make up important discharge pathways; impulses relayed through them are carried down by the reticulobulbar, reticulospinal, and olivospinal tracts. In man the discharge through the rubroreticulospinal pathways is more important than that through the rubrospinal tracts. The red nucleus also sends efferent impulses to the nucleus ventralis lateralis of the thalamus, the frontal cortex, the basal ganglia, the contralateral dentate nucleus, the motor nuclei of the brain stem, and possibly the substantia nigra. The substantia nigra receives a small communication from the globus pallidus (and possibly the putamen) and also receives fibers from the tegmental nuclei and possibly from the red nucleus and subthalamic nucleus. Its efferent impulses go to the globus pallidus and putamen through the comb bundle, and also to the tegmental nuclei. Cortical connections with areas 6, 8, 4s, and 4 have been described.

The basal ganglia and related centers may be considered to have their own reflex arc. Afferent impulses, which ascend through various pathways to the thalamus, go after synapse to the caudate and then to the putamen and globus pallidus. These structures also receive afferent impulses from the frontal cortex. Internuncial fibers connect the nuclear masses. Efferent or effector fibers go from the caudate to the putamen and globus pallidus and from the putamen to the globus pallidus. Striofugal fibers go via the ansa lenticularis and related pathways to the thalamus, hypothalamus, subthalamic nucleus, red nucleus, and substantia nigra, and also to the reticular formation and other lower centers and then, through the rubrospinal, reticulospinal, olivospinal, tectospinal, and the questionable nigrospinal and subthalamicospinal and other descending pathways, to the anterior horn cells, where they synapse. The impulses are then carried along the final common pathway to the individual muscles. Impulses that descend through these tracts may either facilitate or inhibit motor activity and influence the normal balance between the α- and γ-motor systems.

The basal ganglia and the related structures constitute an important efferent system. Their discharges, however, are indirect and take place by way of relays. The extrapyramidal cortex and the basal ganglia discharge to the midbrain nuclei, the red nucleus, tegmentum, and substantia nigra in part, and these latter structures in turn discharge to the brain stem and spinal cord. The tegmentum is an important internode in the discharge of the basal ganglia to lower levels and an important efferent correlation center in which there is an interplay of striatal and cerebellar functioning with a conditioning cortical component.

The connections of the basal ganglia and related structures may represent the original avenues for impulses from higher to lower portions of the nervous system, and pathways from the cortex to the spinal cord, at first indirect, have been short-circuited in the mammal through the evolution of the direct corticospinal system. However, there is a close functional relationship between the cortex, both pyramidal and extrapyramidal, and the basal ganglia, and between the cerebellum, thalamus, and brain stem structures and the basal ganglia. It may not be possible to consider disease of one part of this system complex and overlook the others. Even in disease restricted to the basal ganglia there may be disturbance of cortical, cerebellar, thalamic, and brain stem functions.

With few exceptions the so-called extrapyramidal syndromes are peculiar to man, and because of the failure to produce disturbances in experimental animals sufficiently akin to those of human disease, there is still a lack of clear understanding of the functions and pathophysiology of the structures that are believed to constitute the extrapyramidal level. Consequently, our assumptions regarding the effects of disease of these structures are largely hypothetical. It was believed for many years that the principal functions of the striatum and the pallidum had to do with tone, especially in taking and maintaining postures, and with the control of automatic locomotor reflexes. These structures form a postural background against which voluntary movements are executed, although they are incapable of initiating such movements. They appear to act by programming complex automatic movements. In the lower forms they are also important in movements of flight, fright, defense, and self-protection, as well as in synergistic control. Mammals with the cerebral cortex removed but with the basal ganglia intact can walk, run, and even jump in an effective though automatic manner. However, they lack initiative, spontaneity, and memory. They have few and rudimentary conditioned reflexes, and cannot react in the light of past experience.

There is still much to be learned regarding the specific functions of the individual structures of the extrapyramidal level. Their relationships to each other and to the symptoms which appear in pathologic conditions will be discussed under the clinical manifestations of extrapyramidal disease. There may be various combinations of lesions in which one or another of the nuclear masses may predominate. Some clinical conditions may cause either paralytic or release phenomena consequent to destruction, while others may be irritative and excitatory in nature, and it is often impossible to differentiate the two, or they may coexist. The localization of function in the extrapyramidal system is not as discrete as in the cerebral cortex and, therefore, syndromes produced by disease are often general. However, a degree of localization exists and it is not uncommon to see disorders of this system affecting one extremity or one side of the body more than the other.

PATHOLOGIC PHYSIOLOGY

The pathologic physiology responsible for the motor abnormalities that are associated with disease of the extrapyramidal system has not as yet been fully explained. Much progress has been made in recent years in defining various neurotransmitters, their types of receptors, and systems using the several types. A discussion of these is beyond the scope of this text; however, disturbances in these substances and modalities have influenced our concepts of extrapyramidal diseases, especially Parkinson's disease and the choreas, and promise further understanding. Brief mention of some of these derangements is made with the discussion of the individual diseases later; details are found in neurology and neuropharmacology texts.

The earlier theories concerning extrapyramidal motor abnormalities were based principally on clinical and pathologic studies, and concepts that varied widely were presented. Although Parkinson's disease, perhaps the most characteristic of the extrapyramidal syndromes, was first described in 1817, no anatomic or physiologic basis for the syndrome was suggested. Gowers (1888), Omerod (1890), Anton (1895), and Jelgersma (1909) noted changes in the basal ganglia in chorea, athetosis, and Parkinson's disease, but the first adequate descriptions of the relationship of neurologic symptoms to lesions of the basal ganglia were made in 1911 and 1912 by Alzheimer, Vogt, Wilson, and Lewy. Cecile Vogt demonstrated the involvement of the caudate and putamen in athetosis, and Wilson, in his description of progressive lenticular degeneration (now called hepatolenticular degeneration or Wilson's disease), further clarified the knowledge regarding the functions of the basal ganglia. The epidemic of encephalitis that occurred from 1917 to 1922 brought about detailed demonstrations of lesions of the basal ganglia and the brain stem, although physiologic mechanisms were not explained.

Symptoms of extrapyramidal dysfunction are more apt to occur with mild, diffuse damage to the basal ganglia and related structures than with large circumscribed lesions of any one portion. Neoplasms affecting these structures, for instance, only rarely cause the motor manifestations of extrapyramidal diseases, and it has been observed that tumors characterized by hyperkinesias and abnormalities of tone and posture are usually primarily in parts of the brain other than the so-called extrapyramidal structures. It appears that the symptoms of extrapyramidal disease result from partial rather than complete destruction of the basal ganglia, and they may be produced by slowly degenerating neural lesions capable of producing abnormal discharges; such symptoms often make their appearance long periods of time after an infection or injury. With most diseases of the basal ganglia there are widespread lesions that also involve other areas of the brain, and the lesions may vary from case to case. Furthermore, there is a difference in the manifestations associated with disorders involving the same structures: there may be a resting tremor with rigidity in one case, and choreiform or athetoid movements in another. Most neurologists have been of the opinion that both disturbances in tone and involuntary movements represent either 1) the release of relatively healthy, undamaged efferent neural pathways from the controlling or inhibitory influence of specific nuclear areas, or 2) the disordered function of intact neural structures when their connections with other areas have been interrupted. It may be, however, that abnormal discharges from degenerating neurons are responsible, or imbalance between damaged and intact neural structures with consequent relative excess or deficiency of one or more neurotransmitters. There is no unanimity of opinion regarding either the exact pathophysiology or the nature or exact location of the responsible pathologic changes.

An intimate relationship exists between the functions of certain portions of the cerebral cortex and those of the basal ganglia, and it may be that the activities of the latter are seldom independent of those of the former. Several feedback loops, long and short, go from the cortex to the basal ganglia and back; disturbances of these pathways may trigger various extrapyramidal signs and symptoms. Areas 6 and 4 of the frontal cortex both have direct connections with the extrapyramidal system, and the same may also be true for the so-called suppressor areas (4s, 8, and others), although certain concepts concerning the cortical suppression system and indeed the existence of specific suppressor areas have been questioned. Furthermore, there is a close integration with important midbrain and hindbrain structures. Higher motor centers discharge into and through the reticular formation in the midbrain, pons, and medulla. The ventromedial portion of the medullary reticular formation receives impulses from the cortex and cerebellum and from the basal ganglia by relays, and in turn discharges to the spinal cord; it has an inhibitory effect on lower motor nuclei, and tends to suppress motor activity.

The excitatory mechanism is located in the dorsolateral portion of the medulla and in the reticular formation of the midbrain and pons; this, too, receives impulses from the cortex, cerebellum, and basal ganglia, and facilitates motor responses. These centers, especially those concerned with facilitation, are closely linked with the vestibular system, which plays an important part in the regulation of tone and simple postural and righting reflexes, and in the control of balance between the α- and γ-motor systems. Normally there is an equilibrium between the activities of the suppressor and facilitatory mechanisms and between α- and γ-control, and adjustment between them is necessary for phasic movement and postural activity. When this balance is upset by disease processes or experimentally produced lesions, involving those centers themselves or structures or pathways discharging to them, abnormalities of tone, movement, or posture may appear.

As a consequence, disturbances in tone as well as hyperkinesias and other abnormalities of movement may result from many different alterations of either structure or function. Rigidity, which may result from an abnormal bombardment of the myoneural outflow, may be caused by pallidal lesions that interrupt the normal inhibitory effect of the pallidum on lower reflex arcs, impairment of conduction of impulses from the cortex to the pallidum and other basal ganglia, combined extrapyramidal and pyramidal involvement at capsular levels, interruption of pallidofugal fibers, release of lower centers from vestibular control, impairment of function of suppressor areas, or stimulation of facilitatory centers. Hyperkinesias of various types may be caused by imbalance of the reciprocal innervation between cortical and extrapyramidal centers; interruption at any site of the complex circuitous pathway between the cortex, basal ganglia, lower extrapyramidal centers, cerebellum, thalamus, and cortex; disease of any of the structures entering into this circuit; abnormal rhythmic activity of the reticular formation when it is released from control by a higher center through lesions at mesencephalic or pontine levels; or alteration of the normal balance between the α- and γ-motor systems. Hypokinesia, bradykinesia, and loss of associated movements may be the result of rigidity alone, depending upon the extent or severity of pathologic change; it may be, however, that widespread extrapyramidal involvement interferes with the initiation of or the conduction of impulses for simple automatic activities and movements of association and expression.

CLINICAL MANIFESTATIONS OF DISEASES OF THE EXTRAPYRAMIDAL LEVEL

Information regarding the functions of the basal ganglia and related extrapyramidal structures has been determined more on clinical than on experimental evidence. Diseases of the basal ganglia are common and they comprise some of the more important neurologic entities. Knowledge, however, of the pathologic change responsible for these diseases is fairly recent and is still incomplete.

Disease of the extrapyramidal system is usually chronic and of gradual onset unless due to anoxia, drugs, or toxins. It is manifested by one or more of three principal motor abnormalities: disturbance in tone, derangement of movement, and loss of associated or automatic movements. The disturbance in tone usually takes the form of hypertonicity or rigidity, often "cogwheel" in type (see "Hypertonicity" in Ch. 28). All muscles are affected, and often the muscles of the neck and trunk and the flexors of the extremities are most involved. The derangement of movement is usually a hyperkinesia, which may be patterned or nonpatterned, and may take the form of a tremor or of choreiform, athetoid, dystonic, or other movements described further in Chapter 31. These are independent of voluntary motion and usually disappear during sleep. Often, however, particularly in parkinsonism, there is a decrease in motor activity; this may be manifested by **hypokinesia,** or poverty of movement, **bradykinesia,** or loss of speed and spontaneity of movement, or even **akinesia,** severe deficiency of movement. There is only rarely, however, a severe loss of power or a paralysis, and movements of a volitional or semivolitional character persist unless there is associated corticospinal tract disease. The loss of associated, or automatic, physiologic and expressive movements may give rise to abnormal postures, masklike facial expression, and infrequent blinking. It is probably intimately associated with the disturbances of tone and muscular activity.

In addition to these motor phenomena, there may be emotional changes and mental symptoms of various types — namely, exaggerated responses of anger or pleasure with unmotivated or spontaneous laughing and crying; compulsions, obsessions, depression, or irritability; slowness of thought processes; and manifestations of intellectual deterioration that lead to complete dementia in certain instances. Sensory symptoms are almost never seen unless there is associated involvement of the thalamus or of the sensory pathways. There are no characteristic reflex changes and no pathologic reflexes unless there is associated corticospinal tract involvement. There is no atrophy, and no fasciculations or trophic changes (see Table 21-1, in Ch. 21).

Diseases of the extrapyramidal level are frequently of degenerative or involutional origin, but they may also result from inflammatory or toxic processes, viral disorders, certain intoxications, vascular disease, anoxia, neoplasms, trauma, and disturbances of development. In most lesions that affect the basal ganglia there is a diffuse disease process, with involvement of other parts of the brain as well. It is, therefore, doubtful whether a given symptom is the result of striatal disease or is due to disease elsewhere. The question has also been raised as to whether the disturbances in tone and the hyperkinetic manifestations are release phenomena, resulting from removal of inhibitory mechanisms or loss of control by higher centers, or whether they are manifestations of stimulation or irritation of the basal ganglia.

The most characteristic or most representative of the extrapyramidal diseases are **Parkinson's disease** and the parkinsonian syndromes that occur following encephalitis and as side reactions to the use of phenothiazines and other psychotropic drugs (Fig. 22-4) and toxins. In these disorders various manifestations of the previously discussed three motor abnormalities are evident. There is marked hypertonia, or rigidity, which principally affects the spinal muscles and the proximal and flexor groups of the extremities; occasionally the rigidity is of a cogwheel type. There is a characteristic hyperkinesia with a coarse tremor, sometimes called "pill-rolling." It is fairly rhythmic, gross, from 2 – 6/sec, and may involve the hands, feet, jaw, tongue, lips, and pharynx. It is usually a **resting tremor,** present when the extremity is not voluntarily moved; it usually lessens during voluntary movement and disappears in sleep.

There is slowing of all movements, and there is loss of associated and automatic movements, with masking of the face, infrequent smiling and blinking, loss of swinging of the arms in walking, and micrographia. The gait is slowed and shuffling in character, with a flexed posture of the body and extremities, stooping, propulsion and festination (a tendency to increase the speed and fall forward when walking). If a patient, standing upright, is suddenly pushed either backward or forward, he cannot immediately

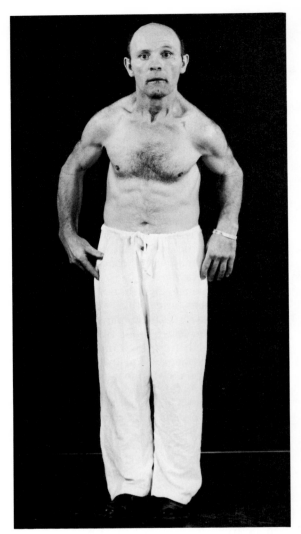

FIG. 22–4. A patient with Parkinson's disease, showing rigidity, masked facies, and typical posture.

contract the muscles necessary for maintenance of equilibrium, and will fall in the direction he was pushed. Because of the rigidity and bradykinesia, strength may seem to be decreased but there is no true loss of power, such as is seen in spinal or corticospinal lesions, in spite of the synonym of **paralysis agitans** for the disorder. The rigidity and bradykinesia, however, may make locomotion and motor activity slow and difficult, and may produce an apparent paralysis that is rigid in type, is not complete, is generalized, and involves movements and not muscles or muscle groups. Under emotional stimulation, however, the extremities can often be used rapidly and effectively. Abnormalities of phonation and articulation are common. There is no atrophy, and no fasciculations, characteristic change in the stretch reflexes, or pathologic reflexes of the type seen in corticospinal tract disorders (see Table 21-1 in Ch. 21). If there is associated corticospinal tract involvement, this may cause reflex changes. There is often exaggeration of the orbicularis oculi and orbicularis oris reflexes (see "Examination of the Reflexes," Ch. 13), and other special reflex phenomena are occasionally elicited (Ch. 39).

The manifestations differ in each case: in some the tremor is the outstanding symptom, in others the rigidity, the bradykinesia, or the loss of associated movements. Associated involvement of the midbrain structures may cause changes in ocular movements and in pupillary reactions, and hypothalamic involvement may cause hyperhidrosis, greasy seborrhea, and somnolence. Dementia is a common late manifestation attesting to more diffuse and widespread involvement of the central nervous system.

Parkinsonian manifestations may also occur as a sequel to encephalitis and may develop following anoxia, trauma, carbon monoxide or manganese poisoning, or from certain organic toxins. Similar syndromes, as well as other more bizarre extrapyramidal manifestations, are observed following the use of the phenothiazine and related drugs. Tremors, rigidity, and athetoid and choreiform movements may also be symptoms of magnesium deficiency. Choreoathetosis may develop during administration of levodopa or dopamine agonists for Parkinson's disease; here the movements appear to be dose-related.

There is not yet universal agreement about the pathologic basis of Parkinson's disease and the parkinsonian syndromes. In the so-called idiopathic variety alterations have been said to occur predominantly in the pallidum and striatum, with loss of ganglion cells, gliosis, and vascular abnormalities, whereas in postencephalitic parkinsonism such changes have been observed more frequently in the substantia nigra. Greenfield and others, however, have observed alterations in the substantia nigra and locus ceruleus — namely, loss of pigmented cells, the presence of hyaline inclusion bodies, lipochrome granules, and neurofibrillary tangles, in both conditions. The pathologic alterations, however, are often widespread, and the site of most damage probably determines whether tremor, rigidity, or loss of associated movements will be most marked. The basic pathophysiology of Parkin-

son's disease was elucidated in 1960 when Ehringer and Hornikiewicz found that there is a deficiency of dopamine in the striatum of patients with this disorder, following which Birkmayer and Hornykiewicz, Barbeau, Cotzias, and others demonstrated that levodopa, a precursor of dopamine, is able to replenish the missing dopamine and bring about temporary relief of symptoms.

Other diseases of the extrapyramidal system show varying degrees of the manifestations previously mentioned. In **Wilson's disease** or **hepatolenticular degeneration,** which has its usual age of onset between the ages of 10 and 20, there are tremors, occasionally rigidity, spasmodic movements of various types, hypertonia leading to contractures, and muscular weakness and wasting. The tremors may be present in the resting state and increased by voluntary action. Most characteristic, however, is a severe tremor of the outstretched upper extremities that has been called a "wingbeating" movement. This is not a true intention tremor, but is most marked with sustained positions. Pathologically there are symmetric degenerations in the lenticular nuclei, together with widespread changes in both the cerebrum and cerebellum, and a nodular cirrhosis of the liver. Wilson's disease is a genetically determined disorder of copper metabolism, inherited in a recessive manner. There is a decrease of ceruloplasmin in the blood and accumulation of copper in brain, liver, and other organs, and the pathologic alterations and symptoms of the disease are probably the result of copper toxicity. The **pseudosclerosis of Strümpell and Westphal** may be identical with Wilson's disease, although some of the patients reported to have had this condition had a later onset of symptoms and more marked mental changes, and may have suffered from a similar but somewhat different disease process.

In **congenital athetosis (mobile spasm)** there are slow, writhing, undulating, twisting movements of the distal portions of the extremities, usually the hands, fingers, and toes, with frequent grimacing. There often is associated spasticity, with increased reflexes and corticospinal signs, and there may be convulsive manifestations. The Vogts have found pathologic changes limited to the caudate and putamen, especially the latter, in these cases. These changes may be due to birth injury, anoxia, hemorrhagic disease of the newborn (erythroblastosis fetalis), intrauterine infections, toxic or inflammatory factors, or primary agenesis; the terms **status marmoratus** and **status dysmyelinatus** have been used in referring to them. Lesions of the precentral cortex may also cause athetosis.

In **dystonia musculorum deformans (torsion spasm,** or **Ziehen – Oppenheim disease)** (Ch. 31) there are slow writhing movements and bizarre grotesque torsions and twistings of the shoulder and pelvic girdles and the trunk; there may be rigidity, scoliosis, and lordosis. In this condition, too, lesions have been described in the striatum and pallidum. Spasmodic torticollis (Ch. 16) in which there is spasm with dystonic movements limited to the cervical muscles, may also on occasion be a striatal disease, in some instances owing to encephalitis.

In the **syndrome of Hallervorden and Spatz** there is a stiffness of all four extremities with tremors, athetoid movements, dysarthria, dementia, and emotional disturbances. Usually the condition begins in childhood and is a familial manifestation. Pathologically there is degeneration with deposition of pigment containing iron and fat in the globus pallidus and reticular zone of the substantia nigra; there also are diffuse cerebral and cerebellar alterations.

In **progressive pallidal degeneration** there is intense rigidity with tremors; pathologically there is atrophy of the globus pallidus.

In **Creutzfeldt – Jakob disease (subacute spongiform encephalopathy)** there is a rapidly progressing mental deterioration in middle life, accompanied by signs of involvement of the extrapyramidal and corticospinal systems and occasionally of the lower motor neurons. The motor symptoms include hyperkinesias, abnormalities in tone, dysphagia, and dysarthria. Pathologically there are spongy and deteriorative changes in the cerebral cortex, the basal ganglia, and other parts of the nervous system. The disorder is transmissible, caused by a "slow virus" or subviral particle or protein called prion by some.

The choreas are also extrapyramidal diseases, but show mainly hyperkinetic phenomena without rigidity — often, rather, with marked hypotonicity. **Sydenham's chorea** is a disease of children or adolescents related to streptococcal infection. There are quick, irregular, involuntary, jerky, asymmetric, nonrhythmic, purposeless movements that are increased by emotional and other stimuli. In **Huntington's chorea** the movements are less jerky, more purposeful, slower, and more gross, with grimacing, twisting, weaving, and lashing; the same movement may be repeated. There is also progressive intellectual deterioration. The disease is inherited as a mendelian dominant with involvement of chromosome 4. The pathologic changes in Sydenham's chorea have never been adequately studied, but diffuse alterations have been described; these may be either degenerative or inflammatory, and seem to affect mainly the striatum and cerebral cortex. In Huntington's chorea there is profound atrophy of the caudate, putamen, and cerebral cortex, with dilation of the lateral ventricles; microscopically there are diffuse degenerative changes in the brain.

In **hemiballismus** there are unilateral flail-like, writhing, twisting, or roiling movements that may be intense and may lead to exhaustion. These follow an isolated lesion, usually vascular in origin, hemorrhagic or occlusive, of the contralateral subthalamic nucleus or its neighboring pathways.

Extrapyramidal manifestations (tremor, rigidity, and loss of associated movements) are seen in the Shy-Drager syndrome, in which they are associated with orthostatic hypotension.

Progressive supranuclear palsy, or **Steele – Richardson – Olszewski syndrome,** is another slowly progressive degenerative disease of adults with extrapyramidal manifestations, eye movement disturbances, and eventual dementia.

Bizarre hyperkinesias are present in such conditions as striatonigral degeneration and corticodentatonigral degeneration in which there are pathologic alterations in the basal ganglia, substantia nigra, and dentate nucleus.

In paramyoclonus multiplex and familial myoclonus epilepsy there are rapid jerky movements resembling the response of a muscle to mechanical stimulation; there is no wasting and there is no disturbance of tone. Similar movements are seen in subacute sclerosing panencephalitis and some of the lipid storage diseases. The pathologic changes responsible for these manifestations are not definitely known, but usually there are diffuse degenerative alterations and often inclusion bodies in the neurons, particularly in the dentate nucleus, substantia nigra, and basal ganglia. As in almost all the diseases described previously, the pathologic changes are widespread and involve many different structures, even though they may predominate in specific areas.

Investigative and surgical approaches of various types have been made in the attempt to relieve the symptoms of extrapyramidal disease, and these have, incidentally, led to a better understanding of the basic pathophysiology of the clinical conditions. It has long been known that either injection of procaine into the involved muscles or section of either the anterior or posterior nerve roots will decrease rigidity, although these measures will not influence tremor. Both of these procedures interrupt either the afferent or efferent pathway of the proprioceptive reflex arc; neither is a suitable or practical treatment procedure. Furthermore, it is also well known that the tremor of parkinsonism is lessened or abolished by a capsular hemiplegia, at least for the duration of the paralysis, but the impairment of motor function may be more incapacitating than the hyperkinesia. On the basis of these clinical observations, surgical measures have been used in an attempt to mitigate the symptoms of diseases. Various technics have been directed to the cerebral cortex, internal capsule, basal ganglia, pallidofugal fibers, and spinal cord.

A number of destructive lesions were used as part of a surgical approach to the relief of symptoms of Parkinson's disease. These included lesions in the nucleus ventralis lateralis or other thalamic nuclei (thalamotomy) by the injection of procaine in oil or alcohol, by electrolysis, by ultrasound, or by freezing technics. These procedures provided a degree of relief of tremor and some of the other symptoms of Parkinson's disease for a variable period of time, usually only a few years. Most of these procedures have been abandoned. More recently efforts to transplant adrenal medullary tissue into the basal ganglion regions have provided a new approach to the surgical management of Parkinson's disease. Their success and longevity remain to be determined.

The advent of effective medical therapy for Parkinson's disease in the form of levodopa and various dopamine agonists and similar substances has obviated the need for surgery to a great extent.

BIBLIOGRAPHY

Adams RD, Victor M. Principles of Neurology, 4th ed. New York, McGraw – Hill, 1989

Adams RD, Van Bogaert L, Van der Ecken H. Striatonigral degeneration. J Neuropathol Exp Neurol 1964;23:608

Barbeau A. L-dopa therapy in Parkinson's disease — A critical review of nine years' experience. Can Med Assoc J 1969;101:191

Birkmayer W, Hornykiewicz O. Der L-Dioxyphenylalanin (Dopa). Effekt bei der Parkinson-Akines. Wien Klin Wochenschr 1961;73:787

Brodal A. Neurological Anatomy in Relation to Clinical Medicine, 3rd ed. New York, Oxford University Press, 1981

Browder J. Section of the fibers of the anterior limb of the internal capsule in parkinsonism. Am J Surg 1948;75:264.

Bucy PC. The surgical treatment of extrapyramidal diseases. J Neurol Neurosurg Psychiatry 1951;14:108.

Cooper JR, Bloom FE, Roth RH. The Biochemical Basis of Neuropharmacology, 5th ed. New York, Oxford University Press, 1986

Cotzias GE, Papavasiliou PS, Gellene R. Medication of parkinsonism — Chronic treatment with L-dopa. N Engl J Med 1969;280:337

Denny – Brown D. The Basal Ganglia and Their Relation to Disorders of Movement. London, Oxford University Press, 1962

Fulton JF, Kennard MA. A study of flaccid and spastic paralyses produced by lesions of the cerebral cortex in primates. Assoc Res Nerv Ment Dis Proc 1934;13:158

Gibbs CJ Jr, Gajdusek DC, Asher DM et al. Creutzfeldt – Jakob disease (subacute spongiform encephalopathy). Transmission to the chimpanzee. Science 1968;161:388

Greenfield JG, Bosanquet FD. The brain-stem lesions in parkinsonism. J Neurol Neurosurg Psychiatry 1953;16:213

Klemme RM. Surgical treatment of dystonia, with report of one hundred cases. Assoc Res Nerv Ment Dis Proc 1942;21:596

Narabayashi H, Okuma T, Shikiba S. Procaine oil blocking of the globus pallidus. Arch Neurol Psychiatry 1956;75:36

Parkinson J. An Essay on the Shaking Palsy. London, Sherwood, Neely and Jones, 1817

Rebeiz JJ, Kolodny EH, Richardson EP Jr. Corticodentatonigral degeneration with neuronal achromatasia. Arch Neurol 1968;18:29

Shy GM, Drager GA. A neurological syndrome associated with orthostatic hypotension. Arch Neurol 1960;2:511

Spiegel EA, Wycis HT. Thalamotomy and pallidotomy for treatment of choreic movements. Acta Neurochir 1952;2:419

Stern G. The effects of lesions in the substantia nigra. Brain 1966;89:449

Vinken PJ, Bruyn GW (eds). Handbook of Clinical Neurology. Vol 6, Diseases of the Basal Ganglia. Amsterdam, North Holland, 1968

Vogt C, Vogt O. Zur Lehre der Erkrankungen des striären Systems. J Psychol Neurol 1920;25:628

Wilson SAK. Progressive lenticular degeneration. A familial nervous disease associated with cirrhosis of the liver. Brain 1912;34:295

Wilson SAK. The old motor system and the new. Arch Neurol Psychiatry 1924;11:385

Yahr MD (ed). The Basal Ganglia. New York, Raven Press, 1976

Chapter 23
THE CORTICOSPINAL (PYRAMIDAL) LEVEL

The corticospinal level of motor integration is also referred to as the **cortical level,** and the **upper motor neuron level.** It must be remembered, however, that it is only one of many motor fiber systems that converge upon the anterior horn cell and the final common pathway, and therefore it is only one of many upper motor neuron levels. It should be stated at the outset that experimental work, not all of which has been accepted by clinicians, has materially altered certain long-accepted concepts of the function of the corticospinal system, its relation to the extrapyramidal system, and the changes that may be caused by disease of either of these systems. It is apparent, however, that the corticospinal level does not function independently. In both the normal state and in the presence of disease it is closely integrated with other levels of motor activity, as well as with a constant stream of incoming sensory impulses. The terms corticospinal (pyramidal) and extrapyramidal have become blurred anatomically, and some anatomists suggest they be abandoned. Clinicians, however, continue to find them useful in the sense that signs and symptoms due to lesions of the direct motor pathways differ from those of the indirect ("extrapyramidal") system. Objections can be raised to the use of the terms corticospinal, pyramidal, or upper motor neuron levels; none fully describe the more voluntary, direct descending motor pathways precisely, but a better term has not come into use.

ANATOMY AND PHYSIOLOGY

The corticospinal level of the motor system has been called the "new motor system." It is found fully developed only in mammals and reaches its highest development in apes and man. In the newborn infant the descending fibers of the corticospinal system have little or no myelin sheathing. The process of myelination starts immediately after birth and is usually complete by the age of two years. Walking and other skilled movements are learned as the pathway matures and myelination progresses. The existence of a motor area in the brain was suggested by Robert Boyle as long ago as 1691. In the 1860s Hughlings Jackson, from a study of focal epilepsy, assumed the presence of an area in the cerebral cortex that governs isolated movements. In 1870 Fritsch and Hitzig found that galvanic stimulation of the exposed frontal cortex of the dog caused movements of the contralateral extremities. In 1873 Ferrier confirmed this work in monkeys, using faradic stimulation, and also produced paralysis by ablation of the excitable region. Further work on localization of function of the cerebral cortex was carried out by Beevor and Horsley. The first recorded electrical stimulation of the human brain was carried out by Bartholow in 1874.

The major motor units of the corticospinal level are situated in the posterior portions of the frontal lobes of the brain. The motor cortex of primates arises in the depths of the rolandic fissure, or central sulcus, and spreads out for a variable distance rostrally over the adjacent precentral or posterior frontal convolution. It extends from the sylvian fissure up to and over the vertex and for some distance on the medial surface of the brain. This area coincides cytoarchitectonically with the area gigantopyramidalis (Campbell's area precentralis, area 4 of Brodmann, and area FA of Economo and Koskinas) (Fig. 23-1).

It was long believed that the descending corticospinal pathway or pyramidal tract consisted mainly of the neuraxes of the Betz cells, or giant pyramidal cells, which are found in the fifth layer of this area. The origin of the name of this pathway, however, is linked with the medullary pyramids and not with the large pyramidal cells of the motor cortex. While there are some 25,000 – 35,000 Betz cells in the precentral cortex, there are about 1,000,000 fibers in the corticospinal tract at the level of the pyramids. It is probable that about 3% of the pyramidal fibers arise from the Betz cells, and they may not be physiologic units but only the larger members of a much more numerous group of corticospinal cells. Fulton, however, stated that excitable properties of area 4 depend largely, if not entirely, upon the integrity of the Betz cells, and that isolated movements disappear when these cells are destroyed and are absent if they are underdeveloped. On the other hand, Walshe stated that it is difficult to regard the Betz cell as a specific morphologic entity, and that it is merely the largest of the pyramidal cells. He believed that the smaller giant cells and the large pyramidal cells in the fifth layer, and possibly even the small pyramidal cells of the third layer of the motor cortex, exert a similar function, and stated that the giant cells probably innervate larger motor units. The larger giant cells may mediate simple movements of the legs and trunk; finer and more complex movements are subserved by the smaller giant cells and the larger pyramidal cells.

Furthermore, it is probable that the parietal lobe (areas 1, 2, 3, 5, 7), areas 6 and 8 of the frontal lobe (Fig. 23-1) and other portions of the brain, including the temporal and occipital lobes and certain subcortical centers, make important contributions to the corticospinal tract; it may also contain some ascending fibers. Because area 4 does not supply as many nuclei in the spinal cord as the pyramidal tract does, there are fewer degenerative changes in the anterior horn cells following cortical ablation than after section of the pyramid.

Closely related to the motor cortex, both anatomically and functionally, is the premotor region, which is also referred to as the extrapyramidal cortex (Fig. 23-2). It is situated just rostral to area 4, and has been termed area 6 by Brodmann. It is similar histologically to the motor cortex but lacks the giant pyramidal cells. Some fibers from area 6 pass to area 4 and then downward with the corticospinal tract; others pass directly downward with the pyramidal fibers and decussate with them. There is probably less complete crossing of the fibers from the premotor cortex than of those from the motor cortex. In addition, the premotor region is in direct communication with the basal ganglia and other portions of the extrapyramidal system and contributes the chief cortical component to them. Laboratory and clinical investigations have also demonstrated the presence of secondary and supplementary motor areas with complete representation of contralateral somatic musculature. The former (secondary motor area) is situated in the parietal operculum, at the foot of the precentral gyrus, and along the upper border of the sylvian fissure; the latter (supplementary motor area), which probably has bilateral representation, is in the paracentral region on the medial surface of the hemisphere, anterior to the motor cortex. There are other, less important and less complete supplementary motor areas, e.g., in the cortex of the insula.

Within the motor cortex there is a definite localization of function. "Centers" have been described that control various activities. A center, however, is not a focus that has the sole control of a specific function, but is the seat of greatest intensity of this function. Skeletal musculature is represented in reverse order upon the contralateral motor area. The center for the larynx and pharynx is lowest, just above the sylvian fissure, and this is followed, in an ascending direction, by centers for the palate, jaw, tongue, mouth, face, eyelids, forehead, neck, thumb, fingers, wrist, elbow, shoulder, thorax, and abdomen. The lower extremities and sacral centers are represented on the medial surface of the hemisphere. It has been stated that the leg areas are represented on the lateral surface with only the sacral centers present on the medial aspect; this was, however, based on evidence from experimental animals. In man the motor centers for the upper extremity extend upward on the lateral surface of the brain as far as its superior border, whereas centers for the thigh and leg are represented on the medial surface of the hemisphere

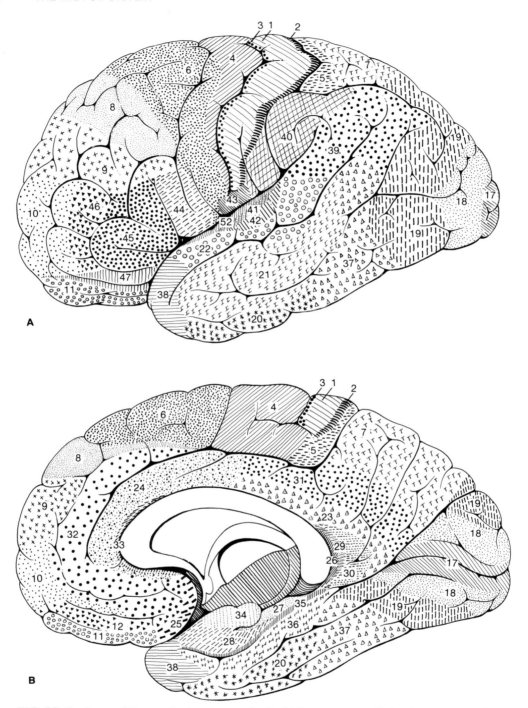

FIG. 23–1. Areas of the cerebral cortex, each of which possesses a distinctive structure. **A.** Lateral surface. **B.** Medial surface. (Modified from Brodmann K: Vergleichende Lokalisationlehre der Grosshirnrinde in ihren Prinzipien dargestellt auf Grund des Zellenbaues. Leipzig, JA Barth, 1919)

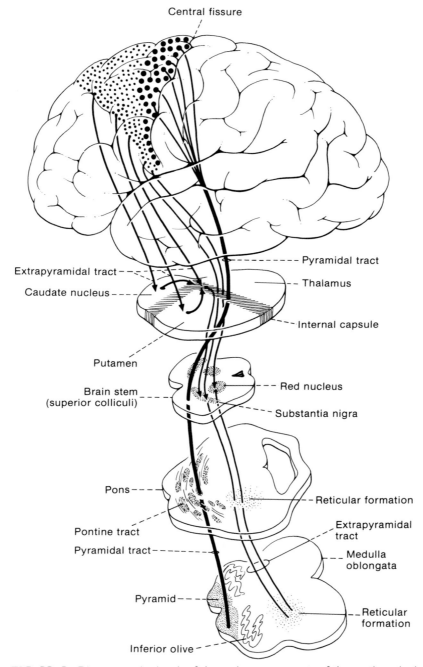

FIG. 23–2. Diagrammatic sketch of the major components of the corticospinal and extrapyramidal systems. (Modified from Benda CE, Cobb S. Med 1942; 21:95)

(Fig. 23-3). The acquisition of speech and other forms of expression and the elaboration of new and complex functions of the upper extremities may have been accompanied by corresponding expansion of cortical areas representing the tongue, mouth, lips, thumb, and fingers, with the result that the cortical representation for the leg has been forced upward and then onto the medial surface of the hemisphere. Areas for the tongue, face, and digits are exceptionally large and are out of proportion with those that control the proximal musculature (Fig. 23-4).

The neuraxes of the motor units in the precentral convolution, or the pyramidal fibers, pass

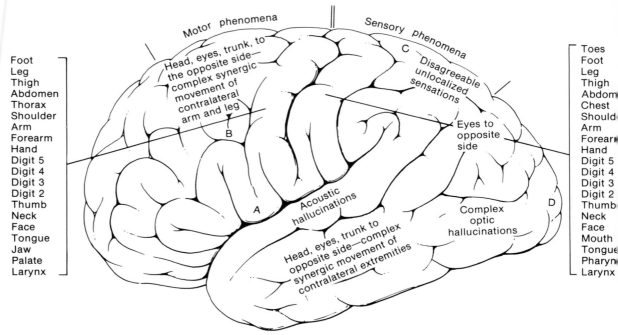

FIG. 23–3. Localization in the cerebral cortex. Principal excitable foci as determined by electrical stimulation. **A.** Chewing and swallowing movements. **B.** Eyes deviate to opposite side. **C.** Sensory aura in opposite leg. **D.** Unformed visual hallucinations. (Modified from Bailey P: Intracranial Tumors, 2nd ed. Springfield IL, Charles C Thomas, 1948)

through the corona radiata into the genu and the anterior two thirds of the posterior limb of the internal capsule (Fig. 23-5). Those to the face and medullary centers are anterior and are followed in a posterior direction by those to the upper extremity, trunk, and lower extremity. At the midbrain level the pyramidal fibers traverse the intermediate three fifths of the cerebral peduncle, with those to the medullary centers in a medial and somewhat dorsal position. The descending neuraxes then pass through the basilar portion of the pons, where they are separated by transverse fibers, and enter the medulla as the pyramidal tract (Fig. 23-6). Those that convey impulses to the pontine and medullary centers are the corticopontine and corticobulbar fibers. The majority of them decussate before synapsing with the specific nuclei, but most of the innervation of brain stem centers is both crossed and uncrossed.

The neuraxes that convey impulses to the spinal cord are the corticospinal fibers. In the caudal portion of the medulla the majority of them (80% – 90%) decussate and descend through the lateral funiculus of the spinal cord in the lateral corticospinal pathway to supply the muscles of the opposite side of the body. Those of the upper extremity cross more rostrally and assume a medial position in the tract. There are individual variations in the percentage of crossed fibers in the lateral corticospinal tracts, and the tracts may contain some uncrossed fibers. In addition they also contain other corticofugal fibers as well as some ascending ones. About 50% of the fibers of the lateral corticospinal tract terminate in the cervical region, 20% in the thoracic area, and 30% in the lumbosacral portion of the cord. The smaller ventral corticospinal tract descends uncrossed in the ipsilateral ventral funiculus and usually does not extend below the midthoracic region; these fibers, too, usually cross before terminating.

The neuraxes carried through these pathways terminate at appropriate levels to supply the motor nuclei of the cranial nerves and the anterior horn cells of the spinal cord. Those to the cord end in the zona intermedia between the anterior and posterior horns, and there is an intercalated neuron between the neuraxis of the corticospinal cell and the anterior horn cell for the majority; a few fibers end directly on the anterior horn cells. Impulses then travel from the

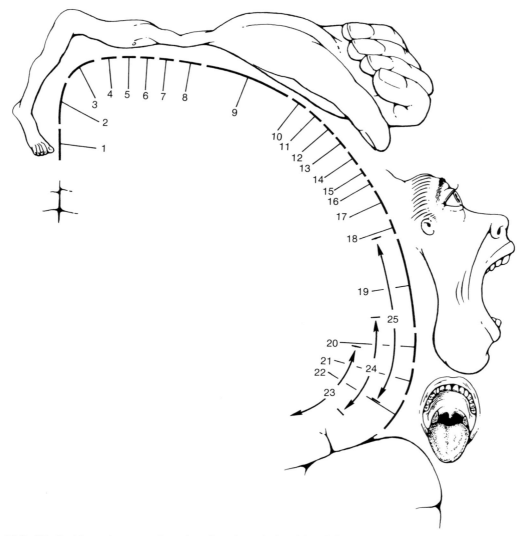

FIG. 23–4. Motor homunculus, showing the relationship of the motor centers to cortical representation. **1.** Toes. **2.** Ankle. **3.** Knee. **4.** Hip. **5.** Trunk. **6.** Shoulder. **7.** Elbow. **8.** Wrist. **9.** Hand. **10.** Little finger. **11.** Ring finger. **12.** Middle finger. **13.** Index finger. **14.** Thumb. **15.** Neck. **16.** Brow. **17.** Eyelid and eyeball. **18.** Face. **19.** Lips. **20.** Jaw. **21.** Tongue. **22.** Swallowing. **23.** Mastication. **24.** Salivation. **25.** Vocalization. (Modified from Penfield W, Rasmussen T: The Cerebral Cortex of Man. New York, Macmillan, 1950)

motor nuclei and anterior horn cells, which together with their neuraxes are the final common pathway, to the neuromuscular junction of striated muscles. A single corticospinal fiber innervates more than one neuron in the spinal cord, and probably some innervate many.

The pyramidal and related motor cells in the cerebral cortex may be considered motor centers, or centers of adjustment, which send effector stimuli through the pathways just described (Fig. 23-7). Receptor impulses of the pyramidal arc

are carried up the spinal cord and brain stem through the various sensory pathways to the thalamus. After synapse in the thalamus, impulses are relayed through the thalamic radiations to the parietal cortex, and then to the motor cells of the cortex, stimulation of which causes muscular activity.

Excitation of the motor cortex (area 4), such as by electrical stimulation or during a jacksonian seizure, causes muscular contractions on the opposite side of the body. Although it is generally

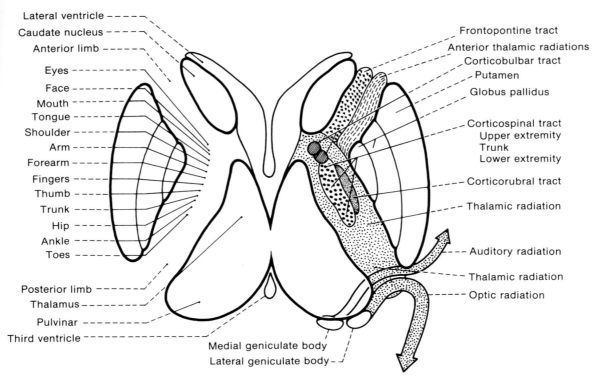

Lateral ventricle
Caudate nucleus
Anterior limb
Eyes
Face
Mouth
Tongue
Shoulder
Arm
Forearm
Fingers
Thumb
Trunk
Hip
Ankle
Toes
Posterior limb
Thalamus
Pulvinar
Third ventricle
Medial geniculate body
Lateral geniculate body
Frontopontine tract
Anterior thalamic radiations
Corticobulbar tract
Putamen
Globus pallidus
Corticospinal tract
Upper extremity
Trunk
Lower extremity
Corticorubral tract
Thalamic radiation
Auditory radiation
Thalamic radiation
Optic radiation

FIG. 23–5. The internal capsule. Anterior aspect is at top of illustration.

accepted that the response is not one of simple contraction of isolated muscles, but one of groups of muscles acting harmoniously, Ruch and others demonstrated that individual muscles as well as movements may be finely represented in the motor cortex. Undoubtedly, however, the response to cortical stimulation is altered by the intensity and frequency of the stimulus and the depth of anesthesia; proprioceptive impulses are also important, and alterations in the posture of a limb modify the response. Stimulation of area 4 causes discrete movements involving principally the digital muscles at the distal joints and the muscles supplied by the cranial nerves. The foci of localization overlap, but areas controlling movements of the thumb, index finger, hallux, and face have the widest distribution and the lowest threshold. Stimulation of the premotor cortex (area 6) also causes a contralateral motor response, but a stronger stimulus is necessary than when area 4 is stimulated. The resulting movements are more complex and consist of slow, synergistic, postural or patterned contractions of a generalized type that involve large muscle groups.

Ablation of the motor cortex causes paralysis, or loss of movement, on the opposite side of the body. This affects principally the distal joints, with less involvement at the proximal joints, and finer volitional movements are abolished. It had generally been accepted that area 4 ablations produce a spastic paralysis with hyperreflexia and no atrophy, which will be described subsequently as the characteristic "pyramidal syndrome." Experimental investigations, however, followed by clinical application in humans, have altered the older concepts of the function of the pyramidal system and their relations to disturbances of motor control, although the entire subject remains controversial. Experimental lesions limited to some portion of the pyramidal tracts or to their cells of origin in the motor cortex, area 4 of Brodmann, yield a syndrome different from that just described. Instead of spasticity and hyperreflexia there is a flaccid motor paralysis, with transient depression of all reflexes and resulting muscular atrophy; the only pathologic reflex responses are the extensor portion of the Babinski sign and Chaddock's sign. There may be transient spasticity at the distal joints.

After complete destruction of the pyramidal cells or of their tracts the signs of Babinski and Chaddock persist and there is an enduring para-

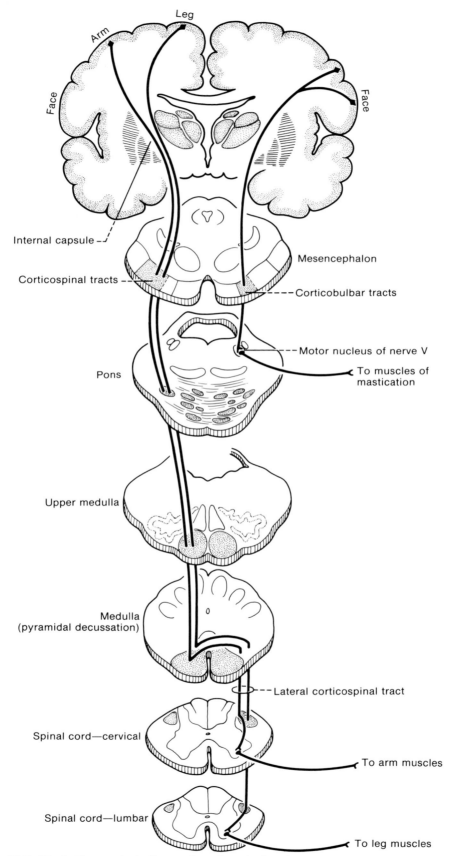

FIG. 23–6. The corticobulbar and corticospinal pathways.

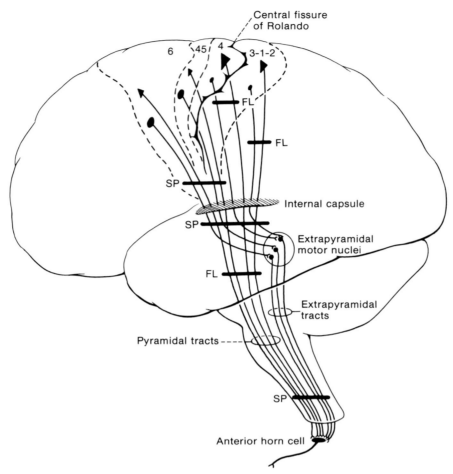

FIG. 23–7. Diagrammatic sketch of corticospinal and extrapyramidal projections from the cerebral cortex. Direct cells of the pyramidal tract are represented in the cortex as triangles, those of the extrapyramidal tract as circles. Size of triangles and circles represent relative number of cells in each cortical area. The letters **SP** indicate site of lesions causing a spastic paralysis, and the letters **FL** indicate site of lesions causing a flaccid paralysis. (Modified from Welch WK, Kennard MA: J Neurophysiol 7:255–268, 1944)

lysis of isolated movements, especially those of the distal joints, but the flaccidity and hyporeflexia tend to disappear with time. All these manifestations are more marked with bilateral extirpation of area 4. Permanent spasticity, a manifestation which in man is usually considered to be due to a lesion of the motor area or the corticospinal tract, was not observed after isolated section of area 4 in experimental animals.

Section of the corticospinal tracts in the cerebral peduncle or in the medulla has also been shown to produce a hypotonic paresis, and damage to the spinal portion of the corticospinal tract in monkeys has caused a hypotonic paresis, decreased deep and superficial reflexes, exagger-

ated associated movements, and atrophy, especially of the distal muscles. Bucy sectioned the intermediate portion of the cerebral peduncle in the human for the relief of hemiballismus and found no motor impairment and no spasticity in the contralateral extremities, only a slight increase in reflexes, and an extensor Babinski response. Several recent reports of lesions in humans confined to the medullary pyramids, verified by imaging and pathologic study, have shown that spasticity can indeed result from these insults eventually.

Ablations of area 6 or its projection fibers in animals, on the other hand, give rise to a contralateral hemiparesis or hemiplegia with increased resistance to passive movement, moderately increased deep reflexes, disturbances of skilled movements, forced grasping, and vasomotor changes. There are also plantar flexor reflexes and the fanning portion of the Babinski sign. The resistance to passive movement is of a rigid type, equal in quantity through all ranges of passive movement and from the beginning to the end of such movement. It is approximately equal in all muscle groups. All these changes, except the disturbance of skilled movement, are transient; all are exaggerated on bilateral extirpation of area 6. Removal of area 6 after removal of area 4 causes a previously flaccid extremity (or one spastic only at the distal joints) to become highly spastic and remain so. There is a loss of voluntary power in the contralateral limbs. Deep reflexes become uniformly exaggerated, there is forced grasping, and both the extensor and fanning Babinski responses appear and remain permanently. Additional removal of the homolateral postcentral gyrus or the contralateral motor area causes increase in the paresis and spasticity.

Other studies are at variance with these observations. Denny–Brown stated that ablations of area 4 lead to only transient defects, but that spasticity always eventually accompanies the paralytic manifestations of such lesions and is most pronounced with total lesions. If area 6 is also removed, there is greater spasticity, with flexion of the elbow and extension of the knee and ankle. Ablation of area 6 alone produces a posture of slight flexion in both upper and lower extremities, with a soft plastic resistance of both flexors and extensors. He suggested that the phenomenon of shock plays a part in the delayed development of spasticity, and that more extensive ablations may be followed by a longer period of flaccidity, before the eventual appearance of spasticity. Furthermore, proprioceptive and other impulses are important to the development of hyperreflexia, the grasp reflex, and increase in tone.

It is difficult to evaluate the disparity in experimental results and the differentiation between some of them and what has long been known as the "pyramidal syndrome" in man, with spasticity, hyperreflexia, and pathologic reflexes, but no resulting atrophy. Most experimental work has been performed entirely on animals, but there has been some investigation on humans, and there have been isolated cases in humans in which it could be definitely established that the pathologic process was limited either to the pyramidal cortex and its pathways or to the premotor cortex and its descending tracts. The hypotonia that has been reported to occur with lesions of area 4 in lower primates is rarely seen in man except as an initial effect. Differences undoubtedly exist between the motor reactions in man and those in experimental animals, and it may be that in many of the reported ablations of area 6 there was some involvement of the true motor cortex. In fact, there is evidence to suggest that the physiologic motor cortex extends far into the so-called premotor area. Lassek noted that there often is little evidence of destruction of pyramidal fibers with lesions of area 4 and in patients who have had a cerebral hemiplegia or hemiparesis, and stated that it is difficult to correlate clinical manifestations with the small amount of degeneration in this pathway. Clinical data derived from evidence of the newer imaging procedures will gradually help to clarify the issues relating to the corticospinal system and its symptomatology.

In addition, there is serious question on the part of neurophysiologists concerning any relationship of the corticospinal complex to spasticity. It is generally believed that such increase in tone may be related more closely to dysfunction of the extrapyramidal rather than the pyramidal portion of the nervous system, or to interruption of corticofugal fibers other than pyramidal in the corticospinal pathway. Spasticity in all probability results from imbalance of the facilitatory and inhibitory centers in the midbrain and brain stem reticular formations, as well as altered balance between the α- and γ-motor systems in the spinal cord. Inhibition of suppressor impulses is followed by enhancement of facilitatory mechanisms. Within the spinal cord those impulses that lead to exaggeration (or reduction in the threshold) of the stretch reflexes, the essential aspect of spasticity, may be carried by the reticulospinal and vestibulospinal rather than the corticospinal tracts.

On the basis of experimental data together with the clinical sources that are accumulating, one can conclude that the corticospinal tract deals with discrete, isolated motor responses, especially with the finer adjustments of voluntary movement of the digits, and that disease of the pyramidal system *per se* results in hypotonia, areflexia, and possibly atrophy. It is recognized that in certain instances vascular and other cerebral lesions may be followed by a paralysis that remains flaccid, with loss of tendon reflexes but with an extensor plantar response. The clinical signs probably follow a lesion limited to some portions of the pyramidal cortex or its descending pathways. The premotor cortex and its pathways are concerned with larger coordinated responses, more stereotyped movements that are partly automatic and involve the trunk and the proximal segments, and postural mechanisms. It contributes the principal cortical components to the extrapyramidal level, and hyperkinesias have been relieved by ablation of area 6.

Hemiplegia in man is generally produced by combined destruction of the motor and premotor components of the upper motor neuron, and there are combinations of the foregoing symptoms, often with severe motor paralysis. In all probability the more violent reactions, such as spasticity and hyperreflexia, overshadow the flaccidity and hyporeflexia. Various pathologic responses — the Hoffmann sign and the forced grasping and finger flexor reflexes in the upper extremity, and Chaddock's sign, together with both the fanning and extensor portions of the Babinski sign — are obtained (Ch. 35). The affected extremities may at first be flaccid with depressed reflexes (either shock or pyramidal tract effects), but spasticity, reflex exaggeration, and vasomotor change may develop within a few days. The various pathologic responses, such as the Babinski, Chaddock, and Hoffmann signs, may remain permanently.

CLINICAL MANIFESTATIONS OF DISEASE OF THE CORTICOSPINAL LEVEL

When considering the manifestations of disease of the corticospinal level, this text will follow those concepts of corticospinal function generally accepted by clinicians, and this level of the motor system will be presumed to consist of the principal efferent corticospinal neurons through which purposive movements are initiated and performed. The corticospinal level not only activates but also integrates highly skilled, refined, discrete movements, although it is by no means the sole cortical mechanism for movement. It is responsible for the initiation of movement of individual muscles and it also causes the inhibition, or graded relaxation, of antagonistic muscles necessary for the performance of skilled acts. By its integrating action individual muscular contractions are correlated into complicated motor reactions; a specific act can be started and then abruptly stopped, following which it may either be resumed or altered for the performance of a different act. Also, along with other cerebral and brain stem mechanisms, it constantly supplies lower centers with tonic impulses of various types that have an inhibiting effect on them.

In disease of the pyramidal cortex or its descending pathways there is a release of this inhibiting effect, and the spinal level is allowed to respond to all stimuli. As a result, responses are exaggerated and there is an excessive, or unbalanced, activity of the lower centers that are normally under cortical control.

Disease of the corticospinal pathway may be caused, as may disease elsewhere in the central nervous system, by birth injury, vascular disease, neoplasms, inflammation, toxins, degeneration, or trauma. Destruction of the neuron or of its neuraxis, whether resulting from involvement of the gigantopyramidal cells themselves, the internal capsule, the cerebral peduncle, the fibers as they pass through the pons or medulla, or the corticospinal tract, produces a definite syndrome. Inasmuch as the corticospinal pathway has an integrating and inhibiting effect upon the lower centers, the essential manifestations of such a lesion consist of a loss of skilled voluntary movements, or impairment of integration of movements, and an overactivity or exaggeration of response of the lower centers.

There is a loss of voluntary movement. This loss of power, instead of being associated with a decrease in tone, is hypertonic, or spastic (see Table 21-1, in Ch. 21). Increased tension of the muscle masses may be felt on palpation and there is increased resistance to passive movement. The paresis is generalized rather than focal; it involves either entire extremities or specific movements, rather than specific muscles. In a lower motor neuron paralysis, for instance, either the short or the long flexor muscles may be paralyzed. When a corticospinal lesion develops, on the other hand, flexion as a whole may be paretic. It may be impossible to flex or extend one finger without flexing or extending them all. If a muscle has many functions, some of these may be affected while others are not impaired.

There is usually no localized atrophy, although there may be some generalized loss of muscle volume, in part owing to disuse, and there may be apparent atrophy in a long-standing paralysis owing to lack of development of the involved part, especially if the responsible lesion is congenital or occurs early in life. If atrophy does occur with corticospinal tract disorders, it usually affects the small muscles of the hand; it progresses rapidly if it appears early, and slowly if it appears late. There are no fasciculations. The muscle stretch reflexes, instead of being lost, are exaggerated, and clonus may be elicited. The superficial reflexes are diminished or absent.

Finally, there are various pathologic reflexes, such as the Babinski sign, which are often termed **pyramidal reflexes** or **upper motor neuron signs** (Ch. 35). Some of the normal associated movements may be lost, but abnormal associated movements are present (Ch. 38). Trophic changes are rarely present, but occasionally one sees edema, desquamation, pigment changes, and a glossy skin.

In a paresis of central origin, which usually takes the form of a hemiparesis, the loss of power has certain characteristics. Involvement of the face is limited to the lower portion although occasionally eyelid closure may be slightly weak, and voluntary movements are affected more than emotional ones. There is often normal movement in response to emotional stimuli. There may be only slight or differential involvement of the muscles innervated by the spinal accessory nerve. There may be slight weakness of the affected side of the tongue, but the throat and jaw muscles function normally. Deglutition, articulation, movements of the trunk, and other acts that have bilateral supranuclear innervation are little affected with a central paresis.

Voluntary, skilled, learned actions are most impaired, and there is loss of the ability to perform fine and isolated acts, especially those of the distal portions of the extremities, with precision and delicacy (Fig. 23-8). Gross movements and those that are habitual or that have little voluntary control are spared. The paresis of the extremities has a characteristic distribution. In the upper extremity the extensor and external rotation muscles are primarily affected, with relative sparing of the flexor and internal rotation muscles; in the lower extremity weakness is most marked in the flexors and internal rotators, with relative sparing of the extensors and external rotators. As a result, the arm is held in a position of adduction, flexion, and slight internal rotation at the shoulder; there is flexion and pronation at the elbow, with flexion of the wrist and fingers. Additional flexion can still be carried out, but there is marked weakness of extension. There is loss of isolated movements of the wrist and fingers, but movements at the elbow and shoulder are less affected. In the lower extremity the leg is extended and adducted at the hip and extended at the knee and ankle. There is an equinus deformity of the foot with plantar flexion and inversion of the foot and toes; there is loss of dorsiflexion and eversion. There is also weakness of flexion at the hip and knee.

The spasticity, or increase in tone (Ch. 28), is most marked in the flexor muscles of the upper limb and the extensors of the lower, and may become more apparent if an attempt is made to ex-

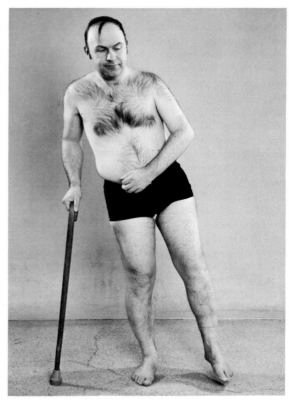

FIG. 23–8. Left hemiparesis of 15 years' duration. The patient circumducts his left leg as he begins walking.

tend the muscles of the upper extremity or to flex those of the lower. Passive motion can be carried out with little difficulty if done through a small range of movement, but resistance increases if an attempt is made to move the extremities through a greater range. On slow movement passive motion may be carried out with little difficulty, but on rapid movement there is a "blocking" and one may at times get a waxing and sudden waning of tone that gives the so-called clasp-knife phenomenon.

One of the most characteristic and common examples of paralysis at the corticospinal tract level is that which occurs following a hemorrhage, thrombosis, or embolism affecting the internal capsule. If the patient is examined soon after the event occurs, flaccid paralysis and areflexia may be observed on the opposite side of the body, but after the period of shock is past the previously described spasticity, typical of "capsular" hemiplegia, becomes apparent. The lesion need not, however, be in the internal capsule, but may be cortical, in the corona radiata, or anywhere along the course of the corticospinal pathway. In the capsular hemiplegia which follows interruption of the blood supply in the distribution of the branches of the middle cerebral artery, the upper extremity is affected more than the face or lower extremity and the hand is affected more than the shoulder. If the involvement is in the distribution of the anterior cerebral artery, the leg is affected more than the face or arm. In brain stem lesions involving the pyramidal pathways, unilateral or bilateral paralysis may result, at times affecting the lower extremities more than the uppers; it may even be crossed.

In spinal cord lesions of sudden onset involving the corticospinal pathways, especially if bilateral, there may also be a period of flaccidity and areflexia accompanying the paralysis below the level of the lesion. This is the period of "spinal shock," which sooner or later gives way, in most instances, to the corticospinal syndrome. Occasionally in spinal lesions a "paraplegia in flexion" develops in which there is flexion at the hips, knees, and ankles instead of extension. This is indicative of a more complete interruption of conduction of descending impulses in the spinal cord. Involuntary flexor spasms make their appearance, they gain in force and frequency, and finally the legs become fully flexed with the knees pressed tightly against the abdominal wall. This syndrome is probably caused by interruption of the vestibulospinal and other extrapyramidal pathways as well as the corticospinal tracts.

The paresis of corticospinal lesions is only occasionally complete; this may result from a variety of factors, and these same mechanisms may be in part responsible for the recovery of function that follows many such lesions. Some of the musculature may have bilateral innervation or there may be incomplete decussation at the pyramids in the medulla; the corticospinal tracts themselves receive impulses from many regions other than the motor cortex, including areas 6, 8, 1, 2, 3, 5, and 7; many of the motor "centers" are widespread and the foci of localization overlap.

The motor and precentral cortex and its neuraxes constitute only one portion of the motor system, and other cortical and subcortical centers are important in muscular activity; both the supplementary and secondary motor cortices may assume function in disease of the corticospinal system. Sensory components are important both in influencing the type and degree of paralysis and in contributing to motor recovery, and the prognosis for return of function is less optimistic if there is significant sensory loss. It has been shown that hemispherectomy in pa-

tients with infantile hemiplegia can result in improvement in convulsions and mental symptoms without increasing the motor deficit. Although removal of a normally developed hemisphere in adults (as for treatment of a neoplasm) is followed by a spastic hemiparesis that principally affects skilled movements at distal joints, such removal in patients who have had a spastic hemiparesis since birth or early childhood is followed by a transient flaccid deficit that later becomes spastic, and the residual weakness is no worse than before the operation and is sometimes less. It is probable, in these patients, that either the normal hemisphere on the opposite side or other cortical or subcortical structures have previously assumed a portion of the function of the diseased area of the cortex.

Irritation of the corticospinal system, especially stimulation of the pyramidal cortex, causes an increased motor response with involuntary movements on the opposite side of the body. This may result in jacksonian convulsive seizures. In the presence of cerebral neoplasms or other pathologic processes there may be a corticospinal type of paresis, together with recurrent jacksonian convulsions in the involved extremities. Section of the pyramidal pathway after it has left the cortex, however, produces only paresis, and convulsions do not occur.

Time, clinical observation, and experimental data have shown that the concept of the "pure" corticospinal lesion must be changed, and that in the classic upper motor neuron lesion there is involvement of both motor and premotor centers. For clinical evaluation it seems justifiable to continue to regard the manifestations of spasticity, hyperreflexia, and pathologic reflexes as signs of involvement of the corticospinal system, but to remember that in certain "pure" pyramidal lesions there may instead be flaccidity, often followed by atrophy. In the presence of the classic upper motor neuron syndrome with spasticity and hyperreflexia there is probably, in most instances, either simultaneous involvement of both the motor (pyramidal) and premotor cortices, or interruption of their projections as they course through the internal capsule and descend into the spinal cord.

BIBLIOGRAPHY

Brodal A. Neurological Anatomy in Relation to Clinical Medicine, 3rd ed. New York, Oxford University Press, 1981

Bucy PC (ed). The Precentral Motor Cortex. Springfield, IL, Charles C Thomas, 1944

Bucy PC. Is there a pyramidal tract? Brain 1957;80:376

Davidoff RA. The pyramidal tract. Neurology 1990;40:332

Denny – Brown D. The frontal lobes and their function. In Feiling A (ed). Modern Trends in Neurology. New York, PB Hoeber, 1951

Denny – Brown D. The Cerebral Control of Movement. Springfield, IL, Charles C Thomas, 1966

Foerster O. The motor cortex in man in the light of Hughlings Jackson's doctrines. Brain 1936;59:135

Fulton JF, Kennard MA. A study of flaccid and spastic paralyses produced by lesions of the cerebral cortex in primates. Assoc Res Nerv Ment Dis Proc 1934;13:158

Jagiella WM, Sung JH. Bilateral infarction of the medullary pyramids in humans. Neurology 1989;39:21

Lassek AM. The Pyramidal Tract: Its Status in Medicine. Springfield, IL, Charles C Thomas, 1954

Paulson GW, Yates AJ, Paltan – Ortiz JD. Does infarction of the medullary pyramid lead to spasticity? Arch Neurol 1986;43:93

Penfield W, Rasmussen T. The Cerebral Cortex of Man: A Clinical Study of Localization of Function. New York, Macmillan, 1950

Powers RK, Marder – Meyer J, Rymer WZ. Quantitative relations between hypertonia and stretch reflex threshold in spastic quadriparesis. Ann Neurol 1988;23:115

Ruch TC, Chang HT, Ward AA Jr. The pattern of muscular response in evoked cortical discharge. Assoc Res Nerv Dis Proc 1947;26:61

Walshe FMR. The problem of the origin of the pyramidal tract. In Garland H (ed). Scientific Aspects of Neurology. Baltimore, Williams & Wilkins, 1961

Wiesendanger M. Pyramidal tract function and the clinical "pyramidal syndrome." Human Neurobiol 1984;2:227

The cerebellum is not primarily a motor organ. Phylogenetically it has developed out of a primary vestibular area, and it is intimately associated with the vestibular system and the various conductors of proprioceptive impulses. Originally its functions were related entirely to the vestibular complex. The cerebellum first reaches major proportions in birds, where it is important in maintaining equilibrium and orientation in space. It reaches its greatest development, however, in mammals which have skilled movements of the extremities. The evolution of the cerebellum parallels the development of the cerebral hemispheres. It has an intimate relationship with corticospinal and extrapyramidal components of motor function as well as with the brain stem reticular formation, and plays such an important part in motor control that one is justified in referring to the "cerebellar level" of motor activity or integration.

ANATOMY AND PHYSIOLOGY

The cerebellum is situated in the posterior fossa of the skull, beneath the occipital lobe of the cerebrum from which it is separated by the tentorium cerebelli. Below and anteriorly it is separated from the posterior aspect of the pons by the fourth ventricle and from the posterior aspect of the medulla and the dura mater covering the atlantooccipital membrane by a dilation of the subarachnoid space, the cisterna magna. From a morphologic point of view it is composed of three parts: a small, unpaired, median portion called the vermis, and two large, lateral masses,

the cerebellar hemispheres, which are connected with each other by the vermis (Figs. 24-1 and 24-2). Both the vermis and the hemispheres are divided, by fissures and sulci, into lobes and lobules.

The cerebellum is made up primarily of white matter which is covered with a thin layer of gray matter, the cerebellar cortex. Within the white matter are situated several gray masses, the cerebellar nuclei. The dentate nuclei, the largest of these, are purse-shaped structures situated within each hemisphere (Fig. 24-3). In the hilus of each dentate nucleus is the emboliform nucleus, and medial to the latter are the smaller globose nuclei which may consist of one or more rounded gray masses. In man these latter two nuclear groups are together called the nucleus interpositus. Within the medullary body of the vermis, at the roof of the fourth ventricle, are the fastigial, or roof, nuclei. Microscopically the cortex is made up of three distinct layers: (1) the outer, nuclear, or molecular layer; (2) the layer of Purkinje cells; and (3) the inner, or granular, layer.

The division of the cerebellum into vermis and hemispheres is a grossly morphologic but not a physiologic one, and the division into lobes and lobules has been classified variously (Fig. 24-4). According to Ingvar, the cerebellum may be divided into three lobes. The anterior lobe, which lies in front of the fissura prima, consists of the anterior portion of the vermis, with some lateral extensions. It is made up of the lingula, lobus centralis, and culmen. The posterior lobe comprises the midline pyramis, uvula, and nodule, with the flocculus and paraflocculus as lateral

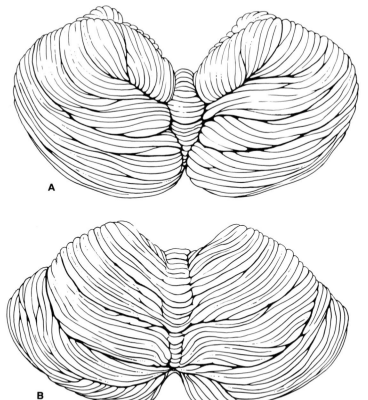

FIG. 24–1. A. Ventral and **B.** Dorsal views of the human cerebellum. See Fig. 24–4 for names of lobes and lobules.

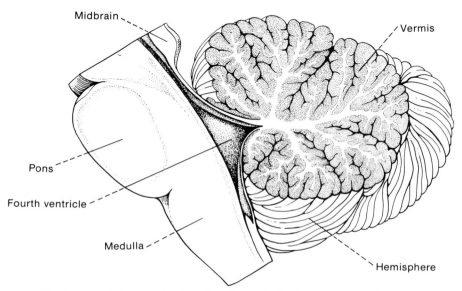

FIG. 24–2. Median longitudinal section through the human cerebellum, pons, and medulla.

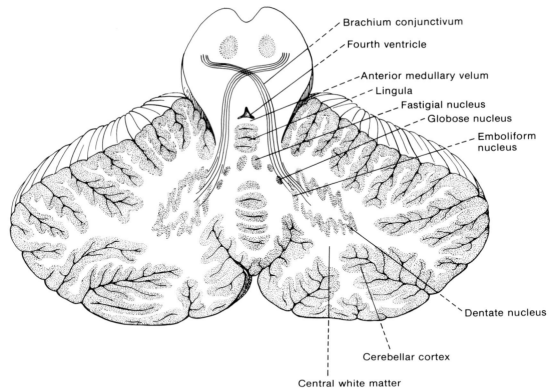

FIG. 24–3. Horizontal section through the human cerebellum showing the arrangement of the cortical gray matter and locations of the nuclei within the white matter.

extensions. The middle lobe is situated between the fissura prima and the prepyramidal sulcus; it consists of lobuli simplex, ansiformis, and paramedianus, along with the declive and tuber, and makes up the major portion of the cerebellum. Within the cerebellar cortex there is also a longitudinal pattern of organization with a certain degree of somatotopic representation. Very roughly speaking, the more medially located portions of the cerebellar cortex interact with the more medially situated areas of the vestibular nuclei, whereas the corresponding lateral areas of the cerebellar and vestibular nuclei also interconnect with each other. Similar relationships exist with cerebellar connections to other parts of the central nervous system.

Using phylogeny and experimental physiology as bases for classification, the cerebellum has been divided into two primary divisions. The vestibular flocculonodular lobe, or archicerebellum, is phylogenetically the oldest part, and its connections are primarily if not entirely vestibular. It receives fibers directly from the eighth nerve and possibly from the vestibular

nuclei, and it discharges to the vestibular nuclei. The corpus cerebelli, from which it is separated by the fissura posterolateralis, may be subdivided into a paleocerebellar and neocerebellar portion. The paleocerebellar portion is the more basal region which communicates with the spinal cord, brain stem, and vestibular centers. It is composed of the anterior lobe and the posterior portion of the posterior lobe. The principal afferent connections of the anterior lobe come from the ventral spinocerebellar tract, although the lingula receives some fibers from the vestibular nuclei and the culmen some corticocerebellar fibers. The discharges are to the vestibular nuclei, brain stem, and spinal cord. The posterior portion of the posterior lobe receives afferent fibers from the dorsal spinocerebellar tract and from the brain stem. The uvula also receives some vestibular fibers; the pyramis and paraflocculus, some corticocerebellar fibers. The posterior portion of the posterior lobe discharges to the brain stem, vestibular nuclei, and spinal cord. The neocerebellar division (middle lobe and anterior portion of the posterior lobe) is in communica-

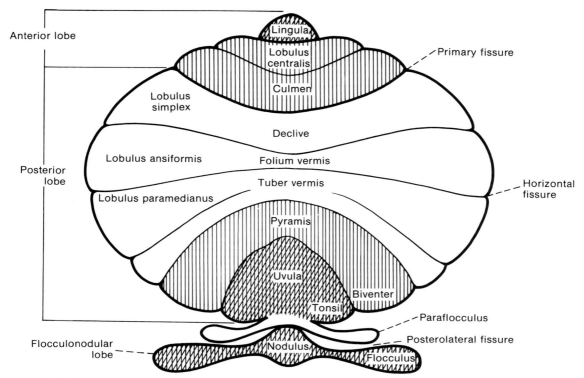

FIG. 24–4. Diagram of the cerebellum showing the lobes and lobules. The middle lobe is the large unshaded area.

tion with the cerebral cortex. It becomes enormously developed in mammals in association with differentiation of the skeletal musculature and growth of the cerebral hemispheres. In primates it is greatly elaborated and overshadows the rest of the cerebellum. Its afferent connections are principally corticopontine, or corticopontocerebellar, although the lobulus simplex receives some spinocerebellar fibers; it discharges through the dentate nucleus to the red nucleus and thalamus, and thus to the cerebral cortex.

The cerebellum is connected with the rest of the central nervous system by means of the three cerebellar peduncles. The inferior cerebellar peduncle, or restiform body, connects the cerebellum with the spinal cord and the medullary centers, and through it go, as ascending fibers, the dorsal spinocerebellar tract, the dorsal and ventral external arcuate fibers from the nuclei gracilis and cuneatus, the olivocerebellar, reticulocerebellar, and vestibulocerebellar pathways, and direct communications from the eighth nerve. The descending, or efferent, pathways are the cerebelloolivary, cerebellospinal, cerebello-

vestibular, and fastigiobulbar fibers. The middle cerebellar peduncle, or brachium pontis, connects the cerebellum with the cerebral cortex, and through it run the pontocerebellar tracts; these are the final neurons of the corticopontocerebellar pathway which comes mainly from the frontal, temporal, and other areas of the cortex to communicate with the contralateral cerebellar hemisphere. The superior cerebellar peduncle, or brachium conjunctivum, contains the principal efferent fibers of the cerebellum, the dentorubral and the dentothalamic pathways. Also contained in it are the ventral spinocerebellar pathway (afferent), fastigiobulbar fibers (fasciculus uncinatus of Russell), and the cerebellotegmental, cerebellotectal, and tectocerebellar tracts.

The afferent fibers are distributed to the cerebellar cortex and are furnished primarily by tracts which enter through the middle and inferior peduncles. Impulses ascend to the granular and molecular layers, but ultimately impinge upon the dendrites of the Purkinje cells, the axons of which pass through the white matter of the hemispheres and are distributed to the cerebellar nuclei, chiefly the dentate nuclei. Two structurally different afferent terminals are found in the cerebellar cortex. **Mossy fibers,** the termination of those neurons which enter the cerebellum through the inferior cerebellar peduncles, especially the direct spinocerebellar, olivocerebellar, and external arcuate tracts, give off many fine collaterals around the cells of the granular layer. The axons of the granular cells enter the molecular layer where they divide and establish synaptic relations with the dendritic expansions of the Purkinje cells. **Climbing fibers**, the terminations of the neurons carried through the brachium pontis, pass out to the molecular layer and divide into collaterals which come into contact with the arborizations of the Purkinje cells. The mossy fibers are thus connected indirectly with a large number of Purkinje cells, whereas the climbing fibers are in communication with only one or two Purkinje cells. The "avalanche" type of conduction from the mossy fibers, whereby certain incoming impulses are distributed to many cells, is an important characteristic of cerebellar function. Thus, on a cellular level, the cerebellum functions somewhat like a computer.

The efferent fibers from the cerebellar cortex and the Purkinje cells are nearly all relayed to the deep nuclei, where the efferent fibers from the cerebellum originate (Fig. 24-5). A small, phylogenetically old bundle, however, the flocculovestibular tract, travels directly from the flocculi to the vestibular nuclei. The fastigial nucleus, the oldest of the cerebellar nuclei, receives afferent fibers from the paleocerebellum and also from the vestibular nuclei and the eighth nerve. Its efferent impulses, many of them crossing in the roof, pass into the brain stem to the vestibular nuclei, especially the lateral one (Deiters' nucleus), and the reticular formation. Some of these go through the inferior peduncle, others (fasciculus uncinatus of Russell) pass with the superior peduncle. The dentate nucleus, the most important of the nuclear masses in terms of clinical function, receives its afferent fibers principally from the Purkinje cells of the neocerebellum; the emboliform nucleus receives impulses from the neocerebellum and the paleocerebellum; and the globose nuclei, principally from the paleocerebellum. All three of these nuclei discharge in the major efferent system of the cerebellum, the brachium conjunctivum, which terminates in the contralateral red nucleus and nucleus ventralis lateralis of the thalamus. Impulses are then relayed to the cerebral cortex.

The functions of the cerebellum were first studied by the analysis of the effects of removing the entire organ. Following extirpation there appears a state similar to that seen in decerebrate rigidity, with opisthotonos, head retraction, tonic extension and abduction of the forelimbs, and clonic movements of the hind limbs. Tremors are also present, and in unilateral ablations there are forced movements toward the side of the lesion. These effects are probably due to the release of postural mechanisms from inhibitory effects normally exercised by the cerebellum. Next deficiency phenomena develop, characterized by weakness, hypotonia, incoordination, and tremor on muscular activity; these resemble the symptoms seen clinically with extensive damage to the cerebellum. Finally there is a gradual recovery, probably explained by the progressive assumption of cerebellar function by the cerebrum or brain stem.

Stimulation of certain areas in the cerebellum is followed by localized motor responses and by either inhibition or facilitation of postural tonus and of cortically and reflexly induced movements; these effects are probably produced by means of impulses which converge on the midbrain and bulbar reticular formations.

From a phylogenetic point of view, the cerebellum is primarily a highly specialized vestibular nucleus. It receives afferent impulses from the labyrinths and vestibular centers, spinal cord, and brain stem (including the reticular formation and olivary bodies), and projects to the vestibular nuclei, vestibular tracts, and reticular formation. It probably also receives fibers from and projects to the vestibular areas in the cerebral cortex. It appears that the cerebellum and vestibular centers function together in the maintenance of equilibrium, the orientation of the organism in space, and the regulation of muscular tone and posture.

In the mammal, however, and especially in man, the cerebellum has many important functions other than those related to equilibrium and tone. It receives proprioceptive impulses from all parts of the body and both motor and sensory impulses from the cerebrum. It either dampens or potentiates and coordinates these impulses, and then passes them on. The histologic structure of the cerebellar cortex indicates that impulses brought into it are built up and strengthened through the "avalanche" method of conduction. The major functions of the cerebellum, from a clinical point of view, are the integration and coordination of somatic reactions. It reinforces and resynthesizes motor impulses and graduates and harmonizes muscular contractions, both in voluntary movement and in the maintenance of posture. Responses are made

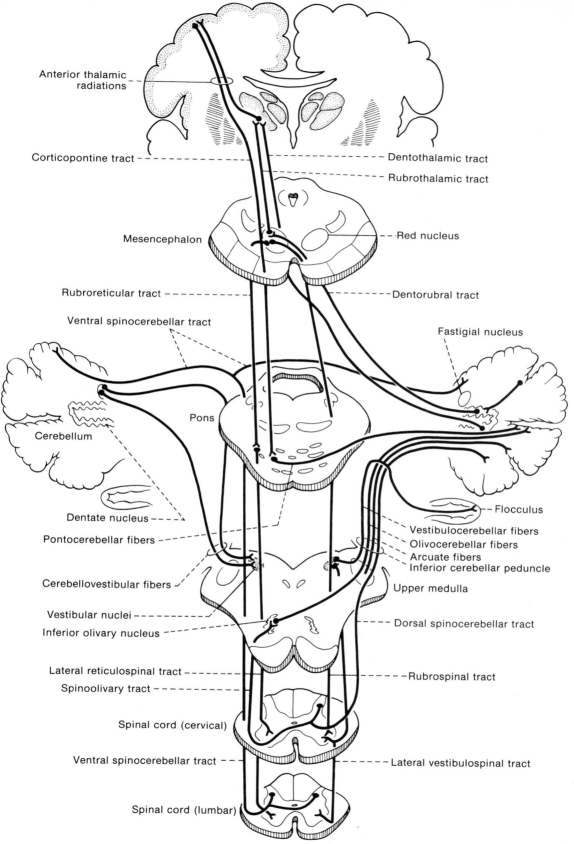

Anterior thalamic radiations

Corticopontine tract

Dentothalamic tract

Rubrothalamic tract

Mesencephalon

Red nucleus

Rubroreticular tract

Dentorubral tract

Ventral spinocerebellar tract

Fastigial nucleus

Pons

Cerebellum

Flocculus

Dentate nucleus

Pontocerebellar fibers

Vestibulocerebellar fibers
Olivocerebellar fibers
Arcuate fibers
Inferior cerebellar peduncle

Cerebellovestibular fibers

Upper medulla

Vestibular nuclei

Inferior olivary nucleus

Dorsal spinocerebellar tract

Lateral reticulospinal tract

Spinoolivary tract

Rubrospinal tract

Spinal cord (cervical)

Ventral spinocerebellar tract

Lateral vestibulospinal tract

Spinal cord (lumbar)

FIG. 24–5. Principal afferent and efferent connections of the cerebellum.

stronger and more certain, and voluntary movements are made smooth and synchronous. The cerebellum is the portion of the brain through which the cerebral motor cortex achieves the synthesis of coordinated units which compose voluntary movements. Thus it plays an important part in all motor functions. Recent investigations conclude that cerebellar structures function in scheduling a sequence of ordered responses prior to the initiation of movement, and that the cerebellum then translates such programmed responses into action. In humans, the lateral portions of the cerebellum appear more involved in timing processes, whereas the medial areas seem to function more in the implementation of responses at the desired time.

In addition, it has also been shown that tactile, auditory, and visual areas exist in the cerebellum. Motor, tactile, visual, and auditory centers in the cerebrum, both cortical and subcortical, project to similar areas in the cerebellum, which in turn project back to the corresponding cerebral areas. The structure thus is neither exclusively vestibular, proprioceptive, nor motor in function, but acts either to diminish or to reinforce both sensory and motor impulses, and is an important modulator of neurologic function. It projects impulses, often indirectly, to each source from which it receives them, and accordingly appears to act as an integrating mechanism that operates through a series of feedback circuits to maintain a desired level of neural activity.

CLINICAL MANIFESTATIONS OF CEREBELLAR DYSFUNCTION

The symptoms of cerebellar disease in man are, on the whole, consistent with those produced experimentally in animals. The principal manifestations are disturbances of muscular coordination and of locomotion and equilibrium (see Table 21-1 in Ch. 21). Voluntary movement is impaired. Muscular strength is normal or slightly decreased and easily fatigued. There is delay both in initiating and in relaxing contractions, and the contractions are of an intermittent and irregular character. The major disturbance, however, can be spoken of in a general way as loss of coordination, loss of control, or ataxia. The ataxia, however, is not specific for cerebellar disease, and lesions in other parts of the nervous system must be excluded before ascribing ataxia to cerebellar disease. Tests of cerebellar function are discussed in Chapter 30. The various aberra-

tions of movement, muscle function, and equilibrium that are seen in cerebellar disease are classified as follows:

Dyssynergy, and **asynergy** refer to the decrease and the loss of the faculty to associate more or less complex movements that have special functions. There is a lack of coordinated action between various groups of muscles or various movements which, as components of an act, are normally associated with the proper degree, harmony, timing, and sequence so that the act can be performed smoothly and accurately. The result is a lack of speed and skill in performing movements which require the synchronous activity of several groups of muscles or of several movements. If the various successive components of the act are not correlated in proper sequence and degree and are not properly grouped together, there is **decomposition of movement** — the act is broken down into its component parts and it is executed in the manner of a robot or puppet.

Dysmetria is the loss of ability to gauge the distance, speed, or power of movement. In lack of judgment of distance, or range, of movement, the act may be stopped before the goal is reached, or the individual may overshoot the desired point. In loss of judgment of rate, or speed, the movement may be carried out too slowly or too rapidly. With inability to gauge force, or power, the act may be carried out with too little or too much power.

Dysdiadochokinesia, or **adiodochokinesis,** is a disturbance in the reciprocal innervation of agonists and antagonists; there is a loss of ability to stop one act and follow it immediately by its diametric opposite. This is also known as impairment of rapid alternating movements. It is seen when the patient attempts alternate successive pronation and supination of the hands, rapid tapping of the fingers, or alternate opening and closing of the fists. Alternate movements are carried out either slowly or irregularly and clumsily. A disturbance in reciprocal innervation is also present in the **Holmes rebound phenomenon,** in which there is a loss of the "check reflex" and a failure of the ability to relax the contraction of the flexors of the forearm and rapidly contract the antagonists, or extensors.

Hypotonia, or **muscle flaccidity** with a decrease in resistance to passive movement of the joints, is often seen in cerebellar disease. The muscles are flabby and assume unnatural attitudes; the parts of the body can be moved passively into positions of extreme flexion or extension. There is a "hypotonic attitude" of the wrists, with a curving, downward flexion when the arms are extended. There have been some reports of the partial alleviation of the hypertonicity of parkinsonism and of congenital spastic paresis by surgical removal of either the dentate nucleus or large portions of the cerebellar hemispheres.

Asthenia, fatigability, and **slowness of movement** may develop. Asthenia refers to a mild degree of weakness. Severe weakness does not occur in lesions affecting the cerebellum alone. The muscles tire easily. Commencement of voluntary movement is delayed, and both the contraction and relaxation phases are abnormally slow.

Abnormal movements, or **hyperkinesias,** are frequent symptoms of cerebellar dysfunction. One most commonly sees an **intention type of tremor** (**active, kinetic,** or **terminal tremor**) which is not present at rest but becomes evident on purposeful movement. When this occurs in the hand, there are coarse, irregular, to-and-fro, jerky movements which increase in amplitude and coarseness as the hand approaches its objective. The movements may involve not only the extremities, but also the head or even the entire body. It has been stated that the hyperkinesias may be due to hypotonia and irregularities of muscular contraction, but these factors do not entirely explain them. There may be, however, other abnormalities of movement, secondary to unsteadiness and incoordination, which may simulate more gross hyperkinesias. The tremors and other movements probably result from involvement of the cerebellar afferent pathways in their connections with the red nucleus and thalamus (dentorubral and dentothalamic pathways, or superior cerebellar peduncle).

Abnormalities of posture and gait with abnormal attitudes and spontaneous deviation of the head and parts of the body may be seen in cerebellar disease. In unilateral cerebellar disease there may be deviation of the head and body toward the affected side, with past pointing of the extremities toward that side. In standing the body is inclined to fall toward the side of the lesion, and in walking there is a deviation toward that side. The outstretched extremities deviate laterally, toward the affected side. There may be a decrease or absence of the normal pendular movement of the arm in walking. In midline, or vermis, lesions the patient may not be able to stand erect and may fall either backward or forward. The gait is staggering, reeling, or lurching in character, without laterality. Abnormal attitudes of the extremities owing to muscular hypotonicity have already been mentioned.

Speech disturbances may be noted, and articulation may be slow, ataxic, slurred, drawling, jerky, or explosive in type, owing to asynergy of the muscles of phonation. The scanning speech of multiple sclerosis and the staccato speech of Friedreich's ataxia are probably the result of cerebellar dysfunction.

Nystagmus and deviation of the eyes may be present with lesions of the cerebellum. The former is encountered frequently, but may differ in type as well as in mechanism of production. Its presence often indicates that the vestibulocerebellar pathways are affected, and thus suggests involvement of either the vermis region or the inferior cerebellar peduncle. On other occasions the abnormal ocular movements may result from involvement of the connections of the cerebellum with other centers rather than actual lesions of the cerebellum itself. They may be caused by pressure on other structures, or what appears to be nystagmus may actually be an ocular expression of cerebellar asynergia. With a lesion of one hemisphere the eyes at rest may be deviated 10° – 30° toward the unaffected side. When the patient attempts to focus his vision elsewhere the eyes move toward the point of fixation with quick jerks, and there are slow return movements to the resting point. The movements are more marked and of greater amplitude when the patient looks toward the affected side. When a tumor of the cerebellopontine angle is present, the nystagmus is coarse on looking toward the side of the lesion and fine and rapid on gaze to the opposite side. Nystagmus is usually not present with parenchymatous cerebellar degenerations. Occasionally, with cerebellar lesions, there is **skew deviation** of the eyes: the eye homolateral to the lesion is turned downward and inward, and the contralateral eye upward and outward.

The **muscle stretch reflexes** are normal or diminished in disease limited to the cerebellum. Occasionally one may note **pendular reflexes.** If the patellar tendon is stimulated while the foot is hanging free, there is a series of to-and-fro movements of the foot and leg before the limb finally comes to rest; this response is normally prevented by the after-shortening of the quadriceps femoris. When hyporeflexia is present, it and the pendular response are probably caused by the hypotonicity of the flexor and extensor muscles and the lack of the restraining effect which they normally exert upon each other when a normal degree of tone is present. The cutaneous reflexes are unaffected.

Rigidity has been said to occur in association with cerebellar lesions. So-called tonic convulsions are often called "cerebellar fits." In these there is sudden rigidity, with extensor hypertonia, often of a decerebrate type, and opisthotonos, accompanied by cyanosis and unconsciousness. The arms are extended at the elbows, flexed at the wrists, and strongly pronated. The legs are extended at the hips, knees, and ankles, and the toes are plantar flexed. While these tonic manifestations have been attributed to cerebellar disease and have been said to occur either on the basis of irritation or secondary to release of postural mechanisms from the normal inhibitory action of the cerebellum, they are probably the result of transient ischemia of higher centers in the brain stem and cerebrum, at times due to pressure.

There is no paralysis or loss of power in lesions of the cerebellum, although the ataxia may be so profound and the asthenia so marked that motor activities cannot be performed. Atrophy and fasciculations do not develop. There are no pathologic reflexes, and even though the cerebellum is a proprioceptive reception center there are no conscious or demonstrable sensory changes when the disease process is confined to the cerebellum. The ataxia and other abnormalities are never limited to specific muscles, muscle groups, or movements, and are apparent in an entire extremity, an entire half of the body, or bilaterally in the head, neck, trunk, or entire body.

LOCALIZATION OF CEREBELLAR DISEASE

At present, evidence of *clinical localization of function* in the cerebellum is inconclusive. There is no cytoarchitectonic evidence of such localization. If it does exist, it is in relation to the efferent rather than the afferent system. Experimental studies have demonstrated syndromes that follow lesions of the three major divisions of the cerebellum, and the usually accepted clinical syndromes correspond to the pathophysiologic alterations produced by these experimental lesions. Recently introduced precise imaging studies, such as computerized tomography and magnetic resonance may further help to define the clinical functions of the various parts of the cerebellum.

Lesions of the flocculonodular lobe, or archicerebellum, give rise to the **vermis,** or **midline syndrome.** There is a large vestibular component to the manifestations, and the symptoms closely resemble those found in vestibular disease. In addition, since the vermis is unpaired and appears to be of importance in the regulation of the axial structures, or those that are bilaterally innervated, coordination of the head and trunk are affected. There are gross postural and locomotor disturbances of the entire body. There is trunkal ataxia with swaying and unsteadiness when standing, and the patient may be unable to maintain an upright position. At times there may be loss of ability even to hold the trunk erect when seated, or to hold the neck and head in a steady and upright position. There is no lateralization and there may be a tendency to fall either backward or forward. The disturbance in equilibrium is especially marked in the gait, which may be characterized by swaying, staggering, and titubation. The patient may reel, in a drunken manner, to either side. There may be little or no particular involvement of the extremities, especially the upper extremities, although all coordinated movements may be poorly performed. There may be unsteadiness of the head, neck, or entire body, and gross impairment of muscle function, but there usually are no tremors. Muscle tone is normal, as are the reflexes. Nystagmus may be present, but often is not marked. Dysarthria, however, is often evident. The most common cause of the complete vermis syndrome is a medulloblastoma of the cerebellum, which occurs by far most frequently in children.

Lesions of the **anterior lobe** of the cerebellum (paleocerebellum) may cause hypertonicity, decerebrate rigidity, and increased stretch reflexes, but some of these signs are probably related to concomitant involvement of the brain stem. There may be gross disturbances of coordination and equilibrium, and nodding and weaving movements of the head and trunk. Alcoholic and carcinomatous (remote effect) degenerations of the cerebellum affect mainly the anterior lobe, and it is involved in such conditions as corticocerebellar and olivopontocerebellar degenerations.

The **syndrome of the cerebellar hemispheres** is essentially that seen in disease of the corpus cerebelli, or neocerebellum. The manifestations are appendicular rather than axial. They are usually unilateral and occur on the side of the diseased hemisphere. There is a gross disturbance of skilled movements of the extremities, and the arm and hand are affected more than the leg and foot, regardless of the area of the hemisphere involved. Distal movements are affected more than proximal and fine movements more than gross ones. Disturbances of isolated movements, with ataxia, dysmetria, dyssynergy, dysdiadochokinesia, hypotonicity, asthenia, and fatigability are present. Movements are performed irregularly, and there may be tremors of an intention type, or other hyperkinesias if the dentate nucleus or its efferent pathways are involved. The muscle stretch reflexes are usually diminished or are of the pendular type.

Posture and gait are not impaired to the extent that is detected in the vermis syndrome, but there may be characteristic changes. There may be swaying and falling toward the side of the lesion, with deviation of the occiput toward that side. The patient may be unable to stand when using only the homolateral foot, but may retain the ability to stand when using only the contralateral foot. He may be unable to bend his body toward the involved side without falling. In walking there may be some unsteadiness, and the patient may deviate or rotate toward the involved side. There may be a "compass gait" toward the involved side (see "Equilibratory Coordination," Ch. 30), and in walking around a chair, whether in a clockwise or a counterclockwise direction, the patient shows a tendency to fall toward the affected side. There may be spontaneous deviation of the extended extremities toward the involved side, with past pointing toward that side. There may be a slurred type of dysarthria, although disturbances of articulation

are more marked in vermis lesions. Nystagmus is a common finding; it is usually horizontal but may be rotatory. It is coarser and slower when the eyes are deviated toward the side of the lesion. The above syndrome is seen most characteristically in hemispheric neoplasms, as in astrocytoma of the cerebellum.

The symptoms of cerebellar disease differ markedly in severity, depending upon the acuteness or the chronicity of the process. If the lesion is acute, the symptoms are profound; if it is slowly progressive, the manifestations of cerebellar deficiency are much less severe. There may be an extensive involvement of the hemispheres without clinical symptoms, and there may be considerable recovery from the effects of an acute lesion. In fact, persons with little remaining cerebellar tissue eventually can function quite well. The symptoms of cerebellar deficiency may be similar regardless of the etiology of the disease process, and whether the lesion is congenital or acquired.

Among the *causes of cerebellar disease* may be included the following: congenital abnormalities such as agenesis or hypoplasia, atresia of the foramina of Luschka and Magendie with enlargement of the fourth ventricle (Dandy–Walker syndrome), or cerebellar involvement associated with platybasia (basilar impression), the Chiari malformations; neoplasms of either the vermis or the hemispheres, or of the brain stem or cerebellopontine angle with secondary cerebellar involvement; trauma, including cerebellar extradural hematoma; acute and chronic infections and toxic disorders and those resulting from prolonged use of certain drugs such as phenytoin; deficiency states; vascular lesions, including intracerebellar hemorrhage and thrombosis of the posterior inferior, anterior inferior, and superior cerebellar arteries; so-called degenerative processes, including the hereditary cerebellar and spinocerebellar ataxias, olivopontocerebellar atrophy, progressive and myoclonic cerebellar dyssynergy, parenchymatous and cortical cerebellar atrophy, Joseph disease, lipid and other storage disorders, and hereditary ataxic polyneuritis (Refsum's syndrome); and demyelinating diseases such as multiple sclerosis. Cerebellar degenerations have also been reported secondary to or associated with alcoholism, hyperpyrexia, carcinomatosis, lymphomas, and oculocutaneous telangiectasia. It must be remembered that on occasion symptoms suggestive of involvement of one cerebellar hemisphere may be encountered with lesions of the opposite cerebral hemisphere, and that under-development or atrophy of one cerebellar hemisphere may be associated with underdevelopment or involvement of the opposite cerebral hemisphere.

Extensive studies have been carried out on experimental animals to investigate the relationship between the cerebellum and motor abnormalities, convulsive episodes, and behavior. It has been shown, on the basis of anatomic and electrophysiologic evidence, that the cerebellum can modify sensory information and motor behavior. As a consequence, chronic stimulation of the cerebellum was carried out for the treatment of both epilepsy and motor disturbances such as cerebral palsy. Low-frequency stimulation was used in the treatment of epilepsy, and higher-frequency stimulation for cerebral palsy. Because of late complications, however, these modes of therapy have become uncommon.

BIBLIOGRAPHY

Aicardi J, Barbosa C, Andermann E et al. Ataxia-oculomotor apraxia: a syndrome mimicking ataxia-telangiectasia. Ann Neurol 1988;24:497

Brodal A. Neurological Anatomy in Relation to Clinical Medicine, 3rd ed. New York, Oxford University Press, 1981

Cooper IS, Amin I, Riklan N et al. Chronic cerebellar stimulation in epilepsy. Arch Neurol 1976;33:559

Dow RS, Moruzzi G. The Physiology and Pathology of the Cerebellum. Minneapolis, University of Minnesota Press, 1958

Fenichel GM, Phillips JA. Familial aplasia of the cerebellar vermis. Possible X-linked dominant inheritance. Arch Neurol 1989;46:582

Fields WS, Willis WD, Jr (eds). The Cerebellum in Health and Disease. St. Louis, WH Green, 1970

Gilman S, Bloedel JR, Lechtenberg R. Disorders of the Cerebellum. Philadelphia, FA Davis, 1981

Greenfield JG. The Spino-cerebellar Degenerations. Springfield IL, Charles C Thomas, 1954

Holmes G. The Croonian lectures on the clinical symptoms of cerebellar disease and their interpretation. Lancet 1922;1:1177, 1231;2:59, 111

Ingvar S. On cerebellar localization. Brain 1923;46:301

Inhoff AW, Diener HC, Rafal RD, Ivry R. The role of cerebellar structures in the execution of serial movements. Brain 1989;112:565

Ivry RB, Keele SW, Diener HC. Dissociation of the lateral and medial cerebellum in movement timing and movement execution. Exp Brain Res 1988;73:167

Landau WM. Ataxic hindbrain thinking: The clumsy cerebellum syndrome. Neurology 1989;39:315.

Larsell O. The cerebellum: A review and interpretation. Arch Neurol Psychiatry 1937;38:580

Masur H, Elger CE, Ludolph AC, Galanski M. Cerebellar atrophy following acute intoxication with phenytoin. Neurology 1989;39:432

Rowland LP (ed). Merritt's Textbook of Neurology, 8th ed. Philadelphia, Lea & Febiger, 1989

Snider RS. Recent contributions to the anatomy and physiology of the cerebellum. Arch Neurol Psychiatry 1950;64:196

Chapter 25
PSYCHOMOTOR COMPONENTS

The final or highest motor level of integration, in the present concept of motor activity, is the so-called psychomotor level. This is the "newest" of all motor levels, and it corresponds to the third level of Jackson — the motor division of the "organ of the mind" — which has its origin in the prefrontal areas of the brain. Cobb refers to it as the "cortical associative" level that involves initiative and memory, in contrast to the "cortical motor" level, which is herein called the corticospinal or pyramidal level. This latter is referred to as the center for voluntary motor activity, but by "voluntary" is meant most highly integrated, rather than actually volitional.

The psychomotor level may be thought of as the portion of the motor system where volitional movements are initiated, but it should be considered both voluntary and involuntary, conscious and unconscious. All purposive movements are initiated and guided in their performance by a constant stream of afferent impulses that reach the cerebral cortex, following which associations take place, so that sensation and motion are interdependent in the performance of voluntary movement. The sensations, however, need not be consciously perceived. Furthermore, at this level of integration, initiative, memory, and symbolization enter into motor activity; memories are called out and previous experiences are used to alter responses to immediate stimuli. Skilled acts can be performed with a high degree of precision, but stereotyped and automatic movements integrated at a lower level and patterned complexes learned earlier in life can be used as part of the response.

It is easily understood that there is a major element of voluntary control of all motor activity; movements may be initiated or stopped, inhibited or exaggerated, or in many ways altered through volitional control. Alterations in tone, changes in posture, contractures, and abnormalities of movement may all be of voluntary origin. In malingering, for instance, a paralysis, hyperkinesis, or abnormality of tone may be simulated on a voluntary basis. Reflexes may even be influenced. There are also, however, alterations in motor power that originate in the psychomotor sphere but are involuntary or unconscious in origin. In hysteria, for example, there may be paralyses, hyperkinesias, changes in tone, contractures, and even resulting deformities and atrophy that are psychogenically initiated but are on an unconscious basis. The paralyses, however, are apparent rather than real, and may simulate other types of loss of power; they are often bizarre in character and fail to conform to a specific organic or anatomic pattern. The tone may be normal or variable, but is often increased. Fasciculations, primary atrophy, and electrical abnormalities are absent, and there is no true ataxia. The reflexes are usually normal, but occasionally there is hyperactivity of both deep and superficial reflexes. There are no pathologic reflexes, and associated movements are normal (see Table 21-1, in Ch. 21). Hyperkinesias, if present, can usually be differentiated from abnormal movements of organic origin. The differentiation between psychogenic disturbances of motor activity, either on a conscious or an unconscious basis, and changes in motor function secondary to organic disease is sometimes difficult (Ch. 55).

The motor manifestations seen in some of the psychoses, such as the psychomotor retardation of the depressed patient, the hyperactivity of the manic, and the bizarre motor phenomena of catatonia and some of the organic psychoses, are also evidences of disturbed function of this level of motor integration, as are the automatisms and abnormal behavior of complex partial epileptic seizures. Finally, the apraxias (Ch. 52), in which there is loss of ability to carry out purposive acts in the absence of paralysis, may be considered disturbances of psychomotor function, regardless of whether the apraxia is motor, sensory, or idiokinetic in type.

The psychomotor level of integration is the highest one in evolutionary development, and is not present in lower forms. It is a motor level, but not purely motor, since in its functioning such factors as association, memory, imitation, and coordination in the volitional sense of the word are brought into play.

SUMMARY

In summing up our knowledge of motor integration, we can see that each of the components of the motor system has its part to play: the myoneural junction, where the motor impulse reaches the muscle fibers; the anterior horn cells in the spinal cord and the motor nuclei in the brain stem, which act as the final common pathway along which all impulses must travel in order to reach expression in the muscles; the simple postural and standing reflexes in the hindbrain and more complex standing and righting reflexes in the midbrain; the coordinating action of the cerebellum; the function of the basal ganglia in locomotor reflexes and automatic movements; the motor and premotor cortex in integration of skilled movements; and finally the association areas in use of experiences and in the conscious and unconscious control of motor activity. No coordinated or integrated action can take place without simultaneous and synchronous action of all, harmoniously playing on the anterior horn cells. In order to appraise the constituent motor functions and the method for examining each, and in order to comprehend intelligently the significance of changes in movement that may occur in disease of the nervous system, we must first appreciate the combined and coordinated action of these individual components of motor activity.

Chapter 26
FUNCTIONS OF THE MOTOR SYSTEM

Motor activity is brought about by the combined and harmonious action of the various component parts of the motor system. Abnormalities of movement may be caused (1) by impairment or loss of function of one or more of the so-called levels of motor integration; (2) by overactivity of the lower centers as a result of their release from the inhibiting action of the higher centers; (3) by irritation, or stimulation, of certain constituent parts; or (4) by partial assumption of function by healthy tissues to compensate for impairment or disease of others. Consequently, the character of change in motor function that occurs in disease is dependent both upon the component level involved and upon the type of pathologic process that affects it. In most instances, however, the so-called levels cannot be examined or even considered individually, for they all act together upon the final common pathway where they are synthesized, oftentimes in a complex fashion. Even though one level may be predominantly affected by a disease process, the resulting change in function can be considered only as it influences motor activity as a whole. The character of the impairment, however, and the portion of the motor system primarily involved, give important information to aid in determining the location and diagnosis of the pathologic process.

There are many constituent functions of motor activity, each of which is influenced to some extent by all of the levels of motor integration. For adequate evaluation of motor functions as a whole each may have to be examined and appraised individually. The most obvious function is motor strength, or power, as exhibited in active movement. If this is impaired there is increased fatigability, decreased dexterity, and abnormalities in the speed and range of movement, with resulting weakness or paralysis, and deformities. There are, however, many other important elements of motor function, namely, muscle tone, or the resistance to passive movement; muscle volume and contour; coordination of movement, including such factors as agility, flexibility, balance, and performance of complex and skilled acts; abnormal movements; posture and gait. Each of these is discussed individually in Chapters 27 through 32; the methods of examination are presented, and the changes that occur in association with disease processes are outlined. Normal and abnormal associated movements are considered in Chapter 38, and defects of purposive movement, or the apraxias, in Chapter 52.

In order to evaluate the above factors most effectively and in order to perform a systematic examination of the various motor functions, special observations and certain tests are indicated. These are described in detail under the individual subjects. A few preliminary generalizations, however, should be remembered. As in the case of the examination of the sensory system, the motor examination is most satisfactory if the subject is alert and his mind is keen. He should understand the procedures and be ready and willing to cooperate. Their purpose and method should be explained to him in simple terms, so that he may comprehend what is expected of him. Pain, discomfort of any type, sedative or narcotic drugs, fatigue, nervous tension, and apprehension all may interfere with the observations. If the patient is in a state of confusion or lowered consciousness, or if his intelligence is impaired or he fails to understand the examiner's terminology, the procedures may be modified. If fatigue and inability to concentrate occur, the examination should be stopped and resumed when the patient is rested. The possibility of conscious or unconscious (malingered or hysterical) changes must always be borne in mind.

During the examination of motor functions the patient should be warm and comfortable. Clothing that interferes with visualization of muscles should be removed. The room should be well lighted. One may first, by inspection, observe the posture and build, muscular development, bulk and symmetry, the position of the body parts at rest, active and passive movements, congenital absence of muscles, presence of deformities, and skeletal abnormalities. The character of the spontaneous active movements should be noted, as well as any abnormal movements. During the examination, however, one relies not only on inspection but also on palpation, to note volume, consistency, contraction, and tenderness, and, to a lesser extent, on percussion. The two sides of the body should be compared, and any asymmetries noted. One should always inquire about handedness before testing motor power. The dominant extremity is normally slightly stronger than its mate.

The examination of motor functions, if carried out adequately and in detail, is a difficult and arduous procedure. It must be painstaking and accompanied by critical evaluation. It requires the knowledge of the action of each muscle and muscle group, and ranges from the testing of a single muscle to the evaluation of complex movements, coordinated functions, and skilled acts. It frequently must include electromyography and nerve conduction studies, and on occasion requires special chemical tests as well as muscle biopsy and histochemical study of muscle.

Chapter 27
MOTOR STRENGTH AND POWER

Motor strength and power indicate the capacity to exert and release force; they involve the expenditure of energy. Of importance are both the power of movement and the strength of contraction, not only of individual muscles, but also of groups of muscles and of movements. Power is sometimes classified as **kinetic,** the force exerted in changing position, and **static,** the force exerted in resisting movement. Both are tested, and in most disease processes both are equally affected. In certain conditions, however, as in the extrapyramidal syndromes, kinetic power may be diminished while static power remains normal. In examining strength and power we are interested especially in voluntary, or active, motility. In general, this is tested in two ways — by having the patient carry out movements against the resistance of the examiner, and by having him resist active attempts on the part of the examiner to move fixed parts. On occasion, however, movements may have to be tested when they are carried out without resistance or even with assistance, and one may only be able to note the power to resist gravity, or may even observe muscle strength when the parts are supported in water. Passive movements may also be tested to note range or limitation of motion. Impairment of strength and power results in **weakness,** or **paresis;** absence of strength, in **paralysis.**

Simultaneous with the testing of strength and power and the observation of their impairment, associated functions and abnormalities must be noted. **Endurance** is the ability to perform the same act repeatedly over a period of time; loss of endurance may be an early manifestation of paresis. Abnormal fatigability may precede other objective manifestations of impairment of energy. The speed, or rapidity, of movement and the range, or amplitude, of motion may be impaired in weakness. If loss of these functions is present, there may be a decrease in the flexibility, or suppleness, of movement, or loss of ability to move the joints through their full range. This may be followed by limitation of movement, contractures, and deformities.

There is a marked individual variation in muscle strength, dependent in part upon body build, early training, and activity. As a result, a *diffuse* deficiency in strength of mild degree may be of little significance but the presence of *local* muscle weakness or paralysis is of great importance, and recognition of such changes has definite localizing value in the diagnosis of peripheral or central nervous system lesions. If weakness is found, one should determine whether it is diffuse or localized. If localized, one should determine whether it is due to involvement of a specific muscle, of various muscles supplied by one nerve or nerve root, of a group of muscles supplied by a certain segment of the spinal cord, of a specific movement involving more than one muscle, or of an entire extremity.

Weakness is manifested not only by loss of power, but also by fatigability, variation in strength on repeated tests, diminished range and rate of movement, loss of coordination, irregularity and clumsiness of motion, tremulousness, loss of associated movements, and lack of ability to carry out skilled acts. Attempts to contract individual muscles may be accompanied by movement of an entire extremity. In comatose states the paretic extremities may be flaillike, and drop when the examiner releases them. In extrapyramidal disease rigidity may interfere with apparent muscle power, and bradykinesia delays the onset of muscle contraction and causes retardation of movement. Hyperkinesias of various types and ataxia may make motor activity difficult. Loss or impairment of motion may also occur with pain, swelling, spasm, local shock, fractures, dislocations, adhesions or ankylosis of joints, contractures of either agonists or antagonists, loss of tendon or muscle sense, hysteria, malingering, and catatonic states.

Motor weakness, if diffuse, may be the result of poor muscular development or inadequate muscular training. On the other hand, diffuse weakness may be found in some myopathies, such as the dystrophies, and in electrolyte disturbances, toxic and deficiency states, and the various types of myositis, in debilitated states due to chronic systemic illness, and to some degree in advanced age. Either localized or diffuse weakness may be a manifestation of myasthenia gravis (or the rare drug-induced myasthenias), in which there is an increased muscular fatigability. Repeated contractions may be followed by such profound fatigue that an apparent paresis develops; similar fatigability follows repeated electrical stimulation (Jolly's reaction). The neostigmine and edrophonium tests may be used to confirm the diagnosis of myasthenia gravis. The subcutaneous injection of 1.5 mg of neostigmine methylsulfate (with 0.6 mg atropine sulfate) is followed by a marked improvement in the asthenia and fatigability and an increase in the strength of the paretic muscles. The patient should be observed at 10 min intervals for a period of 1 hour after the injection. The objective and subjective improvement may be charted. A similar increase in strength follows the intravenous injection of 10 mg of edrophonium chloride, but the improvement starts within 10 sec, and strength may reach its maximum and begin to decline before 5 min have passed. The prompt improvement in function with both of these tests differentiates myasthenia gravis from the myopathies, the myasthenic syndrome of Eaton – Lambert, neurosis, fatigue states, and cranial nerve palsies. Occasionally either quinine sulfate or curare is given first to persons with suspected myasthenia gravis to cause increased weakness before the neostigmine or edrophonium tests are carried out. Such procedures are hazardous, however, and should be considered only in carefully selected patients who are under continuous observation. Determination of acetylcholine

receptor antibody titers in the serum is also a useful diagnostic adjunct for myasthenia gravis.

Focal loss of strength results in either a paresis or a paralysis, in the presence of which one must determine the degree, character, and distribution of the impairment of motor power. The paralysis may involve one muscle, a group of muscles, certain movements, or one or more extremities. A **monoplegia** is the paralysis of one extremity; **diplegia,** of like parts on the two sides of the body; **hemiplegia,** of one half of the body; **paraplegia,** the legs or the lower parts of the body; **quadriplegia** and **tetraplegia,** of all four extremities. **Hemiplegia alternans** affects the upper extremity on one side of the body and the lower extremity on the other side.

When a muscle is maintained in a position of contraction or shortening for a period of time, a contracture may develop: the muscle cannot be stretched to normal limits without considerable pressure and the production of pain. This may be neurogenic, without alteration of muscle tissue, but in most instances there is fibrous replacement of the muscle tissue. Contractures may develop following prolonged spasm of muscles, in association with spastic paralysis (especially if the muscles are not passively stretched at regular intervals), or from the overaction of one group of muscles when unopposed by weakened antagonists. They may result in periarthritic changes, ankylosis of joints, and deformities. Spasm, contracture, and structural fixation of joints may occur simultaneously.

It must be borne in mind that contractures and deformities that resemble them may be the result of many different causes. An equinus deformity of the foot, for instance, may be produced by a foot drop resulting from a peripheral peroneal palsy; by spasm of the gastrocnemius, in a spastic paresis; by a developmental anomaly, such as a congenital clubfoot; or by trauma or arthritis. In the evaluation of contractures and deformities it is important to differentiate between those of neurogenic origin and those due to fractures and other post-traumatic lesions, arthropathies, congenital abnormalities, muscular or tendinous strain or infiltration, habitual postures, occupational factors, or other diseases that cause mechanical difficulty with movement. The periarthritic changes in the shoulder that may develop because of disuse following a hemiplegia must be differentiated from limitation of movement in the shoulder owing to primary articular disease. The ankylosis of the wrist joint associated with a long-standing wrist drop caused by a radial nerve palsy, and the contracture of the fingers occurring with claw hand resulting from an ulnar nerve paralysis, must be differentiated from the deformities seen in arthritis, Volkmann's contracture, Dupuytren's contracture, and so forth. It is important to determine if pain is present on passive movement, and one should make every effort to determine whether limitation or absence of movement is the result of paralysis, pain, muscle spasm, swelling, or fibrous or bony alterations.

EXAMINATION OF MOTOR STRENGTH AND POWER

The evaluation of motor strength and power of various muscle groups and movements is a complicated process and requires a detailed examination. Adequate knowledge of the function of the individual muscles is necessary. Actually, however, the contraction of a single muscle is rarely possible, since others that have similar functions participate in almost every movement. Furthermore, in order for a muscle to contract, its antagonists must relax and the synergistic and fixating muscles must also be brought into play. The predominating action of a single muscle, however, can usually be determined. In addition to the understanding of the action of individual muscles, one must, in the evaluation of motor function, understand the combined action of groups of muscles in the performance of gross movements and comprehend the harmonious and synchronous or consecutive action of muscles in carrying out coordinated acts. The examiner must also be familiar with the peripheral nerve and segmental innervation of each important muscle in order to distinguish peripheral nerve and plexus lesions from those that involve segmental structures. Inasmuch as many muscles are innervated from more than one spinal segment, it is important to remember that involvement of the fibers from one segment does not necessarily mean a complete loss of function of the involved muscles. Certain combinations of motor deficit can point only to a peripheral nerve lesion, others to a plexus or a segmental or root injury. In peripheral nerve lesions muscles or groups of muscles supplied by a particular nerve may be paralyzed, whereas in radicular or segmental lesions parts of muscles innervated by different nerves may be affected. Sometimes these muscles have antagonistic functions.

To test motor power, the various movements at each joint and the strength of each important muscle should be examined individually and its

grade recorded, as far as possible. The patient may be either seated or recumbent. He is instructed to either resist active attempts by the examiner to move fixed parts or to initiate and carry out movements that are resisted by the examiner. Both methods may be used interchangeably, although patients usually comprehend and cooperate better with the former, while initiation of movement by the patient may be the best method of testing weak muscles. The examiner should avoid abrupt application of pressure and should gradually increase the force exerted; cooperative patients maintain a smooth resistance and this "follow-through" continues as the examiner decreases the force exerted and allows the joint to move. Repeated testing may be used to demonstrate the presence of fatigability.

It must always be remembered that there is much individual variation in muscle power and that the muscles on the dominant side are usually somewhat stronger than those opposite. Corresponding muscles on the two sides of the body should always be compared. Fatigue, systemic illness, failure to comprehend the method of testing, and many other factors may result in a false and/or distorted impression of weakness. Much experience may be necessary before an examiner can be certain of his results in determining loss of strength or varying degrees of weakness. While judgment of the force exerted in either initiating or resisting movement is the major criterion in the evaluation of strength or weakness, observation of muscular contraction and palpation are also essential guides, especially if there is a decrease in power. By placing the fingertips over the belly of the muscle or over its tendon one may feel the contraction of the former and the movement of the latter. Even the powerless effort to move a muscle may be accompanied by a synergistic contraction of neighboring or antagonistic muscles, which may be palpated rather than seen, and in feigned paralyses the contraction of the suspected muscles may be felt when the patient is asked to carry out movements with the antagonists. By careful observation one may also judge loss of function of certain muscles by noting the alterations of movement and position and substitution of other movements for paretic ones.

Proper positioning of the patient is necessary in conducting and evaluating tests of muscle strength. The part of the body to be examined is placed in the position that will permit the muscle to act directly and at the same time inhibit as far as possible the action of muscles of similar function. It is important to fix the proximal portion of a limb when the movements of the distal portion are being tested; for instance, the humerus should be fixed when testing pronation, so that the patient does not use his shoulder to compensate for a deficiency in pronation. Paresis may be overlooked when the action of accessory muscles is substituted for that of affected ones. On the other hand, paresis may be mistaken for paralysis if the movement takes place in an unfavorable attitude, as, for instance, the overcoming of the effect of gravity. The biceps and triceps muscles can contract more easily, in the presence of weakness, if the elbow is raised outward to the height of the shoulder so that the forearm can be moved in the horizontal plane. There may be an apparent weakness of grip with a radial nerve palsy if it is tested with the wrist in flexion, but if the wrist is actively or passively extended it can be seen that the flexors of the fingers contract normally. Paresis of muscles must be distinguished from spasm or contracture of antagonists, and involvement of individual muscles or muscle groups from generalized weakness of major portions of the body or predominant paresis of major movement patterns, such as flexion or extension of entire extremities.

The position and attitude of the limbs, the facility, range, speed, endurance, and fatigability of the motor responses, and the regularity of voluntary and spontaneous movements should be observed. If there is a deficiency of motor response, one should note whether it is spastic or flaccid in type. If contractures or deformities are present, the examiner should attempt to determine whether these have a neurogenic origin or are caused by lesions of the bones, joints, tendons, or fascia, or whether several factors are present. Both active and passive movements should be tested and if limitation of movement is accompanied by discomfort or pain, this should be noted. Range of movement may be limited by fibrosis, contractures, or changes at the joints. Weakness and increased tone, however, may also affect range. Speed of movement in itself is not an important criterion; there is a wide individual variation in this, but it is specifically increased in hyperthyroidism and manic states, and decreased in hypothyroidism, depressed states, parkinsonism, fatigue, and various myopathies. Slowness of movement may be the first manifestation of extrapyramidal disease, but a delay in muscular contraction and a retardation of movement may be an early sign of weakness. Abnormalities in regularity of movement usually signify ataxia, tremor, or chorea, but they may also appear when weakness is present. **Motor impersistence** is the inability to sustain

voluntary motor acts that have been initiated on verbal command. It is seen in brain-damaged persons, usually children. Some degree of mental impairment is usually present. It has been said to occur most often with left hemisphere lesions. It may be an apractic disorder.

The motor examination may have to be modified, often with only a rough estimation of function, in various disease states, in confused or stuporous patients, and in infants and young children. In the presence of coma, for instance, assessment of motor function may have to depend upon the presence of spontaneous movements, the position of the extremities, asymmetries of voluntary movements on the two sides, or withdrawal of an extremity in response to painful stimulation. Hemiplegia may be diagnosed in the comatose patient by noting the absence of contraction of the facial muscles on one side following pressure on the supraorbital ridge, the flaillike dropping of the wrist and forearm when the examiner releases them while the flexed elbow is resting on the bed, and the similar extension and external rotation of the thigh and leg when released after having been placed in flexion with the heel resting on the bed (Ch. 54). In infants and young children muscle function may have to be tested largely by observing spontaneous motor activity and by noting the general posture and the position of the extremities when the body is prone, supine, seated, and upright. Resistance to passive movement, the motor response to reflex testing, and palpation may provide indirect evidence of muscle strength.

The testing of motor power in suspected hysteria and malingering may also require special technics. The fact that an apparent weakness is not of organic origin, however, may be suspected from various observations during the motor examination, some of which are as follows: The muscular contractions are poorly sustained and may give way abruptly, rather than gradually, as the patient resists the force exerted by the examiner (so-called **give-way weakness**); there may be absence of follow-through when the examiner withdraws his pressure; there may be an increase rather than a decrease in strength with repeated testing; resistance may be felt in the antagonists when the patient fails to contract the muscles under observation. On occasion functional testing may demonstrate the absence of weakness suspected during the routine test. For example, there may be apparent paresis of either dorsiflexion or plantar flexion of the foot when the patient is examined in the seated or recumbent position, but when he is upright it may be observed that he is able to stand on either the heel or the toe of that foot, and support his entire body in doing so. Weakness of hysterical origin may disappear following the injection of barbiturates or tranquilizers, but mild or latent organic motor deficits may be made more conspicuous by this means.

It is usually possible to evaluate muscle strength and power sufficiently well without recourse to special instruments. The subjective impression of the investigator is usually adequate. Such evaluation, however, is not quantitative; it varies with the experience and ability of the examiner, there is a large subjective element, and there may be disagreement between observers. On occasion, and for special purposes, one may resort to the use of instruments for measuring strength, especially when quantitative determinations are desired. Various dynamometers, myosthenometers, myometers, and ergometers are available. Energy may be measured by weights, spring balances, dial or mercury gauges, strain gauge transducers, or by electrical means. Special instruments can determine the amount of work done per unit of time; this may be useful in assessment of efficiency, fatigue, and response to medication. Quantitative measurements and permanent records are of help in evaluating the progression of a disease process or the recovery of function during regeneration of a nerve lesion, but only if they are used in a consistent, controlled fashion with the patient rested and able to cooperate fully. It must be stated, however, that none of these mechanical devices eliminates the subjective element in testing muscle strength, and that none of them is applicable in testing certain muscle groups, such as the rotators of the shoulder and the back and trunk muscles. With all of them the results are difficult to evaluate in the presence of fixed contractures.

Muscle function may be graded in various ways, but the following is an acceptable classification:

0. No muscular contraction occurs.
1. A flicker, or trace, of contraction occurs without actual movement, or contraction may be palpated in the absence of apparent movement; there is minimal or no motion of joints (0% – 10% of normal movement).
2. The muscle moves the part through a partial arc of movement with gravity eliminated (11% – 25% of normal movement).

3. The muscle completes the whole arc of movement against gravity (26% – 50% of normal movement).
4. The muscle completes the whole arc of movement against gravity together with variable amounts of resistance (51% – 75% of normal movement).
5. The muscle completes the whole arc of movement against gravity and maximum amounts of resistance several times without signs of fatigue. This is normal muscular power (76% – 100% of normal movement).
S. Spasm of muscle occurs.
C. Contracture of muscle.

EXAMINATION OF STRENGTH AND POWER OF SPECIAL MOVEMENTS AND INDIVIDUAL MUSCLES

Detailed discussions of the motor examination of the muscles supplied by those cranial nerves that have motor functions, namely, the oculomotor, trochlear, trigeminal, abducens, facial, glossopharyngeal, vagus, accessory, and hypoglossal nerves, have already been presented. An equally detailed examination should be directed toward the motor functions of the rest of the body. The strength and power of the individual muscles and of movements should be carefully determined, and impairment or loss of function noted. Fortunately many good anatomic texts are available that will assist the examiner in becoming familiar with the principal functions and the innervation of the various muscles. Tables or charts that give this information are also available. These, however, are not too satisfactory, and tabulation is difficult as many muscles have more than one function, and some have opposite functions when extremities are placed in varying positions. Furthermore, there is a difference of opinion regarding the exact innervation of individual muscles, and occasionally there is variable or anomalous innervation. Tables 27-1 through 27-4 give the most generally accepted innervation, from the point of view of both the spinal cord segments and the peripheral nerves, of the more important muscles. No table of muscle functions is given as these are discussed in detail in the text.

A brief outline of the major movements and individual muscles to be tested, and their innervation, follows.

Examination of Movements and Muscles of the Neck

The principal neck movements are those of flexion, extension (retraction), rotation, and lateral deviation (abduction). These functions and their testing have already been mentioned in Chapter 16. The spinal accessory nerve, along with the second, third, and fourth cervical segments, supplies the sternocleidomastoid and trapezius muscles. The former is a flexor and rotator of the head and neck, whereas the latter retracts the neck and draws it to one side. The platysma and the suprahyoid and infrahyoid muscles also aid in flexion. Other muscles that act on the head and neck are as follows: Muscles that support the head and fix the neck and also flex the neck, tilt it to one side, and rotate it are the scaleni anterior, medius, and posterior, and longi capitis and colli. The rectus capitis anterior flexes and rotates the neck, and the rectus capitis lateralis tilts it to one side. Muscles that fix or steady the neck as well as extend it and tilt and rotate it are the splenii capitis and cervicis, semispinales capitis and cervicis, intertransversarii, rotators, and the upper portion of the sacrospinalis (erector spinae), including iliocostalis cervicis and longissimi capitis and cervicis. The spinalis cer-

vicis holds the neck steady and head erect and extends the vertebral column, and the rectus capitis posterior, obliqui capitis, and multifidi extend and rotate the neck. All of these muscles are supplied by branches of the eight cervical nerves (Table 27-1).

In testing the neck movements and muscles the patient should be asked to flex his neck so that his chin rests upon his chest, to extend or retract it as far backward as possible, to rotate it from side to side, and to tilt it lateralward. These are first done against the resistance of the examiner's hand; then the examiner attempts passive movements while the patient resists them. Finally the muscles may be palpated to determine the degree of contraction. Flexion is tested with the patient recumbent; the examiner stabilizes the thorax by placing one hand over the chest, and resists attempted flexion by placing the other hand on the forehead. The contracting muscles can be seen and felt (Fig. 27-1). Extension is examined with the patient prone, the upper chest stabilized, and resistance against the occiput; the contracting muscles can be seen and felt, and the strength of movement can be judged (Fig. 27-2). Rotation and lateral movements can be evaluated by modification of these procedures. It is difficult, if not impossible, to

TABLE 27–1. Innervation of Muscles Responsible for Movements of the Head and Neck

Muscle	Segmental Innervation	Peripheral Nerve
Sternocleidomastoid	Cranial XI; C (1) 2–3	Spinal accessory nerve
Trapezius	Cranial XI; C (2) 3–4	Spinal accessory nerve
Scalenus anterior	C 4–7	
Scalenus medius	C 4–8	
Scalenus posterior	C 6–8	
Longus capitis	C 1–4	
Longus colli	C 2–6	
Rectus capitis anterior	C 1–2	Suboccipital nerve
Rectus capitis lateralis	C 1	Suboccipital nerve
Rectus capitis posterior	C 1	Suboccipital nerve
Obliquus capitis inferior	C 1	Suboccipital nerve
Obliquus capitis superior	C 1	Suboccipital nerve
Splenius capitis	C 2–4 (1–6)	
Splenius cervicis	C 2–4 (1–6)	
Semispinalis capitis	C 1–4	
Semispinalis cervicis	C 3–6	
Spinalis cervicis	C 5–8	
Sacrospinalis	C 1–8	
Iliocostalis cervicis	C 1–8	
Longissimus capitis	C 1–8	
Longissimus cervicis	C 1–8	
Intertransversarii	C 1–8	
Rotatores	C 1–8	
Multifidi	C 1–8	

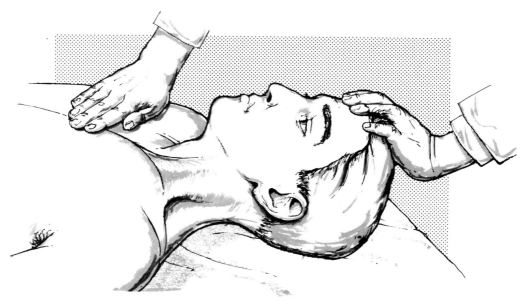

FIG. 27–1. Examination of flexion of the neck. The patient attempts to flex his neck against resistance; the sternocleidomastoid, platysma, and other flexor muscles can be seen and palpated.

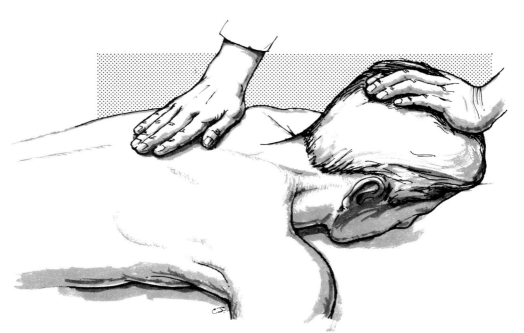

FIG. 27–2. Examination of extension of the neck. The patient attempts to extend his neck against resistance; contraction of the trapezius and other extensor muscles can be seen and felt, and strength of movement can be judged.

test the function of the neck muscles individually, except, of course, for the sternocleidomastoid and trapezius. Furthermore, one can appraise only weakness of movements, not of individual muscles. It must be recalled that conditions other than paralytic ones may affect these movements. Flexion of the neck, with limitation of extension, may be seen in parkinsonian states and cervical spondylosis, retraction in meningitis and meningismus; lateral deviation and rotation in torticollis.

Examination of Movements and Muscles of the Upper Extremities

The responsible muscles and their innervation are given in Table 27-2.

The Shoulder Girdle. Movements of the shoulder girdle are those that take place at the sternoclavicular and acromioclavicular joints. These consist of elevation, depression, retraction, protraction, and rotation of the scapula.

Elevation of the scapula (scapula raised and glenoid cavity tilted upward) is carried out by the trapezius and levator scapulae muscles, assisted by the sternocleidomastoid and the lower portion of the serratus anterior. The trapezius, which is the most important elevator of the scapula and shoulder girdle, is also discussed elsewhere (see "Clinical Examination" in Ch. 16). It is innervated by the eleventh cranial nerve together with the third and fourth cervical segments. The upper fibers elevate, retract, and rotate the scapula and brace the shoulder, especially if the head is fixed. The middle fibers rotate and retract the scapula, and the lower fibers depress it and draw it toward the midline. The trapezius aids in forced respiration, and along with the serratus anterior elevates the abducted arm above the horizontal. The functions of the upper fibers are tested by having the patient elevate or shrug his shoulder against resistance (see Fig. 16-3), and the middle fibers by having him brace and retract the scapula against resistance (Fig. 27-3). Muscle power can be compared with that on the normal side, and muscular contractions can be seen and palpated. In unilateral paralysis of the trapezius the shoulder cannot be elevated and retracted and the arm cannot be abducted above the horizontal. The upper portion of the scapula falls laterally, the inferior angle is drawn medially, and the vertebral border is flared; this abnormal position is accentuated on attempted abduction of the arm, but is decreased on forward elevation. The sagging of the shoulder causes a drooping of the entire arm, and the fingertips on that side are at a lower level than those on the normal side; this can be demonstrated by having the patient place his palms together, slightly downward, in front of his body. The levator scapulae (levator anguli scapulae) draws the scapula upward and rotates it so that the inferior angle approaches the spinal column. It is also tested by observing elevation of the scapula, but it is situated more deeply than the trapezius, and its contraction cannot be seen and only occasionally can be palpated; it is rarely possible to detect weakness of the levator scapulae on clinical examination unless the trapezius is also involved.

Depression of the scapula is carried out by the lower fibers of the trapezius and by the pectoralis minor and subclavius muscles, assisted by the lower part of the pectoralis major and by the latissimus dorsi. The pectoralis minor pulls the scapula downward and rotates it, and also aids in forced respiration. The subclavius depresses the clavicle and the point of the shoulder, carrying them downward and forward. These muscles are both concealed by the pectoralis major and consequently cannot be adequately tested individually. Furthermore, it is difficult to distinguish depression of the scapula from similar or associated movements of the upper arm. The pectoralis major and latissimus dorsi will be discussed under "The Shoulder Joint."

Retraction (adduction) of the scapula (scapula and glenoid cavity tilted backward) is carried out by the rhomboidei major and minor and the middle part of the trapezius, assisted by the latissimus dorsi. The rhomboidei draw the scapula upward and medially toward the spine and rotate it so as to depress the tip of the shoulder. These muscles, too, are situated deep to the trapezius. Their contraction is seen with difficulty and it is rarely possible to detect weakness or paralysis unless the trapezius is also involved. Occasionally, however, if the examiner attempts to push the elbow forward while the patient, with the hand on the hip, retracts the shoulder, the contraction of the rhomboidei can be felt and seen (Fig. 27-4).

Abduction (protraction) of the scapula (scapula and glenoid cavity tilted forward) is carried out by the serratus anterior together with the pectoralis minor and the upper part of the pectoralis major. The serratus anterior (magnus) is supplied by the fifth through the seventh cervical segments through the long thoracic nerve.

TABLE 27–2. Innervation of Muscles Responsible for Movements of the Shoulder Girdle and Upper Extremity

Muscle	Segmental Innervation	Peripheral Nerve
Trapezius	Cranial XI; C (2) 3–4	Spinal accessory nerve
Levator scapulae	C 3–4	Nerves to levator scapulae
	C 4–5	Dorsal scapular nerve
Rhomboideus major	C 4–5	Dorsal scapular nerve
Rhomboideus minor	C 4–5	Dorsal scapular nerve
Serratus anterior	C 5–7	Long thoracic nerve
Deltoid	C 5–6	Axillary nerve
Teres minor	C 5–6	Axillary nerve
Supraspinatus	C (4) 5–6	Suprascapular nerve
Infraspinatus	C (4) 5–6	Suprascapular nerve
Latissimus dorsi	C 6–8	Thoracodorsal nerve (long subscapular)
Pectoralis major	C 5– Th 1	Lateral and medial anterior thoracic
Pectoralis minor	C 7– Th 1	Medial anterior thoracic
Subscapularis	C 5–7	Subscapular nerves
Teres major	C 5–7	Lower subscapular nerve
Subclavius	C 5–6	Nerve to subclavius
Coracobrachialis	C 6–7	Musculocutaneous nerve
Biceps brachii	C 5–6	Musculocutaneous nerve
Brachialis	C 5–6	Musculocutaneous nerve
Brachioradialis	C 5–6	Radial nerve
Triceps brachii	C 6–8 (Th 1)	Radial nerve
Anconeus	C 7–8	Radial nerve
Supinator brevis	C 5–7	Radial nerve
Extensor carpi radialis longus	C (5) 6–7 (8)	Radial nerve
Extensor carpi radialis brevis	C (5) 6–7 (8)	Radial nerve
Extensor carpi ulnaris	C 6–8	Radial nerve
Extensor digitorum communis	C 6–8	Radial nerve
Extensor indicis proprius	C 6–8	Radial nerve
Extensor digiti minimi	C 6–8	Radial nerve
Extensor pollicis longus	C 6–8	Radial nerve
Extensor pollicis brevis	C 6–8	Radial nerve
Abductor pollicis longus	C 6–8	Radial nerve
Pronator teres	C 6–7	Median nerve
Flexor carpi radialis	C 6–7 (8)	Median nerve
Pronator quadratus	C 7– Th 1	Median nerve
Palmaris longus	C 7– Th 1	Median nerve
Flexor digitorum sublimis	C 7– Th 1	Median nerve
Flexor digitorum profundus (radial half)	C 7– Th 1	Median nerve
Lumbricales 1 and 2	C 7– Th 1	Median nerve
Flexor pollicis longus	C 8– Th 1	Median nerve
Flexor pollicis brevis (lateral head)	C 8– Th 1	Median nerve
Abductor pollicis brevis	C 8– Th 1	Median nerve
Opponens pollicis	C 8– Th 1	Median nerve
Flexor carpi ulnaris	C 7– Th 1	Ulnar nerve
Flexor digitorum profundus (ulnar half)	C 7– Th 1	Ulnar nerve
Interossei	C 8– Th 1	Ulnar nerve
Lumbricales 3 and 4	C 8– Th 1	Ulnar nerve
Flexor pollicis brevis (medial head)	C 8– Th 1	Ulnar nerve
Flexor digiti minimi brevis	C 8– Th 1	Ulnar nerve
Abductor digiti minimi	C 8– Th 1	Ulnar nerve
Opponens digiti minimi	C 8– Th 1	Ulnar nerve
Palmaris brevis	C 8– Th 1	Ulnar nerve
Adductor pollicis	C 8– Th 1	Ulnar nerve

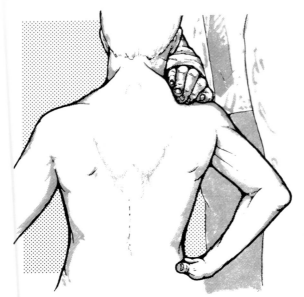

FIG. 27–3. Examination of the trapezius. On retraction of the shoulder against resistance, the middle fibers of the muscle can be seen and palpated.

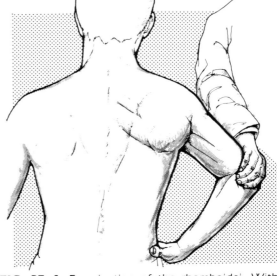

FIG. 27–4. Examination of the rhomboidei. With hand on hip, the patient retracts the shoulder against the examiner's effort to push the elbow forward; the contracting muscles can be seen and palpated.

It keeps the vertebral border of the scapula applied to the thorax and draws the scapula forward and laterally. It rotates the scapula and raises the point of the shoulder, and fixes the scapula while other muscles abduct or flex the arm. Along with the trapezius it abducts the arm above the horizontal and aids in forced respiration. It is tested by forward elevation of the arms and pressure with the palms against some resistance, such as a wall (Fig. 27-5). Normally the medial border of the scapula remains close to the thoracic wall, but with weakness or paralysis of the serratus anterior the inferior angle is shifted medially and the entire vertebral border protrudes posteriorly, away from the thoracic wall, causing the deformity known as "winging" (Fig. 27-6); this is accentuated by the tests just described. Abduction of the arm may cause comparatively little winging, however, which aids in differentiating a serratus anterior palsy from the flaring of the scapula that occurs with weakness of the trapezius.

Rotation of the scapula is carried out by the trapezius, serratus anterior, pectorales, rhomboidei, and latissimus dorsi. It cannot be tested without examining the other functions of these various muscles, and along with depression cannot be distinguished from similar movements at the shoulder joint. In the muscular dystrophies

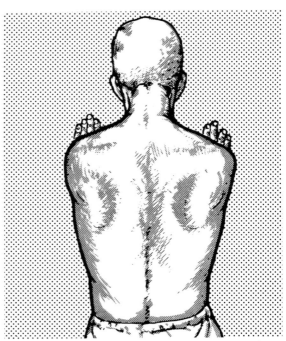

FIG. 27–5. Examination of the serratus anterior. The patient pushes against a wall with his arms extended horizontally in front of him; normally, the medial border of the scapula remains close to the thoracic wall.

there often is weakness of all the shoulder girdle muscles, and if the examiner attempts to lift the patient by grasping his elbows or upper arms or supporting him in the axillae, the shoulders are pushed upward, along the sides of the head, while the trunk remains fixed; the patient is lifted "through the shoulder blades." This is a particularly useful method of evaluating weakness about the shoulder girdle in children who cannot cooperate in formal tests of individual groups of muscles. Bilateral winging of the scapulas is usually present in the dystrophies.

The Shoulder Joint. The principal movements at the shoulder joint are abduction and elevation, adduction, external and internal rotation, and flexion and extension of the upper arm.

The deltoid and supraspinatus muscles, aided by the subscapularis and the upper part of the infraspinatus, are the abductors of the shoulder. The deltoid is the most prominent muscle in the region of the shoulder. It is supplied by the fifth and sixth cervical segments through the axillary nerve, a branch of the posterior cord of the brachial plexus. When this muscle contracts as a whole the arm is abducted (raised laterally) to the horizontal plane. Further abduction, or elevation above the horizontal plane, is carried out by the associated action of the trapezius and the serratus anterior that rotate the scapula and tilt the angle of that bone upward. The posterior fibers of the deltoid also assist in extension and external rotation of the arm, and the anterior fibers in flexion and internal rotation. The anterior and posterior portions, acting together, aid in adduction of the arm. The major function of the deltoid is tested either by noting the ability of the patient to abduct the arm through a range of 15° – 90° against resistance (Fig. 27-7), or by having him abduct the arm to the horizontal level, either laterally or in forward position (the elbow may be either flexed or extended), and resist the examiner's attempt to counteract the abduction. With this latter maneuver it is possible for the examiner to test both sides simultaneously and compare their strength; this may aid in the evaluation of moderate weakness. During contraction of the deltoid the body of the muscle may be seen to stand out and can be palpated. If there is minimal weakness, the patient may be able to abduct the arm voluntarily, but not against resistance; he may move the trunk and raise the tip of the shoulder to aid in the attempt. If the weakness is more profound, active eleva-

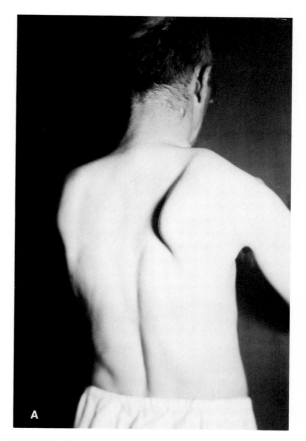

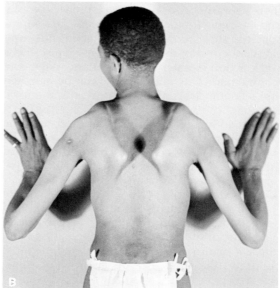

FIG. 27–6. "Winging" of the scapula. **A.** Unilateral winging secondary to paralysis of the right serratus anterior. **B.** Bilateral winging in a patient with muscular dystrophy.

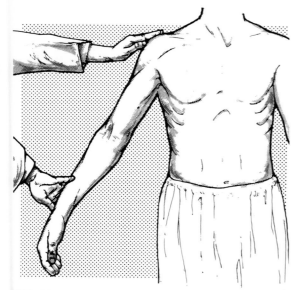

FIG. 27–7. Examination of the deltoid. The patient attempts to abduct his arm against resistance; the contracting deltoid can be seen and palpated.

tion to the horizontal plane may be impossible, but the passively abducted arm can be held up against the force of gravity. In complete paresis no contraction of the muscle is possible. Weakness of the deltoid is easily observed and, if it is caused by a lesion of the anterior horn cells or their neuraxes, atrophy appears quite promptly and fasciculations are often noted. The supraspinatus aids the deltoid in abducting the arm, especially during the initial stages. It also has a weak action in external rotation and extension. Contraction of its muscle belly can be palpated and sometimes seen when the arm is abducted less than 15° against resistance (Fig. 27-8).

The adductors of the shoulder are the pectoralis major and latissimus dorsi, aided by the biceps, triceps, coracobrachialis, the anterior and posterior portions of the deltoid, and the external and internal rotators. The pectoralis major is innervated by fibers from the fifth cervical to first thoracic segments through the lateral and medial anterior thoracic nerves. It is the principal adductor of the arm, and is also a flexor and internal rotator. When the arm is fixed the muscle draws the chest upward, as in climbing; it also assists in raising the ribs in forced respiration. On attempts to adduct the horizontally abducted arm against resistance, the contraction of the sternocostal and clavicular portions of the muscle can be seen and felt (Fig. 27-9). The mus-

cle can also be palpated on flexion of the horizontally abducted arm and when the hands are pressed together while the arms are in a horizontal position in front of the patient. Because of the force of gravity, the arm may hang in adduction even though the pectoralis is weak.

The latissimus dorsi is supplied by the sixth, seventh, and eighth cervical segments through the thoracodorsal (long subscapular) nerve. It adducts and extends the arm and is also a medial rotator. When the humerus is fixed, the latissimus draws the pelvis and the lower part of the trunk forward and upward. When the arm is hanging by the side, it depresses, retracts, and rotates the scapula. It also aids in forced respiration. The muscle may be tested in various ways. If the patient attempts to adduct the horizontally and laterally extended arm against resistance (*i.e.*, to press the arm against resistance while it is extended horizontally), the muscle can be seen and palpated (Fig. 27-10). The muscle belly can also be palpated on coughing and when the patient pushes his arm downward and backward.

External rotation of the arm is carried out principally by the infraspinatus and teres minor muscles, with the associated action of the posterior fibers of the deltoid. The infraspinatus is the chief external rotator; the upper part is also

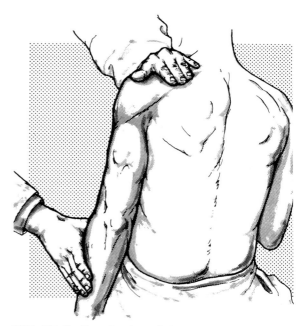

FIG. 27–8. Examination of the supraspinatus. Contraction of the muscle fibers can be felt during early stages of abduction of the arm.

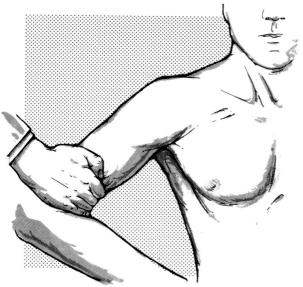

FIG. 27–9. Examination of the pectoralis major. Contraction of the muscle can be seen and felt during attempts to adduct the arm against resistance.

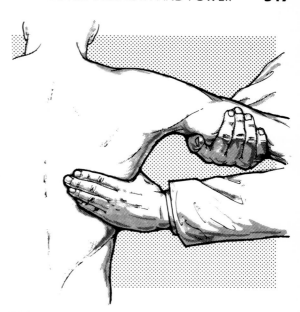

FIG. 27–10. Examination of the latissimus dorsi. On adduction of the horizontally and laterally abducted arm against resistance, the contracting muscle fibers can be seen and palpated.

an abductor, the lower part an adductor. The teres minor acts with the infraspinatus to rotate the arm laterally and is also an adductor. In testing these muscles the patient attempts to move his forearm laterally and backward against resistance, and thus produce external rotation at the shoulder, while the elbow is flexed at an angle of 90° and kept to the side (Fig. 27-11). The contraction of the infraspinatus can usually be felt.

Internal rotation at the shoulder results from contraction of the subscapularis and teres major muscles, together with the action of the anterior fibers of the deltoid, and the latissimus dorsi, pectoralis major, and biceps muscles. The teres major acts as an internal rotator and extensor and aids the latissimus dorsi in adducting the arm. The subscapularis is the chief internal rotator of the arm; it is also an extensor when the arm is at the side and a flexor when the arm is in abduction, and it assists in adduction and abduction. Internal rotation is tested by having the patient carry his arm medially and forward against resistance while the elbow is flexed and at the side.

Flexion of the arm (forward elevation) is carried out by the anterior fibers of the deltoid, and the pectoralis major, subscapularis, coracobrachialis, and biceps muscles. The coracobrachialis flexes the arm at the shoulder and also aids in adduction. The muscles, especially the deltoid

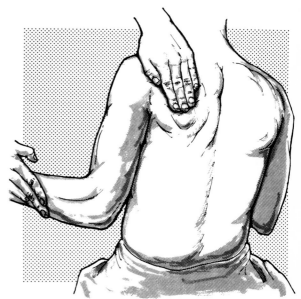

FIG. 27–11. Examination of the external rotators of the arm. On external rotation of the arm while the elbow is flexed and kept close to the body, the contractng infraspinatus muscle can be seen and palpated.

and pectoralis, may be palpated when an attempt is made to flex the arm against resistance. Extension of the arm (backward elevation) is carried out by the posterior fibers of the deltoid, together with the latissimus dorsi, triceps, subscapularis, and teres major muscles. This action can be tested by having the patient attempt extension of the arm against resistance. The specific functions of the individual muscles concerned, however, are better examined by tests discussed in the preceding paragraphs.

The Elbow. The principal movements at the elbow consist of flexion and extension of the forearm at the elbow joint and pronation and supination at the radioulnar joint.

Flexion at the elbow results from contraction of the biceps brachii and brachialis muscles, together with the brachioradialis, extensor carpi radialis longus, flexor carpi radialis, palmaris longus, and pronator teres. The biceps brachii is supplied by the fifth and sixth cervical segments through the musculocutaneous nerve, a branch of the lateral cord of the brachial plexus. It is a flexor of the elbow and also a supinator of the forearm, especially when the latter is flexed and pronated. It also aids in flexion, medial rotation, and adduction of the upper arm. The brachialis is supplied by the same nerve and segments; its only function is flexion of the forearm. The brachioradialis is innervated by fibers from the fifth and sixth cervical segments through the radial nerve. It flexes the forearm when the latter is in semipronation and also acts as a supinator when the arm is extended and pronated. When the forearm is flexed and supinated, it acts as a pronator. The functions of the biceps and brachialis muscles are tested by having the patient attempt to flex the extended and supinated forearm against resistance, or by having the examiner try to extend the forearm while the patient maintains it in flexion. During these maneuvers the contraction of the muscles, especially that of the biceps, can be seen and felt (Fig. 27-12). The brachioradialis is tested by attempts to flex the forearm while it is midway between pronation and supination (thumb up). When resistance is offered to this movement the belly of the muscle stands out prominently and can be palpated (Fig. 27-13). Even when the biceps and brachialis are completely paralyzed, the brachioradialis is still capable of flexion at the elbow, providing the forearm is in semipronation.

The triceps brachii is the principal extensor of the forearm. It is innervated by the sixth, seventh, and eighth cervical segments and possibly

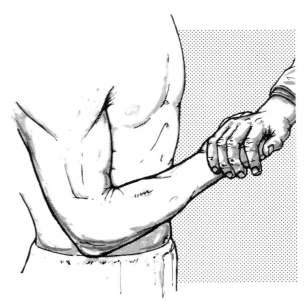

FIG. 27–12. Examination of the biceps brachii. On attempts to flex the forearm against resistance, the contracting biceps muscle can be seen and palpated.

the first thoracic segment through the radial nerve, a branch of the posterior cord of the brachial plexus. It extends the elbow and holds the forearm in extension, and also extends and adducts the upper arm. The anconeus aids the triceps in extension. To test these muscles the arm is abducted to eliminate the action of gravity on the forearm and the forearm is placed in a position midway between flexion and extension. The patient then attempts either to extend the forearm at the elbow or to retain it in the partially extended position against the examiner's resistance (Fig. 27-14). During the movement the contraction of the three bellies of the muscle can be palpated. Simultaneous testing of the two sides gives a comparison of their strength and may aid in evaluating moderate weakness. The triceps is less powerful when the elbow is fully flexed, and slight weakness may be more easily detected if its function is tested in this position. If the triceps is paralyzed, the forearm can assume the position of extension only through the influence of gravity.

Supination results from the contraction of the biceps, brachioradialis (supinator longus), supinator brevis, extensor carpi radialis longus, and extensor and abductor pollicis longus muscles. The biceps is the strongest supinator of the forearm, but its action in this respect is most marked when the forearm is flexed and pronated. The

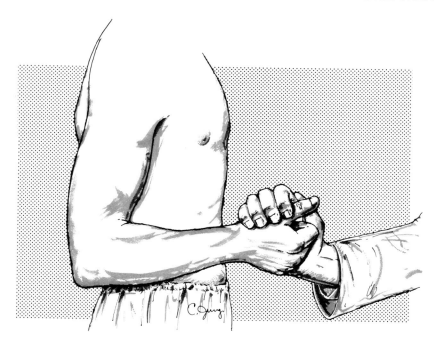

FIG. 27–13. Examination of the brachioradialis. On flexion at the semipronated forearm (thumb up) against resistance, the contracting muscle can be seen and palpated.

brachioradialis acts as a supinator only when the arm is extended and pronated; when the forearm is flexed and supinated it acts as a pronator. The extensor carpi radialis longus functions in a similar manner. The supinator brevis is less powerful as a supinator than the biceps, but it acts through all degrees of flexion and supination.

Supination is tested by attempts on the part of the patient to carry out this movement against the examiner's resistance, or to hold the forearm in supination while the examiner attempts to carry out pronation. The examiner may grasp either the wrist or the back of the hand, or the patient may be asked to grip the examiner's hand.

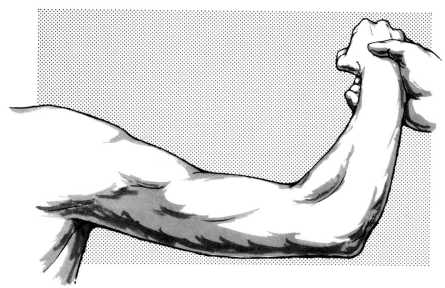

FIG. 27–14. Extension of the forearm. On attempts to extend the partially flexed forearm against resistance, contraction of the triceps can be seen and palpated.

If the aforementioned maneuvers are done while the forearm is in extension, the brachioradialis may be palpated (Fig. 27-15); if while in flexion, the biceps may be palpated. The supinator brevis, one of the deep muscles of the forearm, cannot be adequately palpated.

Pronation is brought about by the action of the pronator teres, also a weak flexor of the forearm, and the pronator quadratus; additional muscles are the brachioradialis, palmaris longus, extensor carpi radialis longus, and flexor carpi radialis. In testing pronation the arm should be externally rotated at the shoulder, and the elbow should be near the trunk. The patient then attempts to carry out pronation against resistance or to hold the forearm in pronation while the examiner attempts to carry out supination (Fig. 27-16), with maneuvers similar to those for supination but in the opposite direction. The effect of gravity should be eliminated.

The Wrist. The principal movements at the wrist are flexion and extension of the hand, together with adduction (ulnar flexion) and abduction (radial flexion).

Flexion, or palmar flexion, of the hand at the wrist is carried out principally by the flexor carpi radialis and flexor carpi ulnaris muscles. The former, supplied by the median nerve, also assists in pronation and in flexion of the forearm and is a weak abductor of the wrist. The latter, supplied by the ulnar nerve, is also an adductor of the wrist and hand. The palmaris longus is also a flexor of the wrist and, in addition, is a weak flexor and pronator of the forearm. Additional muscles aiding in flexion of the hand at the wrist are the flexor digitorum profundus, flexor digitorum sublimis, flexor pollicis longus, and abductor pollicis longus (discussed subsequently). Flexion at the wrist may be tested by attempts to bend the hand toward the forearm

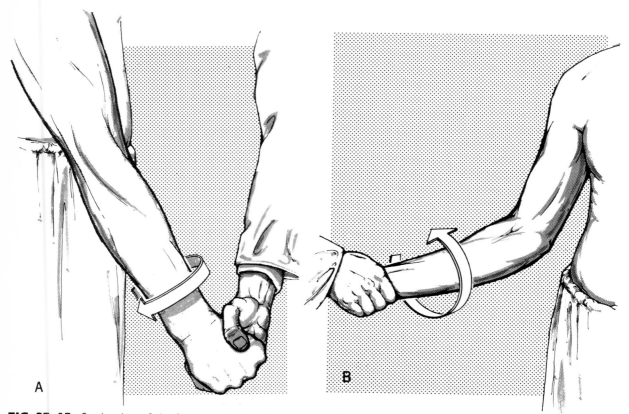

A

B

FIG. 27–15. Supination of the forearm. **A.** On attempts to supinate the extended forearm against resistance, the contracting brachioradialis can be seen and palpated. **B.** On attempts to supinate the flexed forearm against resistance, the contracting biceps can be seen and palpated.

ments through the radial nerve. The extensors carpi radialis longus and brevis also abduct the hand and steady the wrist when the flexors act on the fingers, and the extensor longus is a weak flexor of the forearm and aids in pronation and supination. The extensor carpi ulnaris is also an adductor. In testing these muscles the forearm is placed in pronation (it may be resting on the arm of a chair) and the wrist is partially extended. The patient then either attempts to extend the wrist further against the examiner's resistance, or to hold it in partial extension while the examiner attempts to flex it (Fig. 27-18). The participating muscles and their tendons can be palpated. If the wrist is extended to the ulnar side, the extensor carpi ulnaris can be felt; if toward the radial side, the extensor carpi radialis longus; and if in the midposition, the extensor digitorum communis. Moderate weakness of the extensors results in involuntary flexion at the wrist when the patient attempts to grip his fingers; marked weakness causes a wrist drop, the outstanding symptom of a radial nerve palsy (Ch. 43). Paresis of the extensors of the wrist may also be an early sign of hemiparesis.

Adduction, or ulnar deviation or flexion, at the wrist is carried out principally by the flexor carpi ulnaris and extensor carpi ulnaris muscles, assisted by the flexor pollicis longus; abduction, or radial deviation or flexion, is carried out by the flexor carpi radialis, extensors carpi radialis

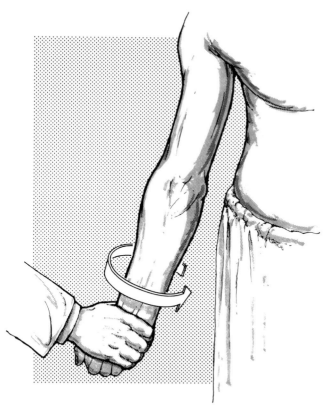

FIG. 27–16. Pronation of the forearm. On pronation of the forearm against resistance, contraction of the pronator teres can be seen and palpated.

against resistance (Fig. 27-17). The motion of both the flexor carpi radialis and flexor carpi ulnaris muscles can be seen and felt, and the contraction of the tendons of both of these muscles together with that of the palmaris longus may be seen. The flexor carpi radialis can be tested individually by having the patient flex his wrist toward the radial side against resistance directed toward the thumb. Function of the flexor carpi ulnaris can be tested by having the patient flex the wrist toward the ulnar side while the examiner presses on the small fingers. Paralysis of the flexors of the wrist does not give rise to any marked deformity, since gravity enables the hand to assume a flexed position.

Extension (dorsal flexion) at the wrist is carried out by the extensor carpi radialis longus, extensor carpi radialis brevis, extensor carpi ulnaris, and extensor digitorum communis, possibly assisted by the other extensors of the thumb and fingers. These muscles are supplied by the sixth, seventh, and eighth cervical seg-

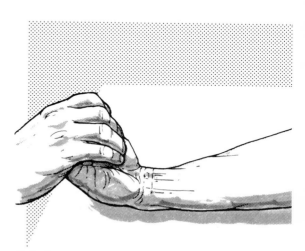

FIG. 27–17. Flexion at the wrist. On flexion of the hand at the wrist against resistance, the tendon of the flexor carpi radialis can be seen and palpated on the radial side of the wrist, and that of the flexor carpi ulnaris on the ulnar side; the tendon of the palmaris longus can also be seen and palpated.

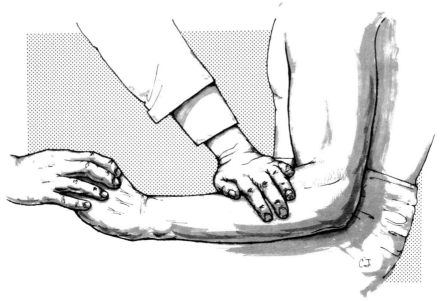

FIG. 27–18. Extension at the wrist. On attempts to extend the hand at the wrist against resistance, the bellies of the extensors carpi radialis longus, carpi ulnaris, and digitorum communis can be seen and palpated.

longus and brevis, abductor pollicis longus, and extensors pollicis longus and brevis. These movements, too, may be tested by carrying them out against resistance.

The Hands and Fingers. Detailed muscle testing is necessary to examine the muscles of the hand and fingers. Innervation is complex, numerous substitution movements are possible, and misinterpretations may be made. The various muscles that supply the hands and fingers must be examined individually for flexion, extension, adduction, abduction, and opposition.

Flexion of the Fingers. The primary action of the flexor digitorum profundus is the flexion of the distal phalanges of the second, third, fourth, and fifth fingers. On continuing its action, however, it also flexes the remaining phalanges of these digits, and finally the hand. The radial half of this muscle is supplied by the median nerve, the ulnar half by the ulnar nerve, the fibers coming from the seventh and eighth cervical and first thoracic segments of the spinal cord. The flexor digitorum sublimis, also supplied by the median nerve, primarily flexes the middle phalanges of the four fingers, but a continuation of its action will result in a flexion of the proximal phalanges of these digits, and finally of the hand at the wrist. The proximal phalanges of the

four fingers are flexed by the interossei and the lumbricales. The former muscles, innervated by the ulnar nerve, also adduct (volar interossei) and abduct (dorsal interossei) the fingers. The interossei and lumbricales together extend the middle and distal phalanges. The two lumbricales on the ulnar side of the hand are innervated by the ulnar nerve, and the two on the radial side of the hand by the median nerve. The flexor digiti minimi brevis flexes and slightly abducts the proximal phalanx of the little finger; two other muscles acting on the little finger are the abductor digiti minimi, which abducts the little finger, flexes its proximal phalanx, and extends the distal phalanges, and the opponens digiti minimi, which flexes, adducts, and slightly rotates the fifth metacarpal. These three muscles are supplied by the eighth cervical and first thoracic segments through the ulnar nerve, as is the palmaris brevis, which wrinkles the skin on the ulnar border of the hand and deepens the hollow of the hand.

When the flexor digitorum profundus is tested the patient resists attempts to extend the distal phalanges of the individual fingers while the middle phalanges are fixed (Fig. 27-19). The flexor digitorum sublimis is tested by having the patient resist attempts to straighten the fingers at the first interphalangeal joints while the proximal phalanges are fixed (Fig. 27-20). For this

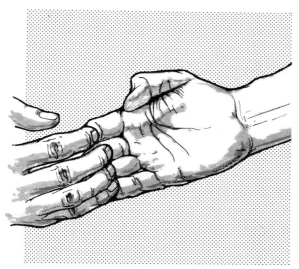

FIG. 27–19. Examination of the flexor digitorum profundus. The patient resists attempts to extend the distal phalanges while the middle phalanges are fixed.

test to be valid the distal phalanges must be completely flaccid and flexion at the proximal interphalangeal joint by the flexor profundus should be eliminated. The function of the interossei and lumbricales in flexion at the metacarpophalangeal joint is tested with the interphalangeal joints in either flexion or extension. When paralysis of these latter muscles is present, there is extension at the metacarpophalangeal joints and flexion of the distal phalanges,

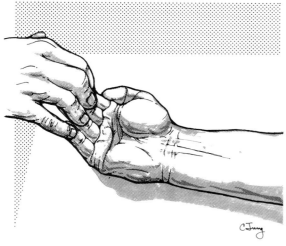

FIG. 27–20. Examination of the flexor digitorum sublimis. The patient resists attempts to straighten the fingers at the first interphalangeal joint.

together with loss of adduction of the fingers. Flexion of the fingers at all joints is necessary to make a fist. The thumb may be in either flexion or extension. The strength of the fist depends not only upon the degree of flexion at the metacarpophalangeal and interphalangeal joints, but also upon the position of the thumb and its ability to flex and to brace the fingers, and upon the synergistic action of the extensor carpi ulnaris and the radial extensors in fixation of the wrist. A firm fist can be made only with the wrist in extension.

Grip, or hand grip, should always be tested and its strength noted. The examiner should not be able to withdraw his fingers from the clenched hand of a person with normal grip strength. For quantitative testing a dynamometer may be used. If successive readings are recorded, fatigability can be gauged; this is of particular importance in myasthenia gravis. On the other hand, with nonorganic weakness, sometimes the strength may appear to increase with repeated testing.

Extension of the Fingers. The extensor digitorum communis extends the proximal phalanges of the second, third, fourth, and fifth fingers, and continuing its action, partially extends the interphalangeal joints and the hand. The extensor indicis proprius extends the proximal phalanx of the index finger and adducts this digit. The extensor digiti minimi extends the little finger. These three muscles are supplied by the sixth, seventh, and eighth cervical segments through the radial nerve. The interossei and lumbricales extend the middle and distal phalanges. To test the action of the extensor digitorum communis on the fingers, the patient is asked to resist attempts to flex the fingers at the metacarpophalangeal joints while the forearm is in pronation and the wrist stabilized; the muscle belly and its tendons can be seen and palpated (Fig. 27-21). The function of the lumbricales and interossei is tested by having the patient attempt to extend the middle and distal phalanges against resistance while the metacarpophalangeal joints are hyperextended and fixed and the proximal interphalangeal joints are partly flexed (Fig. 27-22).

The Thumb and its Muscles. The abductor pollicis longus abducts the thumb and extends it to a slight degree. Continuing its action it flexes and abducts the hand and aids in supination. The extensor pollicis longus extends the terminal

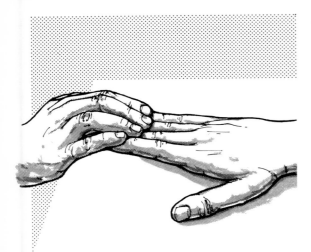

FIG. 27–21. Examination of the extensor digitorum communis. With hand outstretched and interphalangeal joints held in extension, the patient resists the examiner's attempt to flex the fingers at the metacarpophalangeal joints.

When the extensor pollicis longus is tested the patient attempts to extend the thumb at the interphalangeal joint, or attempts to resist passive flexion of the thumb at that joint while the proximal phalanx is immobilized. This can be performed with the palm of the hand down on the table, or with the ulnar edge down at right angles to the table. The tendon can be seen and felt (Fig. 27-23). The extensor pollicis brevis is tested by having the patient attempt extension or resist flexion of the thumb at the metacarpopha-

phalanx of the thumb, and, continuing its action, extends the proximal phalanx and slightly adducts the thumb. It is also an abductor of the hand and an accessory muscle in supination. The extensor pollicis brevis extends the proximal phalanx of the thumb and abducts the thumb. It is also an abductor of the wrist. These three muscles are supplied by the sixth, seventh, and eighth cervical segments through the radial nerve. The abductor pollicis longus is the only flexor of the wrist that is supplied by the radial nerve.

The flexor pollicis longus flexes the distal phalanx of the thumb, and by continuing its action also flexes the proximal phalanx and adducts the thumb; it assists in flexion and adduction of the hand. The flexor pollicis brevis flexes and adducts the proximal phalanx of the thumb and extends the distal phalanx. The abductor pollicis brevis abducts the thumb, flexes the proximal phalanx, and extends the terminal phalanx. The opponens pollicis flexes and adducts the thumb, opposing it to the other fingers. These four muscles are supplied by the median nerve, although the medial head of the flexor pollicis brevis is innervated by the ulnar nerve. The segmental supply is primarily, if not entirely, from the eighth cervical and first thoracic levels. The adductor pollicis adducts the thumb and flexes the first metacarpal bone and the proximal phalanx; it is supplied by the eighth cervical and first thoracic segments through the ulnar nerve.

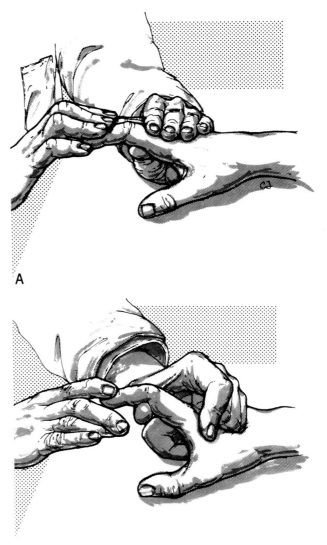

A

B

FIG. 27–22. A and **B.** Extension of the middle and distal phalanges. The patient attempts to extend the fingers against resistance while the metacarpophalangeal joints are fixed.

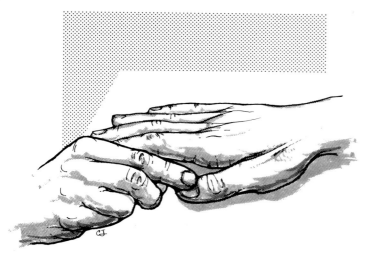

FIG. 27–23. Examination of the extensor pollicis longus. The patient attempts to resist passive flexion of the thumb at the interphalangeal joint; the tendon can be seen and palpated.

langeal joint while the metacarpal bone is immobilized. Again, the tendon can be observed and palpated (Fig. 27-24). On hyperextension of the thumb, especially at both joints, the tendon of the extensors longus and brevis and that of abductor pollicis longus come into full prominence, forming the boundaries of the "anatomic snuff box." In full extension the abductors of the thumb take part. In examining the flexor pollicis longus the patient is asked to resist an attempt to extend the distal phalanx of the thumb while the proximal phalanx is flexed and immobilized and the thumb is in the position of palmar adduction (Fig. 27-25). In testing the flexor pollicis brevis

the patient is asked to flex the proximal phalanx of the thumb and simultaneously extend the distal phalanx.

Abduction, Adduction, and Opposition of the Thumb and Fingers. Abduction of the thumb is carried out in two planes: by moving the thumb in the same plane as that of the palm (radial abduction), and by moving it at right angles to the plane of the palm (palmar abduction). In testing radial abduction the hand may be lying in either pronation or supination on a table or it may be placed, ulnar border

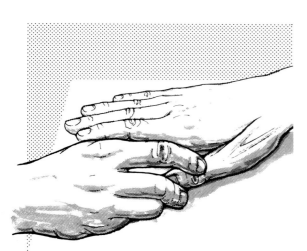

FIG. 27–24. Examination of the extensor pollicis brevis. The patient attempts to resist passive flexion of the thumb at the metacarpophalangeal joint; the tendon can be seen and palpated.

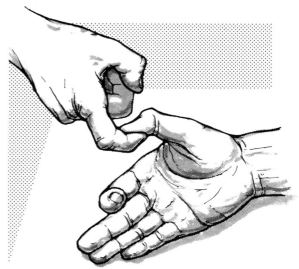

FIG. 27–25. Examination of the flexor pollicis longus. The patient resists attempts to extend the distal phalanx of the thumb while the proximal phalanx is fixed.

down, at right angles to a table. The thumb is then moved lateralward if the hand is horizontal, or upward if the hand is vertical, against resistance. This movement is carried out by the abductor pollicis longus and the extensor pollicis brevis. The tendon of the former muscle can be seen and felt (Fig. 27-26). In testing palmar abduction the thumb is moved at right angles to the palm and inside the radial margin of the hand, against resistance (Fig. 27-27). One may carry this out by placing the hand on a table, dorsal surface down, with a pencil or some other object between the thumb and the palm, the pencil being at a plane at right angles to the hand. The patient then attempts to raise the thumb, against resistance, to a point vertically above its original position, keeping it parallel to the pencil and keeping the thumbnail at right angles to the palm. This latter movement is carried out by the abductor pollicis brevis, along with the abductor pollicis longus, flexor pollicis brevis, and opponens pollicis. In paralysis of abduction the thumb is adducted and falls into the palm of the hand.

Adduction of the thumb is also carried out in two planes: in the plane of the palm (ulnar adduction), and in a plane at right angles to that of the palm (palmar adduction). Ulnar adduction is carried out by having the patient approximate the thumb to the palm in the same plane as the palm, the thumbnail being as nearly as possible

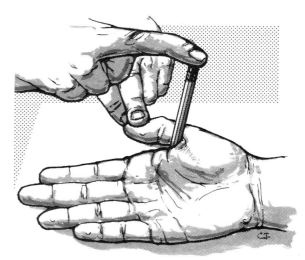

FIG. 27–27. *Palmar abduction of the thumb. The patient attempts, against resistance, to bring the thumb to a point vertically above its original position.*

parallel with the nails of the other fingers (Fig. 27-28). In palmar adduction the thumb is approximated to the palmar aspect of the index finger at right angles to the palm. The thumbnail is at right angles to the nails of the other fingers (Fig. 27-29). In either or both of these tests a piece of paper may be grasped — in the former between the thumb and radial border of the index finger, and in the latter between the thumb and palmar aspect of the index finger —

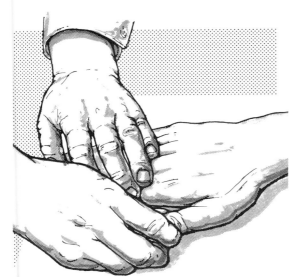

FIG. 27–26. *Radial abduction of the thumb. The patient attempts to abduct the thumb in the same plane as that of the palm; the tendon of the abductor pollicis longus can be seen and palpated.*

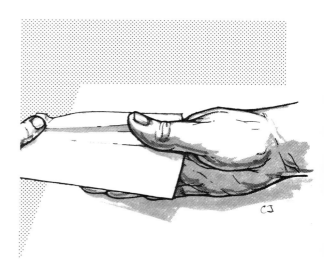

FIG. 27–28. *Ulnar adduction of the thumb. The patient attempts to grasp a piece of paper between the thumb and the radial border of the index finger while the thumbnail is parallel to the nails of the other fingers.*

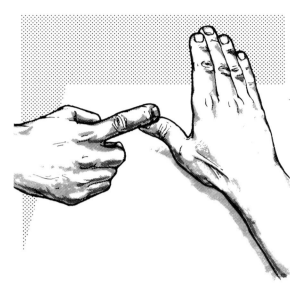

FIG. 27–29. *Palmar adduction of the thumb. The patient, against resistance, attempts to approximate the thumb to the palmar aspect of the index finger; the thumbnail is kept at a right angle to the nails of the other fingers.*

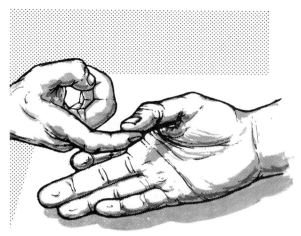

FIG. 27–30. *Examination of the opponens pollicis. The patient attempts, against resistance, to touch the tip of the little finger with the thumb.*

and the patient may try to retain this against the examiner's attempts to withdraw it. The adductor pollicis is the major muscle in both of these acts, especially the former; participating muscles are the first volar interosseous, flexors pollicis longus and brevis, and extensor pollicis longus. When weakness of the adductor is present, the patient attempts to retain the paper between his thumb and index finger by flexion of the thumb at the interphalangeal joint (*signe de journal* of Froment); this may be a significant finding in an ulnar nerve palsy.

Opposition of the thumb is tested by having the patient attempt, against resistance, to touch the tip of the little finger with the thumb against resistance (Fig. 27-30). The thumbnail should remain on a plane parallel to the palm and the palmar surface of the thumb should come in contact with the palmar surface of the little finger. In weakness of the opponens pollicis the patient may be able to oppose the thumb to the index finger or middle finger, but not to the little finger. In testing opposition of the little finger (opponens digiti minimi) the patient is asked to move the extended little finger in front of the other fingers and toward the thumb (Fig. 27-31). This movement is dependent not only on the ability of the little finger to move toward the radial side of the hand, but also on the palmar elevation of the head of the fifth metacarpal. When

opposition is full there is cupping of the palm and rounding of the dorsal metacarpal arch. Opposition of the thumb and little finger may be tested in one maneuver. When both are opposed their extended tips meet and form an arch over the palm (Fig. 27-32). The strength of the combined movement may be gauged by the patient's ability to retain his grasp on a paper that is held between them while the examiner attempts to pull it away, or the examiner may attempt to sep-

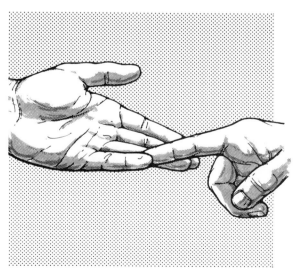

FIG. 27–31. *Examination of the opponens digiti minimi. The patient attempts to move the extended little finger in front of the other fingers and toward the thumb.*

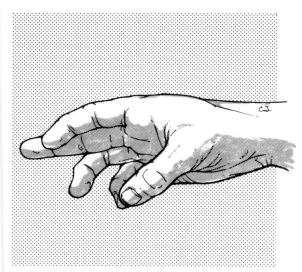

FIG. 27–32. Opposition of the thumb and little finger.

arate the touching tips of the patient's thumb and little finger by pushing a finger or thumb between them. The flexors of the thumb and little finger and the short abductor of the thumb probably enter into these movements.

Adduction of the fingers (volar interossei) is a movement that consists of bringing the fingers tightly together. This may be tested in various ways. While the fingers are abducted and the palm is flat on a table, the patient may try against resistance to adduct the fingers (Fig. 27-33). The degree of functional integrity of the adductors may be tested by having the patient attempt to retain a piece of paper between adjacent fingers while the examiner attempts to withdraw it. The examiner may interpose his fingers with those of the patient and observe the strength of adduction. In testing abduction of the fingers they are fully extended and spread apart and the patient either endeavors to resist the examiner's attempt to bring them together or he attempts to abduct them against resistance (Fig. 27-34). This is largely a function of the dorsal interossei, and the contraction of these muscles can sometimes be felt. Abduction of the little finger is a function of the abductor digiti minimi.

Examination of Movements and Muscles of the Thorax, Abdomen, and Trunk

The examination of the thoracic, abdominal, and trunk muscles (Table 27-3) cannot be evaluated with the detail that is used in the examination of the muscles of the upper extremity. These muscles are large and their action is often combined. As a result it is difficult to evaluate them individually. They should, however, be examined with as much detail as possible.

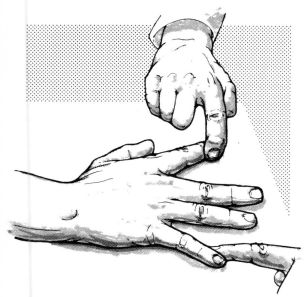

FIG. 27–33. Adduction of the fingers. The patient attempts to adduct the fingers against resistance.

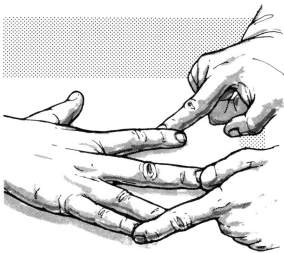

FIG. 27–34. Examination of the abduction of the fingers. The patient resists the examiner's attempt to bring the fingers together.

TABLE 27–3. Innervation of Muscles Responsible for Movements of the Thorax and Abdomen

Muscle	Segmental Innervation	Peripheral Nerve
Diaphragm	C 3–5	Phrenic nerve
Intercostal muscles (internal and external)	Th 1–12	Intercostal nerves
Levatores costarum	C 8–Th 11	Intercostal nerves
Transversus thoracis	Th 2–7	Intercostal nerves
Serratus posterior superior	Th 1–4	Intercostal nerves
Serrratus posterior inferior	Th 9–12	Intercostal nerves
Rectus abdominis	Th 5–12	Intercostal nerves
Pyramidalis	Th 11–12	Intercostal nerves
Transversus abdominis	Th 7–L 1	Intercostal, ilioinguinal, and iliohypogastric nerves
Obliquus internus abdominis	Th 7–L 1	Intercostal, ilioinguinal, and iliohypogastric nerves
Obliquus externus abdominis	Th 7–L 1	Intercostal, ilioinguinal, and iliohypogastric nerves

The Muscles of the Thorax. The thoracic muscles consist of the internal and external intercostals, transversus thoracis, levatores costarum, serratus posterior superior, serratus posterior inferior, and diaphragm. In addition might be included those muscles attached to the sternum, clavicles, and scapulae that act as accessory muscles of respiration; the quadratus lumborum, which draws the last rib downward; and spinal muscles in the thoracic area.

The internal and external intercostals draw the ribs upward and outward and thereby enlarge the thoracic cavity. The internal intercostals may also contract the thorax. Both sets are innervated by the anterior divisions of the twelve thoracic nerves (intercostal nerves). The levatores costarum assist in drawing the ribs upward and bend the spinal column backward and laterally and rotate it. They are innervated by the anterior division of the eighth cervical nerve and the first eleven intercostal nerves. The transversus thoracis is supplied by the second to the sixth or seventh intercostal nerves; it draws the anterior portions of the ribs downward in expiration. The serratus posterior superior is supplied by the first four intercostal nerves; it elevates the ribs to which it is attached and thus aids in inspiration. The serratus posterior inferior is innervated by the ninth to the twelfth intercostal nerves; it draws the lower four ribs downward and outward. The diaphragm is innervated by the third through the fifth cervical segments by

means of the phrenic nerve. The principal muscle of respiration, it is a dome-shaped musculofibrous septum that separates the thoracic from the abdominal cavity.

During quiet inspiration the first and second pairs of ribs are fixed by the resistance of the cervical structures; the last pair by the quadratus lumborum. The other ribs are elevated, and the anteroposterior and transverse diameters of the thorax are increased. The vertical diameter is increased by the descent of the diaphragm. Expiration is effected by the elastic recoil of the walls of the thorax and by the action of the internal intercostals, latissimus dorsi, transversus thoracis, and the abdominal muscles, which push back the viscera previously displaced downward by the diaphragm. In deep inspiration other muscles are brought into action. The first rib is no longer fixed, but is raised with the sternum by the scaleni and sternocleidomastoids, and all the other ribs are raised to a higher level. The shoulders, the clavicles, and the vertebral borders of the scapulas are fixed and the limb muscles and the trapezius, serratus anterior, pectorales, supraspinatus, rhomboidei, latissimus dorsi, levator scapulae, and extensors of the cervical spine are brought into play. There is an increased descent of the diaphragm, the transverse diameter of the upper part of the abdomen is greatly increased, and the subcostal angle is widened. The diaphragm also contracts before and during various expulsive acts such as coughing, sneezing, laughing, vomiting, hiccuping, urination, defecation, and parturition, and it exerts pressure on the abdominal viscera.

Paralysis of the intercostal muscles causes adduction of the costal margins and excessive protrusion of the epigastrium during inspiration. It is difficult to diagnose paralysis of the intercostals, but the presence of respiration that seems to be entirely abdominal with alternate bulging and retraction of the epigastrium may be significant. Furthermore, it may be determined that the intercostal spaces are retracted during inspiration, and that the ribs are not raised and separated.

When bilateral paralysis of the diaphragm is present, the excursion of the costal margins is increased and the epigastrium is retracted during inspiration. The abdomen cannot be protruded. The movable shadow caused by retraction of the lower intercostal region during inspiration (Litten's sign) is absent. The expulsive acts mentioned previously are carried out with difficulty. In unilateral paralysis of the diaphragm the signs are not always easy to demonstrate, but it may frequently be seen during quiet inspiration that the excursion of the costal margin on the affected side is slightly increased, and Litten's sign is absent. Fluoroscopy is a valuable aid to the diagnosis of either unilateral or bilateral diaphragmatic paralysis. If there is either diaphragmatic or intercostal weakness or paralysis, accessory muscles that act in deep inspiration are brought into play, and the patient breathes largely by using his scaleni, sternocleidomastoids, serrati, and pectorales.

The Muscles of the Abdomen. The abdominal muscles are the rectus abdominis, pyramidalis, transversus abdominis, and obliqui. The rectus abdominis flexes the thorax on the vertebral column; it also compresses the abdominal viscera in such acts as defecation and parturition, and aids in forced expiration. It is innervated by the anterior divisions of the fifth to twelfth thoracic nerves (intercostal nerves). The pyramidalis tenses the linea alba; it is innervated by the anterior divisions of the eleventh and twelfth thoracic nerves. The transversus abdominis supports and compresses the contents of the abdomen; it may also contract the thorax and aid in expiration. It is innervated by the lower five or six intercostal nerves and by filaments from the iliohypogastric and ilioinguinal nerves (seventh thoracic through first lumbar segments). The obliquus externus abdominis supports and compresses the abdominal viscera

and assists in expelling their contents; it also depresses the thorax in expiration, flexes the spinal column, and rotates the spinal column toward the opposite side. The obliquus internus abdominis, like the external oblique, supports and compresses the abdominal viscera, depresses the thorax, and flexes the spinal column; it rotates the column to the same side. Both of these muscles are supplied by the anterior divisions of the lower four to six thoracic (intercostal) nerves together with filaments from the iliohypogastric and ilioinguinal nerves (seventh thoracic through first lumbar segments); the external oblique may be innervated only by the intercostal nerves.

In raising the trunk from a supine to a sitting position, the thoracic and lumbar segments of the spine are flexed by the action of the spinal muscles, together with the recti abdominis and the internal and external obliques, which draw the sternum closer to the pubis. In the beginning the flexors of the hips merely serve to fix the pelvis. After the shoulders have been raised about 8 in., the hip flexors contract strongly and bring the trunk to an upright position. If the abdominal muscles are weak, the trunk may be partially erected by the powerful hip flexors, but it is not possible to assume a complete sitting position unless the patient supports himself with his hand or unless his legs are held down by the examiner.

The abdominal muscles may be tensed and tested by having the patient raise his head against resistance (Fig. 27-35), cough, or attempt to rise to a sitting from a recumbent position with the hands held behind the head or the arms folded over the chest (Fig. 27-36). The abdominal muscles will contract and, if the tension of the abdominal musculature is equal on the two sides, the umbilicus will remain in the midline. When there is weakness of the abdominal musculature, these movements are carried out with difficulty, and the patient will raise his legs from the bed on attempting to rise to a sitting position. If the abdominal muscles are paralyzed on one side, the umbilicus is pulled to the normal side during these maneuvers and on inspiration, and the involved side is seen to bulge on coughing and straining. Paralysis of the upper half of the abdominal muscles is associated with downward movement of the umbilicus when the abdominal wall is tensed, and paralysis of the lower half, with upward movement; this is **Beevor's sign.** When bilateral paralysis of the abdomen is present, the umbilicus will be seen to bulge on coughing, raising the head, and attempting to sit up; expiration is affected, forced

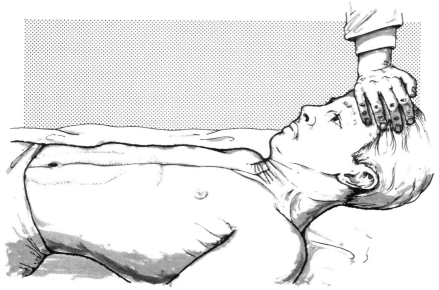

FIG. 27–35. Examination of the abdominal muscles. The recumbent patient attempts to raise his head against resistance.

movements are no longer possible, and urination and defecation become difficult. Palpation is a valuable aid in the examination of the abdominal muscles, and by its means the contracted muscles can easily be distinguished from the relaxed.

The Muscles of the Pelvis. The muscles of the pelvis, including the urinary bladder and the perineal and external genital muscles, are not accessible for the usual clinical testing. The cremaster muscle, which is sometimes classed as an abdominal muscle, is referred to under the cremasteric reflex in Chapter 34. The sphincter ani is mentioned under the anal reflex. The bladder musculature and some of the functions of the genitalia are discussed in Part F, "The Autonomic Nervous System."

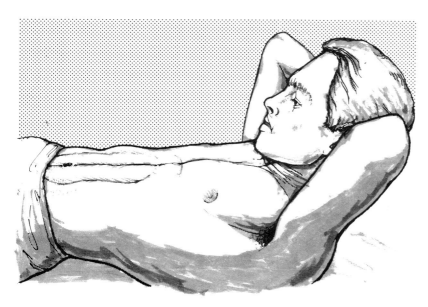

FIG. 27–36. Examination of the abdominal muscles and flexor muscles of the spine. The patient attempts to rise from a recumbent to a sitting position without the use of the hands.

The Muscles of the Spine. The functions of the upper portion of the spinal column have been discussed with the muscles and movements of the neck. Many of the muscles mentioned in that section continue downward and carry out similar functions for the remainder of the spinal column, the principal movements of which are flexion, extension, lateral deviation (abduction), and rotation. The sacrospinalis (erector spinae) and its divisions, the iliocostales dorsi and lumborum and longissimus dorsi, serve, when acting on one side, to bend the spinal column toward that side. When acting on both sides they extend the spinal column. The intertransversarii bend the vertebral column laterally, and when acting on both sides make it rigid. The spinalis dorsi extends the spinal column. The semispinalis dorsi extends the spinal column and rotates it toward the opposite side; they act bilaterally as extensors. The rotatores and interspinales rotate and extend the vertebral column. The quadratus lumborum produces lateral flexion and extension of the vertebral column. All of these muscles are supplied by the posterior and occasionally by the anterior rami of the corresponding spinal nerves. In addition, the abdominal muscles and the flexors of the neck and thigh and levatores costarum participate in extension. The flexors and extensors and rotators of the shoulder as well as those of the hip and the thoracic and abdominal muscles participate in rotation. The shoulder muscles are important in lateral inclination of the spine, and the lateral abdominal muscles and the latissimus dorsi in lateral trunk raising.

The extensors of the spine are tested by having the patient lie in a prone position and attempt to raise his head and shoulders without the assistance of his hands (Fig. 27-37); extension is further tested if he attempts to raise the lower extremities, or if the resistance is applied to the upper thorax. When there is paralysis of the extensors there is a moderate degree of lordosis, which disappears when the patient lies down. In sitting the spinal column has a convex curve, and the patient prevents himself from falling downward by supporting himself with his hands. The flexors are tested by having him rise from a recumbent position to a seated and then a standing position without the use of the hands (see Fig. 27-36). This tests also the flexors of the abdomen and hips. The flexors and extensors of the spine may both be tested by having the patient bend at the wrist, touch his fingertips to the floor, and then resume the erect position. The rotators and lateral flexors of the spine should also be examined.

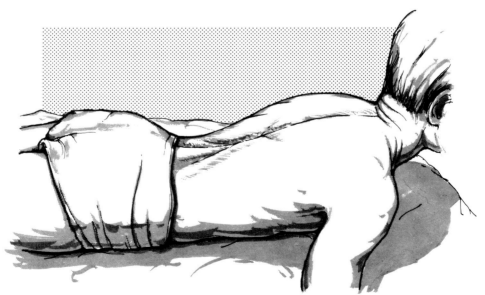

FIG. 27–37. Examination of the extensors of the spine. The patient, lying prone, attempts to raise the head and upper part of the trunk.

Examination of the Movements and Muscles of the Lower Extremities

The movements of the lower extremities are less complex than are those of the upper extremities, and there are fewer substitution movements. As a result there is less chance for error in the assessment of muscle function. It is extremely important, however, to eliminate the effect of gravity in evaluating movements. Table 27-4 lists the pertinent muscles and their innervation.

TABLE 27–4. Innervation of Muscles Responsible for Movements of the Lower Extremities

Muscle	Segmental Innervation	Peripheral Nerve
Psoas major	L (1) 2–4	Nerve to psoas major
Psoas minor	L 1–2	Nerve to psoas minor
Iliacus	L 2–4	Femoral nerve
Quadriceps femoris	L 2–4	Femoral nerve
Sartorius	L 2–4	Femoral nerve
Pectineus	L 2–4	Femoral nerve
Gluteus maximus	L 5–S 2	Inferior gluteal nerve
Gluteus medius	L 4–S 1	Superior gluteal nerve
Gluteus minimus	L 4–S 1	Superior gluteal nerve
Tensor fasciae latae	L 4–S 1	Superior gluteal nerve
Piriformis	S 1–2	Nerve to piriformis
Adductor longus	L 2–4	Obturator nerve
Adductor brevis	L 2–4	Obturator nerve
Adductor magnus	L 2–4	Obturator nerve
	L 4–5	Sciatic nerve
Gracilis	L 2–4	Obturator nerve
Obturator externus	L 2–4	Obturator nerve
Obturator internus	L 5–S 3	Nerve to obturator internus
Gemellus superior	L 5–S 3	Nerve to obturator internus
Gemellus inferior	L 4–S 1	Nerve to quadratus femoris
Quadratus femoris	L 4–S 1	Nerve to quadratus femoris
Biceps femoris (long head)	L 5–S 1	Tibial nerve
Semimembranosus	L 4–S 1	Tibial nerve
Semitendinosus	L 5–S 2	Tibial nerve
Popliteus	L 5–S 1	Tibial nerve
Gastrocnemius	L 5–S 2	Tibial nerve
Soleus	L 5–S 2	Tibial nerve
Plantaris	L 5–S 1	Tibial nerve
Tibialis posterior	L 5–S 1	Tibial nerve
Flexor digitorum longus	L 5–S 1	Tibial nerve
Flexor hallucis longus	L 5–S 1	Tibial nerve
Biceps femoris (short head)	L 5–S 2	Common peroneal nerve
Tibialis anterior	L 4–S 1	Deep peroneal nerve
Peroneus tertius	L 4–S 1	Deep peroneal nerve
Extensor digitorum longus	L 4–S 1	Deep peroneal nerve
Extensor hallucis longus	L 4–S 1	Deep peroneal nerve
Extensor digitorum brevis	L 4–S 1	Deep peroneal nerve
Extensor hallucis brevis	L 4–S 1	Deep peroneal nerve
Peroneus longus	L 4–S 1	Superficial peroneal nerve
Peroneus brevis	L 4–S 1	Superficial peroneal nerve
Flexor digitorum brevis	L 4–S 1	Medial plantar nerve
Flexor hallucis brevis	L 5–S 1	Medial plantar nerve
Abductor hallucis	L 4–S 1	Medial plantar nerve
Lumbricales (medial 1 or 2)	L 4–S 1	Medial plantar nerve
Quadratus plantae	S 1–2	Lateral plantar nerve
Adductor hallucis	L 5–S 2	Lateral plantar nerve
Abductor digiti quinti	S 1–2	Lateral plantar nerve
Flexor digiti quinti brevis	S 1–2	Lateral plantar nerve
Lumbricales (lateral 2 or 3)	S 1–2	Lateral plantar nerve
Interossei	S 1–2	Lateral plantar nerve

The Hip Joint. The movements that take place at the hip are flexion, extension, abduction, adduction, and internal and external rotation.

The principal flexors of the thigh at the hip are the psoas and iliacus muscles. The psoas major is innervated by branches from the trunks of the second, third, and fourth lumbar nerves. The iliacus is innervated by the second, third, and fourth lumbar segments through the femoral nerve. Occasionally there is also a psoas minor that is innervated by branches from the first and second lumbar nerves. These muscles together are often referred to as the iliopsoas. This, acting from above, is the most powerful flexor of the thigh on the pelvis, and conversely, when the thigh is fixed, acting from below it flexes the pelvis and trunk forward upon the femur. The psoas also bends the spinal column laterally and rotates the thigh inward; the iliacus rotates the thigh slightly outward. The two muscles on each side, when acting together, serve to maintain an erect posture by supporting the vertebral column and pelvis on the femurs, and they bend the trunk and pelvis forward. Accessory flexors of the hips are the rectus femoris, adductors magnus, longus, and brevis, sartorius, pectineus, tensor fasciae latae, gracilis, and anterior fibers of the glutei medius and minimus. The iliopsoas may be tested by having the patient attempt to flex the thigh against resistance. This is carried out with the patient in the recumbent position with the knee flexed, the angle between the thigh and the trunk slightly less than 90°, and the leg supported on the examiner's hand. Further flexion is attempted against resistance (Fig. 27–38). Flexion of the hip may also be tested with the patient recumbent and the knee in extension, or with the patient seated and his legs over the edge of the examining table. The flexors of the hip may be examined along with the abdominal muscles by having the patient rise from a recumbent to a sitting position without the assistance of his hands.

The major extensor of the thigh is the gluteus maximus. This muscle, innervated by the fifth lumbar and the first sacral segments through the inferior gluteal nerve, is the most powerful extensor and lateral rotator of the thigh. It not only brings the bent thigh into line with the body, but it also causes the body to assume an erect posture after stooping, and supports the pelvis. It is also an adductor of the thigh, but when the thigh is flexed it is a weak abductor. Acting from below it extends the trunk. Additional extensors are the posterior fibers of the glutei medius and minimus, the lower part of the adductor magnus, the piriformis, obturator internus, and hamstrings. The gluteus maximus is important in climbing steps, jumping, and rising from a chair. When paralysis of the glutei develops, the pelvis is bent forward as the patient attempts to

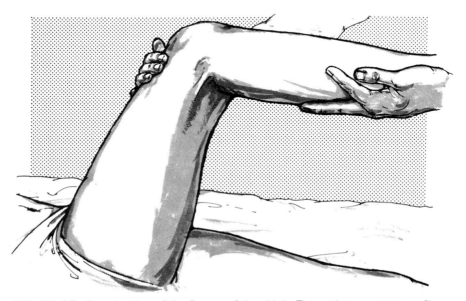

FIG. 27–38. Examination of the flexors of the thigh. The patient attempts to flex the thigh against resistance; the knee is flexed and the leg rests on the examiner's arm.

get out of a chair. To test the function of this muscle the patient lies prone and lifts his lower extremity, flexed at the knee, off the table. Then he attempts to maintain it in this position while the examiner tries to press it back down. The contraction of the muscle can be palpated and can usually be seen (Fig. 27-39). The gluteus maximus can also be tested by having the patient lie on his side and extend the flexed hip, or by having him stand upright from a stooped position. In the muscular dystrophies there is marked weakness of the extensors, and the patient arises from a stooped position by using his hands to "climb up the legs" (Gowers' maneuver, Fig. 21-5).

Abduction at the hip is carried out by the gluteus medius and minimus, piriformis, sartorius, and tensor fasciae latae. The upper fibers of the gluteus maximus and the obturator internus also aid in abduction when the thigh is flexed. The glutei medius and minimus are supplied by the fourth and fifth lumbar and first sacral segments through the superior gluteal nerve. Both are abductors and medial rotators of the thigh and lateral flexors of the pelvis. The anterior portion of the gluteus medius is a flexor and medial rotator, whereas the posterior portion is an extensor and lateral rotator. The anterior part of the gluteus minimus is a flexor, the posterior part an extensor. The piriformis is an abductor, lateral rotator, and weak extensor of the thigh. The sartorius is an abductor, flexor, and lateral rotator of the thigh, and a flexor and medial rotator of the leg.

The tensor fasciae latae makes the fascia lata tense, flexes and abducts the thigh and rotates it medially, and flexes and abducts the pelvis. Abduction is tested by having the patient attempt to move the leg outward against resistance while recumbent with his leg in extension (Fig. 27-40); the gluteus medius and tensor fasciae latae can be palpated. It may also be tested with the patient lying on the contralateral side; the strength of movement can then be evaluated against both gravity and resistance. When paralysis of these muscles is present, the thigh cannot be abducted or rotated medially; during walking the trunk bends toward the affected side, the leg swings inward, and the excessive raising and lowering of the pelvis causes a waddling gait. If the patient stands on the foot on the side of the weak glutei, there will be sagging of the opposite side of the pelvis because of gluteal insufficiency on the involved side.

Adduction of the thigh is principally a function of the three adductors, together with the pectineus, gracilis, quadratus femoris, obturator externus, hamstrings, and the lower fibers of the gluteus maximus. The iliopsoas is also an adductor when the thigh is flexed. The adductor longus is an adductor, flexor, and medial rotator of the thigh. The adductor brevis is an adductor and to a lesser extent a flexor and a lateral rotator. The adductor magnus is the strongest adductor; its superior and middle fasciculi are extensors and lateral rotators of the extended thigh and medial rotators of the flexed thigh. The

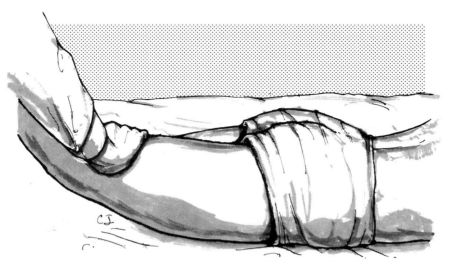

FIG. 27–39. Examination of the extensors of the thigh at the hip. The patient, lying prone with the leg flexed at the knee, attempts to extend the thigh against resistance; contraction of the gluteus maximus and other extensors can be seen and palpated.

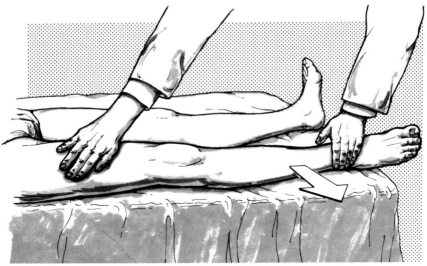

FIG. 27–40. Abduction of the thigh at the hip. The recumbent patient attempts to move the extended leg outward against resistance; contraction of the gluteus medius and tensor fasciae latae can be palpated.

gracilis adducts, flexes, and laterally rotates the thigh; it also flexes the leg and medially rotates the flexed leg. The pectineus is a flexor and adductor of the thigh. The three adductors and the gracilis are supplied by the second, third, and fourth lumbar nerves through the obturator nerve, and the adductor magnus receives an extra branch from the fourth and fifth lumbar segments through the sciatic. The pectineus is supplied by the second, third, and fourth lumbar segments through the femoral nerve. Adduction is tested while the patient is on his back with the legs in extension; he adducts the thigh while the examiner attempts to abduct it. The contraction of the adducted muscles can be palpated (Fig. 27-41). Adduction can also be tested with the

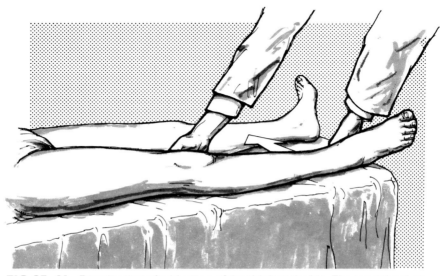

FIG. 27–41. Examination of adduction of the thigh at the hip. The recumbent patient attempts to adduct the extended leg against resistance; contraction of the adductor muscles can be seen and palpated.

patient lying on the homolateral side; the opposite leg is passively raised and supported, and the patient attempts to adduct the thigh against gravity and resistance.

Internal, or medial, rotation of the thigh is carried out principally by the anterior parts of the glutei medius and minimus and the tensor fasciae latae, together with the adductor longus, upper part of the adductor magnus, semitendinosus, and semimembranosus muscles, the lower part of the adductor magnus when the thigh is flexed, and the iliopsoas when the tibia is fixed. To test internal rotation the patient lies prone with the lower leg flexed at the knee. He then attempts to carry the foot laterally, thus rotating the hip medially, while the examiner tries to pull the foot medially. During this maneuver the gluteus medius can be felt to contract (Fig. 27-42). Internal rotation can also be tested with the patient recumbent and his leg either extended or flexed and hanging over the edge of the examining table.

External, or lateral, rotation of the thigh at the hip is carried by the gluteus maximus, obturators internus and externus, gemelli superior and inferior, quadratus femoris, and piriformis, assisted by the adductor brevis, sartorius, gracilis, iliopsoas, posterior part of the gluteus medius, long head of the biceps, and lower part of the adductor magnus. The obturator internus is a powerful lateral rotator of the thigh; it is also an extensor and abductor when the hip is flexed at a right angle. The obturator externus is a powerful lateral rotator and a weak adductor. The gemelli superior and inferior function as essential parts of the obturator internus. The quadratus femoris is a powerful lateral rotator and a weak adductor. The obturator internus is supplied by a special nerve, the nerve to the obturator internus, from the fifth lumbar and the first, second, and third sacral segments. The obturator externus is supplied by the obturator nerve (second to fourth lumbar segments). The quadratus femoris is innervated by a special nerve that is derived from the fourth and fifth lumbar and first sacral nerves. The superior gemellus is supplied by a branch of the nerve to the obturator internus or a branch of that to the quadratus femoris, and the inferior gemellus is innervated by a branch of the nerve to the quadratus femoris.

External rotation is tested by maneuvers similar to those for testing internal rotation, but the patient attempts to carry the foot medially against resistance, thus rotating the hip laterally. If these muscles are paralyzed the entire leg is turned inward.

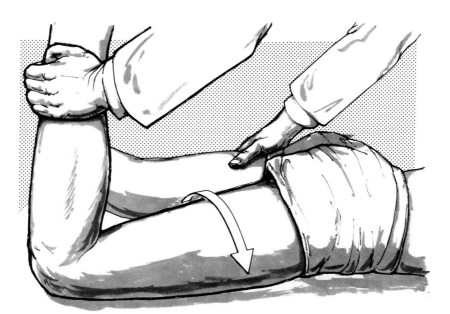

FIG. 27–42. Examination of internal rotation of the thigh. The patient, lying prone with the leg flexed at the knee, attempts to carry the foot laterally against resistance, thus rotating the thigh medially; contraction of the gluteus medius can be palpated.

The Knee Joint. The movements that take place at the knee joint are flexion, extension, and internal and external rotation.

Flexion of the leg at the knee is carried out by the biceps femoris, semimembranosus, semitendinosus, popliteus, gracilis, sartorius, and gastrocnemius muscles. The first three of these muscles are known as the **hamstring muscles.** The biceps femoris flexes the leg, and when the leg is flexed it is a lateral rotator. It also extends and adducts the thigh, and the long head is a lateral rotator of the thigh. The long head, acting from below, assists in extending the trunk upon the thigh. The semimembranosus and semitendinosus muscles flex the leg and act as medial rotators. Acting from below they extend the thigh, or the trunk upon the thigh, and adduct and medially rotate the thigh. The popliteus flexes and medially rotates the leg. These muscles are supplied by branches of the sciatic nerve. The short head of the biceps receives its innervation from the fifth lumbar and first and second sacral segments through the common peroneal nerve, and the long head from the fifth lumbar and first sacral segments through the tibial nerve. The semitendinosus is supplied by the fifth lumbar and first and second sacral through the tibial nerve, and the semimembranosus by the fourth and fifth lumbar and first

sacral through the tibial nerve. The popliteus is supplied by the fifth lumbar and first sacral segments through the tibial nerve.

Flexion at the knee is tested while the patient is in the prone position with his leg in partial flexion. His ability to maintain flexion while the examiner attempts to extend the leg will reveal the strength of the hamstrings. The tendons of the semimembranosus and semitendinosus (medially) and that of the biceps (laterally) can be seen and felt to contract (Fig. 27-43). The patient, lying prone, may be asked to maintain his legs in flexion at right angles at the knee; in weakness of the flexors the leg will fall, gradually or rapidly (leg sign of Barré). If flexion of the knee is tested while the patient is lying supine, the simultaneous flexion at the hip may result in a misinterpretation of the strength of the hamstrings. Furthermore, in this latter position the contraction of the muscles cannot be satisfactorily palpated. The function of the sartorius, which is not only a flexor but a medial rotator of the leg and an abductor, flexor, and lateral rotator of the thigh, may be examined by having the patient attempt to flex his knee against resistance while he is lying supine with the knee moderately flexed and the thigh flexed and rotated laterally. The muscle belly can readily be seen and felt (Fig. 27-44).

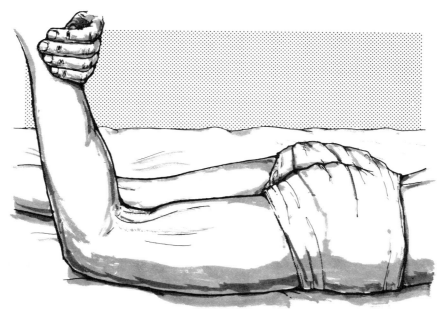

FIG. 27–43. Examination of flexion at the knee. The prone patient attempts to maintain flexion of the leg while the examiner attempts to extend it; the tendon of the biceps femoris can be palpated laterally and the tendons of the semimembranosus and semitendinosus, medially.

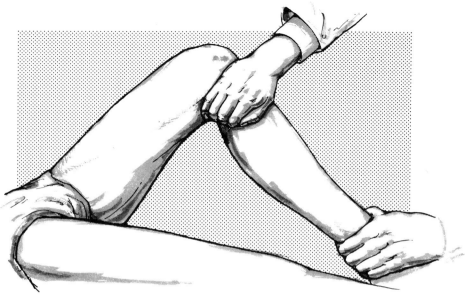

FIG. 27–44. *Examination of the sartorius. With the thigh flexed and rotated laterally and the knee moderately flexed, the patient attempts further flexion of the knee against resistance.*

The quadriceps femoris is composed of four large muscles, rectus femoris, vastus lateralis, vastus medialis, and vastus intermedius, which are united into a common tendon inserted into the upper border of the patella. This group of muscles acts as the extensor of the leg at the knee; its force is three times that of its antagonists, the hamstrings. The rectus femoris, acting from below, also flexes the thigh at the hip and flexes the trunk forward on the femur. These muscles are innervated by the second, third, and fourth lumbar segments through the femoral nerve. The quadriceps is tested when the patient, lying supine, attempts to extend the leg at the knee while the examiner tries to flex it (Fig. 27-45), or attempts to maintain extension against the examiner's resistance. The contraction of the muscle can be seen and palpated. The examiner may use one arm as a fulcrum, placing it beneath the knee, or he may use one hand to palpate the contraction of the quadriceps. The quadriceps may also be tested with the patient seated. Paralysis prevents the leg from being extended, and when it is passively raised it falls back down. If the quadriceps is weak, the patient will have marked difficulty in rising from a kneeling position and in climbing stairs; he can walk backward, but has difficulty in walking forward. With paralysis of the extensors of the leg the oval contour of the thigh, which is nor-

mally in a vertical or upright position when the patient is recumbent, is flattened horizontally. Both the flexors and the extensors of the leg are such powerful muscles that, in the normal individual, it is often not possible for the examiner's hand to overcome either flexion or extension at the knee.

Internal and external rotation at the knee are relatively minor movements. Internal, or medial, rotation is carried out by the semimembranosus, sartorius, popliteus, and gracilis muscles; external, or lateral, rotation by the biceps femoris and tensor fasciae latae. These movements may be tested against resistance.

The Ankle Joint. Movements affecting the ankle joint are plantar flexion and dorsiflexion. Plantar flexion (flexion) of the foot is carried out principally by the gastrocnemius, soleus, and plantaris muscles assisted by tibialis anterior, peroneus longus, peroneus brevis, and flexors digitorum longus and hallucis longus. The first three muscles, sometimes known as triceps surae, also raise the heel, as in walking, and invert the foot, and the gastrocnemius assists in flexing the leg at the knee. They are innervated by the tibial division of the sciatic nerve. The function of these muscles is tested by having the patient attempt to maintain plantar flexion while the examiner offers resistance by means of

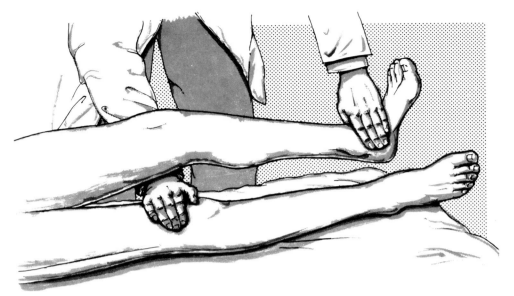

FIG. 27–45. Examination of extension of the leg at the knee. The supine patient attempts to extend the leg at the knee against resistance; contraction of the quadriceps femoris can be seen and palpated.

pressure against the sole of the foot and palpates the contracting gastrocnemius (Fig. 27-46). They may also be evaluated by having the patient stand on his tiptoes. In weakness or paralysis of the plantar flexors the patient is unable to stand on his toes.

Dorsiflexion (extension) of the foot at the ankle is carried out by the tibialis anterior muscle assisted by the peroneus tertius and extensors digitorum longus and hallucis longus. The tibialis anterior is supplied by the fourth and fifth lumbar and first sacral segments through

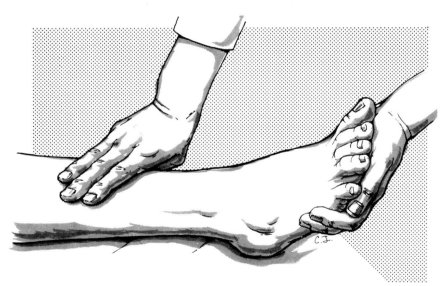

FIG. 27–46. Examination of plantar flexion of the foot. The patient attempts to plantar flex the foot at the ankle joint against resistance; contraction of the gastroc-nemius and associated muscles can be seen and palpated.

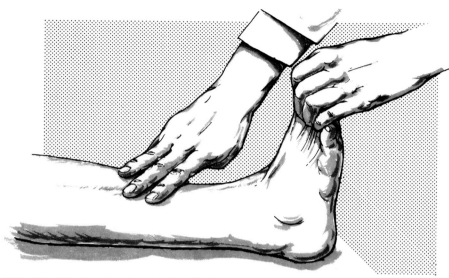

FIG. 27–47. Examination of dorsiflexion (extension) of the foot. The patient attempts to dorsiflex the foot against resistance; contraction of the tibialis anterior can be seen and palpated.

the deep peroneal nerve. In addition to its action as a dorsiflexor of the foot it is an invertor. When the foot is on the ground it tilts the leg forward, as in walking. It is examined by having the patient dorsiflex his foot while the examiner attempts to press down the toes (Fig. 27-47). The contracted muscle can be seen and palpated. Dorsiflexion may also be tested by having the patient stand on his heel and raise the ball of the foot and toes. In paralysis of the dorsiflexors there is a foot drop with often an audible double slap as the toes and then the heel of the foot fall on the ground in walking, and the patient walks with a steppage gait, attempting to raise the depressed toes off the ground by exaggerated flexion at the hip and knee; he is unable to raise the sole of the foot off the ground while standing on his heel.

The Tarsal Joints. Movements at the tarsal joints consist of inversion and eversion. Inversion, and medial deviation or elevation of the inner border of the foot, is carried out by the tibialis posterior assisted by the tibialis anterior, gastrocnemius, soleus, and the flexor digitorum longus and hallucis longus. The tibialis posterior is supplied by the fifth lumbar and first sacral segments through the tibial nerve. It is also a plantar flexor. Inversion is tested by having the patient attempt to elevate the inner border of the plantar-flexed foot against resistance. During this maneuver the tendon of the tibialis posterior

can be seen and felt just behind the medial malleolus (Fig. 27-48).

Eversion, or lateral deviation or elevation of the outer border of the foot, is carried out by the peronei longus, brevis, and tertius and the extensor digitorum longus. The peronei longus and brevis are supplied by the fourth and fifth lum-

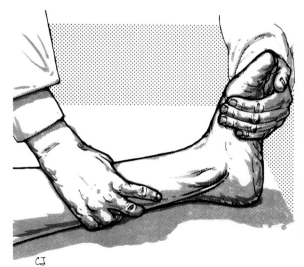

FIG. 27–48. Examination of inversion of the foot. The patient attempts to raise the inner border of the foot against resistance; the tendon of the tibialis posterior can be seen and palpated just behind the medial malleolus.

bar and first sacral segments through the superficial peroneal nerve. They are plantar flexors as well as evertors. The peroneus tertius is supplied by the fourth and fifth lumbar and first sacral segments through the deep peroneal nerve. It is a dorsiflexor as well as an evertor. To test these muscles the plantar-flexed foot is held in a position of eversion while the examiner attempts to produce inversion; the tendons of the peronei longus and brevis, which are situated a little above and behind the external malleolus, can be seen and felt to tighten (Fig. 27-49).

Muscles of the Foot and Toes. Muscle testing of the foot and toes cannot be carried out with as much detail as can that of the hand, since the function of the individual muscles is not so clearly defined. The principal movements are extension (dorsiflexion) and flexion (plantar flexion). With plantar flexion there is cupping of the sole. Abduction and adduction of the toes are minimal.

The extensors of the toes are the extensors digitorum longus and brevis and the extensors hallucis longus and brevis. These muscles are supplied by the fourth and fifth lumbar and first sacral segments through the deep peroneal nerve. The long extensors extend the metatarsophalangeal and interphalangeal joints of the toes and dorsiflex the ankle joint. The extensor digitorum longus is also an evertor. The extensor digitorum brevis, whose most medial and largest belly is the extensor hallucis brevis, aids the long extensor in extending the proximal phalanx of the four medial toes. Dorsiflexion of the toes against resistance may be used as a test for the function of these muscles. The tendons of the long extensors and the belly of the extensor digitorum brevis can be palpated during this maneuver (Fig. 27-50).

Flexion, or plantar flexion, of the toes is carried out by the flexors digitorum and hallucis longus, flexors digitorum and hallucis brevis, and certain of the intrinsic muscles of the sole of the foot. The flexors digitorum longus and hallucis longus are supplied by the fifth lumbar and first sacral segments through the tibial nerve. These muscles flex the phalanges of all five toes, acting chiefly at the distal interphalangeal joints. They also plantar flex the ankle joint and invert the foot. The flexor digitorum brevis, supplied by the medial plantar nerve, acts at the proximal interphalangeal and metatarsophalangeal joints, flexing the middle phalanges on the metatarsals. The flexor hallucis brevis, also supplied by the medial plantar nerve, acts at the metatarsophalangeal joint and

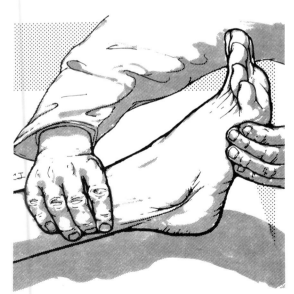

FIG. 27–49. Examination of eversion of the foot. The patient attempts to raise the outer border of the foot against resistance; the tendons of the peronei longus and brevis can be seen and palpated just above and behind the lateral malleolus.

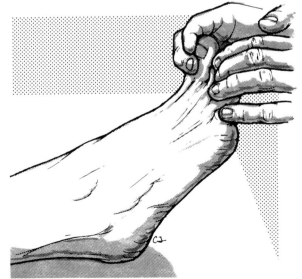

FIG. 27–50. Examination of dorsiflexion (extension) of the toes. On attempts to dorsiflex the toes against resistance, the tendons of the extensors digitorum and hallucis longus and the belly of the extensor digitorum brevis can be seen and palpated.

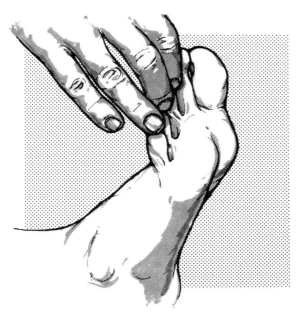

FIG. 27–51. Examination of flexion of the toes. The patient attempts to flex the toes against resistance.

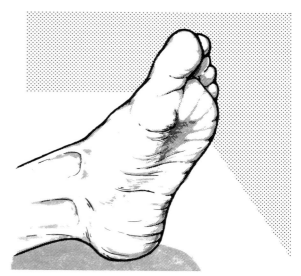

FIG. 27–52. Cupping of the sole of the foot.

flexes the proximal phalanx of the great toe. In this it is aided by the adductor and abductor hallucis. These muscles are tested by having the patient flex the digits and attempt to maintain flexion against resistance (Fig. 27-51).

The intrinsic muscles of the sole of the foot, in addition to the short flexors, are as follows: The quadratus plantae assists the long flexors in flexing the toes; it is innervated by the first and second sacral segments through the lateral plantar nerve. The abductor hallucis abducts and flexes the proximal phalanx of the great toe; it is supplied by the medial plantar nerve. The adductor hallucis adducts and flexes the proximal phalanx of the great toe; it is innervated by the lateral plantar nerve. The abductor digiti quinti flexes and abducts the proximal phalanx of the little toe; the flexor digiti quinti brevis also flexes this phalanx. Both are supplied by the lateral plantar nerve. The lumbricales flex the proximal phalanges of the four lateral toes. The medial one or two lumbricales are supplied by the medial plantar nerve, and the lateral two or three by the lateral plantar nerve. The interossei are innervated by the first and second sacral segments through the lateral plantar nerve. They flex the proximal phalanges; the dorsal interossei are abductors of the toes and the plantar interossei, adductors. Any extensor action of the interossei or lumbricales is questionable.

The testing of these muscles individually is a difficult matter. Abduction and adduction are extremely weak movements, and the long and short flexors are much more powerful in flexion than are the other intrinsic muscles. In fact some of these muscles are more important from a static than an active point of view. The quadratus plantae, adductor hallucis, and flexor digitorum brevis are important in maintaining the longitudinal arches of the foot. The chief function of the abductor hallucis is to maintain the medial longitudinal arch, and that of the abductor digiti quinti and flexor digiti quinti brevis, to maintain the lateral longitudinal arch. These muscles, however, may be tested together by asking the patient to attempt to make a cup of the sole of the foot (Fig. 27-52).

CONCLUSIONS

To recapitulate, in the testing of motor strength and power all of the important muscles should be tested individually. Movements should be tested at all joints, and evidence of paresis or paralysis noted.

It must be recalled that involvement of individual muscles only occurs in lesions of the spinomuscular level or those of the anterior horn cells or the peripheral nerves. The syndromes associated with injuries of the peripheral nerves, plexus involvement, and segmental lesions of the spinal cord are summarized in Part G, "Diagnosis and Localization of Disorders of the Peripheral Nerves, Nerve Roots, and Spinal Cord." In the presence of dysfunction at the myoneural junction and in the myopathies and polymyositis the changes are more general. Lesions of the extrapyramidal and corticospinal complexes, whether cerebral in origin or due to interruption of the descending motor pathways, produce loss of strength and power, but under such circumstances the loss is generalized and involves either entire extremities or gross movements such as flexion and extension of an entire extremity. Cerebellar involvement is not followed by loss of power, but the resulting ataxia may interfere with voluntary movements. So-called psychomotor involvement may be followed by nonorganic paresis — either of a hysterical type or due to malingering. Under such circumstances the paralysis is often somewhat bizarre and does not follow an organic pattern (Ch. 55).

BIBLIOGRAPHY

Aids to the examination of the peripheral nervous system. Medical Research Council memorandum No. 45 (superseding war memorandum No. 7). London, Her Majesty's Stationery Office, 1976

Adams RD, Victor M. Principles of Neurology, 4th ed. New York, McGraw – Hill, 1989

Daniels L, Williams M, Worthingham C. Muscle Testing: Techniques of Manual Examination, 2nd ed. Philadelphia, WB Saunders, 1956

Haymaker W, Woodhall B. Peripheral Nerve Injuries: Principles of Diagnosis, 2nd ed. Philadelphia, WB Saunders, 1953

Hollinshead WF. Functional Anatomy of the Limbs and Back. Philadelphia, WB Saunders, 1951

Joynt RJ, Benton AL, Fogel ML. Behavioral and pathological correlates of motor impersistence. Neurology 1962; 12:876

Kendall FR, Kendall FP. Muscles: Testing and Function. Baltimore, Williams & Wilkins, 1949

Kranz LG. Kinesiology Laboratory Manual. St. Louis, CV Mosby, 1948

Lockhart RD. Living Anatomy: A Photographic Atlas of Muscles in Action and Surface Contours. London, Faber and Faber, 1948

Mayo Clinic and Foundation. Clinical Examinations in Neurology, 5th ed. Philadelphia, WB Saunders, 1976

Oester YT, Mayer JH, Jr. Motor Examination in Peripheral Nerve Injuries. Springfield, IL, Charles C Thomas, 1960

Rowland LP (ed). Merritt's Textbook of Neurology, 8th ed. Philadelphia, Lea & Febiger, 1989

Russell WR. Use of a recording dynamometer in clinical medicine. Br Med J 1954;2:731

Sunderland S. Nerves and Nerve Injuries, 2nd ed. Edinburgh, Churchill Livingstone, 1978

Tourtellotte WW, Haerer AF, Simpson JF, Kuzma JW et al. Quantitative clinical neurological testing. Ann NY Acad Sci 1965;122:480

Van Allen MW. Pictorial Manual of Neurologic Tests. Chicago, Year Book Medical Pub, 1969

Walton J (ed). Disorders of Voluntary Muscle, 5th ed. Edinburgh, Churchill Livingstone, 1988

Wells F. Kinesiology, 2nd ed. Philadelphia, WB Saunders, 1955

Westerberg MR, Magee KR, Shideman FE. Effect of Tensilon in myasthenia gravis. Neurology 1953;3:302

Chapter 28
MUSCLE TONE

Tone, or **tonus,** has been defined as the tension of the muscles when they are relaxed, or as their resistance to passive movement when voluntary control is absent. Muscle itself has complex qualities such as extensibility, contractility, elasticity, ductility, and independent irritability. When a muscle fiber contracts it does so maximally or not at all. Even in apparently relaxed muscles there is a constant, slight, fixed state of tension by which they are held in a given position, resist changes in their length, prevent undue mobility at joints, assure the retention of posture, and are in readiness either to contract or relax promptly when a specific increase or decrease occurs in the total number of impulses delivered to them. This tension is necessary to hold the different parts of the skeleton in their proper relationships throughout the various and frequently changing attitudes and postures of the body. It is greatest in those muscles that maintain the body in an erect position; these are the antigravity muscles, principally the flexors in the upper and the extensors in the lower extremities. Normal muscles, especially those just mentioned, show a slight resistance to passive movement in spite of voluntary relaxation.

The state of continuous tension of muscles is dependent upon the integrity of the muscle tissue, the myoneural junction, the peripheral nerves, the α- and γ- motor neurons and interneurons in the spinal cord, and the central connections. Motor centers on the cerebral cortex and basal ganglia, the facilitatory and inhibitory centers in the midbrain and brain stem reticular formations, the cerebellum, and the vestibular apparatus all supply impulses that influence tone to the motor nuclei in the spinal cord. There is a constant discharge of impulses from the anterior horn cells and that is in part responsible for the comparatively steady contraction of the various fibers that go to make up the individual muscles. No action potentials can be obtained by electromyography, however, from normal muscles at rest in well relaxed subjects, despite the fact that muscle is normally in a state of slight tension. Action potentials appear only with movement and cease at the end of it.

Tone is a reflex phenomenon, and afferent as well as efferent components influence it. Impulses sent through the γ-efferents stimulate the intrafusal fibers in the muscle spindles, which in turn send afferent impulses to the anterior horns of the spinal cord to initiate contraction of muscle by reflex action of the alpha-motor neurons. Muscle is flaccid and behaves as noncontractile tissue when deprived of its motor and sensory supply. When a muscle with normal innervation is passively stretched, its fibers actively resist the stretching and enter into an entire state of increased and sustained tension. First a lengthening reaction takes place, but proprioceptive impulses carried to the nervous system call forth an increase in tension, and a shortening reaction follows. Thus the **stretch reflex** is evident. This is a reaction evoked by the stimulation of the sensory organs in the muscle; it depends for its development on impulses from tension receptors in the muscle itself. It is present at all times; even in apparently relaxed muscle a slight degree of tension is constantly present as long as the muscle innervation is intact; this is normal **tone.** If a muscle is stretched beyond its normal limits by gravity, manipulation, stimulation, or disease, additional tension is developed, and a tonic response takes place. A reflex contraction of the antagonistic muscles may block the attempted contraction of the stimulated muscles. Most types of hypertonicity can be abolished by interruption of either the γ-efferent impulses to the intrafusal fibers or the afferent impulses from the muscle spindles. Selective blockade of the γ-efferents may be produced by either intrathecal or epidural injection of local anesthetics.

An involuntary postural contraction of muscles is necessary for the maintenance of normal positions and attitudes. Tone is the basis or background for posture, and is important in the coordination of movement. Tonic reflexes mediated through the reticular formation, the otolith organs, the vestibular apparatus, and other higher centers are important in maintaining the steady contraction of the antigravity muscles that is necessary to the standing position, as well as to other postural and righting reflexes. Tone may be influenced by disease at various levels of the nervous system. Interruption of the spinal reflex arc abolishes it, but loss of impulses from supraspinal levels that normally inhibit lower reflex centers usually causes an increase in tone. Imbalance of higher facilitatory and inhibitory centers may either decrease or augment tone, and the same is true, but to a lesser degree, of mental states and volitional factors.

EXAMINATION OF TONE

Tone is difficult to appraise. It cannot be measured quantitatively except as a skilled examiner gives his impression in the light of previous experience. Normal muscle shows some slight resistance to passive movement in spite of voluntary relaxation, and it may be difficult to differentiate between this and a slight increase or decrease in tone. Consequently the evaluation of tone is entirely a matter of judgment and can be learned only by repeated trials. Furthermore, inadequate relaxation or slight resistance to passive movement, on either a conscious or unconscious basis, may seriously affect tone and may cause misinterpretations. A tense or apprehensive patient may present voluntary or involuntary resistance to passive movement that may simulate an organic increase in tone.

In testing tone, the examiner should attempt to secure the complete cooperation of the patient, who should be comfortable and relaxed, and have complete confidence in the examiner.

Irrelevant conversation or questioning the patient about unimportant matters during the examination may aid in obtaining adequate relaxation. Observation, especially of the extremities, is the first test. The character of spontaneous movements and abnormalities of posture or of the position of the extremities may indicate changes in tone. Palpation of the muscles, to note their consistency, passive elasticity, firmness, or turgor, is useful, but palpation of the muscle bellies themselves does not alone give a reliable indication of tone. An individual with well-developed musculature may have firm muscles in spite of normal tone. The resting muscles may feel flabby in hypertonic conditions. There may be increased consistency of the muscles in the presence of edema or inflammation; they may feel firm and rubbery in myositis or in muscular dystrophy. With spasm secondary to pain there may also be increased turgor. Palpation is most useful in detecting hypotonicity. Muscle tenderness may also be revealed by palpation, as discussed later in the chapter. Percussion, or stretching the muscle by tapping it, is used in evaluating direct muscular irritability, or idiomuscular contraction, also discussed later. This, however, is not a specific test of tone.

The most important criterion in the examination of tone is the resistance of muscles to passive manipulation when they are relaxed and when voluntary control is absent. In testing tone one examines passive, not active, movement, and notes the degree of tension present on passive stretching of muscles, as well as the extensibility and range of motion. Changes in tone are more readily detected in the muscles of the extremities than in those of the trunk. In testing these the patient is asked to give the arm to the examiner, to relax completely, and to avoid tension. The part is moved passively, first slowly and through a complete range of motion, and then at varying speeds. The examiner may shake the forearm to and fro and note the excursions of the patient's voluntarily relaxed hand; he may brace a limb and then suddenly remove the support; he may note the range of movement of a part in response to a slight blow. The same parts on the two sides of the body are compared to assess differences in tone.

The resistance to movement and the power to maintain postures against external forces are noted, both on slow and rapid motion and on partial and full range of motion. The distribution of the abnormality in tone, i.e., the movement or muscles involved, as well as the type and degree of the change, should be recorded. A limitation of the range of motion, plasticity, the assuming of new positions, pain on movement, defensive spasm, contractures, fibrotic changes, and ankylosis should all be appraised. At times, when surgical procedures are being contemplated for the relief of severe limitation of movement of an extremity, it may be necessary to anesthetize the patient, using general, spinal, or local anesthesia, or to inject drugs such as curare, in order to differentiate between 1) reflex contraction resulting from overactivity of one group of muscles unopposed by weak antagonists and 2) contracture resulting from fibrotic changes in the muscle and tendons.

It is important to remember that tone may be influenced by temperature (cooling increases and heat decreases tone), the speed of passive movement, the presence of synergistic movements, emotional states, and volition. Tone is especially difficult to evaluate in newborn infants, in whom there may be wide variations in apparent tonus on different examinations, in either health or disease.

Careful clinical appraisal is the best criterion of abnormalities in tone. Various mechanical, electronic, and other appliances have been devised for testing tonus. Most of these, however, do not measure pure tone, but rather the resistance of muscle to stretching, muscle consistency, and an admixture of voluntary motion and effects of muscle contraction.

Special methods of examination of tonus are often helpful in the neurologic appraisal. These are most frequently used in evaluation of the rigidity that is a characteristic feature of extrapyramidal disorders, but may also be significant in spasticity and hypotonicity. Some of them are as follows:

The Babinski Tonus Test. The forearms are flexed passively at the elbows while the upper arms are held abducted at the shoulders. When hypotonicity is present there is exaggerated flexibility and mobility, and the elbows can be bent to an angle that is more acute than normal. With hypertonicity there is reduced flexibility of the forearms against the upper arms, and passive flexion cannot be carried out beyond an obtuse angle.

The Head-Dropping Test. The patient lies supine without a pillow and should be completely relaxed, with eyes closed and attention diverted. The examiner places a hand under the patient's occiput, and the other hand briskly raises the head and then allows it to drop. Normally the head drops rapidly into the examiner's hand, but in patients with extrapyramidal rigidity there is delayed, slow, gentle dropping of the head owing to rigidity that principally affects the flexor muscles of the neck. When nuchal rigidity resulting from meningeal irritation is present there is resistance to and pain on flexion of the neck.

Pendulousness of the Legs. The patient sits on the edge of a table with his legs hanging freely. The examiner either extends both legs to the same horizontal level and then releases them or gives both legs a brisk push backward. If the patient is completely relaxed and does not voluntarily suppress or increase movement, there will normally be a swinging of the legs that progressively diminishes in range and usually disappears after six or seven oscillations. In extrapyramidal rigidity there is a decrease in swinging time, but usually no qualitative changes in the response. In spasticity there may be little or no decrease in time, but there is a qualitative change: the movements are jerky and irregular, the forward movement may be greater and more brisk than the backward one, and the movement may not be limited to the anteroposterior plane, but may assume a zigzag character. In hypotonia the response is increased in range and prolonged beyond the normal. In all the aforementioned the abnormality is more apparent if it is a unilateral one.

The Shoulder-Shaking Test. The examiner places his hands on the patient's shoulders and shakes them briskly in both a backward and forward and a rotatory direction. With extrapyramidal disease there will be a decreased range of arm swinging on the affected side. With hypotonia, especially that associated with cerebellar lesions, the range of swinging will be greater than normal.

The Arm-Dropping Test. The patient's arms are briskly raised and then dropped. With increase in tone there is a delay in the downward movement of the arm, while with hypotonicity the dropping is abrupt. A similar maneuver may be carried out, on the recumbent patient, by suddenly lifting and then dropping the extended leg.

Pronation of the Hands. In the presence of hypotonicity, especially that associated with cerebellar lesions or Sydenham's chorea, there is a tendency for the hands to assume a position of pronation; this is apparent when the arms are outstretched horizontally, but is exaggerated when they are raised above the head. On forward elevation of the arms there is a characteristic position of the hands, with flexion at the wrists, hyperextension of the proximal and terminal phalanges, and moderate overpronation. When the arms are elevated above the head there is increased pronation of the forearm, with internal rotation of the shoulders, and as a result the palms are turned outward. This phenomenon differs from the pronation signs of Strümpell and Babinski, in which the response is an abnormal associated movement caused by spasticity of the pronator muscles.

The Pronator Drift Test. With his eyes closed, the standing patient holds both arms outstretched in front of him. The elbows should be fully extended, the wrists extended, and the hands open with the palms up. In the presence of a mild hemiparesis, before significant weakness is apparent, there may be slow pronation of the wrist, slight flexion of the elbow and fingers, and a downward and lateral drift of the hand (Fig. 28-1). These have been said to be the result of a mild increase in tone that is not otherwise apparent. A similar pronation response may also appear with hypotonicity and may be seen with cerebellar lesions and in Sydenham's chorea.

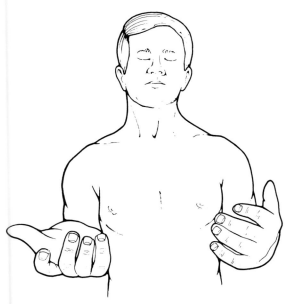

FIG. 28–1. Pronation sign in patient with left hemiparesis.

Myotatic Irritability, Myoedema, and Tenderness

Related to the inspection, palpation, and passive resistance used in the testing of tone is the observation of the so-called **idiomuscular contraction** or **myotatic irritability,** which follows percussion or other mechanical stimulation of muscle. In the normal and normally innervated muscle there is a brief and feeble contraction after it is tapped with a percussion hammer. In many muscles this response may be so slight that it cannot be seen or felt and is observed with difficulty. Myotatic irritability is increased in wasting diseases, such as cachexia and emaciation, and in many diseases of the lower motor neuron. It is increased, by both response to minimal stimuli and acceleration of contraction, in progressive spinal muscular atrophy. Mechanical stimulation may bring out fasciculations. In neuritis, the myotatic irritability may be increased, although the muscle stretch reflexes are diminished. In myositis the irritability may be either increased or decreased, and in the muscular dystrophies it is usually diminished. In myotonia there is a persisting contraction following mechanical stimulation of muscle, and there is hyperexcitability to such stimulation in tetanus and in tetany or certain electrolyte disturbances.

Occasionally, after a muscle is percussed with a reflex hammer, a wave of conduction radiates along the muscle fiber away from the point of percussion. A small ridge or temporary swelling is noted at the point of stimulation and this persists for several seconds. This is known as **myoedema.** It may represent a marked exaggeration of idiomuscular excitability but the basis for its development is poorly understood and swelling of the muscles and surrounding tissues suggest that more than idiomuscular excitability plays a part. The response differs from percussion myotonia or the usual myotatic irritability in which there is a depression rather than a raised area. Myoedema is seen in wasting diseases such as cachexia and emaciation, but if it is looked for, it is occasionally seen in normal individuals.

Muscle tenderness may also be elicited by palpation of the muscles. In the neuritides, especially, squeezing of the muscle masses or the tendons, or even very slight pressure upon them, may cause exquisite pain. Tenderness is also observed in acute poliomyelitis. It is of diagnostic significance in both, especially if accompanied by paresis, flaccidity, and loss of tendon reflexes. A decrease in tenderness, or rather a decrease in deep pain sensation, is noted in tabes dorsalis. An increase in tenderness and a loss of deep pain are sensory rather than motor manifestations, but one may appraise them during palpation of the muscles in the examination of muscle tone. Wide-spread muscle tenderness to palpation may also be noted with inflammatory disorders of the muscles, especially polymyositis and dermatomyositis, while focal muscle tenderness occurs with trauma or overexertion of muscles.

ABNORMALITIES OF TONE

Abnormalities of tone may occur in the presence of disease of any portion of the motor system. Lesions at the spinomuscular level, either in the anterior horn cell, the peripheral nerve, the myoneural junction, or the muscle itself, may affect tone. Involvement of the extrapyramidal complex, the corticospinal level, the vestibular or midbrain centers, or the psychomotor sphere may be followed by alterations in tone. In addition, tonus is influenced by interference with the proprioceptive impulses and their pathways of conduction.

Pathologic conditions may cause either a decrease or an increase in tone. Loss or diminution of tone is classified as **hypotonicity,** and pathologic increase, as **hypertonicity.** There are various subdivisions within these groups. Increased tone, in the form of spasm and contracture, may cause limitation of motion and thus simulate paresis.

Hypotonicity

Hypotonicity, or flaccidity, results from involvement of the spinomuscular level or interference with the proprioceptive pathways, but may also be present with cerebellar lesions and in the choreas. It is characterized by a decrease in or loss of normal tone. The muscle is flaccid and flabby, or soft to palpation. The involved joints offer little or no resistance to passive flexion or extension, even when such movement is carried out rapidly. The excursion at the joint may be normal, but is usually increased; there is absence of a "checking" action on extreme passive motion. The limb cannot steadily maintain positions into which it is brought either actively or passively. If the involved extremity is lifted and allowed to drop, it falls abruptly. A slight blow causes it to

sway through an excessive excursion. The muscle stretch reflexes are usually decreased or absent when hypotonia occurs from lesions at the spinomuscular level. It must be remembered that flaccid paralysis of muscles may be accompanied by spasm or contracture of their antagonists, which may be misleading to the inexperienced examiner. Abnormalities of joint motility, such as the Ehlers-Danlos syndrome, in which there is hyperelastic skin with extreme flexibility of joints, are not necessarily accompanied by a decrease in muscle tone.

If the anterior horn cell or its neuraxis is cut off from the muscle by disease or trauma, the continuous rhythmic impulses that maintain tonus are no longer present, and sustained contraction of the muscle is absent. Thus disease of the spinal and neural portions of the spinomuscular level cause hypotonicity, or flaccidity, of the muscles involved. Among such diseases are poliomyelitis, progressive spinal muscular atrophy, syringomyelia, peripheral neuritis, the Guillain-Barré syndrome, and chronic recurring neuropathies. In spinal shock, which follows abrupt transection of the spinal cord, the activity of the anterior horn cells and the spinal reflexes are temporarily suppressed below the level of the lesion, with resulting flaccidity.

Abnormalities of the muscle itself or of the myoneural junction — i.e., of the muscular and neuromuscular portions of the spinomuscular level — are also accompanied by a decrease in tone. Such is the case in the muscular dystrophies, the benign congenital myopathies, polymyositis, thyrotoxic and carcinomatous myopathy, steroid or other drug-related myopathy, myasthenia gravis, the myasthenic syndrome, and the various types of familial periodic paralysis. A similar decrease in tone may be found in association with metabolic or electrolyte disturbances, malnutrition, debilitating disease, or administration of drugs or poisoning by various toxins that affect the function of the myoneural junction. A large variety of conditions affecting the spinomuscular level may cause the "floppy infant" syndrome with generalized hypotonicity.

Tone is also decreased when the muscles are deprived of their proprioceptive impulses, either by spinal or by neural disease. Thus in tabes dorsalis, in which the proprioceptive pathways are interrupted either in the dorsal root ganglia or in the posterior columns, there is hypotonicity of the muscles with hyperextensibility of the joints. During local anesthesia (peripheral nerve block) and spinal anesthesia (anterior horn cell and nerve root involvement) as well as the deeper stages of general anesthesia (central involvement) there is hypotonicity; sensory as well as motor impulses are interrupted. The association of flaccidity with some lesions of the parietal lobe is probably secondary to disturbances of sensation.

Hypotonicity may occur under other circumstances. It is present with cerebellar disease of various types, but there is no flaccidity of the degree that one finds in disease of the lower motor neurons, and the reflexes are not lost although they may be of the pendular variety. There are no pathologic reflexes. Muscle tone is diminished in chorea, akinetic epilepsy, deep sleep, syncope, states of lowered consciousness, and directly after death. In cataplexy, usually associated with narcolepsy, there are attacks of weakness of the limbs and complete loss of tone, precipitated by emotional stimuli; with narcolepsy there may also be periods of paralysis that develop during relaxation or just before going to or awakening from sleep (**sleep paralysis**). Cataplexy may occur in association with rare midbrain tumors, causing sustained hypotonia. Immediately following a cerebrovascular lesion of abrupt onset there may be flaccid paralysis of the affected parts; this is sometimes referred to as **cerebral shock.** The presence of flaccidity with lesions of the motor cortex (area 4) and its descending pathways, seen in experimental animals and occasionally in clinical states in man, and its relationship to other aspects of motor function, is discussed in Chapter 23. Hypotonicity may also be induced by selective blocking of the γ-efferent fibers and by the administration of drugs that interrupt internuncial motor neuron discharges.

Hypertonicity

Hypertonicity is usually caused by lesions central to the anterior horn cells, or by interruption of impulses from supraspinal regions. It is seen most frequently with dysfunction of the so-called extrapyramidal and corticospinal levels, and is caused by either interruption of impulses that normally inhibit lower centers or imbalance of facilitatory and inhibitory centers, with consequent alteration of the α- and γ-motor neuron balance or lowering of the threshold of the spinal reflexes. It may also be caused by voluntary or unconscious contraction of muscles, reflex contraction, and muscle disease, and may be present with other disturbances of function. The

major types and causes of hypertonicity are discussed.

Extrapyramidal Rigidity. This form of rigidity occurs with lesions of the basal ganglia or of some other portion of the extrapyramidal level of motor function or its connections with the midbrain and brain stem reticular formations. The various pathophysiologic theories for this increase in tone are discussed in Chapter 22. With rigidity of this type there is a state of fairly steady muscular tension that is equal in degree in opposing muscle groups. Therefore, both flexor and extensor muscles in the extremities are involved, with resistance to passive movement in all directions. The actual degree of such resistance is often less than that found with spasticity, but it is present throughout the entire range of motion and is continuous from the beginning to the end of the movement. Furthermore, the resistance is constant whether the extremity is moved slowly or rapidly. There is a continuous increase in stimulation of both agonists and antagonists, and neither group is ever at complete rest. On palpation the muscles may be firm, tense, and prominent.

After being moved the part may retain its new position with the same resistance to movement that was noted in the original position (**plasticity; flexibilitas cerea** or **waxy flexibility**); the extremities may assume awkward postures. This type of hypertonicity is referred to as **lead-pipe resistance.** Often the so-called **cogwheel rigidity** is encountered; there is an intermittent yielding of the muscles to stretching and on passive motion against muscular tension the resistance is interrupted at regular intervals in a jerky fashion. The muscles seem to give way in a series of steps, as if the manipulator were moving a limb attached to a heavy cogwheel or pulling it over a ratchet. This latter phenomenon may be related in part to the tremor that often occurs with rigidity in extrapyramidal disease.

Rigidity of this type is most commonly encountered in Parkinson's disease and in other parkinsonian syndromes (see Fig. 22-4). It appears first in the proximal musculature, then spreads to the distal. All muscles may be affected, but there is predominant involvement of those of the neck and trunk, and the flexors of the extremities. There is associated slowing of the voluntary use of the limbs, in both flexion and extension, but no real paralysis. With repeated active movement there is a gradual decrease in speed and amplitude; this may be brought out by rapid opening and closing of the eyes or mouth, movements of the tongue, or finger-thumb approximation. In addition there is loss of associated movements. Whether the bradykinesia and loss of associated movements are secondary to the hypertonicity or are of central origin and unrelated to the rigidity is still controversial. The rigidity of extrapyramidal disease may be demonstrated by the head-dropping, shoulder-shaking, and similar tests, as well as by noting slowness of starting and limitation of amplitude of movement, loss of pendulousness of the arms and legs, inability to carry out rapid repeated movements and to maintain two simultaneous voluntary activities, and impairment of associated movements, such as swinging of the arms in walking. The rigidity on one side may be exaggerated by active movement of the contralateral limbs.

Similar rigidity may be encountered in various types of encephalopathy, including that due to anoxia, carbon monoxide intoxication, or poisoning by manganese or other toxins; may follow the administration of such drugs as reserpine, phenothiazines and other psychotropic substances; and may be seen in other extrapyramidal syndromes, such as dystonia and athetosis, and in spasmodic torticollis. In some of the corticospinal and extrapyramidal disorders the **gegenhalten phenomenon** is present. This is the stiffening of the limb in response to contact and a resistance to passive changes in position and posture; the strength of the antagonists increases as the examiner uses increasing force to change the position of a limb.

The rigid type of hypertonicity may be relieved, to some extent at least, by injection of local anesthetics into the involved muscles, selective blocking of the γ-efferent fibers, intracarotid injection of barbiturate, or the various surgical procedures discussed in Chapter 22. None of these, however, brings about lasting improvement in rigidity. Pharmacotherapeutic agents (levodopa, dopamine agonists, and related substances) are now used for the relief of rigidity in Parkinson's disease and similar conditions.

Spasticity. This occurs in association with lesions of the so-called pyramidal or corticospinal level of function, and has been ascribed to the loss of, or release from, the normal inhibiting action of the cortex on the anterior horn cells (Ch. 23). Experimentally, however, lesions limited to the pyramidal complex may produce flaccidity, and theories of spasticity indicate that it may result from an imbalance of the inhibitory and facilitatory centers in the midbrain and brain stem reticular formations, with a consequent imbalance of the α- and γ-motor neurons. A lowering of the reflex threshold is a regular feature of spasticity. Spasticity may result from 1) disorders affecting suppressor areas in the cortex or elsewhere, 2) interruption of suppressor impulses to the inhibitory reticular area in the lower brain stem, or 3) enhancement or stimulation of the facilitatory or excitatory reticular areas in the midbrain and brain stem. This leads to facilitatory influx to the spinal cord, conducted by reticulospinal, vestibulospinal, and other pathways, and consequent alteration of the balance between the α- and γ-motor systems. Impairment of the central inhibitory influences that normally reduce spinal stretch reflexes is followed by an exaggerated contraction of muscles that are subjected to stretching, and by an increased resistance to manipulation. For descriptive purposes, however, the term pyramidal or corticospinal will be used for those lesions of the cerebrum and descending pathways that cause spasticity.

Spasticity is a state of sustained increase in tension of a muscle when it is passively lengthened. This tension is caused by an exaggeration of the muscle stretch reflex; there is increased sensitivity to stimulation of proprioceptive receptors within the muscles, and such stimulation causes the shortening reaction to be intensified and the muscular tension to be augmented. This tension may be felt from the beginning of a passive movement and may increase to the extent to which the muscle is lengthened. Passive movement of the extremity may be carried out with comparative freedom if it is done slowly, but attempts at rapid or forceful movement cause tension to appear; there is "blocking," with complete limitation of further movement. Passive movement may also be carried out with little resistance through a limited range of motion, but extremes of movement, such as complete flexion or extension, likewise result in blocking and limitation to further movement. If the limb is left in the new position, it may be maintained there. There may be an elastic, springlike resistance to stretching at the beginning of movement, especially if the part is moved abruptly or suddenly, following which the muscle resists to a certain point and then suddenly relaxes — the phenomenon sometimes referred to as the **clasp-knife** type of resistance. This waxing and waning of resistance distinguishes spasticity from rigidity.

Occasionally spasticity is so marked that the examiner cannot passively move an extremity, although the patient himself may retain a certain amount of ability to move it. Spastic muscles may be hard and unyielding on palpation, but sometimes they are soft and flabby. Usually they feel normal. The degree of firmness depends not so much on the actual amount of spasticity as on the degree of contraction or relaxation at the time of palpation. Completely relaxed spastic muscles show no electrical activity, but minimal stimulation causes an immediate response. No objective means have been devised for the accurate measuring of spasticity, and clinical evaluation is the most reliable criterion. It must be remembered, however, that the range of movement of spastic extremities and the degree of hypertonicity often varies between examinations and with repeated testing.

In the presence of spasticity the muscle stretch reflexes are exaggerated and pathologic reflexes such as the Babinski and Chaddock signs can be elicited. Passive dorsiflexion of the ankle, downward movement of the patella, and occasionally even passive extension of the wrist may cause alternate contraction and relaxation of the agonists and antagonists — the phenomenon called **clonus** (Ch. 35). Forced grasping and tonic perseveration of motion may be evident, and there often are abnormal associated movements. Muscle power is difficult to assess in the presence of severe spasticity.

Diseases that cause paralysis are often characterized by sustained contraction of specific groups of muscles. With hemiparesis or hemiplegia of cerebral origin, for instance, the spasticity is most marked in the flexor muscles of the upper and the extensor muscles of the lower extremity; this causes postural flexion of the arm and extension of the leg, the characteristic distribution in cerebral hemiplegia (see Fig. 23-8). The arm is adducted and flexed at the shoulder, the forearm is flexed at the elbow, and the wrist and fingers are flexed; there may be forced grasping. The lower extremity is extended at the hip, knee, and ankle, and there is inversion with plantar flexion of the foot; there may be marked spasm of the adductors of the thigh. There is more passive resistance to extension than to flexion in the upper extremities, and to flexion than to extension in the lower extremities. With bilateral cerebral lesions the increased tone of the adductors of the thighs is responsible for the **scissors gait** in which one leg is pulled toward the other as each step is taken. In relatively complete spinal cord lesions there may be, rather than extension, violent flexor spasms of the lower extremities, reflexes of spinal automatism, and paraplegia in

flexion. Spasticity is sometimes relieved by selective anterior rhizotomy, peripheral nerve or posterior root section, injection of either alcohol or phenol into the subarachnoid space, or even by section or removal of part or all of the malfunctioning area of the spinal cord (cordectomy or myelotomy). Neuromuscular blocking agents such as curare, decamethonium, and succinylcholine, and internuncial blocking agents and "muscle relaxants" have also proved to be of partial, often temporary therapeutic value.

Catatonic Rigidity. This form is similar in many respects to extrapyramidal rigidity and probably is physiologically related. There is a waxy or lead-pipe type of resistance to passive movement, a cerea flexibilitas, but the posturing, bizarre mannerisms, and mental picture of the schizophrenic state are also seen. It may be possible to mold the extremities into any position, following which they remain in this position indefinitely. Experimental catatonia has been produced in animals by the use of bulbocapnine, epinephrine, and other drugs, and by the production of chemical, metabolic, and other changes.

Decerebrate and Decorticate Rigidity. Decerebrate rigidity is characterized by marked rigidity and sustained contraction of all the extensor (antigravity) muscles, whereas in decorticate rigidity there is flexion of the elbows and wrists with extension of the legs and feet. These are discussed in Chapter 37, "Postural and Righting Reflexes." A similar generalized rigidity or spasticity with neck retraction, or **opisthotonos,** may also occur in meningitis or meningeal irritation, the tonic stage of a convulsive attack, and so-called cerebellar or posterior fossa fits. In all these the hypertonicity and associated symptoms doubtless result from brain stem involvement.

Voluntary Rigidity. This is characterized by a conscious bracing of various muscle groups. This may be done to protect the body against injury, in response to pain, and to perform certain voluntary muscular activities. There is an individual variation in the degree of voluntary rigidity that a patient may present, and it is often difficult to differentiate between factors that are truly volitional and those that are unconscious or involuntary, especially if the hypertonicity is related to excitement, alarm, or fatigue. Tense, apprehensive individuals show increased muscular tension and rigidity at all times, and such persons may have exaggerated muscle stretch reflexes. The exaggeration, however, is one of range of response, and the latent period is not shortened. Heavily muscled individuals often relax less well than others, and in such persons the muscle stretch reflexes may appear to be diminished and be elicited only on reinforcement. The sudden bracing of muscles in response to shock or in checking a fall has as its basis both volitional and unconscious factors.

Involuntary Rigidity. This may be similar to the voluntary variety and difficult to differentiate from it. The unconsciously motivated muscle tension of the apprehensive person who shows exaggerated muscle stretch reflexes may be wide in distribution and long in duration. It may be precipitated by excitement, alarm, or fatigue. On the other hand, an increase in tone of psychogenic origin may be bizarre and may simulate any type of hypertonicity. In so-called major hysteria there may be an extreme degree of generalized rigidity with neck retraction and opisthotonos, the body resting with only the head and heels upon the bed (*arc de cercle*); the manifestation may simulate either decerebrate or catatonic rigidity, and is termed hysterical rigidity.

Reflex Rigidity. Reflex rigidity, or spasm of skeletal muscle, is a response to sensory irritation, usually to pain. It is a state of sustained involuntary contraction accompanied by muscle shortening. By observation, raised, contracted muscles can be noted; on palpation they are firm and resistant. Among the more common examples of reflex spasm of muscles in response to pain are the boardlike abdomen of acute abdominal disorders, rigidity of the neck and back in meningitis, and the localized spasm in the extremities following trauma. The muscle spasm of arthritis may be of similar origin, as may the spasm that is seen in some patients with myositis and the contractures seen in peripheral vascular lesions, such as Volkmann's ischemic contractures. Reflex rigidity may result from sensory stimuli other than pain. Cold, for instance, may call forth generalized hypertonicity. Muscle contracture may follow prolonged spasm. In McArdle's disease muscle spasms, painful cramps, and weakness are brought on by exercise and repeated voluntary contractions; these phenomena are hastened and augmented by ischemia. Similar spasms and cramps occur in paroxysmal myoglobinuria, where they are followed by paresis or even complete paralysis;

during the attacks the affected muscles are edematous, tense, and tender.

Myotonia. In both the congenital and acquired types of myotonia, in myotonic dystrophy (a chromosome 19 disorder), in paramyotonia, and occasionally in myxedema, there is an increase in muscle tone and contraction that is evident on active rather than passive movement; tone is usually normal when the muscles are relaxed. In paramyotonia, and to a lesser degree in the other conditions, a severely increased muscle tone is precipitated by cold. There is tonic perseveration of muscular contraction, and relaxation takes place slowly. Myotonia may be demonstrated in the hand-grip test, in which there is slow relaxation of the hand muscles after a strong grip. Sudden movements may be followed by marked spasm and inability to relax; repetition of movement, however, often brings about ease of relaxation and a gradual decrease of hypertonicity. Electrical stimulation of muscle causes an exaggerated contraction that relaxes slowly (**myotonic reaction**). **Percussion myotonia** may be elicited by mechanical stimulation; abrupt tapping of the thenar eminence with the reflex hammer is followed by opposition of the thumb that persists for several seconds before relaxation begins, and tapping of the tongue, deltoid region, or other muscular masses produces a depression or "dimple" that disappears slowly. The muscles may appear hypertrophic; the muscle stretch reflexes are normal. Strength is usually normal rather than increased but it is decreased in myotonic dystrophy. Myotonia is probably peripheral in origin, and various causes have been hypothesized. Quinine, procaine amide, and phenytoin have been reported to be of some value in reducing the duration of myotonia, although they have no effect on muscle weakness in those myotonic disorders associated with dystrophic changes.

Other Types of Rigidity. Muscular rigidity may also be seen in epilepsy, tetany, and tetanus. In epilepsy there may be generalized rigidity during the tonic phase of the fit. Occasionally there are "tonic fits" with no clonic phase. This type of hypertonicity is of central origin; it may result from temporary interruption of the corticospinal or extrapyramidal pathways or from imbalance of inhibitory and facilitatory centers, or it may be related to decerebrate rigidity.

In tetany there are tonic muscular spasms and also hyperirritability of the muscular and nervous systems to mechanical and electrical stimuli, leading to localized or generalized hypertonicity. The manifestations may be intermittent or continuous; they involve the distal limb segments predominantly, and are usually bilateral. The spasm may be preceded by feelings of stiffness and pain. In the attacks the fingers are closely approximated and are flexed at the metacarpophalangeal joints and extended at the interphalangeal joints; the thumb is extended and adducted; there is flexion at the wrist with flexion and pronation at the elbows. There is plantar flexion of the toes; the sole of the foot is concave, and the ankle is inverted and may be in plantar flexion or dorsiflexion. The term **carpopedal spasm** is used to include both the wrist and ankle flexion — the so-called obstetrical hand and the talipes equinovarus deformity. The muscles of the body, head, and face may be involved, and opisthotonos may result. During the attacks the muscles are rigid and painful. Tapping or mechanical irritation (Chvostek's sign) and electrical stimulation (Erb's sign) show the muscles to be overexcitable, and such stimulation reproduces the spasm, as does pressure over the nerves or arteries (Trousseau's sign). The hypertonicity is probably largely of muscular origin. It is related to disturbances of calcium and phosphorus metabolism and to abnormalities in the acid-base equilibrium of the body, as well as to other metabolic derangements.

In tetanus there is an increase in muscle tone with consequent generalized bodily rigidity. In most instances this first involves the face and jaw muscles, but may affect the abdominal muscles, extremities, and spinal muscles as well, with resulting abdominal rigidity, extensor rigidity, and opisthotonos. Both the prime movers and the antagonists may be hypertonic. Spasm of the muscles of mastication causes trismus, and retraction of the angles of the mouth brings about the so-called risus sardonicus. Muscle spasm may occur spontaneously; voluntary contraction or mechanical, tactile, auditory, visual, or other stimuli may precipitate paroxysms of muscle contraction that increase in intensity and spread to other muscles. Between seizures there is usually some persisting muscular rigidity. The muscle stretch reflexes are grossly exaggerated and a light tap upon a tendon may throw the limb into violent spasms. The toxin of *clostridium tetani* has been determined to be a powerful blocker of acetylcholine release at the presynaptic level.

In the stiff-man syndrome there are painful tonic muscular spasms and progressive rigidity of the muscles of the trunk, neck, abdomen, back, and proximal parts of the extremities. On electromyography there is a constant discharge of normal motor unit potentials simulating what is seen with prolonged volitional contraction of muscles. Pathologically there are nonspecific muscle fiber alterations. The etiology of this syndrome is not known. In a majority of cases the spasms are controlled by the use of diazepam.

A related condition is neuromyotonia, or **Isaac's syndrome.** Some authorities feel that stiff-man syndrome and neuromyotonia overlap. In the latter, however, there is, in addition to stiffness, a constant myokymia that is widespread. Neuromyotonia is at times relieved with phenytoin.

Rigidity, usually generalized, is a feature of the syndrome of malignant hyperthermia, precipitated at times during general anesthesia, and often related to the use of psychotropic medications. The rigidity of malignant hyperthermia responds to the muscle relaxant, dantrolene.

Focal muscle spasms, cramps, and dystonia will be discussed with abnormal movements (Ch. 31).

BIBLIOGRAPHY

Adams RD, Victor M. Principles of Neurology, 4th ed. New York, McGraw – Hill, 1989

Alter M. The digiti quinti sign in mild hemiparesis. Neurology 1973;23:503

Brennan JB. Clinical method of assessing tonus and voluntary movement in hemiplegia. Br Med J 1959;1:767

Brumlik J, Boshes B. Quantitation of muscle tone in normals and in parkinsonism. Arch Neurol 1961;4:399

Gordon EE, Janusko DM, Kaufman LA. Critical survey of the stiff-man syndrome. Am J Med 1967;42:582

Huang CC, Chu NS, Lu CS et al. Chronic manganese intoxication. Arch Neurol 1989;46:1104

Lance JW. The control of muscle tone, reflexes, and movement: Robert Wartenberg Lecture. Neurology 1980; 30:1303

Landau WM. The essential mechanism in myotonia: An electromyographic study. Neurology 1952;2:369

Landau WM. Spasticity and rigidity. In Plum F (ed). Recent Advances in Neurology. Philadelphia, FA Davis, 1969

Landau WM. Spasticity: The fable of a neurological demon and the Emperor's new therapy. Arch Neurol 1974; 31:217

Landau WM, Weaver RA, Hornbein TF. Fusiform nerve function in man. Arch Neurol 1960;3:10

Lorish TR, Thorsteinsson G, Howard FM. Stiff-man syndrome updated. Mayo Clin Proc 1989;64:629

Olafson RA, Mulder DW, Howard FM. "Stiff-man" syndrome. Mayo Clin Proc 1964;39:131

Powers RK, Marder – Meyer J, Rymer WZ. Quantitative relations between hypertonia and stretch reflex threshold in spastic hemiparesis. Ann Neurol 1988;23:115

Rademaker GGJ. On the lengthening and shortening reactions and their occurrence in man. Brain 1947;70:109

Rushworth G. Spasticity and rigidity: an experimental study and review. J Neurol Neurosurg Psychiatry 1960;23:99

Sherrington CS. Postural activity of muscle and nerve. Brain 1915;38:191

Stahl SM, Layzer RB, Aminoff MJ, Townsend JJ et al. Continuous cataplexy in a patient with a midbrain tumor: The limp man syndrome. Neurology 1980;30:1115

Swaiman KF. Pediatric Neurology. Principles and Practice. St. Louis, CV Mosby, 1989

Thompson PD, Berardelli A, Rothwell JC et al. The coexistence of bradykinesia and chorea in Huntington's disease and its implications for theories of basal ganglia control of movements. Brain 1988;111:223

Wartenberg R. Some useful neurological tests. JAMA 1951;147:1645

Yamaoka LH, Pericac – Vance MA, Speer MC et al. Tight linkage of creatine kinase (CKMM) to myotonic dystrophy on chromosome 19. Neurology 1990;40:222

Chapter 29
MUSCLE VOLUME AND CONTOUR

The volume and contour of the individual muscles and the muscle groups give information about the presence of either atrophy or hypertrophy. There is normally an appreciable individual variation in muscular development, but noteworthy changes in the size and shape of the muscle masses, especially if such changes are circumscribed or asymmetric, may be significant in the examination of the motor system, and on occasion are among the earliest signs of motor dysfunction.

Muscle atrophy, or **amyotrophy,** may be defined as the wasting or diminution in size of a part. Atrophy of muscles consists of a decrease in their volume or bulk, and is usually accompanied by changes in shape or contour. In the neurologic examination one is specifically concerned with wasting of muscles secondary to disorders affecting the anterior horn cell, the nerve root(s), the peripheral nerve, or the muscle itself. Atrophy, however, may also result from resection of muscle tendon, deficient blood supply to the muscle, inadequate nutrition, endocrine changes, toxic and infectious factors, and aging.

Muscle hypertrophy is an increase in the bulk, or volume, of muscle tissues. It may be the result of excessive use of the muscles, or it may occur on a pathologic basis. In myotonia congenita there may be what appears to be hypertrophy without significant increase in strength. In the muscular dystrophies there may be pseudohypertrophy due to infiltration of the muscles with fat and connective tissue.

EXAMINATION OF MUSCLE VOLUME AND CONTOUR

Muscle volume and contour are examined and atrophy or hypertrophy appraised by inspection, palpation, and measurement.

By means of inspection the general muscular development of the size of the individual muscles and muscle groups are noted, and special attention is paid to abnormalities in volume and contour and to evidence of atrophy and hypertrophy. Symmetric parts of the two sides of the body should be compared, and the muscular landmarks carefully scrutinized. Any flattening, hollowing, or bulging of the muscle masses should be evaluated. The muscles of the face, shoulder, and pelvic girdles, and distal parts of the extremities — especially the palmar surfaces of the hands, the thenar and hypothenar eminences, and the interosseous muscles — should be examined specifically. One should also at this time make note of congenital absence of or defects in skeletal muscles.

The muscle masses should also be carefully palpated, and their volume, contour, and consistency noted. Normal muscles are semielastic and regain their shape at once when compressed. When myotonia or hypertrophy is present, the muscles are firm and hard; in pseudohypertrophy they appear enlarged but may feel doughy or rubbery on palpation; atrophic or degenerated muscles are soft and pulpy in consistency. Palpation is not a final criterion, however, for degenerated muscles that have undergone fibrous changes may be hard and firm, whereas those that have been overgrown with or replaced by fat may be doughy and rubbery.

To determine the degree of atrophy or hypertrophy, measurements may be essential. A pronounced increase or decrease in the size of muscles may be recognized at first glance, especially when confined to one side of the body, one extremity, or one segment of a limb. If the differences are slight, however, it may be difficult to come to any conclusion from comparison of the corresponding muscles and muscle groups on the two sides of the body by inspection alone, and measurements are necessary. A tape measure, calipers, or an oncometer may be used. The size of the individual muscles and the circumference and size of the extremities are measured and compared. Measurements should all be made from fixed points or landmarks, and the sites — such as the distance above or below the olecranon, anterior superior iliac spine, or patella — should be recorded. The extremities should be in identical positions and in equal states of relaxation or contraction, and similar parts of the body should be examined on the two sides. It is often valuable, also, to measure the length of the limbs.

If either atrophy or hypertrophy is present, the distribution should be noted. The changes may be limited to an individual muscle, to all the muscles supplied by a specific nerve, to those supplied by certain segments of the spinal cord, or to one half of the body, or they may be multifocal, generalized, or diffuse. It must be remembered, however, that there is a great deal of individual variation in muscular development, in part constitutional and in part due to training, activity, and occupation. Certain individuals have small or poorly developed muscles, whereas others show outstanding muscular development. Individuals who do sedentary work, elderly persons, and those with chronic disease may have small muscles without evidence of wasting or atrophy. Athletes may develop physiologic hypertrophic muscles. It is also important to remember that in normal individuals there is some difference in the size of the muscle masses and even of the hands and feet on the two sides of the body. In a right-handed person the right side frequently shows better development.

The appraisal of bulk and contour should be correlated with the other parts of the motor examination, especially with the evaluations of strength and tone. In the atrophies associated with arthritis and disuse there may be a pronounced decrease in volume with little change in strength. In the myopathies, on the other hand, there may be little apparent atrophy in spite of a striking loss of power.

If muscular changes in the form of atrophy or hypertrophy are present, and if there is any question regarding etiology, a muscle biopsy should be considered. This procedure is performed under local anesthesia. The examiner should be certain that the muscle tissue that is removed is obtained from the involved area. However, it is best to obtain the muscle specimen from a moderately involved area; that is, neither from a part of the muscle that has become totally fibrosed, nor from a normally strong portion of muscle. The tissue is examined for microscopic evidence of pathologic change. The size of the individual muscle fibers, the presence or absence of striations, the character of the sarcoplasm, and the appearance and location of the nuclei should be noted; the replacement of muscle tissue by connective or fatty tissue, vascular changes, phagocytic or lymphocytic infiltration, and other pathologic alterations should be determined. The character of the nerve fibers and motor end-plate may also be observed. Special histochemical staining technics are often indicated. The biopsy examination of muscle is valuable in diseases such as myositis, myopathy, trichinosis, other inflammatory conditions, congenital muscle disorders, and at times the dystrophies and other muscle diseases. Examination of the skin and subcutaneous tissues may also give essential information, especially in such conditions as polyarteritis nodosa and dermatomyositis.

Electromyography of the affected muscles usually aids in the differential diagnosis of muscular atrophy. It differentiates between neurogenic and myogenic atrophy, gives objective information on the exact distribution of muscle involvement, helps to decide at which level the lower motor neuron and its peripheral axons are diseased, and aids in the diagnosis of specific disease of muscle and of the myoneural junction.

ABNORMALITIES OF VOLUME AND CONTOUR

Muscular Atrophy

Muscular atrophy may be caused by many processes. The most important varieties are those of neurogenic origin. These must, however, be differentiated from those that are secondary to other etiologic factors. The various types of atrophy are discussed individually.

Neurogenic Atrophy

Under normal circumstances each muscle is being bombarded constantly by a rhythmic volley of motor impulses from the anterior horn cells (Ch. 21). These stimuli are responsible for the trophic state of the muscle. As long as the motor nuclei, their neuraxes, the myoneural junction, and the muscle fibers are in a state of health, the nutrition and tonus of the muscle are maintained. When these impulses no longer reach the muscle, owing to disease of the anterior horn cells or of their neuraxes, certain changes take place. The muscle lies inert and flaccid, and no longer contracts voluntarily or reflexly. There is an alteration in the electrical excitability and in the chemical irritability. All the affected fibers lose weight and decrease in size, and as a result there is wasting or atrophy of the entire muscle mass. Associated with the loss of substance there may be an increase in connective tissue. There may be fibrotic changes, and the atrophied muscle may be infiltrated with fat. This is **neurogenic atrophy.** The more abrupt or extreme the interruption of nerve supply, the more rapid is the wasting. The atrophy may either precede or follow other evidence of muscular dysfunction, such as paralysis and flaccidity. In rapidly progressing diseases the paralysis and flaccidity precede the atrophy, whereas in degenerative and slowly progressive diseases the atrophy precedes the paralysis and flaccidity. If the pathologic process is confined to the anterior horn cells or the spinal cord, the atrophy is segmental in distribution, whereas involvement of the peripheral nerves is followed by wasting of those muscles supplied by the involved nerves or their roots.

Poliomyelitis is characterized by sudden onset and rapid destruction of the anterior horn cells. Atrophy may develop within a short period of time, but it does not appear until after the paralysis. It is segmental in distribution, depending upon the location of the pathologic process within the spinal cord, and the degree of paralysis and atrophy parallels the severity of the disease. Microscopically there is widespread reduction in the size of the paralyzed fibers, but there seldom is any increase in fibrous tissue in relation to the atrophy, and when fibrosis is prominent it is probably related to either contracture or overstretching.

Progressive bulbar palsy, progressive spinal muscular atrophy, and **amyotrophic lateral sclerosis** are wasting diseases in which there is a slow but widespread degeneration of the motor nuclei and the anterior horn cells, causing a progressive muscular atrophy that may appear before paralysis is evident (Fig. 21-3). In these the distribution of the atrophy has been referred to as segmental, but in general the changes are rather diffuse and begin in particular groups of muscles. In progressive bulbar palsy the atrophy is first noted in the muscles supplied by the twelfth, tenth, and seventh cranial nerves; in progressive spinal muscular atrophy of the Aran – Duchenne type it is first seen in the distal musculature — the thenar, hypothenar, and interosseous muscles of the hand, and the small muscles of the foot — and then spreads up the limbs to the proximal parts; in infantile progressive spinal muscular atrophy (Werdnig – Hoffmann paralysis) the atrophy first involves the trunk, pelvic, and shoulder muscles and then spreads toward the periphery. An outstanding manifestation of these syndromes is the presence of fasciculations in the involved muscles (Ch. 31). Microscopically there is much variation in the size of muscle fibers, with groups of atrophic fibers scattered among normal ones, demonstrating differential atrophy of multiple motor units. In the heredofamilial muscular atrophy described by Wohlfart, Kugelberg, and Welander, principally the proximal muscles are affected; because of this distribution and also because of the slow progression of this disorder, it may be mistaken for muscular dystrophy.

Segmental atrophy may also follow focal spinal cord lesions involving the anterior horn cells. The rapidity of the progress depends upon the type of pathologic change. In syringomyelia, where there is a slow degeneration, fasciculations may be seen in the involved muscles.

With isolated lesions of the peripheral nerve roots there is atrophy consequent to interruption of the innervation of muscle. The atrophy follows the paralysis, but with traumatic nerve lesions it may develop within a short period of time. It is limited to the muscle(s) supplied by the involved nerve or nerve root(s). The characteristic distribution of paralysis and wasting seen in some of the more frequently encountered isolated neuritides may be found in Chapter 43. Within one month after denervation there may be a 30% loss of weight in the affected muscle, and a 50% loss within two months; thereafter the atrophy progresses more slowly and replacement by connective tissue and infiltration by fat follows.

In polyneuritis and Guillain – Barré syndrome the atrophy may be more widespread. In polyneuritis the motor changes may vary from slight weakness and wasting to widespread paralysis and atrophy; they are usually greatest in the distal portions of the extremities. The distal atrophy seen in the peroneal or neural type of Charcot – Marie – Tooth disease resembles that of a severe chronic polyneuritis (see Fig. 21-4).

Interruption of the sensory nerve fibers alone does not lead to muscular atrophy, although it is possible that some trophic impulses pass to the anterior horn cells by way of the posterior roots, and atrophy may occasionally appear, after some period of time, with destruction of the posterior roots; this is seen in conditions such as tabes dorsalis. It is probable, however, that either interference with autonomic impulses or disuse may be the actual cause of such atrophy. In addition to motor and sensory neurons, however, there are trophic neurons, of autonomic origin, which have to do with the nutrition and metabolism of muscle and other tissues. In diseases of the lower motor neuron one may find, in addition to muscular atrophy, other trophic changes in the skin and subcutaneous tissues; edema, cyanosis or pallor, coldness, sweating, changes in the hair and nails, alterations in the texture of the skin, osteoporosis, and even ulcerations and decubiti. Interruption of autonomic fibers may be a factor in muscle atrophy, owing to "trophic dysfunction" as well as to loss of vasomotor control. The changes in the skin, nails, hair, and subcutaneous tissues are the result of interruption of the autonomic pathways, vasomotor paralysis, and destruction of the vasoconstrictor fibers. Interruption of the sensory fibers with loss of pain sensation may predispose to ulcerations following trauma and burns. The complete syndrome of peripheral nerve dysfunction, with paralysis and atrophy, sensory impairment, areflexia, and changes in the skin and other tissues is the result of interruption of motor, sensory, and autonomic fibers. There may be extensive trophic changes with ulcerations at the site of anesthetic areas, decubiti, bone changes, and arthropathies.

Lesions of the upper motor neurons are usually not followed by atrophy of the paralyzed muscles, although if such lesions are of long duration, dating from birth or early childhood, there may be a failure of development of the muscles (and other structures, such as bones) in the involved portions of the body that may simulate atrophy. If the onset occurs later in life,

there may be some generalized loss of muscle volume and secondary wasting because of disuse. It is never severe and muscles retain their electrical irritability. Experimentally, however, lesions of the motor cortex (area 4) and the descending corticospinal pathways may be followed by muscular atrophy, and on occasion severe wasting appears with cerebral hemiplegias. The atrophy progresses rapidly if it appears early, and slowly if it appears late. Usually in these cases there are associated trophic and sensory changes, and the wasting may in part be secondary to involvement of the postcentral gyrus or parietal lobe, lesions of which are known to be followed by atrophy of the contralateral portions of the body. The loss of muscle bulk associated with involvement of these latter structures may appear promptly, and the degree of atrophy depends upon the size and character of the lesion and the extent of the hypotonia and sensory change. The distribution is determined by the localization of the process within the parietal lobe. It is most severe if the motor cortex or pathways are involved along with the sensory areas of the brain.

Congenital hemiatrophy, which may involve one side of the face, or the face and the corresponding half of the body, is characterized by underdevelopment, together with progressive atrophy, involving not only the muscles but also the skin, hair, subcutaneous tissues, connective tissue, cartilage, and bone. It may be the result of autonomic nervous system involvement and/or pathologic changes in the cerebrum. There may be underdevelopment of one half of the body secondary to either lack of development or atrophy of the opposite cerebral hemisphere.

Other Varieties of Muscular Atrophy

Myogenic, or **myopathic, atrophy** is that which arises as a result of disease within the muscles themselves and is secondary to specific muscular dysfunction. Atrophy of muscular origin may develop in the myopathies and in the various types of myositis.

Wasting of muscle tissue is an important manifestation of the dystrophies. In these conditions atrophy, flaccidity, and weakness may appear simultaneously. The involvement is predominantly of the proximal rather than the distal musculature; the shoulder and hip girdles are principally affected (see Fig. 21-5). In the pseudohypertrophic type of Duchenne, which usually has its onset in childhood, the pelvic muscles, followed by the shoulder muscles, become weak and atrophic. As the disease progresses there is increasing wasting of all muscles of the shoulders, upper arms, pelvis, thighs, and chest (Fig. 29-1). The calf muscles may appear very large; during the early stages of dystrophy they may feel firm and hard and remain strong. In some patients, however, there may be either a soft doughy, or elastic and rubbery feeling on palpation — the so-called pseudohypertrophy.

The limb-girdle variety, including the scapulo-humeral dystrophy, affects primarily the shoulders and upper arms (Fig. 29-2); occasionally there is pseudohypertrophy of the deltoid and other shoulder muscles. In the Landouzy–Dejerine facioscapulohumeral type the atrophy predominates in the muscles of the face, shoulder girdles, and arms. Distal myopathy, affecting the muscles of the hands and feet, is occasionally seen. Other related conditions include be-

nign congenital hypotonia, and other congenital nonprogressive or slowly progressive myopathies. In myotonic dystrophy the atrophy may be generalized, but is most marked in the facial and sternocleidomastoid muscles. Microscopic examination in the dystrophies reveals marked variation in the size of individual muscle fibers, some being large and others atrophic. Vacuolization and degeneration of the muscle, and infiltration of connective tissue and fat between the muscle fibers, may be seen.

In **myositis,** or **polymyositis,** there is muscular weakness and flaccidity, often symmetric and usually proximal, along with pain, tenderness, and atrophy. The muscles may be flaccid. Microscopically there is a patchy or diffuse inflammatory reaction with cellular infiltrations, proliferation of sarcolemmal nuclei, and degeneration of muscle fibers. Myositis seems to be related to

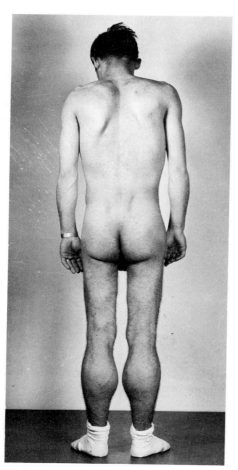

FIG. 29–1. A patient with Duchenne muscular dystrophy, showing pseudohypertrophy of the calf muscles.

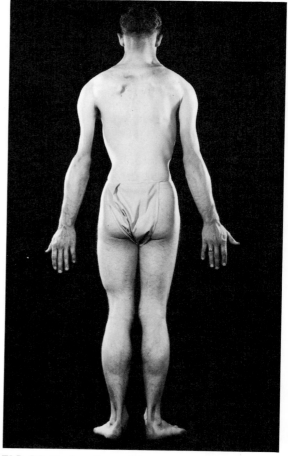

FIG. 29–2. A patient with scapulohumeral muscular dystrophy, showing atrophy of the muscles of the shoulders and upper arms.

dermatomyositis, polyarteritis nodosa, and disseminated lupus erythematosus, as a part of a generalized collagen disturbance. Specific varieties of myositis, such as those associated with carcinoma or with trichinosis and cysticercosis, may also be encountered.

Atrophy of disuse follows prolonged immobilization of a part of the body. It must be differentiated from neurogenic atrophy. Wasting of this type is characterized by shrinkage of the muscle fibers and reduction in the amount of sarcoplasm, but there is no loss of striations, no degeneration of the individual fibers, no changes in the electrical responses of the muscles, and no degeneration of the nerves or their endings. The loss of volume may develop almost as rapidly as that which follows absence of stimulation from anterior horn cells. It is brought about by immobilization and the consequent inability of the muscle to respond to stimuli.

Atrophy of disuse may occur in an extremity that has been in a splint or cast, one that cannot be moved because of joint involvement such as arthritis or periarthritis, or one that is paretic following a cerebral lesion. It also develops in tenotomized muscles, in the skeletal muscles of an individual who has been bedfast for any period of time, and in extremities that are not used owing to hysterical paralysis. In this condition vasomotor and trophic changes are occasionally seen, contractures may develop, and it may be difficult to differentiate between an organic and a psychogenic lesion.

Arthrogenic atrophy may appear in association with joint disease. In rheumatoid arthritis (atrophic arthritis, or *arthritis deformans*) the predominant muscular atrophy is in the region of the involved joints; it is usually most marked in the extensor muscles, and in those proximal to the affected joints. It is more severe and develops more rapidly in acute arthritis. Atrophy of this type may in part be the result of inactivity or disuse, but other suggested causative factors include some reflex influence from the diseased tissues upon the anterior horn cells, possibly secondary to pain and infiltration; muscle spasms; metabolic changes; and involvement of the smaller branches of the motor nerves or of the autonomic nervous system innervation of the atrophic areas.

Nutritional atrophy may occur in a variety of circumstances. A normal blood supply is essential to the nutrition and oxygenation of muscles. Interruption of the blood supply may lead to muscle atrophy as well as to alterations in the skin and other trophic changes. If the atrophy is caused by the interruption of the continuity of a single artery, the changes are found in the distribution of the occluded vessel. In **Volkmann's ischemic contracture** there is atrophy due to loss of nutrition and oxygenation of a group of muscles; this is usually accompanied by trophic changes in the skin and subcutaneous tissues. Atrophy on a nutritional basis may also occur with cachexia and weight loss. The muscle change is usually generalized. Possibly some vitamin deficiency is the most important factor, although deprivation of oxygen, changes in lactic acid content, disturbances of phosphorus and potassium metabolism, etc., are also significant.

Endocrine dysfunction of various types may lead to atrophy and other changes in muscle. In thyrotoxic myopathy there may be weakness, fatigability, and muscular atrophy that may be either localized or diffuse, but the hip and shoulder girdle areas are usually the most severely affected. Coarse fasciculations are often seen in the affected areas. A syndrome of periodic paralysis may also be present with thyrotoxicosis (Ch. 21). With hyperparathyroidism there may be symmetric weakness and associated atrophy; mainly the proximal muscles are affected. Muscular weakness and atrophy are also frequent findings in pituitary cachexia and in Addison's disease. Muscle wasting also occurs with diabetes. The most common syndrome is characterized by distal weakness and atrophy, secondary to a peripheral neuropathy. There are, however, cases with localized, asymmetric atrophy that does not correspond to peripheral nerve distribution. These have been termed **diabetic amyotrophy;** the underlying cause for the atrophy, however, is probably a mononeuritis or radiculopathy. Patients with diabetes may also develop either localized lipodystrophy or areas of focal muscular atrophy following injections of insulin.

Miscellaneous causes of muscular atrophy may include toxic and infectious factors, amyloidosis, senile atrophy, and trauma. In the amyotrophies associated with carcinoma and the reticuloses the atrophy is not dependent upon cachexia or invasion from the primary tumor and the etiology is uncertain, possibly immunologically mediated. Generalized muscle atrophy, often mainly proximal, may develop in association with the administration of some steroids; this "steroid myopathy" usually is reversible upon withdrawal of the drugs. Occasionally atrophy develops in patients with longstanding myasthenia gravis and with periodic paralysis. In Gowers' localized panatrophy there is wasting of all subcutaneous tissues, and in larger areas the muscles may also be involved; this may be related to either hemiatrophy or scleroderma. In adiposis dolorosa (Dercum's disease) the muscles may be replaced with fat.

Muscular Hypertrophy

Hypertrophy of muscles is encountered less frequently than atrophy. Extremely muscular individuals may show pronounced development of certain groups of muscles. This is often found in athletes and holders of heavy industrial jobs, e.g., foundry workers, and may be termed a **functional** or **physiologic hypertrophy.** The occupational history may give relevant information. Hypertrophy of muscles, real or apparent, may be seen in the myotonias. Microscopic examination may show an increase in the diameter of all individual muscle fibers. There is, however, a disproportion between muscle bulk and power, and although the muscles appear strong, they may actually be of only normal strength or even slightly weak. In myotonic dystrophy there is myotonia, with or without hypertrophy, but also atrophy, especially of the facial and sternocleidomastoid muscles. In **hypertrophia musculorum vera** there is enlargement of the muscles, usually those of the limbs, but any area may be affected. The hypertrophy is progressive, but spontaneous arrest usually occurs. The enlarged muscles may have increased strength, or there may be diminished power and ready fatigue. Electrical reactions are normal. There is no pathologic alteration other than increased size of muscle fibers.

DeLange described muscular hypertrophy occurring at birth with associated motor disturbances and mental deficiency. This is not to be confused with the Cornelia DeLange syndrome, which consists of short stature, mental retardation, thin downturning lips, micromyelia, and other congenital defects. Enlarged muscles with reduced strength, fatigability, and slowness of contraction and relaxation may be found in association with hypothyroidism and clinical myxedema; in cretinism and infantile hypothyroidism there may be diffuse muscular hypertrophy (the **Debré – Semelaigne syndrome**). In the early stages of acromegaly there may be genera-lized muscular hypertrophy with increased strength, but in later stages there is weakness and amyotrophy. Edema and inflammation of muscles may simulate hypertrophy.

Congenital hemihypertrophy, which may involve one side of the face, or the face and the corresponding half of the body, is more rare than the corresponding hemiatrophy; there are usually other anomalies of development. Pseudohypertrophy of certain muscle groups is seen in some of the muscular dystrophies, especially the Duchenne variety, where hypertrophic changes occur principally in the calf muscles (see Fig. 29-1). This is not, however, true hypertrophy, but a degenerative change in the muscles, with fatty and connective tissue infiltrations.

BIBLIOGRAPHY

Brooks JE. Disuse atrophy of muscle. Arch Neurol 1970;22:27

DeLange C. Congenital hypertrophy of the muscles, extra-pyramidal motor disturbances and mental deficiency. Am J Dis Child 1934;48:243

Fenichel GM, Daroff RB, Glaser GH. Hemiplegic atrophy: Histological and etiological considerations. Neurology 1964;14:883

Garland H. Diabetic amyotrophy. Br Med J 1955;2:1287

Henson RA, Russell DS, Wilkinson M. Carcinomatous neuropathy and myopathy: a clinical and pathological study. Brain 1954;77:82

Kakulas BA, Adams RD. Diseases of Muscle, 4th ed. Philadelphia, Harper & Row, 1985

Kugelberg E, Welander L. Heredofamilial juvenile muscular atrophy simulating muscular dystrophy. Arch Neurol Psychiatry 1956;75:500

Magee KR, Critchley M. Gowers' local panatrophy and its relation to certain types of insulin lipodystrophy. Neurology 1957;7:307

Magee KR, DeJong RN. Hereditary distal myopathy with onset in infancy. Arch Neurol 1965;13:387

Mulder DW, Bastron JA, Lambert EH. Hyperinsulin neuropathy. Neurology 1956;6:627

Ringnose RE, Jabbour JT, Keele DK. Hemihypertrophy. Pediatrics 1965;36:434

Silverstein A. Diagnostic localizing value of muscle atrophy in parietal lobe lesions. Neurology 1955;5:30

Sunderland S, Lavarack JO. Changes in human muscle after tenotomy. J Neurol Neurosurg Psychiatry 1959;22:167

Walton J (ed). Disorders of Voluntary Muscle, 5th ed. Edinburgh, Churchill Livingstone, 1988

Chapter 30
COORDINATION

Although motor strength and power may be preserved, active movements may be severely affected in diseases in which there is a disturbance of coordination.

In order to perform any movement, but especially a complex act that involves many muscle groups, it is necessary that the agonists, antagonists, synergists, and muscles of fixation be adequately correlated. The agonists contract to execute the movement; the antagonists relax or modify their tone to facilitate it; the synergists reinforce the movement; the fixating muscles prevent displacements and maintain the appropriate posture of the limb. The individual muscles that enter into the act must be associated in proper and harmonious grouping, with synchronous or successive contraction for regulated control of movement. The rate, range, and force of each component part of the act must be regulated. Strength must be steadily maintained. In addition sensory functions, especially those related to proprioception, must be intact. Coordination is defined as the normal use of motor, sensory, and synergizing factors in the performance of movements. All these are necessarily present in the organization of the perfectly executed act.

The cerebellum is essential to synergy and is considered to be the center of coordination. The tests to be discussed are mainly examinations of cerebellar function. It is important to remember, however, that all of the component levels of the motor system enter into the performance of smooth and accurate muscular activity. Paresis due to involvement of the spinomuscular level may interfere with skill and precision. Diseases of the extrapyramidal system may influence control because of rigidity, akinesia or bradykinesia, lack of spontaneity, and loss of associated movements. A corticospinal lesion may cause jerkiness and clumsiness of movement, loss of motor control, and poor integration of skilled acts. Psychomotor disturbances often cause difficulty with coordination, and a hysterical or a malingered derangement may simulate a true ataxia. Weakness and abnormalities of tone of any type may interfere with coordination. In the hyperkinesias there may be irregularity in the timing and excursion of successive movements.

Skilled motor activity is dependent upon all levels of motor integration, but the sensory and vestibular systems play significant roles. Sensory functions, especially proprioception, are essential to the proper correlation of motor acts. Disturbances of the kinesthetic modalities, especially those conveying knowledge of motion, position, and weight, may cause loss of motor control. There may be disturbances of coordination with lesions of the peripheral sensory nerves, dorsal funiculi of the spinal cord, ascending proprioceptive pathways in the brain stem, thalamus, and parietal lobes of the brain. The labyrinths and the vestibular apparatus are intimately connected with the cerebellum and are essential to equilibratory control. Diseases of the vestibular apparatus may be difficult to differentiate from disturbances of cerebellar function.

Diseases of other parts of the nervous system may also cause defects of coordination. The connections between the motor cortex and the cerebellum, the corticopontocerebellar tracts, are important pathways in motor control, and the motor cortex of one cerebral hemisphere is intimately connected with the opposite cerebellar hemisphere. Occasionally, it is difficult to differentiate by clinical examination between signs caused by a lesion of the frontal cortex on one side and those secondary to involvement of the contralateral cerebellar hemisphere. Lesions of the medulla, pons, and midbrain, too, frequently cause disturbances in coordination. In such lesions there may be involvement of the ascending proprioceptive pathways (including the spinocerebellar tracts), the vestibular nuclei and their connections, the corticopontocerebellar fibers, or one or more of the cerebellar peduncles. Only in disease of the cerebellum, however, is coordination markedly disturbed in the absence of other changes in motor or sensory function, or without other evidence of focal nervous system dysfunction. In the strict sense of the word, the term **incoordination** may be assumed to signify lack of accuracy of movement that is not secondary to paresis, abnormality of tone, or the presence of involuntary movements.

Disturbances of coordination may differ in degree and type. There is a definite individual variation in motor control, and in disease processes there may be a variation from slight incoordination to severe ataxia. **Agility** is the ability to carry out skilled movements rapidly. **Flexibility** or **suppleness** is the ability to move joints with ease through their full range. **Balance** is adequately controlled neuromuscular activity resulting from parallel functions of the motor and kinesthetic systems. Disturbances of any of these may lead to clumsiness or awkwardness of movement. **Equilibratory coordination** is the maintenance of balance, especially in the upright position; **nonequilibratory coordination** is concerned with discrete intentional movements of the extremities, mainly the finger motions. **Static ataxia** is the failure of coordination while in the resting state — the extended but otherwise static extremity cannot be held quietly without swaying or oscillating. **Motor, or kinetic, ataxia** appears only on movement. Static ataxia is the more severe, and if it is present there is also motor ataxia; motor ataxia, however, may be present without static ataxia.

The performance of a skilled or complicated act — one that requires higher cerebral control in either the motor or sensory spheres, together with psychic elaboration of the ideational plan before the act is carried out — is considered as an **eupractic function**. The perfect execution of such acts is known as **eupraxia**; a disturbance in the execution of skilled acts is **apraxia**. The eupractic functions and their disturbances will be considered under the cerebral functions in Part H, "Diagnosis and Localization of Intracranial Disease."

EXAMINATION OF COORDINATION

Various special examinations may be carried out in the testing of coordination, but oftentimes a careful observation of the patient during the examination as a whole may give much information. He should be watched while lying, seated, standing, and walking. He should be observed carefully while carrying out both routine and skilled acts. Performance while dressing and undressing, buttoning and unbuttoning clothing, and tying shoelaces should be noted, as should be tremors and hyperkinesias. Any disturbance of postural fixation should be described. He may be asked to carry out simple acts such as writing his name, using simple tools, drinking a glass of water, and tracing lines with a lightweight pen while no support is given at the elbow. General observation of the patient (for example, circumstances just described and while carrying out the actions mentioned) may yield as much information concerning coordination as a detailed clinical examination. This is especially true for infants and children, in whom the examination may have to be limited to simple observation of activity during relaxation and at play and by noting the child's ability to reach for and use toys and objects.

In the detailed testing of coordination one must remember the various portions of the nervous system that may be involved, and their relationship to each other. Tests for coordination may be divided into those concerned with equilibratory and nonequilibratory functions.

Equilibratory Coordination

Equilibratory coordination, or the maintenance of balance and the coordination of the body as a whole, is noted in the examination of station and gait. Only abnormalities characterized by ataxia will be mentioned here; other disturbances are listed in Chapter 32. If an abnormality is present while the patient is resting or in a stationary position, it may be considered as a variety of static ataxia; if while the body as a whole is in motion, as motor, or kinetic, ataxia.

The patient may first be observed while he is lying down or seated; only very gross disturbances of coordination will be apparent. There may be oscillations or unsteadiness of the body even while lying down. The patient may be unable to fix and coordinate the spinal, trunk, pelvic, and shoulder muscles properly, and may lack the ability to maintain a steady seated position; he may sway or fall if seated without support. There may be nodding movements of the head.

It is in the standing position, however, that moderate disturbances of equilibratory coordination first become apparent. The patient is asked to stand with the feet closely approximated, first with his eyes open, and then closed. The position of the body as a whole and that of his feet, shoulders, and head should be noted, as should tremors, swaying, and lurching. In a sensory type of ataxia, especially if conduction of the proprioceptive impulses through the spinal cord is impaired, as in tabes dorsalis, the patient may be able to maintain the upright position while the eyes are open, but when the eyes are closed he sways and tends to fall. This is the **Romberg** sign. He may attempt to prevent the swaying by placing his feet some distance apart, thus standing with a broad base.

Slight swaying with the eyes shut may occur in some normal individuals. In the vermis or middle cerebellar syndrome, which principally affects equilibrium, the patient may have difficulty in standing erect and maintaining a steady position with the eyes either open or closed. He may sway and lurch from side to side or backward and forward, and there may be oscillatory movements of the entire body. He may separate his feet in order to maintain his position. If he falls, it is generally in a backward or forward direction. Even in cerebellar disease, however, the difficulty is somewhat more marked when the eyes are closed. In a unilateral, or hemispheric, cerebellar lesion, or in a unilateral disturbance of vestibular function, the patient will sway or fall toward the involved side. While standing, the patient may tilt the head toward the involved side with the chin rotated toward the sound side, and the shoulder on the involved side is somewhat higher than the other and slightly in front of it.

Various modifications of the postural examination may be carried out. Difficulty with balance may be accentuated if the patient stands with his feet in a tandem relationship — with one heel directly in front of the opposite toes — and especially if he attempts to follow movements with his eyes, not his head. The patient may be given a light push, first toward one side and then toward the other; with a cerebellar hemispheric lesion he will lose his balance more easily when pushed toward the involved side. He may then be asked to stand on one foot at a time. With cerebellar hemispheric lesions he may be unable to maintain his equilibrium while standing on the ipsilateral foot, but may stand without difficulty on the contralateral foot. With involvement of the cerebellar vermis, diffuse cerebral disease, and some toxic states, he may move about as though skating or waltzing. In all of these tests sensory ataxia can be differentiated from predominantly cerebellar ataxia by an accentuation of the difficulty when the eyes are closed; and unilateral cerebellar or vestibular disease from vermis involvement by laterality of unsteadiness. In hysteria there may be a false Romberg sign; there may be marked unsteadiness, but the swaying is at the hips rather than at the ankles.

Coordination of the body as a whole may also be tested by asking the patient to rise from a lying to a seated position without the use of his hands, and from a seated position to an erect one; to bend forward, touch the floor with his hands, and then resume the erect position; to bend the head and trunk as far forward as possible; and to bend from side to side. In rising from the supine position he may fail to press down his lower extremities; consequently he will raise his legs, especially the one on the involved side, instead of lifting his trunk forward. In rising from a seated position he may fail to flex his thighs and to pull his knees and trunk forward, and accordingly will be unable to secure or maintain balance. In bending forward he may be unable to coordinate the functions of the spinal, pelvic, and lower extremity muscles to maintain balance. In bending backward he may fail to flex his knees to prevent falling. In bending from side to side he may have more difficulty with balance on the involved side, and tend to fall toward that side. If the patient attempts to jump on one foot, while the eyes are either open or closed, unilateral ataxia may be demonstrated.

Gait is tested by having the patient walk forward and backward with the eyes open and closed. Disturbances of function that are moderately evident in the evaluation of station may become more marked in the examination of gait. Any swaying, staggering, or deviation should be noted. With a cerebellar vermis lesion the patient will exhibit a lurching, staggering, type of gait (titubation), with the eyes both open and closed, but without laterality. With sensory ataxia the patient may walk fairly well with his eyes open, as long as he is able to watch the floor and surrounding environment, but on closing his eyes he sways and staggers. With a hemispheric cerebellar lesion the patient will stagger and deviate toward the involved side.

These abnormalities of gait can be further amplified by certain variations of the test. The patient may be asked to walk along a straight line on the floor, or he may be asked to **walk tandem**, i.e., by placing one heel directly in front of the opposite toes, with the eyes both open and closed (in some test batteries the patient is asked to walk a beam). The patient next is asked to walk in a sideward direction and overstep, or cross one foot over the other, in doing so. He is also instructed to walk forward and then turn around rapidly, or to walk around a chair, first in a clockwise direction, then counterclockwise. With hemispheric cerebellar lesions there is a deviation of the body, with a tendency to fall toward the involved side, whereas with vermis lesions the ataxia will be as marked toward one side as toward the other.

The difficulties in gait may be accentuated by asking the patient to walk rapidly or to run, by asking him to arise abruptly from a seated position and walk, or by having him stop abruptly on command. In the stepping test he is asked to mark time for 1 min with his eyes closed; with unilateral cerebellar disease he will gradually rotate the axis of his body toward the involved side. An alternate test is carried out by having the patient walk forward and backward eight steps repeatedly with his eyes closed; with hemispheric lesions there will be a gradual turning toward the affected side (**compass gait**). It must be borne in mind, however, that these tests may give abnormal responses with disease of the vestibular complex as well as of the cerebellum, and additional signs must be elicited in order to differentiate between the two.

Nonequilibratory Coordination

In testing nonequilibratory coordination we are concerned with the patient's ability to carry out discrete, oftentimes relatively fine, intentional movements with the extremities. Many elements of coordination should be observed. One should note the patient's ability to control the muscles and movements that normally act in harmony and to associate the various compo-

nents of an act in their proper synchrony, sequence, and degree, so that the act may be carried out smoothly and accurately; disturbances of these functions cause dyssynergy. One should observe the ability to judge and control the distance, speed, and power of an act and its component parts; loss of these results in **dysmetria.** The ability to carry out successive movements and to stop one act and follow it immediately by its diametric opposite should be appraised; difficulty with these functions causes **dysdiadochokinesia,** loss of checking movements, and the rebound phenomenon. Finally, the position of the individual parts of the body should be noted, especially the extremities; and posture-holding, or defective postural fixation, may be diagnostically significant.

It must be recalled that in cerebellar disease there are not only these elements of incoordination, but also hypotonia, asthenia or slowness of movement, and postural deviation, all of which may contribute to the motor disturbance, together with other findings such as dysarthria, nystagmus, tremors of an intention type, usually with an ataxic element, and other abnormal movements. Also, these several abnormalities are not unique to cerebellar disorders, occurring as well with lesions of the cerebellar and vestibular connections. In testing coordination of the upper extremities, various routine or special tests may be carried out. The patient's handedness should be determined, as it is obvious that right-handed individuals show somewhat more awkwardness in carrying out skilled acts with the left hand and vice versa. One should also notice the patient's general motor ability and his agility and skill in carrying out various motor acts. In toxic and fatigue states and with heavy sedation there may appear to be a clumsiness of motor ability that is not normal to the individual.

The **finger-to-nose test** may be carried out with the patient lying, seated, or upright. He is asked to abduct and extend the arm completely, and then to touch the tip of his index finger to the tip of his nose. The test is performed slowly at first, then rapidly, and with the eyes open and then closed. The examiner may place the outstretched extremity in various positions, and have the test carried out in different planes and from various angles. One should note the smoothness and accuracy with which the act is executed, and look for oscillations, jerkiness, and tremor. An intention tremor may be evident during the test, and often becomes more marked and more coarse and irregular as the finger approaches the nose; a resting tremor may disappear during the test. In sensory ataxia the subject may carry out the act without too much difficulty while the eyes are open, but may be unable to find the nose when the eyes are closed, owing to loss of appreciation of position in space. In cerebellar ataxia the difficulty may vary from slight incoordination, with a blundering type of movement, to complete inability to execute the act. With dysmetria the patient may stop before he reaches his nose (hypometria), pause and then complete the act slowly and unsteadily (bradytelokinesia), or either overshoot the mark or bring the finger to the nose with too much speed and force (hypermetria). With dyssynergy the act is not carried out smoothly and harmoniously; there may be irregular stops, accelerations, and deflections, or the act may be decomposed into its constituent parts. If the lesion responsible for the difficulty is confined to one cerebellar hemisphere, the ataxia is limited to that side of the body, or there may be consistent deviation to the ipsilateral side of the nose.

If the finger-to-nose test is carried out against slight resistance, the act is reinforced, and slight ataxia becomes more manifest or latent ataxia evident. The examiner may apply such resistance by placing his fingers on the volar surface of the patient's forearm and exerting slight pressure while the patient moves his arm toward the nose; or by placing a rubber band around the patient's wrist and pulling gently on it during the test. In hysteria or malingering there may be bizarre responses of various types; the patient may appear to be unable to touch the finger to the nose, or he may circle around it from one side to the other with widespread, wandering movements, but eventually approximate it to the very tip of the nose, or he may repeatedly but precisely touch some other part of his face, implying there is no loss of sensation or coordination.

In the **nose-to-finger test** the patient touches the tip of his index finger to his nose, then touches the tip of the examiner's finger, and again touches the tip of his nose. The examiner's finger is moved about during the test, and the patient is asked to touch it when it is held at different sites as well as to vary the rate of performance; in this way distance, speed, and power are all tested, as well as repetitive movements. The examiner may withdraw his finger slowly, and note the patient's ability to follow it accurately while making repeated efforts to touch it.

In the **finger-to-finger test** the patient is asked to abduct the arms to the horizontal, and then bring in the tips of the index fingers through a wide circle to approximate them exactly in the midline. This is done slowly and rapidly and with the eyes first open and then closed. With unilateral cerebellar disease there is deficient abduction; the finger on that side may not reach the midline, and the finger on the normal side crosses the midline to reach it. Also, the arm on the affected side may sag and undershoot, so that the finger on that side will be below the one on the normal side.

The usual test for **dysdiadochokinesia** is carried out by having the patient alternately pronate and supinate his hands, either outstretched or with the elbows fixed to his sides. The movements are performed as rapidly as possible. Any movement, however, that is concerned with reciprocal innervation and alternate action of agonists and antagonists can be used. The patient may be asked to open and close his fists alternately, flex and extend individual fingers rapidly, approximate the tips of the index finger and thumb, or the tip of the flexed index finger against the interphalangeal joint of the extended thumb repetitively and rapidly, tap on a table with his fingertips, pat his hand rapidly against a table top, pat the palm of one hand alternately with the palm and dorsum of the other, or pat the thighs with the palms and dorsa of the hands alternately. Often, patients seem to have problems performing one or more of these tests due to lack of comprehension or other factors unrelated to coordination. The examiner should switch to some of the alternate tests to decide if a coordination problem exists.

A good test for both dysdiadochokinesia and rapid skilled movements is carried out by having the patient touch the tip of his thumb with the tip of each finger rapidly and in sequence; he should be instructed to start with the index finger and proceed to the little finger, repeat with the little finger and proceed to the index finger, repeat with the index finger, and thus carry on the test. Coordination, speed of movement, and fatigue can be established quantitatively by counting the number of times the patient taps a button of a laboratory key counter or similar device in a given period of time. Dysdiadochokinesia of the tongue may be tested by having the patient protrude and retract his tongue or move it from side to side as rapidly as possible.

In all of these tests the rate, rhythm, accuracy, and smoothness of the movements should be noted. Ataxia may be more obvious with rapid alternating contraction of antagonists. With dysdiadochokinesia one act cannot be followed by its diametric opposite; the contraction of one set of agonists and relaxation of the antagonists cannot be followed immediately by relaxation of the agonists and contraction of the antagonists. As a consequence, the test is either carried out slowly, with pauses during transition between the opposing motions, or it is done unsteadily and irregularly, with loss of rhythm. There may be a rapid fatigability: the movements may be executed satisfactorily in the beginning, but after a few attempts they become awkward and clumsy; prolonged attempts may lead to confusion and cessation. The two extremities should be examined at the same time, and the normal compared with the abnormal; with unilateral testing the difficulty may not be very marked on either side, but simultaneous testing may cause accentuation of the abnormality on the affected side. In hemispheric disease of the cerebellum there is ipsilateral dysdiadochokinesia. It is important to remember that in right-handed individuals skilled movements are normally not quite as accurate or rapid on the left side. A diagnosis of dysdiadochokinesia cannot be made in the presence of motor paresis, bradykinesia, or gross sensory changes.

The checking movements of the antagonistic muscles, the ability to contract the antagonists immediately after relaxation of the agonists, and the braking mechanism after the sudden release of a resistance opposite a strong voluntary movement are all evaluated in the **rebound test** of Gordon Holmes. The patient is asked to adduct his arm at the shoulder, flex the forearm at the elbow and supinate it, and clench his fist firmly. The elbow may be supported on a table or it may be held unsupported close to the body. The examiner pulls on the wrist against resistance and then suddenly releases it. In the normal individual the contraction of the biceps and other flexors of the forearm is followed almost immediately by contraction of the triceps, the tendency toward flexion is checked by the rapid action of the antagonists, and the movement of the limb is arrested. In cerebellar disease, on the other hand, when the strongly flexed extremity is suddenly released the individual is unable to stop the contraction of the flexors and follow it immediately by contraction of the triceps. There is loss of the "checking factor." As a consequence the hand flies up to the shoulder or mouth, often with considerable violence. The examiner's free arm should be placed over the patient's face to receive the blow.

The test may be carried out in other ways. Extension of the forearm against resistance may be tested instead of flexion; both arms may be out-stretched in front of the patient, and the examiner may press either down or up on them against resistance, and then suddenly let go. In this way the rebound phenomenon and loss of checking movements can be compared simultaneously on the two sides. It must be stated, however, that the rebound phenomenon of Gordon Holmes is sometimes absent in cerebellar disease, and that it may be present in normal limbs or even exaggerated in spastic limbs. In the absence of spasticity or significant weakness, however, a unilaterally present rebound test has greater significance than a bilaterally present test.

To test **pointing** and **past pointing** the patient and examiner should be opposite each other, either seated or standing. The outstretched upper extremity of each one is held in the horizontal position with the index fingers in contact, or with the patient's index finger placed upon the tip of the examiner's index finger. The patient is then asked to elevate his arm to a vertical position, so that the finger is pointed directly upward, and then return the arm to the horizontal position in such a way that his index finger will again approximate the examiner's. This should be done first with the right arm and then with the left, and should be tried a few times with the eyes open, and then with them closed. Both arms may be tested simultaneously. After the test has been carried out with the patient raising his arm, it may be repeated by having him lower his arm to the vertical position, and then bring it up to the horizontal.

In the normal individual there will be no deviation, but in cerebellar or labyrinthine disease there will be deviation to the involved side, or **past pointing,** more marked with the eyes closed. The more often the test is repeated, the greater will be the deviation. In vestibular disease there is deviation, or past pointing, of both upper extremities toward the involved side; this is also the side that shows the slow component of the patient's nystagmus. In unilateral cerebellar disease there is past pointing toward the side of the lesion, but only in the ipsilateral arm; there may also be displacement in a downward direction. Furthermore, there is no specific correlation between the direction of nystagmus and the direction of the past pointing. Vestibular tests and imaging procedures may be of further aid in this differentiation.

Position-holding in the upper extremities can also be tested, and the static ataxia evaluated. The patient is asked to stand with both arms outstretched in front of him at the horizontal level, and to hold them thus, with the eyes first open and then closed. With unilateral cerebellar disease the ipsilateral arm gradually deviates laterally, owing to predominant activity of the abductor muscles. The arm on this side may also be elevated slightly, owing to overactivity of extensor muscles, or it may be held lower than the normal one, the result of asthenia, hypotonicity, and loss of tonic contraction of the muscles surrounding the joints. Such deviation occurs more promptly and to a greater degree when the eyes are closed; it may be accentuated by having the patient raise his arms to the vertical and then lower them to the horizontal several times. The examiner may tap the patient's outstretched wrists and note the patient's ability to maintain them in position or the amount of deviation that may occur. Normally there should be sufficient resistance to hold the extremities in position, but with cerebellar disease there may be greater displacement than normal; the arm will swing up and down a few times, and there will be a gradual lateral and upward deviation.

If the patient tries to hold a joint rigid while the examiner attempts rhythmic alternate movements, there may be instability and rebound owing to imbalance of antagonistic muscles. If support is suddenly withdrawn from the patient's braced outstretched arms, the one on the side of a cerebellar lesion will fall through a greater angle and develop irregular movements. There is also a characteristic position of the extended hand in cerebellar disease. The wrist is flexed and arched dorsally, the fingers are hyperextended, and there is a tendency toward overpronation. This position is probably associated with the hypotonia. The hand is similar to that seen in Sydenham's chorea. There may be loss of the normal pendular movements of the arms in walking, but in the shoulder-shaking test there is an increase in the range and duration of swinging of the arms, although the movements may be irregular and nonrhythmic.

Other special examinations may be carried out. The patient's judgment of the power and range of movement, as well as accuracy and direction, may be tested by having him make a fist and drive it into the examiner's outstretched palm with as much force as possible. Another test for dysmetria consists in having the patient draw a straight line with a pencil or chalk, starting and stopping at fixed points. He may have difficulty in starting at the correct point and may either stop before he reaches the second point or overshoot the mark. The evaluation of the patient's ability to carry out rapid, skilled, delicate movements with the fingers is often important.

His skill in using tools and scissors may be a valuable criterion. He may be asked to thread a needle, pick up a pin, put a stylus in a hole, use a pegboard, string beads, pour water from one test tube to another, or draw circles on a board or paper. It is true that many of these acts test other motor functions as well as coordination, but they aid in evaluating the latter. Having the patient grab his thumb with the opposite hand when the thumb is held at various levels and positions, tests coordination when the eyes are open as well as proprioceptive sensation when the eyes are closed. With a unilateral cerebellar lesion the patient may underestimate the weight of objects placed in the ipsilateral hand, whereas with an extrapyramidal lesion he may overestimate such objects.

Tests similar to those used with the upper extremities may be applied to the lower extremities. In the **heel-to-knee-to-toe test** the patient is asked to place the heel of one foot on the opposite knee and then push it along the shin in a straight line to the great toe. If there is dysmetria, he will undershoot or overshoot the mark, and in the presence of dyssynergy the movement may be broken down into its constituent parts and the descent along the shin is jerky and unsteady. Intention tremor and oscillations may be evident. In spinal ataxia the patient may have difficulty in locating the knee with the heel, and may grope around for it; there is difficulty in maintaining the heel on the shin, and it may slide off either laterally or medially during its descent. Similar tests of the lower extremities can be carried out by having the patient place his foot on a chair or some other fixed object, or by asking him to kick the examiner's hand with his foot. The rate, range, and force of movements may be tested by having the patient touch the examiner's finger with his great toe; the finger is moved about during the test, and the patient is asked to touch it at various sites as well as to vary the rate of performance. The patient may be asked to draw a circle or a figure 8 with his foot, either with the foot elevated or on the floor; in ataxia the movement will be unsteady and the figure irregular.

Dysdiadochokinesia in the lower extremities is tested by alternate dorsiflexion and plantar flexion of the feet or the toes, tapping the floor or some fixed object with the sole of the foot, or tapping the heel of one foot against the shin of the other leg. Rebound is tested by sudden release on the part of the examiner after he has been resisting either flexion or extension at the knee, hip, or ankle.

Position-holding in the lower extremities can be tested in various ways. The patient, lying supine, is asked to raise his legs in the air, one at a time. If there is ataxia the leg cannot be lifted steadily or in a straight line to a vertical position. There may be adduction, abduction, rotation, oscillations, or jerky movements from one position to another. When the limb is again lowered the patient may throw it down heavily and it may not return to its original position, next to its mate, but may be deviated across it or away from it. The seated patient may be asked to extend his legs without support and attempt to hold them steady; with a unilateral cerebellar lesion there may be oscillations and lateral deviation of the ipsilateral extremity. With cerebellar lesions the extended supported legs show an increased range and duration of pendulousness when they are released or given a brisk push. The patient, lying prone, is asked to bend his knees and maintain the shins in the vertical unsupported position; with unilateral cerebellar disease there may be marked oscillations and lateral deviation of the ipsilateral leg.

In both the upper and lower extremities the patient may be asked to reproduce in one limb the position in which the other has been placed by the examiner. This may be carried out with the tests for position-holding. It is in reality, however, a method of evaluating proprioceptive sensibility rather than coordination.

Under certain circumstances, principally in medical research, there are ataxia test batteries that are used for quantitative testing of ataxia and vestibular function.

Conditions Characterized by Disturbances in Coordination

To ascribe ataxia as a sign of cerebellar disease is an oversimplification. Other causes must first be ruled out, but often the causes are multifactorial involving cerebellar, vestibular, sensory systems, and tracts to and from these areas. In the differential diagnosis of disturbances of coordination it must be recalled that sensory ataxia is always most apparent when the patient's eyes are closed. The disability is the result of impairment of proprioceptive sensibility. The patient may be able to carry out simple and complex acts without too much difficulty if vision can be substituted for kinesthetic sensation, but with the eyes closed there is a marked disability. Such disturbances are found predominantly in posterior column disease, and consequently in such disorders as tabes dorsalis and posterolateral sclerosis. There may also be sensory ataxia with disease of the peripheral nerves, interruption of the proprioceptive pathways in the brain stem, and disease of the parietal lobe.

Cerebellar ataxia is present with the eyes open and closed, although the difficulty may be more marked when the eyes are closed. There are two clearly defined cerebellar syndromes. With the vermis, or midline, syndrome the outstanding symptoms are those of equilibratory coordination, with marked abnormalities of station and gait. In the hemispheric syndrome there is nonequilibratory ataxia, with disturbance in coordination of the ipsilateral extremities, the arm more than the leg. These syndromes and the associated disturbances of function in cerebellar disease are discussed in Chapter 24.

Unilateral vestibular disease may simulate cerebellar involvement, but there is much more subjective vertigo, and postural deviation, kinetic deviation, and nystagmus are present, without a great deal of real dysmetria or dyssynergy. Caloric tests and other studies (see Chapter 14) are of aid in the diagnosis.

In disease of the brain stem there may be interruption of the proprioceptive pathways, involvement of the cerebellar peduncles, disturbance of function of the vestibular nuclei and their connections, or dysfunction of other structures, such as the inferior olivary bodies or the red nuclei, which are allied to the cerebellum in function and intimately connected with it. In multiple sclerosis and Friedreich's ataxia the symptoms may be those of sensory involvement in the spinal cord and brain stem along with cerebellar dysfunction.

Disturbance of function of the contralateral frontal lobe, especially of the motor centers, may cause difficulty in coordination very like that which follows involvement of the ipsilateral cerebellar hemisphere. In fact, especially in the presence of neoplasms, the clinical differentiation between the two may be difficult. However, if the lesion is a cerebral one, hyperactivity of the muscle stretch reflexes, increase in tone, and pathologic reflexes should be expected, while in purely cerebellar lesions one would expect hypotonia, diminished or pendular reflexes, and no pathologic reflex responses. Pressure of a cerebellar neoplasm on the brain stem may cause corticospinal tract involvement, however, which can confuse the picture. One would expect more marked papilledema with a cerebellar (posterior fossa) neoplasm than with a cerebral one, but again this finding cannot always be relied upon.

The modern imaging procedures, such as computed tomography, magnetic resonance imaging, single photon scanning, positron emission tomography, as well as angiography and evoked potential studies play an important part in the localization of lesions in the posterior fossa and the cerebellum; these tests usually differentiate supratentorial from infratentorial processes. Unfortunately, they do not make a diagnosis themselves, nor do they depict the full extent of dysfunction of the central nervous system due to a given pathologic process.

BIBLIOGRAPHY

Angel RW. The rebound phenomenon of Gordon Holmes. Arch Neurol 1977;34:250

Fisher CM. A simple test of coordination in the fingers. Neurology 1960;10:745

Fisher CM. An improved test of motor coordination in the lower limbs. Neurology 1961;11:335

Fregly AR, Graybiel A. An ataxia test battery not requiring rails. Aerospace Med 1968, 39:277

Gilman S, Bloedel JR, Lechtenberg R. Disorders of the Cerebellum. Philadelphia, FA Davis, 1981

Graybiel A, Fregly AR. A new quantitative ataxia test battery. Acta Otolaryngol 1966;6:292

Orrison NW. Introduction to Neuroimaging. Boston, Little, Brown & Co, 1989

Schnitzlein HN, Murtagh FR. Imaging Anatomy of the Head and Spine. Baltimore, Urban and Schwarzenberg, 1985

Wartenberg R. Cerebellar signs. JAMA 1954;156:102

Chapter 31
ABNORMAL MOVEMENTS

Abnormal movements, or **hyperkinesias**, may occur in a variety of forms and under many different circumstances. They are for the most part involuntary contractions of voluntary muscles. Of clinical significance in the diagnosis and localization of disease of the nervous system, they should be carefully observed and described as a part of the examination of the motor system.

Hyperkinesias may involve any portion of the body. They are usually symptoms and signs of disease, not disease entities. They result from involvement of various parts of the motor system — the motor cortex and its descending pathways, basal ganglia, thalamus, subthalamic nucleus, substantia nigra, red nucleus, reticular formation, inferior olivary body, dentate nucleus, other cerebellar structures and their connections, spinal cord, peripheral nerves, or the muscles themselves. They may be of organic origin and related to infectious processes, anomalies of development, or neoplastic changes, or they may be of psychogenic origin. The character of the movement depends on both the site of the lesion and the type of pathologic change. Lesions at different sites sometimes cause identical movements; on the other hand, different pathologic processes that affect one part of the motor system may cause varying hyperkinesias.

In the examination of abnormal movements, the physician should observe their clinical appearance and visible manifestations, analyze the pattern of the movements, and then describe the various components. The following should be carefully noted: (1) the part of the body involved, or the exact location of the movements; (2) the extent of the hyperkinesia, or its distribution as regards part of a muscle, an entire muscle, movement involving joints, or more complex or composite patterns consisting of a sequence of different movements; (3) the pattern, rhythmicity, uniformity, multiformity, and regularity of recurrence — there may be a regular or rhythmic recurrence of activity involving the same muscle or groups, or there may be an irregular pattern of constantly changing motion of different parts; (4) the course, speed, and frequency of each particular movement; (5) the amplitude and force of the motor response; (6) the relationship to posture, rest, voluntary activity or exertion, involuntary activity, and fatigue; (7) the response to heat and cold; (8) the relationship to emotional tension and excitement; (9) the degree that they are increased or controlled by attention; (10) the presence or absence of the hyperkinesias during sleep. If the movements fit into a definite clinical picture, a specific name should be applied to them, but it is better to describe them than to attempt to name them. It may on occasion be possible, from their visible characteristics alone, to determine the site of the responsible lesion and the relationship of lesions at various sites to different forms of involuntary movements. However, in the case of abnormal movements resulting from lesions of the basal ganglia and their connections, it must be acknowledged that the specific anatomic site of the lesion responsible for the movement has not been established and, indeed, it is unlikely that a single specific site exists. Rather, the "lesion" may reflect chemical or transmitter disturbances, often involving several portions of the basal ganglia.

In addition to observation, palpation may be used, especially if the movements are very fine ones limited to individual muscles. Various mechanical, electrical, and other means have been used to record the frequency, rhythmicity, and amplitude of the various hyperkinesias, often in an attempt to evaluate the effects of treatment. These include myography, in which the oscillations are recorded directly, electromyography, and other electronic, photoelectric, and electromechanical devices. A videotaped record may also provide useful information in following the course of the disorder.

In the following discussions, the more important of the hyperkinesias are described in detail.

TREMORS

A tremor is a series of involuntary, relatively rhythmic, purposeless, oscillatory movements that result from the alternate contraction of opposing groups of muscles. Tremors may be of small or large excursion, and may involve one or more parts of the body. A **simple tremor** involves only a single group of muscles and its antagonists. A **compound tremor** involves several groups of muscles and is composed of several elements in combination; this results in a series of complex movements, as, for instance, alternate flexion and extension together with alternate pronation and supination. While the physician is concerned, in the evaluation of tremor, specifically with those muscles having reciprocal innervation, muscles of fixation and synergists also play a part in the movement. Tremors may be apparent on observation during either the resting state or activity, but are often accentuated if the patient is asked to hold his fingers extended and separated and his arms outstretched. Slow movements, writing, and the drawing of circles may also bring them out.

Tremors may be classified in various ways: by location, rate, amplitude, rhythmicity, relationship to rest and movement, etiology, and underlying pathologic change. Also important in their appraisal, however, is the relationship to fatigue, emotion, self-consciousness, heat, cold, and use of medications, alcohol, or street drugs. Tremors may be unilateral or bilateral; they are most commonly seen in the distal parts of the extremities — the fingers or hands — but may also be observed in the arms, feet, legs, tongue, lips, eyelids, jaw, and head. Occasionally they involve the entire body. They may be slow, medium, or rapid in rate. If there are 3–5 oscillations/sec, the tremor is slow; if there are 10–20 oscillations/sec, it is rapid. Tremors may be coarse, medium, or fine in amplitude. They may be either constant or intermittent and either rhythmic or relatively nonrhythmic; a certain amount of rhythmicity is implied, however, in the term tremor.

The relationship of a tremor to either rest or activity may be significant. **Resting** or **static tremors** are present mainly during relaxation, and decrease or disappear with activity. **Motor** or **intention tremors** appear only or mainly with deliberate, willed movement, and may become more marked toward the termination of such movement. **Tension** or **postural tremors** become evident during a volitional increase in muscle tonus, as when the limbs are actively maintained in a certain position. Tremors may be present only with emotional tension or fatigue, or they may be accentuated by these factors. Most organic tremors are accentuated by emotional excitement, and most normal individuals may develop tremors with tension, apprehension, heat, cold, and fatigue. Tremors of the shivering type may be brought on by cold, but identical movements can be produced psychogenically. Many tremors fall into more than one group, as far as the previously described classifications are concerned, and for that reason it is best to discuss the more important varieties individually without attempting to place them into definite categories.

There is a **normal** or **physiologic tremor** present during muscular contraction. This may be brought out by placing a limb in a position of postural tension or by performing voluntary movements at the slowest possible rate. This normal tremor varies from about 8–12 oscillations/sec, with an average of 10 in the young adult; it is somewhat slower in children and in older persons. The frequency for an individual is the same at different sites in the body. The visible tremors of normal persons that are brought out by tension, fatigue, and fright are doubtless accentuations of this physiologic tremor. There have been many theories regarding the source of this tremor. Some investigators indicate that it persists in the absence of muscle innervation and secondary feedback, and therefore conclude that it does not have a neural origin; they have suggested that cardiac and respiratory activity are responsible for it.

Fine tremors are usually rapid (10–20 oscillations/sec). They have been referred to as **toxic tremors**, and the most typical example is that seen in hyperthyroidism. The movements involve principally the fingers and hands. Since they are fine they may be difficult to see, but may be brought out by placing a sheet of paper on the outstretched fingers; the movement of the paper may be apparent even though the fingers are not seen to move. The tremor may be present both at rest and on activity, but it is accentuated by activity as well as by tension and apprehension. Similar tremors are found in association with other toxins such as alcohol, nicotine, and mercury, and with various drugs such as caffeine, bromides, barbiturates, chloral, cocaine, adrenaline, amphetamine, ephedrine, and other stimulants. Fine, rapid tremors may be present in tension and apprehension states and in the neuroses. A fine tremor of the closed eyelids (Rosenbach's sign) is seen in hyperthyroidism and in tense individuals.

Tremors of medium amplitude and rate are often evident in anxiety states and are precipitated by apprehension, fear, and fatigue. They may be present in the absence of disease. They are usually postural tremors, most evident with the hands outstretched, but they are made worse by movement and may interfere with motor activity. They resemble familial tremors. The intention tremors of multiple sclerosis and those encountered in disease of the cerebellum and its connections are usually of medium amplitude and may vary in degree from mild to severe.

Coarse tremors occur in a variety of states; they are usually slow. That of Parkinson's disease is one of the most characteristic. Coarse tremors are also seen in Wilson's disease and other extrapyramidal syndromes. Familial tremors are medium to coarse in amplitude, and those occurring in general paresis and alcoholism may also be coarse, especially if the movements are diffuse, as they are in delirium tremens. The intention tremor of multiple sclerosis may be coarse and irregular, especially when associated with ataxia. Psychogenic tremors and those associated with diseases of the midbrain and cerebellum may also be coarse and slow.

Resting, static, or **nonintention tremors** occur most frequently in diseases of the basal ganglia and the extrapyramidal pathways. The most characteristic tremor of this type is that seen in Parkinson's disease and in the various parkinsonian syndromes. This is a slow, coarse tremor of the compound type. The rate may vary from 2 – 6 oscillations/sec, usually averaging about 4 – 5. The movement in the hand characteristically consists of alternate contractions of agonists and antagonists involving the flexors,

extensors, abductors, and adductors of the fingers and thumb, together with motion of the wrist and arm including flexion, extension, pronation, and supination. As a result there is a repetitive movement of the thumb on the first two fingers, together with the motion of the wrist, which produces the so-called **pill-rolling** or **bread-crumbing tremor**. This tremor is relatively rhythmic and it is of the nonintention type, *i.e.*, it is present with inactivity and may become less marked with activity. It may disappear temporarily while the limb is engaged in a voluntary effort. It is probably incorrect, however, to say that the tremor is present at rest: it is present, or most marked, when the limb is in an attitude of repose or static posture, but it disappears with complete relaxation and sleep. It is independent of voluntary movement and may be temporarily suppressed by such movement. Because of the uniformly alternating movements at regular intervals, it is sometimes called an **alternating tremor**. Occasionally the tremor of Parkinson's disease is of both the intention and nonintention type.

The tremors just described not only involve the hands, but may also affect the feet, jaw, tongue, lips, and head. They may be unilateral at the onset, but in most cases eventually become bilateral. They disappear during sleep and are aggravated by emotional stimuli, fatigue, and anxiety. The associated manifestations of rigidity, loss of associated movements, and bradykinesia may be apparent in the parkinsonian syndromes, but in some patients the tremor is the predominant symptom, whereas in others the rigidity or bradykinesia may be more marked.

As was stated, this type of tremor is seen most characteristically in Parkinson's disease and parkinsonian syndromes but is also seen in extrapyramidal syndromes following carbon monoxide and manganese intoxication and repeated trauma, as in boxers. **Senile tremors** may resemble parkinsonian ones in degree, amplitude, and rate. They, too, are usually present at rest, but may also be increased by activity. They commonly affect the head, jaws, and lips. The movement of the head may be in either an anteroposterior (affirmative) or lateral (negative) direction. The onset occurs much later in life, and there is no associated muscular rigidity or weakness. Probably most senile tremors are tremors of the familial or essential variety (discussed subsequently) that are late in onset.

Motor, kinetic, or **intention tremors** are absent while the individual is resting, but appear with activity. As long as the patient is quiet no tremors are apparent, but when voluntary movements are attempted, as when he brings the tip of his finger to his nose, the tremor becomes evident and may be very marked. It increases with continued movement and as the digit approaches the goal (terminal tremor). This tremor may be of medium amplitude and fairly regular in rhythm, or it may be coarse, jerky, and irregular, especially when associated with ataxia. It is also increased by emotional stimuli and self-consciousness. It may involve the extremities, head, or entire body.

This type of tremor is seen most characteristically in multiple sclerosis, and it is considered to be very suggestive of this disorder although not pathognomonic; the tremor may be of either the medium or the coarse type. It is also seen in Friedreich's ataxia and other types of hereditary spinocerebellar degenerations. These disorders are believed to affect the cerebellar afferent and efferent pathways, especially those pathways connecting the dentate nucleus with the red nucleus and the thalamus, which pass through the superior cerebellar peduncle (brachium conjunctivum). If the disease process is in the cerebellum itself, the hyperkinetic phenomena are apt to be coarse in amplitude, with involuntary jerking movements that are increased by voluntary effort, although there may also be an oscillation of a more regular, rhythmic type in the absence of active innervation. Not only the extremities but also the head or entire body may be affected. These may in part be manifestations of ataxia, dyssynergy, and loss of the steadying effect that the increased tonus of the antagonistic muscles normally affords to voluntary movements. Such hyperkinesias may be termed *ataxic tremors.*

Tension, or **postural, tremors** appear with a volitional increase in muscle tonus, as when the limbs are actively maintained in certain postures. Occasionally they are slightly increased by action, but they usually stop with movement. They are usually absent with complete rest, and become marked when the parts are placed in fixed attitudes. They may be brought out by having the arms and hands outstretched, or by stopping the finger-to-nose test a short distance from the nose and holding the finger in that position. They are finer and more rapid than resting tremors, averaging 8 – 12 oscillations/sec, and are less rhythmic.

Familial tremors are usually of the tension or postural variety, but they also persist or become more exaggerated during volitional movements. They may vary from mild to severe in intensity.

They usually progress very slowly in severity over many years or remain unchanged. Often they begin in the dominant hand. They are absent at rest and are worsened by emotional tension and by the use of the proximal muscles. They usually affect the fingers and hands, but the neck, larynx, and tongue may be affected. They are not accompanied by weakness, rigidity, ataxia, or loss of associated movements. They are temporarily lessened by the ingestion of alcohol and sedative drugs but worsen when the effect of these wears off. They respond more consistently, but incompletely, to beta blockers such as propranolol, and to primidone. When the tremors develop during childhood, adolescence, or late life, they are sometimes referred to as **infantile, juvenile,** or **senile tremors.** Similar tremors, with no associated family history, are called **benign,** or **essential tremors.** These tremors have no known central nervous system pathology.

The tremor of Wilson's disease (progressive lenticular degeneration) may be of various types. There may be a slow, alternating tremor at rest, resembling that of Parkinson's disease, or a tremor that is increased by voluntary action. Most characteristic of the adult variety, however, is a coarse, irregular tremor that may be apparent during movement but is most marked during the maintenance of sustained postural attitudes. There may be violent up-and-down "flapping" movements of the hands and wrists while they are held outstretched, and coarse "wing-beating" movements of the abducted shoulders. In severe cases this may even appear to be present at rest; however, the parts are probably not completely relaxed but under some tension, and the slightest stimulation may elicit the movement.

The term **asterixis** (inability to maintain a fixed posture) has been applied to to-and-fro movements of the hands and fingers that is seen in patients with hepatic and other encephalopathies. This is most effectively elicited by having the patient hold his arms outstretched with fixed extension at the elbow and wrist and abduction of the fingers. If asterixis is present there will be side-to-side movements of the fingers, and flexion-extension movements of the fingers and wrists. These are intermittent, rapid, and arrhythmic. Asterixis has also been reported to occur with overdosage of phenytoin and other medications. Unilateral asterixis has been reported with lesions of the pons and medulla.

Psychogenic tremors are often of medium amplitude, but they may be fine or coarse. They may be present at rest but they are usually accentuated by voluntary movement. They may appear when the part is being held still against the force of gravity, as when the arm is outstretched. They result from the contraction of opposing groups of muscles that are in use in the attempt to keep the extremity in a static position. They are precipitated or aggravated by tension, apprehension, self-consciousness, fatigue, and cold, and markedly so by emotional stress and strain. They may be brought on by fear, anxiety, or sudden fright, and may involve any part of the body. They are seen in hysterical individuals, anxiety states, neurasthenia, and other neuroses and also in almost every person under certain environmental conditions. The tremor of the hand that is accentuated when an individual is being observed closely and the shaking of the knees and tremulousness of the voice that appear when an inexperienced speaker has to address a large audience are common examples of tremors of this type. They may be accentuations of physiologic tremor.

Shivering, or **rigor,** consists of clonic movements of various groups of muscles, principally the masseters but also the muscles of the limbs and trunk. It may be of physiologic or psychologic origin; it is brought out by cold, but also by emotional stimulation. The movements may be inhibited to a certain extent by voluntary contraction of the muscles. Shivering is often accompanied by cutis anserina.

Tremors may occur under a variety of other conditions and may be important manifestations of various pathologic processes. Involvement of the red nucleus is followed by ataxia and tremor on the opposite side of the body. The tremor is said to be coarse, slow, and rhythmic, and is present at rest; it is accentuated by voluntary movement. The so-called **rubral tremor** can be experimentally produced in animals. In Benedict's syndrome there are such tremors along with ataxia contralateral to the lesion, and an ipsilateral third nerve paralysis. The tremor of alcoholism may be of the fine, toxic variety, but it may also be coarse and slow, as in delirium tremens where it averages about 4/sec. The movements may involve the extremities, jaws, lips, face, tongue, or any part of the body. There may be violent tremors of the entire body. Similar tremors may manifest in various withdrawal states from drug or substance abuse. In chronic alcoholism one frequently observes **Quinquaud's sign**: when the patient's fingers, abducted, flexed at the metacarpophalangeal joints, and extended at the interphalangeal joints, are placed vertically in the examiner's

hand, at right angles to the palm, a trembling or wormlike sensation is felt, due to the slight shocks from the repeated up-and-down movements of the individual fingers. Tremors resulting from alcoholism may be extremely variable in type and rhythm and may be influenced or aggravated by emotional stimuli.

In dementia paralytica there may be tremors of the extremities, and characteristically one sees them in the lips (perioral tremors) and tongue. Tremors are often seen in acute infectious states. In spasmus nutans, which occurs in infants from 6 months to 2 years of age, there is a rhythmic nodding or rotatory tremor of the head associated with a fine, rapid, pendular nystagmus. If the eyes are closed the tremor may either increase or decrease, and if the movement of the head is controlled the nystagmus usually increases. Tremors and other abnormal muscular movements may be present with disturbances of magnesium, calcium, sodium, and potassium metabolism, following the ingestion of certain drugs, rarely after head injuries, with some central nervous system infections, and in various rare diseases, such as kuru, which has been described in New Guinea.

FASCICULATIONS AND FIBRILLATIONS

Fasciculations are fine, rapid, flickering or vermicular twitching movements that appear with contraction of a bundle, or fasciculus, of muscle fibers. They are usually not extensive enough to cause movement of joints, except occasionally in the digits. They vary in size and intensity. They may be so faint and small that they but slightly ripple the surface of the overlying skin, or they may be coarse enough to be apparent readily. They are often irregular and inconstant, visible in muscles at one time and not at another. At times they are abundant, at others they require a careful search. They are usually present at rest, but they may be brought out, made more rapid, or intensified by light mechanical stimulation of the muscle or by placing it under tension. They are also brought out by fatigue and cold. They may be seen to course throughout an entire muscle, without causing it to contract as a whole, or they may occur first in one part of a muscle and then in another. Adequate illumination is necessary in order to visualize them, and they may be seen best with oblique lighting or in the peripheral portion of the examiner's visual fields. They may be more difficult to see in women than in men because of the presence of more subcutaneous fat in the former. Occasionally they can be palpated even though invisible to the eye, or they may at times be heard by the use of a stethoscope. Many patients are not aware of the presence of fasciculations, but others may see or feel them, or both. Electromyography can detect their presence even when they cannot be seen.

At one time the terms *fibrillation* and *fasciculation* were used synonymously. **Fibrillations,** however, are contractions limited to a single muscle fiber or to a group of fibers smaller than a fasciculus. They are fine, continuous, tremorlike contractions present in denervated muscle. They are too small to be visible through the skin. Electromyographically these are of short duration (less than 1 or 2 msec) and low voltage (rarely more than 50 microV). **Fasciculations** are contractions of a large group of fibers, or fasciculus, usually constituting a single motor unit supplied by a single anterior horn cell. Such units may vary in size and may be composed of up to 200 individual fibers. Fasciculations are thus much more gross than fibrillations, and can be seen through the intact skin. They may be from 8 – 12 msec in duration, and the discharge is from ½ – 1 mV. Fasciculations and fibrillations are present in sleep. Fasciculations are activated by mechanical stimulation of the muscles, but those resulting from neurologic disease are not significantly affected by emotional or mental activity. They are exaggerated by the administration of cholinergic drugs, and in fact may be produced in normal individuals by such drugs. They are not abolished by spinal anesthesia or peripheral nerve block. They are obliterated by the administration of curare and by the injection of local anesthetics directly into the muscle. Quinidine may also abolish fasciculations.

Fasciculations are seen most frequently, and are of most significance, in association with disorders resulting from degeneration of the anterior horn cells of the spinal cord and the motor nuclei of the brain stem, in such conditions as progressive spinal muscular atrophy, progressive bulbar palsy, amyotrophic lateral sclerosis, and syringomyelia; they disappear by the time atrophy is complete. They are rarely seen in the myopathies; disease processes such as the Guillain – Barré syndrome or poliomyelitis, in which there is an abrupt loss of function of the anterior horn cells and their neuraxes; or in conditions such as polyneuritis, in which the atrophy results from peripheral nerve injury or disease. They are present on occasion, however, in all these conditions, and thus may be found in

poliomyelitis, both in the acute stage and in residually paretic muscles following acute poliomyelitis. They also occur in acute inflammations of the peripheral nerves, compression of the peripheral nerves or nerve roots, from disks, spondylosis, or trauma, myositis, extramedullary and intramedullary tumors of the spinal cord, and states such as thyrotoxic myopathy, uremia, and paraneoplastic neuropathy. They may follow exposure to various heavy metals or other toxins, and at times occur after spinal anesthesia and in completely denervated muscles. Movements resembling fasciculations, as well as tremors, may be detected with disturbances of magnesium, calcium, sodium, and potassium metabolism that affect the muscle or myoneural junction. The exact mechanism and significance of fasciculations and their mode and site of origin are not definitely known.

Fibrillations, which make their appearance about 10 – 20 days after denervation of muscle, are evidence of disordered muscle metabolism secondary to the loss of trophic influence from the anterior horn cells. There is an abnormal irritability of muscle, probably owing to heightened excitability of the sarcolemma or of rapidly conducting portions of the muscle fibers to traces of free acetylcholine in the tissues. Fibrillations may originate in the motor end-plate of a muscle fiber and extend along the course of the fiber. It has been suggested that fibrillations may be synchronized into fasciculations, or contractions of a group of fibers making up one motor unit. The fasciculations that occur in thyrotoxic myopathy and other toxic states may result from an increased concentration of acetylcholine at the myoneural junction or increased sensitivity of the muscle fibers to the transmission of acetylcholine.

Fasciculations that occur with spinal cord neoplasms, ruptured intervertebral disks, and irritation of the nerve root or nerve are probably the physiologic equivalent of the contraction of a group of fibers supplied by a single axon. They may indicate either degeneration or irritability anywhere along the course of the lower motor neuron, from the anterior horn cell to the myoneural junction and the muscle. Their presence may be of value in the localization of disease of the spinal cord, nerve roots, or peripheral nerves.

Fasciculations should be searched for carefully, especially in conditions where there is evidence of muscular wasting. They are most significant when present in conditions such as progressive spinal muscular atrophy and amyotrophic lateral sclerosis, and in these indicate progressive degeneration of the anterior horn cells. They may serve as an index to the severity and prognosis of the disease: if they are numerous, the progress of the disease will probably be rapid. They are usually seen first in the shoulder girdles, upper arms, and chest muscles. They may disappear when atrophy is extensive.

The presence of fasciculations unaccompanied by atrophy, however, does not necessarily indicate the presence of a serious disease process. Spontaneous, benign fasciculations are not infrequently seen in normal persons, and are especially common in medical students and physicians. These may be present at rest or may be brought out by fatigue and tension states. There is no atrophy or evidence of muscular or motor dysfunction, and there are no fibrillations by electromyography. It has been suggested that there may be some underlying biochemical or related abnormality at the myoneural junction that is responsible for these benign fasciculations, or they may be similar to the myokymic movements now to be described.

MYOKYMIA

Myokymias, or **myokymic movements,** are spontaneous, transient or persistent movements that affect a few muscle bundles within a single muscle but usually are not extensive enough to cause movement at a joint. They are not limited to the muscle fibers or fasciculi, and they are somewhat more coarse, more slow and undulating, "worm-like," and usually more prolonged and widespread than fasciculations. They may be caused by irregular discharges spreading to and through various muscle bundles. There is no associated muscular atrophy. They usually are not affected by motion and position. During electromyography there is spontaneous, continuing motor unit activity of resting muscles. Myokymic movements are sometimes referred to as "false fasciculations." If they are quivering and flickering in character, they are commonly known as "live flesh."

Myokymic movements may be of physiologic origin. They may occur in normal individuals after strenuous and unaccustomed exercise, in association with unusual fatigue or exhaustion, or as a transitory occurrence in facial muscles, especially the orbicularis oculi. They may appear during an attempt to maintain contraction of weak muscles and disappear when the muscles are relaxed. They may occur with chilling or when going to sleep. They are most often seen, however, in conditions in which there is weakness or fatigue, such as anemia, debilitating disease, infection, or metabolic disorders. They have been reported in hyperthyroidism and with salt deprivation, uremia, and tetany. They may be a transient result of toxins, having been reported to occur from rattlesnake venom. They are occasionally familial, and frequently develop in individuals undergoing emotional stress. Myokymic movements may be seen, along with fasciculations, in progressive spinal muscular atrophy and the related wasting diseases. Here they probably result from the fatigue that accompanies the weakness and atrophy.

Myokymic movements are occasionally accompanied by cramping and pain; usually there is an associated increase in myotatic irritability. It has been suggested that they are not exaggerated following the administration of neostigmine, and that they are abolished during occlusion of the circulation, appearing again about 3 min after the occlusion is removed. The clinical significance of myokymic movements is doubtful, and they are often found in normal persons with no progressive neuromuscular disease. One might raise the question whether so-called benign or spontaneous fasciculations might not more correctly be termed myokymic movements, especially if they are slightly more coarse and irregular than the usual fasciculations. Myokymic movements and benign fasciculations may well represent similar alterations in muscle physiology.

So-called facial myokymia has been reported to be present in patients with multiple sclerosis, intramedullary brain stem neoplasms, and syringobulbia. Similarly, facial myokymia may develop as part of the Guillain–Barré syndrome. Functional deafferentation of the facial nucleus was postulated as a cause of facial myokymia. It could also be that these movements result from irritation of the facial nerve nucleus or the nerve itself, and might better be called tremors or spasms.

MYOCLONUS

The term **myoclonus** has been used for several differing motor phenomena. In general, however, a myoclonic movement may be defined as a disturbance of neuromuscular activity characterized by abrupt, brief, rapid, lightning-like, jerky, arrhythmic, asynergic, involuntary contractions involving portions of muscles, entire muscles, or groups of muscles regardless of their functional association. The movements may be either single or repetitive, and are similar to those that follow stimulation of a muscle. Myoclonus is seen principally in the muscles of the extremities and trunk, but the involvement is often diffuse and widespread; the contractions may be present in the facial muscles, jaws, tongue, pharynx, and larynx, and may appear symmetrically on the opposite side of the body. They occur at a rate of $10-50$/min, but some varieties are much more rapid. They appear in paroxysms at irregular intervals, during either the resting or active state, and may be activated by emotional, mental, tactile, visual, and auditory stimuli. They may be decreased by voluntary movement and increased during stimulation. They appear during the process of going to sleep, but usually disappear during sleep.

Myoclonic movements, like fasciculations and myokymias, occasionally are too small in degree to cause movement of joints. Usually, however, they affect entire muscles or muscle groups, producing clonic movements of the extremities. They may be so violent that they cause an entire limb to be suddenly thrown out, or they may even throw the patient to the ground. There may be successive or simultaneous involvement of many muscles. Myoclonic movements are not activated by mechanical stimulation or stretching of the muscle and are not affected by neostigmine.

There has been much difference of opinion regarding the pathologic process underlying myoclonic movements. It was once felt that the neural discharge that excites the muscular contraction was confined to the lower motor neuron. Their occurrence in association with various degenerative brain diseases, however, suggests that in most cases involvement of the cerebral cortex, gray matter, thalamus, substantia nigra, basal ganglia, dentate nucleus, cerebellum, or brain stem alone or in combination, is responsible for them. A variety of processes evidently lead to hyperexcitability of the cortex, subcortical structures, or even the lower motor neuron alone. No unique pathologic substrate has been described.

Myoclonic movements may occur in a variety of conditions, and their significance varies. They have been observed in acute and chronic encephalitis, meningitis, toxic and postanoxic states, metabolic disorders, degenerative diseases, and vascular and neoplastic conditions; they have also been reported with lesions of the peripheral nerves, nerve roots, and spinal cord.

They frequently are symptoms of diffuse cerebral degenerative disease, especially in children. They may be of diagnostic significance in the lipidoses, subacute sclerosing panencephalitis, the Hallervorden–Spatz syndrome, Creutzfeldt–Jakob disease, and Wilson's disease. On the other hand, some myoclonias may be benign and without serious significance; others may be psychogenically precipitated. Movements difficult to differentiate from myoclonus may be present in hysteria. Hereditary essential myoclonus is usually a benign disorder, although on occasion there is some impairment of cerebellar function and gradual progression of the symptoms. Benign nocturnal myoclonus is often reported in healthy persons. Paroxysmal kinesogenic myoclonus has also been described. The syndrome of action or intention mycolonus develops as a sequel to cerebral anoxia.

Paramyoclonus multiplex of Friedreich has been described as a disease of adult life coming on after fright, trauma, mental or physical exhaustion, or infection. There are paroxysmal contractions of the limb and trunk muscles, occurring at a rate of $40-50$/min, which are present at rest, are aggravated by emotional stimulation, and disappear on voluntary contraction of the muscles and during sleep. The etiology is not known and some authorities question the existence of this syndrome.

Myoclonic movements are frequently encountered in epilepsy. Many epileptic patients have occasional random myoclonic jerks of the axial or proximal limb musculature; these may appear or increase in frequency immediately prior to a seizure. They occur most frequently in hereditary light-sensitive and reading epilepsy. Massive **myoclonic spasms of infancy** are characterized by frequent, sudden, violent jerking attacks with flexion of the neck and trunk and adduction or abduction and extension of the arms and legs. The body may bend forward and the child may fall to the floor during the attack. These are often associated with systemic biochemical disorders or degenerative brain disease; the prognosis is poor and there may be intellectual and motor deterioration. In **familial myoclonus epilepsy** of Unverricht and Lundborg myoclonic jerkings are present during and between attacks and intensified before the seizure occurs. They may involve the muscles of the extremities, face, tongue, jaw, and pharynx. There is progressive motor and intellectual deterioration. Because Lafora inclusion bodies have been found throughout the central nervous system, as well as in other organs, in some patients with this syndrome, it has been suggested that such cases be called **Lafora's disease.** In **myoclonic cerebellar dyssynergy** there are myoclonic jerkings and progressive cerebellar degeneration; Hunt attributed the movements to atrophy of the dentate nucleus, but his patients also had involvement of other parts of the nervous system.

While it has been stated that myoclonic movements are arrhythmic and diffuse, the term has also been applied erroneously to rhythmic and localized motor phenomena. So-called **palatal (palatopharyngolaryngo-oculodiaphragmatic) myoclonus** is characterized by involuntary movements of the soft palate and pharynx, sometimes of the larynx, eye muscles, and diaphragm, and occasionally of other muscles. It may be unilateral or bilateral. The movements may vary from 50–240/min. They are generally not influenced by drugs or sleep but may be inhibited at first by voluntary effort. The uvula may deviate either upward and downward or to one side; the posterior pharyngeal wall moves laterally, and the larynx moves in an upward and downward direction. If the movements involve the diaphragm or larynx, they may cause a grunting respiratory noise. A clicking sound sometimes accompanies movements of the pharynx, audible to the patient and sometimes the examiner as well. This condition has been associated with lesions of the olivodentatorubro-metencephalic pathways, and there may be hypertrophy of the inferior olivary nucleus or involvement of the olivocerebellar or the central tegmental tracts, cerebellum, or brain stem. This syndrome most often has its onset in late adult life, and has been reported with vascular, neoplastic, inflammatory, and degenerative lesions. Rarely, it disappears cyclically in sleep, or it may subside spontaneously after several years. It may develop in children on a congenital basis. Often no symptoms are present. It has also been referred to as **palatal nystagmus.** Neither myoclonus nor nystagmus is a suitable term, however, as the movement is rhythmic and is actually a tremor.

CHOREA

Chorea is characterized by involuntary, irregular, purposeless, asymmetric, nonrhythmic hyperkinesias. They are spontaneous in onset and are abrupt, brief, rapid, jerky, unsustained, and explosive in character. The individual movements may be discrete, but they are variable in type and location, so that there may be an irregular pattern of multiform, constantly changing movements of different parts of the body that appear at irregular intervals. There is an interruption of harmonious coordination of prime movers, synergists, and antagonists. The movements are present during the resting state but are brought out or increased by activity and tension. They are aggravated by emotional stress and self-consciousness, and usually disappear during sleep. At times they appear purposeful to an observer, but they are actually aimless.

Choreic movements may involve one extremity, one half of the body, or the entire body. They are seen most characteristically in the upper extremities, where they involve principally the distal portions, but may also affect the proximal parts, the lower extremities, the trunk, face, tongue, lips, larynx, and pharynx. There may be repeated twitching and grimacing movements of the face that change constantly in character and location. The patient is frequently unable to hold out his tongue for any length of time, and when asked to protrude it he shoots it out and then jerks it back. The voice may be affected, and there may be abnormal vocalizations, difficulty in maintaining phonation, or aphonia. There may be disturbances of chewing and swallowing. The movements of the hands may interfere with dressing and eating. There is a waxing and waning of the grip of the individual fingers when the patient grasps the examiner's hand; this causes the so-called milking grip. Often the movements may be brought out by asking the patient to carry out two acts at the same time; he can touch his finger to his nose if he does that alone, and he can protrude his tongue alone, but on attempts to do both simultaneously, the jerky movements become noticeable. The hyperkinesias interfere with and distort voluntary movements, and the latter may be sharp, jerky, and unsustained.

In addition to the movements, there is hypotonia of the skeletal musculature. As a result there is little force to the spontaneous movements and there is little resistance to passive movement. The outstretched hands are held with hyperextension of the proximal and terminal phalanges, flexion and dorsal arching of the wrist, and pronation that is increased when the arms are raised above the head. The fingers are separated and the thumb is abducted and droops downward. In association with the hypotonia there is marked fatigability of the skeletal musculature. There is no paralysis, but the constantly repeated hyperkinesias and their interference with voluntary movement and sustained muscular contraction may cause a marked impairment of motor function. The tendon reflexes are of the pendular or "hung" variety.

The most characteristic movements are seen in **Sydenham's chorea,** also known as chorea minor or rheumatic chorea, and known by the laity as St. Vitus' dance. This occurs in childhood and adolescence in relationship to rheumatic fever. It may recur, at times during pregnancy as chorea gravidarum. A cerebral vasculopathy is the assumed cause. The movements may be limited to one extremity or one half of the body, or may be diffuse. Frequently, during or after recovery from Sydenham's chorea a patient may retain minimal choreic movements or may have minor ticlike movements that are difficult to differentiate from chorea. In **Huntington's chorea,** or chronic hereditary chorea, a dominantly inherited condition involving chromosome 4, the onset is usually in adult life and there is steady progression. The movements are similar to those of Sydenham's chorea, but are often somewhat slower, less jerky, and more bizarre, widespread, and violent. They may be seemingly purposeful, and the same pattern may be repeated over and over again. Frequently the larger muscle groups and the proximal portions of the extremities are affected, and there may be repeated shrugging of the shoulder girdle or flaillike movements of the arm. Facial grimacing may be more marked, and there may be twisting and lashing movements that lie between those of chorea and athetosis. Movements of the fingers and hands may be accentuated while the patient is walking. It is accompanied by progressive intellectual deterioration. There is also a form of nonprogressive chorea that is inherited as a recessive trait. Choreic movements are also being reported with a great variety of other conditions. Chorea may be a transient side effect of many medications such as psychotropic agents, phenytoin, antihistamines, amphetamines, levodopa, methylphenidate, and others. It may be a persisting feature of the use and former use of psychoactive drugs as part of the syndrome of tardive dyskinesia. Chorea may occur with inborn errors of metabolism, such as propionic acidemia and hyperuricemia. It has been described with metabolic derangements including nonketotic hyperglycemia and hyperthyroidism. It may be a remote effect of carcinoma or be part of multisystem familial degenerative disorders. Vascular disorders in the form of infarcts of the caudate nucleus, polycythemia, lupus erythematosus, and others have also been described as causes of chorea, as have, rarely, cerebral neoplasms and trauma.

There is no unanimity of opinion regarding the specific location of the pathologic process responsible for all choreic movements. In Huntington's chorea there is atrophy of the caudate nuclei and there is also involvement of the putamen and cerebral cortex, with diffuse degenerative changes in the brain (Fig. 31-1). Clearly, in many cases the "lesion" is merely chemical in nature.

HEMIBALLISMUS

Movements similar to those of chorea are the ballistic movements seen in hemiballism, or hemiballismus. These, too, are involuntary, purposeless movements, but are much more rapid and forceful and involve largely the proximal portions of the extremities. They are continuous, wild, violent, swinging, flinging, rolling, throwing, flaillike movements of the extremities. They are usually unilateral, and may involve one entire half of the body; as a result of their intensity they may cause movement of the entire body. Rarely, they are bilateral. The movements may spare the face and trunk. They are ceaseless during the waking state and disappear only with deep sleep; because of their violence they may lead to exhaustion. Hemiballismus follows an isolated lesion, usually vascular in origin but rarely neoplastic or other, of the contralateral subthalamic nucleus or the neighboring structures or pathways. The prognosis was once considered to be very poor, but patients may recover without residual effects. Tranquilizing and sedative drugs are of therapeutic value. Surgical procedures such as thalamotomy have been used in some refractory cases. Hemiballismus may simulate hemichorea or blend into it at times. Some observers do not separate the two entities.

ATHETOSIS

In athetosis the hyperkinesias are slower, more sustained, and larger in amplitude than those in chorea. They are involuntary, irregular, coarse, somewhat rhythmic, and writhing or squirming in character. They may involve the extremities, face, neck, and trunk. In the extremities they affect mainly the distal portions, the fingers, hands, and toes. The movements are characterized by any combination of flexion, extension, abduction, pronation, and supination, often

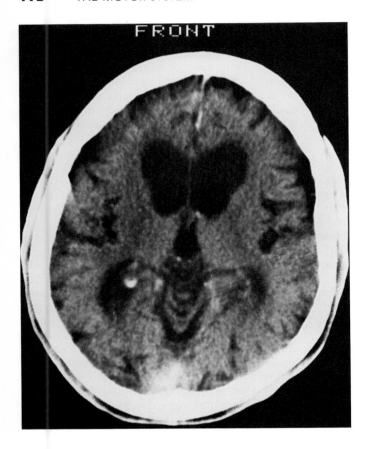

FIG. 31–1. Computed tomogram of the brain of a patient with advanced Huntington's chorea, demonstrating cerebral and caudate atrophy along with ventricular enlargement.

alternating and in varying degrees (Fig. 31-2). Hyperextension of the fingers and wrist and pronation of the forearm may alternate with full flexion of the fingers and wrist and supination of the forearm. Facial grimacing, which is slower and more sustained than in chorea, often accompanies the movements of the extremities, and there may be synkinesias affecting other parts of the body. The hyperkinesias may not be constant or continuous, but may recur in series, intensified by voluntary motion or tension. They disappear in sleep. There is usually associated spasticity or hypertonicity of the musculature, with some paresis. Voluntary movements are disturbed, and coordinated action may be difficult or impossible.

Athetosis is usually of congenital origin and it may be present in association with varying degrees of congenital spastic paraparesis. It may be either unilateral or bilateral. The predominant pathologic changes are in the caudate and putamen, although there may also be cortical involvement. Double athetosis may be associated with status marmoratus or with brain changes resulting from erythroblastosis fetalis, kernicterus, or infantile encephalitis. Acquired athetosis may follow disease or trauma in later life. Many of its causes overlap with those of chorea, and in fact many patients have features of athetosis plus chorea.

Pseudoathetosis has been used to describe similar undulating and writhing movements of the extremities that are more marked when the eyes are closed and are usually unassociated with an increase in muscle tone. Movements of this type occur with lesions of the parietal lobe and such conditions as tabes dorsalis, posterolateral sclerosis, and peripheral nerve disease. They are not true hyperkinesias, but are the result of loss of position sense.

Choreoathetoid movements are those that appear to lie between choreic and athetoid movements in rate and rhythmicity, and may represent a transitional form. They probably result from a pathologic process similar to that causing athetosis, but slightly at variance in location. They may be present with many disorders, including birth injury, Wilson's disease,

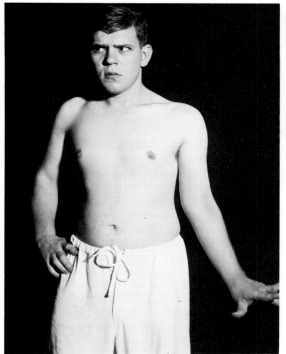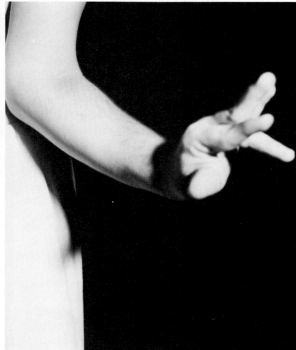

FIG. 31–2. A patient with congenital unilateral athetosis.

liver disease, and ataxia with oculocutaneous telangiectasia. Families with both paroxysmal dystonic choreoathetosis and paroxysmal kinesogenic choreoathetosis have been reported. The latter variety, which is movement-induced, is a form of reflex epilepsy and responds to anticonvulsant medication.

DYSTONIA

In **dystonia** there are movements that are similar in many respects to those seen in athetosis, but they involve larger portions of the body, and there are distorted postures of the limbs and trunk resulting from excessive tone in certain muscle groups. The movements are slow, bizarre, may be grotesque in type, and have an undulant, writhing, twisting, and turning character. They may start distally, usually in the foot, with plantar flexion and inversion, and then spread to the opposite side, the upper extremities, and the trunk, face, and tongue. In advanced cases there are writhing movements of the shoulder muscles, hip girdles, and trunk. The patient twists his spine in a peculiar fashion, bringing about marked torsion of the entire ver-

tebral axis with lordosis, scoliosis, and tilting of the shoulders and pelvis. Dysarthria, facial grimacing, and torticollis (Chapter 16) may be present. The muscles are often in a constant state of hypertonicity, and the muscular contraction itself may cause severe pain. The movements are involuntary but are increased by voluntary activity and emotion. Eventually postures become fixed by contractures, and deformities develop. Denny–Brown preferred to use the term dystonia for the postures assumed by the patient, or the fixed or relatively fixed attitude in association with other disorders of movement, rather than for the hyperkinesia itself. Dystonia rarely may be intermittent or paroxysmal, lasting minutes.

Movements of this type are often manifestations of **dystonia musculorum deformans,** a rare progressive disease that usually begins in childhood. It is most often heredo-familial, inherited either as a dominant or recessive trait, although sporadic cases are encountered. Theoretically the symptoms result from pathophysiologic alterations in the extrapyramidal system, principally in the caudate nucleus and putamen, at times in the thalamus as well. Occasionally, imaging procedures confirm lesions in these structures. In recent years dystonic movements have most frequently been seen after the ingestion of phenothiazine and other psychotropic drugs and as a dose-related symptom of levodopa and dopaminergic drugs. They have also been reported to occur from ingestion of cimetidine. They have also been present in severe athetosis, in Wilson's disease, in Huntington's chorea as it progresses, and with vascular, neoplastic, metabolic, and other disorders affecting the basal ganglia.

In spasmodic torticollis (Ch. 16) there are torsion movements of the head and neck and sometimes of the shoulders that resemble those seen in dystonia. In the beginning the twisting and turning may be intermittent, or present only in paroxysms, but later in the course of the syndrome there is persistent contraction of the involved muscles with resulting deviation of the head.

Focal dystonias of peripheral origin have been described in relation to nerve, plexus, or nerve root trauma and entrapment, at times related to occupational factors. These blend into the disorders listed under cramps.

ORAL – FACIAL DYSKINESIAS

Oral – facial dyskinesias are bizarre movements of the mouth, face, jaw, and tongue that may consist of grimacing, pursing of the mouth and lips, "fish-gaping" movements, and writhing movements of the tongue. These often develop after prolonged use of phenothiazine and other psychotropic drugs, and for this reason are often spoken of as **tardive dyskinesias.** They may, however, occur shortly after the administration of the drug has been started, and they may be associated with the use of other drugs, such as levodopa and dopamine agonists, in which case they are dose-related. Unfortunately, the term tardive dyskinesia is often used for all oral – facial movements, which sometimes develop with no relation to drug use, especially in older people, edentulous persons, and patients with long-standing psychoses. They are sometimes associated with midline cerebellar lesions. Also, drug-induced dyskinesias associated with the use of phenothiazine and other pharmaceutical preparations may take other forms, such as parkinsonian manifestations, chorea, athetoid and dystonic movements, akathisias, and oculogyric crises. Blepharospasm and spastic dysphonia often combine with oral-facial dyskinesias as the so-called **Meige syndrome.**

SPASMS

Spasms are generally organically precipitated contractions of a single muscle or of a group of muscles, often of all the muscles supplied by a single nerve. Clonic spasms are rapid in onset and brief in duration and may be repetitive; they often result in movement of the affected part. Tonic spasms are more prolonged or continuous; they may cause either alteration of position or limitation of movement. Spasms that limit movement may be defensive or protective. A painful, tonic, spasmodic muscular contraction is often spoken of as a cramp. Prolonged spasm may cause reflex rigidity or be followed by muscular contracture.

Spasms are usually of reflex origin and may result from irritation or stimulation at any level from the cortex to the muscle fiber. In most cases, however, they are due to peripheral irritation affecting either muscles or nerves. They may occur in any musculature of the body. They must be differentiated from tics, or habit spasms. Unfortunately the two terms are often used interchangeably.

Pain may cause either tonic or clonic spasms of muscles, especially if the painful stimulus is focal or discrete; this may cause defensive spasm and reflex rigidity. Mechanical irritation may cause local spasm. Associated with the hyperirritability of the nerves and muscles in tetany and tetanus there may be prolonged and characteristic muscle spasm. Muscle spasm and rigidity may also occur on a voluntary basis or in response to fear, excitement, or tension. Most of these phenomena are considered abnormalities of tone rather than muscle spasms, and are discussed in Chapter 28. Spasms may follow injury or irritation of peripheral nerves, especially during the progress of regeneration. They may also result from irritation of motor nuclei in the brain stem or spinal cord or from disease processes within these structures. Finally, they may be produced by irritation of cortical centers in the brain or lesions of descending motor pathways. Some of the more common spasms are now discussed.

Facial spasm usually consists of brief, clonic, repeated contractions of the muscles supplied by one of the facial nerves. The movements may involve the frontalis, corrugator, and orbicularis oculi as well as the muscles of the lower portion of the face. The spasm usually follows a peripheral type of facial palsy, and may develop during the course of recovery. The entire nerve or only certain branches may be affected, and there may be repeated contractions of the various muscles supplied by the involved nerve, with wrinkling of the forehead, closing of the eye, and retraction of the angle of the mouth. If the spasm affects only the orbicularis oculi, it is termed a **blepharospasm.** Facial spasm and blepharospasm may at times be temporarily alleviated by injections of botulinum toxin into the affected muscles. If there is a faulty regeneration of the facial nerve with misdirection of the outgrowth or regenerating fibers, retraction of the mouth may be accompanied by spasm of the orbicularis oculi, or winking may be accompanied by a spasmodic drawing back of the angle of the mouth (see Fig. 13-9). If the movements are tonic, there is facial contracture. Reflex spasm may also result from pain in the involved side of the face, irritation of the facial nerve anywhere along its course, irritation of the facial nucleus by demyelinating, vascular, or neoplastic disorders, or irritations of that portion of the cerebral cortex that controls facial movements (jacksonian manifestations). In the risus sardonicus of tetanus there is a tonic spasm of the facial muscles. Chvostek's sign in tetany is characterized by hyperirritability of the facial nerve and muscles, causing brief spasm on stimulation of them.

Other spasms have been mentioned with other motor cranial nerves. Spasms of the eye muscles may be of either peripheral or central origin. Oculogyric crises may be considered as spasms of upward gaze. In trismus there is a spasm of the muscles of mastication. In tic douloureux the facial muscles may go into spasm as a result of sudden, severe pain. Spasm of the pharynx, larynx, esophagus, or cardia may be of reflex origin, associated with organic disease such as rabies or tetany, or of psychogenic origin. Spasm of the sternocleidomastoid, especially if reflex in origin and not persistent, may cause a torticollis. This, however, is more frequently characterized by a dystonic type of movement (see Dystonia). Glossospasm, or spasm of the tongue, may be of either reflex or psychogenic origin.

Hiccup, or **singultus,** is a brief spasm, or reflex contraction, of the diaphragm, usually associated with adduction of the vocal cords and forcible inspiration of air into the lungs. There is a sudden arrest of inspiration by closure of the glottis; this produces the peculiar respiratory sound. Hiccup may be reflexly excited by stimulation of sensory nerves over a wide area, especially the phrenic or vagus nerves. It may follow irritation of the lower end of the esophagus, gastric distention, irritation of the lungs or pleura, mediastinal or intrathoracic abscesses and tumors, aortic aneurysm, and abdominal irritation or distention. It may also follow central irritation, be part of brain stem vascular disease (lateral medullary syndrome), be associated with changes in the body chemistry (acetonemia or uremia), be a manifestation of encephalitis or other central nervous system disease, or be of psychogenic origin. In intractable cases it may be necessary to perform section of the phrenic nerve.

Spasms may occur in any of the viscera: the stomach, pylorus, small or large intestine, rectum, ureter, bladder, or anal or vesical sphincter. Such spasms may be associated with irritation, pain, inflammation, or other reflex causes. In tabetic crises there is painful spasm of the viscera. Spasm of the bodily musculature, especially if it causes reflex rigidity, may be an important diagnostic criterion in abdominal disease and osteomyelitis. Localized myospasm, or muscular cramps, may occur secondary to vascular insufficiency, fatigue, anoxia, alkalosis, calcium or magnesium deficiency, sodium and potassium imbalance, infection, drug ingestion, and exposure to cold, and in some diseases of muscle, such as McArdle's disease and idiopathic paroxysmal myoglobinuria (Ch. 28). Localized spasm may also be of psychogenic origin; such spasm of the posterior cervical muscles may be responsible for some cases of the so-called tension headache.

Focal jacksonian attacks, especially if they are limited to the face, an arm, a leg, or one half of the body, are manifestations of muscle spasm. Here there is involvement of a group of muscles that are synergistic in function. The movements are clonic in nature, and result from stimulation of the contralateral motor cortex. The characteristic distribution in cerebral hemiplegia — flexion in the upper extremity and extension in the lower — may also be considered as manifestations of spasm. Hypertonicity of the muscles, however, with selective preference for certain groups, secondary to removal of cerebral inhibition, adequately explains this phenomenon. Following transection of the spinal cord there may be mass spasms of the lower extremities. These are essentially reflex in nature and are responses to cutaneous and proprioceptive stimuli that are acting on spinal centers no longer inhibited by higher levels. They are discussed with the reflexes of spinal automatism (Ch. 36).

TICS

In contrast to a true spasm, a **tic** is usually regarded as a **habit spasm** and is considered to be of psychogenic origin. A tic may be defined as a coordinated, repetitive, seemingly purposive act involving a group of muscles in their normal synergistic relationships. Most tics are conditioned reflexes. They are originally precipitated by some physical or emotional stimulus but are perpetuated as a stereotyped, recurrent, relatively involuntary movement. Tics, like spasms, consist of brief contractions of whole muscles or groups of muscles, but are always accompanied by motion of the affected part. They appear suddenly and recur at irregular intervals. They may imitate or resemble true spasms, but are often more or less bizarre or complex. They may be faster and sharper than spasms, and are seemingly purposeful. They are not usually confined to a single muscle or group of muscles, and may involve the opposing action of more than one nerve. They are stereotyped movements and are always reproduced in the same definite pattern. The movements can be controlled to a certain extent by the will. They are often compulsive in nature and they cease during sleep. They are exaggerated by emotional strain and tension; they may become less marked when the patient's attention is diverted. They are often associated with an intolerable mounting tension. Voluntary inhibition causes a state of anxiety that is temporarily relieved by indulgence in a tic.

Tics, or habit spasms, may involve any portion of the body. A blepharospasm, which may originate as a true spasm if associated with irritation of the eye, may persist as a tic after the irritating stimulus has been removed. Habit spasms of the face may be difficult to differentiate from true spasms, but they fail to follow the organic distribution of motor stimulation. For instance, instead of raising of the forehead by the action of the frontalis in association with contraction of the orbicularis oculi, there may be lowering of the eyebrow. Other muscles aside from those supplied by the facial nerve may be brought into action. Spasmodic torticollis may originate as a tic or compulsive movement. Rotatory and shrugging movements of the head and shoulders may be tics, and the muscles of the extremities may be involved. Habit spasms of the abdominal muscles and of the diaphragm may resemble a hiccup or may be characterized by sudden jerking movements and cause motion of the body as a whole; they may be accompanied by grunting or barklike respirations. Multiple tics may persist after chorea. Tics are more often present in children than adults. A **tiqueur** is a person who is subject to one or multiple tics.

Giles de la Tourette's syndrome (*maladie des tics*) is a rare condition that has its onset in childhood, and occurs most frequently in boys, usually in the preadolescent period. It is characterized by the presence of multiple tics, imitative gestures, stereotyped movements, grunts and groans, explosive utterances that frequently are of an obscene nature, and evidence of regressive behavior. The symptoms have been shown to improve with the use of the butyrophenone haloperidol as well as with pimozide. The syndrome has been considered to be of nonorganic origin, but some authorities suggest that it has an organic basis. This syndrome is familial in a minority of cases, but no consistent hereditary pattern has emerged. Dopaminergic overactivity has been advocated as a cause, but the neuropathologic basis is uncertain.

CRAMPS

Cramps may be defined as localized, involuntary, painful contractions of skeletal muscles. They may affect a portion of a muscle, an entire muscle, or groups of muscles that act together synergistically. The contractions are sustained, but usually for only limited periods of time. They may cause movement at joints, which results in contractures for the duration of the cramp.

Most if not all people experience occasional cramps, which may have no known single etiology. They do seem, however, to be precipitated by exertion and by cold. Those that occur during sleep and cause awakening may be precipitated by minor movements during sleep. Abnormalities in muscle metabolism such as those secondary to disturbances in calcium, lactic acid, and the various muscle enzymes may underlie frequent cramps; in McArdle's disease, which occurs in young men, there is a disorder of muscle energy metabolism secondary to phosphorylase deficiency. The muscle contractions that occur in tetanus, tetany, and the stiff-man syndrome are referred to by some authorities as cramps.

The cramps known as **occupational spasms,** such as **writer's cramp** and the spasms of the typist's finger or the violinist's shoulder, are characterized by extreme spasm and tension of certain muscle groups that interfere with specific activities and come on only when the attempt is made to carry out these activities.

In writer's cramp, for example, the muscles of the hand and fingers become rigid and painful as the patient starts to write and his writing becomes illegible. There is no atrophy, weakness, or electromyographic change in the muscles, however, and they can be used normally for other tasks. Similar cramps may occur in telegraphers, pianists, and others. Because they do not appear to have an organic etiology, occupational spasms have been called occupational neuroses. However, they have also been called focal dystonias and treated as such. Probably both organic and nonorganic varieties exist.

HYPERKINESIAS INVOLVING MAJOR PORTIONS OF THE BODY

Convulsive attacks and other involuntary muscular contractions that involve major portions of the body may be regarded as hyperkinesias. Convulsions and the convulsive disorders have been described in detail under the discussion of the neurologic history (Ch. 2). The diagnosis of the convulsive states is considered more at length in Chapter 53. It should be repeated that an accurate description of the convulsive attack, should any be seen, is of paramount importance. In the grand mal or major motor seizure one should note the objective manifestations of the aura, the cry, the tonic and clonic phases of the attack, and the postconvulsion manifestations and behavior. Any suggestions of lateralization or localization should be stressed. Jacksonian, or focal, attacks should be described in detail, noting the site of the first hyperkinetic manifestations and the spread of the motor phenomena. One should also attempt to describe, as accurately as possible, absence seizures, complex partial seizures, akinetic seizures, tonic (so-called cerebellar) epilepsy, status epilepticus, and other equivalents and variants. Fainting, or simple syncope, may be related to epilepsy, and its objective manifestations should be described.

An unusual focal abnormal movement disorder is seen in the **alien hand syndrome,** when automaton-like behavior and excursion of an upper extremity occurs contralateral to a deep frontal and corpus callosum lesion.

Familial hyperkinesias are seen in the syndromes of **hyperekplexia** (pathologic startle response) and **restless legs;** both conditions respond to anticonvulsants and are not invariably familial.

Other generalized disturbances of bodily motility may be seen. Some of these, such as catatonic rigidity, tetanus, and tetany may be regarded as disturbances of tone rather than hyperkinesias, and are described in the discussion of muscle tone. Decerebrate rigidity is also described in Chapter 37, "Postural and Righting Reflexes." Mass movements that follow transection of the spinal cord are discussed in Chapter 36. In meningitis there may be either spasmodic or persistent generalized rigidity with opisthotonos, emprosthotonos, or pleurothotonos. The diagnostic signs of tetany and meningitis are referred to in Chapter 39. **Jactitation,** the to-and-fro tossing of the patient who is acutely ill, and **carphology,** the involuntary picking at the bedclothes by patients in febrile states and conditions of great exhaustion, are indicators of grave illness.

Akathisia is defined as motor restlessness, or the inability to sit still and the irresistible urge to move about. It has been described in Parkinson's disease and related states, but also occurs with agitation and after the ingestion of psychotropic drugs. Children with organic brain damage often are hyperactive, restless, impulsive, and readily distracted.

PSYCHOGENIC HYPERKINESIAS

Psychogenic hyperkinesias, or hysterical movements, are defined as those that do not correspond to any of the previously described types; they are bizarre, change in type from time to time, and are influenced by tension and suggestion. There is no adequate collective name for them. Those most frequently seen are tics, or habit spasms. They may be unconscious and purely involuntary or they may be of compulsive or obsessional origin. Mannerisms are somewhat more complicated and stereotyped and are usually carried out in a more leisurely manner. They may appear only under emotional stress or when the patient is engaged in some particular activity.

Many of the abnormal movements that have been described may occasionally be of psychogenic as well as organic origin, or may be exaggerated by emotion. Convulsions may be precipitated by emotional tension, but attacks that closely resemble major motor seizures may be seen in hysteria. Organic and functional "seizures" can be differentiated by electroencephalographic video monitoring technics. Generalized hypertonicity that resembles that of tetany and tetanus may also be seen in hysteria. In so-called major hysteria there may be neck retraction and opisthotonos with the *arc de cercle.*

Abnormalities of movement of various types may be encountered in mental disease. There may be either overactivity or underactivity, with psychomotor hyperkinesia, hypokinesia, or akinesia. In **parakinesia,** which is usually of psychogenic origin, there is perversion of motor function that results in strange and unnatural movements. This may cause either distortion of movement, with motor manifestations that resemble those seen in chorea and athetosis, or psychomotor dyspraxia, with difficulty in the performance of skilled acts. In manic states there is motor acceleration with increased activity; in depressed states there is lack of initiative with diminished motor activity; in schizophrenia there may be negativism with bizarre mannerisms and sometimes increase in tone; and in childhood schizophrenia there may be rocking, pushing, and circling movements. Various parakinesias are seen in the organic psychoses, and marked motor overactivity in delirium.

If the hyperkinesia defies classification and is too bizarre to be considered of organic origin, it should be described in detail. The possibility that it may be a hysterical conversion phenomenon should be borne in mind.

LOCALIZATION

To sum up the hyperkinesias briefly from the point of view of localization, it may be seen that any of the levels of the motor system, from the motor cortex to the muscle itself, may be involved in their production. Lesions at various sites may be related to different forms of abnormal movement. If one is familiar with the site of the pathologic change that is predominantly responsible for the various types, one may be able to determine the specific localization of the disease process. The lesion itself may not cause the movement, but it may permit intact structures to function in an abnormal manner.

BIBLIOGRAPHY

Adams RD, Foley JM. The neurological disorder associated with liver disease. Assoc Res Nerv Dis Proc 1953;32:198

Adams RD, Victor M. Principles of Neurology, 4th ed. New York,: McGraw – Hill, 1989

Ahronheim JC. Hyperthyroid chorea in an elderly woman associated with sole elevation of T3. J Am Geriat Soc 1988;36:242

Aiger BR, Mulder DW. Myoclonus: Clinical significance and an approach to classification. Arch Neurol 1960;2:600

Albin RL, Bromberg MB, Penney JB, Knapp R. Chorea and dystonia: A remote effect of carcinoma. Movement Disorders 1988;3:162

Altrocchi PH. Spontaneous oral-facial dyskinesia. Arch Neurol 1972;26:506

Andrew J, Fowler CJ, Harrison MJ. Tremor after head injury and its treatment by stereotaxic surgery. J Neurol Neurosurg Psychiatry 1982;45:815

Angelini L, Rumi V, Lamperti E, Nardocci N. Transient paroxysmal dystonia in infancy. Neuropediatrics 1988; 19:171

Appenzeller O, Biehl JP. Mouthing in the elderly: A cerebellar sign. J Neurol Sci 1968;6:249

Banks G, Short P, Martinez AJ, Latchaw R et al. The alien hand syndrome. Clinical and postmortem findings. Arch Neurol 1989;46:456

Biary N, Cleeves L, Findley L, Koller W. Post-traumatic tremor. Neurology 1989;39:103

Biary N, Koller WC. Essential tongue tremor. Movement Disorders 1987;2:25

Biary N, Koller W. Handedness and essential tremor. Arch Neurol 1985;42:1082

Brick JF, Gutmann L. Rattlesnake venom-induced myokymia. Muscle Nerve 1982;5:S98

Brumlik J. On the nature of normal tremor. Neurology 1962;12:159

Bruyn GW, Padberg G. Chorea and polycythemia. Eur Neurol 1984;3:26

Bruyn GW, Padberg G. Chorea and systemic lupus erythematosus. A critical review. Eur Neurol 1984;23:278

Burne JA. Reflex origin of parkinsonian tremor. Experiment Neurol 1987;97:327

Carpenter MB. Athetosis and the basal ganglia. Arch Neurol Psychiatry 1950;63:875

Conn HO. Asterixis in non-hepatic disorders. Am J Med 1960;29:647

Critchley M. Observations on essential (heredofamilial) tremor. Brain 1949;72:113

Darras BT, Ampola MG, Dietz WH, Gilmore HE. Intermittent dystonia in Hartnup disease. Pediatry Neurol 1989; 5:118

Daube JR, Peters JR. Hereditary essential myoclonus. Arch Neurol 1966;15:587

Davis CH Jr, Kunkle EC. Benign essential (heredofamilial) tremor. Arch Intern Med 1951;87:808

Denny – Brown D. The nature of dystonia. Bull NY Acad Med 1965;41:858

Eldridge R, Fahn S. Dystonia. New York, Raven Press, 1976

Farmer TW, Wingfield MS, Lynch SA et al. Ataxia, chorea, seizures, and dementia. Pathologic features of a newly defined familial disorder. Arch Neurol 1989;46:774

Field JR, Corbin KB, Goldstein NB, Klass DW. Gilles de la Tourette's syndrome. Neurology 1966;16:453

Forster FM, Borkowski WJ, Alpers BJ. Effects of denervation on fasciculations in human muscles: relations of fibrillations to fasciculations. Arch Neurol Psychiatry 1946; 56:276

Friedman DI, Jankovic J, Rolak LA. Arteriovenous malformation presenting as hemidystonia. Neurology 1986; 36:1590

Gruener R, McArdle B, Ryman BE et al. Contracture of phosphorylase deficient muscle. J Neurol Neurosurg Psychiatry 1968;31:268

Haerer AF, Currier RD, Jackson JF. Hereditary nonprogressive chorea of early onset. N Engl J Med 1967;276:1220

Herz E. Dystonia. Historical reviews, analysis of dystonic symptoms and physiologic mechanisms involved. Arch Neurol Psychiatry 1944;51:305

Herz E. Dystonia. Clinical classification. Arch Neurol Psychiatry 1944;51:319

Hodge JR. Akathisia: The syndrome of motor restlessness. Am J Psychiatry 1959;116:337

Hoehn M, Cherington M. Spinal myoclonus. Neurology 1977;27:942

Hoogstraten MC, Lakke JP, Zwarts MJ. Bilateral ballism: A rare syndrome. J Neurol 1986;233:25

Hunt JR. Dyssynergia cerebellaris myoclonica. Brain 1921;44:490

Jacobs L, Newman RP, Bozian D. Disappearing palatal myoclonus. Neurology 1981;31:748

Jankovic J, Ford J. Blepharospasm and orofacial-cervical dystonia: Clinical and pharmacological findings in 100 patients. Ann Neurol 1983;13:402

Kempster PA, Brenton DP, Gale AN, Stern GM. Dystonia in homocystinuria. J Neurol Neurosurg Psychiatry 1988;51:859

Klawans HL, Barr A. Prevalence of spontaneous lingual-facial-buccal dyskinesias in the elderly. Neurology 1982;32:558

Koller W, O'Hara R, Dorus W, Bauer J. Tremor in chronic alcoholism. Neurology 1985;35:1660

Kotagal P, Lüders H, Morris HH et al. Dystonic posturing in complex partial seizures of temporal lobe onset: a new lateralizing sign. Neurology 1989;39:196

Lance JW. Action myoclonus, Ramsay – Hunt syndrome, and other cerebellar myoclonic syndromes. Adv Neurol 1986;43:33

Lance JW, Adams RD. The syndrome of intention or action myoclonus as a sequel to hypoxic encephalopathy. Brain 1963;86:111

Layser RB, Rowland LP. Cramps. N Engl J Med 1971;285:31

Lugaresi E, Cirignotta F, Montagna P. Nocturnal paroxysmal dystonia. J Neurol Neurosurg Psychiatry 1986;49:375

Marsden CD, Obeso JA, Zarranz JJ, Lang AE. The anatomical basis of symptomatic hemidystonia. Brain 1985;108:463

Mateer JE, Gutmann L, McComas CF. Myokymia in Guillain – Barré syndrome. Neurology 1983;33:374

Mayeux R, Albert M, Jenike M. Physostigmine-induced myoclonus in Alzheimer's disease. Neurology 1987;37:345

McDaniel KD, Cummings JL, Shain S. The "yips": A focal dystonia of golfers. Neurology 1989;39:192

Montplaisir J, Godbout R, Boghen D, DeChamplain J et al. Familial restless legs with periodic movements in sleep: Electrophysiologic, biochemical, and pharmacologic study. Neurology 1985;35:130

Nath A, Jankovic J, Pettigrew LC. Movement disorders and AIDS. Neurology 1987;37:37

Nathanson M. Palatal myoclonus: Further clinical and pathophysiological observations. Arch Neurol Psychiatry 1956;75:285

Nausieda PA, Grossman BJ, Koller WC, Weiner WJ et al. Sydenham chorea: an update. Neurology 1980;30:331

Obeso JA, Viteri C, Martinez Lage JM, Marsden CD. Toxic myoclonus. Adv Neurol 1986;43:225

Peterson DI, Peterson GW. Unilateral asterixis due to ipsilateral lesions in the pons and medulla. Ann Neurol 1987;22:661

Plant GT, Williams AC, Earl CJ, Marsden CD. Familial paroxysmal dystonia induced by exercise. J Neurol Neurosurg Psychiatry 1984;47:275

Rector WG Jr, Herlong HF, Moses H, 3rd. Nonketotic hyperglycemia appearing as choreoathetosis or ballism. Arch Intern Med 1982;142:154

Rhee KJ, Albertson DE, Douglas JC. Choreoathetoid disorder associated with amphetamine-like drugs. Am J Emergency Med 1988;6:131

Ribera AB, Cooper IS. The natural history of dystonia musculorum deformans. Arch Pediatr 1960;77:55

Richards NR, Barnett HJM. Paroxysmal dystonic choreoathetosis. Neurology 1968;18:461

Romisher S, Felter R, Dougherty J. Tagamet-induced acute dystonia. Ann Emergency Med 1987;16:1162

Sáenz – Lope E, Herranz – Tannaro FJ, Masdeu JC, Chacón Peña, Jr. Hyperekplexia: A syndrome of pathological startle responses. Ann Neurol 1984;15:36

Samie MR, Ashton AK. Choreoathetosis induced by cyproheptadine. Movement Disorders 1989;4:81

Saris S. Chorea caused by caudate infarction. Arch Neurol 1983;40:590

Sax DS, Bird ED, Gusella JF, Myers RH. Phenotypic variation in 2 Huntington's disease families with linkage to chromosome 4. Neurology 1989;39:1332

Schady W, Meara RJ. Hereditary progressive chorea without dementia. J Neurol Neurosurg Psychiatry 1988;51:295

Scherokman B, Husain F, Guetter A, Jabbari B et al. Peripheral dystonia. Arch Neurol 1986;43:830

Schwarz GA, Yaroff M. Lafora's disease: Distinct clinicopathologic form of Unverricht's syndrome. Arch Neurol 1965;12:311

Sethi KD, Ray R, Roesel RA et al. Adult-onset chorea and dementia with propionic acidemia. Neurology 1989;39:1343

Stevens H. Jumping Frenchmen of Maine: Myriachit. Arch Neurol 1965;12:311

Stevens H. Paroxysmal choreoathetosis. Arch Neurol 1966;14:415

Swanson PD, Luttrell CN, Magladery JW. Myoclonus: A report of 67 cases and review of the literature. Medicine 1962;41:339

Waybright EA, Gutmann L, Chou SM. Facial myokymia. Pathological features. Arch Neurol 1979;36:244

Wee AS, Subramony SH, Currier RD. Orthostatic tremor in familial-essential tremor. Neurology 1986;36:1241

Weiner WJ, Nausieda PA, Klawans HL. Methylphenidate-induced chorea: Case report and pharmacologic implications. Neurology 1978;28:1041

Welch LK, Appenzeller O, Bicknell JW. Peripheral neuropathy with myokymia, sustained muscular contraction, and continued motor unit activity. Neurology 1972;22:161

Chapter 32
STATION AND GAIT

The evaluation of the patient's station and gait is an essential part of the examination of the motor system, and the appraisal of these functions may yield much relevant information. The patient's position when standing and his mode of locomotion should not, however, be considered the sole diagnostic criteria, even though they may, at times, be pathognomonic of certain nervous system disorders. They are, nevertheless, important when considered in conjunction with the other neurologic findings.

Reference to the general appearance of the body as a whole was made in Chapter 3, and the gait has been discussed in some detail in the tests for coordination (Ch. 30). The postural and righting reflexes are described in Chapter 37. Posture, however, and locomotion merit individual discussion from a diagnostic point of view, and specific disorders of gait are especially significant.

EXAMINATION OF STATION

Posture is an active neuromuscular process that is dependent upon a number of factors and reflex responses. It is a complicated mechanism, especially in the human, whose biped gait and erect position over a narrow base require more efficient maintenance and control of equilibrium than is necessary in quadrupeds. An involuntary contraction of muscles is necessary for normal positions and attitudes. Tonus, especially of the antigravity muscles, is essential. Centers in the brain stem play a part in controlling the steady contraction of the antigravity muscles that is necessary for the standing position. Righting reflexes and more complex reflexes have as their afferent stimuli proprioceptive impulses from the skeletal muscles as well as labyrinthine and visual impulses. Standing may be considered a postural reflex that is dependent upon reflexes mediated through the medulla and influenced to a marked degree by tonic neck and labyrinthine reflexes. If any of the mechanisms responsible for static or postural reflexes are impaired, normal standing will be impaired. In addition, however, proprioceptive sensations must be mediated from the extremities and trunk, the skeletal system must be intact, the muscles must be functioning normally, and coordination must be adequate. Posture is affected by disturbances of proprioceptive sensation, derangements of muscle power or tone, abnormalities of vestibular function, and dysfunction of the basal ganglia, the cerebellum, and their connections.

Station may be defined as the patient's attitude, or manner of standing. His posture, the position of his body as a whole, and the position of its parts are noted, and any abnormality is observed. The attitude and position of the head, the position of the extremities, and any outstanding skeletal anomalies are significant. The healthy individual stands in the erect position with his head up, chest out, and abdomen in. Abnormalities of station may indicate dysfunction of the skeletal and muscular systems as well as nervous system impairment. Skeletal changes such as kyphosis, scoliosis, lordosis; abnormalities in the position of the head, shoulders, hips, or extremities; and asymmetries, anomalies of development and abnormalities of contour may give diagnostic information. Poor posture may be evidence of inadequate muscular development. In weakness and in debilitated states the patient may need support to stand erect. If the patient is unable to stand, the position of the body should be noted in the seated or the recumbent position. A tendency to lie on one side, drawing up of the knees, and opisthotonos may all be diagnostically significant.

From a neurologic point of view, station is tested by having the patient stand with his feet closely approximated, first with the eyes open and then with the eyes closed. Any unsteadiness, swaying, deviation, or tremor should be noted. Station may be further evaluated by having the patient stand, with the eyes both open and closed, on one foot at a time, on his toes and then his heels, and in a tandem position with one heel in front of the toes of the other foot. He may be given a push to see whether he falls to one side, forward, or backward. Additional tests include having him hop on one foot; mark time; rise from a supine or seated position; stoop and resume the erect position; and bend backward, forward, and to each side. It is often of value to keep a photographic record of the patient's station and posture.

Certain abnormalities of station are pathognomonic of nervous system dysfunction. In diseases of the proprioceptive pathways there is a sensory type of ataxia, and the patient is able to maintain the erect position with the eyes open, but sways or falls when they are closed (**Romberg's sign**). He may attempt to compensate for his unsteadiness by placing his feet some distance apart, in order to stand with a broader base. In cerebellar disease there is swaying with the eyes open and closed, and the patient may have to stand with a broad base. With a vermis lesion the patient may sway backward, forward, or to either side. With hemispheric cerebellar disease and unilateral vestibular involvement he falls toward the affected side. In the **false Romberg test,** seen in hysteria, the patient sways from his hips instead of from his ankles; he may sway through a wide arc and it may seem inevitable that he will fall, but he is usually able to regain his balance and resume the upright position. If he does fall, he does not hurt himself. It may be possible to divert the patient's attention during the Romberg test by having him carry out the finger-to-nose test. In tabes dorsalis or in other syndromes in which there is true sensory ataxia this will be accompanied by increasing unsteadiness; in hysteria the patient

may be able to carry out the test without difficulty.

The attitude and station may give specific information in certain disease syndromes. In hemiparesis there is a characteristic deformity with flexion of the upper extremity and extension of the lower extremity. In Parkinson's disease there is stooping with the head and neck bent forward and the arms and knees flexed. In the muscular dystrophies there is a pronounced lordosis. In depressed states there may be a stooped and dejected appearance; in manic states, an erect domineering position; in schizophrenia the patient may assume bizarre postures that he may hold for long periods of time. Hyperkinesias such as athetoid and choreic movements may become evident while station is being tested.

EXAMINATION OF GAIT

Gait, or the act of walking or locomotion, is an intricate process that is influenced by a number of bodily mechanisms and is the result of the integrity of many different types of reflexes. As with station, the following are needed: simple reflex mechanisms at the spinal cord level; postural and standing reflexes that hold the body erect by increased tone of the antigravity muscles; neck and labyrinthine reflexes for the proper maintenance of tone; righting reflexes to maintain the position of the head, limbs, and trunk; integration of motor function from the cortex; automatic mechanisms mediated by the basal ganglia for posture, tone, associated movements, and synergisms; coordinating functions of the cerebellum; sensory elements, mainly proprioceptive, to inform the individual of the position of the various parts of the body and to give proper spatial orientation.

During walking, the weight of the body is supported by one lower extremity while the other executes the movement of progression. The supporting limb is first fully extended, but the heel is lifted as the center of gravity is advanced. The opposite limb begins the movement of progression as soon as the body weight is transferred to the supporting limb. The weight of the body is then supported for a short interval by the heel of the advancing limb, then by the foot until the heel is lifted and then by the ball of the foot. The normal gait thus represents the heel-toe phases of support and progression. The pelvis rotates slightly to the side of progression. In addition to the movements of the trunk and lower extremities, there are normal associated swinging movements of the upper extremities: as one lower extremity is advanced, the upper extremity of the opposite side advances.

Impairment of the act of walking is found in a wide variety of conditions. Mechanical factors such as diseases of the muscles, bones, tendons, and joints are important. Disorders of the nervous system, however, cause the most significant abnormalities in locomotion, and occasionally the appraisal of the gait alone may reveal the presence and diagnosis of nervous system disease to the practiced eye. Disturbances in gait may follow involvement of any portion of the motor system: the motor cortex and its descending pathways, extrapyramidal complex, cerebellum, anterior horn cells, peripheral motor nerves, or muscles. Abnormalities of the psychomotor level (hysteria and malingering), as well as involvement of the vestibular complex, sensory nerves, posterior columns, and afferent cerebellar pathways, may also cause changes in gait. The evaluation of the gait is important, but it must be appraised along with the other findings.

Gait, like station, is tested with the eyes open and closed. The patient should not only be asked to walk forward, but also backward, sideward, and around a chair. He may be asked to walk on his toes and on his heels; to follow a line on the floor; to walk on a rail; to walk tandem, i.e., to place one heel directly in front of the toes of the other foot; to walk in a sideward direction and to overstep, or cross one foot over the other, in doing so; to walk forward and turn rapidly; to walk forward and backward repeatedly six to eight steps with the eyes closed; to walk slowly, then rapidly, then run; to climb stairs. He may be asked to rise abruptly from a chair, stand erect, walk, stop suddenly, and turn quickly on command (**Fournier's test**).

When appraising the gait one should note the position of the body as a whole and also the freedom of movement, position of the extremities, inclination of the pelvis and thighs, supporting and progression movements of the legs and feet, size and speed of the individual steps, swinging of the arms, and associated movements of the eyes, head, and trunk. One should notice whether the patient walks steadily or unsteadily, watches the ground, assumes a broad base, deviates the body, drags or slaps the feet, or uses any accessory muscles. At times it may be necessary to observe the gait while the patient is assisted in walking or walks with the aid of a cane, crutches, braces, or other apparatus. Some information regarding the gait may be derived from listening to the patient walk. There is a flopping sound to the gait of a person with a foot drop, a dragging or a scraping in spasticity, and a stamping in ataxia. It may be valuable to note the worn places in the patient's shoes. A videotape often aids in interpretation, and also affords a permanent record. It is necessary to recall that there are marked individual variations in gait: each individual has his own gait, which is characteristic to the point that he may be recognized by it. There may even be an inheritance of the characteristics of gait, and children may walk like their parents. Persons in certain occupations may develop special types of gaits — those of the sailor and cowboys are well known.

There are certain mechanical disturbances in gait that may be confused with disorders of neurologic origin. If the skin of the feet is inflamed or irritated by calluses, blisters, or chilblains, or if there are painful hyperesthesias of the feet due to vascular disease or neuropathy, there may be an abnormality in gait that is characterized chiefly by a shortened phase of support. Pain caused by relaxation of the metatarsal arches may result in a similar abnormality of gait. Relaxation of the longitudinal arches causes flat feet, often with a peculiar slapping, everted gait. Myositis of the calf or gluteal muscles may cause limping or shuffling on one or both sides as a result of pain. Arthritis may cause difficulties with gait that are secondary to both pain and deformity. Intense pain in the calf muscles interferes with gait in lumbar stenosis and in intermittent claudication. The latter is usually associated with vascular disease in the lower extremities; the pain increases as walking is continued and is relieved following a brief period of rest. In pregnancy, ascites, and abdominal tumors there may be a lordosis that resembles that seen in the muscular dystrophies. With dislocation of the hips there may be a waddling that is suggestive of the dystrophic gait. Marked stooping in ankylosing spondylitis may resemble that of parkinsonism. Other skeletal, muscular, and orthopedic dysfunctions may simulate nervous system disease.

There are various abnormalities of gait that are of diagnostic importance in neurologic disease. Some of them may even be considered as pathognomonic of certain disease processes. The more important and more characteristic of these are described. On occasion two or more of these may be present simultaneously.

The Gait of Weakness

It must be recalled that illness of any duration may be followed by some abnormality in locomotion. This so-called gait of weakness is not characteristic of any specific neurologic disease or of focal nervous system damage, but inasmuch as it may be confused with other gaits, especially the ataxic and hysterical varieties, it should be mentioned. The gait of weakness is seen most frequently in wasting and debilitating diseases of long duration, but it may be present in association with an acute illness of any severity. It may, for instance, be apparent after a short period of confinement to bed or after a brief febrile episode. It is characterized mainly by unsteadiness and the wish for support. The patient staggers and sways from side to side with a suggestion of ataxia. He may appear anxious to lean on chairs for support or to brace himself against a wall. He moves slowly and his knees may tremble. If the difficulty is marked, he may fall.

Ataxic Gaits

There are two types of ataxic gait — that resulting from sensory ataxia, and that associated with disease of the coordinating mechanisms. Elements of both disturbances may contribute to gait abnormalities in the same person.

The Gait of Sensory Ataxia. This is caused most frequently by interruption of the proprioceptive pathways in the spinal cord. It is commonly encountered in posterolateral sclerosis, multiple sclerosis, and tabes dorsalis. It is often referred to as the **gait of spinal ataxia.** It may also be seen in conditions such as peripheral neuritis and in brain stem lesions where there is interference with the conduction of kinesthetic sensations. The ataxia is caused by impairment of the senses of position and motion of the parts of the body, especially of the joints, muscles, and tendons of the feet and legs, and by a loss of spatial orientation. The patient is no longer aware of the position of his lower extremities in space, or even of the position of the body as a whole, if visual impulses are not correlated with proprioceptive ones. Locomotion may not be abnormal when the patient walks with his eyes open, but if involvement is at all marked it will be noted that the gait is irregular and jerky, and that the patient walks with a broad base. He throws out his feet and comes down first on the heel and then

on the toes with a slapping sound, or "double tap." The phase of progression is lengthened as increased time is necessary to execute the muscular movements required to place the feet on the floor. The patient watches his feet and keeps his eyes on the floor while walking. When the eyes are closed the feet seem to shoot out, the staggering and unsteadiness are increased, and he may be unable to walk. The double tap, by which the hypotonic feet are stamped or brought down noisily in two places, may be so characteristic that the trained observer may suspect the condition by hearing the patient walk. However, the gait of bilateral foot drop may superficially resemble this double-tapping gait.

The Gait of Cerebellar Disorder. The gait of cerebellar disease is caused by involvement of the coordinating mechanisms in the cerebellum and its connecting systems. It is characterized by ataxia that is present with the eyes both open and closed, but even here it is increased somewhat when the eyes are closed. With a vermis or midline lesion there is a staggering, unsteady, irregular, lurching, titubating, wide-based gait, and the patient may sway to either side, backward, or forward. He is unable to walk tandem or follow a straight line on the floor. Tremors and oscillatory movements of the entire body may be noted. This gait, in an exaggerated degree, is seen also in acute alcoholism and drug intoxications.

In disease localized to one cerebellar hemisphere or its connections or in unilateral vestibular disease, there is persistent swaying or deviation toward the involved side. As the patient attempts to walk a straight line or to walk tandem he turns toward the side of the lesion. When walking around a chair, in either a clockwise or a counterclockwise direction, he consistently falls toward the side of the lesion. When walking a few steps backward and forward there may be evidence of the "compass" deviation (Ch. 30).

Spastic Gaits

There are also two types of spastic gait — that associated with unilateral and that with bilateral involvement of the corticospinal pathways.

The Gait of Spastic Hemiparesis. The gait of spastic hemiparesis is seen most frequently following a cerebral vascular lesion, but it may be caused by any lesion that interrupts the corticospinal innervation to one half of the body. There is a spastic hemiparesis contralateral to the lesion, with increased tone, increased reflexes, and a characteristic distribution of weakness. The upper extremity shows marked paresis of extension and is held in flexion and adduction at the shoulder, flexion at the elbow, and flexion at the wrist and interphalangeal joints. The lower extremity shows marked paresis of flexion and is held in extension at the hip and knee, with plantar flexion of the foot and toes (see Fig. 23-8). There is a resulting equinus deformity of the foot, with shortening or contracture of the Achilles tendon, and the lower extremity on the involved side is functionally slightly longer than that on the normal side. When walking the patient holds his arm tightly to the side, rigid and flexed; he extends it with difficulty, and does not swing it in a normal fashion. He holds his leg stiffly in extension and flexes it with difficulty. Consequently the patient drags or shuffles his foot and scrapes the toes. With each step he may tilt the pelvis upward on the involved side to aid in lifting the toe off the floor and may swing the entire extremity around in a semicircle from the hip, or **circumduct** it. The phase of support is shortened because of weakness and the phase of progression is lengthened owing to spasticity and slowing of movement. The sound produced by the scraping of the toe, as well as the wear on the shoe at the toe, may be quite characteristic. The patient may be able to turn toward the paralyzed side more easily than toward the normal side. He may walk in a sideward direction toward the paralyzed side without difficulty, since the opposite, or normal, foot is approximated without scraping. When walking toward the normal side, however, the opposite, or paralyzed leg is dragged and that foot scrapes as it approaches the normal foot. In patients with a very mild hemiparesis, loss of swing of the affected arm may be a significant diagnostic finding. Dragging or scraping of the foot may be apparent only with fatigue.

The Gait of Spastic Paraparesis. The gait of spastic paraparesis is encountered in congenital spastic diplegia, or Little's disease, with incomplete dysfunction of the spinal cord, and related conditions. In these there is spastic paresis of both lower extremities, with less marked or no involvement of the upper extremities. In addition to the extensor deformity of the lower limbs with equinus position of the feet and shortening of the Achilles tendons, there usually is pronounced obturator, or adductor, spasm. As a result the patient walks with a bilateral stiff, shuffling type of gait, dragging his legs and scraping his toes; in addition there is adduction of the thighs, so that the knees may cross, one in front of the other, with each step. This produces the **scissors gait.** The steps are short and slow; the feet seem to stick to the floor. Swaying and staggering may suggest an element of ataxia, but usually there is no true loss of coordination. The shuffling, scraping sound, together with worn areas at the toes of the shoes, may be characteristic.

The Spastic – Ataxic Gait

In many diseases of the nervous system, especially in the posterolateral sclerosis of pernicious anemia and in multiple sclerosis, there is involvement of both the corticospinal and the proprioceptive pathways, with a resulting spastic – ataxic gait.

The amount of ataxia or of spasticity, or the predominance of one over the other, depends upon the site of the predominant pathologic change. The ataxia may be of either the cerebellar or the spinal type. In pernicious anemia it is predominantly the latter; in multiple sclerosis it may have both sensory and cerebellar origin. In amyotrophic lateral sclerosis there may be a bilateral foot drop as well as spasticity, and this may result in an abnormality in walking that may suggest a spastic – ataxic gait.

The Parkinsonian Gait

In the various extrapyramidal syndromes, especially Parkinson's disease and other parkinsonian states, there is an abnormality of gait that is characterized by rigidity, bradykinesia, and loss of associated movements. The gait is slow, stiff, and shuffling; the patient walks with small, mincing steps. There is a characteristic posture with an associated bodily deformity. The patient is stooped, with his head and neck forward and his knees flexed; the upper extremities are flexed at the shoulders, elbows, and wrists, but the fingers may be extended at the interphalangeal joints (see Fig. 22-4). This stooped position causes a forward shifting of the center of gravity, with a tendency to fall forward when walking (**propulsion**), as well as to increase the speed when walking (**festination**). There is difficulty in initiating movements, apparent when the patient gets out of a chair or starts to walk, in stopping, and in carrying out two actions simultaneously. The patient may move *en bloc* and turn about slowly, making small steps in order to do so. Loss of associated movements may be manifested by absence of normal arm swinging in walking; this interferes with speed and balance. Tremors may become more marked while walking. In some cases there is profound akinesia, with little ability to move. Occasionally the parkinsonian manifestations are unilateral.

Marche à Petits Pas

In patients with cerebral or spinal disturbances of various types, there may be an abnormality of gait called *marche à petits pas*, which bears some resemblance to that seen in Parkinson's disease. Locomotion is slow, and the patient walks with very short, mincing, shuffling, somewhat irregular footsteps. There is often a loss of associated movements. This type of gait often is part of the syndrome of **normal pressure hydrocephalus** but may also occur with other types of hydrocephalus. It is often associated with signs and symptoms of dementia and loss of urinary sphincter control in normal pressure hydrocephalus. The same constellation of findings is typical of the syndrome of multi-infarct dementia. Imaging procedures can differentiate these conditions. In some patients with *marche à petits pas*, there are bizarre manifestations, such as dancing or hopping movements. There may be generalized weakness of the lower extremities or of the entire body, the patient fatiguing easily.

Apraxia of Gait

Apraxia of gait is the loss of the ability to use the lower limbs properly in the act of walking, although there is no demonstrable sensory impairment or motor weakness. It is seen in patients with extensive cerebral lesions, especially of the frontal lobes. The patient cannot carry out purposive movements with the legs and feet, such as making a circle or kicking an imaginary ball. In rising, standing, and walking there is difficulty in initiating movements, and the automatic sequence of composite movements is lost. The gait is slow and shuffling, with short steps. The patient may have difficulty in lifting his feet from the floor, or he may raise them without

advancing them. In addition, perseveration, hypokinesia, rigidity, and stiffness of the limb in response to contact (gegenhalten) are often seen.

The Steppage Gait

The steppage gait appears in association with foot drop and is caused by weakness or paralysis of dorsiflexion of the foot and/or the toes. The patient either drags his foot in walking or, in attempting to compensate for the foot drop, lifts his foot as high as possible to keep the toes from scraping the floor. Thus there is an exaggerated flexion at the hip and the knee; the foot is thrown out and the toe flops down with a characteristic sound before either the heel or the ball of the foot strikes the floor. The phase of support is shortened. The patient is unable to stand on his heel, and when he stands with his foot projecting over the edge of a step, the forefoot drops.

The steppage gait may be unilateral or bilateral, and it may result from any of a number of disorders. Perhaps the most common cause is paralysis of the tibialis anterior and/or extensors digitorum and hallucis longus. Lesions of either the common or deep peroneal nerve, of the fourth lumbar through first sacral spinal segments or roots, or of the cauda equina may cause such a paresis. Foot drop and steppage gait may also be present with poliomyelitis, progressive spinal muscular atrophy, amyotrophic lateral sclerosis, Charcot – Marie – Tooth disease, and peripheral neuritis. In many of these conditions the difficulty may be bilateral. If the steppage gait is associated with peripheral neuritis, there is usually sensory as well as motor involvement, and the gait may be complicated by the presence of pain, dysesthesias, and paresthesias, so that support of the body is distressing. The gait under such circumstances may be one of deliberation and hesitation, with a shortened phase of support and prolonged phase of progression.

The Dystrophic Gait

The dystrophic gait is seen in the various myopathies in which there is weakness of the hip girdle muscles. It is most characteristic of muscular dystrophy, but may be present also with myositis and other diseases of the spinomuscular level that affect these muscles. The patient stands and walks with a pronounced lordosis, and in walking there is a marked waddling because of difficulty in fixing the pelvis. The patient walks with a broad base and shows an exaggerated rotation of the pelvis, rolling or throwing his hips from side to side with every step to shift the weight of the body. This compensatory lateral movement of the pelvis is due in large part to weakness of the gluteal muscles. In addition, the patient has marked difficulty in climbing stairs, and he often needs a handrail so that he may pull himself up with his hands. He is also unable to rise from a lying to a seated position without assisting himself with his hands, "climbing up on himself" by placing his hands first on his knees and then on his hips to brace himself (see Fig. 21-5). A waddling type of gait is also seen in association with dislocation of the hips.

Gaits Associated With Various Pareses and Paralyses

The most characteristic of these is the steppage gait, already mentioned, but other pareses may cause other anomalies. With paralysis of the gastrocnemius and soleus muscles the patient is unable to stand on his toes, and the heel comes down first in walking. This may cause a shuffling gait that is devoid of spring. With paresis of the hamstring muscles, there is weakness of flexion at the knee. In paralysis of the quadriceps femoris muscles, as in a femoral neuritis, there is paralysis of extension at the knee; the patient is unable to extend the leg while seated, is unable to climb or descend stairs or rise from a kneeling position without bracing the knee, has to walk by holding the knee stiffly, and tends to fall if the knee bends. He has less difficulty in walking backward than forward. If the deep peroneal nerve is injured below the point where branches are given off to the tibialis anterior and the extensor digitorum longus, there may be only weakness of dorsiflexion on the great toe. In paralysis of the superficial peroneal nerve there is loss of eversion, and the patient walks on the outer aspect of the foot. Lesions of the sciatic nerve and its larger branches may cause varying types of gait anomalies.

Gaits Associated With Various Hyperkinesias

In conditions such as Sydenham's chorea, Huntington's chorea, other forms of transient or persisting chorea, athetosis, and dystonia muscu-

lorum deformans the abnormal movements may become more marked while the patient is walking, and the manifestations of the disease more evident. Not only are the hyperkinesias apparent, but also the changes in power and tone that accompany them. In Sydenham's chorea the jerky, purposeless movements may be observed, as well as the hypotonia with the characteristic hypotonic hand (see "Chorea," Ch. 31). In Huntington's chorea the gait may be grotesque or dancing, and may appear histrionic. In athetosis the distal movements and in dystonia the proximal movements may be marked during walking, and in both there are accompanying grimaces. In postencephalitic states there may be hopping and jumping elements in the gait.

Gaits Associated With Psychoses

In various psychotic processes there are characteristic changes in the gait. The depressed patient is stooped and slowed in walking. The manic patient is overactive and erect. In schizophrenia various abnormalities may be noted, especially if there are catatonic manifestations.

Gaits Associated With Various Organic Diseases

Many other abnormalities of gait may be found in association with muscular, skeletal, and orthopedic abnormalities with secondary nervous system involvement. These will not be mentioned in detail here, although some of them have significance in the neurologic examination. The gait of lumbosacral nerve root irritation is quite characteristic, for example. The patient may walk with a list to the involved side in order to prevent stretching of the roots; he is bent forward and toward the side of the lesion and drops his pelvis on that side. On other occasions the trunk may be inclined toward the opposite side; a scoliosis may result from attempts to keep the weight on the sound limb, and the pelvis is tilted so that the affected hip is prominent and elevated. There is loss of the normal lumbar lordosis owing to involuntary spasm of the low back muscles. The patient walks with small steps; if the pain is severe, he avoids complete extension of the hip and knees and places only the toes on the floor, since dorsiflexion of the foot aggravates the pain. He often uses a cane to keep from bearing weight on the involved leg.

Hysterical Gaits

Individuals with hysteria or other abnormalities in the psychomotor sphere may show various derangements of station and gait. They may be unable either to stand or to walk despite the absence of paralysis. Tests for power, tone, and coordination may be normal if carried out while the patient is lying down. The gait is nondescript and bizarre, and may show variations from the normal that do not conform to a specific organic disease pattern. It is often irregular and changeable, with elements of ataxia, spasticity, and other types of abnormality. There are superfluous movements, and often marked swaying from side to side. The patient may appear to be falling, but is usually able to regain his balance without doing so. If he does fall, it is in a theatrical manner without injury to himself. The gait may suggest the presence of a monoparesis, hemiparesis, or paraparesis, yet the limbs can be used in an emergency. It may show skating, hopping, dancing, or zigzag characteristics; the legs may be thrown out wildly, or there may be a tendency to kneel every few steps. Tremulousness of the extremities or ticlike or compulsive features may be present. Although the patient cannot walk forward, he may be able to walk backward or to one side or to run without difficulty. The bizarre movements often require more coordinative reactions than normally necessary. The term **astasia – abasia** has been given to this type of gait disturbance. These words, however, actually mean "inability to stand and walk," and it is better to use the term **hysterical dysbasia** for the difficulty with gait, and the term **stasibasiphobia** in referring to fear of standing or walking.

BIBLIOGRAPHY

Abd EL, Naby S, Hassanein M. Neuropsychiatric manifestations of chronic manganese poisoning. J Neurol Neurosurg Psychiatry 1965;28:282

Brain R. Posture. Br Med J 1959;1:1489

Fisher CM. Hydrocephalus as a cause of disturbance of gait in the elderly. Neurology 1982;32:1358

Gilman S. Gait disorders. In Rowland LP (ed). Merritt's Textbook of Neurology, 8th ed. Philadelphia, Lea & Febiger, 1989

Koller WC, Trimble J. The gait abnormality of Huntington's disease. Neurology 1985;35:1450

Kotsoris H, Barclay LL, Kheyfets S, Hulyalkar A et al. Urinary and gait disturbances as markers for early multi-infarct dementia. Stroke 1987;18:138

Kremer M. Sitting, standing, and walking. Br Med J 1958;2:63

Martin JP. A short essay on posture and movement. J Neurol Neurosurg Psychiatry 1977;40:25

Meyer JS, Barron DW. Apraxia of gait: A clinicophysiological study. Brain 1960;83:261

Saunders JBDM, Inman VT, Eberhart HD. The major determinants in normal and pathological gait. J Bone Joint Surg (Am) 1953;35:543

Soelberg Sørensen P, Jansen EC, Gjerris F. Motor disturbances in normal pressure hydrocephalus. Special reference to stance and gait. Arch Neurol 1986;43:34

PART E
The Reflexes

The investigation of the reflexes is often considered to be the most important part of the neurologic examination. In fact, the cursory neurologic appraisal that is carried out by the inexperienced observer or by one not familiar with neurologic technics is frequently limited to an evaluation of the pupillary and the biceps, triceps, patellar, and Achilles reflexes. It must be stressed, however, that although the examination of the reflexes is essential in the adequate appraisal of a patient with disease of the nervous system, it constitutes only one portion of the neurologic investigation. The reflexes can be evaluated only when considered as a part of the entire picture — including the sensory appraisal and the examination of cranial nerves and of motor function.

The reflexes are significant for many reasons. In the first place, alterations in their intensity and character may be the earliest and most subtle indications of a disturbance in neurologic function. Furthermore, the testing of the reflexes is the most objective procedure of the neurologic examination. In the sensory appraisal the physician relies largely upon the patient's voluntary responses, and the evaluation of muscle strength, tone, and coordination also necessitates voluntary cooperation. The reflexes, it is true, may be reinforced or decreased voluntarily and in nonorganic disease, but they are under voluntary control to a lesser extent than most other parts of the neurologic examination, and abnormalities of the reflexes are difficult to simulate. They are not as dependent upon the attention, cooperation, or intelligence of the patient, and consequently can be evaluated in confused individuals, those of low intelligence, infants and children, and stuporous and comatose patients, when other tests cannot be performed. The integrity of the motor and sensory systems can sometimes be appraised more adequately by the examination of the reflexes than by other means.

A reflex is an invariable adaptive response to the stimulation of a sense organ, which involves the use of a center of adjustment and of the conductors necessary to connect this center with the appropriate receptor and effector apparatus. It is often mechanically induced, but exceptions occur. In other words, a reflex is any action performed involuntarily as the result of an impulse or impression that is transmitted along afferent fibers to a nerve center, thence to efferent fibers, and then calls into action certain cells, muscles, or organs. The response may be motor, sensory, or visceral, depending upon the type and intensity of the stimulus, the sensory organ stimulated, and the cells or organs that respond. Although most reflexes are involuntary and relatively independent of consciousness, the individual is usually aware of their presence during or after the response.

An intact sensory system and an intact motor system are needed for a normal reflex response, and knowledge of both sensory and motor functions is necessary to an understanding of reflex action. The stimulus is received by the receptor, which may be a sensory ending in the skin, mucous membranes, muscle, tendon, or periosteum, or, in special types of reflexes, in the retina, cochlea, vestibular apparatus, olfactory mucosa, gustatory bulbs, or viscera. The stimulation of the receptor initiates an impulse that is carried along the primary conductor, the afferent (sensory) nerve, and then is transmitted to the central nervous system. There a synapse takes place with the intercalated neuron, which relays the impulse to the center of adjustment, the cell body of the efferent neuron. The secondary conductor, the neuraxis of the efferent neuron, transmits the impulse to the effector, the cell, muscle, gland, or blood vessel that then responds. A disturbance in function of any of the above parts of the reflex arc — the receptor, sensory nerve, intercalated neuron, motor unit, efferent nerve, or effector apparatus — will cause a break in the reflex arc and a consequent decrease or loss of the reflex.

Although monosynaptic and polysynaptic reflexes can be differentiated by experimental technics, few of the reflexes that are investigated clinically are as simple as the primitive response to a stimulus just described. All parts of the nervous system are intimately connected, and it is rare for one part to react without affecting or being affected by other parts. Almost immediately upon entering the central nervous system the afferent nerve divides into ascending and descending branches. These, as collateral fibers, arborize with motor cells at higher and lower levels on the same and opposite side. Association pathways may carry the impulse to the cerebral cortex for either reflex or voluntary modification of the response. The more complex reflex acts are accomplished through a mechanism that provides for connections between the various segments on the same and opposite sides of the spinal cord, brain stem, and brain. The more complex the reflex, the greater the number of the associated neurons and mechanisms that are used.

Innervation of one muscle group is accompanied by inhibition of the antagonist muscle group (Sherrington's law of reciprocal innervation); if by reflex action the extensors of a limb are contracted, the flexors are relaxed. The response may be increased gradually to a maximum when the stimulus is prolonged; this is brought about by activation of a progressively larger number of motor neurons and is known as **recruitment.** If the strength of the stimulus is increased, the excitatory process also spreads to a greater number of neurons; this phenomenon is called **irradiation.** Reflexes are under cerebral control, and may be increased by removal of cerebral inhibition as well as by overstimulation of the reflex centers. Exceptions are the cutaneous reflexes, which are often diminished or absent when cerebral influences are interrupted.

Reflex activity is essential to the normal functions of the human body. Every striated muscle contracts on direct mechanical, electrical, voluntary, and reflex stimulation. The body and its constituent parts draw away from injurious stimuli — nociceptive reflexes. Reflex activity is important in maintaining the body in its daily environment, in sustaining an upright position, in standing and walking, and in movement of the extremities. It is an integral part of the response to visual, gustatory, auditory, and vestibular stimulation. It is essential to metabolism and to the functions of the viscera. All involuntary and many voluntary acts are reflex in nature.

Reflexes have been named in various ways: some according to the site of elicitation or the part of the body stimulated; some according to the muscles involved or the part of the body that responds; some according to the ensuing movements, the joint upon which it acts, or the nerves involved. Many carry the names of one or more individuals who are said to have first described them.

Some hundreds of reflexes have been identified. Many of them are not important for clinical diagnosis and it is necessary to study only the more essential ones. Inasmuch as all the reflexes cannot be tested in the routine neurologic examination, and many have no clinical importance, only the more important ones will be described. The majority of these are muscle responses; the muscle involved rather than the site of stimulation is most important.

When a muscle with normal innervation and with normal tissue is passively stretched, its fibers react by resisting the stretch, and they enter into a state of increased and sustained tension, or contraction. This may be caused by gravity, manipulation, and other factors, but in reflex responses the contraction results from stimulation of the sensory organs in the muscle, either di-

rectly or indirectly through a stimulus applied to its tendons, the bone to which it is attached, or the overlying skin. Either direct or indirect stimulation of any muscle results first in a lengthening reaction, but then the proprioceptive impulses carried to the nervous system from sensory organs within the muscle itself call forth an increase in tension, and a shortening reaction, or contraction, follows. A sudden stimulus, such as a brief, sharp impact, is followed by an immediate response, with a pull exerted longitudinally through the muscle. Some muscles react more strongly than others. The extensor muscles of the thigh and leg, for instance, which are important in standing and walking, react more promptly and strongly than the flexor muscles. The flexor excitation is damped out rapidly by inhibiting impulses from higher centers; if these inhibiting influences are removed, there is an increase in reflex activity.

The stretch reflex response to direct stimulation occurs in every striated muscle and continues for a period even after stimulation has ceased. In fact there is an increased muscular response to direct stimulation for a short time after the nerve supply has been severed. This phenomenon is known as **idiomuscular** or **myotatic irritability.** Myotatic irritability may persist until atrophy has taken place. As a consequence, direct stimulation of muscle tissue has little value in neurologic diagnosis, except to determine myotatic irritability. The reflex responses that have diagnostic value are the indirect ones. An exception is in the detection of myotonia, where there is a prompt contraction but a delayed relaxation of the muscle directly percussed. Myotonia usually is not observed after indirect stimulation via the tendon.

The student should thoroughly understand the important reflexes and why they are tested. He should learn how to elicit them, their relationship to disease symptoms, their significance, and the diseases with which they may be associated or by which they may be altered in any way. He should be aware that their presence or absence and the ease with which they are elicited depend on many factors, including the conditions under which they are tested. Furthermore, he should be familiar with the responding muscles and their functions; with the innervation, not only of the muscle involved but also of the site of stimulation and with the center in the brain, brain stem, or spinal cord that is involved in the reflex activity. In the routine neurologic examination the degree of activity of the reflexes is evaluated by observation and palpation. In carrying out investigative procedures, however, various technics have been employed to quantitate the degree of muscular response and the time consumed in contraction and relaxation. Apparatus used for such measurements include the electromyogram and other electronic, electromagnetic, and photoelectric recording devices that register the speed, duration, and pattern of reflexes. With the exception of the electromyogram, these complex technics for studying reflexes are predominantly used for research and are rarely necessary for clinical diagnosis.

Reflexes may be classified in various ways, and there is necessarily a certain amount of overlapping in the different categories. For the purpose of the present discussion, the following groups are considered: muscle stretch reflexes, superficial (cutaneous) reflexes, corticospinal tract responses, reflexes of spinal automatism, postural and righting reflexes, associated movements, "frontal release" signs, and miscellaneous neurologic signs, including those of basal ganglion involvement, meningeal irritation, and tetany. Organic, or visceral, reflexes are described in Part F, "The Autonomic Nervous System." Cerebral reflex activities that are concerned with vision, hearing, etc., are discussed with these respective functions. **Conditioned,** or **acquired, reflexes** are those in which, as the result of certain experiences, a specific response may be called forth by an indifferent stimulus: they depend upon the integrity of the cerebral cortex, are developed through training and association, and cannot be considered with the other reflexes. At the present time they have little diagnostic implication, but play a role in therapy when behavioral modification, biofeedback, and other such technics are used. Emotional reflexes, too, involve higher cortical functions; they also have little relationship to the neurologic examination.

Chapter 33
THE MUSCLE STRETCH REFLEXES

The muscle stretch reflexes are those that are elicited in response to application of the stimulus to either tendons or periosteum, or occasionally to bones, joints, fascia, or aponeurotic structures. They are often incorrectly called tendon or periosteal reflexes. It is the muscle stretch that elicits the reflex; the tendon is a convenient location to apply the stimulus. Because the stimulus is mediated through the deeper sense organs such as the neuromuscular and neurotendinous spindles, they may be referred to as the proprioceptive reflexes. They are all, however, muscle stretch reflexes and are produced by the indirect stimulation of muscles and the calling forth of a response to a sudden stretch imposed upon them. They are not evoked by direct stimulation of muscle tissues. The term **deep reflex** has also been used for muscle stretch reflexes.

The muscle stretch reflexes are best tested by the use of a rubber percussion hammer, although other objects may also be used. A soft rubber hammer is most desirable, for the pain that may follow a blow with a hard hammer may interfere with the response. The stimulus should be quick and direct, and should be a threshold one, and no greater than necessary. The patient should be comfortable and relaxed. The part of the body to be tested should be in a position for optimal muscular response. Because the amount and briskness of the reaction depend largely upon the state of tone in the muscles, they should usually be in a state of slight tension or contraction. In order to compare the reflexes on the two sides of the body, the position of the extremities should be symmetric. The reflexes may be examined even

though the patient is unconscious. For an accurate determination the examiner should feel as well as see the contraction, by placing one hand over the muscle that responds. He should notice both the presence of the reflex and the degree of activity. The latter is estimated by the speed and vigor of the response, the range of movement, and the duration of the contraction. Reflex response times can be quantitated electronically, but this type of evaluation is reserved for research activities.

Reflexes may be classified as absent, sluggish or diminished, normal, exaggerated, and markedly hyperactive. For the purposes of clinical note-taking some neurologists grade them numerically, as follows: O = absent; + = present but diminished; ++ = normal; +++ = increased but not necessarily to a pathologic degree; ++++ = markedly hyperactive, often with associated clonus. The response should always be compared on the two sides of the body; unequal reflexes may be as significant as either increased or absent reflexes. Reflexes may be charted in several ways, for example, as shown in Table 33-1, or as in Fig. 33-1.

As far as possible the muscle stretch reflexes should be named by the muscles involved in the response rather than the site of stimulation or the nerve involved. For the purpose of classification they will be divided as follows: reflexes supplied by the cranial nerves, reflexes of the upper extremities, reflexes of the trunk, and reflexes of the lower extremities. The innervation of the reflexes is stated with the description of each reflex. The muscle stretch reflexes innervated by the cranial nerves have been discussed

TABLE 33-1. METHOD OF RECORDING THE COMMONLY TESTED MUSCLE STRETCH REFLEXES.*

	Right	Left
Biceps	2+	2+
Triceps	2+	2+
Brachioradialis	2+	2+
Patellar	2+	2+
Achilles	2+	2+
Plantar	↓	↓

*Grades 0 to 4+ (see text) used for all but plantar reflex, which is down (↓, normal), absent (0), or up (↑, abnormal). Other reflexes must be added and charted as needed.

in detail in Part C, "The Cranial Nerves" under the heading of the respective cranial nerves.

MUSCLE STRETCH REFLEXES OF THE UPPER EXTREMITIES

The biceps, triceps, brachioradialis, and finger flexor reflexes are the most important muscle stretch reflexes in the upper extremity.

The Biceps Reflex. The arm is held in a relaxed position, with the forearm midway between flexion and extension and in slight pronation. The position is obtained most satisfactorily if the patient's elbow is resting in the examiner's hand. The examiner places his thumb or finger over the biceps tendon and taps the thumb with a reflex hammer (Fig. 33-2). The major response is a contraction of the biceps muscle with flexion of the forearm. Inasmuch as the biceps is also a supinator of the forearm, there is often a certain amount of supination. If the reflex is exaggerated, the reflexogenous zone is increased and the reflex may even be obtained by tapping the clavicle. Also, in exaggeration of this reflex there may be associated flexion of the wrist and fingers and adduction of the thumb. The sensory supply of this reflex is through the midcervical nerves, and the motor supply to the biceps is through the musculocutaneous nerve (fifth and sixth cervical segments). The reflex center is at the fifth and sixth cervical segments.

The Triceps Reflex. This reflex is elicited by tapping the triceps tendon just above its insertion on the olecranon process of the ulna. The arm is held midway between flexion and exten-

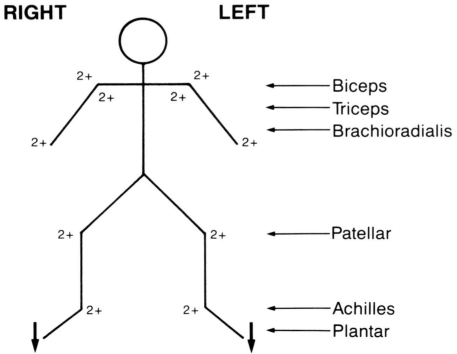

FIG. 33–1. Alternate method of recording the commonly tested muscle stretch reflexes. For grading see text and Table 33–1.

following stimulation at the olecranon. This response appears when the arc of the triceps reflex is damaged, as in lesions of the seventh and eighth cervical segments; in such cases the stimulus calls forth a flexion response, with the contraction of the biceps being unopposed by the triceps muscle.

The Brachioradialis (Radial Periosteal or Supinator) Reflex. If the styloid process of the radius is tapped while the forearm is in semiflexion and semipronation, there will be flexion of the forearm, together with supination (Fig. 33-4). The supination is more marked if the forearm has been extended and pronated, but there is less flexion. If the reflex is exaggerated there is associated flexion of the wrist and fingers, with adduction of the forearm. The principal muscle involved is the brachioradialis, and it can be stimulated not only at its tendon of insertion on the lateral aspect of the base of the styloid process of the radius, but also along the lower one third of the lateral surface of the radius or at its tendon of origin above the lateral epicondyle of the humerus. The innervation of this reflex is through the radial nerve (fifth and sixth cervical segments). In the presence of corticospinal tract involvement or other conditions causing reflex hyperactivity with, in addition, a lesion of the fifth cervical segment or its neuraxes, there may be contraction of the flexors of the hand and fingers without flexion and supination of the fore-

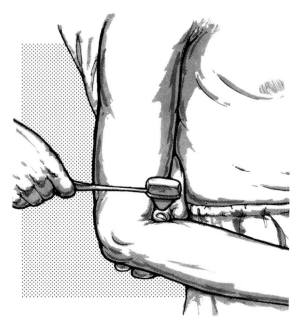

FIG. 33–2. *Method of obtaining the biceps reflex.*

sion, and it may be rested on the examiner's hand or on the patient's thigh (Fig. 33-3). The response is one of contraction of the triceps muscle, with extension of the forearm. The sensory and motor innervations are through the radial nerve (sixth through eighth cervical segments), and the center is in the lower cervical portion of the spinal cord. The so-called **paradoxical triceps reflex** consists of a flexion of the forearm

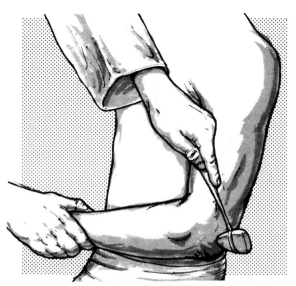

FIG. 33–3. *Method of obtaining the triceps reflex.*

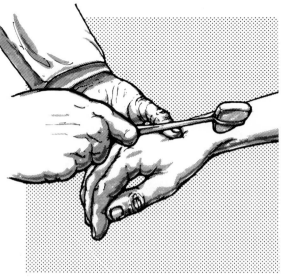

FIG. 33–4. *Method of obtaining the brachioradialis reflex.*

arm. This is termed **inversion of the radial reflex.**

The biceps, triceps, and brachioradialis reflexes should be obtained without difficulty in normal individuals. The following reflexes of the upper extremities may be elicited only to a slight extent in normal persons. If they are conspicuous, one can assume the presence of a general reflex exaggeration.

The Finger Flexor Reflex (Wartenberg's Sign).

To elicit the finger flexor reflex, the patient's hand is in partial supination, resting on a table or a solid surface, and the fingers are slightly flexed. The examiner places his middle and index fingers on the volar surface of the phalanges of the patient's four fingers, and taps his own fingers lightly with the reflex hammer (Fig. 33-5). The response is one of flexion of the patient's four fingers and the distal phalanx of the thumb. The reflex may be reinforced by having the patient bend his fingers as the blow is being applied. The nerve supply, as in the wrist flexion reflex, is through the median and ulnar nerves (sixth cervical through first thoracic segments). This reflex is difficult for the inexperienced examiner to elicit, but Wartenberg considered it one of the most important reflexes in the upper extremity. Forced grasping and the Hoffmann and Trömner signs, which are pathologic variations of this response, will be described with the corticospinal tract signs.

The Scapulohumeral Reflex.

Tapping over the vertebral border of the scapula, either at the tip of its spine or at its base near the inferior angle, is followed by retraction of the scapula. This is done principally through the action of the rhomboidei major and minor, which are innervated by the dorsal scapular nerve (fourth and fifth cervical segments). There may be associated elevation of the scapula and adduction and external rotation of the humerus through the action of the trapezius, latissimus dorsi, infraspinatus, and teres minor.

The Deltoid Reflex.

Tapping over the insertion of the deltoid muscle at the junction of the upper and middle third of the lateral aspect of the humerus is followed by a contraction of the muscle with resulting abduction of the upper arm. The sensory and motor supply to this reflex are through the axillary nerve (fifth and sixth cervical segments).

The Pectoralis Reflex.

With the patient's arm in midposition between abduction and adduction, the examiner places his finger as nearly as possible on the tendon of the pectoralis major muscle near its insertion on the chest of the greater tubercle of the humerus (Fig. 33-6). Tapping the finger is followed by abduction and slight internal rotation of the arm at the shoulder. The contraction of the muscle may be felt

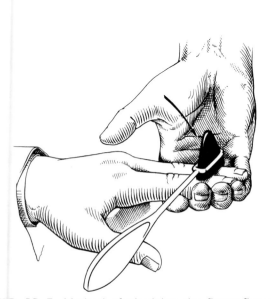

FIG. 33–5. Method of obtaining the finger flexor reflex.

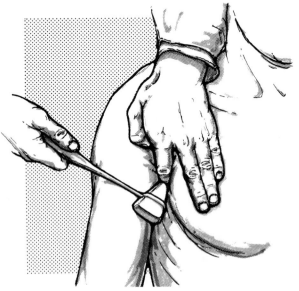

FIG. 33–6. Method of obtaining the pectoralis reflex.

but not seen in the normal individual. This reflex is innervated by the lateral and medial anterior thoracic nerves (fifth cervical through first thoracic segments).

The Latissimus Dorsi Reflex. With the patient prone and his arm abducted and in slight external rotation, the examiner places his fingers on the tendon of the latissimus dorsi near its insertion in the intertubercular groove of the humerus, and taps his finger with the reflex hammer. This is followed by abduction and slight internal rotation of the shoulder. This reflex is innervated by the thoracodorsal (long subscapular) nerve (sixth through eighth cervical segments).

The Clavicle Reflex. In patients with reflex hyperactivity in the upper extremities, a tap over the lateral aspect of the clavicle is followed by extensive contraction of various muscle groups in the upper limb. There are individual variations, but normally the response should be the same on each side. This is not a specific reflex, but is an indication of the spread of reflex response. It is useful in comparing the reflex activity of the two upper limbs.

The Pronator Reflex. If either the styloid process of the ulna or the posteroinferior surface of the ulna is tapped while the forearm is in semiflexion and the wrist in semipronation there will be pronation of the forearm, often with adduction of the wrist. There may also be flexion of the wrist and fingers. The same response may be obtained by stimulating the palmar surface of the lower aspect of the radius, which causes brief supination followed by pronation. The major muscles participating in this response are the pronators teres and quadratus, and the innervation is through the median nerve (sixth cervical through first thoracic segments). This reflex may be exaggerated early when corticospinal tract lesions develop.

The Wrist Extension Reflex. Tapping of the extensor tendons of the wrist while the forearm is pronated and the wrist is hanging down may be followed by a contraction of the extensor muscles and extension at the wrist. This reflex is supplied by the radial nerve (sixth through eighth cervical segments). Under certain circumstances one may get flexion of the wrist and fingers on tapping the dorsum of the carpometacarpal area. This is known as the carpometacarpal, or carpophalangeal, reflex of Bechterew,

and is discussed with the corticospinal tract signs.

The Wrist Flexion Reflex. Tapping the flexor tendons of the wrist on the volar surface of the forearm at or above the transverse carpal ligament when the hand is in supination and the fingers are slightly flexed is followed by a contraction of the flexor muscles of the hand and fingers. This reflex is innervated by the median and perhaps the ulnar nerves (sixth cervical through first thoracic segments). This is also known as the **hand flexor reflex.**

The Thumb Reflex. Tapping of the tendon of the flexor pollicis longus muscle just above the tendon of the pronator quadratus is followed by flexion of the distal muscles of the thumb. This reflex is supplied by the median nerve (sixth cervical through first thoracic segments).

MUSCLE STRETCH REFLEXES OF THE TRUNK

The muscle stretch reflexes of the trunk are obtained only to a minimal extent or not at all in normal individuals.

The Costal Periosteal Reflex. Tapping the lower rib margins, the costal cartilages, or the xiphoid process of the sternum of the supine patient with the reflex hammer is followed by contraction of the upper abdominal muscles and slight excursion of the umbilicus toward the site of stimulation. If either the rib margins or costal cartilages are stimulated, there is an oblique deviation of the umbilicus upward and laterally, and if the xiphoid process is tapped, there is an upward deviation of the umbilicus. These reflexes are innervated by the upper intercostal nerves (fifth through ninth thoracic segments).

The Abdominal Muscle (Deep Abdominal) Reflexes. The abdominal muscle reflexes are muscle stretch reflexes obtained on brisk stretching of the muscles and they are elicited at many places on the abdominal wall; there are many methods of testing them. The examiner may tap the abdominal wall overlying the muscles, but better results are obtained if he stretches the muscles slightly by pressing on them with a tongue blade or ruler, and then taps this briskly with a reflex hammer. He may also use an index finger to press on the muscles, or insert the finger in the umbilicus to effect the same result, and then tap the finger. The response is a prompt contraction of the muscles, and a deviation of the umbilicus toward the site of the stimulus. The reflex is reinforced by slight contraction of the abdominal wall, which may be accomplished by having the patient cough, attempt to raise his head against resistance, or make a slight attempt to rise. The innervation is by the anterior divisions of the fifth through twelfth thoracic nerves (intercostal nerves), as well as the ilioinguinal and iliohypogastric nerves. The abdominal muscle reflexes are present to only a minimal extent in normal persons, and are most significant if they are exaggerated or if there is dissociation between the deep and superficial abdominal reflexes (the latter are described in Chapter 34). The two should not be confused. If the deep abdominal reflexes are brisk when the superficial abdominal reflexes are absent, a corticospinal tract lesion is suspected.

The Iliac Reflexes. Tapping over the iliac crest is followed by contraction of the lower abdominal muscles. This reflex is innervated by the lower intercostal nerves (tenth through twelfth thoracic degments).

The Symphysis Pubis Reflexes. Tapping over the symphysis pubis is followed by a contraction of the abdominal muscles and a downward movement of the umbilicus. The reflex should be tested with the patient recumbent and with his abdominal muscles relaxed and his thigh in slight abduction and internal rotation. If a unilateral stimulus is applied by tapping 1½ – 2 cm from the midline, there is not only the "upper response" just described, but also a "lower response," or **puboadductor reflex,** with contraction of the adductor muscles of the thigh on the side stimulated, and some flexion of the hip. This latter response is also seen if the reflex is exaggerated. The symphysis pubis reflex is innervated by the lower intercostal, ilioinguinal, and iliohypogastric nerves (eleventh and twelfth thoracic and upper lumbar segments).

The costal periosteal, iliac, and symphysis pubis reflexes may be considered as manifestations of the deep abdominal muscle reflexes in which the stimulus is directed toward the site of insertion.

The Back Reflexes. With the patient lying prone, the sacral and lumbar areas of the spine are tapped. The reflex response consists of contraction of the erector spinae muscles. The innervation is through the thoracic, lumbar, and sacral nerves.

MUSCLE STRETCH REFLEXES OF THE LOWER EXTREMITIES

The Patellar (Quadriceps) Reflex. The patellar, or quadriceps, reflex, usually called the **knee jerk,** is characterized by contraction of the quadriceps femoris muscle, with resulting extension of the leg, in response to a stimulus directed toward the patellar tendon. A firm tap on the tendon draws down the patella and stretches the muscle. This is followed by contraction of the muscle. If the reflex activity is brisk, the contraction is abrupt and strong and the amplitude of the movement is large.

This reflex may be elicited in various manners. It is often tested with the patient seated in a chair with his feet resting on the floor. The examiner places one hand over the quadriceps femoris muscle and with the other hand taps the patellar tendon just below the patella. In this way the examiner can palpate the contraction of the muscle and observe the rapidity and range of response (Fig. 33-7); he can also compare the responses on the two sides. If the patient is lying in bed, the examiner should partially flex the knee by placing one hand beneath it and then tap the tendon (Fig. 33-8). The responses on the two sides can be compared if he lifts both knees simultaneously, supporting them on his forearm as the patient's heels rest lightly on the bed, before tapping the tendons. Many examiners test the patellar reflex by having the patient sit on the edge of a table with his legs hanging over the edge in such a manner that his feet do not touch the floor, or by having the patient sit with one leg crossed over the other and tapping the patellar tendon of the superior leg. In these various ways the *range* of response can be noted, but inasmuch as it is more important to note the *speed* of response, *i.e.,* the duration of the latent period between the time of the stimulus and the resulting response, the better procedure is to palpate the quadriceps.

If the patellar reflex is exaggerated, there may be not only extension of the leg, but also adduction of the thigh, which on occasion is bilateral. There may be a bilateral extensor response. Also, if the reflex is exaggerated, the response may be obtained by stimulation not only of the patellar tendon but also of the tendon of the quadriceps femoris muscle just above the patella, the **suprapatellar** or **epipatellar reflex.** The tendon

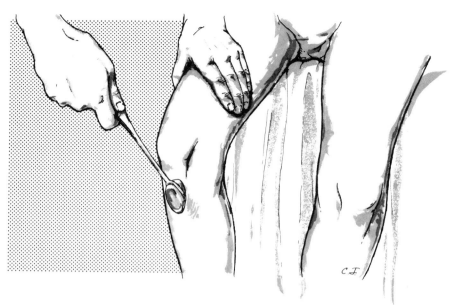

FIG. 33–7. *Method of obtaining the patellar (quadriceps) reflex with the patient seated.*

can be tapped directly, or, with the patient recumbent, the examiner can place his index finger on the tendon and tap the finger or push down the tendon. Contraction of the quadriceps causes a brisk upward movement of the tendon, together with extension of the leg (Fig. 33-9). In marked exaggeration of the patellar reflex one may elicit patellar clonus (Ch. 35). Absence of the patellar reflex is known as **Westphal's sign.** An **inverted patellar reflex** may be seen with lesions of the nerve or nerve roots supplying the quadriceps: tapping the patellar tendon here results in contraction of the hamstrings and flexion of the knee. The patellar reflex is innervated

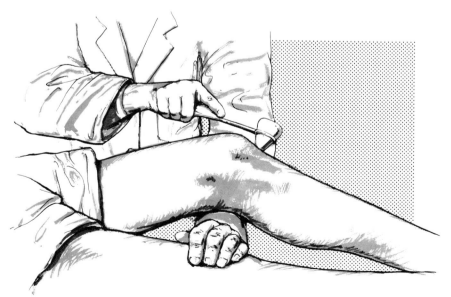

FIG. 33–8. *Method of obtaining the patellar (quadriceps) reflex with the patient recumbent.*

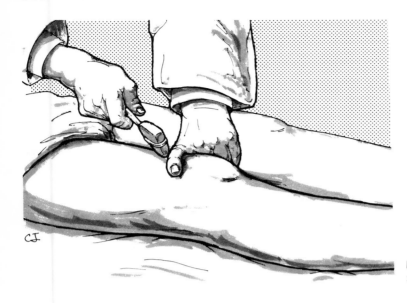

FIG. 33–9. Method of obtaining the suprapatellar reflex.

by the femoral nerve (second through fourth lumbar segments).

The Achilles (Triceps Surae) Reflex. The Achilles, or triceps surae, reflex, or the **ankle jerk,** is obtained by tapping the Achilles tendon just above its innervation on the posterior surface of the calcaneus. This is followed by contraction of the posterior crural muscles, the gastrocnemius, soleus, and plantaris, with resulting plantar flexion of the foot at the ankle. If the patient is seated or is lying in bed, the thigh should be moderately abducted and rotated externally, the knee should be flexed, and the foot should be in moderate inversion; the examiner should place one hand under the foot to produce moderate dorsiflexion at the ankle (Fig. 33-10). If the reflex is obtained with difficulty, the patient may be asked to press his foot against the examiner's hand in order to tense the tendon. If it cannot be elicited in this manner, the patient should be asked to kneel on his knees on a chair, preferably on a soft surface, while the feet project at right angles; the Achilles tendons are percussed while the patient is in this position (Fig. 33-11). The reflex may also be obtained while the patient is lying prone with his feet in moderate dorsiflexion. If either of these two latter positions is used, the responses on the two sides may be compared with ease. Some exami-

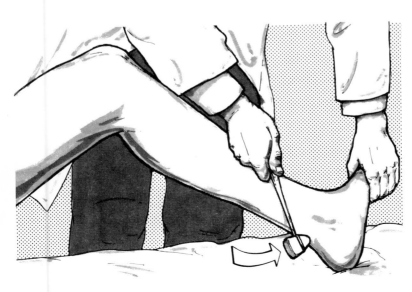

FIG. 33–10. Method of obtaining the Achilles (triceps surae) reflex with the patient recumbent.

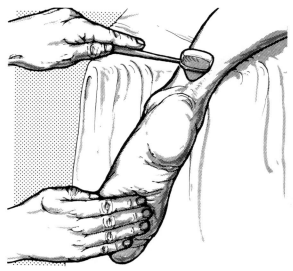

FIG. 33–11. Method of obtaining the Achilles (triceps surae) reflex with the patient kneeling.

ners prefer to obtain the Achilles reflex by tapping the ball (sole) of the foot.

If the Achilles reflex is exaggerated, it may be elicited by tapping other areas of the sole of the foot, the **medioplantar reflex,** or by tapping the anterior aspect of the ankle, the **paradoxical ankle reflex.** In more marked exaggeration spontaneous clonus may be obtained when the tendon is tapped. Although the Achilles reflex, when carefully elicited, should be present in normal individuals, it tends to be diminished with age and its absence in elderly individuals is not necessarily of clinical significance. The Achilles reflex is innervated by the tibial nerve (fifth lumbar through second sacral segments).

The patellar and Achilles reflexes are the most important muscle stretch reflexes in the lower extremities. The following reflexes are less significant. The response may be minimal or even absent in normal individuals. Their exaggeration strongly suggests the presence of corticospinal tract disease.

The Adductor Reflex. With the thigh in slight abduction, either the medial epicondyle of the femur is tapped in the vicinity of the adductor tubercle, or the medial condyle of the tibia is stimulated. The response is a contraction of the adductor muscles of the thigh and inward movement of the extremity. If the reflex is exaggerated, there may be crossed, or bilateral, adduction. This reflex is mediated through the obturator nerve (second through fourth lumbar

segments). An adductor response can also be obtained, if there is exaggeration of the reflex, by tapping the spinous processes of the sacral or lumbar vertebrae while the patient is in a seated position (the **spinal adductor reflex**) or by tapping the crest or the superior spines of the ilium. The puboadductor reflex has been described with the symphysis pubis reflex.

The Internal Hamstring (Semimembranosus and Semitendinosus, or Posterior Tibiofemoral) Reflex. This reflex is elicited by stimulating the tendons of the semitendinosus and semimembranosus muscles just above their insertions on the posterior and medial surfaces and medial condyle of the tibia. This is best done with the patient in the recumbent position, the leg abducted and partially externally rotated, and the knee slightly flexed. The examiner's fingers are placed over the lower portions of the muscles and their tendons on the medial aspect of the leg just below the knee, and the fingers are tapped with the reflex hammer. The response is an increased flexion of the leg, with slight internal rotation of the leg. This reflex is supplied through the tibial portion of the sciatic nerve (fourth lumbar through second sacral segments).

The External Hamstring (Biceps Femoris, or Posterior Peroneofemoral) Reflex. This reflex is elicited by stimulating the tendon of the biceps femoris muscle just above its insertion on the lateral side of the head of the fibula and the lateral condyle of the tibia. With the patient either recumbent or lying on the opposite side, and with the leg in moderate flexion at the knee, the examiner places a finger over the tendon of the biceps femoris muscle on the lateral aspect of the leg just below the knee, and taps the finger (Fig. 33-12). The response consists of a contraction of the muscle with resulting flexion of the knee and moderate external rotation of the leg. The reflex may also be elicited by tapping the head of the fibula; this is known as the **fibular reflex.** The nerve supply for the long head of the biceps is the same as that for the posterior tibiofemoral reflex, through the tibial portion of the sciatic nerve, but the short head of the biceps is supplied by the common peroneal portion of the sciatic nerve (fifth lumbar through second or third sacral segments).

The Tensor Fasciae Latae Reflex. This reflex is tested by tapping over the tensor fasciae latae muscle at its origin near the anterior supe-

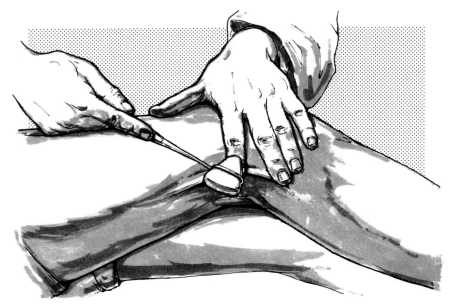

FIG. 33–12. Method of obtaining the biceps femoris reflex.

rior iliac spine; the patient is in the recumbent position. The response consists of slight abduction of the thigh. This reflex is innervated by the superior gluteal nerve (fourth lumbar through first sacral segments).

The Gluteus Reflexes. Tapping the lower portion of the sacrum or the posterior aspect of the ilium near the origin of the gluteus maximus muscle is followed by a contraction of this muscle, with extension of the thigh. This reflex is best tested with the patient in the recumbent position, but with his weight on the opposite side so that there is moderate flexion of the ipsilateral thigh; it may also be elicited with the patient in the prone position. The reflex is innervated by the inferior gluteal nerve (fifth lumbar through second sacral segments). A **gluteus medius reflex** may on occasion be elicited by stimulating the anterior portion of the iliac crest near the site of origin of the muscle. The response is one of slight abduction and medial rotation of the thigh. The innervation is the same as that of the tensor fasciae latae reflex (superior gluteal nerve), and the response is almost identical; it may not be possible to differentiate these two reflexes.

The Extensor Hallucis Longus Reflex. With the patient recumbent, the examiner exerts moderate pressure with his finger on the dorsal surface of the terminal phalanx of the great toe.

Tapping the finger is followed by extension of the toe, which may be felt more readily than it is seen. This reflex is innervated by the deep peroneal nerve (fourth lumbar through the first sacral segments). It may be absent with herniation of the nucleus pulposus between the fourth and fifth lumbar bodies.

The Tibialis Posterior Reflex. Tapping the tendon of the tibialis posterior just above and behind the medial malleolus is followed by inversion of the foot. This reflex is best examined with the patient prone and the foot, in a neutral position or in slight eversion, extended beyond the edge of the bed. The leg should be supported by the examiner and slightly flexed at the knee. This reflex is innervated by the tibial nerve (fifth lumbar through first sacral segments). It may be absent if there is herniation of the nucleus pulposus between the fourth and fifth lumbar vertebral bodies, but it is difficult to obtain in the normal individual, and to be significant its absence must be unilateral.

The Peroneal Reflex. With the patient's foot plantar flexed and inverted, the examiner presses a finger firmly over the distal ends of the first and second metacarpal bones. A brisk tap to the finger is followed by eversion and dorsiflexion of the foot. The reflex response consists of contraction of muscles supplied by the deep and superficial peroneal nerves (fourth lumbar through first sacral segments), and is absent with lesions of the respective nerve roots.

The Plantar Muscle Reflexes. There are numerous reflexes in which the response is flexion of the toes. These are difficult to elicit in normal individuals, are of limited clinical significance, and are of importance only when exaggerated. They are discussed with the corticospinal tract responses in Chapter 35.

INTERPRETATION OF THE MUSCLE STRETCH RELFEXES

The reflexes just described are the most important of the muscle stretch reflexes. All are not of equal significance, however, and not all can be elicited in the normal individual. The most valuable for clinical diagnosis are the biceps, triceps, brachioradialis, patellar, and Achilles reflexes (see Table 33-1); under most circumstances one should be able to elicit these in every normal person. Some studies indicate that 3% – 10% of normal people with no other evidence of disease of the nervous system may show the absence of one or more of these reflexes. In general, however, the significant stretch reflexes are rarely absent in normal persons if the technic of eliciting them is adequate. They are present even in premature infants at 33 weeks' gestation in the vast majority of cases.

While the statement has been made that the degree of activity of the muscle stretch reflexes depends upon the speed and vigor of reaction, the range of movement, and the duration of the contraction, it is the speed of reaction, or the duration of the latent period between the time that the stimulus is applied and the time that the response occurs, that is the most important factor for clinical evaluation of disease states. It may be perceived more accurately by palpation than by vision.

The adequate evaluation of the reflex response obviously depends upon experience. Each examiner must come to his own conclusions, based upon previous impressions, the type of stimulus used, the intensity of the stimulus, the position of the part at the time the reflex is being tested, the general condition of the patient, the environmental surroundings, and other factors, by far the most important being the diligence and practice expended in learning the technics. The appraisal depends upon the individual interpretation of the examiner. There is no standard, and there is a certain amount of normal variation in reflex activity. What is normal for one individual may be an increased or a decreased response for another. In some persons the reflexes are lively, in others they are sluggish. Under normal circumstances the reflexes should be equal on the two sides — if equal, they are probably not pathologic unless there is either marked diminution or marked increase of response.

REINFORCEMENT OF THE REFLEXES

In certain individuals the reflexes may appear to be markedly diminished, or even absent, although no other evidence of nervous system disease is present. This is apt to be the case in muscular or athletic individuals with firm, well-developed muscles, or in tense, apprehensive persons who may be bracing their muscles either voluntarily or without being aware of doing so. Under such circumstances it may be necessary to use reinforcement in order to elicit the reflexes. In carrying out reinforcement, an attempt is made to divert the patient's attention and thus relax the muscles.

Reinforcement may be carried out according to the method of Jendrassik: On testing the patellar reflexes the patient is asked to hook the flexed fingers of the two hands together, placing the palmar surfaces of the fingers of one hand against the palmar surfaces of the other, and to attempt to pull them apart at the time the reflex is being stimulated (Fig. 33-13). He may be asked to clench his fists, to grasp firmly the arm of the chair or the side of the bed, or to clench one of the hands or the arm of the examiner. Reinforcement may also be carried out by having the patient look at the ceiling and cough at the time the reflex is being tested. The examiner can frequently divert the patient's attention merely by talking to him while testing the reflexes, discussing his illness with him, or asking him irrelevant questions. The patient may be asked to take a deep breath, count, read aloud, or repeat verses while the reflexes are being examined. A sudden loud noise, a painful stimulus elsewhere on the body, such as the pulling of a hair, or a bright light flashed in the eyes, may also be a means of reinforcement. Mechanisms involved in reflex reinforcement are probably active at several levels; supraspinal, fusimotor, and long-loop components have been identified.

Procedures other than distraction are also helpful in reinforcing the muscle stretch reflexes. A slight increase in tension of the muscle groups

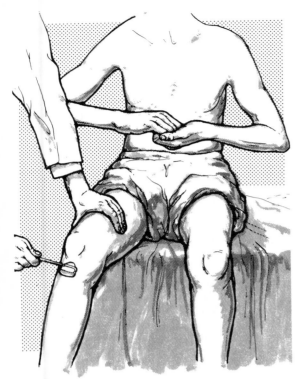

FIG. 33–13. Method of reinforcing the patellar reflex.

being tested may reinforce the reflex response. The patient may tense the quadriceps by pushing the ball of the foot against the examiner's hand while the patellar reflex is being elicited; the gastrocnemius may be tensed by pushing the ball of the foot against the floor or against the examiner's hand while the Achilles reflex is being tested. By means of these technics the amplitude of the reflex may be increased or an otherwise latent reflex may be obtained. Reflexes that are normal on reinforcement, even though they cannot be obtained without reinforcement, may be considered normal reflexes.

ABNORMALITIES OF THE MUSCLE STRETCH REFLEXES

If there is abnormality of the muscle stretch, or deep, reflexes, the response is manifested by either hypoactivity or hyperactivity. In hypoactivity the response varies from a diminished or sluggish one to complete absence of the reflex. When reflexes are hyperactive, varying degrees of increased speed and vigor of response, exag-

geration of the range of movement, decrease in threshold, extension of the reflexogenous zone, and prolongation of the muscular contraction are evident. The pathologic conditions in which these various changes occur are discussed in the following sections. Table 33-2 summarizes the patterns of reflex responses seen with lesions at various sites.

Diminution to Absence of the Muscle Stretch Reflexes

When hypoactivity of the reflex is present there is a sluggish response and/or a diminution in the range of response. An increase in the intensity of the stimulus may be necessary to elicit the reflex, or repeated blows may be necessary, for a single stimulus may be subliminal. Muscle stretch reflexes are absent if they are not obtained even with reinforcement.

Diminution of the reflexes results from an interference with the conduction of the impulse through the reflex arc, and absence indicates interruption of the reflex arc. Such changes may be associated with dysfunction of the receptor, afferent pathway, intercalated neuron, motor unit, efferent pathway, or effector apparatus. Interference with the sensory pathway may be caused by the following conditions: lesions of the sensory nerves (*e.g.*, sensory neuritis), involvement of the posterior roots (radiculitis), affections of the dorsal root ganglia (tabes dorsalis), dysfunction of the posterior columns of the spinal cord (tabes dorsalis, posterolateral sclerosis). Syringomyelia and other intramedullary lesions may interfere with the function of the intercalated neuron. Involvement of the motor unit and pathway may be associated with numerous conditions: lesions of the motor nucleus or anterior horn cell (poliomyelitis, progressive spinal muscular atrophy, syringomyelia), affections of the anterior nerve roots and motor nerves (radiculitis, motor neuritis), dysfunction of the myoneural junction (myasthenia gravis, myasthenic syndromes). With peripheral nerve lesions the reflexes may not return until a major portion of motor function has recovered. Sometimes there is persisting areflexia following nerve root lesions and peripheral neuropathies, even after complete return of both motor and sensory functions. In myasthenia gravis the reflexes are absent only when there is extensive involvement with failure of muscular contractions, and in familial periodic paralysis they are absent only temporarily. With

TABLE 33-2. REFLEX PATTERNS

Site or type of Lesion	Muscle Stretch Reflexes	Superficial Reflexes	Cortico-spinal Tract Responses	Reflexes of Spinal Automatism	Associated Movements
Myoneural junction	Normal or decreased	Normal	Absent	Absent	Normal
Muscle	Usually decreased	Normal	Absent	Absent	Normal
Peripheral nerve or anterior horn cell	Decreased to absent	Decreased to absent	Absent	Absent	Normal
Corticospinal tract	Hyperactive (especially in speed of response)	Decreased to absent	Present	Present (associated extrapyramidal involvement)	Pathologic associated movements present
Extrapyramidal system	Normal; occasionally slightly increased or decreased	Normal or slightly increased	Absent	Absent	Normal associated movements absent
Cerebellum	Decreased pendular	Normal	Absent	Absent	Normal
Psychogenic	Normal or increased (especially in range of response)	Normal or increased	Absent	Absent	Normal or bizarre

diseases of the motor apparatus, or the muscles, such as the myopathies and myositis, the reflexes may persist until the atrophy or muscular involvement is too extensive to allow a muscular contraction. In muscular dystrophy the proximal reflexes disappear early, but the distal reflexes may persist until later progression of the disease.

The muscle stretch reflexes may also be either diminished or absent in various other conditions. Although they may be increased in the earlier stages of coma, they are absent in deep coma, narcosis, and heavy sedation. They are often absent in deep sleep. They are characteristically absent during nerve block, caudal anesthesia, and spinal anesthesia. They are absent in spinal shock following a sudden transverse lesion of the spinal cord, but reappear below the level of the lesion after a period of 3 – 4 weeks, and usually become hyperactive (see "Spinal Shock," Ch. 36). In fact they may be present in extensive spinal cord lesions in spite of complete loss of sensation. They are often absent in Adie's syndrome (presumably due to impaired function of the large spindle afferents), a symptom complex also characterized by tonic pupils with impaired reaction to light. The reflexes are diminished and often lost in asthenic states and severe toxic and metabolic disorders of the central nervous system.

In myxedema there is a prolongation of both the contraction and relaxation times, especially the latter; the reflex time returns to normal with treatment of the hypothyroid condition. Some observers have stated that careful measurement of reflex time is an accurate test of thyroid function, but others have failed to confirm this, and it must be recalled that slow contraction and relaxation times may also occur with other conditions, including lower motor neuron disease, in which there is decreased activity. A delay in relaxation is also often found in some myotonic disorders. In diabetic neuropathy there may be either prolongation of the reflex time or decrease or absence of the reflexes before there is other evidence of nervous system involvement. In porphyria there may be absence of some of the reflexes; those that remain may be elicited only following repeated stimulations. There may be prolonged relaxation of reflexes in anorexia nervosa. They may be either diminished or lost in the presence of increased intracranial pressure, especially in posterior fossa tumors. In exhaustion following extreme exertion they may be diminished or absent.

In paraplegia in flexion (Ch. 36) it may not be possible to obtain the deep extensor reflexes, even though the neurologic status would suggest that there should be reflex hyperactivity; this condition is caused by spasm of the antagonist, or flexor, muscles, and the flexor muscles are hyperactive. In severe states of spasticity and rigidity it may not be possible to obtain the muscle stretch reflexes. The reflexes may be increased in the early stages of a peripheral neuritis, especially if there is pain, possibly owing to the irritability of the afferent nerves, but they disappear after the pathologic changes in the nerves have become more definite. The reflexes may appear to be absent in neurologic disorders in which there is marked spasticity with contractions and in diseases of the joints characterized by inflammation, contractures, and ankylosis. Here their absence is apparent rather than real, and is due to lack of motility at the joint or pain on moving the joint; careful observation may show that a muscular contraction takes place even though there is no movement at the joint. In parietal lobe lesions there may be an increase in threshold and a slowness of response, but an increased excursion.

Hyperactivity of the Muscle Stretch Reflexes

Hyperactivity of the muscle stretch reflexes is characterized by the following changes: a decrease in the reflex threshold, and increase in the speed of response (a decrease in the latent period), exaggeration of the vigor and range of movement, prolongation of muscular contraction, extension of the reflexogenous zone (or zone of provocation), and propagation of the reflex response. A minimal stimulus may evoke the reflex, and reflexes that are not normally obtained may be elicited with ease. There may be a wide zone or areas for effective stimulation in neighboring structures, and application of the stimulus to sites at some distance from the usual one may cause the response: the patellar reflex may be elicited by tapping the surface of the tibia or the dorsum of the foot, and the biceps and other arm reflexes by tapping the clavicle or scapula. The response may involve adjacent or even contralateral muscles, and the contraction of one muscle may be accompanied by contraction of others. Contraction of the biceps or brachioradialis may be accompanied by flexion of the fingers and adduction of the thumb; extension of the leg may be accompanied by adduction of the thigh, or there may be bilateral extension of the legs. One stimulus may be followed by repeated contractions and relaxations, owing to repeated volleys of discharges, so that clonus may be obtained. The muscle stretch reflexes are exaggerated in association with an increase in the tone of the contracting muscles.

The muscle stretch reflexes are increased with lesions of the corticospinal or pyramidal system (using the terms in their accepted clinical sense). Spasticity and exaggeration of the muscle stretch reflexes have, in the past, been felt to be the result of interruption of impulses from the pyramidal cortex and loss of the inhibiting effect of this portion of the motor system on the anterior horn cells. It is probable, however, that these changes are due to involvement of a variety of structures in the descending motor pathways at cortical, subcortical, midbrain and brain stem levels as well as in the spinal cord. Disturbances are thus not limited to the traditional corticospinal or pyramidal tract, with reticulospinal, vestibulospinal, and other descending tracts being affected to various degrees. Spasticity results from a lowering of the reflex threshold due to dysfunction of some or all of the structures and pathways mentioned. From a clinical point of view, however, the term *pyramidal* or *corticospinal* continues to be used in referring to the site of involvement as well as the ensuing change in function.

A lesion at any level of the corticospinal system, then, and/or other related upper motor neuron components, from the motor cortex to just above the segment of origin of a reflex arc, will be accompanied by spasticity and exaggeration of the muscle stretch reflexes. Not only are existing reflexes increased in the aspects described previously, but latent ones and those that are normally elicited with difficulty may be obtained with ease. In hemiplegia resulting from a cerebral lesion, the characteristic distribution is that of flexion of the upper extremities, with more marked weakness of the extensors, and of extension of the lower extremities, with more marked weakness of the flexors. Consequently the flexor reflexes are exaggerated to a greater degree in the upper extremities, and the extensor reflexes in the lower. The reflexes may be present in spinal cord lesions in spite of the apparent absence of sensation. If the spasticity is too marked, however, the resulting contractures may interfere with the reflex response. This may be the case in paraplegia in flexion, but on the other hand the increased tone of the flexor muscles probably causes absence of the extensor reflexes.

The muscle stretch reflexes are also increased in the early stages of stupor, anesthesia, and narcosis. They are exaggerated in tetany, tetanus, and poisoning with strychnine and other stimulants, owing to increased irritability of both the nerves and the muscles. Cold and exercise may increase the reflex response, although extreme exercise may be followed by areflexia. The reflexes may be increased in the early stages of a neuritis, possibly because of the increased irritability of the nerve fibers, but they disappear after the pathologic changes have fully developed. The muscle stretch reflexes may be increased if the tone of the opposing muscles is diminished; consequently the patellar reflex may be hyperactive if there is weakness of the hamstrings. They are often increased in hyperthyroidism, and the speed of the response is diminished when the thyroid overactivity is decreased.

Exaggeration of the muscle stretch reflexes may also be found in psychogenic disorders, such as neurosis and hysteria (see Table 33-2), and in states of anxiety, fright, and agitation. The reflexes vary in these conditions; they may be normal, or they may be decreased owing to voluntary or involuntary tension of the antagonistic muscle, but they are most frequently increased. The hyperactivity may be marked, but it is an exaggeration not in the speed of the response but in the excursion or range of response. The foot may be kicked far into the air and held extended for a time after the patellar tendon is tapped, but the response takes place slowly and relaxation is equally slow. There is often a bilateral response with a jerking of the entire body when the reflexes are tested. There is no increase in the reflexogenous zone in psychogenic lesions, and although there may be irregular repeated jerky movements (spurious clonus), no true clonus is present. Furthermore, there are no other signs of organic disease of the corticospinal system.

In lesions of the extrapyramidal system there are no consistent changes in the muscle stretch reflexes (see Table 33-2). The response depends to a certain degree upon muscular tonicity and the amount of rigidity that is present. Usually the reflexes are slightly exaggerated, owing to increased tension of the muscles, but this is not a consistent finding, and the rigidity may cause retardation, diminution, or absence of the reflexes. In diseases of the cerebellum the reflexes are often somewhat diminished (see Table 33-2), perhaps as a part of the hypotonicity and the loss of the reflex contraction of the antagonists. Frequently, however, they are of the pendular variety: if the patellar reflex is tested while the foot is hanging free, there may be a series of jerky to-and-fro pendular movements of the foot and leg before the limb finally comes to rest. This increased swinging may also be the result of hypotonia of the extensor and flexor muscles and a lack of the restraining influence they normally exert on each other. Normal aftershortening of the flexors is absent. The pendular response may also be observed in chorea, but here more frequently one finds "hung" reflexes: if the patellar tendon is tapped while the foot is

hanging free, the leg may be held in extension for a few seconds before relaxing, owing to prolonged contraction of the quadriceps. Furthermore, in chorea the response may not be obtained until the stimulus has been applied a number of times.

BIBLIOGRAPHY

Abraham AS, Atkinson M, Roscoe B. Value of anklejerk timing in the assessment of thyroid function. Br Med J 1966;1:830

Barraquer – Bordas L. On the zone of provocation of the deep muscle reflexes. Acta Psychiatr Belg 1956;31:227

Berlin L. A peroneal muscle stretch reflex. Neurology 1971;21:1177

Boyle RS, Shakir RA, Weir AI, McInnes A. Inverted knee jerk: A neglected localising sign in spinal cord disease. J Neurol Neurosurg Psychiatry 1979;42:1005

Bronish FE. The Clinically Important Reflexes. New York, Grune & Stratton, 1952

Clare MH, Landau WM. Fusiform function. Part V. Reflex reinforcement under fusiform block in normal subjects. Arch Neurol 1964;10:123

Delwaide PJ, Toulouse P. Facilitation of monosynaptic reflexes by voluntary contraction of muscle in remote parts of the body. Mechanisms involved in the Jendrassik manoeuvre. Brain 1981;104:701

Gassel MM, Diamptopuolos E. The Jendrassik maneuver. II. An analysis of the mechanism. Neurology 1964;14:640

Impallomeni M, Kenny RA, Flynn MD, Kraenzlin M et al. The elderly and their ankle jerks. Lancet 1984;1:670

Kuban KCK, Skouteli HN, Urion DK, Lawhon GA. Deep tendon reflexes in premature infants. Ped Neurol 1986;2:266

Lance JW, De Gail P. Spread of phasic muscle reflexes in normal and spastic subjects. J Neurol Neurosurg Psychiatry 1965;28:328

Miyasaki M, Ashby P, Sharpe JA, Fletcher WA. On the cause of hyporeflexia in the Holmes – Adie syndrome. Neurology 1988; 38:262

Pavlov IP. Conditioned reflexes: An investigation of the physiological activity of the cerebral cortex. Anrep GV (trans). London: Oxford University Press, 1927

Reinfrank RF, Kaufman RP, Wetstone SJ et al. Observations of the Achilles reflex. JAMA 1967;199:59

Stakenburg M. A reflex hammer for accurate measurement of reflex latency. Electroencephalogr Clin Neurophysiol 1979;46:613

Stam J, Speelman HD, van Crevel H. Tendon reflex asymmetry by voluntary mental effort in healthy subjects. Arch Neurol 1989;46:70

Schwartz RS, Morris JGL, Crimmins D et al. A comparison of two methods of eliciting the ankle jerk. Aust NZ J Med 1990;20:116

Teasdall RD, van den Ende H. A note on the deep abdominal reflex. J Neurol Neurosurg Psychiatry 1982;45:382

Wartenberg R. The Examination of Reflexes: A Simplification. Chicago, Year Book Medical Pub, 1945

Chapter 34
THE SUPERFICIAL (CUTANEOUS) REFLEXES

The superficial reflexes are those that are elicited in response to the application of a stimulus to either the skin or mucous membrane. Certain of these reflexes are associated with the individual cranial nerves and have been described in Part C, "The Cranial Nerves." Others with visceral components are discussed in Part F, "The Autonomic Nervous System." In the present classification will be included only the cutaneous reflexes — those superficial reflexes that may be elicited by stimulation of the skin, usually by a tactile stimulus such as a light touch or a scratch. A painful stimulus such as a prick or a pinch may call forth a defense reaction. These reflexes are not muscle stretch reflexes in the sense of the deep reflexes, but are skin–muscle responses. Inasmuch as the stimulus is a superficial one, they are sometimes known as exteroceptive reflexes, but probably the deep pressure or proprioceptive endings are also stimulated. These reflexes respond more slowly to the stimulus than do the deep reflexes, their latent period is more prolonged, they fatigue more easily, and they are not as consistently present as the muscle stretch reflexes.

THE SUPERFICIAL REFLEXES OF THE UPPER EXTREMITIES

The Palmar Reflex. Gentle stroking across the palm of the hand is followed by a flexion of the fingers or a closing of the hand. The thickness of the skin over the palm interferes with the ease with which this reflex may be obtained, and it is not found to an appreciable extent in normal individuals beyond the first few months of life. It is of clinical significance only in its pathologic state, the grasp, or forced grasping, reflex, to be discussed with the corticospinal tract responses of the upper extremities. The sensory and motor innervation of this reflex is through the median and ulnar nerves (sixth cervical through first thoracic segments).

The Scapular and Interscapular Reflexes. These reflexes are elicited by scratching or irritating the skin over the scapula or in the interscapular space. There is a contraction of the scapular muscles and a retraction and sometimes an elevation of the scapula. There may be associated adduction and external rotation of the arm. These cutaneous reflexes are related to the deep scapulohumeral reflex (Ch. 33), and the innervation is similar.

THE SUPERFICIAL ABDOMINAL REFLEXES

Gentle stroking of the abdomen or scratching it with a blunt object is followed by homolateral contraction of the abdominal muscles and retraction or deviation of the linea alba and umbilicus toward the area stimulated. These reflexes should be tested with the patient recumbent and the abdominal wall thoroughly relaxed. The arms should be at the sides, and the head should rest on a soft pillow to avoid tension of the abdominal musculature. Sometimes the reflex is obtained most satisfactorily at the end of expiration. A blunt point such as a match stick, split tongue blade, or wooden applicator is a satisfactory stimulus. If the object is too blunt, there may be no response, and a painful stimulus may call forth a defense reaction rendering the response unreliable. Too firm a stimulus may elicit the abdominal muscle stretch reflex (Ch. 33). The state of tonicity of the recti abdominis muscles and the position of the linea alba and the umbilicus should be noted, and any deviation should be recorded.

The abdominal reflexes have been subdivided as follows (Fig. 34-1):

The Epigastric Reflex. A stimulus directed from the tip of the sternum toward the umbilicus, or from the breast or costal margin diagonally toward the umbilicus, is followed by a contraction of the upper abdominal muscles with dimpling and drawing in of these muscles. There usually is no retraction of the umbilicus. This reflex is innervated by the intercostal nerves from the fifth through the seventh thoracic segments.

The Upper Abdominal, or Supraumbilical, Reflex. This is elicited by stimulating the skin of the upper abdominal quadrants, usually in a diagonal fashion, downward and outward from the tip of the sternum, or in a horizontal fashion, starting externally and going medially. There is a contraction of the abdominal musculature and a diagonal deviation of the umbilicus, upward and outward, toward the site of the stimulus. This reflex is innervated by the inter-

costal nerves from the seventh through the ninth thoracic segments.

The Middle Abdominal, or Umbilical, Reflex. Stimulation of the skin of the abdomen at the level of the umbilicus, either by a horizontal stimulus, starting externally and proceeding medially, or by a vertical stimulus along the lateral abdominal wall at the level of the umbilicus, is followed by a lateral deviation of the linea alba and umbilicus. This reflex is innervated by the intercostal nerves from the ninth through the eleventh thoracic segments.

The Lower Abdominal (Infraumbilical or Suprapubic) Reflex. This is elicited by stimulating the skin of the lower abdominal quadrants, either diagonally in an upward and outward direction from the region of the symphysis pubis, or horizontally, starting externally and proceeding medially. There is a contraction of the abdominal muscles and a diagonal deviation of the umbilicus toward the site of the stimulation. This reflex is innervated by the lower intercostal and the iliohypogastric and ilioinguinal nerves (eleventh and twelfth thoracic and upper lumbar segments).

Bechterew's Hypogastric Reflex consists of a contraction of the lower abdominal muscles in response to stroking the skin on the inner surface of the homolateral thigh.

These reflexes may be difficult to obtain or evaluate in ticklish individuals. They may be absent in acute abdominal disorders (**Rosenbach's**

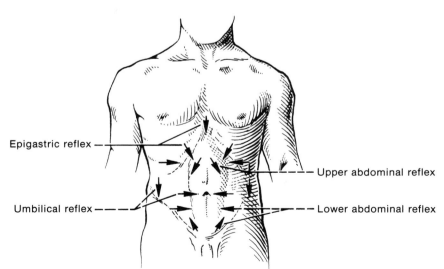

FIG. 34–1. Sites of stimulation employed in eliciting the various superficial abdominal reflexes.

sign) and abdominal or bladder distention, in obese persons and those with relaxed abdominal walls, and in women who have borne children. They may be absent on one side owing to the presence of an old abdominal incision. The latency is longer and the response is slower in children and elderly individuals than in young adults. Diminution or absence of the superficial abdominal reflexes is not significant under the above circumstances, but their absence in young individuals, especially those with good muscular development, is definitely pathologic. Dissociation of the reflexes, with absence of superficial and exaggeration of deep abdominal reflexes or of other muscle stretch reflexes, is a significant finding. If there is diminution of the reflex response, the reflex may fatigue easily; it may be elicited once or twice and then disappear. If the reflexes are diminished or absent, the lower abdominal reflex is usually affected first. In unilateral abdominal paralysis one may get an inversion of the abdominal reflexes with deviation of the umbilicus to the opposite side.

THE SUPERFICIAL REFLEXES OF THE LOWER EXTREMITIES

The Cremasteric Reflex. This reflex is elicited by stroking the skin on the upper, inner aspect of the thigh, from above downward, with a blunt point, or by pricking or lightly pinching the skin in this area. The response consists of a contraction of the cremasteric muscle with homolateral elevation of the testicle. This reflex may be absent in elderly males, in individuals who have a hydrocele or varicocele, and in those who have had orchitis or epididymitis. The innervation is through the first and second lumbar segments (ilioinguinal and genitofemoral nerves). This reflex is not to be confused with the **scrotal reflex,** a visceral reflex, which is characterized by a slow, vermicular contraction of the dartos on applying a cold object to it or on stroking the perineum.

The Gluteal Reflex. A contraction of the gluteal muscles may follow stroking the skin over the buttocks. The gluteus maximus is innervated by the inferior gluteal nerve (fourth lumbar through second sacral segments), and the skin of this area is innervated by the cutaneous branches of the posterior rami of the lumbar and sacral nerves.

The Plantar Reflex. Stroking the plantar surface of the foot from the heel forward is normally followed by plantar flexion of the foot and toes (Fig. 34-2). There is some individual variation in the response, with both flexor and extensor components present, and some variability dependent upon the site of maximal stimulation. Stroking of the posterior and lateral portions of the foot is followed by maximal plantar flexion, whereas stimulation of the anterior and medial portions, especially the ball of the great toe, may cause brief extension, more marked in the great toe than the foot. The dominant response, however, except when the ball of the great toe is stimulated, is one of plantar flexion, and with repeated stimulation the normal pattern is one of flexion. This reflex is innervated by the tibial nerve (fourth lumbar through first or second sacral segments). The predominant flexion response is the normal one after the first 12 – 18 months of life but, like the palmar reflex, is of more significance when it is present in its pathologic variation (the Babinski sign, which is described with the corticospinal tract responses of the lower extremities). The normal response may be difficult to obtain in individuals with plantar callosities, and in ticklish persons there may be a voluntary withdrawal with flexion of the hip and knee, but in every normal individual there is a certain amount of plantar flexion of the toes on stimulation of the sole of the foot. If the short flexors of the toes are paralyzed or if the

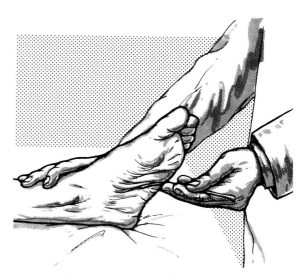

FIG. 34–2. *Method of obtaining the plantar reflex.*

flexor tendons have been severed accidentally, however, an extensor response may occur; this may be termed an inversion of the plantar reflex of peripheral origin. A tonic plantar reflex, characterized by a slow, prolonged contraction, has been described as a sign of frontal lobe and extrapyramidal involvement.

THE SUPERFICIAL ANAL REFLEX

The internal anal sphincter reflex is discussed under "Autonomic Nervous System Reflexes," in Chapter 41. There is, however, a cutaneous anal reflex that consists of a contraction of the external sphincter in response to stroking or pricking the skin or mucous membrane in the perianal region. This reflex is innervated by the inferior hemorrhoidal nerve (second through fourth or fifth sacral segments).

ABNORMALITIES OF THE SUPERFICIAL REFLEXES

The effect of lesions at various sites on the superficial reflexes is summarized in Table 33-2. The superficial reflexes, like the deep reflexes, are either diminished or absent in the event of a disturbance in the continuity of the reflex arc: In the afferent nerve, motor center, or efferent nerve. The superficial reflexes, however, especially the abdominal and cremasteric reflexes, have a special significance when their absence is associated with an exaggeration of the deep reflexes (**dissociation of reflexes**) or when they are absent in instances where signs of corticospinal tract involvement are elicited. The superficial reflexes have, in addition to a spinal reflex arc, a superimposed cortical pathway. Impulses ascend through the spinal cord and brain stem to the parietal areas of the brain and have connections with the motor centers of the cortex. Efferent impulses then descend either in the corticospinal pathways or in intimate association with them. As a consequence, an interruption of the reflex arc at a higher level, or a lesion anywhere along the corticospinal pathway, will usually cause either diminution or absence of these reflexes. This change is on the side of the body contralateral to the lesion if the lesion is above the pyramidal decussation, and is homolateral if the lesion is below the pyramidal decussation. This dissociation of reflexes, or absence of superficial reflexes in the presence of exaggerated deep reflexes, is a significant finding in corticospinal tract disease. Dissociation of abdominal reflexes alone (diminution or loss of the superficial ones and hyperactivity of the deep ones) may be of diagnostic importance. It must be stated, however, that occasionally with apparent corticospinal tract disease the superficial abdominal reflexes are intact, and such may be the case in congenital spastic paraparesis and even certain transverse lesions of the spinal cord.

The abdominal reflexes are also absent in deep sleep, surgical anesthesia, and coma, and in the presence of violent emotions such as fear. They are absent in newly born infants and appear after about 6 months to 1 year; their appearance may be dependent upon the myelination of the corticospinal tracts, which is not complete at birth. Apparent abdominal reflexes, which are elicited in about one third of the infants examined, differ from the normal adult response: they are characterized by a diffuse reaction, often with associated movement of the legs. It must always be borne in mind that both the abdominal and the cremasteric reflexes may be absent in persons without neurologic disease. It has been said that absence of the abdominal reflexes is pathognomonic of multiple sclerosis; this, however, is not a characteristic of the disease itself, but of the spinal cord or corticospinal tract involvement that is so frequently a part of the disorder. Fatigability of the abdominal reflexes has been said to be an early sign in multiple sclerosis and other corticospinal tract disorders, including hemiplegia.

The superficial reflexes, including the abdominal reflexes, are occasionally moderately exaggerated in parkinsonism and other extrapyramidal disorders. It has been suggested that this increase results from involvement of a center at the level of the midbrain that normally inhibits the superficial reflexes. The abdominal reflexes may also be increased, often to a marked degree, in tension states and neuroses. On occasion this overactivity is so extreme that the umbilicus is said to "chase the pin" when the stimulating instrument is drawn in a circular manner over the surface of the abdomen. This may have diagnostic significance, because in both corticospinal tract disease and psychogenic states the muscle stretch reflexes may be exaggerated, although the type of increase is different; in psychogenic disorders the superficial reflexes may also be increased, whereas they are decreased in corticospinal tract disease. The superficial reflexes are normal with cerebellar lesions.

It is advisable to interpret changes in the superficial reflexes in the light of all other findings on the neurologic examination and related imaging and electrodiagnostic studies. Definite signs of corticospinal tract disturbance (Chapter 35) are of greater importance than decrease or absence of superficial reflexes.

BIBLIOGRAPHY

Grimby L. Normal plantar response: Integration of flexor and extensor reflex components. J Neurol Neurosurg Psychiatry 1963;26:39

Lehoczky T, Fodors T. Clinical significance of the dissociation of abdominal reflexes. Neurology 1953;3:453

Madonick MJ. Statistical control studies in neurology. 8. The cutaneous abdominal reflex. Neurology 1957;7:459

Magladery JW, Teasdale RD, French JH, Busch ES. Cutaneous reflex changes in development and aging. Arch Neurol 1960;3:1

Chapter 35
CORTICOSPINAL (PYRAMIDAL) TRACT RESPONSES

With disease of the corticospinal or pyramidal system (in the usually accepted clinical sense — see Ch. 23), certain abnormalities are found in the reflex pattern. This is true whether the disease process is in the motor cortex itself, the projection fibers, or anywhere along the descending tracts. The superficial reflexes may be decreased or absent, and the muscle stretch reflexes are exaggerated (see Table 33-2). If the hyperactivity of the latter is sufficiently great or if muscle tonus is markedly increased, there is also a pathologic response in the form of **clonus** — a series of rhythmic involuntary muscular contractions induced by the sudden passive stretching of a muscle or tendon. An autonomous central generator has been postulated to produce clonus, but self-reexcitation of stretch reflexes has also been implicated. At times this clonus is spontaneous and will develop with the slightest stimulus; it may be produced merely by placing weight on the toes and actively dorsiflexing the foot at the ankle. On other occasions it may have to be brought on by special maneuvers. Clonus occurs most frequently at the ankle, knee, and wrist, but it may be obtained elsewhere.

Ankle clonus consists of a series of rhythmic alternating flexions and extensions of the foot at the ankle; it follows stretching of the triceps surae, and is the result of repeated contractions of this muscle. It is sometimes produced by attempts to elicit the Achilles reflex, but is easiest to obtain if the examiner supports the leg, preferably with one hand under the knee or the calf, grasps the foot from below with the other hand, and quickly dorsiflexes the foot while maintaining pressure on the sole at the end of the move-

ment (Fig. 35-1). The leg and foot should be well relaxed, the knee and ankle in moderate flexion, and the foot slightly everted.

Patellar clonus consists of a series of rhythmic up-and-down movements of the patella. It follows stretching the quadriceps, and is the result of repeated contractions of this muscle. It may appear in the process of eliciting the patellar or suprapatellar reflex (see Fig. 33-9). It is most easily elicited, however, if the examiner grasps the patella between his index finger and thumb and produces a sudden, sharp, downward displacement of this structure. The leg should be in extension and relaxed as much as possible.

Clonus of the wrist or of the fingers may be produced by a sudden passive extension of the wrist or fingers. Clonus of the jaw occurs occasionally.

Varying degrees of clonus may be obtained. Transient (exhaustible, nonsustained, or abortive) clonus is significant, although sustained clonus is usually indicative of a more profound corticospinal tract dysfunction. Transient clonus, however, is not always indicative of organic disease of the central nervous system and may be found in other conditions, either organic or psychogenic, in which there is general hyperactivity of the reflexes. A true clonus must be differentiated from a false or spurious one, which is always indicative of psychogenic disorders. **False clonus,** also termed pseudoclonus, is not only poorly sustained but also irregular in rate, rhythm, and excursion. At the ankle a true clonus can usually be stopped by a sharp passive plantar flexion of the foot or of the great toe,

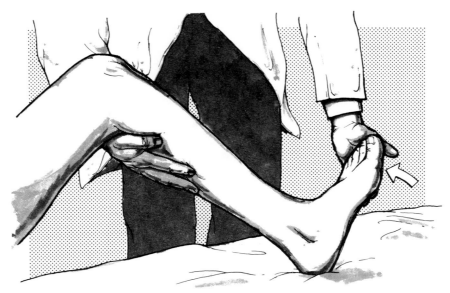

FIG. 35–1. Method of eliciting ankle clonus.

whereas false clonus is not altered by such a maneuver.

In addition to such changes, lesions of the corticospinal system are characterized by the presence of certain pathologic reflex responses not found in the normal individual. Some of these are actually exaggerations, perversions, or abnormal manifestations of muscle stretch and superficial reflexes that are normally present; the response may occur on the basis of decrease in threshold, increase in stimulus, or extension of the zone of provocation. Others are closely allied to postural reflexes and associated movements or are related to primitive defense reflexes that are normally suppressed by cerebral inhibition but are released when the lower motor neuron is separated from the influence of the higher centers. In most instances they appear to be the result of involvement of the descending extrapyramidal pathways from the premotor cortex as well as the descending corticospinal fibers from the motor cortex, but they are generally known as corticospinal or pyramidal tract responses. For the purposes of classification the corticospinal tract responses of the upper and lower extremities are considered separately.

CORTICOSPINAL TRACT RESPONSES IN THE UPPER EXTREMITIES

The corticospinal tract responses in the upper extremities are less constant, more difficult to elicit, and usually less significant diagnostically than those found in the lower extremities. A great deal of confusion exists concerning the names and the reflexes themselves, with many variations and modifications of the same response. Those of most frequent occurrence and of most clinical significance follow. These responses occur only with lesions above the fifth or sixth cervical segments of the spinal cord.

The Grasp (Forced Grasping) Reflex

This is a flexor response of the fingers and hand following stimulation of the skin of the palmar surface of the fingers or hand. There are four variations and modifications: (1) If the examiner's fingers are introduced into the patient's hand, especially between the thumb and forefinger, or if the skin of the palm is stimulated gently, there is a slow flexion of the digits. The patient's fingers may close around the examiner's fingers in a gentle grasp that can be relaxed upon command. This is the **simple grasp reflex,** an exaggeration of the normal palmar reflex. (2) If the patient's flexed fingers are gently extended by the fingers of the examiner, they will flex against the examiner's fingers. This is the **"hooking" response.** Inasmuch as stretching of the flexor muscles initiates this effect, it could be considered a pathologic variation of the finger flexor reflex as well as the palmar reflex. (3) If the simple grasp response is marked, the examiner will note that as he tries to withdraw his fingers the force of the patient's grasp increases and there is loss of ability to relax it voluntarily or on command. The grip may be so firm that the patient can be lifted from the bed by the examiner. This is known as **tonic perseveration,** or the **forced grasping reflex,** and is a part of the counterholding, or gegenhalten, phenomenon, in which muscle contraction develops in response to contact and as a resistance to changes in position and posture. The strength of grasp becomes exaggerated with attempts to withdraw the examiner's hand or to extend the patient's fingers passively. (4) The sight of the observer's hand near but not touching the patient's hand, or even a very light touch on the patient's hand between the thumb and forefinger while his eyes are closed, leads him to move his hand in such a way as to facilitate grasping the examiner's fingers, sometimes with a sequence of rhythmic reaching movements. This is termed the **groping response.**

These responses may be part of the normal postural or body righting reflexes. They are present from birth and begin to diminish at the age of 2 – 4 months. They may be so marked in the infant that the child can be suspended by his own grasp. In older individuals these reflexes are inhibited by the action of the pyramidal and premotor cortices and occur only as release phenomena. They may persist in children with birth injuries, developmental disturbances, motor difficulties of cerebral origin, and mental deficiency. In adults they may be present in patients with spastic hemiplegia of cerebral origin, but are found more frequently in those with extensive neoplastic or vascular lesions of the frontal lobes or with cerebral degenerative processes. These responses are usually contralateral but occasionally are ipsilateral, and are believed to indicate predominant involvement of the premotor region, although the motor area is probably affected as well. They may also be present in comatose patients, and have been reported in association with lesions of the posterior fossa, probably secondary to increased intracranial pressure. In experimental neurophysiology of primates, in which forced grasping can be tested, grasping comes on immediately after the removal of the premotor area, but it does not persist. It becomes permanent after removal of both areas 4 and 6. Whereas the grasping responses are exaggerations of normal reactions and occur as release phenomena, the groping response is a somewhat more complicated reaction that is modified by visual and tactile integration at the cortical level. Many neurologists would classify these reflexes with the so-called frontal release signs or primitive reflexes rather than with the corticospinal tract responses.

The Hoffmann and Trömner Signs and the Flexor Reflexes of the Fingers and Hand

To elicit the **Hoffmann sign** the examiner supports the patient's hand, dorsiflexed at the wrist, so that it is completely relaxed and the fingers are partially flexed. The middle finger is partially extended and either its middle or distal phalanx is grasped firmly between the examiner's index finger and thumb. With a sharp, forcible flick of his other thumb, the examiner nips or snaps the nail of the patient's middle finger, causing a forcible increased flexion of this finger by sudden release (Fig. 35-2). If the Hoffmann sign is present, this is followed by flexion and adduction of the thumb and flexion of the index finger, and sometimes flexion of the other fingers as well. The sign is said to be incomplete if only the thumb or only the index finger responds. An alternate method of performing this same test is that described by **Trömner** in which the examiner holds the patient's hand in relaxation by grasping either the proximal or middle phalanx of the partially flexed middle finger between his thumb and index finger. With the middle finger of the other hand he taps the volar surface of the distal phalanx of the middle finger (Fig. 35-3). The response is the same as that in the Hoffmann sign and either manner of testing may be used. Sometimes both are referred to as the Hoffmann test, but they should be differentiated.

These signs are variations in the technic of eliciting the **finger flexor reflex** (see Fig. 33-5), and when present indicate hyperactivity of the muscle stretch reflexes. They are often called corticospinal tract signs, and when positive are said to indicate the presence of a lesion of the corticospinal system above the fifth or sixth cervical segment. They are not necessarily pathologic, however, and may be present with in-

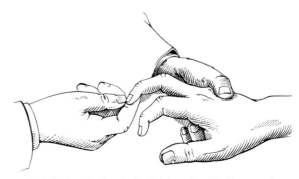

FIG. 35–2. Method of eliciting the Hoffmann sign.

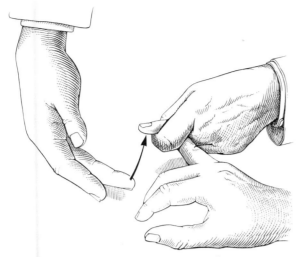

FIG. 35–3. *Method of eliciting the Trömner sign.*

creased muscle tonus and generalized reflex hyperactivity associated with tetanus, tetany, anxiety, and tension states. An incomplete Hoffmann sign is encountered fairly frequently in healthy persons. It can be stated, however, that a very active, complete Hoffmann or Trömner sign, especially if unilateral or if associated with other abnormalities of the reflexes or with a history of nervous system disease, is certainly suggestive if not diagnostic of corticospinal tract involvement.

Many other flexor reflexes of the fingers and hand have been described and have been referred to as corticospinal tract responses. Most of these are variations or exaggerations of the finger flexor reflex, which may be barely perceptible in normal persons, or of this response together with the wrist flexion reflex. Some may be related to forced grasping. Probably, like the Hoffmann sign, they show the presence of reflex hyperactivity, but if unilateral or associated with other reflex changes may suggest corticospinal tract involvement. They are not used frequently in the routine neurologic examination because many are elicited with difficulty and found only in isolated cases.

In the **Rossolimo of the hand,** flexion of the fingers and supination of the forearm follow either percussion of the palmar aspect of the metacarpophalangeal joints or tapping the volar surface of the patient's fingertips. Flexion of the fingers and hand may follow not only stimulation of the flexor tendons on the volar surface of the forearm, but also percussion of the dorsal aspect of the carpal and metacarpal areas (the

Mendel – Bechterew of the hand, or the **carpometacarpal** or **carpophalangeal reflex** of Bechterew), or tapping the dorsum of either the hand or the fingers. Flexion of the wrist and fingers appears with an exaggerated brachioradialis reflex, and with inversion of this reflex there is such flexion with flexion and supination of the forearm. The **thumb-adductor reflex of Marie – Foix** consists of adduction and flexion of the thumb, sometimes with flexion of the adjacent digits and more rarely with extension of the little finger, in response to either superficial stroking of the palm of the hand in the hypothenar region, or scratching the ulnar side of the palm.

The same response is also obtained in the following maneuvers: In the Foxe reflex by pinching the hypothenar region; in the Oppenheim sign by rubbing the external surface of the forearm; in the Schaefer sign by pinching the flexor tendons at the wrist; in the Gordon flexion sign by squeezing the muscles of the forearm. The ulnar adduction reflex of Pool consists of adduction of the thumb on stimulating any portion of the palm that is innervated by the ulnar nerve.

Extensor Reflexes of the Fingers and Hand

Hand flexion may be followed by extension of the fingers and hand, or extension responses may occur instead of flexion. In addition to forced grasping, an extension reaction of the fingers and hand following dorsal stimulation has been described in the newborn. In the **Chaddock wrist sign** either pressure or scratching in the depression at the ulnar side of the tendons of the flexor carpi radialis and palmaris longus muscles at the junction of the forearm and wrist, or pressure on the palmaris longus tendon, is followed by flexion of the wrist and simultaneous extension and separation of the digits. At times the response may follow irritation of almost any part of the skin on the ulnar side of the volar aspect of the forearm as high as the elbow. In the **Gordon extension sign** extension and occasionally fanning of the flexed fingers follow pressure on the radial side of the pisiform bone. In the **extension-adduction reflex of Dagnini** percussion on the radial aspect of the dorsum of the hand is followed by extension and slight adduction of the wrist. In the **Bachtiarow sign** stroking downward along the radius with the thumb and index finger is followed by extension and slight adduction of the thumb. In the **tonic extensor reflex of the digits** described by

Vernea and Botez superficial stimulation of the dorsum of the fingers of patients with a grasp reflex is followed by tonic extension of the fingers; this may be followed by the grasp response. These reflexes, too, have been said to indicate lesions of the corticospinal system, but like the flexor reflexes are evidence of reflex hyperactivity and suggest corticospinal tract involvement only if they are unilateral or associated with other reflex changes. These reflexes, although they are unique and interesting, probably have little clinical significance.

Other Corticospinal Responses of the Upper Extremities

The Palmomental Reflex of Marinesco – Radovici. This is manifested by contraction of the ipsilateral mentalis and orbicularis oris muscles in response to stimulation of the thenar area of the hand. There is wrinkling of the skin of the chin and slight retraction and sometimes elevation of the angle of the mouth. The reflex may be elicited by scratching with a blunt point over the eminence from the wrist to the proximal phalanx or in the opposite direction, or by tapping this area. This sign is sometimes present with corticospinal tract disease, but may also be found with frontal lobe lesions and diffuse cortical involvement (see Chapter 39, "Frontal Release Signs"). It is occasionally present in normal persons, especially those who are anxious and apprehensive; it is absent in peripheral facial palsy and may be exaggerated in central facial paresis. If the response is a marked one, there may be wide zones for effective stimulation, including the hypothenar area of the hand. Contraction of the mentalis muscle in response to stroking of the palmar surface of the thumb is the **pollicomental reflex.** The localizing value and clinical significance of these reflexes are limited.

The Klippel – Feil Sign. This sign consists of involuntary flexion, opposition, and adduction of the thumb on passive extension of the fingers when there is some degree of contracture in flexion.

The Leri Sign. To test for this sign the examiner holds the patient's supinated and slightly flexed forearm in one hand, and with the other forcibly flexes the patient's fingers and wrist. In normal persons this maneuver is accompanied by contraction of the biceps muscle and flexion of the forearm, and there may also be adduction of the upper arm. This response is absent with lesions of the corticospinal system; this absence is known as the Leri sign. Associated flexion at the elbow may be increased with frontal lobe lesions.

The Mayer Sign. The patient's hand is held in the examiner's hand, palm up, with the fingers slightly bent and the thumb in slight flexion and abduction. The examiner places slow but firm pressure on the proximal phalanges of the fingers, especially the third and fourth fingers, flexing them at the metacarpophalangeal joints and pressing them against the palm. In normal persons this is followed by adduction and opposition of the thumb with flexion at the metacarpophalangeal joint and extension at the interphalangeal joint. This response is absent in corticospinal tract lesions, and its absence is known as the Mayer sign. It is occasionally absent in normal individuals, but such absence should be bilateral. It is also absent in hypotonia and peripheral nerve lesions. It is increased in meningitis and may be exaggerated in brain tumors, especially if located in the frontal lobes.

The normal response in both the Leri and Mayer signs may be difficult or impossible to elicit in individuals without nervous system disease. Consequently these signs may have little clinical significance.

The Bending Reflex. The Mayer and Leri phenomena are probably related to postural reflexes and associated movements. Seyffarth described a similar phenomenon, which he called the bending reflex: Forced passive palmar flexion of the wrist is accompanied by flexion of the elbow in normal subjects. Attempted passive extension of the elbow during its phase of flexion reinforces the bending reflex and causes it to spread to the shoulder muscles. With frontal lobe lesions the associated contraction of the proximal muscles is greatly increased and can be obtained even with passive radial flexion of the wrist.

The Sign of the Forearm. Stroking the radial aspect of the semiflexed and semipronated forearm is followed, in the normal individual, by further flexion of the forearm and radial elevation of the hand. In lesions of the corticospinal system there is flexion of the forearm without elevation of the hand, while in psychogenic hyperactivity of the response the elevation of the hand may be more marked than the flexion of the forearm.

The Nociceptive Reflexes of Riddoch and Buzzard.

In corticospinal tract lesions characterized by hemiplegia, painful stimulation by scratching, pricking, or pinching of the ulnar aspect of the palmar surface of the hand or the fingers, the inner surface of the forearm or arm, the walls of the axilla, or the upper part of the chest will result in mass flexion movements of the upper extremity, with abduction and external rotation of the shoulder, and flexion of the elbow, wrist, and finger joints. In quadriplegia, especially if due to a high cervical lesion, the same type of stimulus evokes an extensor response characterized by elevation, retraction, adduction, and internal rotation of the ipsilateral shoulder, extension of the elbow, pronation of the forearm, flexion of the wrist, and hyperextension and adduction of the fingers, with overlapping of the extended fingers and adduction of the thumb in extension. The flexor response is most easily elicited by stimulation of the hand or forearm, whereas the extensor response is most easily initiated by a stimulus to the upper arm or axillary wall. These are considered to be associated postural reactions related to the reflexes of spinal automatism.

Some of the corticospinal tract responses described here, as for instance the grasp reflex, are seen only in instances where the disease process is extensive. Many of them are related to each other and are merely different modes of eliciting the same response. Some may be found in nonorganic as well as in organic states. The responses that are obtained must be evaluated not on the basis of the individual sign, but as a part of the entire reflex picture.

CORTICOSPINAL TRACT RESPONSES IN THE LOWER EXTREMITIES

The corticospinal tract responses in the lower extremities are more constant and more clearly defined than those in the upper limbs and may be elicited with more ease. As is also the case with the upper extremity reflexes, however, there is a great deal of confusion of names and reflexes, and many of the so-called reflexes are merely variations in the method of eliciting the same responses, or modifications of the same reflex. The most important of these responses may be classified as (1) those characterized in the main by dorsiflexion of the toes, and (2) those characterized by plantar flexion of the toes. There are, in addition, a few miscellaneous responses.

Corticospinal Responses Characterized in the Main by Extension (Dorsiflexion) of the Toes

The Babinski Sign

In the normal individual, stimulation of the plantar surface of the foot is followed by plantar flexion of the toes (see Fig. 34-2). The response is usually a fairly rapid one, the small toes flex more than the great toe, and the reaction is more marked when the posterior and lateral aspects of the plantar surface are stimulated. This is the normal plantar reflex, a superficial reflex innervated by the fourth lumbar through the first or second sacral segments by means of the tibial nerve. In disease of the corticospinal system there is an inversion of this reflex, the **Babinski sign** or **extensor plantar response.** Stimulation of the plantar surface of the foot, under such circumstances, is followed by dorsiflexion of the toes, especially of the great toe, together with a separation or fanning of the toes (Fig. 35-4). The two essential manifestations were described separately by Babinski as the *phénomène des orteils* (the dorsiflexion of the toes) and the *signe de l'éventail* (the fanning). In addition, especially if the response is marked, there is dorsiflexion at the ankle, with flexion at the knee and hip, and possibly slight abduction of the thigh. These associated movements are brought about by contraction of the anterior tibial, hamstring, tensor fasciae latae, and related muscles. They are a part of the spinal defense reflex mechanism. The contraction of the tensor fasciae latae has been referred to as **Brissaud's reflex.** The dorsiflexion of the toes may be the only visible effect, but the contraction of the thigh and leg muscles is always present and can be detected by palpation.

The Babinski sign is elicited by stimulating the palmar surface of the foot with a blunt point, preferably a match stick, a toothpick, a wooden applicator, a broken tongue blade, or the tip of a key. Some examiners use a fingertip or the thumbnail. The stimulus should be a threshold one, and as light as possible, but if no response is obtained, progressively sharper objects and firmer applications may be used. Both tickling, which may cause voluntary withdrawal, and pain, which may bring about a reversal to flexion as a nociceptive response, should be avoided. The stimulus is directed from the heel forward, usually stopping at the metatarsophalangeal joints, and both the inner and outer aspects of the sole should be tested. If the response is difficult to obtain, it may be elicited more readily by

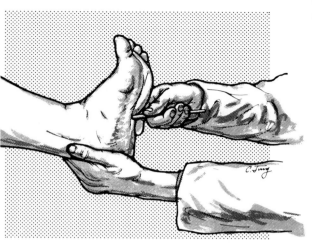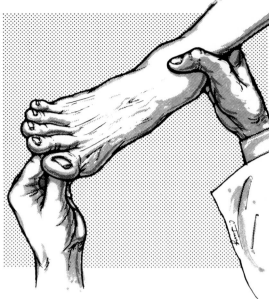

FIG. 35–4. Method of eliciting the Babinski sign.

stimulating the lateral aspect of the sole, often continuing along the metatarsal pad from the little to the great toe. The patient should be well relaxed, and it is best to have him lie in the recumbent position with his hips and knees in extension and his heels resting on the bed. If he is seated, the knee should be extended, with the foot held either in the examiner's hand or on his knee. The response may sometimes be reinforced by rotating the patient's head to the opposite side. It may be inhibited when the foot is cold and increased when the foot is warm although a cold stimulus has been used to evoke the response. It may be abolished by flexion of the knee, and in 50% of cases, is abolished by placing an Esmarch bandage around the leg.

The characteristic response is one of slow, tonic, sometimes clonic, dorsiflexion of the great toe and the small toes with fanning, or separation, of the toes. Occasionally, however, there is a rapid but brief extension at first, which is followed by flexion, or predominant flexion followed by extension. There may be only extension of the great toe, or extension of the great toe with flexion of the small toes. Either dorsiflexion or fanning may occur separately. Occasionally brief flexion of the great toe precedes extension. There may be flexion of the hip and knee with no movement of the toes. The response may depend in part upon the site and intensity of the stimulus. With repeated stimulation of the sole the extensor movement may decrease and then disappear. The phenomenon may also show itself in *formes frustes*, which are also significant. For instance, there may be no response whatever to plantar stimulation; this is of consequence if it is known that there is no lower motor neuron lesion to cause paralysis of either extension or flexion, and no lesion of the peripheral nerves. If there is paralysis of the dorsiflexors, there may be no Babinski response even though one is expected. These variations and incomplete responses are sometimes referred to as "equivocal Babinski signs." They are all significant, and the examiner should describe the response rather than make an arbitrary statement that the Babinski sign is either present or absent.

The response to plantar stimulation may be difficult to evaluate, especially when the plantar surface of the foot is overly sensitive. There may be voluntary withdrawal, which consists of rapid flexion of the ankle, knee, and hip. With plantar hyperesthesia, often present with peripheral neuritis, there may also be a reflex withdrawal that interferes with evaluation of the response. Under such circumstances it may be necessary to hold the foot at the ankle. With thick plantar callosities it may be necessary to intensify the stimulus. In individuals with cavus deformities of the feet and with high arched feet, such as are encountered in Friedreich's ataxia, the response is difficult to evaluate because of the presence of some dorsiflexion of the toes. In instances where the reflex is pronounced there may be either contralateral or bilateral responses, with an increase in the reflexogenous zone (a widening of the receptive field), so that the phenomenon may be obtained by stimulation of other than the usual sites. These alternate sites of stimulation will be mentioned with the other dorsiflexion responses in this chapter and with the spinal defense reflexes in Chapter 36. Occasionally there is a "spontaneous Babinski" following manipulation of the foot; in infants and children it is sometimes brought out by rapid removal of the sock or shoe. In patients with extensive corticospinal tract disease dorsiflexion of the great toe and often of the other toes may follow either passive extension of the knee or passive flexion of the hip and knee, and sometimes the toes are held in a constant position of dorsiflexion and fanning.

False responses, or "pseudo-Babinski signs" may occur in the absence of corticospinal tract disease. The voluntary withdrawal in overly sensitive individuals, the response in plantar hyperesthesia, and the reactions from too strong a stimulus may give an appearance of a Babinski sign. In athetosis and chorea there may be a false response due to the hyperkinesia. If the short flexors of the toes are paralyzed, there may be an inversion of the plantar reflex of peripheral origin. All of these should be remembered when describing the response. In most instances, however, there is no contraction of the hamstring muscles in association with a "pseudo-Babinski sign." Also, it has been said that pressure over the base of the great toe will inhibit the withdrawal extensor response, but will not eliminate the extension associated with corticospinal tract disease.

The Babinski sign has been called the most important sign in clinical neurology. It is considered to be one of the most significant indications of disease of the corticospinal system at any level from the motor cortex through the descending pathways. It is not obtained following destruction of the pyramidal system in lower primates and there is an altered plantar response with such lesions in intermediate primates, but an extensor response appears with involvement of the pyramidal system in higher forms. Experiments have suggested that lesions of the motor or pyramidal cortex (area 4 of Brodmann) and its descending pathways are followed by the extensor response together with the Chaddock sign, whereas lesions of the premotor cortex (area 6 of Brodmann) and its descending pathways are followed by the fanning response, together with

the Hoffmann sign, forced grasping, and the Rossolimo sign. In lesions of both the motor and premotor systems, there is a more vigorous extensor response, together with fanning. The results of these studies, however, are not conclusive, although they are useful in the analysis of clinical problems. As has been mentioned in the discussion of the corticospinal system, however, for clinical diagnosis it is appropriate to consider the pyramidal or corticospinal system in the clinically accepted sense, assuming that in most instances of disease of the nervous system, involvement of the premotor cortex and its connections is also present.

The Babinski sign may be an indication of a disturbance of the corticospinal pathway, but not necessarily an interruption. It may be produced following suppression as well as destruction of somatic nerve activity. It is occasionally elicited in persons with no other evidence of corticospinal tract disease and in a small percentage of individuals who show no other evidence of nervous system involvement. It may be the only residual sign of previous disease.

If the basal ganglia and the corticospinal tract are both destroyed, there is no extensor response. In all probability an intact basal ganglion system is essential to its production. It has never been demonstrated unequivocally in lesions of the basal ganglia alone, and its presence in certain extrapyramidal syndromes, such as Parkinson's disease, suggests associated corticospinal tract involvement. Occasionally, however, for reasons not well understood, it may not be possible to elicit the Babinski sign in patients with paraplegia or other diseases affecting the corticospinal pathways, even though other signs of upper motor neuron involvement (spasticity, hyperactive muscle stretch reflexes, and clonus) are present. On the other hand, there may be a crossed extensor response or bilateral Babinski signs following unilateral stimulation in some patients with bilateral cerebral or spinal cord disease.

It must be remembered, however, that the extensor response may at times be found in other conditions in which it is not possible to demonstrate pathologic changes in the corticospinal system. The extensor response has been said to be the normal one in the newborn infant, response to plantar stimulation gradually assuming its flexor form at 6 – 18 months, or by 2 years of age. More recent studies, however, claim that 93% or even more of normal newborns have a flexor plantar response and suggest that the presence of a Babinski sign even at birth is abnormal.

In individuals with delayed maturation resulting from birth injuries or with developmental disturbances, motor difficulties of cerebral origin, or mental deficiency, the assumption of the normal plantar response is much delayed, and if there are persisting motor defects the Babinski sign never disappears. Yakovlev found that prolonged physical exhaustion or a 14-mile march will result in the development of a Babinski sign in 7% of otherwise normal individuals. Investigation showed that those who develop a Babinski sign under such circumstances had learned to walk or talk late or were deficient intellectually; many had a history of premature birth or infantile convulsions. In all probability they had prenatal, natal, or neonatal alterations in the nervous system, especially of the corticospinal centers and pathways, as a result of developmental abnormalities, premature birth, birth injury, or acute disease of the nervous system in early infancy, with a resulting deficiency in myelination, and it was this, rather than locomotion or exertion *per se* that was responsible for the development of the Babinski sign. The ease with which the response is brought on following exertion is an index of the degree of the abnormality. In a few instances a Babinski sign has been observed in patients whose reactions were brought on or reverted to the infantile stage by hypnosis.

The Babinski sign may also be obtained in states of unconsciousness. It is sometimes present in profound sleep; it may be obtained in deep anesthesia and narcosis, in drug and alcohol intoxication, following electroconvulsive therapy, in coma secondary to metabolic disturbances, in post-traumatic states, and in other conditions where there is complete loss of consciousness. It is found in the postconvulsive stage of epilepsy, where it has been used as a criterion of the organicity of the seizures; it is rarely present, however, except during the period of unconsciousness, and is probably a manifestation of the coma or, especially if unilateral, a focal sign pointing to the underlying disease process. In Cheyne–Stokes respirations the extensor response may appear during the period of apnea, whereas in the phase of active respiration the normal reflex in seen. Recovery from deep anesthesia or from coma caused by drug intoxication, such as barbiturate poisoning, is accompanied by the disappearance of the Babinski sign, appearance of the superficial reflexes, and gradual return of the muscle stretch reflexes to normal. The Babinski sign may be obtained in normal individuals following injection of scopolamine or barbiturates in sufficiently large doses, and a latent Babinski phenomenon may be brought out following the injection of a smaller amount. The injection of physostigmine in physiologic doses may abolish a Babinski sign.

Other Dorsiflexion Responses

There are many other corticospinal tract responses in the lower extremities that are characterized by dorsiflexion of the toes. In fact, there are so many modifications that they cannot all be mentioned. Some are merely evidence of an increase in the reflexogenous zone, and thus may denote responses from different parts of the receptive field; others, however, are important in that they can be elicited in cases where, for some reason, the plantar surface of the foot cannot be stimulated. Some of these modifications are as follows:

The **Chaddock sign** is elicited by stimulating the lateral aspect of the foot with a blunt point such as that used to elicit the Babinski sign. The stimulus is usually applied under and around the external malleolus in a circular direction, but may also be applied to the lateral aspect of the foot, below the malleolus, from the heel forward to the small toe. The **Oppenheim sign** is elicited by applying heavy pressure with the thumb and index finger to the anterior surface of the tibia, mainly on its medial aspect, and stroking down from the infrapatellar region to the ankle. The response is a slow one and usually occurs toward the end of stimulation. The **Gordon sign** is obtained by squeezing or applying deep pressure to the calf muscles. The **Schaefer sign** is produced by deep pressure on the Achilles tendon. The **Bing sign** is elicited by pricking the dorsum of the foot with a pin. The **Moniz sign** follows forceful passive plantar flexion at the ankle. The **Throckmorton sign** is produced by percussing over the dorsal aspect of the metatarsophalangeal joint of the great toe just medial to the tendon of the extensor hallucis longus muscle. The **Strümpell phenomenon** follows forceful pressure over the anterior tibial region. The **Cornell response** is elicited by scratching the dorsum of the foot along the inner side of the extensor tendon of the great toe. **Gonda** and **Allen** independently described a sign that is elicited by forceful downward stretching or snapping of the distal phalanx of either the second or fourth toe; and **Allen** and **Cleckley** described one that is produced by a sharp upward flick of the second toe or by pressure applied to the ball of the toe. Gonda has stated that if the response is difficult to obtain, the examiner may flex the toe slowly, press on the nail, and twist the toe and hold it for a few seconds.

Szapiro has described a method of reinforcing the extensor response by adding proprioceptive to exteroceptive stimulation: He presses against the dorsum of the second through fifth toes, causing firm passive plantar flexion, while stimulating the plantar surface of the foot. Similar reinforcement may be brought about by performing two procedures simultaneously (*e.g.*, testing for the Oppenheim sign while stroking the plantar surface of the foot). In all of the tests mentioned, those in which the stimuli are primarily proprioceptive are more apt to be followed by a slow, tonic response, while those that are mainly exteroceptive cause a brief, rapid extension.

These various signs, some of which are elicited by cutaneous stimuli, others by deep pressure, and still others by either passive or active motion, are in all probability incomplete homolateral mass flexion withdrawal responses, related to the reflexes of spinal automatism (Ch. 36). They are modifications of the **Marie – Foix sign,** a part of the spinal defense mechanism, which consists of dorsiflexion of the ankle and flexion at the hip and knee in response to squeezing the toes or strongly plantar flexing the toes or the foot. In all, the pathologic response is extension of the toes, especially of the great toe. Fanning of the toes, if it does occur, is less marked, as is flexion at the hip and knee. The Babinski sign is probably the most delicate, the first to be evident in the presence of disease, and the one that occurs most frequently, but it is occasionally possible to elicit one or more of the others when the Babinski sign cannot be obtained. The Chaddock sign is next in frequency. It may be that a more extensive lesion is necessary for the production of the Oppenheim or Gordon sign than for the Babinski or Chaddock. As previously mentioned, it is occasionally of value to try two maneuvers simultaneously, such as the Babinski and Oppenheim or the Babinski and the Gordon, to bring forth a latent extensor response by means of reinforcement.

Corticospinal Tract Responses Characterized by Plantar Flexion of the Toes

In the newborn infant there is a **grasp reflex** in the foot as well as in the hand, and tonic flexion and adduction of the toes may occur in response to a light pressure on the plantar surface of the foot, especially its distal portion. This disappears by the end of the first year, but it may persist in infants with birth injuries and retarded development. It may be found in adults, along with the hand grasp reflex, in disease of the opposite frontal lobe.

In addition to the superficial plantar reflex, there is a **plantar muscle reflex** consisting of contraction of the flexor muscles of the toes with flexion of the toes following sudden stretching. This response is barely, if at all, perceptible in normal persons, but is present with reflex hyperactivity and, therefore, with corticospinal tract lesions. There is also a group of reflexes, often called **pyramidal tract signs of the lower extremities,** in which the pathologic response is one of plantar flexion of the toes rather than dorsiflexion, in contrast to the Babinski sign. These probably are all manifestations or exaggerations of the plantar muscle reflex, and as such are comparable to the variations of the finger flexor reflex in the upper extremities. They are found in corticospinal tract lesions, but on the other hand their presence may indicate merely a functional hyperactivity of the reflexes. The two to be described first are the most important of the group.

The **Rossolimo sign** is elicited by tapping the ball of the foot, percussing the plantar surface of the great toe, tapping or stroking the balls of the toes, or giving a quick, lifting snap to the tips of the toes (Fig. 35-5). The test should be carried

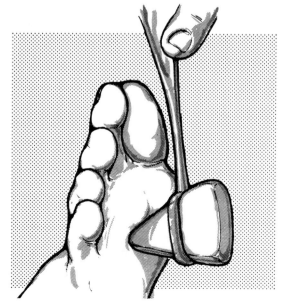

FIG. 35–5. *Method of eliciting the Rossolimo sign.*

out while the patient is lying in the recumbent position with his leg extended. The **Mendel – Bechterew,** or **dorsocuboidal, sign** is elicited by tapping or stroking the outer aspect of the dorsum of the foot in the region of the cuboid bone, or over the fourth and fifth metatarsals. This is also known as the **tarsophalangeal reflex.** Following both of these maneuvers there is only slight dorsiflexion of the toes or no movement whatever in the normal individual. There is a quick plantar flexion of the toes, especially of the smaller ones, in the presence of corticospinal tract disease. These signs may occur early in the disease process, and consequently may have significant diagnostic import. They are especially valuable if the Babinski response cannot be obtained owing to paralysis of the dorsiflexors of the toes. They may, however, be elicited in the presence of reflex hyperactivity, which may render them unreliable if found alone. Often they are not obtained in definite corticospinal tract disease, which limits their

value in clinical practice. The Mendel – Bechterew is found less frequently than the Rossolimo and is a less valuable sign.

There is some difference of opinion regarding the relative diagnostic value of these signs as compared with the Babinski sign. Some observers express the belief that the former occur earlier, are more definite and reliable, and consequently are better diagnostic criteria, while others feel that the Babinski sign is by far the more important and reliable. Their relative diagnostic value probably depends largely upon the individual examiner's experience and interpretation. Landau has suggested that there is no real difference in the significance and pathophysiology of the extensor and flexor reflexes, and that the former is actually a hyperactive flexor response.

Plantar flexion of the toes may also be elicited by application of the stimulus to other portions of the foot and ankle. Bechterew found that percussion of the middle of the sole or of the heel was followed by a plantar flexion response. In

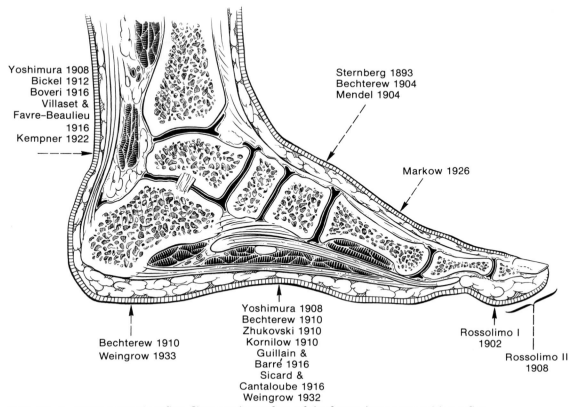

Yoshimura 1908
Bickel 1912
Boveri 1916
Villaset &
Favre–Beaulieu
1916
Kempner 1922

Sternberg 1893
Bechterew 1904
Mendel 1904

Markow 1926

Bechterew 1910
Weingrow 1933

Yoshimura 1908
Bechterew 1910
Zhukovski 1910
Kornilow 1910
Guillain &
Barré 1916
Sicard &
Cantaloube 1916
Weingrow 1932

Rossolimo I
1902

Rossolimo II
1908

FIG. 35–6. Plantar muscle reflex: Sites on the surface of the foot where a tap with a reflex hammer will be followed by flexion of the toes. Names of authors who described these reflexes and dates of publication are shown. (Modified from Wartenberg R: Arch Neurol Psychiatry 52:359–382, 1944)

the **medioplantar reflex of Guillain and Barré** and the **heel reflex of Weingrow** there is plantar flexion with fanning of the toes on tapping the midplantar region of the foot or the base of the heel. The **antagonistic anterior tibial reflex of Piotrowski** is characterized by plantar flexion of the ankle and sometimes of the toes when the belly of the anterior tibial muscle is tapped. The **paradoxical ankle reflex of Bing** consists of plantar flexion of the foot on tapping the anterior aspect of the ankle joint. Some of these correspond to the accessory methods of eliciting the Achilles reflex, and may indicate a spread of the reflexogenous zone. They are mainly, however, manifestations or exaggerations of the plantar muscle reflex (Fig. 35-6). They are found in corticospinal tract lesions, but may indicate reflex hyperactivity. These latter reflexes have less diagnostic value than the Rossolimo and Mendel – Bechterew signs.

Miscellaneous Corticospinal Tract Responses in the Lower Extremities

The following responses may occasionally be elicited: In the **adductor reflex of the foot,** stroking the inner border of the foot, not the sole, from the great toe to the heel, is followed by a contraction of the posterior tibial muscle with resulting adduction, inversion, and slight plantar flexion of the foot. This is often known as **Hirschberg's sign.** It is innervated by the tibial nerve (fourth lumbar through first sacral segments). If the response is contralateral or bilateral it is known as the **Balduzzi sign.** In **von Monakow's sign,** stroking of the lateral margin of the foot is followed by eversion and abduction of the foot.

BIBLIOGRAPHY

Adie WJ, Critchley M. Forced grasping and groping. Brain 1927;50:142

Babinski J. Sur le réflexe cutané plantaire dans certaines affections organiques du système nerveux central. Comp Rend Soc Biol 1896;3:207

Babinski J. Du phénomène des orteils et de sa valeur sémiologique. Sem Méd 1898;18:321

Babinski J. De l'abduction des orteils (signe de l'éventail). Rev Neurol 1903;11:728, 1205

Blake JR, Jr, Kunkle EC. The palmomental reflex: A physiological and clinical analysis. Arch Neurol Psychiat 1951;65:337

Brain R, Wilkinson M. Observation on the extensor plantar reflex and its relationship to the functions of the pyramidal tract. Brain 1959;82:297

Chaney LB, McGraw MD. Reflexes and other motor activities in newborn infants. Bull Neurol Inst (NY) 1932;2:1

Cody FW, Richardson HC, MacDermott N, Ferguson IT. Stretch and vibration reflexes of wrist flexor muscles in spasticity. Brain 1987;110:433

Dohrmann CJ, Nowack WJ. The upgoing great toe: Optimal method of elicitation. Lancet 1973;1:339

Estañol B. Temporal course of the threshold and size of the receptive field of the Babinski sign. J Neurol Neurosurg Psychiatry 1983;46:1055

Fradis A, Botez MI. The groping phenomena of the foot. Brain 1958;81:218

Fujiki A, Shimuzu A, Yamada Y et al. The Babinski reflex during sleep and wakefulness. Electroencephalogr Clin Neurophysiol 1971;31:610

Fulton JF, Keller AD. The Sign of Babinski: A Study of the Evolution of Cortical Dominance in Primates. Springfield, IL, Charles C Thomas, 1932

Grimby L. Pathological plantar response: Disturbances of the normal integration of flexor and extensor reflex components. J Neurol Neurosurg Psychiatry 1963;26:314

Hogan GR, Milligan JE. The plantar reflex in the newborn. New Engl J Med 1971;285:502

Landau WM, Clare MH. The plantar reflex in man, with special reference to some conditions where the extensor response is unexpectedly absent. Brain 1959;82:321

Landau WM. Clinical definition of the extensor plantar response. New Engl J Med 1975;285:1149

McGraw MB. Development of the plantar response in healthy infants. Am J Dis Child 1941;61:1215

Nathan PW, Smith MC. The Babinski response: A review and new observations. J Neurol Neurosurg Psychiatry 1955;18:250

Powers RK, Campbell DL, Rymer WZ. Stretch reflex dynamics in spastic elbow flexor muscles. Ann Neurol 1989;25:32

Riddoch G, Buzzard EF. Reflex movements and postural reactions in quadriplegia and hemiplegia, with especial reference to those of the upper limb. Brain 1921;44:397

Seyffarth H, Denny – Brown D. The grasp reflex and the instinctive grasp reaction. Brain 1948;71:109

Swaiman KF. Pediatric neurology. Principles and Practice. St. Louis: CV Mosby, 1989

Walsh EG, Wright GW. Patellar clonus: An autonomous central generator. J Neurol Neurosurg Psychiatry 1987;50:1225

Walshe FMR. The Babinski plantar response, its forms and its physiological and pathological significance. Brain 1956;79:529

Wartenberg R. The Babinski reflex after fifty years. JAMA 1947;135:763

Yakovlev PI, Farrell MJ. Influence of locomotion on the plantar reflex in normal and in physically and mentally inferior persons: Theoretical and practical implications. Arch Neurol Psychiatry 1941;46:322

Chapter 36

REFLEXES OF SPINAL AUTOMATISM

The reflexes of spinal automatism are also termed **defense reflexes.** Like the corticospinal tract signs described in the last chapter, they become manifest when the inhibiting action of the higher centers has been removed, and thus indicate, in part at least, a release from such inhibition. These reflexes, while present only in pathologic states in humans and higher animals, are phylogenetically and ontogenetically related to responses seen in lower forms. They are also clinical homologues of reflexes seen in "spinal" and decerebrate animals.

FLEXION AND EXTENSION DEFENSE REFLEXES IN THE LOWER EXTREMITIES

The Flexion Spinal Defense Reflex (Babinski). This reflex, also known as the reflex of spinal automatism (Marie), and as the pathologic shortening reflex, reflex flexor synergy, the withdrawal reflex, and the *réflexe* or *phénomène des raccourisseurs*, is, in a manner of speaking, an exaggeration of the Babinski response. As stated in Chapter 35, the Babinski response consists of dorsiflexion and fanning of the toes together with a certain amount of dorsiflexion at the ankle and flexion of the knee and hip, and possibly abduction of the hip. These latter movements result from contraction of the anterior tibial, hamstring, tensor fasciae latae, iliopsoas, and related maucles. The contraction of the tensor fasciae latae is sometimes referred to as **Brissaud's reflex.** If the Babinski response is marked, there is a spread of the reflexogenous

zone so that the response may be obtained not only by stimulation of the plantar surface of the foot but also by stimulation of the dorsum of the foot and the anterior surface of the tibia, or by a painful stimulus to any part of the foot, toes, or leg. Also, if the response is marked and results from a spinal lesion that is partially or completely transverse, it is obtained not only on the side stimulated, but also on the contralateral side.

In normal individuals a painful, or nociceptive, stimulus to the lower portion of the body may be followed by a withdrawal of the legs; this is a quick movement, brief in duration, and while it is characterized by flexion at the hip and knee, there is rarely dorsiflexion at the ankle and there is usually plantar flexion of the toes. When lesions of the spinal cord are present, especially if they are transverse or nearly complete, stimulation below the level of the lesion calls forth the **flexion spinal defense reflex,** or **reflex of spinal automatism,** with flexion at the hip and knee, dorsiflexion at the ankle, and usually dorsiflexion at the great toe and dorsiflexion and fanning of the small toe. The response may be bilateral and is then called the crossed flexor reflex. It may appear to be a voluntary spontaneous movement, but is slower and more tonic than the voluntary response.

This reflex may be evoked by any type of stimulus, but most frequently by an uncomfortable or nociceptive one. Pricking, scratching, or pinching the skin on the dorsal aspect of the foot or ankle, heat, cold, or deep pressure, may initiate the response, as may squeezing the toes or extreme passive plantar flexion of the toes or foot (the **Marie – Foix sign**). At times it may be initiated by moving the foot, testing reflexes, touching the skin lightly, or even by the weight of the bedclothes. It may be elicited by stimulation of either cutaneous or proprioceptive endings, or by stimuli from the viscera (such as distention of the bladder), at any site below the level of the lesion. The upper border of the reflexogenous zone usually corresponds to the lower limit of the spinal cord lesion, and thus may be important in localization. A stronger or more powerful stimulus usually is needed to elicit the responses near the level of the lesion than to obtain it lower down. A painful stimulus above the level of the lesion, however, may cause voluntary movements of the upper part of the body that may be followed by a reflex response of the lower portion; this has been called a "false withdrawal reflex."

The flexion spinal defense reflex appears in patients in whom there has been a partial or a complete isolation of the lower levels of the spinal cord from the rest of the central nervous system. It is found most characteristically in association with injuries, compression, and vascular lesions of the spinal cord. It may be regarded as a protective mechanism against noxious stimuli applied to the lower portions of the body. At times patients may mistake these seemingly spontaneous but actually reflex movements of the lower limbs in response to minimal stimuli for evidence of a return of function and improvement.

Various modifications of the flexion spinal defense reflex may be obtained. The most important of these are listed.

The Uniphasic Reaction. In complete transverse lesions of the spinal cord the only response is flexion of the limbs, as described, with flexion at the hips and knees and dorsiflexion of the ankles and toes. There is never extension. This is termed the **uniphasic motor reaction.** A fixed flexion may result in paraplegia in flexion.

The Biphasic Reaction. If the spinal lesion is not completely transverse, the flexion response may be transient, and followed by extension. This is the **biphasic motor reaction.** If the lesion is incomplete, one may also get a paraplegia in extension, with transient flexion reflexes but a position of extension of the paretic extremities.

The Mass Reflex. The flexion spinal defense reflex may be accompanied in certain instances by muscular contractions of the abdominal wall,

by evacuation of the bladder and bowel, and by sweating, reflex erythema, and pilomotor responses below the level of the lesion. This is termed the **mass reflex of Riddoch.** It is seen in relatively complete transverse spinal lesions after the period of spinal shock has passed. It indicates severe spinal cord injury. The reflexogenous zone may be extended to the bladder, so that distention of the bladder may precipitate the entire reflex complex. Priapism and even ejaculation may be a part of the response. The mass reflex may at times be used in therapy in the retraining of bladder function.

The Crossed Extensor Reflex. Stimulation of the foot or leg on one side may cause flexion of that extremity with an extension response in the other lower extremity. This is the **crossed extensor reflex,** or *phénomène d'allongement croisé*, sometimes known as **Philippson's reflex.** It is similar to the crossed extensor reflex of the "spinal" animal. Clinically, it is usually present in patients with partial or incomplete spinal cord lesions, but has been observed when transection of the cord seems complete. Occasionally in premature or newborn infants, strong pressure in the inguinal regions may produce what resembles a crossed extensor reflex, with flexion of the ipsilateral and extension of the contralateral hip and knee.

The Extensor Thrust. When pressure is applied to the foot of the passively flexed leg, extension may take place. This is known as the **extensor thrust.** Similar extension may occur if the leg paralyzed by a spinal lesion is placed in a position of flexion, and the skin in the lumbar or perineal area or in the adductor region of the thigh is pinched (**réflexe des allongeurs**). The extension may be followed by flexion. At times alternate extension and flexion occur, producing a stepping or marching movement of the two limbs. These manifestations usually occur only in patients with incomplete lesions, and are usually elicited in cases of paraplegia with extensor rigidity.

FLEXION AND EXTENSION DEFENSE REFLEXES IN THE UPPER EXTREMITIES

If the spinal lesion is above the sixth cervical segment of the cord, one may occasionally elicit either flexion or extension defense reflexes in the upper as well as the lower extremities. These have been described under the corticospinal tract responses of the upper extremities as the nociceptive reflexes of Riddoch and Buzzard (Ch. 35).

SPINAL SHOCK

A complete or relatively complete spinal lesion, if abrupt in onset, is followed immediately not only by complete paralysis and anesthesia below the level of the lesion, but also by complete loss of tone and absence of all reflexes, both deep and superficial. This is spinal shock, which is usually transient in duration. The loss of tone and depression of the reflexes are probably the result of a disturbance of the fusiform (γ-efferent) system, which functions to regulate the sensitivity of the muscle stretch receptors. This disturbance of fusiform function results from loss of normal spinal cord activity, which is partially dependent on continual tonic discharges from higher centers, including those relayed through the vestibulospinal and reticulospinal pathways. After a period of time the muscle stretch reflexes appear, but in an exaggerated form, and pathologic responses become manifest as the period of spinal shock subsides. This is usually after an interval of from 3 weeks to one month. If infection has developed, a severe urinary tract infection or infected decubitus ulceration, for example, the period of spinal shock is prolonged. The later development of an infectious process, especially if it is a severe one with associated septicemia, may be followed by the recurrence of a syndrome clinically if not physiologically identical with spinal shock. Spinal shock is most frequently encountered in conditions in which the spinal cord lesion has an abrupt onset, as in the traumatic, infectious, or vascular varieties of transverse myelopathy, and it is only rarely seen in slowly progressive lesions such as tumors of the spinal cord, multiple sclerosis, and posterolateral sclerosis. Spinal shock terminates earlier and the corticospinal tract responses and defense reactions become manifest sooner with incomplete than with complete transverse lesions.

PARAPLEGIA IN FLEXION

In certain patients with transverse involvement of the spinal cord the frequently repeated and easily elicited flexion defense reflexes result in involuntary flexor spasms that occur with increasing frequency. This terminates eventually in a so-called **fixed flexion reflex,** with a permanent state of flexion of the hips and knees and dorsiflexion of the ankles and toes. The exaggeration of the flexor reflex holds the limbs in a position of flexion for longer and longer intervals until they can no longer be actively or even passively extended. The legs and thighs may be completely flexed, so that in the severest cases the knees press against the abdominal wall. This is termed **paraplegia in flexion.** The slightest stimulus, even the weight of the clothes or bedclothes or the sudden uncovering of the legs, may elicit the flexion response, until finally a permanent flexion occurs. Even after the development of a fixed flexion reflex, any additional stimulus may aggravate the degree of flexion. Secondary contractures develop at the joints.

Paraplegia in flexion is most frequently encountered in traumatic and infectious myelopathies and multiple sclerosis, but it may result from extramedullary and intramedullary neoplasms of the spinal cord, posterolateral sclerosis, vascular disorders, and other spinal cord affections. Its presence indicates the existence of a relatively complete interruption of the descending impulses and an approach to a complete separation of the levels of the spinal cord below the lesion from the higher levels. This flexion position of the lower extremities is in contradistinction to the extension position that usually occurs with supraspinal lesions. However, paraplegia in flexion has occasionally been reported with diffuse cerebral lesions.

Although it has been said that paraplegia in flexion occurs as a result of release from the inhibiting action of the pyramidal cortex, it never appears in lesions limited to the corticospinal pathways. The patellar and Achilles reflexes may be absent and it may not be possible to obtain clonus. The hamstring reflexes, on the other hand, may be present and exaggerated. This would suggest that the increase in tone is present only in the flexor muscles, or in the flexor muscles in excess of that in the extensor muscles, in contrast to the usual picture in corticospinal tract disease. It is probable that in addition to the corticospinal pathway, the vestibulospinal and other efferent extrapyramidal pathways are interrupted. The extensor tone derived from the vestibular centers in the reticular formation is lost, and flexor tone predominates.

Paraplegia in flexion is obviously disabling and painful. Its presence makes nursing care difficult and may hasten the development of decubiti. Attempts to change the paraplegia from a spastic to a flaccid one have met with only varying degrees of success. Medical treatment, using neuromuscular and internuncial blocking agents, has thus far met with little success, although newer pharmacologic agents that may be of help are being developed. Injection of alcohol, phenol, or other substances into the subarachnoid space has been of help in the experience of some investigators. Surgical approaches have included freeing the ends of the severed spinal cord from cicatricial tissue, either anterior or posterior rhizotomy or both, and midline myelotomy. Varying degrees of relief have been afforded by these procedures. The development of paraplegia in flexion may be avoided by good nursing care, prevention of the development of decubiti, adequate attention to bladder dysfunction, and avoidance of excessive stimulation to the extremities.

PARAPLEGIA IN EXTENSION

Paraplegia with extensor rigidity usually results from corticospinal lesions in the cerebrum or in the corticospinal pathway above its decussation in the medulla, but may be present with spinal lesions. There is increased tone of both extensor and flexor muscles, but the spasticity predominates in the extensors. As a result there is hyperactivity of the extensor reflexes (patellar and Achilles), and clonus may be obtained. There is tonic extensor spasm of the lower limbs, with the legs in adduction and slight internal rotation. This syndrome has been said to be the result of incomplete transection of the spinal cord, with predominant involvement of the corticospinal pathways. It has, however,

been observed in patients with complete transverse myelitis. It is probable that neither the reflexes nor the position of the extremities indicates the severity of the lesion. All possible combinations of flexion and extension reflexes may occur in the same patient, and the response may depend less upon the flexor or extensor tone than on the intensity, duration, and site of stimulation. Strong, brief, and distal stimuli are more apt to elicit flexion, and mild, prolonged, and proximal ones, extension. Flexion paraplegia is most frequent with severe and relatively high lesions, but the flexor predominance may change to extensor predominance.

BIBLIOGRAPHY

Head H, Riddoch G. The automatic bladder, excessive sweating and some other reflex conditions, in gross injuries of the spinal cord. Brain 1917;40:188

Macht MB, Kuhn RA. The occurrence of extensor spasm in patients with complete transection of the spinal cord. N Engl J Med 1948;328:311

Marshall J. Observations on reflex changes in the lower limbs in spastic paraplegia in man. Brain 1954;77:290

Pollock LJ, Boshes B, Finkelman I et al. Spasticity, pseudo-spontaneous spasms, and other reflex activities late after injury to the spinal cord. Arch Neurol Psychiatry 1951;66:537

Riddoch G. The reflex functions of the completely divided spinal cord in man, compared with those associated with less severe lesions. Brain 1917;49:264

Scarff JE, Pool JL. Factors causing muscle spasm following transection of the cord in man. J Neurosurg 1946;3:285

Weaver RA, Landau WM, Higgins JF. Fusiform function. Part II. Evidence of fusiform depression in human spinal shock. Arch Neurol 1963;9:127

Yakovlev PI. Paraplegia in flexion of cerebral origin. J Neuropathol Exp Neurol 1954;13:267

Chapter 37
POSTURAL AND RIGHTING REFLEXES

The postural and righting reflexes constitute a complex group of reactions that have more significance in experimental than in clinical neurology. They, and abnormalities of them, have little application to neurologic diagnosis except in the examination of infants. A comprehension of them, however, is important to an understanding of the regulation of posture, the establishment and maintenance of the upright position, and the orientation of the body and its parts in space.

Posture (Ch. 32) is largely reflex in origin. Involuntary muscular contraction is necessary for the maintenance of the erect posture and normal position. Tonus, especially in the antigravity muscles, is essential. There are important postural mechanisms in the hindbrain that cause slow and prolonged muscular responses. The vestibular apparatus, especially the lateral (Deiters') nucleus, induces a steady contraction of the antigravity muscles and is essential to the erect, or upright, position.

Standing may be thought of as a postural reflex that depends upon stimuli and motor impulses mediated through the medulla but influenced by the cerebral cortex. The essential afferent impulses are largely proprioceptive ones. Any interference with any of the mechanisms responsible for localized, segmental, or generalized static or postural reflexes will cause an interference with the act of normal standing. The orientation of the head and body in space and the ability to maintain the head in a definite relationship to the body are faculties possessed by all intact vertebrates. The decerebrate animal is incapable of righting itself. It cannot resume its normal posture after being placed in an abnormal position.

The orientation of the body in space, the orientation of the head in space, the position of the head in relation to the trunk, the appropriate adjustment of the limbs and eyes to the position of the head, the ability to rise from a recumbent position, and the sustained modification of the position of one or more parts of the body involve a series of complex reflex mechanisms. These various functions are called into action by the following impulses: stimuli discharging from receptors situated in the labyrinthine apparatus, principally the utricle, but also the semicircular canals and the saccule if motion is involved; proprioceptive impulses from the deep tissues — the muscles, the tendons, and joints of the neck, trunk, limbs, and body wall; tactile (exteroceptive) impulses arising in the skin of the body surface and limbs; visual stimuli from the retina. Impulses from these various sources act upon the head, neck, trunk, and extremities. Inasmuch as the integrity of these stimuli is essential to the erect posture and as they aid in righting the head and body, the responses to them are known as **standing and righting reflexes.** The center for simple postural and standing reflexes is probably situated in the brain stem, and that for the more complex standing and righting reflexes in the midbrain. The center for the visual righting reflex is probably in the cerebral cortex, but the eyes, working on the midbrain in coordination with the hindbrain, set up a train of reflex responses that cause a prone animal to look up, sit up, and then stand in quick, smooth succession, and to maintain its equilibrium and upright position in part by the use of visual stimuli. The communication between the midbrain centers and the vestibular complex — the medial longitudinal fasciculus — is essential to the integrity of the righting reflexes.

Postural reflexes are made up of local static, segmental static, and general static reactions. In all of them the responses are tonic ones. Local static reflexes are those that are confined to one limb. Either proprioceptive or exteroceptive stimuli may set up a reflex response whereby a previously mobile limb becomes rigid. They may provoke extensor rigidity and convert the limb into a pillar of support. Segmental static reactions are those in which a stimulus to one extremity affects the fellow extremity on the opposite side, as in the crossed extensor reflex (Ch. 36). General static reactions have to do with reflexes that arise in one segment but affect muscles innervated by other segments. They may involve the head, the neck, all four extremities, or the entire body. They include righting reactions and statotonic reflexes.

Righting reactions are complex and involve five separate types of reflexes: labyrinthine righting reflexes acting upon the neck muscles, neck righting reflexes acting upon the body, body righting reflexes acting upon the head, body righting reflexes acting upon the body, and optical righting reflexes acting upon the head and body.

The stimuli that call forth the labyrinthine righting reflexes arise in the otoliths of the utricles and to a lesser extent of the saccules; these organs respond to changes of the position of the head and have an influence on body tone. The utricles increase the tone of the bodily musculature as a whole bilaterally and that of the neck muscles ipsilaterally. Such changes are the result of alterations in the position of the head or the body. If the body is tilted, stimuli from the otolith organs act on the neck muscles and the head is rotated in such a manner that it maintains an upright position. If the head is turned, there is increased tone in the neck muscles on the side toward which the face is directed. The response of the labyrinths to movement, especially to rotatory movement and acceleration, is a function of the semicircular canals, and it is discussed with the kinetic labyrinthine reflexes.

The stimuli involved in the neck righting reflexes originate in the muscles, tendons, and other deep structures of the neck. These are mediated through the upper two or three cervical nerves and segments, and possibly through the spinal accessory nerve. They act principally on the head, but through the head act on the body as a whole. If the head is rotated toward one side, the pelvis is tilted slightly toward the opposite side, following which the shoulders and then the hips are turned in the same way that the head is turned.

The stimuli involved in the body righting reflexes acting upon the head and body originate in the deeper tissues, principally the skeletal muscles, of the trunk, body wall, and extremities. These proprioceptive impulses are carried to the medulla, probably to centers in the vestibular nuclei.

The visual, or optic, righting reflexes are probably integrated in the cerebral cortex, but the impulses are mediated by the midbrain and the vestibular centers. When the eyes are turned, the head and body are also turned toward the object on which the attention is directed. Vision does play a large part in posture, but even though vision may be absent there is no impairment of posture or of body righting if the other mechanisms concerned with these functions are intact. On the other hand, in conditions in which there is loss of proprioceptive sensibility, as in tabes dorsalis, this deficiency may be compensated for in part by the use of the eyes.

The statotonic or attitudinal reflexes include the tonic labyrinthine and neck reflexes that act upon the limbs and those that act upon the eyes. The former influence the tone of the skeletal muscles and thereby maintain the different parts of the body in an attitude appropriate to a given position of the head. The labyrinthine reflexes influence the tone of the extensor muscles, which is the same (increased or decreased) in all four extremities. The influence of the neck reflexes is usually in an opposite direction in the upper and lower extremities. The centers for these reactions are in the vestibular nuclei and the upper cervical segments of the spinal cord. The tonic labyrinthine and neck reflexes that act upon the eyes result in changes in eye movements in association with changes in the position of the head; the center for these is situated between the vestibular and ocular nuclei.

Kinetic labyrinthine reflexes are those that result from actual movements of the head or body. The afferent impulses concerned with these have their receptors in the labyrinths, especially in the semicircular canals, and the centers are in the vestibular nuclei. They are discussed with the physiology of the labyrinth (Ch. 14).

The postural and righting reflexes are difficult to demonstrate clinically, and our knowledge concerning them has come largely from experimental neurology. Certain observers object to any attempt to apply them specifically in the human being because of the difference between the type of response found clinically in the upright biped and that experimentally in the quadruped. The postural and righting reflexes, or their homologues, do, however, play an important part in the nervous system function of the human. Righting reflexes can be demonstrated in the very young by movements of the head with passive movements of the body. In the normal adult there is a conjugate deflection of the eyes in association with movement of the head, and a deviation of the arms in the direction of passive rotation of the head. In certain of the extrapyramidal disturbances the normal reactions to sudden passive tilting of the body are lost along with loss of postural reflexes, and the patient is unable to adjust the body and its parts to changes in position. There may also be **gegenhalten,** a stiffening of a limb in response to contact and a resistance to changes of position and posture.

The reflexes that help to maintain posture are said to become gradually somewhat less effective with advancing age. Dysfunction of the postural reflexes in the elderly may contribute to the likelihood of falls in these persons.

Postural and righting reflexes have special importance in understanding pathologic reflex responses such as the grasp reflex, the Babinski sign, and reflexes of spinal defense and spinal automatism; supporting, placing, and hopping reactions; normal and abnormal associated movements; the Brudzinski sign; and the characteristic position of the limbs seen in certain nervous system affections. They are characterized by modifications of position and tonus, more or less sustained and usually of one or more segments of the body, rather than by brief muscular contractions. While they do not, in themselves, have a great deal of application to neurologic diagnosis, special modifications of these responses may be seen on occasion, and may constitute valuable diagnostic criteria.

POSTURAL AND RIGHTING REFLEXES IN INFANCY AND CHILDHOOD

There are a number of responses related to the postural and righting reflexes that aid in the evaluation of normal and abnormal development in infancy and childhood. Some of the more important of these are the following:

The Moro Reflex. This is the body **startle reflex.** Any sudden stimulus, such as a loud noise, a quick movement directed toward the body, a blow on the bed close to the body, a tap on the abdomen, or a bright light suddenly directed toward the eyes, is followed by abduction and extension of all four extremities and extension of the spine, with extension and fanning of the digits except for flexion of the distal phalanges of the index finger and thumb; this is followed in turn by flexion and adduction of the extremities. This reflex is present during the first 3 months of life; during the next 2 months there may be only extension and abduction of the arms and jerking of the knees; then the response gradually disappears, probably with the development of myelination. Children with motor deficits of cerebral origin may show the reflex in a fully developed form for years; the response may be unilateral if only one side is affected.

Landau Reflex. This may be demonstrated in normal infants during the first 1 or 2 years of life. If an infant is held in the examiner's hand in the prone position so that the body is parallel with the floor, there is dorsiflexion of the head with extension of the vertebral column, so that the body assumes an arc with the convexity downward. Passive ventroflexion of the head while the body is in the above position causes flexion of the vertebral column and of the arms and legs, and the body assumes the shape of an arc with the convexity upward. If the child is placed in the recumbent position, there is ventroflexion of the neck, with flexion of the vertebral column, arms, and legs. This is probably a combination of otolith and tonic neck reflexes. When the neck is extended by means of the otolith reflexes, the tonic neck reflexes bring the limbs and body into an appropriate position of extension, and when the neck is flexed, the back and limbs are flexed.

Tonic Neck Reflexes. In the decorticate state, changes in the position of the head relative to the position of the body result in reflex modifications of the tonus and posture of the limbs. When the jaw is passively turned toward the side or the head is bent toward one shoulder, there is increased extensor tonus on that side and increased flexor tonus on the opposite side (Fig. 37-1). The arm on the side toward which the jaw is turned becomes rigid and goes into extension, and the leg may go into extension as well. On the opposite side the arm goes into flexion and the leg may also flex. The flexor tonus is

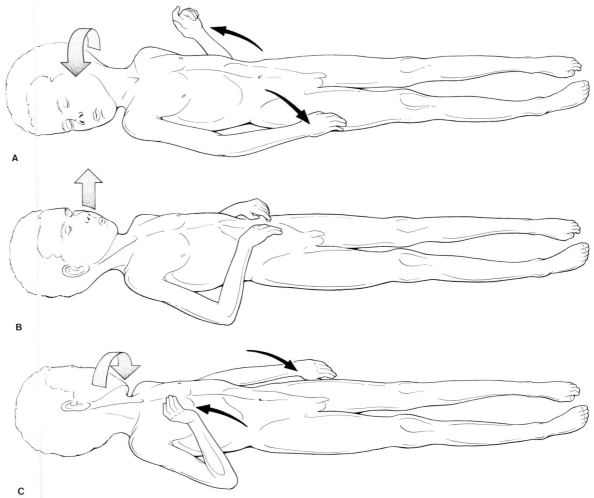

FIG. 37–1. Tonic neck reflexes in a patient with a suprasellar cyst. **A.** Turning of the head to the right produces increased extensor tonus on that side and flexion of the opposite arm. **B.** Characteristic attitude of patient with legs in full extension and arms in semiflexion. **C.** Turning of the head to the left produces increased extensor tonus on that side and flexion of the right arm. (Modified from Davis LE: Arch Neurol Psychiatry 13:569–577, 1925)

not so great as the extensor tonus, but there is no relaxation of the flexed muscles and the grasp reflex may be elicited on the side of the flexion. The extension is usually accompanied by supination, the flexion by pronation. If the head and neck are flexed, the arms flex and the legs go into extension. If the head and neck are extended, the arms extend and the legs go into flexion. Pressure over the vertebra prominens results in relaxation of all four limbs.

These manifestations are reflex responses to afferent stimuli arising from the neck muscles, and also to labyrinthine stimuli. Tonic labyrinthine reflexes, which are similar responses, may be obtained by carrying out similar maneuvers after section of the cervical nerve roots. Reflexes of this type are often found in an incomplete form in normal infants, but they disappear by the age of 4 – 6 months. In pathologic states they may be present in older children in a complete or incomplete form, and they are sometimes found with disease processes of the upper brain stem, usually with fairly diffuse lesions such as basilar meningitis or acute encephalopathy, but occasionally with vascular and neoplastic lesions at the midbrain level. The patient lies with the arms semiflexed over the chest and the legs in extension, but turning, flexion, or extension of the head causes the responses just described. These reflexes probably indicate a "high" decerebration, or decortication, possibly at the thalamodiencephalic level. They may be present and contribute to the associated movements found in spastic hemiplegia and cerebral diplegia.

The Parachute Response. The parachute response appears in infants at the age of 8 or 9 months and persists. To elicit it, the infant is held suspended in a prone position and then is suddenly thrust in a head-first direction toward the examining table or floor. When the response is present the arms immediately extend and adduct slightly and the fingers spread out as if to attempt to break the fall. The response does not depend upon vision, since it may be obtained in blindfolded children. Asymmetry of the response indicates unilateral upper extremity weakness or spasticity. Absence of the response is seen in severe motor disorders and dementia.

The Neck Righting Response. This is a variation of the tonic neck reflex. With the infant in the supine position, its head is turned toward one side. A positive response results in rotation of the shoulder, trunk, and pelvis toward that side, occasionally followed by a turn of the entire body. The reflex becomes evident at about the time the tonic neck reflexes disappear and can be obtained in nearly all infants by the age of 10 months; it disappears at about the time the child can arise directly without first turning on his abdomen. The response should be approximately equal on each side.

The Hand–Mouth Reflex of Babkin. Pressure on the palm of the hand in premature and newborn infants is followed by opening of the mouth, flexion of the neck, and sometimes closing of the eyes and flexion of the forearm. The response is easiest to elicit and most pronounced if the stimulus is bilateral. Except in infants with retarded development this reflex disappears by the third or fourth month of life.

The Placing Reaction. The placing reaction is obtained by holding the infant vertically and in a position in which the dorsum of each foot touches the underside of the examining table. The infant should place each foot on the top of the table. The response usually disappears by the end of the first year of life, when voluntary movements make it difficult to interpret. It persists in children with motor deficits, and in

them may be related to the reflexes of spinal automatism.

Supporting and Stepping Reactions. If the infant is held vertically and its feet are allowed to make firm contact with the top of the examining table, there will be simultaneous contraction of opposing muscles to fix the joints of the lower extremities. This is usually followed by automatic stepping or walking movements in which the infant places one foot in front of the other. These responses are usually present at birth and gradually disappear as the infant develops increasing voluntary motor power.

DECEREBRATE AND DECORTICATE RIGIDITY

Sherrington, in 1898, found that prepontine section of the brain stem induces a heightened reflex tonus of the extensor, or antigravity, muscles of the limbs and vertebral columns. This is followed by a state of exaggerated posture characterized by continuous spasm, sustained contraction, and marked rigidity of the skeletal muscles, predominantly the extensors. There is opisthotonos, all four limbs are stiffly extended, the head is erect, and the jaws are closed. The arms are internally rotated at the shoulders, extended at the elbows, and hyperpronated, with the fingers extended at the metacarpophalangeal joints and flexed at the interphalangeal joints. The legs are extended at the hips, knees, and ankles, and the toes are plantar flexed. The position is an exaggeration or caricature of the normal standing position. The muscle stretch reflexes are exaggerated, the tonic neck and labyrinthine reflexes are retained, and the righting reflexes are abolished. This phenomenon is known as **decerebrate rigidity.**

Decerebrate rigidity follows transection of the brain stem at any level between the superior colliculi (anterior quadrigeminal bodies) or the decussation of the rubrospinal pathway and the rostral portion of the vestibular nuclei, and the integrity of the vestibular nuclei is essential for the continuance of the picture. It is abolished by section of the vestibulospinal pathways, and probably results from release of the vestibular nuclei from higher extrapyramidal control. These nuclei must be intact, but isolated from the midbrain. If one-half of the brain stem has been severed, the rigidity is homolateral. This suggests that the syndrome must result from interruption of some extrapyramidal pathways that have already decussated at this level. The intrinsic activity of the vestibular portion of the reticular formation, no longer modified by higher centers, produces a continuous discharge of impulses to the spinal cord. The facilitatory region of the lateral pontine tegmentum is either unchanged or increased in activity, whereas the suppressor region of the medial pontine tegmentum is depressed. The opisthotonos and extreme rigidity that are sometimes present in patients with basilar meningitis, hydrocephalus, and neoplasms and other lesions of the posterior fossa may be clinical features of decerebrate rigidity. Brain stem dysfunction causing manifestations of decerebrate rigidity may occasionally be caused by supratentorial mass lesions.

In contrast to decerebrate rigidity is **decorticate rigidity.** This is characterized by flexion of the elbows and wrists with extension of the legs and feet. The causative disease is usually higher than that causing decerebrate rigidity and may even be cortical. Often there is widespread, diffuse disease. Two varieties of anatomic decerebration have been described, both associated with upper brain stem damage. That produced by high infarction of the brain stem usually causes marked intorsion of the arms, whereas that produced by damage through the intercollicular area causes less intorsion.

BIBLIOGRAPHY

Byers RK. The functional significance of persistent tonic neck reflexes in fixed brain lesions. Trans Am Neurol Assoc 1953;78:207

Cary JH, Crosby EC, Schnitzlein HN. Decorticate versus decerebrate rigidity in subhuman primates and man. Neurology 1971;21:738

Davis LE. Decerebrate rigidity in man. Arch Neurol Psychiatry 1925;13:569

Evans OB. Manual of Child Neurology. New York, Churchill Livingstone, 1987

Fiorentiono MR. Reflex Testing Methods for Evaluating C.N.S. Development. Springfield, IL, Charles C Thomas, 1963

Goldstein K, Landis C, Hunt WA et al. Moro reflex and startle pattern. Arch Neurol Psychiatry 1938;40:322

Halsey JH, Downey AW. Decerebrate rigidity with preservation of consciousness. J Neurol Neurosurg Psychiatry 1966;29:350

Magnus R. Some results of studies in the physiology of posture. Lancet 1926;2:531, 585

Magnus R, De Kleijn A. Die Abhängigkeit des Tonus der Extremitätenmuskeln von der Kopfstellung. Pfluegers Arch 1912;145:455

McGraw MB. The Moro reflex. Am J Dis Child 1937;54:240

McNealy DE, Plum F. Brainstem dysfunction produced by supratentorial mass lesion. Arch Neurol 1962;7:10

Paine RS, Brazelton TB, Donovan DE et al. Evolution of postural reflexes in normal infants and in the presence of chronic brain syndromes. Neurology 1964;14:1036

Parmelee AH, Jr. The hand – mouth reflex of Babkin in premature infants. Pediatrics 1963;31:734

Pollock LJ, Boshes B, Zivin I et al. Body reflexes acting on the body in injuries to the spinal cord. Arch Neurol Psychiatry 1955;74:527

Rademaker GGJ. On the lengthening and shortening reactions and their occurrence in man. Brain 1947;70:109

Robertson RCL, Pollard C, Jr. Decerebrate state in children and adolescents. J Neurosurg 1955;12:13

Sherrington CS. Decerebrate rigidity, and reflex coordination of movements. J Physiol 1898;22:319

Thomas A, Chesney Y, Saint-Anne Dargassis S. The Neurological Examination of the Infant. London, National Spastics Society, 1960

Weiner WJ, Nora LM, Glantz RH. Elderly inpatients: postural reflex impairment. Neurology 1984;34:945

Certain voluntary movements have a tendency to be accompanied by other unintentional or involuntary responses, the **associated,** or **synkinetic, movements.** These are defined as automatic movements or activities that alter or fix the posture of a part of the body when some other portion of the body is brought into activity by voluntary effort; or as automatic modifications of the attitude of certain parts of the body as a reflex response to the volitional motion of some other portion. These associated movements may be considered, to a certain extent, as postural or righting reflexes that have a peculiarly widespread distribution. They may be clinical homologues of movements seen in decerebrate animals. Inasmuch as they are motor responses, in many instances abnormal ones, they might be considered in the discussion of the motor system rather than the reflexes, but their physiologic relationship to various reflex responses and their correlation with various abnormalities in the reflexes are reasons for their inclusion in the present section. The associated movements that accompany or follow voluntary (or involuntary) motion, however, should be differentiated from those alterations in movements that accompany or follow reflex synergistic movements, although it may be difficult to distinguish between them.

PHYSIOLOGIC ASSOCIATED MOVEMENTS

Associated movements are more complex manifestations of motor function than the simple reflexes, but are more primitive than voluntary movements. They are probably initiated and largely controlled by the extrapyramidal level and its connections, although the corticospinal system does play a part in their occurrence. Many associated movements are present physiologically; in fact they play a part in all normal motor activity. The physiologic or cooperative functions of the antagonists, synergists, and muscles of fixation in any motor response may be considered associated movements, as may the successive or synchronous activity of the component parts of any coordinated or complex motor act. Generally, however, the term is used for more widespread responses. Among the more common of the normal associated movements, which are involuntary accompaniments of all normal voluntary (and involuntary) motor acts, are the following: pendular swinging of the arms when walking; alterations of the muscles of facial expression when talking; facial contortions or grimaces with violent exertion; movements of the head and neck with movements of the eyes; contraction of the frontalis muscle with elevation of the eyes; turning of the eyes, head, or body in response to vestibular or auditory stimulation; normal extension of the wrist with flexion of the fingers; generalized bodily accompaniments of yawning, stretching, coughing, and mental efforts. In certain pathologic states these normal associated movements may be diminished or disappear; in others they may be exaggerated, and abnormal associated movements may be present. Table 33-2 correlates the site of a lesion with the pattern of associated movements. The normal associated movements are lost in diseases of the extrapyramidal system, especially in the parkinsonian syndrome, where masking of the facial expression and absence of swinging movements of the arms when walking are prominent manifestations. With lesions of the corticospinal system, on the other hand, especially those of cerebral origin, there may be a number of associated movements that are not present in normal persons.

The associated movements that are not usually present in the normal individual are discussed in the following paragraphs.

PATHOLOGIC ASSOCIATED MOVEMENTS

Abnormal or pathologic associated movements are usually expressions of activity in paretic groups of muscles that are stimulated by active innervation of other groups. They may be present at all times, be brought out by special examinations, or become evident only during physical activity or periods of emotional stress. They are generalized and coordinated movements, and seen predominantly in disease of the corticospinal pathway, mainly in organic hemiplegia. They are automatic, spontaneous, involuntary modifications of the posture of certain parts of the body, usually accompanying vigorous voluntary movements of another part, and occur on the hemiplegic side, probably as a result of the release of the structures that normally modify the postural adjustments of the body. They are slow, forceful accessions of hypertonus in certain muscles of the already spastic parts that lead to the adoption of new postures. They have a longer latent period than primary movements. The greater the spasticity, the greater the extent and duration of the associated movements.

Generalized Associated Movements

Generalized associated or synkinetic movements are seen in hemiplegia of cerebral origin, where they tend to produce the characteristic position of the extremities (see Fig. 23-8). The upper limb is held in a position of flexion of the fingers and wrist, flexion and pronation at the elbow, and flexion and adduction at the shoulder; the paralysis of the extensors is more marked than that of the flexors. The lower extremity is held with extension at the hip and knee and plantar flexion at the ankle and toes, and with more marked paralysis of the flexors. These characteristics are increased with exertion. Straining and attempts to grip with the paretic hand may cause an increase in the spasticity, with increased flexion of the wrist, elbow, and shoulder; this is sometimes accompanied by associated facial movements on the involved side. The new posture may be maintained until the grip is relaxed. Involuntary movements such as yawning, coughing, and stretching may also increase the tonus and cause the affected arm to extend at the elbow, wrist, and fingers, remaining rigidly in this new attitude until the yawn passes off. This response may arouse in the patient or his friends false hope of improvement. Tonic neck reflexes may also influence these generalized associated movements. Turning the head toward the hemiplegic side may cause increased extensor tonus on that side, and turning it to the normal side may be followed by either increased flexor tonus on the paretic side or flexion of the arm and extension of the leg.

Symmetric (Imitative or Contralateral) Associated Movements

In the normal infant there is a certain tendency for movements of one limb to be accompanied by similar involuntary movements of the opposite limb; this disappears as coordination and muscle power are acquired. These movements may persist to a certain extent in children, in whom they most frequently occur in the form of transient **mirror movements,** or involuntary imitative movements of the contralateral portions of the body; they may be present only as mirror writing. Similar movements are sometimes observed in adults who are in the process of acquiring new patterns of movement or who are exerting excessive physical or mental effort. If these manifestations persist to any marked degree, they should be considered pathologic. Mirror movements usually disappear or become milder at adolescence. They may persist in persons with brain injuries, disturbances of cerebral development, and dysplasias of the upper portion of the spinal cord; under such circumstances there are usually associated abnormalities of motor function, tone, and reflexes, and the movements should be termed pathologic imitative ones. Occasionally, persisting mirror movements are familial, inherited as a simple dominant trait; these are not accompanied by other signs of neurologic disease.

In certain neurologic disorders, forceful voluntary movements of one limb may be accompanied by identical involuntary movements of the same limb on the opposite side. These are pathologic manifestations or exaggerations of the physiologic associated mirror movements. They are usually identical, imitative phenomena, and are most often present in patients with organic hemiplegia. They are usually seen in the paretic limb when the opposite healthy one is forcibly moved, although occasionally such movements may appear in the healthy limb on extreme attempts to move the affected extremity (especially in extrapyramidal disease). They appear particularly when the patient exerts himself to carry out a quick or strenuous movement. Thus, in squeezing the examiner's hand with the healthy hand the paretic hand is seen to flex, and in smiling there may be an exaggerated response on the paretic side. Any forceful movement on the normal side may be followed by a similar but slow tonic duplication of the movement on the paretic side. There may be a spreading of the response, continuing to the previously described generalized associated movements with assumption of the characteristic positions. The symmetric movements may be influenced by the generalized ones. If the patient clenches his normal hand while his head is straight, flexion of the paretic hand may be accompanied by flexion and adduction of the paretic arm. If the head is turned to the paretic side, flexion may be replaced by extension, and if the head is turned to the normal side, flexion and adduction of the paretic arm may be increased.

Imitation synkinesias by themselves have little localizing significance, occurring with lesions in various portions of the neuraxis. Their value in neurologic assessment is in conjunction with other findings. A disorganization of the sensory lemniscal system at any level is said to underlie imitation synkinesias, ultimately causing loss of particular functions in the principal cortical motor neurons.

Coordinated Associated Movements

Coordinated associated movements are involuntary movements of synergistic muscle groups that may accompany a voluntary movement of a paretic limb. They are exaggerations or perversions of ordinary synergistic and cooperative movements, and may be classified into three groups, as follows: (1) movements, not present normally, which accompany movements of a paretic limb; (2) contralateral coordinated associated movements; and (3) associated movements,

normally present, which are abolished in cerebral hemiplegia. These responses are useful in the differentiation between organic and hysterical hemiplegia.

Coordinated Associated Movements in the Paretic Limb

Coordinated associated movements that accompany voluntary motion of involved extremities in patients with cerebral hemiparesis are characterized by a spread of response from one muscle or group of muscles to others. They alter the position of the part and lead to the adoption of new postures. They do not appear in the normal individual or in hysteria.

The Finger Sign, or Interosseous Phenomenon, of Souques. Active elevation and extension of a paretic arm is followed by involuntary hyperextension and abduction of the fingers.

Wartenberg's Sign. Active flexion of the terminal phalanges of the four fingers of a paretic hand about a firm object, or against resistance offered by the examiner's fingers similarly flexed, is followed by adduction, flexion, and opposition of the thumb. In a normal extremity the thumb remains in abduction and extension.

Strümpell's Pronator Sign. Active flexion of a paretic forearm is followed by pronation and flexion of the hand. If this sign is tested by the patient bringing the hand to the shoulder, the dorsum of the hand strikes the shoulder and the palm is forward. If the forearm is flexed in supination or is passively flexed and supinated by the examiner, it immediately assumes a position of pronation.

Pronation Signs. The patient holds his arms and hands outstretched horizontally in front of him, with the hands supinated (palms upward) and fingers and thumb extended. He is asked to stand in this position with his eyes closed. If there is unilateral weakness, the hand will go into partial pronation. There may also be some downward and lateral drift of the hand and some flexion at the elbow and internal rotation at the shoulder (see Fig. 28-1). This is an early sign of corticospinal tract weakness, but it may also appear with hypotonicity and may be seen in Sydenham's chorea and cerebellar lesions.

Additional pronation phenomena have been described by Babinski and Wilson. In the former the palmar aspects of the hands are held in approximation with the thumbs up and are then jarred or shaken; the paretic hand falls into a position of pronation. In the latter there is pronation of the forearm along with internal rotation at the shoulder when the arms are elevated above the head; as a result the palm turns outward. Pronation also occurs on the paretic side when the arms are actively abducted with the forearm in supination or when the arms are passively abducted with the forearm in supination and then suddenly released.

The Radialis Sign of Strümpell. Attempts to close the fingers or to make a fist on the paretic side are accompanied by dorsiflexion of the wrist.

Flexion Response of the Forearm. Flexion of the hips and knees to the squatting position causes increased flexion of the paretic forearm. Flexion of the forearm is also increased by flexion and decreased by extension of the neck.

The Quadrupedal Extensor Reflex. On leaning forward or bending over, as if to place the hands on the floor, the flexed hemiparetic arm goes into a position of extension.

The Trunk – Thigh Sign of Babinski, or Combined Flexion of the Trunk and Thigh. The patient lying recumbent with his legs abducted attempts to rise to a sitting position while holding his arms crossed in front of his chest. In the normal individual the legs remain motionless and the heels are kept pressed down. In corticospinal hemiparesis there is flexion of the thigh in association with flexion of the trunk; as a result there is an involuntary elevation of the paretic limb, and the heel is raised from the bed (Fig. 38-1). The toes may spread out in a fanlike fashion. The normal limb is either not elevated or raised slightly but not as high as the paretic one. In paraparesis both legs are raised. In hysteria the normal leg is elevated, or neither leg is raised. The sign may also be elicited if the patient attempts to sit up from a recumbent position with his legs hanging over the edge of the bed; on doing this the thigh is flexed and the leg extended on the paretic side.

Combined Extension of the Trunk and Thigh. The patient, seated on the edge of an examining table and holding on to the edge of the table with his hands, is asked to lean backwards as far as his arms will stretch. In the normal individual there is no change in the position of the dependent feet and legs, but in corticospinal paresis there is extension of the thigh and leg with flexion of the foot in association with extension of the trunk.

The Combined Flexion of the Thigh and Leg Sign of Neri. The patient, in a standing position, is asked to bend forward as far as possible. In the normal individual the knees remain in extension, but in corticospinal tract lesions there is flexion at the knee (Fig. 38-2). If the patient, lying recumbent, raises his legs alternately, the normal leg remains straight but the paretic leg flexes at the knee. This may also be elicited by passively flexing the hip with the leg in extension.

Hoover's Sign. When a patient, in a recumbent position, flexes the thigh and lifts one leg, there is a downward movement of the other one. The examiner may evaluate this by placing his hands beneath the patient's heels, or it may be tested quantitatively by placing a manometer bulb or a small scale under the heel. In hemiparesis of cerebral origin and with other organic causes for weakness of one lower extremity, this downward pressure of the contralateral

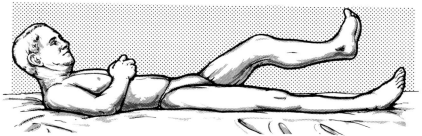

FIG. 38–1. Trunk–thigh sign in patient with left hemiparesis.

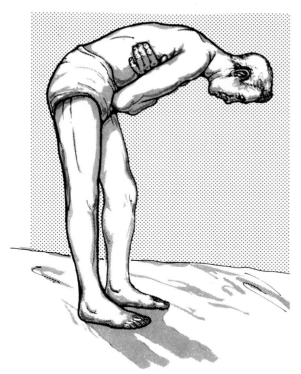

FIG. 38–2. *Combined flexion of the thigh and leg in a patient with left hemiparesis.*

heel is accentuated when the patient attempts to raise the paretic leg, and is also present, although to a less marked degree, in the paretic leg as the patient raises the normal leg. In hysterical or feigned weakness this phenomenon is absent in the normal leg when the patient attempts to raise the seemingly paretic one, although it may be maintained in the paretic one when he raises the normal leg (a normal associated movement). Increased downward pressure of the contralateral normal leg also occurs when a patient with low back pain (*e.g.*, from lumbosacral radiculitis) attempts to raise the painful limb.

The Tibialis Sign of Strümpell. Sharp, voluntary flexion of the thigh on the abdomen and of the leg on the thigh is followed by involuntary dorsiflexion and inversion of the paretic foot. The patient is unable to flex the hip and knee without dorsiflexing the foot (Fig. 38-3). This response is accentuated if the movement is carried out against resistance. In addition to the aforementioned movement, there may also be dorsiflexion of the great toe or of all the toes. This sign may also be tested by flexion of the leg on the thigh while the patient is in the prone position (Fig. 38-4). In the normal individual flexion of the thigh and leg is accompanied by plantar flexion of the foot.

Abduction Response at the Hip Joint. If a patient with weakness resulting from a corticospinal tract lesion stands erect and marks time, there is an abduction movement at the hip joint as the hip and knee on the paretic side are flexed.

The Coughing Sign of Huntingdon. Coughing and straining are followed by flexion at the hip and extension at the knee and consequent elevation of a paretic lower extremity.

The Reinforcement Sign of Babinski. When the patient is seated with his legs hanging free from the examining table, forceful pulling of the flexed fingers of one hand against those of the other is accompanied by extension of the leg on the paretic side.

The Klippel–Feil sign, the Marie–Foix phenomenon, and the reflex responses of Riddoch, Buzzard, and others are sometimes classified as

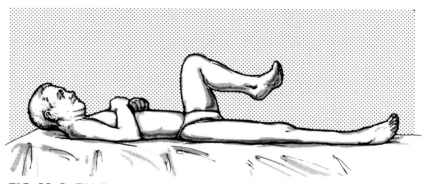

FIG. 38–3. *Tibialis sign in a patient with left hemiparesis.*

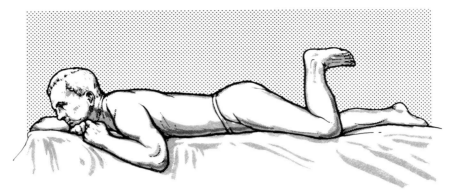

FIG. 38–4. Tibialis sign elicited with the patient in the prone position.

abnormal associated movements. Although related to the spinal automatisms they are also found in patients with cerebral hemispheric lesions. Insamuch as they are all characterized by a response to a specific stimulus, they are described with the corticospinal tract responses (Ch. 35) rather than with the associated movements.

Contralateral Coordinated Associated Movements

Coordinated associated movements in which the response is a contralateral one are similar to the symmetric associated movements, but the response is not always an imitative one and may involve muscles other than those used in the primary movement.

Brachioradial Response. Extension of the flexed elbow on the normal side, especially if it is extended by the examiner against the patient's resistance, is followed by flexion of the elbow on the paretic side.

Associated Contralateral Contraction of the Triceps. In normal individuals flexion of the biceps muscle in one arm is associated with contraction of the contralateral triceps and extension of the opposite arm. In hemiparesis resulting from organic lesions this contralateral extension is present in the normal arm on forceful flexion of the paretic arm, but absent in the paretic arm on flexion of the normal arm.

Sterling's Sign. Active adduction of the shoulder on the normal side against resistance is accompanied by adduction of the shoulder on the paretic side.

Raimiste's Leg Sign. If the examiner opposes forceful attempts at abduction or adduction of the leg on the normal side, the paretic leg will carry out a movement identical with that attempted on the normal side. This is evaluated with the patient in the recumbent position and the lower extremities abducted. As the patient attempts to adduct the sound leg against resistance the paretic leg goes into adduction, and the two will be drawn together. As he attempts abduction, the paretic leg also abducts.

Loss of Coordinated Associated Movements

Certain coordinated associated movements that are normally present are abolished in corticospinal lesions. Some of these are responses to active or voluntary movement, whereas others follow passive movement of the parts. Normal associated and automatic movements, such as swinging of the arms in walking and synergistic movements used in rising and sitting down, are also lost in disorders of the extrapyramidal system, especially parkinsonian syndromes.

The Platysma Sign of Babinski. In normal individuals a contraction of the platysma muscle can be seen and palpated when the person opens his mouth as widely as possible or flexes his chin against his chest. In corticospinal hemiparesis the platysma on the weak side fails to contract when the patient opens his mouth forcibly or grimaces. If resistance is offered to either opening the mouth or flexion of the chin against the chest, contraction of the platysma will be apparent only on the normal side. Obviously, the platysma also fails to contract in a peripheral lesion of the facial nerve.

The Phenomenon of Grasset and Gaussel. The normal individual, when in the recumbent position, can raise either leg separately or can raise both simultaneously. In corticospinal lesions he may still be able to raise either one separately, but cannot raise them simultaneously. If he first raises the paretic one, it falls back heavily as soon as he attempts to raise the normal one or if the normal one is passively raised; this is the result of inability to steady the pelvic muscles on the paretic side. On the other hand, if he first raises the normal one and then the paretic leg is passively raised, the sound one remains elevated and is held in place by the fixed pelvic muscles on that side.

The Leri Sign. This consists of absence of normal flexion at the elbow on passive flexion of the wrist and fingers. It has been listed as one of the corticospinal tract responses of the upper extremities.

The Mayer Sign. This consists of absence of normal adduction and opposition of the thumb with flexion at the metacarpophalangeal joint and extension at the interphalangeal joint when the fingers are passively flexed. It is also discussed with the corticospinal tract responses of the upper extremities.

The Grip Sign. With the examiner's fingers inserted into the contracted hand of the patient, grip is relaxed when the hand is passively flexed on the forearm, but is increased as the hand is extended.

CHANGES IN MOTOR FUNCTION

The following changes in motor function, most of which may be considered abnormalities of the associated movements, are also found in organic hemiparesis and other motor disturbances, principally those of the corticospinal system. They usually present only when other signs of involvement of this system are apparent.

The Babinski Tonus Test. This is a method of evaluating tone and is described in Chapter 28.

The Bechterew Sign. The arms are flexed at the elbow, passively raised to the level of the shoulder, and then suddenly released. In normal individuals the arm will "hang" in midair for a moment or two and then drop. In corticospinal system lesions the arm will hang longer and the dropping will be retarded. In flaccid paralyses and psychogenic lesions, on the other hand, the arm will drop precipitously.

Raimiste's Arm Sign. The patient's elbow is placed on a table and the hand and forearm are held upright by the examiner. When the sound hand is released it remains upright, but when the paretic hand is released it reflexes on the forearm to an angle of about 130°. This is a sign of flaccidity rather than spasticity, but may be present immediately after the onset of an organic hemiparesis.

The Pronation Sign of Neri. With the patient recumbent, his upper extremities are extended and pronated on the examining table. When the forearm is flexed and supinated by the examiner the paretic arm returns to pronation. This is similar in many respects to the Strümpell and Babinski pronator phenomenon.

The Leg Sign of Barré. With the patient prone, the knees are flexed to a right angle and the patient is asked to maintain that position. A normal individual can do so without difficulty. If there is corticospinal paresis, the weak leg will fall, slowly or rapidly depending upon the severity of the paralysis, notwithstanding the fact that the posterior thigh muscles may be seen to be contracting more vigorously on the paretic than on the normal side.

Claude's Sign of Reflex Hyperkinesia. Reflex movements of either extension or retraction may appear following a painful stimulus to an extremity, even though the part may seem totally paralyzed.

The Leg and Knee Dropping Tests. With the patient recumbent, the hips and knees are flexed until the posterior angle of the knee joints is about 45°, and the heels are resting on the table. When a corticospinal tract lesion is present, the affected heel will slide downward so that the leg and thigh go into extension and the latter into external rotation and abduction, and the foot assumes a position of plantar flexion and eversion.

BIBLIOGRAPHY

Archibald KC, Weichec CF. A reappraisal of Hoover's test. Arch Phys Med Rehabil 1970;51:234

Arieff AJ, Tigay EL, Kuntz JF, Larmon WA. The Hoover sign. Arch Neurol 1961;5:673

Cambier J, Dehen H. Imitation synkinesia and sensory control of movement. Neurology 1977;27:646

Fisher CM. Symmetrical mirror movements and left ideomotor apraxia. Trans Am Neurol Assoc 1963;88:214

Green JB. An electromyographic study of mirror movements. Neurology 1967;17:91

Gunderson CN, Solitaire GB. Mirror movements in patients with Klippel – Feil syndrome. Arch Neurol 1968;18:675

Haerer AF, Currier RD. Mirror movements. Neurology 1966;16:757

Hoover CF. A new sign for the detection of malingering and functional paralysis of the lower extremities. JAMA 1908;51:746

List CF. Peculiar types of reflex-synergias observed in comatose patients. J Nerv Ment Dis 1936;83:381

Wartenberg R. Diagnostic Tests in Neurology. Chicago, Year Book Medical Pub, 1953

Chapter 39
MISCELLANEOUS NEUROLOGIC SIGNS

Miscellaneous neurologic signs, some of them reflexes, some closely related to the defense and postural reflex mechanisms, and others more varied in nature, are elicited in certain diseases of the nervous system. The more important ones are listed in this chapter.

SIGNS OF EXTRAPYRAMIDAL DYSFUNCTION

Disorders of the basal ganglia or of the extrapyramidal system are characterized by the following changes: Disturbances in tone, usually of a rigid type; derangement of movement, usually hyperkinesia, but occasionally bradykinesia or akinesia; and loss of normal associated movements. Some of the specific methods of investigating and evaluating hypertonicity and impairment of associated movements are the Babinski tonus, head dropping, pendulousness of the legs, shoulder shaking, and arm dropping tests described in Chapter 28. Also present are slowness of initiating movements, inability to carry out rapid movements, loss of ability to maintain two simultaneous voluntary motor activities, and often gait disturbances. There are no very characteristic changes in the reflexes. The muscle stretch reflexes may be slightly exaggerated, owing to increased muscular tension, but this is not a consistent finding, and they may be retarded, diminished, or absent owing to the marked increase in tonus or to contractures. There are no corticospinal tract responses in classic disorders affecting only the extrapyramidal system.

Some of the reflexes that are believed to indicate both corticospinal and premotor disease, especially those that are sometimes present with diffuse cerebral involvement, may be elicited when there is extrapyramidal dysfunction. These include hyperactivity of the orbicularis oculi (Myerson's sign) and oris reflexes (Ch. 13), and the forced grasping and palmomental reflexes (Ch. 35). In addition, there are a few reflexes that are not easily elicited, which indicate extrapyramidal involvement. Although of limited clinical significance, they will be briefly described.

The Tonic Plantar Reflex. This reflex is present when stroking the sole of the foot is followed by slow flexion and adduction of the toes and distal part of the foot that persists for a minute or two. This response has been attributed to prefrontal and extrapyramidal involvement, and may be contralateral, ipsilateral, or bilateral with respect to the lesion.

Soderbergh's Pressure Reflex. This reflex is present when a slow muscular contraction follows firm stroking of certain bony prominences. For example, if the ulna is stroked in a downward direction, there may be flexion of the three outer fingers, and if the radius is firmly stroked, there may be flexion of the thumb.

The Little Toe Reflex of Puusepp. This reflex is characterized by a slow abduction of the little toe in response to light stroking of the outer border of the foot.

The Schrijver – Bernhard Reflex. This reflex is present when percussing the anterior surface of the leg or tapping the skin over the tibia or anterior leg muscles just below the knee is followed by plantar flexion of the toes. The **Lomadtse sign,** which consists of plantar flexion of the toes on pressure over the anterior aspect of the tibia, is similar. These are both called **distant toe flexor reflexes.**

Souques' Leg Sign. When a patient, seated in a chair, is suddenly pushed backward, the legs normally extend in an attempt to counteract loss of balance. Absence of this extension of the legs is Souques' leg sign; it is found in advanced striatal disease, and is in reality a loss of associated movements.

SIGNS OF MENINGEAL IRRITATION

Signs of irritation of the meninges are most frequently elicited in association with inflammatory involvement of the meningeal tissues, as in bacterial meningitis. They may also, however, be secondary to the presence of foreign material in the subarachnoid space, as in subarachnoid hemorrhage, or with administration of drugs, contrast material, and at times spinal anesthetics. They may also be associated with increased spinal fluid pressure, as in aseptic meningitis and meningismus. The objective manifestations are usually secondary to either displacement of the intraspinal structures or variations in tension on the inflamed and hypersensitive spinal roots, as discussed later. The symptoms and signs of meningeal irritation are varied and depend upon the severity of the process. Among the more common are the following: Headache with pain and stiffness of the neck; irritability, hyperesthesia, sensitivity of the skin, photophobia, and hyperacusis; fever, chills, and other manifestations of infection; nausea and vomiting; confusion, delirium, coma, or convulsions; carphology, or involuntary plucking at the bedclothes; paralytic phenomena; and characteristic cerebrospinal fluid changes. In addition there are certain objective diagnostic criteria, known as signs of meningeal irritation. The outstanding of these are listed.

Nuchal (Cervical) Rigidity. Nuchal rigidity is probably the most widely recognized and frequently encountered sign of meningeal irritation, and the diagnosis of meningitis is rarely made in its absence. It is characterized by stiffness and spasm of the neck muscles with pain on attempts at voluntary movement. There is also resistance to passive movement. Resistance to passive flexion may be so great that the physician is unable to place the patient's chin upon his chest; there may be resistance to extension and rotatory movements as well. The degree of rigidity varies: There may be only slight resistance to passive flexion, or marked spasm of all the neck muscles. Rigidity particularly affects the extensor musculature, however, and flexion may be impossible while hyperextension can be readily carried out; rotatory and lateral movements may also be preserved. If the rigidity of the extensor muscles is marked, there may be retraction of the neck, and even the neck and spine, into a position of opisthotonos.

The only instances in which nuchal rigidity is not found in association with meningitis may be in fulminating or terminal cases, in deep coma, or in disease of very young infants. It must be remembered that nuchal rigidity may also be a manifestation of cervical arthritis and myositis, cervical adenopathy, retropharyngeal abscess, trauma, and other disease processes within the neck, and rigidity may also appear in association with severe infections such as pneumonia and typhoid fever, and with extrapyramidal disorders.

Resistance to Movement of Legs and Back. The patient lies with his legs drawn up; there is flexion of the thighs on the pelvis and of the legs on the thighs. He resists passive extension of the legs. On rising from a supine to a sitting position he supports himself by placing his hands behind him and pressing them against the bed (**Amoss' sign**).

Kernig's Sign. Kernig's sign has been described variously and tested in many different ways. Kernig described it as an involuntary flexion at the knee when the examiner attempts to flex the thigh at the hip while the leg is in extension. It is more commonly elicited, however, by flexing the thigh of the recumbent patient to a right angle, and then attempting to extend the leg at the knee. This passive extension at the knee is accompanied not only by pain and resistance due to spasm of the hamstring muscles, but also by limitation of extension. Full extension of the leg is impossible if the hip is in flexion (Fig. 39-1). According to some definitions, Kernig's sign is positive if the leg cannot be extended at the knee to over 135° while the hip is flexed. In **Lasègue's sign,** which is similar, an attempt is made to flex the thigh at the hip while

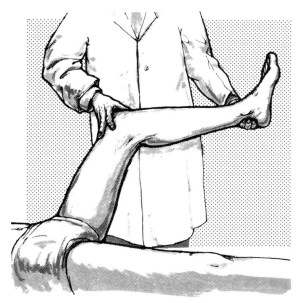

FIG. 39–1. Method of eliciting Kernig's sign.

the leg is held in extension. When positive, this sign is also accompanied by pain in the sciatic notch and resistance to movement. Both Kernig's and Lasègue's signs, as well as the nerve-stretching modifications of the latter (Ch. 47), are positive in meningitis, probably owing to stretching of and tension on the irritated nerve roots and meninges, but both are also positive with irritation of the lumbosacral nerve roots or plexus resulting from a ruptured intervertebral disk or other causes. In the latter conditions, however, the signs are usually unilateral, whereas in meningitis they are bilateral.

Bikele's Sign. This consists of resistance to extension of the elbow when the arm is elevated at the shoulder, and is similar to Kernig's sign in that it is positive on stretching irritated nerve roots. With the patient seated, the forearm is flexed at the elbow and the arm is abducted, elevated, and externally rotated, or is moved upward and backward at the shoulder to a maximal degree. The examiner then attempts passively to extend the forearm at the elbow. The sign is positive if there is resistance to such extension. This sign is also seen in brachial plexus neuritis, probably more frequently than in meningitis.

Brudzinski's Neck Sign. Passive flexion of the head on the chest is followed by flexion of both thighs and legs, so that both lower extremities may be strongly flexed on the pelvis. The

test is carried out by placing one hand under the patient's head and forcibly flexing the neck while placing the other hand on his chest to prevent elevation of the body. Occasionally there is flexion of the arms as well, and there may be fanning of the toes. This sign has been said to represent a tonic neck reflex in a partially decerebrate state, but, like the other meningeal signs, may be a result of tension on the nerve roots. There may be absence of flexion of the thigh and leg on one side in conditions where meningeal irritation and cerebral hemiplegia are present simultaneously.

Brudzinski's Contralateral Leg Signs. Passive flexion of one hip, especially if the hip is flexed while the knee is in extension, is accompanied by flexion of the opposite hip and knee. The same result may be obtained by passive extension of the leg at the knee after the thigh has been flexed to a right angle (Kernig's maneuver). In the **Brudzinski reciprocal contralateral leg sign** one leg and thigh are flexed while the other leg and thigh are extended; when the flexed limb is lowered the contralateral extended one will go into flexion.

Brudzinski's Cheek Sign. Pressure against the cheeks on or just below the zygoma is accompanied by a reflex flexion at the elbows with an upward jerking of the arms.

Brudzinski's Symphysis Sign. Pressure on the symphysis pubis is followed by flexion of both lower extremities.

Guillain's Sign. Pinching of the skin over the quadriceps femoris muscle or squeezing the muscle on one side is followed by flexion of the contralateral hip and knee.

Edelmann's Great Toe Phenomenon. Flexion of the thigh at the hip while the leg is extended at the knee is followed by dorsiflexion of the great toe. This sign may be present in cerebral edema as well as in meningeal irritation.

Various attempts have been made to explain the signs described here. Muscular rigidity, motor irritation, increased intracranial pressure and distention of the meninges, tonic neck reflexes, and crossed reflexes have been suggested as underlying mechanisms. It is probable, however, that in the main the various maneuvers that are carried out produce displacements of the intraspinal structures with changes in tension in the inflamed and hypersensitive spinal nerve roots. O'Connell expressed the belief, based on anatomic observations, that the resulting signs may be postures designed to minimize tension in the inflamed roots, muscle spasms designed to limit movement productive of such tension, or movements designed to produce maximum relaxation in nerve roots rendered tense by some test maneuver.

SIGNS OF TETANY

The clinical manifestations of tetany include spasm and tonic contractions of the skeletal muscles, principally the distal muscles of the extremities. There may be contraction of muscles of the wrist, hands, and fingers, with resulting carpal spasm (the so-called obstetrical or accoucheur's hand), and of the muscles of the foot and toes, causing pedal spasm (Ch. 28). There is hyperirritability of the entire peripheral nervous system, as well as the musculature, to even minimal stimuli. Involvement of the sensory nerves may cause paresthesias in the hands, feet, and perioral region. There may be irritability of the facial muscles and convulsions. These changes are related to disturbances of calcium and phosphorus metabolism and to abnormalities in the acid-base equilibrium of the body; these may be verified by various biochemical examinations. In tetany, however, certain neurologic signs may be present that aid the physician in making a diagnosis on the basis of the clinical examination alone. They are more easily obtained if the patient first hyperventilates for a few minutes. The more important of these are listed.

Chvostek's Sign. Tapping over the point of emergence and division of the facial nerve just anterior to the ear, with either the finger or a percussion hammer, is followed by a spasm or a tetanic, cramplike contraction of some or all of the muscles supplied by the ipsilateral facial nerve. Two points for stimulation have been described. One is just below the zygomatic process of the temporal bone and in front of the ear; the other is midway between the zygomatic arch and the angle of the mouth. Sometimes the response may be elicited merely by stroking the skin in front of the ear. The sign is minimal if only a slight twitch of the upper lip or the angle of the mouth results; it is of moderate degree if there is movement of the ala nasi and the entire corner of the mouth; it is maximal if the muscles of the forehead, eyelid, and cheek also contract. This is

in reality a trigeminofacial reflex, although the afferent impulse may be a proprioceptive one carried through the facial nerve. When the response is marked, however, the muscles supplied by the trigeminal nerve may also respond. Chvostek's sign is the result of a hyperirritability or hyperexcitability of the motor nerves, in this instance the facial nerve, to mechanical stimulation. It is an important sign in tetany, but is occasionally found in other conditions in which there is increased reflex irritability, such as in lesions of the corticospinal tract. It is also present in a majority of neonates and disappears during childhood.

Trousseau's Sign. Compression of the arm by squeezing or constricting it with the hand, a tourniquet, or a sphygmomanometer cuff is followed first by paresthesias of the fingers that progress centripetally over the hand and forearm, then by twitching of the fingers, and finally by cramping and contraction of the muscles of the fingers and hand with the thumb strongly adducted and the fingers stiffened, slightly flexed at the metacarpophalangeal joints, and clustered about the thumb — the so-called **accoucheur's hand.** There may be a latent period of ½ – 4 min. Similar pressure around the leg or thigh will be followed by a pedal spasm. It has been suggested that the response may result from pressure on either the nerve trunks or the arteries. It is probable that occlusion of the arteries causes ischemia of the nerve trunks, and this in turn increases the excitability of the nerves. A modification of this is carried out in the **von Bonsdorff technic,** in which a sphygmomanometer cuff is placed over the arm and is kept moderately inflated for about 10 min. It is then removed and the patient is told to hyperventilate. Typical tetanic spasm occurs much earlier in the previously ischemic arm than in the other arm.

The Pool – Schlesinger Sign. Tension on the brachial plexus by forceful abduction and elevation of the arm while the forearm is extended is followed by tetanic spasm of the muscles of the forearm, hand, and fingers. Tension on the sciatic nerve by forceful flexion of the thigh on the trunk while the leg is extended is followed by spasm of the muscles of the leg and foot.

Schultze's Sign. Mechanical stimulation of the protruded tongue, (*e.g.,* by tapping it with a percussion hammer) is followed by a transient depression or dimpling at the site of stimulation.

A similar phenomenon is evident in patients with myotonia or myotonic dystrophy.

Kashida's Thermic Sign. This consists of the development of hyperesthesias and spasms after the application of either hot or cold irritants.

Escherich's Sign. There is an increased reaction to stimulation of the oral and lingual mucosa, and contractions of the lips, masseters, and tongue follow percussion of the inner surface of the lips or percussion of the tongue.

Hochsinger's Sign. Pressure on the inner aspect of the biceps muscle causes spasm and contraction of the hand. It is possible that in carrying out this maneuver one compresses the brachial artery, and this sign may be a variation of Trousseau's sign.

The Peroneal Sign (Lust's Phenomenon). Tapping over the common peroneal nerve as it winds around the neck of the fibula is followed by dorsiflexion and eversion of the foot.

FRONTAL RELEASE SIGNS

The terms **frontal release signs** and **primitive** (or **atavistic**) **reflexes** are used for responses that are present in some patients with advanced organic dementias, diffuse encephalopathies (metabolic, toxic, postanoxic), normotensive hydrocephalus, post-traumatic states, neoplasms, and cerebral degenerations, and that are usually diffuse but often affect primarily the frontal lobes or the frontal association areas. The significance of these release signs or primitive reflexes has been hotly debated. Some authorities claim they are normal phenomena of advancing age; some even state that these signs are as common in control subjects as in patients with severe neurologic disease. A consensus is gradually emerging, suggesting that any single one of these primitive reflexes may be present in persons without severe central nervous system dysfunction, but that the presence of a combination of several such signs is correlated with grave central nervous system disease. The likelihood of the appearance of primitive reflexes appears to increase with the duration and severity of chronic brain disorders, but not in a linear fashion. The primitive reflexes do not have great localizing value, suggesting instead the presence of diffuse and widespread dysfunction of the hemispheres.

Exaggeration of the muscle stretch reflexes is often present with widespread cerebral disease, and often corticospinal tract responses, such as the grasp reflexes of the hand and foot, and the Hoffmann, Trömner, and Babinski signs, are present. Among the additional responses are those described here. Many of these, too, are exaggerations of normal reflex responses while others are responses that are normally found in infants and disappear in childhood or during maturation but that return in cerebral disease.

The **orbicularis oculi**, or **glabellar**, **reflex** is normally present in adults. If, however, repeated stimuli are directed to the glabella, the blink response normally stops after the first few taps. In corticospinal tract disease, extrapyramidal disease, and diffuse cerebral disease the reflex is exaggerated and continues to be present with repeated stimuli (Myerson's sign).

The **orbicularis oris reflex** may be exaggerated in diffuse cerebral disease, and it often can be elicited by a minimal tap to either the upper or lower lip or even by sweeping a tongue blade briskly across the lips. If such stimulation produces puckering and protrusion of the lips, the response is known as the **snout reflex.**

The **sucking reflex** is normally present in infants, in whom stimulation of the lips is followed by sucking movements of the lips, tongue, and jaw. This reflex disappears after infancy, when sucking becomes a voluntary rather than reflex phenomenon. It, like the snout reflex, is present in some patients with diffuse cerebral disease, in whom testing for the orbicularis oris reflex causes not only puckering and protrusion of the lips, but also sucking and even tasting, chewing, and swallowing movements. This exaggerated response is also known as the **Atz, mastication,** or "**wolfing" reflex.** When present it may be elicited by lightly touching, striking, or tapping the lips, stroking the tongue, or stimulating the palate. When it is grossly exaggerated there may be automatic opening of the mouth, and smacking and chewing movements, even when the object fails to touch the lips but is only brought near to them.

The **head retraction reflex** is a quick, involuntary backward jerk of the head that follows a brisk tap to the upper lip while the head is bent slightly forward. This is normally absent in adults but may be elicited in some patients with bilateral supracervical lesions of the corticospinal pathway and in those with diffuse cerebral disease.

In the **palmomental reflex** there is ipsilateral contraction of the mentalis and orbicularis oris muscles following stimulation of the thenar area of the hand. This is present with corticospinal tract and diffuse cerebral disease, but also is present in a significant number of normal persons.

While the primitive reflexes are not of lateralizing significance, some patients who have bilateral grasp responses also exhibit the phenomenon of **self-grasping,** with one hand grasping the contralateral forearm. When this sign is present unilaterally it suggests a contralateral frontal or parietal lobe lesion. It can also be found to occur bilaterally, when it has no localizing value.

BIBLIOGRAPHY

Bakchine S, Lacomblez L, Palisson E, Laurent M et al. Relationship between primitive reflexes, extrapyramidal signs, reflective apraxia and severity of cognitive impairment in dementia of the Alzheimer type. Acta Neurol Scand 1989;79:38

Gossman MD, Jacobs L. Three primitive reflexes in parkinsonism patients. Neurology 1980;30:189

Herman E. The tonic plantar reflex and its localizing significance. J Nerv Ment Dis 1952;116:933

Hoffman E. The Chvostek sign: A clinical study. Am J Surg 1958;96:33

Huber SJ, Paulson GW. Relationship between primitive reflexes and severity in Parkinson's disease. J Neurol Neurosurg Psychiatry 1986;49:1298.

Isakov E, Sazbon L, Costeff H, Luz Y et al. The diagnostic value of three common primitive reflexes. Eur Neurol 1984;23:17

Jacobs L, Gossman MD. Three primitive reflexes in normal adults. Neurology 1980;30:184

Kugelberg E. Neurologic mechanism for certain phenomena in tetany. Acta Neurol Psychiatry 1946;56:507

Maertens de Nordhout A, Delwaide PJ. The palmomental reflex in Parkinson's disease. Comparisons with normal subjects and clinical relevance. Arch Neurol 1988;45:425

Marti – Vilalta JL, Graus F. The palmomental reflex. Clinical study of 300 cases. Eur Neurol 1984;23:12

Marx P, Reschop J. The clinical value of the palmomental reflex. Neurosurg Rev 1980;3:173

O'Connell JEA. The clinical signs of meningeal irritation. Brain 1946;69:9

Ropper AH. Self-grasping: a focal neurologic sign. Ann Neurol 1982;12:575

Simpson JA. The neurological manifestations of idiopathic hypoparathyroidism. Brain 1952;75:76

Thorner MW. Modification of meningeal signs by concomitant hemiparesis. Arch Neurol Psychiatry 1948;59:485

Toomey JA. Stiff neck and meningeal irritation. JAMA 1945;127:436

Wartenberg R. The signs of Brudzinski and Kernig. J Pediat 1950;37:697

PART F

The Autonomic Nervous System

The nervous system is essential not only in the adjustment of the organism as a whole to its environment, but also in the regulation and coordination of the vital processes. In general, these latter functions are below the conscious level and are not subject to voluntary control. Their nervous integration is accomplished by means of reflex phenomena of varying degrees of complexity. The neurologic regulation of the smooth muscles and glands, which include the muscles of the blood vessels and viscera, the striated muscle of the heart, and the endocrine complex, is carried out by a portion of the nervous system that is somewhat distinct, both centrally and peripherally, from that which carries common sensation and supplies voluntary striated musculature. The neural components that control the regulation of the vital functions constitute what has been known as the autonomic, vegetative, sympathetic, or involuntary nervous system. It must be stressed, however, that it is not a separate nervous system. The autonomic and the voluntary portions are two aspects of a single integrated neural mechanism and are closely interrelated both centrally and peripherally. They are interdependent. The central regulatory structures are closely connected, and autonomic fibers are present in every peripheral spinal nerve and in most cranial nerves.

The autonomic nervous system in general is less available for clinical testing and routine examination than the voluntary nervous system, that part of the neural mechanism that has to do with somatic rather than visceral functions. The intimate correlation, however, between the voluntary and involuntary nervous elements, the interrelations between the conscious and the unconscious, and the presence of many syndromes that are predominantly of autonomic origin make the examination of this portion of the nervous system, as far as it can be performed, an essential part of the neurologic examination.

Chapter 40
ANATOMY, PHYSIOLOGY, AND PHARMACOLOGY OF THE AUTONOMIC NERVOUS SYSTEM

An understanding of the anatomy and physiology of the autonomic nervous system is essential to a comprehension of the reasons for and methods of examining it and also to a clear conception of the clinical syndromes that result from pathologic involvement of its constituent parts. These subjects will be discussed separately for the peripheral autonomic nervous system and for the regulatory structures in the central nervous system.

THE PERIPHERAL AUTONOMIC NERVOUS SYSTEM

The autonomic nervous system consists of a series of cerebrospinal nuclei and nerves with widely distributed ganglia and plexuses that subserve the vegetative functions of the body. In its peripheral connections the system is characterized by a series of synaptic junctions that are situated outside the central nervous system. From anatomic and physiologic points of view there are two primary divisions: (1) the parasympathetic or craniosacral division and (2) the sympathetic, orthosympathetic or thoracolumbar division. This classification is based on the point of outflow from the central nervous system, the distribution of peripheral ganglia, the general antagonism in physiologic effects on visceral tissues, most of which receive innervation from both divisions, and the response to pharmacologic agents. Each peripheral division of the autonomic nervous system is characterized by a two-neuron chain and consists of two anatomic elements: The preganglionic neuron terminates

in a peripheral ganglion, and then the postganglionic neuron, or neuron of the second order, carries impulses to their destination in the viscera. No impulse goes directly to an organ of termination. Although the two divisions can be designated anatomically as the craniosacral and the thoracolumbar portions, or outflows, the clinically favored terms are **parasympathetic** and **sympathetic systems,** or **divisions.** The latter nomenclature is used in this book.

The Anatomy of the Parasympathetic Division

The parasympathetic division (craniosacral or mesencephalic-medullary-sacral outflow) is composed of the visceral efferent fibers of the oculomotor, facial, glossopharyngeal, and vagus nerves, and bulbar portions of the accessory nerve, together with fibers arising in the second, third, fourth, and possibly the fifth sacral segments of the spinal cord. It has also been suggested that vasodilator fibers in the dorsal roots are related to the parasympathetic division or have important affinities with it. The parasympathetic nerves are characterized anatomically by relatively long preganglionic fibers that end in terminal or peripheral ganglia near or on the viscera they supply, and by short postganglionic fibers that arise in proximity to or within the viscus innervated. One preganglionic fiber usually synapses with only one postganglionic neuron. The portions of the parasympathetic division are widely separated, but because of anatomic characteristics, similarity in function, and similar pharmacologic responses, they are classified as parts of one system rather than as separate cranial, bulbar, and sacral divisions.

The anatomy of the cranial portions of the parasympathetic division is discussed with the individual nerves (Part C, "The Cranial Nerves"), but will be briefly reviewed. The tectal, or mesencephalic, portion consists of the parasympathetic nuclei and roots of the oculomotor nerve. The nuclear centers are the Edinger–Westphal nuclei, the medial portions of which are sometimes called the anterior median or medial nuclei. Preganglionic fibers course via the inferior division of the third nerves to the ciliary ganglia, and postganglionic fibers are carried by the short ciliary nerves to the ciliary muscles and the sphincter of the pupil.

The bulbar, or medullary, portion consists of the parasympathetic nuclei and roots of the seventh, ninth, tenth, and eleventh cranial nerves. Preganglionic fibers of the facial nerve arise in the superior salivatory and related nuclear masses. Some are carried by the chorda tympani and lingual nerve to the submaxillary ganglion and ganglion cells in the hilum of the submaxillary gland, with postganglionic fibers to the submaxillary and sublingual glands and the mucous membrane of the mouth and tongue. Others are carried by the greater superficial petrosal and vidian nerves to the sphenopalatine ganglion, with postganglionic fibers continuing to the lacrimal gland and the mucosa of the orbit, nose, posterior portion of the pharynx and soft palate, and the upper portion of the buccal cavity.

Preganglionic fibers of the glossopharyngeal nerve arise in the inferior salivatory nucleus and are carried through the tympanic and lesser superficial petrosal nerves to the otic ganglion; then postganglionic fibers go via the auriculotemporal branch of the fifth nerve to the parotid gland, and with the facial nerve to the mucous membrane of the posterior and inferior portions of the pharynx and buccal cavity. Other preganglionic fibers of the glossopharyngeal nerve along with preganglionic fibers of the bulbar portion of the accessory, and principally of the vagus nerve arise in the dorsal efferent nucleus and terminate in ganglia situated near, on, or in the various viscera supplied by these nerves, including the heart, bronchioles, and gastrointestinal tract. The fibers to the heart terminate in the small ganglia of the heart wall, especially the atrium, from which postganglionic fibers are distributed to the musculature. The preganglionic fibers to the esophagus, stomach, small in-testine, and greater part of the large intestine terminate in the extensive myenteric (Auerbach) and submucous (Meissner) plexuses, from which postganglionic fibers are distributed to the smooth muscles and glands of these organs. A cranial outflow of the parasympathetic division to the pituitary stalk innervating the posterior lobe of the pituitary gland has been suggested.

The sacral parasympathetic fibers arise from cells in the intermediolateral portion of the sacral spinal cord. They travel through the second, third, fourth, and possibly the fifth sacral nerves, and are collected into the nervi erigentes, or pelvic nerves, which proceed to the pelvic plexuses and their branches. Postganglionic fibers may be carried from these plexuses to the pelvic viscera, but most preganglionic fibers continue to small ganglia on or near the viscera where synapses occur and postganglionic fibers pass into the musculature of these organs. The sacral nerves supply the bladder, descending colon, rectum, anus, and genitalia.

The Anatomy of the Sympathetic Division

The sympathetic division, or thoracolumbar out-flow, is composed of preganglionic fibers that arise from cells in the intermediolateral columns of the eighth cervical or first thoracic through the first two or three lumbar segments of the spinal cord. The fibers exit through the ventral roots of the corresponding segmental nerves (Fig. 40-1). Whether, in man, the eighth cervical segment and root contribute to the sympathetic division, or whether the uppermost cells lie between the eighth cervical and first thoracic segment and make their exit with the first thoracic nerve root remains uncertain. The termination of these fibers is threefold: (1) in the paravertebral ganglionic chain, (2) in the prevertebral plexuses and collateral ganglia, and (3) occasionally in terminal ganglia (Fig. 40-2). The postganglionic fibers go to the viscera. The sympathetic differs from the parasympathetic division in that the preganglionic fibers are often short and terminate on ganglia some distance from the viscera they supply, and the postganglionic fibers are longer than those of the parasympathetic division. Also, one preganglionic fiber may synapse with many postganglionic neurons.

The paravertebral, vertebral, or central ganglionic chain, or sympathetic ganglionic trunk, consists of two elongated plexuses, each com-

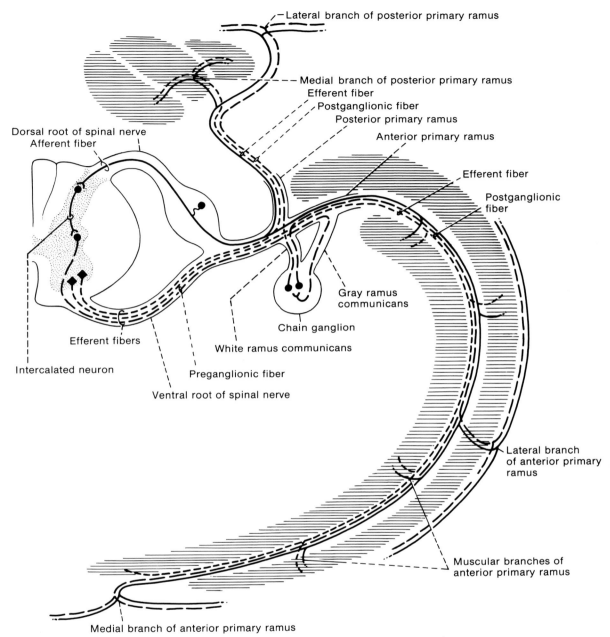

FIG. 40–1. Segmental spinal nerve showing the course of motor, sensory, and preganglionic and postganglionic sympathetic fibers.

posed of a series of ganglia that are usually segmentally arranged and that are bound together by ascending and descending nerve fibers. The preganglionic fibers leave the spinal cord and traverse its ventral root and the mixed spinal nerve to reach the anterior primary ramus. Then they leave the proximal part of this ramus as

finely myelinated fibers (white rami communicantes) and enter the ganglionic chain. They may synapse immediately or may ascend or descend to a higher or lower level before synapsing. The postganglionic fibers are unmyelinated (gray rami communicantes). On reaching the anterior primary ramus they separate into

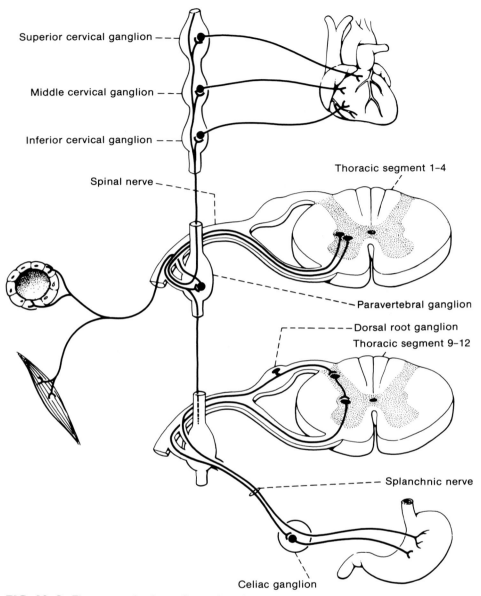

Superior cervical ganglion

Middle cervical ganglion

Inferior cervical ganglion

Spinal nerve

Thoracic segment 1–4

Paravertebral ganglion

Dorsal root ganglion
Thoracic segment 9–12

Splanchnic nerve

Celiac ganglion

FIG. 40–2. The sympathetic outflow, showing connections with the paravertebral ganglionic chain, splanchnic nerves, and collateral ganglia.

two groups, one extending with the anterior primary ramus, the other joining the posterior primary ramus. The sympathetic trunks have from 22 to 24 ganglia and extend from the level of the second cervical vertebra to the coccyx. There are 3 cervical, 10 to 12 thoracic, 4 lumbar, and 4 to 5 sacral ganglia. The chains usually join at the level of the coccyx in an unpaired coccygeal ganglion.

The cervical portion of the sympathetic chain consists of the superior, middle, and inferior cervical ganglia. These innervate structures within the head, upper extremities, and thorax. The superior cervical ganglion, the largest, is opposite the second and third cervical vertebrae and behind the internal carotid artery. It is primarily supplied by the first four thoracic segments. The internal carotid nerve, a direct prolongation of this ganglion, gives rise to postganglionic fibers. It supplies filaments to the internal carotid artery and terminates as the internal carotid and cavernous plexuses. Anterior branches from the ganglion form plexuses around the middle meningeal and external carotid and maxillary arteries.

The sympathetic innervation of the ciliary ganglia travels through the long ciliary nerves from the cavernous plexus. The sphenopalatine ganglion is supplied by the internal carotid plexus through the deep petrosal and vidian nerves. The otic ganglion receives its sympathetic innervation from the plexus around the middle meningeal artery, and the submaxillary ganglion from that around the external maxillary artery. There are other connections from the superior cervical ganglion to other cranial nerves and the upper four cervical nerves, the pharyngeal plexus, the carotid sinus and body, the heart, and the superior cardiac nerves. The middle cervical ganglion communicates with the fifth and sixth cervical nerves to begin the middle cardiac nerve and other branches to the thyroid gland. The inferior cervical ganglion communicates with the seventh and eighth cervical nerves to form the inferior cardiac nerve and nerves to the blood vessels.

The thoracic portion of the sympathetic trunk rests against the heads of the ribs. Occasionally the first thoracic ganglion is blended with the inferior cervical ganglion to form the stellate ganglion. The upper five ganglia provide branches to the cardiac and pulmonary plexuses. It may be that most sympathetic innervation to the heart is transmitted directly from these ganglia, not via the cervical sympathetic chain. The abdominal portion of the sympathetic trunk is situated in front of the vertebral column along the medial margin of the psoas major muscle, and the pelvic portion is in front of the sacrum, medial to the anterior sacral foramina. The fused ganglion in front of the coccyx is known as the ganglion impar. All of these ganglia send gray rami communicantes to the corresponding spinal nerves and many branch to the various plexuses and collateral ganglia. The postganglionic fibers terminate on blood vessels, sweat glands, and other smooth muscle and glandular structures.

Branches of the lower seven thoracic ganglia unite to form the three splanchnic nerves that penetrate the diaphragm and supply the abdomen and the pelvic viscera. These branches are white in color and primarily carry preganglionic fibers that pass through the ganglia without synapse and terminate in the prevertebral plexuses or the collateral ganglia. They do, however, contain a few postganglionic fibers that pass through the more distant plexuses without synapse to reach the viscera. The greater splanchnic nerve is formed by branches of the fifth through the ninth or tenth thoracic ganglia; it terminates in the celiac ganglion. The lesser splanchnic nerve is formed by branches of the ninth, tenth, and sometimes the eleventh thoracic ganglia; it ends in the aorticorenal ganglion. The lower splanchnic nerve arises from the last thoracic ganglion; it ends in the renal plexus.

Within the thoracic, abdominal, and pelvic cavities are aggregations of nerves and ganglia known as the prevertebral plexuses and their collateral ganglia. These are composed of both parasympathetic and sympathetic fibers. The parasympathetic fibers are preganglionic and may synapse in the plexuses or go through without synapse to terminal ganglia. The sympathetic fibers, mainly from the splanchnic nerves, primarily synapse in the plexuses. From these plexuses branches are given off to the thoracic, abdominal, and pelvic viscera.

The cardiac plexus is situated at the base of the heart, and is divided into a superficial portion that lies in the concavity of the aortic arch and a deep portion between the aortic arch and the trachea. Both are supplied by the cardiac branches of the vagus nerves and the cardiac nerves arising from the cervical sympathetic ganglia; they also receive fibers from the thoracic sympathetic ganglia. Branches reach the anterior and posterior coronary plexuses. The cardiac plexuses also communicate with the anterior and posterior pulmonary and the esophageal plexuses, all supplied by the vagus nerve as well as the thoracic sympathetic ganglia.

The celiac plexus is the largest of the three sympathetic plexuses. Situated in the abdomen at the level of the upper part of the first lumbar vertebra, it lies behind the stomach and omental bursa, in front of the crura of the diaphragm and the abdominal aorta, and between the adrenal glands. It is composed of the two celiac ganglia that are supplied by the greater splanchnic nerve and filaments from the right vagus nerve, and the aorticorenal ganglia, which receive the lesser splanchnic nerves. Secondary plexuses arising from or connected with the celiac plexus are the phrenic, hepatic, splenic, superior gastric, adrenal, renal, spermatic or ovarian, superior mesenteric, inferior mesenteric, colic, sigmoid, superior hemorrhoidal, and abdominal aortic. The superior (anterior) gastric plexus and the hepatic plexus also receive branches from the left vagus nerve. The renal and inferior mesenteric plexuses and their branches are also supplied by the lowest splanchnic nerve. All may receive some innervation from the lumbar sympathetic chain.

The hypogastric plexus is situated in front of the last lumbar vertebra and the promontory of the sacrum, between the two common iliac arteries. It is formed by the union of many elements from the aortic plexus and the lumbar sympathetic chain, together with some fibers from the inferior mesenteric plexus. It is divided into the two pelvic plexuses formed by fibers from the hypogastric plexus, preganglionic sympathetic fibers from the second, third, and fourth sacral nerves, and a few filaments from the sacral sympathetic ganglia. Branches are distributed to the pelvic viscera and the internal and external genitalia through the middle hemorrhoidal, vesical, prostatic, vaginal, and uterine plexuses.

The Physiology of the Peripheral Autonomic Nervous System

The autonomic nervous system governs the activities of cardiac and smooth muscle, including the smooth muscle of the blood vessels, and the functions of most glandular structures, including the functions of sweating and digestion. Although a few people seem capable of voluntarily altering heart rate, body temperature, and some aspects of metabolism, the autonomic nervous system is concerned with those processes that normally are beyond voluntary control and for the most part beneath consciousness. It regulates such important functions as respiration, circulation, digestion, temperature adjustment, and metabolism, all vital to normal existence, and combats forces acting from within or without that would tend to cause undesirable changes in the normal function of the body. Cannon used the term **homeostasis** for the ability of the body as a whole to meet changing conditions in its external or internal environment by autonomic adjustments. By homeostasis the constancy of the internal environment of the body and the uniformity and stability of the organism are maintained. During muscular exercise, for instance, there is an augmented blood supply with increased metabolism of skeletal muscle, and a shift of blood volume from one part of the body to another. The increased venous return to the heart is accommodated by reflex acceleration of the heart, peripheral vasoconstriction, and a

consequent rise in blood pressure that is immediately countered by increased activity of the aortic and carotid sinus reflexes. In addition there is bronchiolar dilation to allow for a greater respiratory exchange to meet the oxygen demand, together with cessation of peristalsis, and closing of the sphincters.

The viscera of the body receive a dual autonomic supply; they are innervated by both the parasympathetic and sympathetic divisions. In general these two divisions are antagonistic and reciprocal in their reaction, but there are definite exceptions, and on occasion their functions are correlated rather than antagonistic.

In a number of respects the functions of the parasympathetic division are not as clearly defined as those of the sympathetic division. It supplies special structures, such as the pupils, salivary glands, heart, lungs, gastrointestinal tract, bladder, and portions of the genital system. The structures innervated by the parasympathetic division are partially under the regulation of the motor cortex and may be subject to some degree of voluntary control. In certain parasympathetic functions, as in bladder, rectal, and genital activity, movements of striated musculature are closely correlated with those of smooth muscle. The parasympathetic division is essential to life and the conservation of energy. It controls anabolic, excretory, and reproductive functions, and conserves and restores bodily resources and energy.

The sympathetic division, on the other hand, supplies all portions of the body. Its functions are catabolic and directed toward the utilization of energy. It prepares the organism for either activity or flight, and mobilizes the resources of the body for combat. It acts whenever rapid adjustment to the environment is required. It accelerates the heart, dilates the coronary vessels, increases the arterial blood pressure, empties the blood reservoirs, dilates the bronchi, liberates glucose, and inhibits gastrointestinal activity. It is an emergency protective mechanism that tends to adapt the individual to changes that have taken place in his environment. It temporarily lessens fatigue. It is called into action under emotional stress and causes the individual to react strongly to stimuli of rage and fear.

The functions of the parasympathetic and sympathetic divisions in the innervation of the respective organs and tissues of the body are most easily understood by considering these structures individually and noting the reciprocal or the coordinating action of this dual supply. When both innervate a single organ, the parasympathetic acts largely through the smooth muscle of the organ itself; the sympathetic also acts through the medium of circulation and vasomotor tone.

The Eye

The parasympathetic division stimulates the sphincter of the pupil and causes constriction of the pupil, or miosis. It is generally considered that the sympathetic division stimulates the dilator of the pupil and causes mydriasis. However, some investigators believe there is little if any dilator muscle in the iris, and that the pupillary diameter is influenced almost entirely by parasympathetic activity and is dependent upon the contraction and relaxation of the constrictor musculature. They believe that the sympathetic division influences the size of the pupil only through the medium of the blood vessels of the iris.

The parasympathetic division also stimulates the ciliary muscle. Contraction of the circular fibers of this muscle causes relaxation of the ciliary zonule and decrease in the tension of the lens capsule; this is followed by an increase in the convexity of the lens to adjust the eye for near vision. The sympathetic division supplies the tarsal muscles and the orbital muscle of Müller. The tarsals are smooth muscle sheets in the upper and lower eyelids; that in the upper lid aids in the elevation of the eyelid. The muscle of Müller, in the lower forms at least, keeps the globe of the eye forward in the orbit. It is questionable whether the sympathetic causes relaxation of the ciliary muscle for distance vision, but it may aid in flattening the lens by producing contraction of the radial fibers of the ciliary muscle.

Stimulation of the parasympathetic nerves causes miosis and accommodation for near vision, whereas paralysis produces mydriasis and loss of accommodation. Stimulation of the sympathetic nerves causes mydriasis, widening of the palpebral fissure, and tension of the muscle of Müller, sometimes with exophthalmos; paralysis produces miosis, pseudoptosis, and sometimes enophthalmos, along with facial anhidrosis and vasodilation, resulting in Horner's syndrome.

The Lacrimal and Salivary Glands

The parasympathetic division supplies secretory and vasodilator impulses to the lacrimal and salivary glands and to the mucosal glands of the orbit, nose, pharynx, and mouth. The sympathetic division supplies secretory and vasoconstrictor impulses to the salivary glands. Stimulation of the parasympathetic nerves is followed by lacrimation and the formation of a copious amount of thin, watery saliva. Stimulation of the sympathetic nerves is followed by the formation of a scant supply of thick, viscid saliva. Destruction of the parasympathetic nerves causes diminution of lacrimation and salivation, but destruction of the sympathetics causes little change in these functions.

The Skin Structures

The sympathetic division stimulates the arrectores pilorum muscles and irritation of the sympathetic nerves results in a pilomotor response, or cutis anserina. The sympathetic division also supplies secretory impulses to the sweat glands, and stimulation of the sympathetic fibers results in an excess secretion. Paralysis of the sympathetics results in absence of both the pilomotor response and sweating. The parasympathetic division does not supply either the pilomotor muscles or sweat glands. It should be stressed, however, that although the sweat glands are innervated by fibers that belong to the postganglionic sympathetic system, their function is modified by drugs that influence the parasympathetic division. These nerves are, therefore, cholinergic rather than adrenergic in neural transmission.

The Blood Vessels

The parasympathetic and sympathetic innervation of the various blood vessels of the body is not adequately understood. Histologic investigations have demonstrated that the arterioles, capillaries, and veins are supplied mainly by fibers of the sympathetic division that reach the vessels through somatic nerves given off at segmental intervals. The density of sympathetic innervation varies with the location and size of the vessels. The medium and small-sized vessels have the densest innervation. α-(constrictor) adrenergic fibers are the predominant variety but some β-(dilator) fibers are also present. The sympathetic division supplies vasomotor fibers to the entire arterial system with the possible exception of the coronary arteries. This is most evident in the cutaneous, muscular, and splanchnic vessels. Section of the sympathetic trunk, as in Horner's syndrome, causes marked vasodilation and flushing of the skin and mucous surfaces, and stimulation of the sympathetics causes pallor of the skin and shrinkage of the mucous membranes. The administration of epinephrine or other sympathomimetic drugs results in vasoconstriction and raising of the blood pressure.

Opinion differs concerning the effect of the parasympathetic division on blood vessel caliber; it may either supply general vasomotor impulses, or supply such impulses only to specific structures. Vasodilator fibers carried by the facial and glossopharyngeal nerves innervate the lacrimal, salivary, and associated mucous glands; vasodilator fibers in the sacral nerves supply the helicine arteries. It has been postulated that parasympathetic vasodilator fibers reach the peripheral vessels through the dorsal spinal roots, but there is no definite evidence that much of the peripheral vascular system has reciprocal innervation or has a separate innervation stimulating vasodilation. The sympathetic division alone is felt to influence the diameter of the vessels through increase and decrease in tone. Adrenaline has a dual action on adrenergic blood vessel receptors; it causes vasoconstriction when the α-receptors are stimulated, and vasodilation when the β-receptors are stimulated, the effect depending on which vascular bed is involved. The dilation of the vessels that follows stimulation of the sensory nerves is probably the result of antidromic efferent conduction through those nerves; such efferent impulses are essential to the axon reflex.

The cerebral and meningeal vessels are constricted by the sympathetic and possibly dilated by the parasympathetic division. Stimulation of the sympathetic division, however, causes only partial constriction, or perhaps constriction followed by dilation. The branches of the external carotid artery may respond differently than the branches of the internal carotid. In migraine, where there is constriction followed by dilation of certain arteries, especially the dural and temporal branches of the external carotid artery, this dilation is not relieved by sympathomimetic drugs but is relieved by ergotamine tartrate, a sympathetic depressant.

The helicine arteries are constricted by the sympathetic division and are very definitely dilated by the parasympathetic, their stimulation resulting in relaxation of their tone and engorgement of the corpora cavernosa.

The coronary arteries are constricted by parasympathetic stimulation and dilated by sympathetic impulses.

That the veins as well as the arteries have efferent vasomotor nerves is demonstrated by the therapeutic response to lumbar sympathetic block in the treatment of thrombophlebitis.

The Heart

Stimulation of the parasympathetic division results in a reduction in heart rate, decreased output, diminished conduction at the atrioventricular bundle, and sometimes changes in rhythm such as atrioventricular block or vagal arrest. In general the parasympathetic inhibits and depresses the activity of the heart, slows the beat, and weakens contraction. Stimulation of the sympathetic division results in acceleration of the cardiac rate, increased output, augmented conduction of the atrioventricular bundle, and occasionally changes in rhythm characterized by ventricular extrasystoles, paroxysmal tachycardia, or atrial or ventricular fibrillation, together with a secondary rise in blood pressure. Section of the vagus causes tachycardia. Stimulation of the vagus, as in the oculocardiac reflex, causes slowing of the heart rate and may be of value in the treatment of paroxysmal tachycardia.

The Blood Pressure

The sympathetic division, through its constricting effect on the blood vessels, especially the splanchnic arteries, together with the acceleration of the heart rate, is important in the regulation of blood pressure. The administration of epinephrine or other sympathomimetic drugs will raise the blood pressure, and section of the splanchnic nerves and of other portions of the sympathetic complex was used for the treatment of essential hypertension prior to modern drug therapy. Stimulation of the parasympathetic division may produce some lowering of the blood pressure, possibly due in part to a reduction of cardiac rate and output, and partly, but questionably, the result of vasodilation. The drop in blood pressure is much less, however, than the degree of elevation that follows sympathetic stimulation.

The Respiratory System

The bronchial musculature is contracted and the bronchi and bronchioles constricted by the action of the parasympathetics, which also stimulate the bronchial secretion. The sympathetic division to a lesser extent dilates the bronchi and bronchioles; it probably reduces bronchial secretion by means of vasoconstriction of the arteries supplying the bronchial mucosa, although it may be an inhibitor to the bronchial glands. The symptoms of asthma, the result of bronchial constriction and edema and increased secretion, may be relieved either by drugs that diminish parasympathetic function or by those that stimulate the sympathetic division.

The Gastrointestinal System

In general the parasympathetic division increases the tone and motility of the gastrointestinal tract, relaxes the sphincters, and causes an increased secretion of the various glandular structures, thus aiding the various functions of the gastrointestinal system, including defecation. The sympathetic division decreases the tone and motility, contracts the sphincters, and may inhibit some of the glandular structures.

The supply to the salivary glands has been mentioned. In the esophagus the parasympathetic division stimulates peristalsis, whereas the sympathetic causes contraction of the cardiac sphincter. In the stomach the parasympathetic division causes increased peristaltic activity and increased secretion of the gastric glands, with, as a rule, relaxation of the pyloric sphincter. The sympathetic division causes a decrease in motility, contraction of the pyloric sphincter, and possibly inhibition of gastric secretion. It has a less important role than the parasympathetic division in gastric physiology and secretion, but does decrease the vascularity of the stomach wall. Vagotomy, used in the treatment of peptic ulcer, decreases both the tonus and motility of the stomach and the secretion of hydrochloric acid.

In the intestines the parasympathetic division also causes an increase in motility, tone, and peristalsis, with, in general, relaxation of the sphincters, including the anal sphincter, and an increase in secretion of the mucosal glands. The sympathetic innervation causes decreased peristalsis, contraction of the sphincters, and possibly inhibition of secretions. The parasympathetic supply to the intestines is carried by the vagus nerve as far as the descending colon, and below this by the sacral nerves. Drugs that stimulate structures innervated by postganglionic cholinergic nerves increase peristalsis; those that inhibit structures innervated by such nerves decrease it. Defecation is a function of the parasympathetics, and a defecation center has been postulated in the sacral portion of the spinal cord. Some investigators believe that the sympathetic division has comparatively little significance in the innervation of the intestine and its sphincters, and it probably is less active than the parasympathetic, but it does play a part. Vagotomy has also been used in the treatment of ulcerative colitis and regional enteritis. The external anal sphincter, composed of striated muscle, is innervated by the pudendal nerve from the first through the fourth sacral segments.

The parasympathetic division stimulates bile production in the liver and also contraction of the gallbladder and bile ducts, and the sympathetic may cause relaxation of these structures. The parasympathetic system also causes increased secretion by both the pancreatic acini and islets; the sympathetic may have no effect on these structures. The parasympathetic division thus not only aids in digestion by stimulation of the external secretion of the pancreas but also decreases the glucose content of the blood by production of insulin. The sympathetic nervous system, on the other hand, stimulates glycogenolysis in the liver, raises the glucose content of the blood, and may cause glucosuria. The parasympathetic plays no known part in these latter functions.

The Ureter and Bladder

The parasympathetic division supplies the bladder through the pelvic nerves from the second, third, and fourth sacral segments, with postganglionic fibers to the musculature, partly from the pelvic and vesical plexuses but mainly from small ganglia in or on the bladder wall (Fig. 40-3). It increases the tone and motility of the ureter and causes contraction of the detrusor muscle of the bladder with relaxation of the trigone and internal sphincter. It thus promotes micturition and stimulates emptying of the bladder. The sympathetic division also supplies these structures through fibers that originate in the lower thoracic and upper lumbar segments of the spinal cord and terminate in the hypogastric and vesical plexuses, from which postganglionic fibers go to the bladder musculature. It has been demonstrated that both α- and β-adrenergic receptors are present in the bladder and urethra.

When stimulated, the sympathetic division decreases the tone and mobility of the urethra, relaxes the detrusor, and contracts the trigone or internal sphincter, thereby impeding or inhibiting micturition. Stimulation of the parasympathetic system causes micturition, and stimulation of the sympathetic system causes retention. The activity of the sympathetic nervous system,

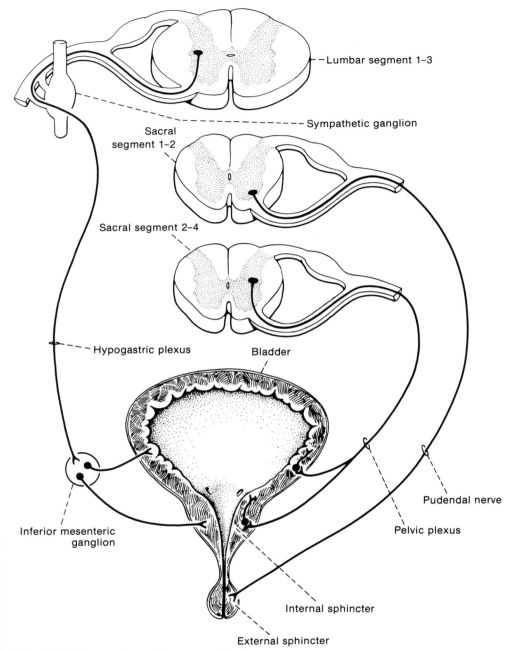

FIG. 40–3. Innervation of the urinary bladder.

however, is much less marked than is that of the parasympathetic division, and section of the former seems to have little effect on the musculature of the bladder. The exact function of the sympathetic division in urination in the normal individual is not understood. It is probable that its influences relate primarily to sexual func-tions, affecting urinary and bladder function indirectly and performing this activity by inhib-iting detrusor contraction during ejaculation. Section of the parasympathetic nerves, on the other hand, is followed by bladder paralysis. The smooth muscle of the bladder, however, also has inherent rhythmicity.

The voluntary nervous system, through the pudendal nerve from the second through the fourth sacral segments, is motor to the striated musculature of the external sphincter and the accessory muscles of the perineum. It is essential to voluntary initiation and control of micturition. This nerve also carries sensation from the bladder, although there is probably an autonomic afferent component as well, carried through both the pelvic and hypogastric nerves.

The Genital Organs

Both the parasympathetic and sympathetic divisions are necessary to sexual activity. Erection depends on a normal parasympathetic division and is the result of engorgement of the corpora cavernosa by dilation of the helicine arteries, or possibly by relaxation of their vascular tonus. Tonic contraction of the transverse perineal, bulbocavernosus, and ischiocavernosus muscles also contributes to erection, and maintains erection by interference with the return of the blood. All of these phenomena follow excitation of vasodilator and muscle reflex centers in the sacral portion of the spinal cord (erection center). Engorgement is in part related also to inhibition of vasoconstrictor centers in the lumbar cord. Stimulation of the sympathetic system, on the other hand, causes constriction of the arteries and subsidence of erection.

Ejaculation consists of two functions—emission, and ejaculation in the restricted sense. Emission is caused by contraction of the smooth muscle of the internal genitalia with delivery of semen to the membranous urethra. This is mediated by stimulation of the sympathetic division, which causes a reflex peristalsis of the ampulla of the ductus deferens, seminal vesicles, and ejaculatory ducts, and contraction of the smooth muscle of the prostate. It has been suggested that an emission center is present in the lumbar portion of the spinal cord. Ejaculation of the fluid through the urethral canal, or expulsion of the seminal fluid, is carried out by means of the parasympathetic division, which stimulates clonic spasms of the ischiocavernosus and bulbocavernosus muscles. The sympathetic division also stimulates contraction of the dartos muscles. A lesion of the parasympathetic causes impotence due to failure of erection and ejaculation, whereas overactivity of the parasympathetic causes priapism. A lesion of the sympathetic division causes impairment of ejaculation, resulting from failure of the spermatozoa to reach the urethra. Overactivity of the sympathetic division causes weak erections and premature ejaculations.

Stimulation of the parasympathetic division causes increased vaginal secretions, erection of the clitoris, and engorgement of the labia minora. The effect of the two divisions on the uterus is variable. The parasympathetic may have little influence, although it may stimulate contraction of the pregnant uterus. The sympathetic system causes contraction of the uterus during pregnancy and may produce either stimulation or inhibition of the nonpregnant uterus. It does stimulate contraction of the fallopian tubes, uterus, and Bartholin's glands at orgasm.

Other Functions

Stimulation of the sympathetic division causes secretion of epinephrine. This effect may be the result of activity at the postganglionic neuron rather than at the adrenal medulla itself, and consequently may be a cholinergic function, even though a part of the sympathetic physiology. The parasympathetic division may inhibit secretion of epinephrine. Stimulation of the sympathetic division causes contraction of the splenic capsule and emptying of the blood reservoirs.

The Pharmacology of the Peripheral Autonomic Nervous System

Much of our knowledge regarding the physiology of the autonomic nervous system has been acquired from information about the action of various pharmacologic substances upon the individual portions of the system. There has been a great proliferation of knowledge in regard to neurotransmitters, including those affecting the autonomic nervous system. Much of this material is beyond the scope of a book dealing with the clinical examination and is covered in excellent references. There are now also known to be at least two subtypes of adrenergic (sympathetic) receptors, alpha and beta, and probably several more. Certain drugs tend to stimulate either the parasympathetic or sympathetic divisions, and other drugs depress or inhibit them. These drugs mimic the effects of nerve stimulation and depression. As the two divisions of the system are in many ways antagonistic, drugs stimulating or depressing one part may, indirectly, cause decreased or increased activity of the other. Some of these agents act at the autonomic ganglia and others act directly upon the autonomic effector cells, the smooth muscle cells or glands. These variabilities in site of action and response are useful not only in understanding the action of the constituent parts, but also in examination and therapy.

Before discussing these various drugs individually, it is necessary to elaborate somewhat on the chemical mediation of nerve impulses. Loewi, in 1921, found that stimulation of the vagus nerve produced or liberated a substance at the myoneural junction that had the same effect as vagus stimulation when it was applied to certain cells and organs. This he called *vagus substance* or *parasympathin.* Loewi, Cannon, and others also found that stimulation of sympathetic fibers liberated a substance that had an action similar to that of epinephrine.

The substance liberated by stimulation of the parasympathetic nerves is now known to be the neurotransmitter **acetylcholine.** It acts as the chemical mediator of the excitatory process that is initiated by parasympathetic nerve impulses. It is split by the action of acetylcholinesterase, a specific enzyme present in the blood and tissues of the body, to choline and acetic acid. Physostigmine and related drugs inactivate the cholinesterase and prolong and intensify the action of acetylcholine. Acetylcholine has two modes and sites of action: (1) It stimulates the ganglion cells (both parasympathetic and sympathetic) when present in low concentrations, and depresses them when present in high concentrations. In this respect it acts similarly to the effects of nicotine, and this is called its **nicotinic** action. It has a like effect on voluntary muscles. (2) It also stimulates the autonomic effector organs (smooth muscle and glands) innervated by the parasympathetic nervous system. In this respect it acts similarly to muscarine, and this is called its **muscarinic** action.

The epinephrine-like substance that is produced or released at the myoneural junction by the stimulation of the sympathetic nerves was first called *sympathin* by Cannon. It is the chemical mediator of the excitatory processes that are initiated by sympathetic nerve impulses at neuroeffector junctions. It differs, however, from epinephrine in certain respects. Epinephrine has both excitatory and inhibitory effects, sympathin also has both, but they are separable. Evidence has accumulated that sympathin is identical with norepinephrine.

Parasympathetic and sympathetic nerve impulses reproduce the peripheral effects of acetyl-choline and norepinephrine. They are either stimulated or inhibited by the action of drugs. The demonstration that acetylcholine acts as a chemical transmitter of impulses for nerves other than postganglionic parasympathetic nerves suggested that it might be better to classify nerves physiologically rather than anatomically. Therefore the term **cholinergic** is used for all nerves that release acetylcholine at their terminals. These include not only all postganglionic parasympathetic nerves but also all autonomic preganglionic fibers, whether parasympathetic or sympathetic, together with the postganglionic sympathetic nerves to sweat glands and certain blood vessels and the somatic nerves to skeletal muscles. The term **adrenergic** is used for those nerves that release sympathomimetic chemicals. These include all postganglionic sympathetic fibers except those to the sweat glands and certain blood vessels. The adrenergic transmitter is norepinephrine, but epinephrine itself is also an adrenergic substance.

The drugs that act upon the autonomic nervous system may be classified as those that act at the autonomic ganglia and those that act at the myoneural junction. It must be stressed, however, that all these drugs affect cells and not nerve endings. Drugs that act upon the cells of the autonomic ganglia act on both parasympathetic and sympathetic ganglia. Inasmuch as their action is related to that of acetylcholine, they affect cells innervated by preganglionic cholinergic nerves. Most of these drugs have a similar action on skeletal muscles.

The principal drug that stimulates cells innervated by preganglionic cholinergic nerves is the neurotransmitter **acetylcholine.** This, in its nicotinic action, stimulates all autonomic ganglion cells innervated by preganglionic parasympathetic and sympathetic nerves and also cells innervated by all cerebrospinal somatic nerves to skeletal muscle fibers. Other esters of choline, such as methacholine, carbachol, and bethanechol, have a similar action but are not as readily susceptible to destruction by acetylcholinesterase and therefore are less evanescent in effect. They have a greater muscarinic than nicotinic action. Physostigmine, neostigmine, and certain organic phosphate compounds also stimulate the autonomic ganglion cells. They do not, however, act on the effector organs, but produce cell responses by virtue of their ability to inhibit acetylcholinesterase, preventing it from destroying the acetylcholine that is produced at the cholinergic nerve endings. They aid the muscarinic action of acetylcholine on smooth muscle, glands, and heart, and its nicotinic action on the autonomic ganglia and skeletal muscles. Nicotine in low concentrations also stimulates ganglion cells. Edrophonium, while primarily a curare antagonist at the skeletal myoneural junction, also has actions resembling those of acetylcholine.

Certain drugs depress or block the action of cells innervated by preganglionic cholinergic nerves: Nicotine in high concentrations prevents the response of ganglion cells to preganglionic nerve stimulation (*i.e.*, it stimulates, then depresses ganglion cells) and blocks synaptic transmission through autonomic ganglia by acting on ganglion cells to make them unresponsive to acetylcholine. Acetylcholine, the choline esters, and the inhibitors of acetylcholinesterase have a similar effect in high concentrations. Curare and the various preparations of **d**-tubocurarine raise the threshold to acetylcholine and prevent ganglion cells and muscles from responding to nerve stimulation, although they have a greater effect on skeletal muscle than on sympathetic ganglion cells. Their mode of action is similar to that of nicotine.

The drugs that act upon the autonomic effector cells do not act peripherally on autonomic nerves, but through performing their function at the myoneural junction and gland cells, act directly on muscles and glands. These may be divided into drugs that affect the parasympathetic division and those that affect the sympathetic divisions.

Drugs Affecting the Parasympathetic Division

Drugs that act on structures innervated by the postganglionic cholinergic nerves act upon all postganglionic parasympathetic nerves together with postganglionic sympathetic nerves that go to sweat glands and certain blood vessels. Those that act as stimulants are called **parasympathomimetic drugs.** These include acetylcholine and the other choline esters mentioned previously that have a muscarinic action on effector cells. The inhibitors of cholinesterase — physostigmine, neostigmine, benzpyrinium, and the organic phosphate compounds — produce similar effects. Other drugs that act directly on the effector cells in a highly selective manner are pilocarpine, muscarine, and arecoline. Muscular and glandular responses to these chemicals occur even after complete nerve degeneration.

Drugs that inhibit structures innervated by postganglionic cholinergic nerves are atropine, scopolamine, hyoscyamine, and many related synthetic drugs. They do not inhibit the nicotinic actions of acetylcholine, but specifically block all muscarinic effects, whether they are excitatory or inhibitory in nature. The site of action is the effector cells directly and not the nerve endings.

Drugs Affecting the Sympathetic Division

Drugs that act on structures innervated by postganglionic adrenergic nerves act upon all postganglionic nerves except those to sweat glands and certain vascular beds. Those that act as stimulants are called **sympathomimetic drugs.** These include epinephrine, norepinephrine, ephedrine, amphetamine, and numerous related synthetic drugs. These act directly on smooth muscle and glandular cells even when the effector organ is denervated. Cocaine also possesses sympathomimetic properties and potentiates the action of epinephrine but not of the other sympathomimetic drugs. A number of synthetic substances have been developed that inhibit or block adrenergically mediated impulses. Both α-blockers and β-blockers exist, counteracting the effects at the two types of adrenergic receptors. Such blockers play important roles in selective inhibition of certain adrenergic functions such as elevation of blood pressure.

Effects of Parasympathomimetics and Sympathomimetics

The therapeutic action of these drugs is well known. The parasympathomimetic drugs cause slowing of the heart, increased peristalsis, urgency of urination, pupillary constriction, and increased salivation and lacrimation. Through their action on the sweat glands and cutaneous vessels innervated by the sympathetic division they cause perspiration and increased heat and redness of the skin due to vasodilation. Those that inhibit the action of the parasympathetic division cause pupillary dilation, tachycardia, diminished salivation, decreased peristalsis, decrease in bronchial secretions, dilation of the bronchi and bronchioles, and, through their action on the sweat glands and blood vessels, diminished perspiration. The sympathomimetic drugs cause tachycardia, increased blood pressure, pupillary dilation, pilomotor response, bronchial dilation, and general vasoconstriction. The adrenergic inhibitors have already been mentioned in the preceding paragraph.

The Afferent Functions of the Peripheral Autonomic Nervous System

The visceral reflex arc obviously must have its afferent side. In addition to the efferent nerves supplied by the autonomic nervous system, general visceral afferent fibers are found in many of the cranial nerves and in the thoracolumbar and sacral autonomic nerves. These fibers convey impulses arising in smooth muscle and glandular structures and conduct sensations of spasm, distention, fullness, pressure, and pain from the viscera.

The afferent fibers conducting impulses from the viscera to the central nervous system have cell bodies in the cerebrospinal ganglia, as do the somatic afferent fibers. Opinions differ concerning the existence of any anatomic or physiologic differentiation between the visceral and the somatic afferent nerves. The distinction between them may be one of peripheral distribution rather than fundamental morphologic or functional significance. The controversy is largely one of terminology and classification. Many authorities express the belief that the visceral afferent fibers are not actually part of the autonomic nervous system, but merely travel with its efferent fibers. The mode of conduction through the spinal cord and the central connections of impulses conducting visceral sensation do not differ from those carrying somatic sensation. Despite the controversy regarding the existence of afferent functions of the autonomic nervous system, its sensory connections are important in the mediation of certain impulses from the viscera, in visceral reflexes, and in the syndromes of reflex or referred pain.

Primary clinical testing of the sensory functions of the afferent fibers carried with the autonomic nerves cannot be executed effectively, and the types of visceral sensations that can be tested may also be carried by somatic nerves. This problem and the subject of referred pain are discussed in detail in Chapter 7.

THE CENTRAL REGULATION OF AUTONOMIC FUNCTION

The peripheral autonomic nervous system is under the control of higher centers at all levels of neuronal integration. The anatomy and physiology of the autonomic nervous system and its disturbances of function cannot be discussed without consideration of those centers in the cerebral cortex, hypothalamus, midbrain, brain stem, and spinal cord that regulate and influence the function of its peripheral components. The most important of these centers is the hypothalamus.

The Hypothalamus

The hypothalamus (Fig. 40-4) lies in the ventral portion of the diencephalon just below the thalamus, and in immediate topographic relation with the pituitary gland, or hypophysis. It forms the greater part of the floor and part of the lateral wall of the third ventricle. From a strictly anatomic point of view it includes the optic chiasm, neurohypophysis (posterior pituitary), infundibulum, pars supraoptica, tuber cinereum, and mammillary bodies, but from a physiologic point of view the first three structures are not included. The pars supraoptica (nucleus supraopticus) is situated slightly above the optic chiasm. The mammillary bodies are a pair of small spheric masses of gray matter situated close together in the interpeduncular space rostral to the posterior perforated substance. They form the caudal portion of the hypothalamus. The tuber cinereum is an elevated gray area rostral to the mammillary bodies; it forms the rostral part of the hypothalamus. Beneath the hypothalamus a hollow, conical process, the infundibulum, projects downward and forward and is attached to the posterior lobe of the hypophysis; it is also called the stalk of the pituitary gland.

The boundaries of the hypothalamus are not sharply defined. Anteriorly it passes without specific demarcation into the basal olfactory and preoptic areas, and caudally it is continuous with and merges into the central gray matter and tegmentum of the midbrain. Laterally it is continuous with the subthalamic region, but superiorly it is separated from the thalamus proper by the hypothalamic sulcus. The region immediately above and anterior to the optic chiasm and extending to the lamina terminalis and anterior commissure is called the preoptic area; although this belongs to the diencephalon, it is usually considered with the hypothalamic centers. The entire area measures only about 14 × 18 × 20 mm and weighs only 4g.

The hypothalamus is composed of numerous nerve cells, not uniformly distributed but arranged into six more or less definite regions or nuclear groups, which are subdivided as follows:

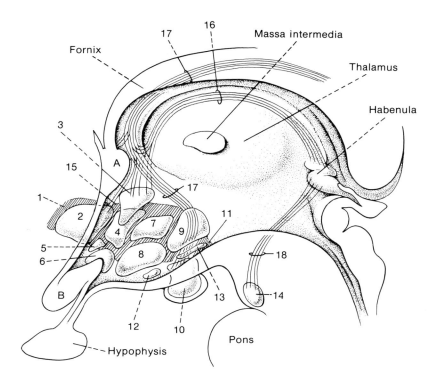

FIG. 40–4. Diagrammatic sketch of the human hypothalamus. **A.** Anterior commissure. **B.** Optic nerve. **1.** Lateral preoptic area (permeated by the median forebrain bundle). **2.** Medial preoptic area. **3.** Paraventricular nucleus. **4.** Anterior hypothalamic area. **5.** Suprachiasmatic nucleus. **6.** Supraoptic nucleus. **7.** Dorsomedial hypothalamic nucleus. **8.** Ventromedial hypothalamic nucleus. **9.** Posterior hypothalamic area. **10.** Medial mammillary nucleus. **11.** Lateral mammillary nucleus. **12.** Premammillary area. **13.** Supramammillary area. **14.** Interpeduncular nucleus. **15.** Lateral hypothalamic area. **16.** Stria habenularis. **17.** Fornix. **18.** Habenulopeduncular tract.

1. The preoptic region lies above and anterior to the optic chiasm and below the anterior commissure. It contains the medial and lateral preoptic areas.
2. The anterior group of nuclei, or rostral or supraoptic middle region, lies above the optic chiasm and is continuous anteriorly with the preoptic region. This region contains two principal cellular masses. The supraoptic nucleus lies immediately above the optic chiasm at the anterior aspect of the optic tract. The paraventricular nucleus is a flat plate of cells lying against the ependymal lining of the third ventricle and between the wall of the third ventricle and the column of the fornix; it is situated above the supraoptic nucleus. Other groups of cells in the region are the nucleus suprachiasmaticus, the nucleus supraopticus diffusus, and the anterior hypothalamic area.
3. The middle group, or tuberal or infundibular middle region, occupies the middle portion of the tuber cinereum. It is composed of the dorsomedial hypothalamic nucleus, the ventromedial hypothalamic nucleus, the dorsal hypothalamic area, the posterior hypothalamic area, and the perifornical area.

4. The lateral group, or region, occupies the lateral part of the tuber cinereum and includes both the lateral hypothalamic area and the nuclei tuberis lateralis.
5. The posterior group, or caudal or mammillary region, includes the premammillary area, the supramammillary area, and the mammillary bodies, containing the medial and lateral mammillary nuclei and the nucleus intercalatus. The posterior hypothalamic area is sometimes placed in this region.
6. The periventricular region contains many cellular masses that form the substantia grisea centralis. Included in this area are the nucleus periventricularis preopticus and the nucleus periventricularis arcuatus.

In spite of its small size, the hypothalamus has extensive and complex fiber connections, some organized into definite bundles or tracts, others diffuse and difficult to trace. There are elaborate interdiencephalic communications. The hypothalamus receives impulses from olfactory and general sensory tracts, hippocampal and temporal lobe cortices, amygdala, limbic system, basal ganglia, subthalamic nucleus, thalamus, and midbrain reticular formation, and from the frontal cortex either directly or indirectly through the thalamic nuclei. It communicates with the anterior thalamic nuclei, posterior lobe of the hypophysis, tegmental nuclei, and reticular formation of the midbrain and brain stem, and by means of descending pathways either directly or indirectly with the preganglionic autonomic centers of the brain stem and spinal cord. In the midbrain these descending pathways occupy both the central and tegmental portions. In the pons they are concentrated in the tegmental area. In the medulla they are chiefly in the lateral portion of the reticular formation. The descending lateral tectotegmentospinal tract, carrying pupillodilator fibers, and the lateral reticulospinal pathway to the sweat glands of the face are near the periphery. The ventral reticulospinal pathway, that innervates the sweat glands and controls vasodilation and temperature regulation of the body and extremities, is more medial.

Within the spinal cord the descending autonomic fibers are in the anterolateral fasciculus. They may be widely distributed but are primarily in the reticulospinal tracts, mainly uncrossed but also crossed, with a decussation occurring both in the brain stem and at spinal cord levels. Some fibers, especially those subserving bladder control, are in close proximity to the corticospinal tracts. Impulses carried through these pathways terminate at appropriate levels in the intermediolateral column of the spinal cord.

The hypothalamus is concerned primarily with receiving the visceral, or interoceptive, impulses, correlating them, and discharging them to appropriate visceral efferent centers. This is the region of the brain where highly organized visceral functions are integrated, and from which the outflow to the respective organs has its origin. The hypothalamus is important in the regulation of the peripheral autonomic nervous system and the various functions necessary for the maintenance of a normal internal environment in the body. This is accomplished primarily by means of reflexes that are mediated by the hypothalamus and descend through crossed and uncrossed pathways into the brain stem and spinal cord to activate the cells of the parasympathetic and sympathetic divisions of the nervous system at appropriate levels.

The hypothalamus is closely related anatomically and functionally to the pituitary. The two structures are interdependent. While the latter may have some trophic influence over the former, it is also dependent upon it, and intact vascular and neural connections between the two are essential for a steady output of pituitary hormones. Consequently, the hypothalamus plays an important role in the central regulation of the endocrine glands, including the thyroid, pancreas, adrenals, and gonads. A great proliferation of knowledge is continuing to take place in regard to central endocrine control, and the new discipline of neuroendocrinology is now advanced to the point where entire texts are devoted to it. In relation to a discussion of the hypothalamus and its functions, the following hormone releasing factors need to be mentioned. Others may be identified in the future. Vasopressin and oxytonin originate in the **neurohypophysis,** the supraoptic and paraventricular nuclei. Corticotropin-releasing factor originates mainly from the paraventricular nucleus. Gonadotropin-releasing hormone is produced in the arcuate nucleus, as is prolactin-releasing factor. Growth hormone-releasing factor and somatostatin (inhibits release of growth hormone) derive from the posterior arcuate, ventromedian, premammillary, periventricular, and paraventricular parts of the hypothalamus. Thyrotropin-releasing factor is produced by many hypothalamic nuclei, except for those in its posterior portion.

Among the visceral functions under control of the hypothalamus are body temperature regulation; basal metabolism; water, glucose, and fat metabolism; cardiovascular regulation including adjustment of the blood pressure and circulation; control of respiration; regulation of bladder functions; influence over sexual activity; and endocrine correlation in general. It has been stated that the hypothalamus is the seat of the emotions. It is probably, however, the motor center for emotional expression, and one of the stations concerned with emotional balance. Primitive pseudoaffective reactions take place when it is released from higher control. It is also important in the control of the sleep cycle.

Localization of function within the hypothalamus is not fully understood. Experimental work has given conflicting information. This is easy to understand when it is remembered that the entire area weighs only 4g out of an average brain weight of about 1200g. Most knowledge regarding hypothalamic function has been obtained from experimental neurology and neurophysiology. Information has been gathered as a result of electrical and chemical stimulation of the hypothalamus, and additional data have been obtained from clinical observation of patients with lesions in the hypothalamic area. Definite functions have been attributed to certain regions or nuclear masses as a result of information from either stimulation or destruction.

A fairly specific topographic orientation for the two divisions of the autonomic nervous system seems to exist. The posterior and lateral hypothalamic nuclei (and the ventromedial nuclei) apparently influence sympathoadrenal stimulation and the regulation of sympathetic outflow and vasomotor control. Stimulation of these areas results in an increase of heart rate, decrease in the caliber of blood vessels, increase in blood pressure, dilation of the pupils, erection of hair, and increase in rate and amplitude of respirations, with inhibition of secretions and movements of the intestine and bladder. The increased metabolic and somatic activity is characteristic of states of emotional stress, combat, or flight. The nuclei of the posterior hypothalamus are also responsible for the massive reaction of "sham rage" that occurs in animals when this region has been released from higher control. Destruction of the posterior nuclei of the hypothalamus and the mammillary bodies produces emotional lethargy, abnormal sleepiness, reduction in heart rate, and a fall in body temperature and general metabolic activities, owing to reduction of general visceral and somatic activities.

The nuclei of the anterior and medial hypothalamic regions, consisting of the anterior and midline hypothalamic nuclei and the tuber cinereum, are concerned with control of parasympathetic activity. Stimulation of these areas results in increased vagal and sacral autonomic activity with reduction of the heart rate, vasodilation, increased salivation and lacrimation, increased motility and tonus of the intestinal and bladder walls, and increased gastric secretion. Lesions of this region may cause gastric disturbances with atony and hemorrhagic erosions of the mucosa of the stomach and intestines.

The relationship of the various nuclear masses to the regulation of metabolic functions is clinically important. The supraoptic nuclei regulate water metabolism, and destruction of them or of the supraopticohypophyseal tract results in diabetes insipidus. There is associated degeneration of the posterior pituitary nuclei and the nerves in the pituitary stalk. Destruction of the tuber region results in disturbances in carbohydrate and fat metabolism, with hyperglycemia and the adiposogenital syndrome. Ablation of the paraventricular nuclei causes hypoglycemia and abnormal sensitivity to insulin. Hyperthermia may result from involvement of the rostral part of the anterior hypothalamic nuclei; this is associated with mechanisms for heat loss, including sweating, vasodilation, and in animals panting. Hypothermia may follow involvement of the posterior nuclei; this is associated with mechanisms for heat production and conservation, including vasoconstriction, increased visceral and somatic activity, and shivering. Disturbances in sleep regulation and hypersomnia may occur secondary to involvement of the posterior hypothalamic nuclei and mammillary bodies. The medial hypothalamus governs satiety and the lateral portions are responsible for appetite; lesions of the former lead to obesity, and of the latter, failure to eat.

The Cortex

The hypothalamus receives communications, either directly or indirectly, from various portions of the cerebral cortex. Both experimental and clinical evidence indicates that these cortical areas comprise a suprasegmental level for the integration of autonomic functions and the maintenance of a constant internal environment for the body. The term "visceral brain" has been applied to the **limbic system.** Authorities differ as to just how many structures are included in the so-called limbic system. The limbic lobe, or gyrus fornicatus, is composed of the cingulate gyrus, isthmus, hippocampal gyrus, and uncus, but closely related are the subcallosal and retrosplenial gyri, pyriform area, hippocampus, and various subcortical structures including the amygdala and septal nuclei. The insula, medial portion of the temporal lobe, and medial and posterior orbital gyri are also closely allied, although not actually a part of the limbic system. The hypothalamus receives discharges from all these structures, as well as from certain frontal and temporal lobe areas.

No separate cortical centers for parasympathetic and sympathetic control have been established with certainty, and the character of the reaction that follows either stimulation or destruction of these areas is dependent upon the general physiologic state of the organism. It has been suggested, however, that the orbital gyri may be related to vagal function and that various portions of the limbic system may be closely related to sympathetic function. There is an extensive overlapping between autonomic and somatic motor representation, and the topographic relationship between cortical areas influencing specific autonomic functions and those regulating corresponding somatic functions is a close one, with interrelations between the two systems. Thus, lacrimation is observed on stimulation of the eye fields, and salivation on stimulation of the motor representation of the face and tongue. Pupillary dilation follows stimulation of area 8 and constriction occurs after stimulation of area 19. Understandably, correlation exists between somatic and vegetative functions in both the motor and sensory areas of the central nervous system, with the hypothalamus, at least in part, under the control of the cerebral cortex.

Experiments indicate that a large variety of autonomic functions are influenced by the cerebral cortex. This is demonstrated more easily by stimulation than by ablation. In addition to lacrimation and salivation, sweating, piloerection, and alterations in cardiovascular, respiratory, gastrointestinal, vesical, and other functions may be demonstrated. These functions are partially controlled by the cortex, which acts as a basis for conditioned and visceral reflexes. Subcortical section of the frontal lobe has interfered with the inhibitory and excitatory autonomic centers in the cortex, resulting in overaction of the autonomic nervous system in response to direct stimulation.

That some important functions are influenced by the cortex has been suggested but not conclusively proved. Gastrointestinal representation is probably in the medial aspect of the frontal lobe and in the limbic system. Stimulation results in increased tone and peristalsis in the stomach and intestines, and increased secretion of digestive ferments. Ablation is followed by a decrease in motility, which may lead to stasis and intussusception, and morbid hunger often develops. Olfactory and gustatory hallucinations, smacking or licking of the lips, tasting and swallowing movements, and epigastric sensations follow irritation of the medial aspect of the temporal lobe, the hippocampus, and the amygdala. Centers regulating both voluntary and autonomic control of the bladder are probably situated in the region of the paracentral lobule and just anterior to it, extending medially and inferiorly into the anterior portion of the cingulate gyrus. Here there is a complicated neurologic mechanism involving somatically innervated sphincters and autonomically innervated viscera. Stimulation of this area is followed by contraction of the bladder. A lesion of one paracentral lobule brings about transient loss of bladder control, and bilateral lesions are followed by severe disturbances of both urination and defecation.

Electrically provoked penile erection in primates has followed stimulation of the anterior cingulate gyrus, medial and lateral preoptic areas, putamen, and other sites in the brain. Among the other autonomic phenomena that may be influenced by these various cortical systems are the following: cardiovascular control, including regulation of blood pressure and heart rate; respiratory rate and rhythm; appetite; vasomotor and temperature regulation. Abnormal affective and emotional responses, fear, and aggressive behavior may be lessened by interrupting the connections between these cortical areas and the thalamus and hypothalamus (Ch. 49).

The anatomic pathways responsible for these reactions are not precisely known. For the most part, perhaps, the impulses are relayed to the hypothalamus, either directly or indirectly through the thalamus, but there may also be projection pathways to the autonomic centers in the brain stem and spinal cord that travel in the lateral columns in close relationship with the corticospinal pathways. The sensory portions of the cerebral cortex play a part in relaying impulses to the motor areas; it is well known that visual, auditory, and other stimuli that call forth emotional responses may cause variations in autonomic reactivity with changes in circulatory and respiratory function, bladder disturbances, either sweating or anhidrosis, and pupillary dilation. Although intellectual functions are under the control of the neopallium, affective behavior is under the influence of the limbic system and its connections, and emotional expression is dependent upon the integrating function of this latter portion of the cortex and the hypothalamus. Affective reactions, however, may produce responses of both the autonomic and somatic nervous systems, probably through integration between autonomic centers in the cortex and hypothalamus, and motor centers, largely extrapyramidal, in the cortex and basal ganglia.

The Midbrain and Brain Stem

The autonomic nuclear centers of the oculomotor, facial, glossopharyngeal, and vagus nerves, which are situated in the midbrain and brain stem, have already been mentioned in the discussions of the cranial nerves and of the peripheral autonomic nervous system. There are, however, other autonomic centers, principally of a reflex nature and probably under the influence of the hypothalamus, which are situated in these areas of the nervous system. The most important are as follows: a vasomotor center that exerts an influence in vasodilation and vasoconstriction and consequently on blood pressure regulation; a center regulating heart rate; and a respiratory reflex center. These are probably situated in the reticular formation of the medulla near the floor of the fourth ventricle and in close association with the dorsal efferent nucleus of the vagus nerve. Inhibitory and facilitatory centers in the midbrain and medulla may enhance inhibitory and facilitatory functions of the hypothalamus. Pressure on the medulla may cause serious disturbances in respiration, heart rate, and blood pressure. Other subsidiary reflex centers influencing pupillary size, gustatory responses, sudomotor activity, piloerection, gastrointestinal function, micturition, and bladder tone may also be located in the brain stem.

BIBLIOGRAPHY

Adams RD, Victor M. Principles of Neurology, 4th ed. New York, McGraw – Hill, 1989

Andrew J, Nathan PW. Lesions of the anterior frontal lobes and disturbances of urination and defecation. Brain 1964;37:233

Appenzeller O. The Autonomic Nervous System: An Introduction to Basic and Clinical Concepts, 2nd ed. Amsterdam, North Holland, 1976

Cannon WB. Bodily Changes in Pain, Hunger, Fear and Rage. New York, D Appleton & Co, 1915

Fields WS, Guillemin R, Carton CA (eds). Hypothalamic – hypophysial Interrelationships. Springfield, IL, Charles C Thomas, 1956

Gillilan LA. Clinical Aspects of the Autonomic Nervous System. Boston, Little, Brown & Co, 1954

Goodman L, Gilman A (eds). The Pharmacological Basis of Therapeutics, 4th ed. New York, Macmillan, 1970

Hess WF. Diencephalon: Autonomic and Extrapyramidal Functions. New York, Grune & Stratton, 1954

Kuntz A. The Autonomic Nervous System, 4th ed. Philadelphia, Lea & Febiger, 1953

Lapides J, Diokno AC. Urine transport, storage, and micturition. In Lapides J (ed). Fundamentals of Urology. Philadelphia, WB Saunders, 1976

Loewi O. Über humorale Übertragbarkeit der Herznervenwirkung. Pflueger's Arch 1921;189:239

Maclean PD, Ploog DW. Cerebral representation of penile erection. J Neurophysiol 1962;25:29

Martin JB, Reichlin S. Clinical Neuroendocrinology, 2nd ed. Philadelphia, FA Davis, 1987

Palumbo LT. Management of Disorders of the Autonomic Nervous System. Chicago, Year Book Medical Pub, 1955

Pick J. The Autonomic Nervous System: Morphological, Comparative, Clinical and Surgical Aspects. Philadelphia, JB Lippincott, 1970

Reichlin S, Baldessarini RJ, Martin JB. The Hypothalamus. New York, Raven Press, 1977

White JC, Smithwick RH, Simeone FA. The Autonomic Nervous System: Anatomy, Physiology, and Surgical Application, 3rd ed. New York, Macmillan, 1952

Chapter 41
EXAMINATION OF THE AUTONOMIC NERVOUS SYSTEM

The examination of the autonomic nervous system provides valuable information in neurologic diseases, and the examiner should be familiar with the important methods of evaluation. Evidence of dysfunction of this portion of the neurologic complex may provide important clues to the diagnosis and localization of disease of the nervous system. Certain routine procedures should be carried out in every neurologic appraisal. Other, more complex, tests are reserved for patients in whom specific autonomic dysfunction is suspected.

THE GENERAL OBSERVATION OF THE PATIENT

Valuable information about the functional state of the autonomic nervous system may be obtained from the general observation of the patient (Ch. 3). The physique and habitus, body build, state of nutrition, deformities, and abnormalities of configuration are important criteria. Special emphasis should be paid to the following aspects of the physical examination:

Endocrine Status. Evidence of endocrine imbalance such as dwarfism, gigantism, acromegaly, cretinism, and other signs of dysfunction of the pituitary, pineal, thyroid, adrenal, or sexual glands can be related to disease of the autonomic nervous system. The degree of physical development, including sexual maturity, is also important.

The Regulation of Vital Processes. The temperature of the extremities and of isolated portions of the body should be noted, as well as the body temperature. Either generalized or local changes in temperature regulation and heat production may be detected. The examiner should take the blood pressure in each arm with the patient recumbent, seated, and standing and should note the rate and regularity of the pulse and the respiratory rate and rhythm.

The Skin and Mucous Membranes. Evidence of autonomic dysfunction may be seen in the skin and mucous membranes. If a change in color, such as pallor, erythema, flushing, or cyanosis, is present, the examiner should determine whether it is localized, limited to the extremities, or generalized. Changes in color with alterations of position may be diagnostic criteria. Variations in the texture, consistency, and appearance of the skin include glossiness, hardness, thickening, wasting, scaling, seborrhea, looseness or tightness, oiliness, and moistness or dryness. Urticaria, generalized or localized edema, trophedema, myxedema, dermatographia, vesicles, bullae, perforating ulcers, and decubiti should be noted.

Perspiration. Disease of the autonomic nervous system may be characterized by any of the following: Excessive perspiration, decreased perspiration, anhidrosis, and localized changes in sweating.

The Hair and Nails. Hypertrichosis, hypotrichosis, abnormal distribution of hair, localized alopecia, abnormal brittleness, color change, and either localized or premature graying of the hair may be significant. Important abnormalities of the nails include brittleness, striations, fissuring, and cyanosis.

The Extremities. Examination of the extremities is important in the appraisal of the autonomic system. The development, color, and temperature of the extremities as a whole, the character and pulsation of the arteries, and the effect of changes in position should be evaluated. By these criteria conditions such as erythromelalgia, acrocyanosis, Raynaud's syndrome, and Buerger's disease may be diagnosed.

Salivation and Lacrimation. The secretory responses of the salivary and lacrimal glands to physical and psychic stimulation may provide information about autonomic nervous system dysfunction.

Fat Metabolism. Obesity, wasting, lipodystrophy, and adiposis dolorosa are seen in autonomic dysfunction. The localization of wasting and the bodily distribution of the adipose tissue should be noted. Other metabolic disorders must be evaluated by special tests to be described.

The Bones and Joints. Changes in bone structure and development, and arthropathies of various types, may result from diseases of the autonomic nervous system.

Evidence of Localized Autonomic Nervous System Involvement. The presence of specific and focal changes, such as Horner's syndrome, in which ipsilateral partial ptosis and miosis and focal loss of sweating give evidence of a localized lesion in the autonomic nervous system.

AUTONOMIC NERVOUS SYSTEM REFLEXES

Many reflexes of importance in the neurologic examination are essentially autonomic responses. Some may be classified as mucous membrane and orificial reflexes, others as true visceral reflexes. All, however, are smooth muscle and glandular responses. Accordingly, the reaction is slower than that which takes place in striated muscle reflexes. In many instances,

however, the smooth muscle response is accompanied by contraction of striated muscle.

The autonomic nervous system reflexes that are functions of various cranial nerves are discussed with the individual nerves (Part C, "The Cranial Nerves"). Among these are the pupillary, lacrimal, salivary, sneeze, sucking, cough, vomiting, carotid sinus, and oculocardiac reflexes. In many of these responses other portions of the autonomic nervous system take part besides those innervated by the cranial nerves, but the visceral components of the individual nerves play a major function.

There are other reflex responses, largely of autonomic origin, which may be assessed in the neurologic evaluation. The most important of these are the following:

The Subcostogastric, or Cutaneogastric, Reflex. Gentle stroking of the skin over the left costal margin is followed by contraction of the gastric musculature. This response may be observed by either palpation or auscultation over the stomach. The reflex is not reliable unless 3 or 4 hours have elapsed since the last meal.

The Rectal, or Defecation, Reflex. Either distention of the rectum or stimulation of the rectal mucosa is followed by contraction of the rectal musculature. This reflex is innervated principally by the sacral autonomic fibers (second, third, and fourth sacral segments); it is evaluated in colonmetrography.

The Internal Anal Sphincter Reflex. Contraction of the internal sphincter of the anus may be observed on introduction of the gloved finger into the anus. This reflex is supplied by postganglionic fibers of the sympathetic division through the hypogastric plexus (presacral nerves). If it is lost, the anus does not close immediately after stimulation. The internal anal sphincter reflex should be differentiated from the superficial anal reflex (Ch. 34).

The Vesical Reflex. Either distention of the bladder or stimulation of the bladder mucosa is followed by contraction of the detrusor muscle, with relaxation of the trigone and internal sphincter. This reflex is supplied largely by the sacral autonomic fibers (second through fourth sacral segments). The various responses to bladder stimulation and distention are discussed under the subject of cystometry.

The Urethral Sphincter Reflex. This consists of the gripping of a sound as it is introduced into the urethra.

The Scrotal Reflex. Application of a cold object to the scrotum, perineum, or inner thigh or trunk is followed by a slow, vermicular contraction of the dartos musculature. The same response may follow stroking of the skin of the perineum or pricking the perineal region with a sharp object. The contraction of the dartos does not cause elevation of the testicle, and this reflex should not be confused with the cremasteric reflex (Ch. 34).

The Bulbocavernosus Reflex. Stroking, pricking, or pinching the dorsum of the glans penis is followed by contraction of the bulbocavernosus muscle and the urethral constrictor, which may be palpated when a finger is placed on the perineum behind the scrotum with pressure on either the bulbous or membranous portion of the urethra. There is also a contraction of the external anal sphincter, which may be felt if a gloved finger is placed in the anus. This reflex is supplied by the third and fourth sacral nerves.

The Genital, Sex, Ejaculatory, or Coital Reflex. Stimulation from either the cerebrum or the periphery may be followed by erection of the penis and sometimes by ejaculation. Erection is a function of the sacral autonomic division and is supplied by the second through the fourth sacral nerves, whereas ejaculation is in part a function of the thoracolumbar autonomic division and is principally supplied by the lumbar nerves. A pathologic exaggeration of this response is seen as part of the mass reflex, and a spinal defense reflex accompanied by priapism and occasionally ejaculation may follow stimulation of either the glans penis or the skin of the penis.

The Mass Reflex. This is a variation of the spinal defense reflex and consists of dorsiflexion of the toes and feet, flexion of the knees and hips, and, in addition, involuntary micturition and defecation, sweating, and vasomotor changes to the level of the lesion. There may be priapism and ejaculation.

Emotional Reflexes. Laughter consists of a deep inspiration followed by a series of short, jerky expirations that may be accompanied by laryngeal sounds. Weeping is an analogous phenomenon, accompanied by sobs and usually by lacrimation. Lacrimation may occasionally accompany laughter. Both are elicited by cortical stimuli and by emotions. Laughing may appear as a response to tickling, and weeping as a response to pain. Precipitate, unmotivated, or excessive laughter or weeping may occur in the presence of cerebral lesions that affect the corticospinal tracts or frontal lobes (and possibly the thalamus) bilaterally. This phenomenon is seen principally in the syndrome of pseudobulbar palsy (Ch. 18).

Sweating, the pilomotor response, the vasomotor response, and reflex erythema may all be considered reflex phenomena involving a reaction to stimulation of sudorific glands, smooth muscle, or blood vessels. The mode of eliciting these responses is, however, somewhat more complex than that used in testing the simple reflexes, and consequently they are considered as special tests of autonomic function.

SPECIAL TESTS OF AUTONOMIC FUNCTION

In addition to the general observation of the patient and the eliciting of the autonomic nervous system reflexes, there are several special tests and examinations of importance in the evaluation of the autonomic nervous system. These are not carried out in every neurologic examination, but the examiner should be familiar with them since they are often essential to the diagnosis of specific lesions of individual portions of the autonomic nervous system. Some of the more useful tests are listed. No single test assesses the entire spectrum of either parasympathetic or sympathetic activity.

Sweat Tests

These are important objective tests of autonomic function. The production of sweat, or perspiration, is a function of the sympathetic division of the autonomic nervous system. The efferent neurons are situated in the intermediolateral columns of the thoracic and lumbar portions of the spinal cord; the preganglionic fibers go to the sympathetic chain ganglia, and the postganglionic fibers are carried by the peripheral nerves to the sweat glands. Paradoxically, however, these postganglionic sympathetic nerves are cholinergic rather than adrenergic. Sweating is produced by drugs such as acetylcholine and pilocarpine, which are classed as parasympathomimetic, and is decreased by atropine, scopolamine, and other drugs that inhibit structures innervated by postganglionic cholinergic nerves.

The sweat test is simple to perform and the results may be observed over the surface of the entire body. The chronologic appearance of perspiration at different sites and quantitative differences may be noted, and photographs or video recordings may be made at any stage of sweat development. Various methods of color determination of sweating include the following: (1) Iodine in oil is painted on the skin and the painted areas are dusted with starch powder, which turns bluish black in the presence of iodine and moisture. (2) The skin is painted with a solution of ferric chloride and then dusted with tannic acid powder, which turns black in the presence of iron and moisture. (3) A saturated alcoholic solution of cobalt chloride, which turns pink when moist, is painted on the skin, or cobalt blue papers are applied to it. (4) Absorbent paper impregnated with silver nitrate and potassium chromate is applied to the skin; the chloride in the sweat reacts with the silver nitrate to form silver chloride. (5) The skin is dusted with quinizarin (1,4-dihydroxyanthraquinone), which is a grayish violet when dry, but becomes deep purple when moistened. The moisture on the skin may also be evaluated by palpation or measured with a hygrometer or sudometer, and it is often possible to see the droplets of sweat on the skin, especially on the papillary ridges of the fingers, with the use of the +20 lens of the ophthalmoscope.

Various diaphoretic procedures may be used. Thermoregulatory, or "heat" sweating is produced by the use of external heat after the ingestion of hot fluids and aspirin. Large electric bakers or cradles are placed over the patient, the open ends covered with woolen blankets; or an electric heat cabinet may be used. The action is a central one, presumably from the stimulation of the thermoregulatory sweating centers in the hypothalamus, and perspiration is called forth over the entire body. It remains to be clarified whether thermoregulatory sweating results from a rise in blood temperature that in turn activates areas of the central nervous system responsible for thermal regulation, or whether a peripheral heat-sensitive receptor is present, reflexly activating the central areas. Perhaps both mechanisms are present. Since the impulses are carried to the sweat glands via the thoracicolumbar sympathetic fibers and then via the pe-

ripheral nerves, this test is particularly valuable in examining lesions of either of these.

Emotional sweating is also produced centrally and corresponds to the spontaneous hyperhidrosis of normal and neurotic persons. It may be elicited by emotional stimuli, intellectual strain, or painful cutaneous sensation. Emotional sweating varies in distribution from thermoregulatory sweating — it tends to be localized to the palms, axillas, and soles — and is characterized by more individual variation in response. It may be assessed by the galvanic skin response or by other means.

Drug-induced sweating is produced by the subcutaneous injection of 5 mg of pilocarpine hydrochloride. It acts peripherally, stimulating the glands innervated by postganglionic cholinergic fibers. The response is more variable than that to heat, and the resulting perspiration may be irregular and spotty. The reaction may be facilitated by loosely covering the part of the body to be tested with a blanket to inhibit excessive evaporation and loss of body heat. There is an individual variation in the sweating response. The test is less reliable than the response to heat and has only a limited diagnostic value. Spinal reflex sweating is seen only in certain pathologic conditions, such as transverse lesions of the spinal cord, and represents a part of the mass reflex of spinal automatism. It may be elicited by various nociceptive impulses applied below the level of the lesion.

Gustatory sweating is produced by the introduction of spiced or highly seasoned foods into the mouth. It is valuable only in tests on the face. The response is elicited with difficulty in the normal individual, and is absent in peripheral lesions of the trigeminal nerve. It is exaggerated in certain pathologic conditions, such as the auriculotemporal and chorda tympani syndromes.

The tests for thermoregulatory sweating are the only ones of these procedures that have some application in clinical neurology. They may aid in the diagnosis of intramedullary lesions and partial or transverse lesions of the spinal cord (a "sweat level," however, is not as accurate as a sensory level in localization of spinal cord lesions). They may also give helpful information in the diagnosis of lesions of the lower brain stem, the sympathetic outflow or fiber pathways, or the peripheral nerves. A simple bedside test may be used to demonstrate the borders of sympathetic denervation related to loss of sweating: a spoon is drawn over the skin; the spoon pulls smoothly over dry (sympathectomized) skin but irregularly and unevenly over moist, perspiring skin. Sweat tests may serve as an index of the completeness of nerve section or sympathectomy (see Fig. 42-1).

Examination of the sweat itself is useful in the diagnosis of cystic fibrosis. An abnormality in the function of the eccrine sweat glands in this disease causes the sweat to contain increased amounts of sodium, chloride, and potassium, and to have increased electrical conductivity.

The Pilomotor Response

Piloerection is also a function of the sympathetic division of the autonomic nervous system. Stimulation of the sympathetic nerves causes contraction of the arrectores pilorum muscles and erection of the cutaneous hairs, known as cutis anserina or "goose flesh." The response may be elicited with ease, but it is inconstant and transient and cannot be demonstrated adequately on the hands or feet. Piloerection may be provoked by gentle stroking of the skin, tickling, scratching with a sharp object, or the application of cold. Ice, cotton soaked in alcohol or ether, or a methyl chloride spray may be used. Piloerection is elicited best at the nape of the neck, in the axillas, on the abdominal wall, and at the upper border of the trapezius. The patient should be in a warm room, since cold influences the response. It may be helpful to warm the body before the application of a cold stimulus. It must be remembered that emotional stimuli may also provoke piloerection.

The reaction appears slowly, after a latent period of 4 – 5 sec; it is complete or at its maximum in 7 – 10 sec and lasts 15 – 20 sec. It first occurs at the site of stimulation and then spreads slowly and widely. If a massive stimulus is used, such as chilling the neck with ice, pinching the skin in the cervical region or at the upper border of the trapezius, tickling or scratching the axilla, or applying cold to the axilla or the abdominal wall, the response takes about ½ min to become manifest and lasts for 1 or 2 min. This is seen best on the trunk and the extensor surfaces of the extremities; symmetric parts of the body should be observed. If one side of the body is stimulated, the response is ipsilateral, but if the midline is stimulated, it is bilateral.

Piloerection is absent in lesions that involve the descending autonomic pathways in the brain stem and spinal cord, sympathetic trunk, preganglionic and postganglionic fibers, and peripheral nerves. It is abolished below transverse spinal lesions, and the descending reaction to a massive stimulus stops at this level. Occasionally, after spinal shock has passed, piloerection is seen as part of the mass reflex of spinal automatism. It must be admitted, however, that the pilomotor response has little diagnostic value; besides giving only limited and indirect information, it is difficult to measure and is inconstant and transient.

The Vasomotor Response

This test is based upon the facts that vasodilation causes flushing of the skin and vasoconstriction is followed by pallor. When the sympathetic division of the autonomic system is interrupted, paralysis of vasoconstriction develops, with resulting temporary vasodilation and flushing. The pallor that follows slight pressure on the skin disappears sooner in involved than in normal areas. The test may be carried out by warming the surface of the body with towels wrung out of very hot water. In transverse spinal lesions there is vasodilation with flushing, redness, and an increase in skin temperature below the level of the lesion. The vasodilation will be most marked at the upper level of the vasoparalytic lesion; a distinct zone of hyperemia on the skin, corresponding to the upper limit of the sensory zone of hyperalgesia, may develop. The hyperalgesic and hyperemic areas indicate the level of root involvement and the uppermost point of the spinal cord lesion. The warming of the skin may be followed by suddenly chilling it with towels wrung out of ice water. A decrease in the vasoconstrictor response to cold may develop below the level of a spinal lesion.

As is true in the case of the pilomotor response, the vasomotor test depends upon several factors and affords only limited and indirect information; it is difficult to evaluate and is often not reliable. More important than the observation of vasodilation or vasoconstriction, which are not easily measured and often difficult to interpret, is the quantitative determination of skin temperature (see below).

Reflex Erythema

Stimulation of the skin by stroking it with a blunt point is followed by focal vasodilation. There is first a local reaction, seen as a red line along the site of stimulation, which is followed in about ½ min by a spreading flush, or flare, on each side of the scratch. Depending upon the in-

tensity of the stimulus and individual susceptibility, the site of stimulation becomes elevated,
with the development of a welt, or wheal, sometimes with a white line in its center. This response is considered to be dependent upon the
axon reflex and the liberation of histamine, and
is similar to that which follows the intradermal
injection of histamine (see following). It disappears after interruption of cutaneous nerves and
below transverse spinal cord lesions. It has little
diagnostic value.

Exaggeration of reflex erythema is called *dermatographia.* This phenomenon is present whenever the sympathetic influence is diminished. It
is marked in individuals with overactivity of the
parasympathetic division and in those with
labile autonomic nervous systems or with evidence of sympathetic and parasympathetic imbalance. It has been reported to be observed to a
marked degree in individuals with psychophysiologic disorders. It is often present, however, in
people with no evidence of any general or
neurologic disease. It may also occur on an allergic basis and as a reaction to chemical and thermal stimuli. It has no diagnostic value other than
indicating either imbalance or hypersensitivity
to the chemicals associated with autonomic
function.

The Histamine Flare

The intradermal injection of 0.1 ml of a 1:1000
solution of histamine phosphate (0.1 mg) is followed, in the normal person, by the immediate
development of focal erythema and pain at the
injection site. This is followed by the appearance
of a spreading flush, or flare, which reaches its
maximum in about 10 min, and the development of a wheal at the site of injection. The response is noted at 1, 5, and 10 min after the
injection and should be compared to that of a
similar control injection on another part of the
body. The reaction is similar to that which is produced by stroking the skin with a blunt point.
An intact arterial circulation and an intact axon
reflex seem necessary for the development of
the flare. The histamine flare may be useful in
the diagnosis of peripheral nerve lesions, but the
blood supply as well as the nerve supply must be
intact. The reaction is absent with complete section of a peripheral nerve and diminished with
partial section. It is decreased or absent below
the level of a transverse spinal lesion. In hysterical anesthesia the reaction is present but painless; in malingering it is present and painful. The

response is markedly diminished in children
with familial dysautonomia.

Skin Temperature Studies

The determination of the skin temperature is an
important part of the examination of the autonomic nervous system. The vasomotor tonus is
reflected in the surface temperature of the body,
and interruption of the sympathetic division
with resulting vasodilation is followed by a rise
in temperature. Conversely, stimulation of the
sympathetics with consequent vasoconstriction
is accompanied by a fall in surface temperature.
Quantitative skin temperature determinations
can be made and are more accurate and objective than the observation of flushing and pallor.
Not only may the continuity of the sympathetic
pathways be evaluated by such determinations
made in the resting state, but valuable additional
information may be obtained by noting the response to peripheral nerve and sympathetic
block, spinal and general anesthesia, warming or
cooling of different portions of the body, and the
use of autonomic blocking drugs. Determinations are made with the use of a differential ther-
mocouple, and the temperature of corresponding areas of the body is compared. Infrared
thermographic methods may also be used. Slight
differences may be measured, but the results are
relative and not absolute, and repeated observations may be necessary. Because the skin temperature is influenced by that of the surrounding
environment, studies should be carried out in a
room of constant temperature and humidity,
and the patient may have to be placed in the
room an hour before testing.

A lesion of the sympathetic division, whether
affecting the descending pathways, cells in the
intermediolateral columns, preganglionic fibers,
sympathetic trunk, postganglionic fibers, or peripheral nerves, is followed by temporary vasodilation, redness, and increase in skin temperature. The temperature of the involved portion of
the body is higher than that of the remainder of
the body during the resting state. In addition it
rises more rapidly and to a greater extent when
either the body as a whole or an unaffected portion of the body is heated, and decreases more
slowly and to a lesser extent when either the
body or an unaffected portion is cooled. This
state lasts only a short time. When the walls of
the vessels regain tone, they again contract, for
when denervated they are hypersensitive to the
epinephrine that is normally circulating in the

blood. The skin of the involved areas·becomes cold and pale, and even cyanotic if the circulation stagnates. The cutaneous vessels fail to respond to stimuli from other areas, and either warming or cooling other parts of the body fails to cause flushing, pallor, sweating, piloerection, or changes in skin temperature in the involved area. This is particularly evident in the distal portions of the extremities.

Owing to the wider distribution and extensive overlapping of preganglionic fibers, warmth and redness persist longer and vasomotor disturbances are less marked with interruption of preganglionic than of postganglionic fibers. However, section of the preganglionic fibers gives more permanent relief in conditions characterized by spasm of cutaneous vessels, since after section of the postganglionic fibers the denervated vessels become more sensitive to circulating epinephrine and related substances, and they again contract. If only the sensory nerves are divided, flushing, pallor, and temperature changes occur in the anesthetic areas in response to warming or cooling of other parts of the body. In hemiplegia the state of the cutaneous vessels, and consequently the temperature of the skin, may vary. It may be warmer or cooler than normal but is usually the latter, in part owing to inactivity or disuse; the vasomotor responses are unchanged.

Skin temperature studies can be useful in the diagnosis of lesions of the sympathetic division, in determining the level of a transverse spinal lesion, in delineating the extent of a peripheral nerve lesion, in the preoperative appraisal of the continuity of sympathetic pathways, and in the differential diagnosis of Raynaud's and Buerger's diseases, peripheral atherosclerosis, and other vascular diseases of the extremities. That is, they aid in differentiating circulatory disorders characterized by sympathetic overactivity and vasoconstriction from those characterized by disease of the vessels themselves or of the vessel walls, with organic obstruction and reduction in the vessel lumens. The various modifications of skin temperature evaluations are listed.

The Resting State. When lesions of the sympathetic division develop there is temporary vasodilation and a rise in skin temperature, followed by vasoconstriction and a fall in temperature in those areas supplied by the nerves of fibers involved. These may be compared with the corresponding normal areas of the body. With transverse lesions of the spinal cord there is a temporary increase followed by a fall in temperature below the level of the lesion. With vascular disease of the extremities, whether the result of vasospasm or of organic obstruction, the skin temperature is lower than in the corresponding normal extremities.

Diagnostic Block of Peripheral Nerves or of Sympathetic Ganglia. Specific peripheral nerves or sympathetic ganglia are injected with local anesthetic. The temperature of the portion of the body innervated by these nerves and ganglia is studied before and after injection, and is also compared with corresponding intact areas of the body. The injection blocks the vasomotor fibers, and in the normal person a moderate rise in skin temperature in the involved area of the body results. If there has been a previous interruption of the continuity of the sympathetics, no change will be detected. If the temperature of the area being tested has been below normal or below that of the corresponding normal portion of the body as a result of sympathetic overactivity or vasospasm, it will promptly return to normal. If it has been decreased as a result of obstruction of the lumens of peripheral vessels, there will be no change. However, in conditions such as Raynaud's disease there may be an element of obstruction, and in Buerger's disease there may be some spasm. Nevertheless, this procedure can be useful in the differential diagnosis of these conditions, peripheral atherosclerosis, and other circulatory disturbances. Diagnostic block is also used as a preoperative test to determine the degree of vasodilation that will result from surgery of the sympathetics.

Spinal and General Anesthesia. General anesthesia is followed by a generalized rise in surface temperature and spinal anesthesia by a rise in that portion of the body affected by the anesthetic agent, both the result of sympathetic paralysis. In vasospastic disorders a rise in temperature of the involved limbs occurs; no change develops if there is organic obstruction of the vessels.

Heating or Cooling of the Body or Extremities. The entire body may be warmed by exposure to higher temperatures through the use of external heat or foreign-body protein injection (*e.g.,* typhoid vaccine), or it may be cooled by exposure to lower temperatures. More frequently in testing, however, portions of the body are heated or cooled. If evaluating temperature changes in the feet is indicated, the hands may either be warmed by immersing them in warm water or placing them in a heat cabinet, or cooled by immersing them in cold water. If the hands are to be examined, the feet may be either warmed or cooled. In the normal individual distant portions of the body respond to such warming or cooling of other portions. In vasospastic conditions a normal, though sometimes delayed, response is obtained in the involved extremities; in organic circulatory disturbances there is little or no response. With interruption of the sympathetic pathways, except immediately after the interruption, the cutaneous vessels of the affected areas fail to respond to warming or cooling of other portions of the body, but warming or cooling the involved areas is followed by similar temperature changes elsewhere in the body, probably through the medium of the temperature of the blood acting on higher centers.

Autonomic Blocking Agents. Various chemical blocking agents may be used in the examination of the autonomic nervous system, as discussed under "Pharmacologic Tests" later in this chapter. The determination of the skin temperature before and after the administration of these drugs can provide valuable diagnostic information.

Determination of Skin Resistance

Section of a peripheral nerve is followed by a significant and permanent increase in the resistance of the portion of skin supplied by that nerve to the passage of a minute, imperceptible current, whereas stimulation of a peripheral nerve is followed by a decrease in skin resistance. The autonomic component of the nerve is the important factor in this resistance, since areas deprived of autonomic supply show a greatly increased resistance even though the other components of the peripheral nerves are intact. The change seems to be correlated with the function of the sweat glands, since the resistance is low if the sweat glands are active and is high if they are inactive, and the degree of resistance compares closely to results obtained in the sweating test. Vasodilation may also play a part.

Skin resistance is measured by means of the dermometer. Various types of instruments have been used. That described by Richter consists of a microammeter with a range of 0 – 100 microamps, a 4½-V battery, and a 1000-ohm potential divider. Two electrodes are used; one is attached to the earlobe and the other to the area of the skin to be examined. The current from the battery passes from one electrode to the other, completing a circuit through the body of the patient and the microammeter. The potential divider regulates the amount of current that flows from the battery through the patient's body when the potential is fixed, and the amount of current registered on the ammeter depends upon the resistance of the patient's skin. The response may be registered on an oscillograph and recorded. With these instruments one can outline changes in resistance over the surface of the body without needing the cooperation of the patient. The procedure is a simple one that can be checked by independent observers.

Skin resistance is increased during sleep, physical inactivity, and absence of emotional excitement. It is high over scar tissues and with lesions of the peripheral nerves and the autonomic nervous system. Skin resistance is determined by local changes such as abrasions and wounds of the skin, by irritation of the skin, and by muscular effort or emotional excitement. Dermometry has most value in the neurologic appraisal if it is used in the diagnosis of lesions of the peripheral nerves and the autonomic nervous system. The findings may be compared with those of the motor and sensory examinations; in peripheral nerve lesions the changes in skin resistance correspond closely with motor and sensory alterations.

By determination of skin resistance spinal, nerve root, and peripheral nerve lesions can be localized. In nerve lesions one can differentiate partial from complete involvement and detect early signs of regeneration. Hysteria and malingering may be distinguished from organic disease. Dermometry also provides an objective, practical way to study the autonomic nervous system, to determine the sympathetic components of the peripheral nerves, and to demonstrate changes in function of the autonomic system. By its use the continuity of the sympathetic division may be measured quantitatively. Stimulation of the sympathetic division causes a decrease in resistance, whereas sympathetic depression is followed by increased resistance. Sympathetic dermatomes, which compare closely to sensory dermatomes (see Fig. 5-10c) may be outlined. Dermometry may also be used to determine the level of a transverse lesion of the spinal cord, since an increase in skin resistance is found below the level of such a lesion. A transection above the first thoracic segment (or above the thoracolumbar outflow), however, is followed by increased resistance over the entire body, whereas no increase follows a lesion below the second lumbar segment.

Various modifications of the determination of skin resistance have been carried out in neurologic diagnosis. The galvanic skin reflex to light cutaneous stimulation may give an objective differentiation between organic and hysterical anesthesias. There is no change in skin resistance of an intact portion of the body when an anesthetic area is stimulated, but a normal reflex is elicited on stimulation of an area of hysterical anesthesia. Skin potentials have been used to demonstrate visceral pain; there is an increase in the potential of the dermatomes that correspond to a painful organ. The dermometer has also been used to investigate emotional reactions. The decrease in the resistance of the skin following psychic stimuli has been called the psychogalvanic reflex, and the instrument used for the determination of this, the psychogalvanometer. The psychogalvanometer is part of the polygraph, an instrument for the simultaneous recording of respiratory movements, pulse, blood pressure, and skin resistance. Alterations in these may reveal emotional reactions that are of use in detecting deception.

Heating Test

Exposure to environmental heat (sunbaths, and hot tubs) as well as internal heat (elevations of body temperature) may aggravate the symptoms of multiple sclerosis (weakness, paresthesias, blurred vision, and diplopia). These symptoms are reversed by cooling. Consequently an exacerbation of symptoms following immersion in a hot tub bath is suggestive of the diagnosis of multiple sclerosis. This is not specific for the disease, however, since it appears, though less frequently, in other diseases as well. Theoretically defective myelin may render some pathways in the nervous system more vulnerable to the influence of heat.

Block of Peripheral Nerves and Sympathetic Ganglia

Local anesthetic block of peripheral nerves, nerve roots, and sympathetic ganglia may be used preoperatively to prognosticate the effect of surgical procedures for the relief of causalgia and other painful disorders of autonomic origin. Such block may also be performed in association with skin temperature studies, sweat tests, and dermometry to determine the continuity of autonomic fibers. It is especially valuable when used with skin temperature studies to detect the amount of vasodilation that follows interruption of the sympathetic fibers, and may aid not only in the differential diagnosis of vascular diseases of the extremities, but also in prognosis.

Plethysmography

By means of an oscillometer or plethysmograph one may measure arteriocapillary tension and determine the expansile pulsation of an extremity at any desired level; thus it may be possible to differentiate between vasospasm and arterial obstruction. Doppler blood flow studies accomplish the same aims.

The Cold Pressor Test

Stimulation of the vasomotor center by cold with resultant rise in blood pressure may be used in the diagnosis of hypertension. The sphygmomanometer cuff is applied to one arm while the other hand and arm are immersed in water of about 4° C. Blood pressure readings are taken every 30 – 60 sec until the highest reading is reached. This is termed the index of response. The arm and hand are then removed from the cold water and readings are taken every 2 min until the basal level is reached. In the normal individual there is a slight rise in both systolic and diastolic blood pressure, with a fall to normal within 3 min after the stimulus is removed. A response of more than 20 mm Hg systolic, and more than 15 mm Hg diastolic, is considered significant. In hypertension there is a greater and more prolonged rise, with a delayed fall; this effect disappears after the administration of tetraethyl-ammonium chloride. There is also increased vasopressor reactivity in patients with cerebral atherosclerosis.

Other Tests of Circulation

Postural effects on blood pressure may be tested by recording with the patient recumbent and erect. More precise evaluation is possible with the use of a tilt table. With orthostatic hypotension due to sympathetic failure the systolic and diastolic blood pressure values fall on assumption of the vertical position.

The blood pressure and pulse responses to Valsalva's maneuver may be studied, but this procedure requires an indwelling arterial catheter for recording the pressure.

Changes in heart rate with respiration, alteration of body posture, exercise, or drugs can also be noted and recorded as part of autonomic assessment. The parasympathetic innervation of the heart may be tested by the so-called diving reflex in response to immersion of the face in water.

Pharmacologic Tests

Although the autonomic nervous system does not lend itself to as complete clinical testing as does the voluntary nervous system, certain information regarding its function may be obtained by inference, especially by noting the effect of drugs that either stimulate or depress its component parts. It may be of diagnostic value to determine the relative irritability of the sympathetic and parasympathetic divisions and to note the effect of both autonomic stimulants and depressants in the relief of symptoms. The injection of 1 mg of epinephrine may produce tachycardia, elevation of the blood pressure, hyperpnea, pallor, tremor, restlessness, feelings of anxiety; and sometimes hyperglycemia and glycosuria. Because the denervated smooth muscle of arterial walls is hypersensitive to epinephrine, injection of this drug may cause striking vasoconstriction after complete degeneration of the sympathetic nerves, especially after a postganglionic operation. The injection of pilocarpine gives little information about parasympathetic overactivity, although sensitive individuals may react with intestinal cramping, perspiration, increased salivation, and muscular fasciculations. The injection of 0.5 – 1 mg atropine may be followed by a decrease in salivation and of perspiration as well as tachycardia. The response to these drugs is variable, however, and gives little pertinent information about the activity of the autonomic nervous system except for their effect on the relief of clinical symptoms. Atropine, belladonna, methantheline, and related drugs decrease spasm of the stomach and bowel. These same drugs and the sympathomimetic compounds decrease bronchiolar spasm; vasodilation and edema of the mucosa may be relieved by the sympathomimetic drugs. Physostigmine and neostigmine aid in the control of paralytic ileus. Contraction of the reflex bladder and uninhibited bladder may be lessened by the use of atropine, and the atonic bladder and colon may be aided by the use of neostigmine. Pilocarpine and related drugs are used in the sweat test. Tolazoline and phentolamine cause vasodilation and may relieve the pain of Raynaud's disease and related conditions.

Various autonomic blocking agents or other drugs acting on the autonomic nervous system are of value in the diagnosis of pheochromocytoma (Ch. 42).

Numerous drugs acting upon the autonomic nervous system have been synthesized in recent years; these may be used both in diagnosis and treatment. Autonomic blocking agents of various types can be used to differentiate between vasospasm and arterial obstruction in the diagnosis and treatment of vascular disease of the extremities. Many of the drugs used in the treatment of essential hypertension have autonomic blocking effects. Other autonomic nervous system stimulants and depressants are used in the treatment of dysrhythmias and other abnormalities of cardiac function. Autonomic drugs are used in both the diagnosis of the various types of neurogenic bladder and in the treatment of vesical dysfunction. Bronchodilators and decongestants are essential to the treatment of bronchial asthma, and other drugs acting on the autonomic system are important in the treatment of abnormalities of gastrointestinal function. Vasopressor agents are used for the treatment of shock and hypotensive states.

Cystometry

The cystometric examination is one of the few clinical diagnostic procedures that can actually test visceral function. In addition to determining the motility of the bladder, one can evaluate enteroceptive or visceral sensory functions by noting reactions to hot and cold water, painful stimulation, and distention. The results, when recorded and charted, constitute the cystometrogram. To perform the procedure, there are various types of cystometers; the water-drip type is the simplest. The patient is first requested to empty the bladder. Following urethral catheterization, sterile water is instilled into the bladder at the rate of 1 ml/sec. The normal individual can perceive hot and cold water and can sense distention of the bladder. The first desire to void develops after about 175 – 250 ml of water have been introduced. Normally, no uninhibited voiding contractions of the detrusor are detected even when the patient begins to feel uncomfortable.

The bladder can accommodate to increased amounts of fluid up to its limits of distention. The intravesical pressure varies between 1 and 15 cm of water. The pressure of the empty bladder is $1-2$ cm, and that of a bladder containing 100 ml of fluid may not be over $6-8$ cm. The act of micturition can be elicited with ease and maintained without straining. It may be initiated and stopped at will. There is complete control of the sphincters at all times.

Bethanechol supersensitivity tests may be performed by giving 2.5 mg of this drug subcutaneously. Bethanechol stimulates cells innervated by parasympathetic nerves, mainly at the neuromuscular junction. In the normal adult the intravesical pressure response to stretching is increased by $2-15$ cm of water at $20-30$ min after the injection. If the rise is less than 15 cm of water, the patient does not have significant neurogenic disease of the bladder. If the rise exceeds 15 cm of water the patient has a neurogenic bladder that can be due to a lesion at the central nervous system level or at the sensory or motor peripheral arcs, or a combination of them.

Careful observation of bladder sensation to pain and temperature, of pressures at which the first desire to void and painful distention occur, of the timing and character of the urinary stream, and of bladder capacity and residual urine provides information about bladder dysfunction that is of value in neurologic diagnosis. Further data may be obtained by electromyography of the bladder wall and by monitoring the activity of the internal and external sphincters. Because micturition and continence also depend upon the closely coordinated activities of the bladder, urethra, and periurethral striated muscle, it is also essential to know the dynamics of the levator ani and of the muscles of the urogenital diaphragm during the storage and evacuation phases of bladder function. Measurement of the function of these muscles can be accomplished by electromyography, and this may be done along with cystometry and electromyography of the bladder muscles in the assessment of the neurogenic bladder. The various types of abnormalities of function are discussed in Chapter 42. Although local disease and psychic factors may also influence the picture, the cystometric and related examinations are important objective means of examining the autonomic nervous system.

Colonmetrography

Procedures similar to those used in the cystometric examination enable one to evaluate the effect of the autonomic nervous system in the control of function of the gastrointestinal tract or, specifically, of the colon. It is also possible to make simultaneous manometric recordings of the contraction and relaxation of the internal and external anal sphincters. These procedures are not used as frequently as cystometry and are somewhat more difficult to appraise.

Miscellaneous Tests

In the diagnosis of diseases of the central and peripheral autonomic nervous systems, including those with and without associated endocrine dysfunction, many other examinations and laboratory procedures give important and sometimes necessary information. Among these may be mentioned the following. Radiologic determination of the motility of the gastrointestinal tract after the administration of some radiopaque substance such as barium or bismuth; determination of the secretory function of the gastric mucosa before and after the administration of food, histamine, or alcohol; measurement of salivary secretion and lacrimation; observation of the effect of either spinal anesthesia or autonomic blockade in megacolon; arteriography; glucose tolerance studies; determination of fluid intake, output, and balance; measurement of blood electrolytes; studies of the diuretic response to intravenous hypertonic saline solution and to nicotine in the diagnosis of diabetes insipidus; the determination of eosinophil response to the injection of epinephrine, insulin, and corticotropin; blood chemistry studies of various types; assays of estrogen, androgen, pituitary follicle-stimulating hormone, growth hormone, and prolactin; determinations of plasma levels of catecholamines and enzymes such as epinephrine, norepinephrine, and dopamine hydroxylase, and of 3-methoxy-4-hydroxymandelic acid and homovanillic acid, vasopressin and renin; urinary excretions of catecholamines, aldosterone, the mandelic and vanillic acids mentioned above; determinations of 17-ketosteroids, and 17-hydroxycorticosteroids and changes in them after the administration of corticotropin; and radioactive iodine uptake and other thyroid function tests.

The availability of radioimmunoassay technics and newer physiologic knowledge have generated a variety of test procedures designed to evaluate hypothalamic-pituitary function. Many of these provoke the discharge of pituitary hormones. Not all of the reported stimulation tests (or their many modifications) have proved to be equally reliable, but the selected use of several of them may be of aid in the confirmation and localization of pituitary and other endocrine disorders. Among these are included tests of corticotropin stimulation following the injection of insulin, vasopressin or corticotropin, or either injection or oral ingestion of metapyrone; tests of gonadotropin stimulation following the injection of gonadotropin-releasing hormone or human chorionic gonadotropin or the oral ingestion of clomiphene; and tests of pituitary stimulation following the injection of insulin, arginine, or thyrotropin-releasing hormone, injection or ingestion of chlorpromazine, or the ingestion of levodopa. Assays, some available only on a research basis, have also been developed for the measurement of the hormone-releasing factors secreted by the hypothalamus (Ch.40).

BIBLIOGRAPHY

Bors E, Comarr AE. Neurological Urology: Physiology of Micturition, Its Neurological Disorders and Sequelae. Baltimore, University Park Press, 1977

Bradley WE. Cystometry and sphincter electromyography. Mayo Clin Proc 1976;51:329

Côté LJ. Neurogenic orthostatic hypotension. In Rowland LP (ed). Merritt's Textbook of Neurology, 8th ed. Philadelphia, Lea & Febiger, 1989

Darrow CW. Neural mechanisms controlling the palmar galvanic skin reflex and palmar sweating: A consideration of available literature. Arch Neurol Psychiatry 1937;37:641

Gautschy B, Weidmann P, Gnädinger MP. Autonomic function tests as related to age and gender in normal man. Klin Wochenschr 1986;64:499

Gold EM. Hypothalamic-pituitary function tests: Current status. Postgrad Med 1977;62:105

Grenell RG, Burr HS. Surface potentials and peripheral nerve injury: A clinical test. Yale J Biol Med 1946;18:517

Guttman SA. Use of furmethide in testing sweat secretion in man. Arch Neurol Psychiatry 1944;51:568

Hines EA Jr, Brown CE. The cold pressor test for measuring the reactibility of the blood pressure: Data covering 571 normal and hypertensive subjects. Am Heart J 1936;11:1

Jacobs HS, Nabarro JD. Tests of hypothalamic-pituitary-adrenal function in man. Q J Med 1969;38:475

Jasper HH, Robb P. Studies of electrical skin resistance in peripheral nerve lesions. J Neurosurg 1945;2:261

Kahn EA. Direct observation of sweating in peripheral nerve lesions. Surg Gynec Obstet 1951;92:22

Lapides J, Diokno AC. Urine transport, storage, and micturition. In Lapides J (ed). Fundamentals of Urology. Philadelphia, WB Saunders, 1976

List CF, Peet MM. Sweat secretion in man. I. Sweating responses in normal persons. Arch Neurol Psychiatry 1938;39:1228

Loeser LH. Cutaneous histamine reaction as a test of peripheral nerve function. JAMA 1938;110:2136

Polinski RJ, Kopin IJ, Ebert MH, Weise V. Pharmacologic distinction of different orthostatic hypotension syndromes. Neurology 1981;31:1

Rakoff J, Vandenberg G, Siler TM et al. An integrated direct functional test of the adenohypophysis. Am J Obstet Gynecol 1974;119:358

Redlich FC. Organic and hysterical anesthesia: A method of differential diagnosis with the aid of the galvanic skin reflex. Am J Psychiatry 1945;102:318

Richter CP. Instructions for using the cutaneous resistance recorder, or "Dermometer," on peripheral nerve injuries, sympathectomies, and paravertebral blocks. J Neurosurg 1946;3:181

Smith AA, Dancis J. Response to infused histamine in familial dysautonomia: a diagnostic test. J Pediat 1963;62:889

Smith AA, Dancis J. Exaggerated response to infused norepinephrine in familial dysautonomia. N Engl J Med 1964;470:704

Tsementzis SA, Hitchcock ER. The spoon test: A simple bedside test for assessing sudomotor autonomic failure. J Neurol Neurosurg Psychiatry 1985;48:378

Wang GH. The Neural Control of Sweating. Madison, University of Wisconsin Press, 1964

Winkelmann RK, Wilhelmj CM, Horner FA. Experimental studies on dermatographism. Arch Dermat 1965;92:436

Ziegler MC, Lake CR, Kopin IJ. Deficient sympathetic nervous response in familial dysautonomia. N Engl J Med 1976;294:630

Chapter 42
DISORDERS OF THE AUTONOMIC NERVOUS SYSTEM

The disorders of autonomic function are complex, varied, and difficult to classify. It is not the purpose of this volume to give a detailed description of diseases or of the various syndromes and clinical entities that may be encountered, or to give an outline of differential diagnosis. Brief mention, however, of some of the more characteristic disorders of autonomic function will assist in understanding the physiology of the autonomic nervous system, the reasons for the various diagnostic procedures, and the alterations in function that occur in disease.

DISORDERS OF FUNCTION OF THE PERIPHERAL AUTONOMIC NERVOUS SYSTEM

Lesions of the peripheral portions of the autonomic nervous system are usually manifested by a deficiency or loss of function of one of the divisions of the system, often with an apparent increase in function of the reciprocal division. Occasionally, however, irritation of one division may result in an increased activity of that portion. In general a lesion of the parasympathetic division, the individual fibers of which are supplied to special structures, is manifested by focal changes, whereas a lesion of the sympathetic division causes more generalized changes. With loss of function of the constituent portions of the parasympathetic division there may be mydriasis, paralysis of visual accommodation, diminution of lacrimal and salivary secretion, cardiac acceleration, bronchial dilation, gastrointestinal atony with decreased secretion, spasm of the sphincters, bladder atony, and impotence. These symptoms are increased by the administration of atropine and relieved, if paralysis is not complete, by the administration of physostigmine and similar drugs. The sympathomimetic drugs, which stimulate the antagonistic sympathetic division, may also increase the symptoms.

A lesion of the sympathetic division may cause vasodilation, anhidrosis, loss of piloerection, reflex erythema, fall in blood pressure, bradycardia, pupillary constriction, bronchial constriction, and impairment of ejaculation. The effect on gastrointestinal and bladder functions is less definite. These symptoms are increased by further inhibiting the action of the sympathetics or by stimulating the parasympathetics, and relieved, if the paralysis is not complete, by the administration of sympathomimetic drugs. Such diminution or loss of sympathetic function may be caused either by brain stem or spinal lesions that affect the descending sympathetic pathways, or by involvement of the intermediolateral cell groups, the preganglionic fibers, the sympathetic ganglia, the postganglionic fibers, or the peripheral nerves.

Following a transverse spinal cord lesion above the eighth cervical or first thoracic segment, loss of sympathetic function of the entire body results, and if it is complete and interferes with vital functions such as respiration and cardiac function, it is incompatible with life. If partial, it may only cause loss of sweating, piloerection, and vasoconstriction of the face and body. A partial lesion at the eighth cervical and upper thoracic levels, especially if it involves only the intermediolateral cells, may affect only sympathetic fibers to the head and neck, causing anhidrosis, vasodilation, and Horner's syndrome. With a transverse lesion at any level of the thoracic or upper lumbar spinal cord there is loss of sympathetic function below the level of the lesion, with anhidrosis, vasodilation, loss of piloerection, and increase in skin temperature. Later there is vasoconstriction with a decrease in temperature; sweating and piloerection may reappear in an exaggerated form as part of the spinal defense reflex. Impairment of bowel, bladder, and sexual functions may also be present, and occasionally orthostatic hypotension or transient hypertension precipitated by bladder or bowel distention. Changes in the body protein and electrolytes, osteoporosis, testicular atrophy, altered excretion of 17-ketosteroids, and occasionally gynecomastia may develop. There are no changes in sympathetic function with lesions below the third lumbar segment, and only the sacral parasympathetics and somatic nerves are affected.

With lesions of the mixed spinal nerves there are also sympathetic changes characterized by loss of sweating, piloerection, and vasoconstriction. With severe involvement there may be extensive alterations in the skin and subcutaneous tissues, described subsequently. In severe neuropathies, such as the autonomic neuropathy that may be present with diabetes, there sometimes are more extensive deficits, with a neurogenic bladder, impotence, bowel incontinence or nocturnal diarrhea, orthostatic hypotension, and neurogenic arthropathy. The sympathetic nerves have been sectioned in the treatment of Raynaud's disease, causalgia, hypertension, and other conditions, and to relieve the pain of angina pectoris and pancreatitis.

The various disorders of function that may follow lesions of the peripheral autonomic nervous system can be comprehended most satisfactorily by listing the tissues, organs, and systems innervated and the dysfunction that may occur in each. In some of the conditions listed the dysfunction may have a central as well as a peripheral basis, but the peripheral involvement usually predominates.

The Eye

A lesion of the Edinger – Westphal nucleus, the anterior median (medial) nucleus of the oculomotor nerve, the preganglionic fibers to the ciliary ganglion, or the postganglionic fibers causes paralysis of the sphincter of the pupil and/or paralysis of accommodation for near vision. Irritation has the opposite effect. Paralysis of the sympathetic fibers to the eye results in miosis, ptosis, pseudoptosis, and either real or apparent enophthalmos, *i.e.*, a Horner's syndrome; there may be associated anhidrosis of the side of the face and conjunctiva. This latter complex may follow involvement of the descending autonomic pathways in the brain stem or cervical portion of the spinal cord, the spinal cord at the junction of the eighth cervical and upper thoracic segments, the preganglionic fibers, the cervical sympathetic ganglion chain, or the postganglionic fibers as they follow the carotid artery into the cavernous plexus and then enter the long ciliary nerves. Cocaine (2% – 5%), which causes dilation of a normal pupil, fails to dilate the pupil of a Horner's syndrome. If the lesion causing the syndrome is a postganglionic one, there may be denervation supersensitivity and an increased response to epinephrine. Stimulation of the sympathetic division may cause mydriasis, widening of the palpebral fissure, and exophthalmos. Pupillary changes may also follow cortical stimulation and destruction.

The Lacrimal and Salivary Glands

A lesion of either the superior or inferior salivary nuclei or their descending fibers, or involvement of the submaxillary, sphenopalatine, or otic ganglia or their postganglionic fibers, will cause a decrease in the amount of salivation and in the amount of mucous secretion in the nose, mouth, and pharynx, together with a decrease in lacrimation. Stimulation of these structures increases these secretions. Dysfunction of the sympathetic division causes little disturbance in these functions, although its stimulation is followed by the formation of thick, viscid saliva. Salivation is stimulated reflexly by olfactory, gustatory, psychic, and other stimuli mediated through the hypothalamus and/or cortex, and may be inhibited centrally. Lacrimation may be either stimulated or inhibited by central effects. The syndrome of "crocodile tears" is characterized by lacrimation on taking food into the mouth.

The Skin Structures

The arrectores pilorum muscles, the sweat glands, and probably the vasomotor fibers of the cutaneous blood vessels are innervated entirely by the sympathetic division. Interruption of sympathetic pathways is followed by loss of pilomotor responses, anhidrosis, and vasodilation. Stimulation has the opposite effect. So-called trophic disorders involving the skin, mucous membranes, hairs, nails, and subcutaneous tissues are frequently encountered in diseases of the sympathetic division and are important in neurologic diagnosis and localization. They are not the result of impairment of innervation to ectodermal tissues alone, but are probably influenced to a great extent by the vasomotor system. In addition to motor and sensory impulses, the peripheral nerves carry autonomic impulses. These function in vasomotor control and thus in nutrition to the skin, mucous membrane, and underlying tissues. Their integrity is essential to the normal physiology and metabolism of these structures, and when their continuity is impaired metabolic changes take place. The resulting abnormalities of function are called **trophic changes.** The more important ones are as follows:

With lesions of the peripheral nerves pronounced changes often develop in the cutaneous structures and sometimes in the mucous membranes. The skin may become smooth, thin, cold, white, and glossy, with atrophy of the subcutaneous tissues. It may become hard, with a leathery appearance, or thick and scaly. Instead of pallor there may be flushing, erythema, cyanosis, or other types of discoloration. Changes in sweat secretion take place, usually in the form of hypohidrosis or anhidrosis, but occasionally as hyperhidrosis. Seborrhea, or oiliness, is sometimes present. Either hypotrichosis or hypertrichosis may occur. The nails become brittle and ridged. These changes are either localized or diffuse.

With lesions of the dorsal root ganglia, especially with inflammatory conditions such as herpes zoster, vesicles and bullae develop in the cutaneous distribution of the specific nerve roots. With transverse lesions of the spinal cord there is anhidrosis with loss of piloerection, redness, and hyperthermia below the level of the lesion. Later there is vasoconstriction with hypothermia, cyanosis, and mottling; abnormal sweating and piloerection may reappear as part of the spinal defense reflex.

With central lesions such as hemiplegia of cerebral origin the involved extremities may be warmer or colder than normal (usually the latter). Cyanosis, dependent edema, and circulatory insufficiency may develop. With cortical involvement there may be an exaggerated pilomotor response on the hemiplegic side. With hypothalamic lesions there may be alopecia

areata, vitiligo, and poliosis or premature graying. In postencephalitic states there may be increased secretion of the sebaceous glands; the skin of the face is greasy and there is marked seborrhea of the face and scalp.

Neurotrophic or perforating ulcers, such as decubiti (bed sores), may develop with the various spinal and peripheral nerve lesions, especially if sensory as well as trophic impulses are interrupted. Pressure over an anesthetic area elicits a flare. If the pressure is not relieved, local anemia occurs and the blood supply to the area is interrupted. This leads to destruction of the deeper layers of the epidermis, and the development of vesicles due to collection of serum between the papillary layer of the dermis and the epidermis. On further pressure the structures of the dermis are also destroyed, with sloughing and the development of an area of necrosis that extends both peripherally and into the deeper structures. Extensive ulcerations may develop owing to the deficient blood supply and the absence of nutrient impulses from the central nervous system; these areas of necrosis, or ulcerations, heal slowly and become infected with ease. These develop at sites of pressure, most frequently over the sacrum, buttocks, trochanters, heels, and malleoli. They are found in severe peripheral nerve lesions, advanced syringomyelia, congenital malformations, and other extensive spinal cord lesions. In tabes dorsalis there may be painless perforating ulcers of the toes and feet (**mal perforant**), probably the result of dorsal root ganglion involvement. In syringomyelia and myelodysplasia the patient may cut or burn himself without experiencing pain; the resulting lesions heal poorly and become infected easily. Syringomyelia accompanied by painless ulcerations of the fingers is called **Morvan's disease;** the term **main succulente** is used if there is edema with lividity and coldness of the hand. When sensory loss in the hands is severe, the fingernails may become thickened, riddled and clawlike. Perforating ulcers of the mouth and nasal septum may be found in association with syphilis and cranial nerve lesions.

Edema of the skin may occur under a variety of circumstances, often the result of autonomic nervous system involvement. In urticaria there is localized edema with erythema. In **angioneurotic edema (Quincke's disease)** localized pruritic swellings, single or multiple, may involve large portions of the body. The manifestations may occur in attacks and may involve the respiratory passages. There is an allergic factor.

In **hereditary trophedema (Milroy's disease)** there is swelling of the lower exremities. In **myxedema** there is a nonpitting edema of the skin. In **hemiedema** there is swelling of one half of the body. Edema is a frequent manifestation of trophic lesions, and is found in the paretic extremities in both lower motor neuron, or peripheral, and upper motor neuron, or central, paralysis. Generalized edema, of course, is usually the result of cardiac or renal disease. If there is any tendency toward edema, it will develop first in paretic extremities.

Color and pigment changes of various types may be noted. Pallor, flushing, and cyanosis have been mentioned. In cases of circulatory insufficiency these vary with change of position. **Vitiligo,** or **leukoderma,** is a patchy loss of pigmentation of unknown origin. Vasodilation and contraction, reflex erythema, and dermatographia contribute to color alterations.

Other varieties of skin changes may be seen in disease of the autonomic nervous system, as well as in clinical entities in which the exact mechanism is not known but an autonomic factor is suspected. **Scleroderma** is a thickening of the skin with atrophy of the subcutaneous tissues. The skin is hard, shiny, and leathery. There may be anhidrosis and alopecia; this may be generalized or diffuse. Localized scleroderma is known as **morphea.** When present on the forehead and extending vertically beyond the hairline, it has been called **en coup de sabre.** Scleroderma may be secondary to syringomyelia, or hemiatrophy, or may occur as a disease entity. It is often a manifestation of collagen diseases. Either trophic changes or hypertrophy of the skin may occur in leprosy.

The Sweat Glands

Disorders of sweat secretion vary in type. Generalized hyperhidrosis is rare; it may be relieved somewhat by drugs such as atropine. Some individuals have a tendency toward spontaneous hyperhidrosis, which tends to be localized to the palmar surfaces of the hands and fingers, the plantar surfaces of the feet and toes, the axillas, and the forehead. Such persons may show excessive sweating when under tension or in cold weather, but the palms and soles may remain relatively dry in warm weather when the entire body is perspiring profusely. Hyperhidrosis is also a symptom of hyperthyroidism and of familial dysautonomia (Riley-Day syndrome), and either hyperhidrosis or spontaneous sweating

occurs with some cerebral lesions. After certain segments of the body have been rendered anhidrotic by sympathectomy there may be a compensatory increase in sweating in other areas. Both familial and congenital anhidrosis are rare, and are usually associated with congenital absence of the sweat glands as a part of hereditary ectodermal dysplasia. Anhidrosis may also occur with hereditary neuropathy and it may be a manifestation of orthostatic hypotension due to neurologic disease. Both segmental hypohidrosis and progressive anhidrosis due to progressive sudomotor denervation have been reported with Adie's syndrome.

Focal loss of sweating may be associated with lesions of the central autonomic pathways, the intermediolateral cells, the preganglionic or postganglionic sympathetic fibers, or the mixed peripheral nerves; this may be surrounded by a zone of increased sweating. Interruption of the reticulospinal pathway in the brain stem or the cervical portion of the spinal cord causes ipsilateral loss of sweating on the face, often a part of Horner's syndrome (Fig. 42-1). Interruption of the ventral reticulospinal pathway causes ipsilateral loss of thermoregulatory sweating on the body below the lesion; there may be hyperhi-

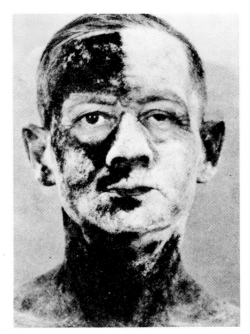

FIG. 42–1. Changes in sweat secretions (dark color signifies perspiration is present) in a patient with left-sided Horner's syndrome. (List CF, Peet MM. Arch Neurol Psychiatry 1938; 40:27).

drosis at the level of involvement. With transverse myelopathy the sweat response may return below the lesion after the period of spinal shock has passed, and may be evident in the spinal defense reflex. There may be a "sweat level," with thermoregulatory sweating above the lesion and spinal reflex sweating below it. Excessive spinal sweating below a transverse lesion may be relieved by sympathectomy. Abnormal gustatory sweating develops secondary to faulty nerve regeneration in the auriculotemporal and chorda tympani syndromes. Gustatory sweating has also been reported following cervicothoracic sympathectomy, and a few cases of hereditary gustatory sweating have been observed.

The Blood Vessels

All the arteries except the coronary arteries are constricted by the action of the sympathetic division. The parasympathetic division is believed to constrict the coronary vessels, and it does dilate the helicine arteries and some of the arteries supplying specific structures, but is not an effective vasodilator in general. Paralysis of the sympathetic division causes peripheral vasodilation of the cutaneous vessels. This may not persist, however, since the denervated muscle may become abnormally sensitive to the epinephrine-like substances normally circulating in the blood, and vasoconstriction may follow. Sympathetic stimulation causes vasospasm.

There is a group of trophic disorders in which the pathologic alterations are primarily in the blood vessels. Many are disorders of the autonomic nervous system manifested chiefly through peripheral vascular involvement while some of them are primary vascular diseases with associated autonomic involvement, but in every one of them there is some evidence, primary or secondary, of involvement of the vasomotor system. Trophic changes do not occur in all. In some there is evidence of vasospasm (Raynaud's disease), in others of vasodilation (erythromelalgia), and in still others of organic obstruction (atherosclerosis and Buerger's disease). The more important ones are listed.

Raynaud's Disease. This is a disorder developing primarily in young women. It most frequently involves the fingers and hands but may affect the toes, tips of the ears, and nose, spreading to involve larger areas. The manifestations are often symmetric. There is abnormal sensitivity to cold, and on exposure to cold, attacks of "local syncope" are induced. Starting with the digits and spreading proximally, the extremities first become cyanotic, then red, and then cold, pale, and numb. After a period of time they again become cyanotic, and then red, hot, and painful. Repeated attacks lead to trophic changes in the digits, ulcerations, and gangrene. Examination shows that the skin temperature is below normal. There is no pallor on elevation or rubor on dependency, but cyanosis and pallor follow exposure to cold. The arterial pulsations are normal. It is believed that cold, emotional stimuli, and other factors cause hyperactivity of the sympathetic division with resulting vasospasm and ischemia. As the disease progresses, changes may appear in the vessel walls. Parasympathomimetic drugs as well as vasodilators have been used in treatment. Protection against cold is important. Effective, though not invariable, relief has been obtained by preganglionic sympathectomy, with consequent vasodilation.

Syndromes similar to Raynaud's disease have been described following trauma and in individuals who work with pneumatic drills or riveting hammers. This latter condition has been known as spastic anemia, white fingers, pneumatic hammer disease, and traumatic vasospastic disease. The exposure to rapid vibration is believed to be an etiologic factor. This condition probably blends into the so-called carpal tunnel syndrome, due to trauma from pressure on the median nerve at the wrist, or from edema.

Acrocyanosis. This disorder bears some resemblance to Raynaud's disease. The hands and less frequently the feet are persistently cold, blue, and sweaty. Exposure to cold intensifies these changes, which begin at the wrist and proceed distally. There may be some puffiness of the fingers. Pain is not a symptom of consequence, and trophic changes and gangrene never develop. The syndrome is believed to be the result of increased tone of the cutaneous arterioles due to hypersensitivity to cold, with consequent local asphyxia.

Acroparesthesia. A slowly progressive disorder that is most often found in women of middle age, this is characterized by numbness and crawling or tingling sensations in the extremities, usually the hands, often associated with pain, slight pallor or mottling of the skin, hyperesthesia, hyperalgesia, and coldness. The symptoms usually occur at night. The syndrome may be due to pressure on the brachial plexus and artery at the thoracic outlet, or even to more distal vascular and nerve compression (carpal tunnel syndrome).

Erythromelalgia (Weir Mitchell's Disease). This is a rare condition of middle life that is characterized by paroxysmal or periodic reddening and severe burning pain and swelling in one or more of the extremities, usually the feet. The attacks, which seldom last more than a few hours, are accompanied by hyperalgesia and sweating of the part. The symptoms are brought on by warmth, excitement, or dependency of the part, and are relieved by rest, cold, or elevation. The skin temperature is elevated; there are no color changes with change of position. Trophic changes may develop in the skin or nails, but no ulcerations occur. The symptoms are believed to be due to vasodilation or to be a result of hypersensitivity of the cutaneous pain fibers to warmth and tension.

Buerger's Disease (Thromboangiitis Obliterans). This condition usually occurs in middle aged males, most frequently in the lower extremities. One of the early symptoms is intermittent claudication, but later there is pain at rest as well as during exercise. There is either rubor or cyanosis of the extremities on dependency, and pallor on elevation. The arterial pulsations are diminished in half the cases, and the skin temperature is low in all. Ulcerations and gangrene may develop. Early in the disease there is hyperactivity of the vasomotor nerves, and at this time vasodilators and even sympathectomy may afford relief. Later there is an organic obstruction of the arteries and to a lesser extent of the veins. The vessels become stiff and hard, the adventitia is thickened, and there is an increase in connective tissue in the media, with narrowing of the lumens, a diminution of the blood flow, and a tendency toward thrombosis.

Peripheral Atherosclerosis. Usually occurring in the older age group, this condition may also cause intermittent claudication as an early symptom, probably the result of relative anoxia of the muscles secondary to narrowing of the arteries and a deficiency in blood supply. Signs of vascular obstruction occur, with a tendency toward ulcerations and gangrene. There is rubor on dependency and pallor on elevation, but there are rarely color changes on exposure to cold. The skin temperature is low, arterial pulsations are diminished, and the sclerotic changes in the vessels may be palpated or may be visualized by roentgenography and angiography. The circulatory status may also be assessed by Doppler blood flow studies.

Causalgia. This is occasionally known as reflex sympathetic dystrophy, but authorities still disagree on the identity of the two conditions. Following injury or irritation of a peripheral nerve, usually the median nerve but occasionally other nerves in the upper extremity or the sciatic nerve in the lower extremity, a syndrome develops that is characterized by pain and by vasomotor and trophic disturbances. The injury may have been slight and the pain is out of proportion to the severity of the trauma. The patient complains of a severe, burning pain, first in the distribution of the involved nerve but later radiating peripherally. The pain is made worse by motion, emotional stimuli, exposure to temperature changes, even very light pressure, and even by air currents. There is marked hyperesthesia of the involved extremity. Accompanying the pain are vascular and trophic changes that consist of redness, a glossy skin, coldness, edema, hyperhidrosis, and changes in the hair and nails. There may be either vasoconstriction with lowering of the temperature of the affected part or vasodilation with elevation of the temperature.

The symptoms are doubtless associated, at least in part, with sympathetic dysfunction. The pain may be caused by self-perpetuating activity within the autonomic reflex arcs long after the precipitating process is gone, or it may be brought about by efferent sympathetic discharges from the hypothalamus that cause direct stimulation of afferent fibers near the site of injury. Other proposed causes include "cross-talk" or ephaptic transmission of nerve fibers. Local anesthetic injection of the sympathetic ganglia supplying the painful area may afford temporary benefit, and in some cases permanent relief follows a complete preganglionic sympathectomy. A preoperative block may help one to predict the results of sympathectomy. The operation is most effective if done early; if the syndrome has been present for a long time, associated psychic changes or secondary hyperirritability of central areas may render the prognosis grave. Blocking agents and vasodilators may also give temporary relief, and some cases have been treated by posterior cordotomy with section of the long intersegmental fibers that lie close to the substantia gelatinosa of Rolando, but the results are often poor.

Sudeck's Atrophy. Also known as post-traumatic osteoporosis, peripheral trophoneurosis, reflex sympathetic dystrophy, and chronic posttraumatic edema, this is a poorly understood syndrome that develops occasionally after trauma. The trauma is often mild, and usually to the distal portions of the extremities. There is local pain, swelling, and often trophic changes in bone. In some cases local anesthetic injection and sympathectomy are followed by relief of symptoms.

The Shoulder – Hand Syndrome. This is also poorly understood and is questionably even a syndrome; however, it is a fairly common problem. Some patients, following myocardial infarction, hemiplegia, or prolonged immobilization of the shoulder consequent to trauma, arthritis, or bursitis, develop severe shoulder pain that is intensified by either active or passive movement. This often leads to further restriction of movement. In time trophic changes may develop in the bones about the shoulder (osteoporosis), and if the immobility persists there may be pain in the hand as well, with vasomotor alterations, edema, trophic changes in the skin and bone, and muscle atrophy. The development of these changes may be prevented, and the symptoms often relieved, by means of passive, assisted active, and active movement of the shoulder, especially if begun early in the course of the disorder.

Trench Foot (Immersion Foot). Following prolonged soaking in cold water or exposure to cold, together with constriction by shoes and other clothing, the toes become white and cold, and sometimes cyanotic and even gangrenous. At the outset the peripheral arteries are contracted, but later they are relaxed, with resulting edema accompanied by paresthesias, pain, and excoriations. The normal vasomotor responses are absent.

Manifestations similar to those of the just-described syndromes may be present with disorders that do not primarily affect the peripheral autonomic nervous system or the blood vessels. These include central lesions such as hemiplegia, metabolic and hormonal disturbances, blood dyscrasias, the collagen and related disorders, and the effect of drugs or toxins such as ergot. In all of the conditions in which there are symptoms and signs of impaired blood supply to the extremities, the degree of impairment may be evaluated by noting color changes and reactive hyperemia with alterations in the position and temperature of the part, and by oscillome-

try, plethysmography, Doppler blood flow studies, skin temperature studies, and other tests described in Chapter 41.

Migraine and other types of cephalgia are in part at least of vascular origin and are associated with disturbances of the autonomic supply to the extracranial and intracranial vessels. The pain is believed by many to be the result of dilation of certain extracranial and dural arteries, especially the temporal and middle meningeal branches of the external carotid artery, with stimulation of the neighboring neural plexuses. It has been postulated that the preceding prodromal symptoms may be the result of an earlier vasoconstriction, possibly of cerebral arteries. In a large percentage of patients the pain is relieved by the early administration of the ergot class of drugs. In cluster headache, which may also respond to this class of drugs, the attacks of pain are believed to be caused by dilation of the intracranial arteries at the base of the brain, especially the cerebral and pial branches of the basilar and internal carotid arteries. Parasympathetic hyperactivity has been proposed as a cause for parts of the cluster headache syndrome. Other varieties of headache, including those associated with fever, may also result from distention of the intracranial arteries, and still other types may be caused by tension on, displacement or inflammation of, or traction on the arteries of the brain and meninges as well as contraction of cervicooccipital muscles.

The Heart

Interruption of the cardioinhibitory fibers that are conducted from the dorsal efferent nucleus through the vagus nerve to the cardiac ganglia on the heart wall causes acceleration, whereas stimulation of the vagus brings about reduced heart rate, decreased cardiac output, diminished conduction at the auriculoventricular bundle, and sometimes auriculoventricular block or vagal arrest. In a lesion of the vagus nerve both the oculocardiac and carotid sinus reflexes are lost. Stimulation of the sympathetic division produces increased conduction at the atrioventricular bundle, cardiac acceleration, increased output, and sometimes ventricular extrasystoles, paroxysmal tachycardia, and either atrial or ventricular fibrillation. Injection of epinephrine directly into the heart muscle has been used in the treatment of sudden cardiac arrest.

When abnormalities of the autonomic system are present, there may be tachycardia, bradycardia, or abnormalities of rhythm. Bradycardia often has diagnostic value or serious prognostic significance in increased intracranial pressure; it may be the result of hypothalamic involvement, but it more frequently follows pressure on the cardiac center in the medulla as a result of herniation of the medulla into the foramen magnum. Sudden death following spinal puncture may be due to cardiac arrest on such a basis. Paroxysmal tachycardia may be caused by heart disease, or it may occur on a reflex basis or in association with emotional stimuli. It is sometimes stopped by pressure on the eyeballs, by means of the oculocardiac reflex. Heart block is usually a symptom of organic disease of the heart, but in Stokes-Adams attacks there may be cardiac arrest due to stimulation of the inhibitory fibers to the heart. If the carotid sinus reflex is hyperactive, pressure on the neck may bring about slowing or temporary arrest of the heart, a fall in blood pressure, and sometimes syncope and convulsions.

The vasovagal attacks described by Gowers are characterized by palpitation, precordial distress, respiratory arrhythmia, disturbances in gastrointestinal motility, and syncope. They were once thought to result from vagal stimulation. Vasovagal syncope is now considered to be simple fainting. Loss of consciousness usually develops when the systolic blood pressure falls to 70 mm Hg or less. It has been suggested that stress, in certain individuals, causes sudden pooling of blood in the muscles. This brings about a decrease in cerebral blood flow and consequent syncope. The exact mechanism underlying syncope, however, remains to be determined. Vasovagal syncope can occur in normal individuals subjected to strong emotional experiences that induce vasodilation, such as anxiety, fatigue, hunger, or severe pain after injury.

The relationship of the autonomic nervous system to the pain of angina pectoris has been the subject of a great deal of discussion. It is believed that the pain is the result of ischemia of the cardiac musculature secondary to spasm of the coronary arteries. The impulses are, however, conducted with the autonomic nerves to the middle and inferior cervical ganglia. This pain has been relieved by either injection or section of the middle and inferior cervical and the upper thoracic sympathetic ganglia. It cannot be stated whether the relief is the result only of interruption of the afferent impulses or also of blocking of the motor impulses. The sympathetic division is believed to exert vasodilator rather than vasoconstrictor effects on the coronary vessels, however, so that one may assume that the relief follows interruption of the sensory pathways. Similar results may be obtained by section of the posterior nerve roots. Constriction of the coronary arteries in response to dilation of the stomach or pain in the abdomen is termed the viscerocardiac reflex.

The Blood Pressure

The blood pressure is increased by the action of the sympathetic division, which causes constriction of the blood vessels, and it may be slightly decreased by the action of the parasympathetic division. Sympathetic stimulants and vasopressor drugs are used in the treatment of shock and hypotensive states. The height of the blood pressure is regulated largely by the hypothalamus and by the tonic activity of the vasomotor center situated in the medulla. The control is not, however, entirely autonomic, since it is also influenced reflexly and by changes in the hydrogen ion concentration of the blood. There are other subsidiary vasomotor centers in the intermediolateral columns of the spinal cord. With focal intracerebral lesions and increased intracranial pressure there may be either a rise or a fall in blood pressure. In paraplegic patients bladder distention may cause hypertension.

Surgery of the sympathetic nervous system, largely section of the splanchnic nerves, was once used quite extensively in the treatment of essential or so-called malignant hypertension. There is still a great deal that is not understood about hypertension and about the physiologic effects of these operative procedures — whether they decrease the blood pressure by vasodilation of the splanchnic area, elimination of excessive adrenal secretion, dilation of the renal vessels, or humoral changes. Furthermore, it is known that hypertension may have both neurogenic and psychogenic components. These operative procedures, however, were definitely valuable and did contribute one of the major advances to the surgery of the autonomic nervous system, although they now have largely been supplanted by various types of drug therapy. Among the pharmacologic agents used in the treatment of hypertension are those that act centrally such as reserpine, vasodilators such as hydralazine, ganglionic and other blocking agents, especially the beta receptor blockers of sympathetic impulses, angiotensin converting enzyme inhibitors, and diuretics. These and other drugs, used alone or in combinations, have been so successful that they have virtually replaced surgical treatment of essential hypertension.

Pheochromocytomas are tumors arising in the chromaffin tissue of the sympathetic nervous system, most frequently in the adrenal medulla. They produce and release amines, predominantly norepinephrine and epinephrine. These substances cause either intermittent or continuous elevation of the blood pressure and concomitant symptoms such as headache, hyperhidrosis, and peripheral vasoconstriction. The presence of such a tumor may be diagnosed by the intravenous administration of phentolamine, and also by the injection of tyramine, histamine, and glucagon, all of which cause a drop in the elevated blood pressure. It must be remembered, however, that these pharmacologic tests are not without risk to the patient. The diagnosis can also be made by the presence of increased amounts of catecholamines and products of their metabolism in the blood and urine, and by imaging studies.

In the syndrome of **orthostatic hypotension** there is an abrupt fall in both the systolic and diastolic blood pressure with resulting syncope as soon as the patient assumes an upright position. There is no compensatory tachycardia, sweating, or pallor. There is a deficiency in the release of norepinephrine and epinephrine with resulting instability of vasomotor reflexes. This may be idiopathic in origin, but specific etiologies include adrenal insufficiency, severe autonomic neuropathies such as diabetic neuropathy, tabes dorsalis, prior sympathectomy that has abolished vasopressor reflexes, and the use of sympatholytic drugs and catecholamine-depleting agents. Familial cases have been reported. Shy and Drager and others have described a progressive disorder affecting both the peripheral autonomic and central nervous system and characterized by orthostatic hypotension, anhidrosis, urinary and fecal incontinence, impotence, ocular palsies, distal wasting and neuropathy, rigidity, and tremor. Some authorities find pathologic distinctions between pure idiopathic orthostatic hypotension, a predominantly postganglionic disorder, and Shy-Drager syndrome, mainly preganglionic. Norepinephrine levels can differentiate the two conditions somewhat. Orthostatic hypotension is also seen with striatonigral degeneration, another multisystem degenerative disorder, and with dopamine beta-hydroxylase deficiency.

The Respiratory System

In bronchial asthma there is constriction of the bronchial musculature with swelling of the mucous membrane, increased secretion of thick mucus, and subsequent dyspnea. Many of these manifestations may be relieved 1) by the use of atropine and related parasympathetic depressants that decrease both constriction and secretions, 2) by epinephrine and related drugs that decrease secretions by vasoconstriction and may have some bronchodilator effect, and 3) by the antihistamine drugs. Stimulation of the carotid sinus may cause reflex inhibition of respiration and even apnea.

The rate and rhythm of respiration are controlled through both the central and autonomic nervous systems. The respiratory center is situated in the medulla and is influenced by neural and chemical stimuli and by changes in acid-base balance. Abnormalities of breathing, such as Cheyne – Stokes respiration, occur secondary to alterations of central respiratory control.

The Gastrointestinal System

The relationship of the autonomic nervous system to visceral disease of the gastrointestinal tract is varied and complex. Increases in tonus, in peristalsis, and in secretion are usually evidence of parasympathetic overactivity, whereas atonia may be the result of sympathetic overactivity. These manifestations may be symptoms of either organic or psychogenic disorders. Often the two are difficult to differentiate, and psychogenic mechanisms may terminate in organic disease.

In cardiospasm there may be spasm of either the esophageal musculature or of the cardiac sphincter. The beneficial effect of atropine in certain cases would suggest that, in those cases at least, parasympathetic activity, probably with spasm limited to the esophageal musculature, is the important factor. In peptic ulcer disease there is increased motility of the gastric musculature and increased secretion of hydrochloric acid. Vagotomy aids in the treatment of peptic ulcers, causing a reduction of gastric motility as well as a decrease in the volume and acidity of the gastric secretions. In both spastic constipation and mucous colitis there is hyperperistalsis with increased intestinal secretion. The symptoms may be alleviated by the use of parasympathetic blocking drugs and on occasion by vagotomy.

On the other hand paralytic ileus may be relieved by the use of neostigmine or similar drugs.

In Hirschsprung's disease, or congenital megacolon, there is dilation of the large intestine, once thought to be due either to abnormal activity of the sympathetics or to decreased activity of the parasympathetics. It is known, however, that the pathologic segment is not the dilated portion of the colon, but rather a distal narrowed segment in which the myenteric (Auerbach's) plexus is deficient or absent. Lumbar sympathectomy was once recommended for the treatment of this disorder, but it is now apparent that successful therapy is possible only by removal of the spastic aganglionic segment. Parasympathetic stimulants such as neostigmine may be of some therapeutic value in mild cases.

Intussusception with invagination of one portion of the intestine into another may be caused by increased peristalsis associated with overactivity of the parasympathetics. Congenital hypertrophic pyloric stenosis may be produced by the deficient inhibition of the pylorus, from either a deficiency of the parasympathetics or an overactivity of the sympathetics. The so-called nervous dyspepsias with hyperacidity, excessive gastric contraction, and pylorospasm may result from sympathetic and parasympathetic imbalance.

The stimulus for defecation consists of stretching of the walls of the rectum by the accumulation of fecal material. When this reaches a certain stage, rhythmic contractions develop and the internal sphincter relaxes; the external sphincter, however, which is under voluntary control, may for a while prevent the escape of feces. The parasympathetic plays a larger part than the sympathetic in defecation, and the latter probably acts only to inhibit the movements of the bowel during the accumulation of its contents. Lesions of the spinal cord that involve either the sacral segments or the descending pathways, and lesions of either the cauda equina or the pelvic nerves, depress the tone and rhythmic contraction of the rectum, with resulting constipation. Defecation may be possible through the action of the levator ani and the abdominal muscles. If the sphincters are toneless, there may be rectal incontinence; the rectal and anal reflexes are lost. In lesions that involve the cerebral centers or descending pathways, or in longstanding disease, the sphincters may regain some tone and reflex activity. These manifestations are better understood in the bladder than in the rectum, but they are comparable in the two structures.

The Bladder

Bladder musculature has tonicity, rhythmicity, and is able to retain without discomfort either small or large amounts of urine; contractions can be stimulated either reflexly or voluntarily. Vesical function is a complex mechanism that involves both the autonomic and the voluntary nervous systems, and disorders of bladder function may follow lesions of the paracentral lobule, hypothalamus, descending pathways in the spinal cord, pre- or postganglionic parasympathetic nerves, or pudendal nerve. It is difficult to differentiate between disorders of function that are entirely autonomic in origin and those with associated voluntary nervous system involvement; these will be considered together. The various disturbances of vesical function may be appraised by cystometry (Ch. 41).

The bladder acts as a reflex organ and contracts in response to a stretch reflex. The afferent impulses are carried to the sacral portion of the spinal cord, and stimulation of efferent centers causes contraction of the detrusor muscle and relaxation of the internal sphincter. There is probably a center in the lumbar spinal cord that produces a contraction of the internal sphincter and allows distention of the bladder and retention of urine. In the baby the bladder is purely reflex in function, but with the maturation of the cerebral cortex and the completion of myelination an inhibitory control over this reflex is developed, with voluntary regulation of the external sphincter. For normal micturition the parasympathetic arc, sympathetic arc, and spinal pathways must be intact, and cerebral inhibition and control of the external sphincter must be normal.

Symptoms of bladder dysfunction are often among the earliest manifestations of nervous system disease. Frequency, urgency, precipitate micturition, massive or dribbling incontinence, difficulty in initiating urination, urine retention, and loss of bladder sensation may occur. The term **neurogenic bladder** has been used for the various types of vesical dysfunction that are caused by lesions of the nervous system. The principal types of neurogenic bladder dysfunction are listed.

The **uninhibited neurogenic bladder** (Fig. 42-2) shows the least variation from the normal.

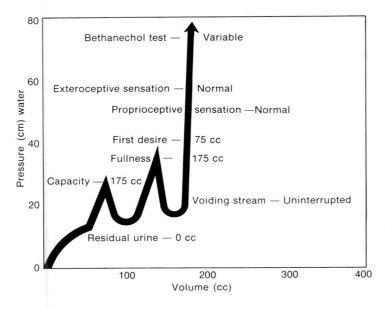

FIG. 42–2. Cystometrogram of the uninhibited neurogenic bladder. (Modified from Lapides J, Diokno AC: Urine transport, storage and micturition. In Lapides J (ed): Fundamentals of Urology. Philadelphia, WB Saunders, 1976)

This type of bladder dysfunction occurs in mental deficiency, cerebral palsy, enuresis in adults, early diffuse brain damage, cerebral lesions affecting the dominant hemisphere, hemiplegia, and early multiple and posterolateral sclerosis. It is characterized by a more or less infantile type of reaction. There is a loss of the cortical inhibition of reflex voiding, while tone remains normal, so that when the bladder is distended it contracts in response to the stretch reflex. There is frequency, urgency, and incontinence not associated with dysuria. Hesitancy may precede urgency. Bladder sensation is usually normal. Several rhythmic uninhibited contractions of the detrusor may take place before bladder capacity is reached and the final emptying contraction occurs. These contractions coincide with the patient's awareness of an urge to void, but micturition does not take place until a contraction occurs that is of sufficient intensity to empty the bladder; then the patient urinates precipitously. Up to this point, however, normal voluntary control is possible. There is no residual urine. The results of the bethanechol supersensitivity test are variable, but uninhibited contractions may occur at small volumes. The number of uninhibited contractions may be reduced by the use of atropine, propantheline, or similar drugs.

The **reflex neurogenic bladder** (Fig. 42-3) occurs with widespread disease of the spinal cord in which both the descending autonomic tracts to the bladder and the ascending sensory pathways are interrupted above the sacral segments of the cord. Thus, it occurs in patients with transverse myelitis, advanced multiple sclerosis, neoplasms, and traumatic and vascular lesions sufficiently extensive to cause a functional transection of the spinal cord. Extensive brain lesions may also cause the development of a reflex neurogenic bladder. All sensation to the bladder is lost; the patient cannot feel heat, cold, or distention. The bladder capacity is small. Micturition is reflex and involuntary. The patient cannot either initiate or stop urination in a normal way, and micturition is precipitous. There are rhythmic uninhibited contractions during filling. The patient may become aware of the presence of a full bladder by autonomic reflexes activated by distention of the bladder — these include sweating, pilomotor phenomena, increased spasticity, and a feeling of fullness in the abdomen — and he may be able to initiate urination by pinching the skin in the perineal region or pressing over the abdomen or bladder. The bladder may empty as part of the mass reflex of spinal automatism. The residual urine volume is variable. In the bethanechol supersensitivity test, reflex contractions occur at small volumes. Drug therapy is not available.

The **autonomous neurogenic bladder** (Fig. 42-4) is one without external innervation. It is caused by lesions of the sacral portion of the spinal cord, the conus medullaris or cauda equina, the motor or sensory roots of the second, third, and fourth sacral nerves, or the peripheral nerves. It occurs with neoplastic, traumatic, inflammatory, and other lesions of the conus medullaris, cauda equina, or sacral nerve roots,

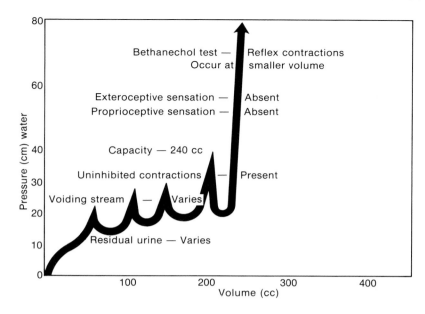

Bethanechol test —   Reflex contractions
          Occur at   smaller volume

Exteroceptive sensation —   Absent
Proprioceptive sensation —   Absent

Capacity — 240 cc

Uninhibited contractions   — Present

Voiding stream   — Varies

Residual urine — Varies

FIG. 42–3. Cystometrogram of the reflex neurogenic bladder. (Modified from Lapides J, Diokno AC: Urine transport, storage and micturition. In Lapides J (ed): Fundamentals of Urology. Philadelphia, WB Saunders, 1976)

and with congenital anomalies such as spina bifida. There is destruction of the parasympathetic supply. Sensation is absent and there is no reflex or voluntary control of the bladder; contractions occur as the result of stimulation of the intrinsic neural plexuses within the bladder wall. There are no sustained contractions of the detrusor as a whole, and no emptying contractions. During filling, however, there are minor inherent contractions of individual muscle groups, and at the height of one of these there may be emptying, which is never complete. There may

be a high intravesical pressure, and the amount of residual urine is large, but the bladder capacity is not greatly increased. On neurologic examination saddle anesthesia and absence of the bulbocavernosus reflex are found. Patients with this type of bladder dysfunction may have incontinence on coughing or straining. Voiding is usually brought about by increasing the intraabdominal pressure, and there may be dribbling as a result of the high intravesical pressure. The desire to void is made known by abdominal discomfort. Cystometry shows absence of sensa-

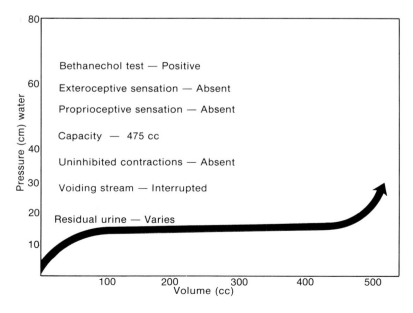

Bethanechol test — Positive

Exteroceptive sensation — Absent

Proprioceptive sensation — Absent

Capacity — 475 cc

Uninhibited contractions — Absent

Voiding stream — Interrupted

Residual urine — Varies

FIG. 42–4. Cystometrogram of the autonomous neurogenic bladder. (Modified from Lapides J, Diokno AC: Urine transport, storage and micturition. In Lapides J (ed): Fundamentals of Urology. Philadelphia, WB Saunders, 1976)

tion, variable capacity and residual urine, and no contractions of the detrusor. The bethanechol supersensitivity test is markedly positive. Treatment consists of teaching the patient to empty his bladder as completely as possible by manual external pressure and increased intraabdominal pressure.

The **sensory paralytic bladder,** also known as the atonic neurogenic bladder (Fig. 42-5), is found with lesions that involve the posterior roots or posterior root ganglia of the sacral nerves or the posterior columns of the spinal cord. This type of bladder is present in patients with tabes dorsalis, posterolateral sclerosis, multiple sclerosis, diabetic autonomic neuropathy, and related conditions. Sensation is absent, and there is no desire to void. There may be distention, dribbling, and difficulty both in initiating micturition and in emptying the bladder. There is low intravesical pressure and a large capacity, with absence of waves of contraction, and a large amount of residual urine. Voiding may be brought about by straining. There is incontinence of an overflow type. Cystometry reveals diminished to absent sensation, no uninhibited contractions, and a bladder of large capacity with a large amount of residual urine. The bethanechol supersensitivity test is positive. The bulbocavernosus reflex is absent. Bethanechol is helpful in treatment.

The **motor paralytic bladder** (Fig. 42-6) develops when the motor nerve supply to the bladder is interrupted. Among the etiologies are poliomyelitis, polyradiculoneuritis, neoplasm, trauma, and congenital anomalies. The bladder distends and decompensates, but sensation is normal. The patient complains of painful distention and inability to initiate urination. If the condition becomes chronic the symptoms are similar to those of obstructive uropathy. The cystometrogram shows normal exteroceptive and proprioceptive sensation and a normal cystometric curve. No contractions of the detrusor are observed and the patient cannot initiate micturition. The residual urine and bladder capacity vary with each individual. Saddle sensation is normal and the bulbocavernosus reflex may or may not be present. The bethanechol supersensitivity test is negative in the acute case and positive in the chronic case.

With spinal cord lesions, especially those of severe degree and sudden onset, such as traumatic myelopathies, there is at first marked urinary retention during the period of spinal shock. Reflex activity is absent; the bladder is atonic and may become markedly distended, with overflow incontinence. Later it becomes autonomous in function, owing to reflex contraction from the plexuses in the bladder wall. If the patient develops a spastic paraplegia, there will be

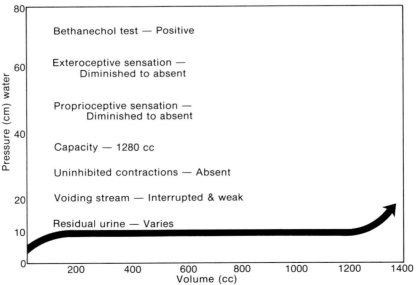

FIG. 42–5. Cystometrogram of the atonic (sensory paralytic) neurogenic bladder. (Modified from Lapides J, Diokno AC: Urine transport, storage and micturition. In Lapides J (ed): Fundamentals of Urology. Philadelphia, WB Saunders, 1976)

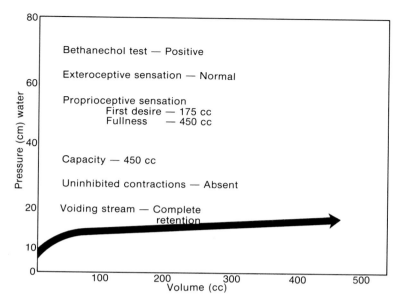

FIG. 42–6. Cystometrogram of the motor paralytic neurogenic bladder. (Modified from Lapides J, Diokno AC: Urine transport, storage and micturition. In Lapides J (ed): Fundamentals of Urology. Philadelphia, WB Saunders, 1976)

a reflex bladder with small capacity and precipitate micturition. The paralyzed bladder not infrequently becomes infected, and chronic infection leads to contraction of the viscus and often to continual dribbling. There may be calculus formation.

With cerebral lesions there may be incontinence at the onset of the lesion, owing to abolition of inhibitory control, or there may be retention with distention of the bladder and overflow incontinence. The mental apathy associated with frontal lobe lesions may lead to involuntary micturition. Vesical dysfunction may be associated with disease of either the corticospinal or extrapyramidal motor systems. Drugs such as hyoscine and related synthetic compounds used in the treatment of some parkinsonian syndromes occasionally cause retention, especially in elderly patients, and some of the tranquilizing and muscle-relaxing drugs occasionally cause enuresis. Both urinary retention and incontinence may have a psychogenic origin. There are many causes, both organic and nonorganic, for nocturnal enuresis in childhood and adolescence.

Local disease in the bladder or urethra may be manifested by symptoms similar to those associated with neurogenic dysfunction, and often, especially in elderly males with prostatic enlargement, it may be difficult to differentiate between the neurogenic manifestations and those due to local disease. In prostatism, with long-standing obstruction and resulting decompensation of the detrusor, bladder sensation may be decreased, the stream is slow and difficult to initiate, there is a high residual volume, and the patient must strain in order to void. Following inflammation of the bladder wall there are also irritative symptoms such as urgency, frequency, and pain on distention.

Surgery of the autonomic nervous system has not contributed significantly to the treatment of neurogenic bladder dysfunction. Blocking or section of the sacral nerves has been used on occasion to relieve retention caused by bladder contraction, and both anterior and posterior rhizotomy have been used to abolish spasm and change a contracted bladder to an autonomous one, with variable results. Electrical stimulation of the bladder wall and the use of an electronic implant have been tried for the treatment of bladder problems associated with spinal cord lesions. Atropine, propantheline, and similar drugs may depress the motor impulses and thus give some symptomatic relief in patients with uninhibited irritable bladders by decreasing frequency and precipitancy, while bethanechol, neostigmine, and similar substances may be of some help in controlling the retention of the sensory paralytic bladder. Imipramine has been helpful in the treatment of childhood enuresis.

Genital Functions

A lesion of the parasympathetic division causes impotence with failure of erection and ejaculation, whereas stimulation of the parasympathetics may cause priapism. With lesions of the sympathetics, or following the administration of certain adrenergic blocking agents, there may be impairment of ejaculation, because the spermatozoa fail to reach the urethra, although erection and orgasm may be preserved. With sympathetic overactivity there are ejaculatio praecox and spermatorrhea, with weakness of erection due to contraction of vasoconstrictor muscles, and hastened flow of spermatozoa due to stimulation of the reflex peristalsis in the seminal vesicles and ducts. Priapism may also result from lesions of the spinal cord above the lumbar level; not only may there be erection, but the coital, or ejaculatory reflex may be increased to such a degree that the slightest stimulus to the penis will result in ejaculation. The physiologic basis of penile tumescence during so-called REM (rapid eye movement) sleep is not known.

Loss of both libido and potency may follow cerebral lesions and the administration of cerebral depressant and autonomic blocking drugs. Antihypertensive drugs such as clonidine, guanethidine, methyldopa, spironolactone, chlorthalidone, reserpine, and the thiazide diuretics may either cause impotence or interfere with ejaculation in men. Disturbances of libido, erection, and ejaculation may also be associated with the use of sedatives, phenothiazines, and other tranquilizers, tricyclic antidepressants, monoamine oxidase inhibitors, and other antipsychotic drugs. Patients with partial complex seizures or temporal lobe neoplasms, especially if they involve the anterior portion of the lobe, often have a decrease in sexual activity and potency. In diabetic neuropathy, retrograde ejaculation may precede the development of impotence: because the internal vesical sphincter does not close, semen goes into the bladder rather than externally through the urethra. Disorders of sexual function in women as related to the autonomic nervous system are less specific, but the same drugs that interfere with erection and ejaculation in men may cause failure to reach orgasm in women. Division of the lumbar sympathetic chain and resection of the superior hypogastric plexus have been carried out for the relief of dysmenorrhea.

DISORDERS OF CENTRAL AUTONOMIC REGULATION

In disorders of function that involve predominantly the central regulatory centers concerned with the autonomic nervous system, signs and symptoms are generalized rather than focal. Some of them are referable to specific visceral systems; others are more diffuse. Clinical literature as well as experimental data relating to the hypothalamus and to disorders arising from the injury or disease of its parts has increased rapidly, and many characteristic syndromes have been described. There may be disturbances of sleep, abnormalities of temperature regulation, changes in carbohydrate and water metabolism, dysfunction of fat metabolism, or respiratory abnormalities, together with, in many instances, behavioral abnormalities and personality changes. Many of the hypothalamic syndromes that are encountered clinically are residuals of encephalitis or are associated with neoplasms. The hypothalamus is, however, under the influence of the cortex, and it may be difficult to distinguish between cortical and diencephalic manifestations. Furthermore, cortical stimulation may be followed by autonomic changes such as pupillary dilation and tachycardia that also occur in response to pain and fright. In addition, manifestations arising from the secondary reflex centers in the midbrain and brain stem and those from the higher centers may be difficult to differentiate, because of the close functional relationship between these centers.

Symptoms referable to general vegetative functions and to the various visceral systems constitute some of the more important manifestations of disorders that involve predominantly the cerebral centers of autonomic regulation. Some of the more important of these are listed. Selye has used the term "adaptation syndrome" as the sum of all nonspecific systemic reactions of the body that ensue upon long-continued exposure to stress. When the organism is subjected to sudden or excessive stress there is first the alarm reaction, during which the blood pressure and temperature fall and the blood sugar level first rises and then falls. This causes the pituitary, or hypophysis, and the adrenals to secrete an excess of hormones to combat these changes and preserve the welfare of the body, and there is a reversal of the aforementioned changes during the stage of resistance. If stress is continued too long, the body succumbs to the effects of excesses of these hormones, originally produced for an emergency defense against stress, and the stage of exhaustion follows. The hypothalamus and the pituitary and adrenal glands are the integrators of the body's defenses against stress, and the symptoms of reaction to stress are essentially those of autonomic imbalance.

Disturbances of Temperature Regulation

Either hypothermia or hyperthermia may result from hypothalamic involvement. Temperature regulation takes place not only through an elevation or fall in the body temperature, but also by means of the physical concomitants of vasodilation, vasoconstriction, sweating, and shivering. Hyperthermia may result from involvement of the tuberal region, and especially of the supraoptic nuclei or the rostral portion of the anterior hypothalamic area. It is associated with sweating, vasodilation, and other mechanisms for heat loss. Hyperthermia is a common symptom with third ventricle tumors, and may follow cerebral trauma or surgery; terminal hyperthermia is a frequent manifestation of cerebral disease. Hypothermia is associated with mechanisms for heat production and conservation, including vasoconstriction, increased visceral and somatic activity, and shivering. It may follow involvement of the posterior hypothalamic area and the mammillary bodies, or of the caudal portion of the lateral hypothalamus. With destruction of the anterior portion of the hypothalamus there is loss of the ability to regulate against heat, and with destruction of the posterior portion there is loss of the ability to regulate against cold.

Disturbances of Water Metabolism

The hypothalamus is closely related anatomically and physiologically to the posterior lobe of the hypophysis. It is probable that the central nervous system regulates water metabolism through the posterior lobe, where antidiuretic hormone is produced. Lesions of the brain of many types may be followed by either decrease, increase, or inappropriate secretion of antidiuretic hormone. Lesions of the supraoptic nuclei or the supraopticohypophyseal tract are followed by diabetes insipidus with polydipsia and polyuria (Fig. 42-7). This involvement is accompanied by degeneration of the nerves in the pituitary stalk and of the nuclei in the posterior lobe of the pituitary. There is a resulting abnormality of fluid balance, with a marked increase in the fluid intake and output, owing to a deficiency of antidiuretic hormone. Diabetes insipidus is a common symptom of tumors in the parasellar region, of encephalitis, and of meningitis, and may develop following intracranial surgery or cerebral trauma. It can also be congenital. There

may be associated manifestations of hypothalamic dysfunction. The condition should be differentiated from the polyuria caused by diabetes mellitus, psychogenic polydipsia, hypercalcemia, and chronic renal disease. The symptoms may be relieved by the administration of vasopressin or posterior pituitary extract, either by injection or by nasal insufflation.

Water intoxication may also be related to hypothalamic dysfunction, and may be caused by either excessive or inappropriate secretion of antidiuretic hormone. Other etiologies include renal insufficiency and sodium depletion, and it is sometimes either iatrogenic or self-induced, often in emotionally disturbed persons. Inappropriate secretion of antidiuretic hormone manifests as a disturbance of blood osmolality. Plasma antidiuretic hormone is elevated abnormally; the osmolality gradually decreases. When the sodium levels, the critical component, fall below 120 meq/L the patient begins to lose attentiveness and gradually heads toward a comatose state as the sodium declines. Inappropriate antidiuretic hormone secretion occurs with a large variety of hemispheric and hypothalamic lesions, and also as a remote or side effect of distant neoplasms and drugs.

Disturbances of Glucose Metabolism

Hyperglycemia with glycosurea, a syndrome resembling diabetes mellitus, may result from lesions of the tuberal region, whereas hypoglycemia with abnormal sensitivity to insulin may follow lesions of the paraventricular nuclei. Hyperglycemia has also been reported in association with lesions in the region of the fourth ventricle, but this is probably the result of damage to the descending hypothalamic pathways or of secondary hypothalamic involvement. The hypothalamus has a general regulatory effect over the autonomic nervous system and over the endocrine system. Consequently, stimulation of the areas concerned primarily with sympathetic regulation may cause glycogenolysis in the liver with resulting hyperglycemia, and stimulation of those centers concerned primarily with parasympathetic regulation may cause increased formation of insulin with hypoglycemia. Emotional hyperglycemia and glycosuria may be related to hypothalamic activity. Through its central regulatory effect on the hypophysis, thyroid, liver, pancreas, and adrenal cortex the hypothalamus functions further in the regulation of carbohy-

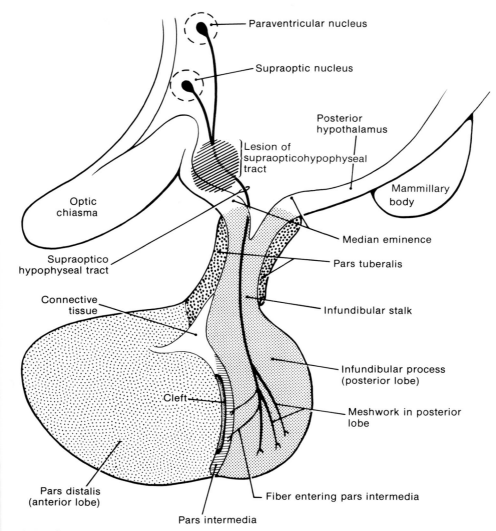

FIG. 42–7. *Longitudinal section through the human hypothalamus and hypophysis.*

drate metabolism. Symmetric lesions of the lateral nuclei at the level of the tuberal nuclei or of the region rostral and lateral to the tuber cinereum in experimental animals have prevented the appearance of hyperglycemia and glycosuria following pancreatectomy. On the other hand, degenerative changes in the paraventricular nuclei have been reported in diabetes mellitus and following pancreatectomy.

Disturbances of Fat Metabolism

The **Fröhlich,** or **adiposogenital, syndrome** was the first hypothalamic syndrome to be described. This disorder usually occurs in boys and

is characterized by disturbances of fat metabolism together with sexual underdevelopment. There is obesity of feminine distribution, often with girdles of fat about the pelvis. Associated manifestations include gynecomastia, underdevelopment of the external genitalia, and retardation of development of the secondary sexual characteristics. There may be underdevelopment of the bony skeleton. This syndrome was originally thought to have a pituitary origin, but it is usually caused by a neoplasm of the nuclei in the middle portion of the hypothalamus. The **Laurence – Moon – Biedl syndrome** is characterized by obesity, hypogenitalism, mental retardation, polydactylism, and pigmentary degeneration of the retina; it is an inherited disorder.

The adiposogenital features may be secondary to hypothalamic involvement, and a deficiency of cells in the tuberal nuclei has been noted. **In hyperostosis frontalis interna (Morgagni's syndrome)** there may be endocrine changes and obesity. Other disturbances of fat metabolism that may be secondary to hypothalamic involvement are **lipodystrophy** and **adiposis dolorosa.** The former is a generalized or a focal wasting of fatty tissues, especially of the face, upper extremities and upper part of the body, with sparing of the pelvis and lower extremities. The latter, also known as **Dercum's disease,** is characterized by the presence of large, painful deposits of fat over the shoulders, arms, and legs. Through the endocrine system (discussed subsequently) the hypothalamus may play a part in the obesity and other disturbances of fat metabolism that occur with disorders of the pituitary and thyroid glands. Extreme wasting may also occur with hypothalamic and endocrine disorders.

Disturbances of Circulation, Cardiovascular Regulation, and Blood Pressure Equilibrium

Through its regulatory effect upon the autonomic nervous system, the hypothalamus plays an important part in the regulation of circulation, heart rate and rhythm, and blood pressure. Stimulation of the posterior and lateral hypothalamic nuclei causes vasoconstriction, an increased heart rate, and a rise in blood pressure, whereas stimulation of the anterior and midline hypothalamic nuclei and the tuber cinereum produces vasodilation and a reduction in heart rate.

The cerebral cortex also has a regulatory effect upon blood pressure and heart rate, and is important in the central control of vasomotor tone. Edema, cyanosis, variations in the caliber of the blood vessels, and temperature changes in the extremities may follow cerebral lesions. In cerebral hemiplegia the temperature of the affected extremities is often first elevated, owing to temporary vasodilation, and then lowered, owing to paralysis of reflex vasodilation. The edema resulting from hemiplegia of cerebral origin is usually mild and may be associated in part with disuse and dependency. If there is any tendency toward development of edema, as the result of cardiac involvement or renal disease, the edema occurs first in the paretic extremities. The edema that is seen in hemiplegia may on occasion be al-

leviated by treatment of associated cardiac or renal disease. It may be that the cerebral lesion merely tends to localize the actual or potential edema to the paretic extremities, but most authorities believe that in certain instances the circulatory disturbances and edema of the hemiplegic limbs do have a cerebral origin.

Abnormalities of heart rate and blood pressure also follow lesions of the secondary reflex centers in the medulla. Pressure on the medulla associated with increased intracranial pressure may cause a marked bradycardia and either an elevation or a decline in the blood pressure. This often has serious prognostic significance. Disturbances of blood pressure are discussed earlier in this chapter, under disorders of the peripheral autonomic nervous system.

Hematopoiesis may also be in part under the influence of the hypothalamus, and polycythemia has been described in association with hypothalamic lesions, especially those involving the hypophyseotuberal region. The presence of an erythrocyte regulatory center in the hypothalamus has been suggested.

Disturbances of Respiration

Abnormalities of the rate, rhythm, and amplitude of respiration, such as hyperpnea, apnea, Cheyne–Stokes respiration, Biot's breathing, and air hunger, may be caused by central, probably hypothalamic, involvement. Hiccuping and yawning are often associated with hypothalamic disease. In postencephalitic states there frequently are bizarre abnormalities of breathing and respiratory tics. Respiration is also influenced by the cortex and is regulated in part by the secondary reflex center in the region of the dorsal efferent nucleus of the vagus nerve. Alterations in the electrolyte and carbon dioxide content of the blood may affect this center, and herniation of the medulla into the foramen magnum may cause respiratory arrest by pressure on it.

Disturbances of Gastrointestinal Function

The hypothalamus is the center concerned with integration and correlation of visceral impulses. Olfactory, gustatory, and other types of stimuli that come into this region call out various types of visceral responses. Lesions of the hypothalamus and its connections can cause accelerated gastrointestinal motility, increased secretion, hypersalivation, and excessive hunger (bulimia or hyperphagia), or they can cause decreased motility and secretion, dry mouth, and decreased appetite. Bulimia is an important symptom of the Klüver-Bucy syndrome of bilateral temporal lobe dysfunction; it may also be present with other cerebral disorders. The **Kleine – Levin syndrome** consists of periodic attacks of hypersomnia accompanied by bulimia, irritability, behavioral changes, and uninhibited sexuality. It usually occurs in young males. A hypothalamic abnormality is suspected, although the basic etiology is unknown. Lesions of the anterior and midline nuclei may cause gastric atony, increased gastric secretions, mucosal hemorrhages, and gastric ulcerations, and also esophageal and intestinal ulcerations and intussusception. Such phenomena may also be associated with cortical lesions, involvement of the medullary centers, and vagal irritation. Projectile vomiting is often associated with increased intracranial pressure, probably the result of pressure on medullary centers. The epigastric aura of epilepsy and the gustatory and olfactory hallucinations and smacking and tasting movements of complex partial seizures are caused by cortical discharges. So-called abdominal epilepsy and migraine may also be caused by cortical discharges. Marasmus and anorexia nervosa may in some instances be associated with hypothalamic lesions.

Disturbances of Bladder Function

Although the hypothalamus undoubtedly plays an important part in bladder function, not much is known concerning the clinical manifestations of vesical disturbances in hypothalamic disease. The relationship of the cerebrum, especially the paracentral lobules, is better known. The types of bladder dysfunction that follow cerebral lesions have been described earlier in this chapter.

Disturbances of the Sleep Cycle

The hypothalamus, especially its posterior portions, including the mammillary bodies, is important in the maintenance of normal sleep rhythm, and hypothalamic lesions may cause hypersomnia, inversion of the sleep cycle, or insomnia. Stimulation of the posterior hypothalamus has been reported to cause hypersomnia and also arousal and wakefulness. It is difficult, however, to isolate the part that the hypothalamus plays in the regulation of sleep from that of the closely adjacent and even overlapping ascending reticular activating system and the diffuse thalamocortical projection system (Ch. 50). The hypersomnia and other abnormalities of sleep that have been reported with hypothalamic lesions may not result from lesions of this structure alone, but also, or instead, may be due to involvement of the midbrain reticular system, or to interruption of the pathways from the cortex to the hypothalamus, or the mammillary peduncle or the mammillotegmental tract.

Hypersomnia is found in acute encephalitis, post-traumatic states, increased intracranial pressure, Wernicke's syndrome, intoxication by barbiturates and other soporifics, and brain tumors, especially those in the region of the third ventricle. Inversion of the sleep cycle may also occur in encephalitis. **Narcolepsy** and **cataplexy** have been described in association with lesions of the posterior hypothalamus, but in nearly all cases the mechanism for the excessive sleepiness and the associated components of narcolepsy — cataplexy, sleep paralysis, and hypnagogic hallucinations — remains unknown. A hereditary predisposition has been described. It has been suggested that the hypersomnia of the Klein-Levin syndrome is due to hypothalamic disturbances. So-called activated or paradoxical sleep (Ch. 54), which is accompanied by rapid eye movements, a low-voltage electroencephalographic pattern, dreaming, and motor inhibition, probably has its origin in the reticular formation.

Disturbances of Sexual Function

Sexual infantilism may occur as an isolated phenomenon or as a part of Fröhlich's and other syndromes. It is a manifestation of damage to the nuclei in the middle portion of the tuberal region. Sexual precocity has been described as a characteristic symptom of the pineal syndrome; the hypothalamus, however, is the critical site for lesions causing pubertas praecox, and it is probably due to pressure on or involvement of the ventromedial and lateral tuberal nuclei and mammillary bodies. Both sexual infantilism and sexual precocity may be manifestations of dysfunction of the endocrine glands, especially the pituitary, gonads, and adrenal glands; such changes may be secondary to underlying hypothalamic involvement. Increased libido, decreased libido, impotence, amenorrhea, hypermenorrhea, and other manifestations of sexual dysfunction are sometimes partly hypothalamic in origin. The somatic manifestations of the orgasm may be due to hypothalamic stimulation.

Disturbances of the Emotions

The hypothalamus is the center that reinforces and coordinates the neural and humoral mechanisms of emotional expression. When the posterior portion of the hypothalamus is released from control by higher centers of the brain, a complex of primitive pseudoaffective reactions takes place. This phenomenon can be exhibited in experimental animals by the production of "sham rage," with pupillary dilation, increased pulse rate and blood pressure, piloerection, and other signs of sympathetic activity. These physical manifestations suggest that an intense emotional reaction is taking place, but there may be merely a motor expression of rage without a change in affect. Similar manifestations have been produced by stimulation of the posterior and lateral hypothalamic areas and by bilateral removal of the frontal or temporal lobes. Abnormal affective and emotional reactions, fear, and aggressive behavior, however, may also be lessened by interruption of the pathways connecting various cortical areas in the frontal and limbic lobes with the thalamus and hypothalamus.

In **autonomic,** or **diencephalic, epilepsy** there are paroxysmal attacks characterized by flushing, lacrimation, perspiration, salivation, contraction and dilation of the pupils, pilomotor disturbances, either chills or hyperthermia, changes in pulse rate and blood pressure, gastrointestinal disturbances, urinary incontinence or frequency, abnormalities of respiration, and occasionally loss of consciousness. These symptoms have been attributed to hypothalamic stimulation. Similar autonomic symptoms occur in complex partial seizures originating elsewhere.

The physical concomitants of emotion, namely, tachycardia, tachypnea, elevation of the blood pressure, perspiration, flushing, piloerection, and various disturbances of gastrointestinal function, are in reality manifestations of hypothalamic function with secondary visceral effects. It has been found that anxiety, resentment, and anger are accompanied by increased adrenergic substances in the blood, whereas tension and possibly fear are associated with increased cholinergic chemicals. In emotional disturbances associated with psychopathologic states these adrenergic and cholinergic responses are exaggerated. In many of the neuroses the symptoms are largely somatic, or vegetative, in nature, and are similar to the physical symptoms encountered in various emotional states. Those referable to the cardiorespiratory system include tachycardia, palpitation, dyspnea, irregular respiration, and pain in the chest. Those referable to the gastrointestinal tract consist of gaseous indigestion, pain, nausea, vomiting, pylorospasm, hyperacidity, spastic constipation, flatulent constipation, and diarrhea. Those referable to the genitourinary system include frequency, dysuria, impotence, lack of libido, amenorrhea, and frigidity. The symptoms of the anxiety neuroses or of normal individuals during periods of stress, namely, tension, palpitation, hyperpnea, nausea, frequency, mydriasis, cold hands and feet, dry mouth, and variable blood pressure, are often the result of hypothalamic stimulation. All are symptoms of autonomic imbalance, and may be of central origin. Many disease syndromes such as hypertension, coronary artery disease, hyperthyroidism, peptic ulcer disease, spastic constipation, ulcerative colitis, migraine, bronchial asthma, and arthritis may have definite psychosomatic correlations. The hypothalamus plays a large part in their development, either primarily or secondarily, even though its relationship to the disease process and the correlation between the organic process and the psychogenic manifestations are not known.

There is also evidence suggesting that disturbances of function of the hypothalamus and of the limbic, septal, and related areas of the brain may bear a causal relationship to the development of certain psychiatric syndromes. Lesions of the anterior portion of the hypothalamus tend to produce excitement, whereas posterior lesions may be accompanied by lethargy, indifference, depression, and possibly even catatonic manifestations. Stimulation of these areas, both in experimental animals and man, may cause emotional responses as well as signs of autonomic nervous system activity. Abnormal recordings have been obtained from electrodes implanted in the septal region of schizophrenic patients. Certain drugs and toxins that act upon the hypothalamus and the reticular formation can cause hallucinations and other symptoms of mental disease, whereas other drugs that act upon these same areas can relieve many of the symptoms associated with the psychoses.

Regardless of the actual or proved relationship of the autonomic nervous system, and especially of the hypothalamus and its cortical influences, to psychiatric disorders, it must be assumed that it has a close relationship to the emotional state and its abnormalities. Whether or not one's emotional life is determined by the functional activity and balance of the hypothalamus and the autonomic nervous system, it can be stated without doubt that many physical symptoms occurring in normal and pathologic emotional states are those of autonomic nervous system activity. Changes in personality varying from depression to manic states and the major psychoses may be in part related to hypothalamic dysfunction. Interruption of the pathways between the frontal cortex and the thalamus and hypothalamus has been used in the past for treatment of certain psychotic states.

Disturbances of Endocrine Function

The hypothalamus is closely related, both anatomically and functionally, to the hypophysis, or pituitary gland. It produces vasopressin and oxytocin, which are stored in the posterior lobe of the pituitary, and secretes the various hormone-releasing factors acting on the anterior lobe. Consequently abnormalities of hypothalamic function may have a close relationship to the various disturbances of endocrine function.

With disease of the pituitary gland there are signs and symptoms of either overactivity or underactivity of the gland itself, and symptoms and signs of target gland dysfunction, as well as associated hypothalamic disturbances. Either hyperactivity of the pituitary or an eosinophilic adenoma of the anterior lobe can cause gigantism or acromegaly. With an adenoma of the chromophobe cells there are generalized endocrine changes, with obesity, diminished metabolism, impotence or decreased sexual desire in the male, and amenorrhea in the female. An adenoma of the basophilic cells along with elevated blood cortisol levels and corticotropin levels causes **Cushing's syndrome,** with obesity, hypertension, amenorrhea, hypertrichosis, polycythemia, and weakness. Similar symptoms may be present with neoplasms of the adrenal glands, ovaries, and testicles, and with involvement of the paraventricular nuclei of the hypothalamus. Deficiency of the pituitary in a child may cause **Lorain's syndrome,** or dwarfism. A deficiency of either growth hormone or growth-hormone releasing factor may contribute to dwarfism or small stature. In the **Prader – Willi syndrome** the releasing factor is deficient. In **Simmonds' disease,** or **pituitary cachexia,** atro-

phy of the pituitary causes symptoms of adrenocortical, gonadal, and thyroid deficiency, with anorexia, weakness, emaciation, loss of sexual functions, and premature aging. In **Sheehan's syndrome,** or ischemic necrosis of the anterior lobe of the pituitary following childbirth or severe postpartum hemorrhage, the symptoms are similar, but appear more rapidly. Hypophysectomy, or complete ablation of the pituitary, has been carried out in the treatment of severe diabetes mellitus, diabetic retinopathy, and advanced carcinomatosis of the breast and ovaries.

The nuclei of the hypothalamus regulate the internal secretions of the thyroid, adrenal, and other glands by production of the hormone-releasing factors mentioned earlier. The hypothalamus, either directly or through the pituitary, may play a part in the development of either hyperthyroidism or hypothyroidism. Lesions of the hypothalamus may affect the islet cells of the pancreas, causing either diabetes mellitus or hyperinsulinism with hypoglycemia. The effect on the sexual glands may be direct, rather than through the pituitary, and may cause sexual precocity, impotence, amenorrhea, deficient development of primary or secondary sexual characteristics, and sexual infantilism.

MISCELLANEOUS DISTURBANCES OF AUTONOMIC FUNCTION

There are other disturbances of function that seem to be related, in part at least, to abnormalities of the autonomic nervous system. These cannot, however, be attributed specifically to either peripheral or central lesions.

Allergic Disturbances

The predominant autonomic manifestations of allergy are vasodilation and exudation. In cutaneous manifestations, such as urticaria, eczema, and angioneurotic edema, there is exudation. In hay fever and allergic rhinitis there is vasodilation, with hypersecretion of the mucous membranes and lacrimal glands. In asthma there is spasm of the bronchial musculature together with vasodilation and mucosal exudation. Many of these manifestations are alleviated by the use of parasympathetic depressants, sympathomimetic drugs, and antihistamine compounds. There is also a close relation between anaphylaxis and the autonomic nervous system.

Trophic Disorders

In addition to trophic disorders that involve the skin and blood vessels there are trophic disturbances of autonomic origin that affect the bones, joints, and muscles. They are usually associated with lesions of the motor or sensory nerves or both, but involvement of the autonomic, or trophic, fibers is responsible for the pathologic changes.

Trophic changes involving the bones and joints were once seen most frequently in tabes dorsalis. They occasionally develop in association with syringomyelia, spinal cord tumors and other spinal lesions, and in diabetic neuropathy and other types of peripheral neuropathy. There is first an osteoporosis accompanied by an abnormal brittleness of the bones that may lead to spontaneous fractures, but the most characteristic changes are those in the joints. There are secretory disturbances of the synovia with swelling of the joints, destruction of joint surfaces and ligaments, atrophy of cartilage or bone, and often painless intraarticular fractures and dislocations; this is known as **Charcot's arthropathy.** With posttraumatic and other peripheral nerve lesions there may be osteoporosis (**Sudeck's atrophy** or **reflex sympathetic dystrophy**). Osteoporosis, osteomalacia, and osteitis fibrosa cystica may occur with parathyroid dysfunction.

Primary atrophy of the muscle is a result of disease of the voluntary motor system. In disease of the autonomic nervous system, however, there may be muscle atrophy associated with trophic changes in the skin and subcutaneous tissues. In **Volkmann's contracture,** or **ischemic paralysis,** there is muscle atrophy due to loss of nutrition and decreased oxygenation of the muscles, and this may be accompanied by changes in the skin and subcutaneous tissues, with cyanosis, coldness, edema, fibrous change in the subcutaneous tissue, etc. Later there is fibrous transformation of the muscles and tendons, with resulting deformities. These changes are out of proportion to the involvement of the motor and sensory nerves.

Either **hemiatrophy** or **hemihypertrophy** may involve one half of the face or one half of the face and body. There is atrophy of the skin, subcutaneous tissues, muscles, and bones. There may be alopecia and scleroderma in the atrophic areas. However, many cases are not accompanied by symptoms suggesting autonomic nervous system dysfunction, and the cause of hemiatrophy and hemihypertrophy remains unknown.

Other Disorders of the Autonomic Nervous System

Familial Dysautonomia. Familial dysautonomia, or the **Riley – Day syndrome,** is inherited as an autosomal recessive trait and is virtually limited to persons of Ashkenazi Jewish extraction. It is a rare disease of infancy and childhood. Manifestations associated with autonomic nervous system dysfunction include excessive perspiration, reduced lacrimation, peripheral vascular disturbances, postural hypotension, erratic temperature control, blotchy skin, and disturbed swallowing reflex. In addition there are other neurologic abnormalities including areflexia, poor coordination, hypogeusia, dysarthria, relative indifference to pain, and corneal anesthesia, and also emotional lability, retardation of physical and psychologic development, and absence of fungiform papillae on the tongue. Pathologic alterations have been found in the peripheral autonomic nervous system and in the spinal cord. A variety of tests give abnormal results in familial dysautonomia. There is little or no reaction to the intradermal injection of histamine and an exaggerated hypertensive response to the injection of norepinephrine and related drugs. Urinary excretion of 3-methoxy-4-hydroxymandelic acid is low, while excretion of homovanillic acid is normal or slightly elevated. Patients show no increase in plasma norepinephrine levels after rising from the recumbent position, standing, or performing isometric exercises, and less than the normal rise in plasma dopamine hydroxylase after assuming an upright position and after performing isometric exercises.

Autonomic Visceral Neuropathy. Certain peripheral neuropathies that are severe in degree may affect the autonomic nerves also, and cause an autonomic visceral neuropathy. This syndrome is found most often in diabetic neuropathy, but may also be present in alcoholic and familial amyloid neuropathies and other severe and long-standing polyneuropathies. The following abnormalities may be present: Involvement of the skin and subcutaneous tissues, with anhidrosis, loss of pilomotor and vasomotor control, abnormal texture and consistency of the skin, dependent edema, and loss of the histamine flare response; gastrointestinal abnormalities including achlorhydria, gastric retention, disturbed motility of the gastrointestinal tract, and either diarrhea or constipation; genitourinary symptoms including disturbances of bladder and sphincter control, either incontinence or retention, and impotence; orthostatic hypotension; and lesions of bones and joints, including the development of Charcot's arthropathy. The pupillary abnormalities frequently found in diabetic patients (miosis, anisocoria, sluggish response to light) are also evidence of autonomic, mainly sympathetic, neuropathy. Pathologic alterations have been found in both preganglionic and postganglionic fibers as well as in the sympathetic chain in persons with diabetic autonomic visceral neuropathy.

Syndromes of acute autonomic neuropathy and of "pure pandysautonomia" have been described, but their clinical manifestations have not been thoroughly reported and no pathologic confirmation is as yet available. Further delineation of these entities is necessary. An experimental autonomic neuropathy has been induced in rabbits immunized with human sympathetic ganglia.

The syndrome of autonomic dysreflexia or hyperreflexia is occasionally seen in patients with a transverse lesion of the spinal cord. It is an exaggeration of the reflex of spinal automatism and is usually precipitated by overdistention of the bladder. There is increased flexion at the hips and knees, hyperhidrosis, penile erection, marked rise in the blood pressure, and reflex headache. There is often an increase in the intracranial pressure, and intracranial hemorrhage has occurred during an episode. The symptoms can be controlled by the use of α-adrenergic blocking agents such as phentolamine.

BIBLIOGRAPHY

Adams RD, Victor M. Principles of Neurology, 4th ed. New York, McGraw – Hill, 1989

Alio J, Hernandez I, Millan A, Sanchez J. Pupil responsiveness in diabetes mellitus. Ann Ophthalmol 1989;21:132

Anderson M, Salmon MV. Symptomatic cataplexy. J Neurol Neurosurg Psychiatry 1977;40:186

Appenzeller O. "Pure pan-dysautonomia": A newly discovered syndrome. CA Med 1972;117:18

Appenzeller O, Arnason BG, Adams RD. Experimental autonomic neuropathy: An experimentally induced disorder of vasomotor function. J Neurol Neurosurg Psychiatry 1965;28:510

Appenzeller O, Richardson EP Jr. The sympathetic chain in patients with diabetic and alcoholic polyneuropathy. Neurology 1966;16:205

Bannister R, Ardill L, Fentem P. Defective autonomic control of blood vessels in idiopathic orthostatic hypotension. Brain 1967;90:725

Biaggioni I, Goldstein DS, Atkinson T, Robertson D. Dopamine-beta-hydroxylase deficiency in humans. Neurology 1990;40:370

Bradley WE, Rockswold GL, Timm GW, Scott FB. Neurology of micturition. J Urol 1976;115:481

Brouwer B. Positive and negative aspects of hypothalamic disorders. J Neurol Neurosurg Psychiatry 1950;13:16

Cushing H. Papers Relating to the Pituitary Body, Hypothalamus and Parasympathetic Nervous System. Springfield, IL, Charles C Thomas, 1932

DeJong RN. The neurologic manifestations of diabetes mellitus. In Vinken PJ, Bruyn GW, Klawans HL (eds). Handbook of Clinical Neurology. Vol 27. Metabolic and Deficiency Diseases of the Nervous System. Amsterdam, North Holland, 1976

Drummond PD. Autonomic disturbances in cluster headaches. Brain 1988;111:1199

Echlin F, Owens FMR, Wells WL. Observations on "major" and "minor" causalgia. Arch Neurol Psychiatry 1949;62:183

Ellenberg M. Retrograde ejaculation in diabetic neuropathy. Ann Intern Med 1966;65:1237

Fisher C, Ingram WR, Ranson SW. Diabetes insipidus and the neurohormonal control of water balance: A contribution to the structure and function of the hypothalamico-hypophysial system. Ann Arbor, MI, Edwards Brothers, 1938

Fogelson MH, Rorke LB, Kaye R. Spinal cord changes in familial dysautonomia. Arch Neurol 1967;17:103

Garland H, Sumner D, Forman RP. The Kleine – Levin syndrome. Neurology 1965;15:1161

Gellhorn E. Analysis of autonomic hypothalamic functions in the intact organism. Neurology 1956;6:335

Green JD. Neural pathways to the hypophysis. In Fields WS, Guillemin R, Carton CA (eds). Hypothalamic-Hypophysial Interrelationships. Springfield, IL, Charles C Thomas, 1956

Heath RG (ed). Studies in Schizophrenia: A multidisciplinary Approach to Mind – Brain Relationships. Cambridge, MA, Harvard University Press, 1954

Hemingway A, Price WM. The autonomic nervous system and regulation of body temperature. Anesthesiology 1968;29:693

Johnson RH, Lambie DG, Spalding JMK. The autonomic nervous system. In Joynt RJ (ed). Clinical Neurology. Philadelphia, JB Lippincott, 1989

Kleeman CR, Fichman MP. The clinical physiology of water metabolism. N Engl J Med 1967;277:1300

Kurchin A, Adar R, Mozes M. Gustatory phenomena after upper dorsal sympathectomy. Arch Neurol 1977;34:619

Kursh ED, Freehafer A, Persky L. Complications of autonomic dysreflexia. J Urol 1977;118:70

Lapides J. Cystometry. JAMA 1967;201:618

Lewis P. Familial orthostatic hypotension. Brain 1964;87:719

Mclean PD. The limbic system ("visceral brain") and emotional behavior. Arch Neurol Psychiatry 1955;73:130

Martin JB, Travis RH, Van den Noort S. Centrally mediated orthostatic hypotension. Arch Neurol 1968;19:163

Masserman JH. The hypothalamus in psychiatry. Am J Psychiatry 1942;98:633

Mayfield FH. Causalgia. Springfield, IL, Charles C Thomas, 1951

Olsson Y, Sourander P. Changes in the sympathetic nervous system in diabetes mellitus: A preliminary report. J Neurovis Relat 1968;31:86

Plum F, Colfelt RH. The genesis of vesical rhythmicity. Arch Neurol 1960;2:487

Poussaint AF, Ditman KS. A controlled study of imipramine (Tofranil) in the treatment of childhood enuresis. J Pediatr 1965;67:283

Riley CM, Day RL, Greeley DM et al. Central autonomic dysfunction with defective lacrimation. I Report of five cases. Pediatrics 1949;3:468

Ross AT. Progressive selective sudomotor denervation: A case with coexisting Adie's syndrome. Neurology 1958;8:809

Seddon H. Volkmann's ischemia. Br Med J 1964;1:1587

Selye H. The general adaptation syndrome and diseases of adaptation. J Clin Endocr 1946;6:117

Shy GM, Drager GA. A neurological syndrome associated with orthostatic hypotension. Arch Neurol 1960;2:511

Solitare GB, Cohen GS. Peripheral nervous system lesions in congenital or familial dysautonomia. Neurology 1972;15:321

Tahmoush AJ, Malley J, Jennings JR. Skin conductance, temperature, and blood flow in causalgia. Neurology 1983;33:1483

Thomashefsky AJ, Horwitz SJ, Feingold MN. Acute autonomic neuropathy. Neurology 1972;22:251

Young RR, Asbury AK, Adams RD. Pure pan-dysautonomia with recovery. Trans Am Neurol Assoc 1969;94:355

PART G

Diagnosis and Localization of Disorders of the Peripheral Nerves, Nerve Roots, and Spinal Cord

To make an accurate neurologic diagnosis the physician must not only establish the presence of a lesion, but also, if possible, must localize the lesion accurately in either the central or the peripheral nervous system. Following this, attempts to determine the nature and etiology of the process are essential. Disorders of the nervous system may affect either its peripheral portions — the individual nerves and the nerve roots; or its central portions — the cerebrospinal axis, including the spinal cord, brain stem, midbrain, cerebellum, and cerebrum. Neurologic localization depends upon the determination of the exact site or sites of involvement of the nervous system.

To localize a lesion of the peripheral nerves one must know the anatomy and physiology of the nerves. Accurate delineation of the site of involvement depends upon specific sensory, motor, trophic, vasomotor, and reflex changes. This is also true of the nerve roots and of the larger nerve trunks in the major plexuses. To localize a lesion within the spinal cord one must be familiar not only with the cross-sectional anatomy of the cord, the cellular distribution in the gray matter, and the principal ascending and descending fiber pathways in the white matter, but also with the details of the longitudinal anatomy and the segmental supply of the sensory, motor, and autonomic functions.

The discussions that follow deal with the approaches to localization employed in the clinical examination of the patient at the bedside or in the office. Great progress has been made in recent years in electrodiagnostic and imaging tests that can help to delineate and localize lesions further in the central and peripheral portions of the nervous system. These tests cannot replace the neurologic examination; they supplement it. Their description, indications, and usefulness are found in texts devoted to the various studies. In regard to the peripheral nerves, nerve roots, and spinal cord, electromyography, nerve conduction studies, and somatosensory evoked potential studies can help to localize and qualitatively identify lesions. Nerve conduction studies specifically address disturbances of the peripheral nerves up to the nerve roots, identifying blocks, disruption of conduction, or slowing of conduction of motor and sensory fibers in various neuropathies. Electromyography helps in the delineation of disorders of the anterior horn cells and their respective motor units by detecting electrical signs of degeneration such as fibrillations and abnormal motor unit potentials. Sensory evoked potentials can help further to identify disturbances of conduction proximally at various levels of the neuraxis. Finally, the imaging procedures, especially computed tomography and magnetic resonance studies, supplemented at times by myelography and spine roentgenograms, help to visualize structural lesions, distortions, deteriorations, and other pathologic processes affecting the spinal cord, the nerve roots and plexuses, and their environment. The most effective use of these and other tests comes after the most precise clinical localization has been made by the neurologic examination.

Chapter 43
DISORDERS OF THE PERIPHERAL NERVES

ANATOMY, PHYSIOLOGY, AND PATHOPHYSIOLOGY OF THE PERIPHERAL NERVES

A typical peripheral nerve has mixed functions. That is, it conducts sensory, motor, and autonomic impulses. The anatomic, physiologic, and clinical characteristics of the cranial nerves are discussed individually in Part C, "The Cranial Nerves." The peripheral spinal, or segmental, nerves are considered in the present part.

The motor components of the peripheral nerves arise in the anterior horn cells of the spinal cord and travel in the converging filaments of the ventral spinal root. They are ultimately distributed to striated muscles. The sensory components arise in the various receptors or endorgans; they have their cell bodies in the dorsal root ganglia and enter the spinal cord through the dorsal roots. The ventral and dorsal roots unite to form the mixed spinal nerve. After this has passed through the intervertebral foramen it divides into anterior and posterior primary branches or rami. These rami subdivide to supply muscular and sensory structures (see Fig. 40-1). The autonomic components of the twelve thoracic and upper two or three lumbar segments of the spinal cord (sympathetic division) arise from the cells in the intermediolateral column. They exit with the ventral roots of the corresponding segmental nerves and traverse the mixed spinal nerve to reach the anterior primary ramus. Here they split off from the proximal part of this ramus as finely myelinated fibers (white rami communicantes) and enter the ganglionated sympathetic chain. The postganglionic fibers are unmyelinated (gray rami communicantes); on reaching the anterior primary ramus they split into two groups, one going with the anterior and the other with the posterior primary ramus. Other autonomic fibers, both those of the parasympathetic division and those from the prevertebral plexuses and collateral ganglia, join the mixed nerves peripherally, although fibers of the sacral portion of the parasympathetic division enter the mixed nerves with the ventral roots.

The posterior primary rami are smaller than the anterior ones. They supply the dorsal structures of the body, including the skin of the posterior surfaces and the longitudinal muscles associated with the axial skeleton. The anterior primary rami are really continuations of the mixed nerves. They supply the ventral and lateral muscles and the skin of the ventrolateral aspects of the body. In the region of the extremities they form the plexuses that innervate the limbs. The anterior primary rami of the thoracic segments of the spinal cord are continued as the intercostal nerves. The lack of correspondence between the spinal segments and their emerging fibers and the spinous processes of the vertebrae is discussed elsewhere (Ch. 5 and Fig. 5-11).

Disorders of the peripheral nerves are characterized by diminution or loss of certain functions and/or by disturbances of function. These changes are secondary either to impairment or interruption of the conduction of impulses through the nerves, or to irritation.

Diminution or loss of function may involve interference with both efferent and afferent impulses. Interference with conduction of efferent impulses causes motor and autonomic changes. Motor changes are characterized by paresis or paralysis of certain muscles or muscle groups. This paresis is focal, is often complete for the muscles involved, and is hypotonic, or flaccid, in character. It may be accompanied or followed by atrophy, abnormal findings on electromyographic examination, and a decrease in motor nerve conduction velocities, and eventually in pathologically identifiable changes in the nerve itself and in the muscles innervated. Autonomic changes result in sudomotor, pilomotor, and vasomotor paralysis, with dryness of the skin, vasodilation, and loss of piloerection. Later there may be cyanosis, edema, secretory and temperature disturbances, and trophic changes in the skin, subcutaneous tissues, hair, and nails, and sometimes in the blood vessels, bones, and joints. Involvement of either parasympathetic or sympathetic fibers that mediate specific visceral and other impulses may cause widespread disturbances of autonomic function. Interference with the conduction of afferent impulses produces impairment or loss of pain, temperature, tactile, pressure, and proprioceptive sensibility, along with slowed or absent sensory nerve conduction and evoked potentials. Interference with the conduction of either efferent or afferent impulses may cause a loss of reflexes.

Disturbances of function may also involve either efferent or afferent impulses. They may be caused by irritation, incomplete loss of conduction, or partial assumption of function by intact elements. Disturbances in the function of motor impulses may produce muscular twitchings (fasciculations), muscle spasm, or reflex rigidity. Abnormal function of efferent autonomic impulses causes alterations of sweating, vasomotor changes, glossy skin, and edema. Disturbances of function of the afferent fibers produce spontaneous pain, paresthesias, phantom sensations, and abnormal responses to heat and cold.

Nerves may be injured by trauma to the neuron or its neuraxis, or by pressure, chemical, thermal, or toxic influences, interruption of blood supply, infectious processes, or deficiency of substances normally required for nerve metabolism. Injuries to nerves may vary in degree and extent, and are classified variously. Complete division of a peripheral nerve is known as **neurotmesis.** There is an interruption of continuity in all essential structures, with complete loss of conduction of both efferent and afferent impulses. This leads to complete and permanent degeneration of the nerve. In **axonotmesis** the

function of the axons, or nerve fibers, is lost, with resulting peripheral degeneration of the conducting structures of the nerve, but the supporting tissues, the epineurium and endoneurium, are preserved. Spontaneous recovery may occur, and during regeneration the nerve fibers follow their original channels. In **neurapraxia** there is a transient block or interruption of continuity resulting from compression or blows by blunt instruments. This is a minimal lesion that does not produce complete paralysis and is not accompanied by peripheral degeneration, although there may be some loss of myelin; recovery is rapid and complete.

Most if not all peripheral nerves of any size are myelinated. When such a nerve is cut or severed from its cell body, certain changes take place, and there is **Wallerian degeneration** distal to the point of transection. The myelin sheath swells, retracts, becomes fragmented, and breaks down into lipoid material. The neurofibrillae of the axon become swollen and fragmented. The neurilemmal sheaths of Schwann multiply; the sheath hypertrophies and fills up the space formerly occupied by the myelin, and the cells assume phagocytic activity. Within 1 – 3 months the fibers and myelin have completely disappeared, and the motor end-plates have degenerated. The neurilemmal sheath and the connective tissue septa of the nerve are left. The proximal segment of the nerve degenerates for only a short distance. If the injury is close to the cell body, the latter may undergo chromatolysis. Regeneration, if it takes place, proceeds distally from the central stump, and the growing fibers penetrate the scar tissue and enter the empty sheath. Functional maturation of the axonal pathway (myelination and restoration of fiber diameter) proceeds more slowly than regrowth of the axis fibers. Regeneration is facilitated by suturing the nerve. The rate of growth varies with different nerves, and atrophy of muscle has an adverse effect on restoration of function. If tissue is interposed and there is some obstruction to regeneration, or if the nerve has been completely severed, a neuroma may develop at the distal end of the proximal segment. Regeneration of any clinical importance does not take place within the central nervous system.

There is a difference in the diameter of the various nerve fibers, and this is accompanied by a variability in the rate of conduction of impulses and in the refractory period, and by a difference in vulnerability to various types of injury. The greater the diameter of the fibers, the faster the speed of conduction. The A group is the largest and its fibers are most susceptible to anoxia and pressure. The group is subdivided into α-, β-, γ-, and δ-fibers. The α-fibers are the largest, about 16 μ in diameter; the smallest, the δ- fibers, are 1 – 2 μ in diameter and carry fast pain impulses. The B group of small myelinated fibers (about 3 μ) are found in the autonomic nervous system. The smallest unmyelinated C fibers are 0.3 – 1.3 μ in diameter. They carry "second" or slow pain. Cocaine, which blocks the conduction of the smaller fibers first, causes loss of sensation in the order of slow pain, cold, warmth, fast pain, touch, and position. Pressure, which blocks the conduction of the large fibers first, causes loss of sensation in the order of position, vibration, pressure, touch, fast pain, cold, warmth, and slow pain, followed by vasomotor paralysis.

The diagnosis and localization of peripheral nerve lesions depends upon the recognition and delineation of changes in function. Diminution or loss of function produces changes that are more outstanding and more apparent objectively than changes resulting from disturbances of function. To determine the presence of involvement of peripheral nerves, and to ascertain the site, one must use portions of the neurologic examination that have already been described. It is important to recognize the nerve or nerves involved, to estimate the degree of damage, and to determine whether the dysfunction is progressing or lessening, and whether spontaneous recovery may be expected or surgical treatment is required. It is necessary to be familiar with the peripheral nerve, plexus, and nerve root supply to the individual muscles and to cutaneous areas in order to differentiate between peripheral nerve, plexus, radicular, and spinal cord lesions.

The sensory examination must be performed carefully and completely (Part B, "The Sensory System"), and the examiner should be familiar with the cutaneous distribution of the more important peripheral nerves (Fig. 5-6). There may be loss or diminution of all types of sensation. The exteroceptive sensations are more important than the proprioceptive ones, especially in lesions restricted to the smaller nerves or to the individual branches of the larger nerves, but with extensive involvement the proprioceptive changes are also significant. There may be areas of anesthesia, hypesthesia, or hyperesthesia corresponding to the sensory distribution of the nerves involved. One must, however, bear in mind the individual variation in areas supplied

by the peripheral nerves (Fig. 5-7), and the algesic overlap (Fig. 5-8). Occasionally there is a spread of the sensory loss beyond the field of the injured nerve. With incomplete and irritative lesions there may be either paresthesias or pain. The latter may be dull, sharp, steady, or intermittent, but is often stabbing or lancinating in character. Pain and numbness may be present simultaneously. The nerves themselves may be hyperalgesic and sensitive, or tender to pressure, and the associated muscles and tendons may show tenderness to pressure. Tender areas along the course of affected nerves have been called **Valleix's points.** Pain in the distribution of a single nerve or group of nerves may be relieved by section of the nerves involved or by injection of local anesthetic or alcohol; to prevent regeneration the nerve should be sectioned central to the dorsal root ganglion.

The motor examination is directed especially toward the recognition of loss or impairment of function of specific muscles or muscle groups. The examiner should be familiar with the nerve supply of the individual muscles, and should test the muscles for active motor power (Ch. 27, Tables 27-1 through 27-4). In addition it is important to note tone, volume and contour, hyperkinetic phenomena, contractures, and abnormalities of position. The electromyographic and nerve conduction velocity determinations are often of great importance in outlining the extent, location, and severity of involvement.

Special tests of autonomic nervous system function are sometimes indicated. Trophic changes such as dryness of the skin, and abnormalities in its texture, cyanosis, hyperhidrosis, hypertrichosis, loss of hair, brittle nails, ulcerations, slow healing, and edema should always be noted.

The muscle stretch and superficial reflexes must be tested, as well as appropriate autonomic nervous system reflexes. Palpation of the involved nerves is an important part of the examination. The size, tenderness, and consistency should be noted, and abnormalities of contour, irritability, thickening, and atrophy or hypertrophy evaluated. There may be pain on passive stretching of the nerves. In the hypertrophic neuritis of Dejerine and Sottas and other rare conditions there is hyperplasia of the involved nerves. Neuromas and neurofibromas are often palpable. Tenderness of the muscles and tendons may be associated with nerve tenderness. Occasionally both muscle and nerve biopsies give pertinent information. In peripheral involvement of the cranial nerves special methods of examination are carried out (Part C, "The Cranial Nerves").

There are syndromes of interruption, compression, contusion, concussion, and irritation of the peripheral nerves. In **complete interruption** of the continuity of a nerve there is an immediate, complete paralysis of all muscles supplied by it. This is followed by loss of tone and progressive atrophy. Spasm and overactivity of the antagonistic muscles may cause contractures. There is also an immediate, complete anesthesia, with absence of pain when pressure is applied to the nerve distal to the lesion. Autonomic functions disappear. Reflexes, both muscle stretch and superficial, are lost if either the afferent or efferent portion of the arc traverses the involved nerve, but muscular irritability may be increased. There usually is no pain. With **partial interruption** there often is clinical evidence of complete loss of function for a period of time after the injury, following which the intact fibers resume normal conduction of impulses. The injured fibers may not regain their functions, and irritative phenomena and trophic changes may appear. The objective findings vary according to the degree and site of injury; motor, sensory, or autonomic changes may predominate.

In the syndrome of **compression** there may be either complete or incomplete paralysis, with variable sensory changes. Tone is preserved; atrophy, reflex changes, and pain may or may not be present. If the compression is abrupt but is relieved promptly, there will be progressive recovery of function. On the other hand, compression by callus formation or scar tissue, and entrapment at a point where a nerve goes through a fibrous or osseofibrous tunnel or changes its course over a fibrous or muscular band, may cause progressive impairment leading to complete loss of function. In **contusion** there is rupture of the fibers within a nerve trunk, with or without hemorrhage. Mild contusions are manifested by incomplete loss of function with progressive recovery; severe ones may cause complete loss of function. **Concussion** is a term signifying temporary derangement of nerve function, partial or complete, without detectable histologic changes. It is most often used to describe cerebral trauma rather than peripheral nerve injuries.

In the syndrome of **irritation** there are variable motor and sensory changes accompanied by pain and hyperesthesia. Tone is preserved, idiomuscular reflexes are increased, and trophic changes may be pronounced. Irritation is usually associated with partial injury, compression, or contusion. Syndromes of irritation are most frequently encountered in the median, tibial, and sciatic nerves. The pain varies in intensity and degree; either heat or cold may increase it.

During regeneration the autonomic fibers are restored first, as shown by improvement in the color and texture of the skin. There may be a return of sensory function before motor regeneration. Protopathic sensations, those mediating gross or poorly localized pain and pressure, return first, whereas the epicritic qualities of tactile discrimination and localization, focal pain sensation, and joint sensibility return later. This view is not universally accepted, and the initial return of sensation may be the result of sensory overlap from the ingrowth of fibers from adjacent uninjured nerves. There may be faulty localization of sensory stimuli during regeneration. The muscles first become painful to pressure, then atrophy is arrested and tone is restored, and finally motor power returns. Those muscles nearest the site of injury or of repair recover first. A careful evaluation of sensory, motor, and autonomic changes may give valuable information about regeneration. **Tinel's sign,** a tingling of the distal portion of a limb on pressure or percussion over the site of a divided nerve, is an early sign. It is elicited most satisfactorily by means of gentle taps with a single finger. The most peripheral point at which this tingling is elicited may be taken roughly as the site to which the fibers have regenerated. Tinel's sign is believed to indicate the presence of young axis cylinders in the process of regeneration. It is considered by many authorities, however, to have doubtful significance; it is often absent, and is sometimes present in spite of complete division of a nerve. Absence of Tinel's sign probably has no diagnostic value; if the sign is present, and if it is found to be advancing peripherally from a nerve lesion, one may assume that regeneration is taking place.

The rate of nerve regeneration is a somewhat disputed subject. It is usually stated that peripheral nerves regenerate at a speed of approximately 1 mm/day, or about 1 in/month. The rate of functional maturation may be more rapid in the early stages of regeneration, and slower in the terminal or distal stages of recovery. The rate is probably not dependent upon fiber size, but on the type and severity of the injury. Neurotization, or nerve growth, proceeds more rapidly than maturation, or return of function. Regeneration is more rapid after simple axonal disruption (axonotmesis) than after complete interruption followed by nerve suture, but under both circumstances the regenerating fibers advance at a progressively diminishing rate.

It may not be possible to tell at the outset, or on the basis of a single examination, whether there has been compression, physiologic interruption without loss of continuity, contusion, partial interruption, or anatomic severance of a nerve. It is often difficult to decide, without repeated examinations, whether degeneration or regeneration is taking place. It is much easier to recognize what nerve or nerves are affected than to ascertain how severely a nerve is injured, whether it will recover spontaneously, or whether an anatomic interruption exists that requires surgical treatment. The sparing of some of the muscles supplied by the involved nerve indicates an incomplete lesion, but this does not necessarily imply the possibility of recovery. On the other hand, a complete loss of function due to pressure or contusion may be followed by rapid, complete recovery. Serial electromyographic and nerve conduction studies can help establish the completeness of lesions and contribute to assessment of early recovery, if any.

LESIONS OF THE PERIPHERAL NERVES

The term **neuritis** is used to denote damage to peripheral nerves regardless of etiology, although many physicians prefer the term **neuropathy** if the damage is not of infectious origin. Involvement of a single peripheral nerve is referred to as **mononeuritis** (or **mononeuropathy**); such focal lesions usually have a mechanical origin. Nerves may be injured by direct trauma such as bullet, cutting, stab, or crushing wounds; severance or tearing from fractures, dislocations, or birth injuries; damage during surgical operations; rupture by either blunt or sharp objects, or injections of drugs or other substances. They may be injured indirectly by crushing, *e.g.,* from a cast or crutch; entrapment; compression by callus formation, scar tissue, tumors, or abscesses; malposition of part of the body during sleep or anesthesia; sudden stretching of an extremity; dislocation of a major joint; or a combination of pressure and stretching in certain positions and occupations. Compression, if sufficient in degree and duration, may lead to degeneration as a result of ischemia; so-called tourniquet paralysis may be caused by either mechanical pressure or ischemia. Stretching of a nerve beyond the limit of physiologic

elasticity causes damage to the epineural vessels, with focal ischemic changes in the nerve fibers. More extensive stretching causes rupture of the perineurium, herniation of the endoneurium, and necrosis of the nerve fibers. Tumors of the peripheral nerves (neuromas, neurofibromas, fibroblastomas, neurofibrosarcomas) may interrupt the continuity of the nerves. **Entrapment neuropathies** are special forms of pressure neuropathy in which nerve injury results from compression by neighboring anatomic structures. The history is essential in determining the etiology of an isolated nerve lesion.

Peripheral nerve involvement is most frequently seen in the extremities, and the physician must be familiar with the sensory distributions, motor supply, and reflex innervation of the major nerves. It is important to remember that the various toxic, infectious, metabolic, deficiency, and vascular disturbances that may cause polyneuritis (see under "Multiple Neuropathy" later in this chapter) may render individual nerves more susceptible to damage by such insults as pressure and stretching. The peripheral nerve lesions encountered following coma and carbon monoxide intoxication may be caused by anoxia superimposed on pressure and vascular insufficiency, and chronic alcoholism, malnutrition, and diabetes may be contributing factors in neuropathies following coma or apparently caused by compression. Trauma of various types, however, is the precipitating cause of most instances of mononeuritis. The major manifestations encountered with involvement of those nerves that are especially vulnerable to mechanical injury are presented in the following discussion.

The Upper Extremities

The Long Thoracic Nerve

This nerve is derived from the fifth through the seventh or eighth cervical segments. It supplies the serratus anterior muscle. It may be injured by continued muscular effort with the arm held above the shoulder, or by pressure from carrying heavy objects or packs on the shoulder, or by supraclavicular or axillary wounds. Involvement of this nerve causes paralysis of the serratus anterior muscle, with resulting winging of the scapula (see Fig. 27-6).

The Axillary Nerve

The axillary or circumflex nerve is derived from the fifth and sixth cervical segments through the posterior cord of the brachial plexus and winds around the neck of the humerus. It supplies the deltoid and teres minor muscles, and transmits sensation from the surface of the upper and outer aspects of the arm. It may be injured by pressure in the axilla, fracture or dislocation of the head of the humerus, perforating wounds, or direct blows against the shoulder; it is commonly affected by the neuritis that follows foreign protein injections. When an axillary nerve lesion is present, there is paralysis of abduction and weakness of external rotation of the arm; the patient is unable to raise his arm to the horizontal plane. There is also some weakness of flexion, extension, and internal rotation. There is anesthesia involving a small area on the upper third of the outer surface of the arm.

The Suprascapular Nerve

This nerve is derived from the fifth and sixth cervical segments through the upper trunk of the brachial plexus. It innervates the supraspinatus and infraspinatus muscles. It may be entrapped as it passes beneath the transverse scapular ligament. The symptoms include pain in the shoulder and weakness and wasting of the supraspinatus and infraspinatus muscles. The symptoms may be relieved by division of the ligament.

The Musculocutaneous Nerve

This nerve is derived from the fifth, sixth, and seventh cervical segments through the lateral cord of the brachial plexus. It innervates the biceps, brachialis, and coracobrachialis muscles, and transmits sensation from the lateral aspect of the forearm extending from the elbow to the thenar eminence. It is not frequently injured. In a musculocutaneous lesion there is weakness of flexion of the forearm if the latter is in supination, and marked weakness of supination. The semipronated forearm can still be flexed by the brachioradialis. There is a relatively small area of anesthesia on the lateral surface of the forearm. The biceps reflex is diminished or absent.

The Radial (Musculospiral) Nerve

This nerve is the largest branch of the brachial plexus and is a continuation of its posterior cord. It is derived from the fifth cervical through the eighth cervical or first thoracic segments. After separating from the other nerves of the plexus, it winds about the humerus in the musculospiral

groove. In the antecubital fossa it divides into its terminal (deep and superficial) branches. It supplies the triceps; the anconeus that functions with the triceps; the brachioradialis; the extensors carpi radialis longus, carpi radialis brevis, carpi ulnaris, digitorum communis, digiti quinti proprius, and indicis proprius; the long and short extensors and the long abductor of the thumb; and the supinator brevis. It transmits sensory impulses from the dorsal aspect of the forearm, wrist, hand, and radial fingers (excluding the middle and distal phalanges), and from the radial aspect of the thenar eminence. Radial nerve paralysis is one of the most common peripheral nerve palsies. The nerve may be affected anywhere along its course. It is commonly injured by pressure in the axilla by a crutch, the back of a chair ("Saturday night palsy"), or dislocation of the shoulder. It may be involved in fractures of the humerus or radius, or in perforating wounds. It may be compressed by callus formation after fracture of the humerus or by pressure just above the wrist, or its branches may be compressed (Fig. 43-1). Radial nerve paralysis is a frequent manifestation of lead neuropathy.

The outstanding manifestation of a radial nerve paralysis is the loss of extension and abduction of the wrist, fingers, and thumb, with, as a result, a characteristic wrist drop. The flexors of the fingers are not impaired, but there is weakness of grip because the patient cannot completely flex his fingers with the wrist in flexion, owing to weakness of the synergists. Extension of the interphalangeal joints is preserved. In the characteristic syndrome the forearm is pronated; the thumb is adducted, flexed, and opposed, and the wrist and fingers are flexed (Fig. 43-2). This deformity is best seen if the forearm is flexed at the elbow. If the lesion is above the nerve supply to the brachioradialis, this muscle is also affected, and there is weakness of flexion of the semipronated forearm, but only slightly impaired supination. In a lesion still higher, there is also involvement of the triceps, so that there is paralysis of all the extensors of the forearm, wrist, and fingers. The sensory manifestations of a radial nerve paralysis are variable and often minimal, owing to overlapping of cutaneous nerves (see Fig. 5-7). The anesthetic area is usually limited to the dorsum of the thumb, although it may involve the dorsum of the radial half or two-thirds of the hand, the first interosseous space and the index finger, and the dorsum of the adjacent proximal phalanges. Trophic changes are minimal. The triceps and

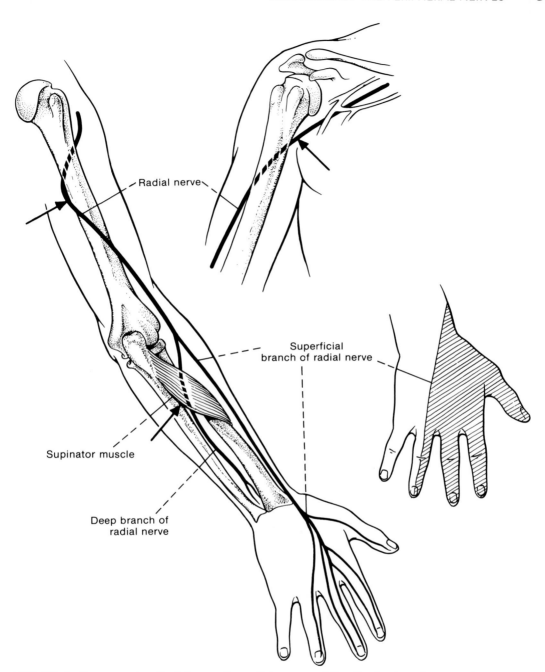

FIG. 43–1. Common sites for injury to the radial nerve and the distribution of sensory loss with a radial nerve lesion.

brachioradialis reflexes may be lost. The function of the brachioradialis is usually spared in plumbism.

Entrapment of the deep radial (posterior interosseous) nerve or compression by a tumor where it passes through the supinator muscle

just below the elbow may cause progressive paralysis and atrophy of the extensor muscles of the wrist and fingers but no wrist drop, since the extensors of the wrist are spared. There are no sensory changes. There is usually pain and tenderness in the region of the elbow. Neuropathy

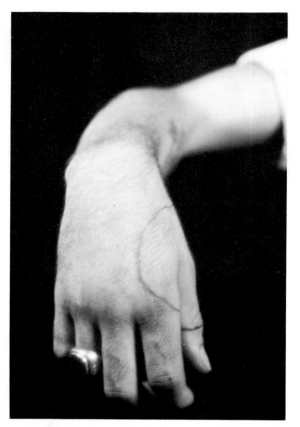

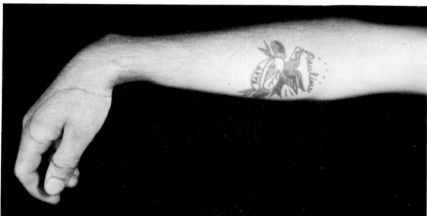

FIG. 43–2. Wrist drop secondary to radial nerve palsy. Sensory deficit in this instance involved the shaded area only.

of the superficial radial nerve will cause pain and alterations of sensation in its distribution; it may be injured with cuts or other types of trauma at the wrist, or it may be compressed by stenosing tenosynovitis of the tendon sheaths of the abductor pollicis longus and extensor pollicis brevis muscles.

The Median Nerve

This nerve arises from two roots, one from the medial and one from the lateral cord of the brachial plexus. Its fibers are derived from the sixth or fifth and sixth cervical through the first thoracic segments. Its motor fibers supply the pronators teres and quadratus, the flexors carpi radialis and digitorum sublimis, the radial half of the flexor digitorum profundus, the palmaris longus, the flexors pollicis longus and pollicis brevis (lateral head), the abductor pollicis brevis, the opponens pollicis, and the two or three radial lumbricales. It transmits sensory impulses from the radial half of the palm of the hand, the palmar surfaces of the thumb and the index and middle fingers, the palmar aspect of the radial half of the ring finger, and the dorsal aspect of the middle and distal phalanges of the index and middle fingers and radial half of the ring finger. The median nerve is well protected by soft tissues, and accordingly is injured less frequently than either the radial or the ulnar nerve. It may, however, be involved in dislocations of the shoulder, injuries of the elbow joint, fractures of the humerus or radius, perforating wounds of the arm or the palmar surface of the wrist, pressure on the arm or forearm, or compression in the forearm or at the wrist (Fig. 43-3).

The most obvious motor manifestations in a median nerve lesion are paralysis of flexion of the wrist, thumb, and radial fingers, loss of grip, loss of pronation, and inability to oppose or approximate the thumb and fingertips. Although flexion at the wrist is impaired and flexion of the distal phalanges of the index and middle fingers is markedly impaired, the proximal phalanges can still be flexed. Loss of ability to flex the distal phalanx of the index finger, without a bone or tendon lesion to account for it, is a pathognomonic sign. The wrist is supinated and drawn to the ulnar side. The thumb lies adducted and extended; it cannot be either opposed to the tip of the little finger or abducted at right angles to the palm (palmar abduction), and the terminal phalanx cannot be flexed (Fig. 43-4). Many of the lost movements, except for flexion of the distal phalanx of the index finger and movements of the thumb, can be substituted by muscles supplied by the ulnar nerve. There is no substitution for palmar abduction, and comparison of this movement on the two sides, while the fingertips are held together at an angle of 90°, is an important test of median nerve function.

If the lesion is in the upper portion of the forearm or higher, the pronators are paralyzed and the arm is in supination; there may be some weakness of abduction of the wrist. If it is lower, only the flexor pollicis longus, the portion of the flexor digitorum profundus to the index finger, and the pronator quadratus are affected; there is no sensory involvement. There is difficulty in making flexion movements of the distal phalanx

of the thumb and index finger; this is known as the **anterior interosseous nerve syndrome.** Owing to the atrophy of the thenar and other muscles and the resulting deformity, a median nerve paralysis is said to result in a simian hand, or "monkey paw." The sensory changes involve the radial side of the palm, including the inner aspect of the thumb, the index and middle fingers, and the radial half of the ring finger. They are less complete on the dorsum of the hand than on the palmar surface, and usually involve only the distal (or middle and distal) phalanges of the index and middle fingers, and sometimes part of the thumb and radial half of the ring finger (see Fig. 5-8). There are no significant reflex changes. Median nerve paralysis is often accompanied by vasomotor and trophic changes and by intractable, burning pain of causalgia, especially if the lesion is an incomplete one. The skin may be flushed, cyanotic, and either wet or dry; the nails are brittle or striated, and there may be changes in hair growth.

The **carpal tunnel syndrome** (which has also been called median thenar neuritis, and partial thenar atrophy) is caused by compression of the nerve as it passes under the transverse carpal ligament at the wrist (Fig. 43-5). Numbness, burning paresthesias, and pain of the wrist, hand, and palmar aspects of the fingers are the first symptoms. These often awaken the patient at night. Later there is weakness, which is most pronounced in the abductor pollicis longus, causing loss of palmar abduction of the thumb. The opponens and short flexor may also be affected, and thenar atrophy develops. Objective sensory changes may be absent. Motor conduction latencies across the carpal tunnel are usually slowed; thus, nerve conduction studies are helpful in the diagnosis of carpal tunnel syndrome. This syndrome may be caused by synovitis, tumor, trauma, thickened ligaments, or rheumatoid or gouty arthritis, or may be associated with systemic disease such as myxedema. It is a common occupational neuropathy resulting from certain frequently repeated movements at the wrist. It occurs in women more frequently than in men, is often bilateral, and is probably the most common cause of so-called acroparesthesias. Temporary or transient cases are common, for example in women with edema or during late stages of pregnancy. More severe cases may be relieved by section of the transverse carpal ligament or removal of a neuroma or ganglion that is compressing the nerve.

The anterior interosseous nerve is the largest branch of the median nerve. It typically supplies

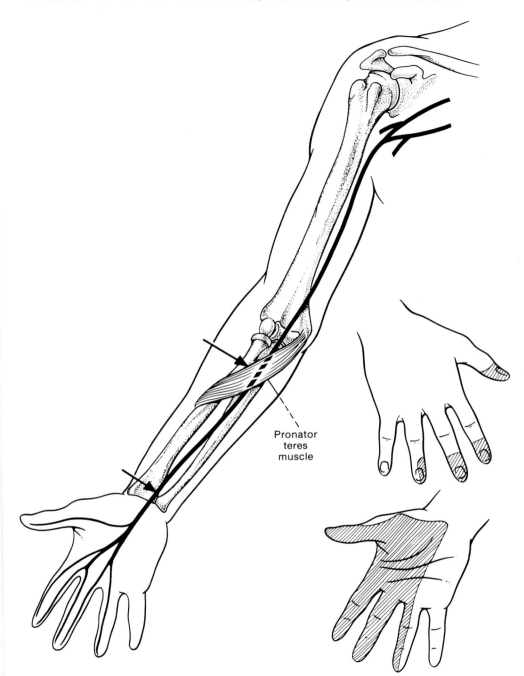

Pronator
teres
muscle

FIG. 43–3. Common sites for injury to the median nerve and the distribution of sensory loss with a median nerve lesion.

the flexor digitorum profundus to the index finger, flexor pollicis longus, and pronator quadratus. When it is paralyzed, the patient is unable to flex the distal interphalangeal joint of either the thumb or index finger, and as a result the tip of the thumb cannot be approximated to the tip of the index finger. There are no sensory changes. This nerve may be injured in penetrating wounds of the forearm or during open reduction of a fracture of the midportion of the

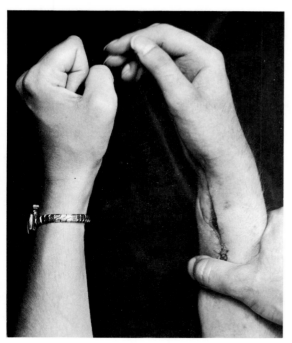

FIG. 43–4. *Motor changes secondary to a lesion of the median nerve, showing loss of flexion of the distal phalanges of the radial fingers.*

the first thoracic segments. It innervates the flexor carpi ulnaris, ulnar half of the flexor digitorum profundus, adductor pollicis, medial head of the flexor pollicis brevis, palmaris brevis, interossei, ulnar lumbricales, and the muscles of the hypothenar eminence—the abductor, opponens, and flexor digiti quinti brevis. It supplies sensation to the dorsal and palmar aspects of the ulnar side of the hand, including the little finger and the ulnar half of the ring finger. The ulnar nerve may be affected by either acute or minor but repeated trauma at the elbow or wrist, or by perforating wounds along its course. It is probably traumatized more often than any other peripheral nerve. An ulnar nerve paralysis may be a late sequel of fractures or dislocations at the elbow; the symptoms develop after the nerve has been damaged by callus formation and fibrous adhesions. This has been termed a **tardive ulnar palsy.**

Either the superficial (sensory) or deep (motor) fibers of the ulnar nerve, or both, may be compressed as the nerve passes through the cubital tunnel in the lateral aspect of the wrist. The resulting syndromes consist of sensory findings, motor findings, or both. The cause may be trauma, constricting fibrous bands, or extrinsically arising compressive masses. Localization

radius. There may also be entrapment by fibrous or tendinous bands.

The **pronator syndrome** consists of compression or entrapment of the median nerve in the proximal forearm at the point where it passes through the two heads of the pronator teres; it affects both motor and sensory components of the nerve. The sensory manifestations are the same as those experienced in the more common carpal tunnel syndrome, but in addition to the thenar muscle weakness and atrophy, there are also varying degrees of weakness of the long flexors of the first three digits and the short flexors of all digits, along with tenderness over the pronator teres muscle and the proximal part of the thenar eminence. Treatment consists of exploration and excision of constrictive bands. Entrapment of the median nerve by a distal humeral supracondylar spur and associated ligament has been described but is rare in occurrence.

The Ulnar Nerve

This nerve is derived from the medial cord of the brachial plexus and receives its supply from the eighth or seventh and eighth cervical through

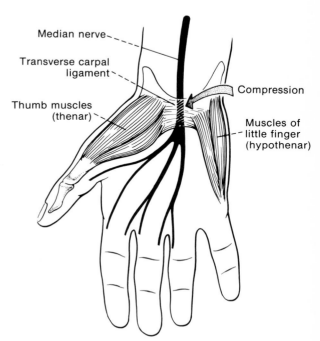

FIG. 43–5. *Diagrammatic sketch of the wrist, showing the relationship of the median nerve to the transverse carpal ligament.*

Median nerve

Transverse carpal ligament

Thumb muscles (thenar)

Compression

Muscles of little finger (hypothenar)

of the compressed segment of the nerve is aided by nerve conduction studies. The treatment is exploration and release of restricting anomalies.

In an ulnar nerve involvement flexion and adduction of the wrist and fingers are impaired, and the hand is turned radialward. Extension of the distal phalanges and flexion of the proximal ones, especially of the two ulnar fingers, are lost; adduction and abduction of the fingers are impaired; and adduction of the thumb and abduction and opposition of the little finger are lost. The *signe de journal* (Ch. 27) is present. The grip, especially that of the ulnar fingers, is weak. Atrophy of the hypothenar eminence develops and, to a lesser extent, of the thenar eminence; the palm is hollowed, and the interosseous spaces are deeply grooved. There is hyperextension of the fingers at the metacarpophalangeal joints and flexion at the interphalangeal joints, especially those of the two ulnar fingers. The resulting deformity of the hand is called **main en griffe** or **claw hand** (Fig. 43-6). Although the abductor of the little finger is paralyzed, this finger may assume a position of abduction when the fingers are extended, owing to action of extensor muscles. Sensory changes are found on the little finger and the ulnar half of the ring finger (see Fig. 5-8). There are no important reflex abnormalities, and usually no trophic changes. The claw deformity is less marked with a lesion above the elbow, since with paralysis of the flexor digitorum profundus there is less flexion of the distal phalanges. With paralysis of the deep palmar branch of the ulnar nerve, usually caused by prolonged pressure on the hypothenar eminence, there is weakness and atrophy that affects the adductor pollicis and interossei more than the hypothenar muscles, without sensory change.

Combined median and ulnar paralyses are not rare, and when present there is a complete claw hand. A Volkmann's ischemic contracture of the forearm may simulate a combined median and ulnar paralysis. Similar deformities may be seen in Charcot-Marie-Tooth disease, progressive spinal muscular atrophy, and amyotrophic lateral sclerosis.

The Thorax

The Phrenic Nerve

This is one of the major motor nerves of the cervical plexus and is the principal respiratory nerve of the body. It is derived from the third through the fifth cervical segments. It is mainly motor, innervating the diaphragm, but it also

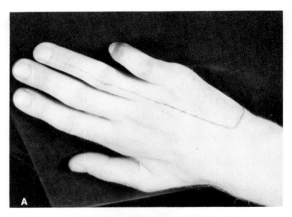

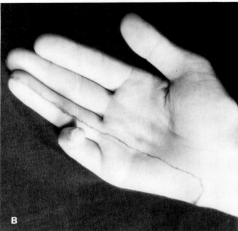

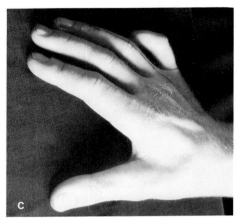

FIG. 43–6. Motor and sensory changes in a lesion of the ulnar nerve. **A.** View of dorsum of the hand. **B.** Palmar aspect. **C.** Oblique view.

carries some sensory filaments from the diaphragm, pericardium, parts of the costal and mediastinal pleura, and the extrapleural and extraperitoneal connective tissues. It may be injured by neoplasms or penetrating wounds. In the past it was sectioned to produce unilateral diaphragmatic paralysis in the surgical treatment of pulmonary tuberculosis. Unilateral paralysis of the diaphragm causes few or no symptoms; the liver and spleen may be elevated on the affected side, the excursion of the costal margins is slightly increased. Litten's sign is absent, and fluoroscopic examination shows relative immobility of one half of the diaphragm. With bilateral paralysis there is dyspnea on the slightest exertion, a scaphoid abdomen that does not protrude on expiration, absence of Litten's sign, increased excursion of the costal margins, retraction of the epigastrium on inspiration, overactivity of the accessory respiratory muscles, and difficulty in coughing or sneezing.

The Lower Extremities

The Femoral Nerve

The femoral nerve is the largest branch of the lumbar plexus. It arises from the posterior divisions of the anterior primary rami of the second, third, and fourth lumbar segments. It supplies the iliacus, pectineus, sartorius, and quadriceps femoris muscles. Through its sensory branches, the intermediate (anterior) and medial cutaneous nerves and the saphenous nerve, it transmits sensation from the anterior and medial aspect of the leg to the ankle. The femoral nerve may be involved in pelvic tumors, psoas abscesses, fractures of the pelvis and upper femur, pressure, aneurysms of the femoral artery, and bullet or stab wounds; it is commonly affected in diabetic mononeuritis, and may be injured during labor or abdominal or pelvic surgery (Fig. 43-7). With injury to this nerve there is complete loss of extension of the leg at the knee and there is some weakness of flexion at the hip. Walking forward and climbing stairs is done with difficulty, although the patient may walk backward with ease. It is necessary for the patient to walk with the leg stiff, and if the knee bends the patient may fall. Injury to the posterior divisions of the anterior primary rami of the second to fourth lumbar segments within the pelvis or abdomen will also affect the function of the psoas major, with loss of flexion of the thigh. With lesions of the femoral nerve the patellar reflex is lost and there is anesthesia of the anterior and medial aspects of the thigh and the medial aspect of the leg. The saphenous nerve, which supplies the skin over the medial or anteromedial aspect of the leg, may be injured during operations on varicose veins or by trauma to or operations on the knee.

The Obturator Nerve

This nerve arises from the lumbar plexus by fusion of the anterior divisions of the anterior primary rami of the second through the fourth lumbar segments. It supplies the adductor muscles of the thigh, the gracilis, and the obturator externus, and transmits sensation from a small area on the medial aspect of the thigh. Injuries to this nerve are rare, but when they occur there is weakness of adduction and external rotation of the thigh, with a small area of anesthesia over the inner surface of the thigh. In the **Howship–Romberg** syndrome, caused by pressure on the obturator nerve by an obturator hernia, there is pain in the medial aspect of the thigh and knee.

The Lateral Femoral Cutaneous Nerve

This nerve is supplied by the posterior divisions of the anterior primary rami of the second and third lumbar segments. It is entirely afferent and transmits sensation from the skin of the anterolateral aspect of the thigh. Involvement of this nerve, usually where it passes under or through the inguinal ligament just medial to the anterior superior iliac spine, or where it pierces the fascia lata, is followed by hypesthesia, sometimes with painful paresthesias, in its cutaneous distribution. The underlying etiology of this syndrome, known as **meralgia paresthetica,** is probably some anatomic variant in the course of the nerve, but the precipitating causes are increased intraabdominal pressure, pregnancy, obesity, trauma, pressure by a belt or truss, occupational postures requiring prolonged hip flexion, diabetes mellitus, debilitating disease, or toxins, infections, and other causes of peripheral neuritis. It has been reported as a complication of inguinal herniorrhaphy.

The Common Peroneal Nerve

The common peroneal nerve is formed by a fusion of the upper four posterior divisions of the sacral plexus (fourth lumbar through second sacral segments). It innervates the short head of the biceps femoris muscle and divides to form the superficial and deep peroneal nerves. Through the lateral sural cutaneous nerve, it transmits sensation from the lateral and posterolateral aspects of the upper portion of the leg. The peroneal anastomotic branch joins the medial sural cutaneous branch of the tibial nerve to

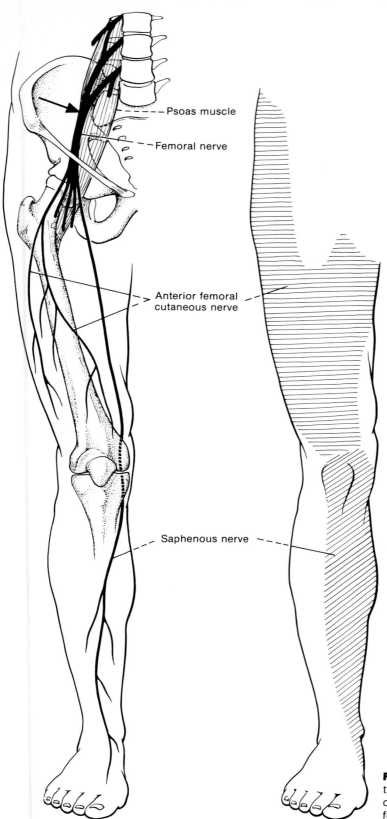

Psoas muscle

Femoral nerve

Anterior femoral
cutaneous nerve

Saphenous nerve

FIG. 43–7. Common sites for injury
to the femoral nerve and distribution
of sensory loss with a lesion of the
femoral nerve and its branches.

form the sural nerve; this transmits sensation from the posterolateral aspects of the leg and ankle, and the lateral aspects of the heel and foot.

The superficial peroneal nerve is supplied by the fourth and fifth lumbar and first one or two sacral segments of the spinal cord. It innervates the peronei longus and brevis muscles and transmits sensation from the skin on the anterolateral aspect of the leg and ankle and the dorsum of the foot. After interruption of this nerve the foot can no longer be everted. Dorsiflexion is possible, but during the process the foot becomes inverted. The sensory changes follow the cutaneous distribution of the nerve. The deep peroneal nerve has the same general segmental supply. It innervates the tibialis anterior, peroneus tertius, extensors hallucis longus and brevis, and extensors digitorum longus and brevis. It also transmits sensation from the skin in the region of the first interosseous space. In a lesion of this nerve there is loss of dorsiflexion of the foot and toes, with a characteristic foot drop and a resulting steppage, or slapping, gait. The patient is unable to stand on his heel and raise the sole of the foot; he attempts to raise the depressed toes off the ground by exaggerated flexion at the hip and knee. The sensory changes are characteristic.

Either the superficial or deep peroneal nerve may be injured by trauma, stretching, or other causes. The common peroneal nerve is very vulnerable to injury, especially where it winds around the neck of the fibula. It may be affected by penetrating wounds, pressure subsequent to fracture of the head of the fibula, compression from a tightly applied plaster cast, or pressure from sitting with the legs crossed, from kneeling, or from assuming bizarre postures in certain occupations (Fig. 43-8). Recent loss of weight may increase the susceptibility of the nerve to damage from pressure, as may alcoholism, diabetes, malnutrition, and other causes of peripheral neuritis. The nerve is commonly affected in lead neuropathy. If the common peroneal nerve is injured, the sensory and motor changes correspond to the distributions of both the superficial and deep branches. The sensory function of the lateral sural cutaneous and sural nerves may or may not be affected, but the innervation to the biceps femoris is usually spared. A foot drop associated with a peroneal palsy (Fig. 43-9) should be differentiated from the deformity of the foot seen in Friedreich's ataxia, as well as from that which occurs in Charcot – Marie – Tooth disease.

The Tibial Nerve

The tibial nerve is the larger of the two terminal branches of the sciatic nerve. It is formed by a fusion of all five of the anterior divisions of the sacral plexus (fourth lumbar through second or third sacral segments). This nerve supplies the long head of the biceps femoris, and the semimembranosus, semitendinosus, gastrocnemius, popliteus, soleus, plantaris, tibialis posterior, and flexors digitorum and hallucis longus muscles and, through the medial and lateral plantar nerves, the plantar flexors of the toes and the small muscles of the foot. Through the sural nerve, formed by a junction of the medial sural cutaneous nerve (tibial) and the anastomotic branch of the common peroneal, it transmits sensation from the posterolateral aspects of the leg and ankle and the lateral aspects of the heel and foot. Calcaneal nerves supply the posterior and medial aspects and plantar surface of the heel, and the medial and lateral plantar nerves, the plantar surface of the foot. If the tibial nerve is injured, there is loss of the functions of these muscles, with anesthesia over the plantar and lateral aspects of the foot, the heel, and the posterolateral aspects of the leg and ankle. The patient is unable to plantar flex or invert the foot, or to flex, adduct, or abduct the toes. He cannot stand on his toes. Trophic changes and causalgic pain may be present. The Achilles reflex is lost. Injuries to this nerve are relatively infrequent because of its deep location and protected course, but it may be involved in lesions in or below the popliteal space. Compression of the nerve as it passes behind the medial malleolus and deep to the flexor retinaculum may cause burning pain and sensory loss in the toes and sole of the foot and paresis or paralysis of the small muscles of the foot; this has been called the **tarsal tunnel** syndrome.

The Sciatic Nerve

The common peroneal and tibial nerves are fused within the pelvis to form the sciatic nerve, the largest nerve in the body. Rami from the tibial trunk supply the semimembranosus and semitendinosus muscles and the long head of the biceps; a branch also goes to the adductor magnus. Rami from the common peroneal trunk go to the short head of the biceps. Serious injury to the main trunk of the sciatic nerve results in loss of function of both the common peroneal and tibial nerves. This is uncommon, but if it occurs there is complete paralysis of all the muscles

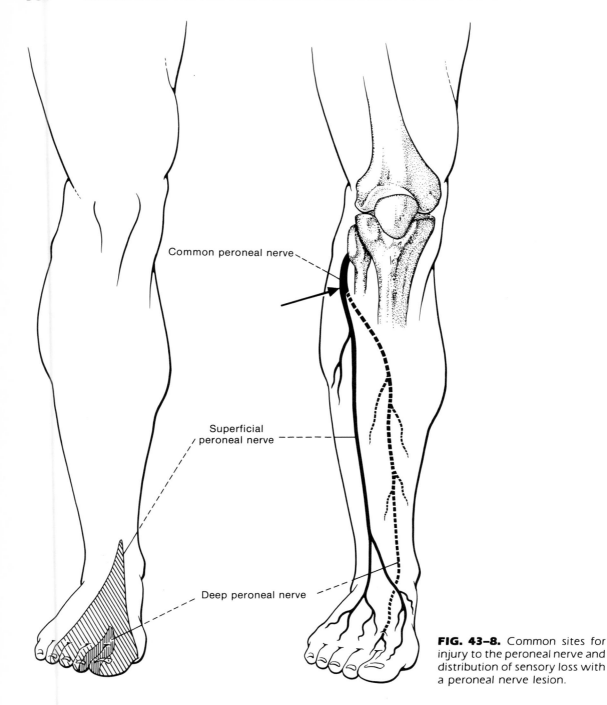

Common peroneal nerve

Superficial peroneal nerve

Deep peroneal nerve

FIG. 43–8. Common sites for injury to the peroneal nerve and distribution of sensory loss with a peroneal nerve lesion.

of the foot, and anesthesia of the foot and all but the anteromedial aspect of the leg. Flexion at the knee is also greatly impaired, the only muscles participating in this movement being the sartorius and gracilis. Ability to flex and extend the ankle and toe joints and the powers of inver-

sion and eversion of the foot are lost. The patient cannot stand on either his heel or his toes. Trophic disturbances and causalgic pain are frequent. The sciatic nerve may be injured in pelvic fractures, dislocations of the hip, tumors, stab or gunshot wounds, dystocia, traction in breech presentations, or intragluteal injections into the nerve. Specific syndromes of sciatic irritation and dysfunction are discussed in Chapter 47.

Lesions of Other Peripheral Nerves

Peripheral nerves other than those that have been mentioned may occasionally be implicated in isolated neuritides. Brief mention may be made of some of the less common syndromes of peripheral nerve involvement.

Truncal neuropathy, with sensory disturbances and abdominal hernia, may be a complication of diabetes mellitus.

The iliohypogastric nerve arises from the first lumbar nerve. It is mainly a sensory nerve, but sends a few filaments to the transversus abdominis and the obliquus internus abdominis, and sometimes to the obliquus externus abdominis. The lateral cutaneous branch is distributed to the skin of the gluteal region, behind the lateral cutaneous branch of the twelfth thoracic nerve; the anterior cutaneous branch transmits impulses from the skin of the hypogastric region, just above the symphysis pubis. With a lesion of this nerve there may be pain or sensory changes in these areas.

The ilioinguinal nerve is also a branch of the first lumbar nerve. Like the iliohypogastric nerve, it is mainly sensory but supplies a few filaments to the transversus abdominis and obliquus internus abdominis and occasionally to the obliquus externus abdominis. It transmits sensation from the skin of the upper and medial part of the thigh, as well as from the upper part of the root of the penis and the scrotum in the male, and the mons pubis and the labium majus in the female. Lesions of the ilioinguinal nerve cause pain and loss of sensation in these areas.

The genitofemoral nerve arises from the first and second lumbar nerves. Its external spermatic branch supplies the cremaster muscle and transmits sensation from a portion of the skin of the scrotum, and its lumboinguinal branch transmits sensation from a small area on the anterior surface of the upper part of the thigh.

The superior gluteal nerve arises from the posterior divisions of the fourth and fifth lumbar and first sacral nerves. It innervates the gluteus medius, gluteus minimus, and tensor fasciae latae muscles. The inferior gluteal nerve arises from posterior divisions of the fifth lumbar and the first and second sacral nerves, and innervates the gluteus maximus. With a lesion of the former nerve, occasionally damaged by intra-

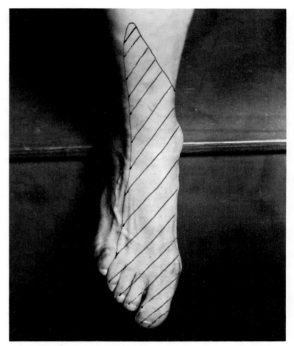

FIG. 43–9. Right peroneal palsy.

gluteal injections, there is weakness of abduction and internal rotation of the thigh; with a lesion of the latter there is impairment of extension of the thigh.

The posterior femoral cutaneous nerve is supplied by the posterior divisions of the first and second sacral nerves and the anterior divisions of the second and third sacral. It transmits sensation from the posterior aspect of the thigh and upper leg. Its gluteal branches supply the skin of the lower gluteal region; the perineal branches are distributed to the upper and medial aspect of the thigh; the inferior pudendal branch supplies the skin of the perineal region together with the scrotum in the male and the labium majus in the female.

The pudendal nerve arises from the anterior divisions of the second, third, and fourth sacral nerves. Its branches are as follows. The inferior hemorrhoidal nerve is distributed to the external anal sphincter and to the skin and mucosa about the anus. The perineal nerve divides into muscular and posterior scrotal (or labial) branches; the former supply the bulbocavernosus, ischiocavernosus, and other perineal muscles, together with the external vesical sphincter; the latter transmit sensation from the scrotum in the male and the labium majus in the female. The dorsal nerve of the penis (or clitoris) supplies the corpus cavernosum and the skin and mucous membrane of the dorsum of the penis (or clitoris), including the glans. The pudendal nerve also transmits sensation from the bladder. Isolated lesions of these individual nerves are rare.

Multiple Neuropathy

The neuropathies that have been described are conditions in which single peripheral nerves are affected. They are usually caused by trauma or pressure. When more than one nerve is affected, the term multiple neuropathy is used. Two varieties of multiple neuropathy are described as follows:

In **mononeuritis multiplex** there is simultaneous involvement of more than one nerve — usually two or three in different parts of the body. By definition it is differentiated from polyneuropathy, in which the function in the distal branches of most peripheral nerves is disturbed to varying degrees. In mononeuritis multiplex the involved nerves are usually seriously affected with localized paralyses and disturbances of sensation. Some of the causes for this are exposure to toxins, diabetes mellitus, collagen disease, especially polyarteritis nodosa, allergic and autoimmune responses, and certain infections including Lyme disease, acquired immune deficiency syndrome, and others.

Polyneuritis, or **polyneuropathy,** is a widespread process affecting predominantly the nerves in the distal portions of the extremities. Although specific nerves may be affected, as shown by nerve conduction determinations, there is a generalized disturbance in function of many nerves, varying in degree but clinically most severe in their distal portions. As a result, the changes may be diffuse and widespread rather than focal. Involvement may be predominantly sensory, motor, or mixed, depending to some degree on the etiology of the polyneuropathy. It may also be primarily axonal or demyelinating in character. The sensory disturbances may be characterized by pain, paresthesias, hyperesthesias, or anesthesia. The impairment of sensation is often confined to the distal portion of the extremities; there is a peripheral blunting of sensation for the entire part, without a well-delineated border. This may simulate a glove or stocking distribution, but the gradual change and the presence of tenderness and hyperpathia in the hypesthetic zone are important in diagnosis. There may be profound impairment of proprioceptive sensations. The motor changes may vary from slight weakness to extensive paralysis with atrophy and deformities, and are also most marked in the distal portions of the extremities. Electrical testing may show decrease in the conduction velocities of both motor and sensory nerves. Autonomic changes may be absent or minimal, but occasionally they are profound, and may even be responsible for bladder, bowel, and related dysfunction (Ch. 42). The peripheral nerves and the muscles and tendons may be tender to pressure, and there is often cutaneous hyperesthesia and hypersensitivity, especially of the soles of the feet, in spite of an elevated sensory threshold. In hypertrophic interstitial polyneuritis and leprosy, and sometimes in amyloid neuritis, the affected nerves are thickened and palpable.

Among the numerous causes for polyneuritis are the following: exposure to or ingestion of toxic substances, both organic and nonorganic; numerous drugs and antineoplastic agents; deficiency states (including alcoholism), especially deficient intake or absorption of the B complex vitamins (thiamine, niacin, pyridoxine, and cyanocobalamin); infections (diphtheria, leprosy, viral and nonspecific systemic infections including acquired immune deficiency syndrome); metabolic disorders (diabetes, hyperinsulinism, porphyria, electrolyte and acid-base disturbances, uremia); collagen diseases (polyarteritis nodosa, disseminated lupus erythematosus); vascular insufficiency and ischemia; allergy (serum neuritis and postinfectious neuritis); genetic disorders (Charcot – Marie – Tooth disease, hypertrophic interstitial neuritis, hereditary ataxic polyneuropathy, hereditary sensory neuropathy); neoplastic infiltrations (carcinoma, leukemia, lymphomas); and other causes that are difficult to classify, such as that for noninfiltrating neuritis associated with carcinomatosis; for the neuritis associated with amyloidosis, sarcoidosis, myeloma, cryoglobulinemias, and gammopathies; and for those developing with exposure to cold and after irradiation. Under many circumstances more than one etiologic factor may be implicated.

Neuralgia

The term neuralgia is used for the syndrome that is characterized by pain in the distribution of certain nerves in the absence of objective signs of dysfunction. There are no motor, reflex, or sensory changes, and there are said to be no pathologic changes of nerve structure. Neuralgias may be reflex phenomena, secondary to some irritative, toxic, or infectious factor. Occasionally a detailed examination may show some minimal evidence of nerve dysfunction. Trigeminal, glossopharyngeal, and sphenopalatine neuralgia are discussed elsewhere (Ch. 12 and Ch. 15). Brachial, occipital, cervical, intercostal, crural, obturator, sciatic, and other neuralgic syndromes have been described.

BIBLIOGRAPHY

Adams RD, Victor M. Principles of Neurology, 4th ed. New York, McGraw – Hill, 1989

Aids to the Examination of the Peripheral Nervous System. Medical Research Council Memorandum No. 45 (superseding War Memorandum No 7). London, Her Majesty's Stationery Office, 1976

Brain WR, Wright AD, Wilkinson M. Spontaneous compression of both median nerves in the carpal tunnel. Lancet 1947;1:277

Clein LJ. Suprascapular entrapment neuropathy. J Neurosurg 1975;43:337

Dyck PJ, Karnes J, Bushek W, Spring E et al. Computer assisted sensory examination to detect and quantitate sensory deficit in diabetic neuropathy. Neurobehav Toxicol Teratol 1983;5:697

Dyck PJ, Low PA, Stevens JC. Diseases of peripheral nerves. In Joynt RJ (ed). Clinical Neurology. Philadelphia, JB Lippincott, 1989

Dyck PJ, Thomas PK, Lambert EH, Bunge R. Peripheral Neuropathy, 2nd ed. Philadelphia, WB Saunders, 1984

Esposito GM. Peripheral entrapment syndromes of the upper extremity. NY State J Med 1972;72:717

Favill J. Outline of the Spinal Nerves. Springfield, IL, Charles C Thomas, 1946

Gutmann E, Gutmann L, Medawar PB, Young JZ. Rate of regeneration of nerve. J Exp Biol 1942;19:14

Halperin JJ, Luft BJ, Anand AK et al. Lyme neuroborreliosis: central nervous system manifestations. Neurology 1989;39:753

Haymaker W, Woodhall B. Peripheral Nerve Injuries. Principles of Diagnosis, 2nd ed. Philadelphia, WB Saunders, 1953

Kopell HP, Thompson WAL. Peripheral Entrapment Neuropathies. Baltimore, Williams & Wilkins, 1963

Lyons WR, Woodhall B. Atlas of Peripheral Nerve Injuries. Philadelphia, WB Saunders, 1949

Magee KR. Neuritis of the deep palmar branch of the ulnar nerve. Arch Neurol Psychiatry 1955;73:200

Miller RG, Kiprov DD, Parry G, Bredesen DE. Peripheral nervous system dysfunction in acquired immunodeficiency syndrome. In Rosenblum ML, Levy RM, Bredesen DE (eds). AIDS and the Nervous System. New York, Raven Press, 1988

Morris HM, Peters BH. Pronator syndrome: Clinical and electrophysiologic features in seven cases. J Neurol Neurosurg Psychiatry 1976;39:461

Mulder DW. Diagnosis and management of mononeuropathies. Postgrad Med 1964;36:321

Nakano KK, Lundergan C, Okharo MM. Anterior interosseous nerve syndromes: Diagnostic methods and alternative treatments. Arch Neurol 1977;34:477

Paine KWE. Tardy ulnar palsy. Can J Surg 1970;13:255

Parry GJ, Floberg J. Diabetic truncal neuropathy presenting as abdominal hernia. Neurology 1989;39:1488

Rowland LP (ed). Merritt's Textbook of Neurology, 8th ed. Philadelphia, Lea & Febiger, 1989

Satran R. Dejerine – Sottas disease revisited. Arch Neurol 1980;37:67

Seddon HJ (ed). Peripheral Nerve Injuries. London, Her Majesty's Stationery Office, 1954

Seddon HJ, Medawar PB, Smith H. Rate of regeneration of peripheral nerves in man. J Physiol 1943;102:191

Spinner M. The anterior interosseous nerve syndrome. J Bone Joint Surg 1970;52:84

Sunderland S. Rate of regeneration in human peripheral nerves: Analysis of the interval between injury and the onset of recovery. Arch Neurol Psychiatry 1947;58:251

Sunderland S. A classification of peripheral nerve injuries producing loss of function. Brain 1951;74:491

Sunderland S. Nerves and Nerve Injuries, 2nd ed. Edinburgh, Churchill Livingstone, 1978

Wadsworth TG, Williams JR. Cubital tunnel external pressure syndrome. Br Med J 1973;1:662

Chapter 44
DISORDERS OF THE NERVE ROOTS

The subjective and objective manifestations of nerve root involvement are similar to those of peripheral nerve involvement, but the distribution of the changes is somewhat different. The sensory manifestations, both the disturbances of function such as pain and paresthesia, and the areas of anesthesia, hypesthesia, and hyperesthesia, are confined to dermatomes, or those cutaneous areas supplied by specific cord segments, dorsal roots, or ganglia. Owing to the overlap of sensory supply by the nerve roots, it may not be possible to map out an area of sensory loss in a lesion involving only one nerve root. There is also some individual variation in the nerve root distributions, both motor and sensory. The motor changes are also dependent upon the radicular or segmental innervation of the muscles, rather than their peripheral nerve supply, and are found in the myotomes, or those groups of muscles supplied by specific spinal segments and their ventral roots. Owing to the fact that most muscles are supplied by more than one segment of the spinal cord, and thus by more than one nerve root, there may be no discernible motor change in instances where there is involvement of only one nerve root.

The pain and hyperesthesia of nerve root origin are termed **radicular** in distribution. If the pain is bilateral and symmetric, involving the trunk, it is called **girdle pain.** Radicular pain is often increased by movement and by actions such as coughing, sneezing, and straining, which either increase the intraspinal pressure or cause stretching of the nerve roots. It is often lancinating in character and is usually intermit-

tent, but occasionally is constant. Pain of nerve root origin may be relieved by section of the nerve roots central to the dorsal root ganglia, or by spinal anesthesia, intraspinal injection of alcohol, or caudal anesthesia.

Radicular involvement may be caused by many processes. These include extramedullary spinal cord lesions such as ruptured intervertebral disks, extradural tumors and abscesses, and arachnoiditis; extramedullary but intradural neoplasms; compression of the spinal column with pressure on the nerve roots by neoplasms, trauma, or infectious processes affecting the vertebrae; and inflammatory, autoimmune, and other processes involving the dorsal root ganglia and nerve roots (radiculitis). Occasionally muscle spasm alone causes nerve root compression.

Tumors of the cervical portion of the spinal cord, especially extramedullary ones, and herniated intervertebral disks in the cervical region are among the most common causes of radicular pain in the neck and upper extremities and motor changes and sensory abnormalities in the distribution of the cervical nerve roots; usually there is no vasomotor dysfunction. The pain may be increased on coughing or straining, or with certain head movements. Because of the limited space between the spinal cord and the vertebral bodies and the fixed position of the cord, midline protrusions of the intervertebral disks produce symptoms that resemble those of spinal cord tumors, with segmental sensory changes and compression of the ascending and descending pathways that may result in a spastic paraplegia.

Lateral protrusions cause monoradicular syndromes; these occur most frequently between the fifth and sixth and between the sixth and seventh cervical vertebrae, with pressure on the sixth and seventh cervical roots, respectively. Radicular pain, tenderness, stiffness of the neck, alterations in the reflexes, objective and subjective changes in sensation in the distribution of the involved roots, and weakness, atrophy, and fasciculations of the muscles in the involved myotomes are the principal manifestations. With compression of the sixth cervical root the pain is mainly on the radial side of the forearm, with paresthesias of the index and middle fingers, weakness of the biceps, brachioradialis, and wrist extensor muscles, and diminution or loss of the biceps and brachioradialis reflexes. With involvement of the seventh cervical root the pain is on either the dorsal or volar aspect of the forearm, with paresthesias of the index and middle fingers, predominant weakness of the triceps, and diminution or loss of the triceps reflex. With involvement of the eighth cervical root the pain is in the ulnar aspect of the forearm, with paresthesias of the ring and little fingers and weakness of the small muscles of the hand. The pain of cervical nerve root irritation may simulate that of coronary artery disease. A syndrome of unilateral ventral pressure, with cord compression but without radicular symptoms, has also been described.

Symptoms similar to those described may also be present with cervical spondylitis and spondylosis, in which there is both foraminal narrowing and spinal cord compression. They have also been reported in association with rheumatoid arthritis and Paget's disease. After flexion — extension injuries of the neck (often referred to as whiplash injuries) that may occur in vehicular rear-end collisions, the major trauma is to the muscles and fasciae of the neck, but if there is damage to the cervical spine there may also be symptoms and signs of nerve root irritation and even of spinal cord compression. Similar symptoms may also appear with developmental anomalies. Roentgenography, computed tomography, or magnetic resonance imaging, myelography, and electromyography may be necessary in order to differentiate the various syndromes.

In herpes zoster, a viral infection affecting predominantly the dorsal root ganglia, there is a severe, burning pain in the distribution of one or more dermatomes. This is followed shortly by the development of vesicles in the cutaneous distribution of the involved root and ganglion (Fig. 44-1). A residual pain, referred to as postherpetic neuralgia, may remain after the disappearance of the vesicles. There may be hyperpathia in the involved area in spite of hypesthesia. Motor involvement is rare. Symptomatic herpes zoster may accompany systemic infections, leukemic or neoplastic infiltrations, or inflammatory involvement of the vertebrae or nerve roots. With tabes dorsalis there are inflammatory changes in the dorsal roots and ganglia and in the posterior funiculi of the spinal cord. There may be radicular pains, sometimes in a girdle distribution. Sensory changes are characterized by loss of proprioceptive sensation and a delayed cutaneous pain response, and autonomic changes are common. There is a loss of reflexes with hypotonia, but no actual loss of motor power. In polyradiculoneuritis (Landry – Guillain – Barré syndrome) there are motor, sensory, and reflex changes similar to those found in polyneuritis, but the involvement is more extensive. The high protein content of the cerebrospinal fluid gives evidence of change within the subarachnoid space, and microscopic examination reveals involvement of the nerve roots and dorsal root ganglia, with an ascending, or axonal, degeneration of the anterior horn cells. Nerve conduction studies are helpful, showing early randomly distributed axonal blocks in peripheral nerves. In **hereditary sensory neuropathy** there are profound sensory disturbances, both superficial and deep, with ataxia, areflexia, and trophic disturbances, but little motor dysfunction; the pri-

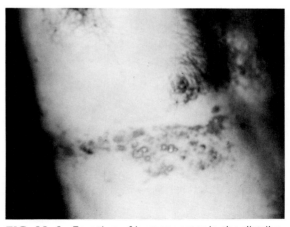

FIG. 44–1. Eruption of herpes zoster in the distribution of the right sixth thoracic nerve root.

mary pathologic changes are in the dorsal root ganglia. In **hereditary ataxic polyneuropathy (Refsum's syndrome)** there are visual and auditory symptoms, electrocardiographic abnormalities, and elevation of the protein content of the cerebrospinal fluid, in addition to ataxia, peripheral nerve manifestations, and abnormalities of phytanic acid metabolism. There is thickening with infiltrations of the peripheral nerves, but the nerve roots are also affected and there is axonal degeneration within the central nervous system.

Nerve root involvement in the lumbosacral region is discussed in Chapter 47.

BIBLIOGRAPHY

DeJong RN. The Guillain – Barré syndrome: Polyradiculoneuritis with albuminocytologic dissociation. Arch Neurol Psychiat 1940;44:1044

Denny – Brown D. Hereditary sensory radicular neuropathy. J Neurol Neurosurg Psychiat 1951;14:237

The Guillain – Barré Study Group. Plasmapheresis and acute Guillain – Barré syndrome. Neurology 1985;35:1095

Keegan JJ. Relations of nerve roots to abnormalities of lumbar and cervical portions of the spine. Arch Surg 1947;55:246

Refsum S. Heredopathia atactica polyneuritiformis. Acta Psychiatr Scand 1946;(suppl) 38:9

Sobue G, Senda Y, Matsuoka Y, Sobue I. Sensory ataxia. A residual disability of Guillain – Barré syndrome. Arch Neurol 1983;40:86

Involvement of the major nerve plexuses, such as the cervical, brachial, and lumbosacral plexuses, may produce changes in sensory and motor functions that differ somewhat in distribution from those caused by peripheral nerve involvement, and also from those associated with radicular lesions.

THE CERVICAL PLEXUS

The cervical plexus is formed by the anterior primary rami of the upper four cervical nerves. There are connections with the superior cervical sympathetic ganglion and the spinal accessory and hypoglossal nerves. The plexus is situated on the side of the neck, behind the sternocleidomastoid and in front of the levator scapulae and scalenus medius muscles. The cutaneous branches supply the skin on the lateral occipital portion of the scalp, the greater part of the auricle, the angle of the jaw, the neck, and the supraclavicular region and upper thorax through the lesser and greater occipital, great auricular, cutaneous cervical, and supraclavicular nerves (see Fig. 12-3). Muscular branches supply the scalenus medius and levator scapulae, diaphragm, many of the vertebral muscles, and in part the sternocleidomastoid, trapezius, and infrahyoid muscles. There are communications with the tongue musculature and the suprahyoid muscles. Injuries to the cervical plexus are infrequent, but any of the individual nerves may be damaged by penetrating wounds, operative trauma, or disease of or trauma to the cervical vertebrae. Involvement of cutaneous branches is

apparent from sensory changes; irritation of them may cause cervicooccipital neuralgia or headache. Interruption of motor branches causes weakness, paralysis, and atrophy of specific muscles; irritation may cause spasm of the neck or diaphragm. Rigidity of the neck in meningitis and diseases of the cervical vertebrae and muscles may be a protective reflex mechanism. The method of examining the various muscles supplied by the cervical plexus and the changes resulting from weakness and paralysis are described in Part D, "The Motor System," and under the discussion of the eleventh and twelfth cranial nerves.

THE BRACHIAL PLEXUS

Lesions of the brachial plexus cause motor and sensory syndromes involving the muscles of the upper extremities that differ somewhat from those that follow lesions of the individual nerves. The brachial plexus is formed by the anterior primary rami of the four lower cervical nerves and the greater part of the first thoracic (Fig. 45-1). The fifth and sixth cervical rami unite to form the upper trunk; the seventh cervical forms the middle trunk, and the eighth cervical and first thoracic form the lower trunk. The trunks are situated in the supraclavicular fossa just distal to the scalenus anterior muscle. Each of the trunks divides into an anterior and a posterior division, from which the three cords are derived. The lateral cord is formed by the anterior divisions of the upper and middle trunks (anterior primary divisions of the fifth, sixth, and seventh cervical

571

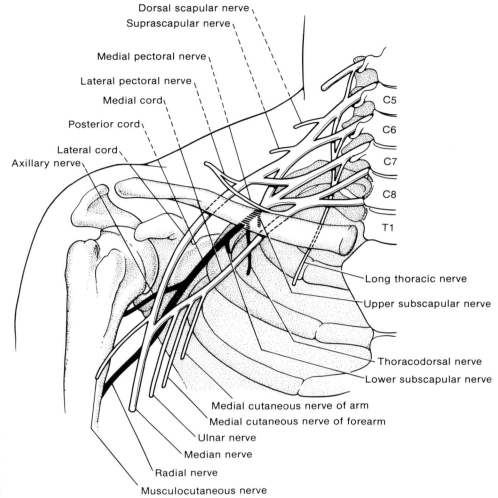

FIG. 45–1. Brachial plexus showing its various constituents and their relationship to structures in the region of the upper chest, axilla, and shoulder.

nerves); the medial cord is formed by the anterior division of the lower trunk (eighth cervical and first thoracic nerves); the posterior cord is formed by the posterior divisions of all these trunks and nerves. The divisions are situated deep to the middle third of the clavicle and extend just beyond the lateral border of the first rib. The cords are in the axilla. The lower trunk is immediately behind the subclavian artery, and all three cords approximate the axillary artery.

The fifth cervical ramus, with the fourth, gives off the dorsal scapular nerve to the rhomboidei and in part to the levator scapulae; the fifth through the seventh or eighth cervical rami give off the long thoracic nerve to the serratus anterior; the fifth cervical ramus also sends a twig to

the phrenic nerve, and the fifth through the eighth cervical rami send branches to the scaleni and longus colli muscles. The upper trunk gives off the suprascapular nerve to the supraspinatus and infraspinatus muscles, and the nerve to the subclavius. From the lateral cord issues the lateral anterior thoracic nerve to the pectoralis major; from the medial cord arise the medial anterior thoracic nerve to the pectorales major and minor and the medial antibrachial and brachial cutaneous nerves; from the posterior cord originate the subscapular nerves to the subscapularis and teres major and the thoracodorsal nerve to the latissimus dorsi. The terminal branches of the posterior cord are the axillary and radial nerves; the terminal branches of the lateral cord are the musculocutaneous nerve and the lateral component of the median nerve; the terminal branches of the medial cord are the ulnar and the medial component of the median nerve. There may be marked anatomic variations of the brachial plexus. In the "prefixed" plexus a large component of the fourth cervical nerve may be included, and less of the first thoracic; in the "post-fixed" plexus there are no components of the fourth cervical, but the entire first thoracic and even a part of the second thoracic may be included.

The upper arm type of brachial plexus palsy (**Erb's palsy,** or **Erb – Duchenne paralysis**) follows injury to the fifth and sixth cervical roots, the upper trunk, or sometimes the upper and middle trunks. It may be caused by traction on the head or shoulder, blows or falls against the head or shoulder, stab wounds, or obstetric injury, especially in the delivery of the after-coming head in a breech presentation. There is paralysis of the deltoid, biceps, brachialis, brachioradialis, and sometimes the supraspinatus, infraspinatus, and rhomboideus muscles. The arm hangs limp at the side of the body, in adduction and internal rotation, and the forearm is in extension, pronation, and medial rotation. The patient is unable to abduct or externally rotate the arm or to flex or supinate the forearm. The biceps reflex is lost. There is little sensory change because of overlapping of the peripheral nerve distributions, but there may be partial anesthesia of the outer aspect of the arm, forearm, and hand (fifth and sixth cervical segments). Transient signs of upper brachial plexus injury may follow prolonged wearing of a military brace in soldiers and also has been reported as a result of wearing a heavy backpack or rucksack.

The lower arm type of brachial plexus palsy (**Dejerine – Klumpke syndrome**) follows injury to the eighth cervical and first thoracic roots, lower trunk, or medial cord. It may be associated with tumors or other pathologic changes of the apex of the lung, fracture of the clavicle or cervical rib, aneurysm of the arch of the aorta, fracture or dislocation of the head of the humerus, a sudden upward pull on the arm, or other injuries from below. Traction on the arm or shoulder or hyperabduction with or without dislocation of the shoulder may also cause the syndrome. There is paralysis of the muscles supplied by the ulnar nerve and to a lesser extent of those supplied by the median nerve, with sensory changes in the distribution of these nerves, or along the inner border of the arm, forearm, and hand (eighth cervical and first thoracic segments).

There is loss of flexion of the wrist and fingers, weakness of the small muscles of the hand, and weakness of grip. Edema, trophic changes, and a Horner's syndrome may be present. Paralysis of the flexors of the wrist and fingers results in a claw hand. A middle arm type of brachial plexus palsy has been described, but is rare; there is weakness of the extensors of the forearm, wrist, and fingers, and there may be sensory changes corresponding to the distribution of the radial nerve.

In lesions of the posterior cord of the brachial plexus there is involvement of the muscles supplied by the axillary and radial nerves, and to a lesser extent of those supplied by the subscapular and thoracodorsal nerves, with loss of abduction and rotation at the shoulder, extension of the forearm, extension of the wrist and fingers, and supination; there may be paralysis of the thumb muscles. The triceps and brachioradialis reflexes are lost. There is anesthesia in the distribution of the axillary and radial nerves. Lesions of the lateral cord cause paralysis of the biceps, brachialis, and coracobrachialis muscles, and of all supplied by the median nerve except the intrinsic muscles of the hand. Lesions of the medial cord cause paralysis of the muscles supplied by the ulnar nerve and of the small muscles of the hand supplied by the median nerve. Infraclavicular lesions cause involvement of the cords of the brachial plexus; fractures and dislocations of the humerus are often responsible. In total brachial plexus palsy there is a flaccid paralysis of the entire arm, the only remaining movement being weak adduction. The hand, forearm, and arm are totally anesthetic except for a small area near the axilla that is supplied by the intercostobrachial nerve. There may be trophic changes and a Horner's syndrome. Owing to individual variations in the brachial plexus, together with variability in the types of injury, there are many incomplete syndromes and a wide range of resulting symptoms.

A number of syndromes have been described in which the symptoms and signs are the result of abnormal compression of the brachial plexus, its constituents, or the subclavian or axillary vessels in the thoracic outlet (or inlet). These may be referred to as cervicobrachial neurovascular compression syndromes. The most characteristic of these is the **scalenus syndrome,** in which a cervical rib, a hypertrophied scalenus anterior muscle, or both may exert pressure on the nerve trunks of the brachial plexus and compress the subclavian artery and vein. Two varieties have been described; the superior type, with pressure on the upper trunk of the brachial plexus by the tendons of origin of the scalenus anterior, and the lower type, which is more frequent, with compression of the lower trunk by the tendons of insertion of the muscle. The outstanding symptom is pain in the outer and anterior shoulder region that radiates into the supraclavicular area and into the arm and hand, on either the ulnar or radial side, or both. It may radiate into the neck, scapula, shoulder, or thoracic wall. The pain often is worse at night, and is increased by recumbency, turning the head toward the unaffected side, downward traction on the arm and shoulder, and pressure on the scalenus muscle, which is tender and painful to palpation (especially at its site of insertion on the first rib). It may be relieved by abduction of the arm. Paresthesias, especially of the thumb and fingers, are common, but objective sensory changes may be minimal. Motor alterations, too, may not be marked; if present they consist of weakness of the hand and finger muscles. Occasionally there is atrophy of the interossei and the thenar and hypothenar muscles. The alterations, both sensory and motor, are most marked in the areas and muscles supplied by the ulnar nerve, but those innervated by the median and even the radial nerve may also be affected. Vascular and autonomic changes include either pallor or cyanosis, subjective coldness and decreased skin temperature, alterations in sweating, edema of the arm and hand, and sometimes even thrombosis of digital arteries and gangrene of the affected fingers. There may be an associated aneurysm of the subclavian artery. The radial pulse may be diminished or obliterated by various maneuvers and diagnostic procedures described later in this chapter, and the brachial blood pressure may be lower on the affected side. Section of the hypertrophied scalenus anterior muscle or its fibrous connections or removal of the cervical rib may bring about relief of symptoms. The scalenus and related thoracic outlet syndromes are not as common as formerly believed. Many of the symptoms, and some of the signs, attributed to these conditions are also found in persons with carpal tunnel syndrome and other compression neuropathies. Before surgical correction is contemplated, these compression syndromes must be localized further with the aid of nerve conduction studies, evoked potential testing, and, at times, angiography.

Other neurovascular compression phenomena that cause symptoms and signs are as follows: In the **costoclavicular syndrome** there is a narrowed space between the clavicle and first rib, with pressure on the brachial plexus and subclavian artery and/or vein as they pass through this aperture; this is accentuated by depression or retraction of the shoulder. The symptoms may be relieved by resection of the first rib. In the **subcoracoid – pectoralis minor** (or **hyperabduction**) **syndrome,** hyperabduction of the arm causes pressure on the stretched vascular structures as they pass posterior to the pectoralis minor muscle and under the subcoracoid process. The symptoms have been relieved by the resection of the pectoralis minor tendon. Other anomalies in the muscular or skeletal development of the thoracic outlet or the shoulder girdle, as well as sequelae of trauma, may cause similar symptoms. Pain, paresthesias, and motor changes in the hands resembling those described previously may also be caused by involvement of the cervical portion of the spinal cord and its emerging nerve roots, as in cervical spondylosis.

Similar symptoms may be associated with other conditions. In **paralytic brachial neuritis (neuralgic amyotrophy,** or **Parsonage – Turner syndrome)** there is a sudden onset of severe pain in the region of the shoulder, followed by extensive paralysis of the shoulder musculature with resulting atrophy of muscles supplied by certain branches of the brachial plexus, as well as sensory changes, but usually no vascular symptoms. The pain gradually subsides as the muscle atrophy supervenes. The etiology of the syndrome is not known. Occasionally a brachial plexus neuritis develops following the injection of foreign proteins. The arm is often maintained in a posture of flexion and adduction at the shoulder, presumably to minimize traction on the brachial plexus.

In **brachial plexus neuralgia** there may be pain without objective sensory or motor changes; this may have an obscure etiology or a reflex origin associated with arthritic changes, periarthritis, myositis, or bursitis. If these are present, there may be localized tenderness and limitation of motion at the shoulder joint. Lesions of the lung apex, especially superior pulmonary sulcus tumors, may cause symptoms resembling the lower type of compression, or those of a lower arm type of brachial plexus palsy; there is often a Horner's syndrome. Subacromial bursitis, arthritis of the cervical spine, an abnormal first rib, cervicodorsal scoliosis, postural defects, a ruptured supraspinatus tendon, spinal cord tumors, herniated intervertebral disks, arthritis or periarthritis of the shoulder, fibrositis, myositis, synovitis, and Raynaud's disease should also be considered in the differential diagnosis of the scalenus syndrome. In the so-called shoulder-hand syndrome there may be pain, atrophy, autonomic changes, and osteoporosis of the hand associated with pain and disuse of the shoulder. This may occur secondary to such varied factors as disease in the region of the shoulder joint, disuse following fracture or paralysis, pressure on the cervical nerve roots or brachial plexus, and myocardial infarction (see Ch. 42).

Special diagnostic procedures may be of aid in the differentiation of certain of the aforementioned syndromes. In the **Adson test** the patient is asked to inspire, hold his breath, and hyperextend his neck. Then the head is passively turned as far as possible, first toward one side and then the other. With the scalenus syndrome there may be accentuation of the pain and weak-

ening or obliteration of the radial pulse, accompanied by a drop in blood pressure in the arm, when the head is turned toward the unaffected (or sometimes the affected) side. The pulse may disappear on both sides with turning of the head in either direction, but there is a longer lag in its return on the affected side. During the maneuver a bruit may develop that is heard best in the supraclavicular space. In the **Allen test,** also positive with the scalenus syndrome, the pulse is diminished on the affected side when the arm is elevated to 90° and rotated externally with the elbow at a right angle, and the head turned forcibly to the nonaffected side. In the **hyperabduction test** the arm is passively hyperabducted and may also be placed in a position of posterior extension. In most normal subjects there is a decrease or weakening of the radial pulse with such a maneuver, but in the hyperabduction syndrome it is obliterated with greater

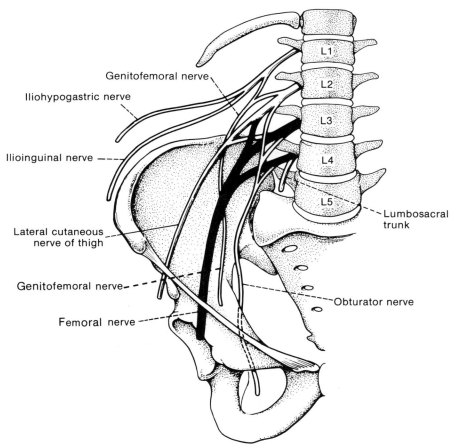

FIG. 45–2. Constituents of the lumbar plexus.

ease than is normal. This test also often produces pain of a radicular nature in patients with paralytic brachial neuritis. In the **shoulder bracing test** the shoulder is passively retracted and depressed; with the costoclavicular syndrome the radial pulse on the affected side is decreased more readily than in the normal subject. Forced depression or downward traction of the arm and shoulder causes increased pain in the presence of a scalenus syndrome, and there is tenderness and pain on pressure over the scalenus anterior muscle. In the **foraminal compression test** the neck is hyperextended and flexed laterally toward the affected side, following which downward pressure is applied to the top of the head. With a laterally herniated intervertebral disk or extramedullary mass the radicular pain is produced or aggravated. Similarly, this radicular pain may be relieved by the **neck traction test,** in which the examiner, grasping both sides of the patient's head, exerts strong upward traction. It must be stressed that these various maneuvers may aid in diagnosis, but are not as reliable as a detailed history and thorough neurologic examination.

THE LUMBAR PLEXUS

The lumbar plexus is formed by the anterior primary rami of the first three lumbar nerves and a part of the fourth, and it may receive a contribution from the twelfth thoracic nerve (Fig. 45-2). It gives off the iliohypogastric, ilioinguinal, genitofemoral, lateral femoral cutaneous, obturator, accessory obturator, and femoral nerves, together with the nerves to the psoas muscles and the lumbosacral trunk to the sacral plexus. There are also collaterals from the first through the fourth lumbar rami to the quadratus lumborum and intertransversarii. The plexus is situated in the substance of the psoas major muscle, in front of the transverse processes of the lumbar vertebrae. Injuries to the lumbar plexus are relatively uncommon, but they may occur in association with fractures or dislocations of the vertebrae,

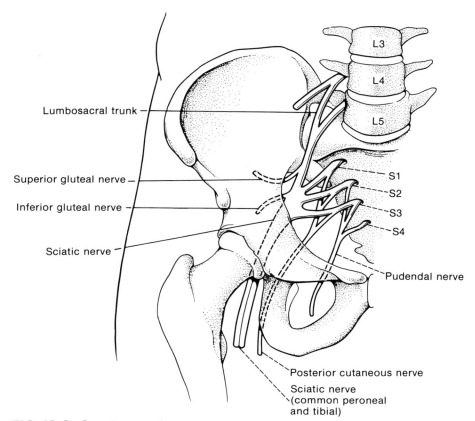

FIG. 45–3. Constituents of the sacral plexus.

penetrating wounds, Pott's disease, psoas abscesses, or pressure from pelvic tumors. Infectious processes or metastatic infiltrations may also affect it. One observes more frequently, however, either radicular symptoms resulting from involvement of the individual rami, or lesions of the constituent nerves. Pain or sensory change in the distribution of these nerves has localizing value. Imaging procedures may be needed to identify mass lesions of this and the sacral plexuses.

THE SACRAL, PUDENDAL, AND COCCYGEAL PLEXUSES

The sacral or lumbosacral plexus shows a great deal of variability. It is formed by the anterior primary rami of the fourth lumbar through the third sacral segments (Fig. 45-3). It lies against the piriformis muscle on the posterior wall of the pelvis. From it are given off various cutaneous branches together with the superior and inferior gluteal nerves, the nerves to the quadratus femoris, obturator internus, and piriformis, and the sciatic nerve. Injuries to the sacral plexus are uncommon, but lesions of the roots or of the primary rami are followed by disabilities of segmental distribution. The individual nerves are frequently involved in lesions of the cauda equina.

Pressure on and irritation of the lower lumbar and upper sacral nerve roots are among the most common causes of low back pain with lumbosacral radiation. Lesions causing such pain are discussed in Chapter 47. The pudendal and coccygeal plexuses and their branches are rarely involved in specific injuries.

BIBLIOGRAPHY

Adson AW, Coffey JR. Cervical rib: A method of anterior approach for relief of symptoms by division of the scalenus anticus. Ann Surg 1927;85:839

Falconer MA, Weddell S. Costoclavicular compression of subclavian artery and vein: Relation to scalenus anticus syndrome. Lancet 1943;2:539

Hershel HC Jr, Razzuk MA. Management of thoracic outlet syndrome. N Engl J Med 1972;286:1140

Keshishian JM, Smyth NPD. Thoracic outlet syndrome: Diagnosis and management. Ann Thorac Surg 1970;9:931

Lain TM. The military-brace syndrome. J Bone Joint Surg 1969;51:557

Naffziger HC, Grant WT. Neuritis of the brachial plexus mechanical in origin: The scalenus anticus syndrome. Surg Gynecol Obstet 1938;67:722

Rowland LP (ed). Merritt's Textbook of Neurology, 8th ed. Philadelphia, Lea & Febiger, 1989

Spurling RG. Lesions of the Cervical Intervertebral Disc. Springfield, IL, Charles C Thomas, 1956

Walshe FMR. Nervous and vascular pressure syndromes of the thoracic inlet and cervico-axillary canal. In Feiling A (ed). Modern Trends in Neurology. New York, PB Hoeber, 1951

Waxman SG. The flexion-adduction sign in neuralgic amyotrophy. Neurology 1979;29:1301

White HH. Pack palsy: A neurological complication of scouting. Pediatrics 1968;41:1001

Winsor T, Brow R. Costoclavicular syndrome: Its diagnosis and treatment. JAMA 1966;106:109

Wright IS. The neuromuscular syndrome produced by hyperabduction of the arms. Am Heart J 1945;29:1

Yoss RE, Corbin KB, MacCarty CS et al. Significance of symptoms and signs in localization of involved root in cervical disk protrusion. Neurology 1957;7:673

Chapter 46

DISORDERS OF THE SPINAL CORD

The spinal cord is an elongated, nearly cylindrical portion of the nervous system that is continuous with the medulla above and ends in a conical extremity, the conus medullaris (Fig. 46-1). It is situated within the vertebral canal. From the apex of the conus medullaris a delicate filament, the filum terminale, descends to the periosteum of the posterior surface of the first segment of the coccyx. The spinal cord is slightly flattened in an anteroposterior direction. An anterior median fissure and a posterior median sulcus divide it into two symmetrical halves. The posterior nerve roots enter the posterolateral sulcus, and the anterior nerve roots make their exit at the anterolateral sulcus. The parenchyma of the spinal cord consists of an H- or butterfly-shaped core of gray matter, containing nerve cells. This is surrounded by tracts of longitudinally arranged nerve processes, mainly myelinated, which carry ascending and descending impulses; these constitute the white matter. Within the center of the gray matter and running throughout the entire length of the cord is a minute remnant of the central canal consisting of a single layer of ependymal cells.

The cellular elements in the gray matter are arranged in functional groups (Fig. 46-2). Those in the anterior horn supply motor impulses to striated muscles. The cells in the medial portion of the anterior horn (nuclei dorsomedialis and ventromedialis) supply trunk muscles. The central cells in the cervical region supply the diaphragm and the muscles innervated by the spinal accessory nerve (nuclei phrenicus and accessorius), whereas those in the sacral region supply the perineal muscles (nucleus centralis).

The lateral cells, present only in the cervical and lumbosacral enlargements, supply the extremities (nuclei ventrolateralis, dorsolateralis, and retrodorsolateralis). The cells in the lateral horn belong to the autonomic nervous system; the intermediolateral cells in the thoracic and upper lumbar segments supply preganglionic nerves of the sympathetic division, and the lateral cells in the sacral area supply preganglionic parasympathetic fibers. The cells in the dorsal portion of the gray matter are nuclei of termination of the afferent neurons. The stellate cells (substantia gelatinosa of Rolando) and dorsal funicular cells (nucleus proprius dorsalis) are present throughout the entire extent of the cord, and receive exteroceptive impulses; the nucleus dorsalis of Clarke is present from the eighth cervical through the third lumbar segment; it receives proprioceptive impulses and gives rise to the dorsal spinocerebellar tract.

The fiber pathways in the white matter are in part crossed and in part uncrossed (see Fig. 46-2). Afferent impulses enter the fasciculus dorsolateralis (Lissauer's tract). The descending pathways carry impulses from higher centers; these terminate in spinal cord nuclei on which they have regulatory and inhibitory functions. The ascending pathways carry sensory impulses of various types from the extremities, trunk, or neck to higher centers. The principal tracts in the dorsal funiculus are the fasciculus gracilis and cuneatus, which carry uncrossed proprioceptive and tactile impulses to the respective nuclei in the medulla, and then, after decussation, to the thalamus. Ascending pathways in the lateral and ventral areas are the lateral and ventral spino-

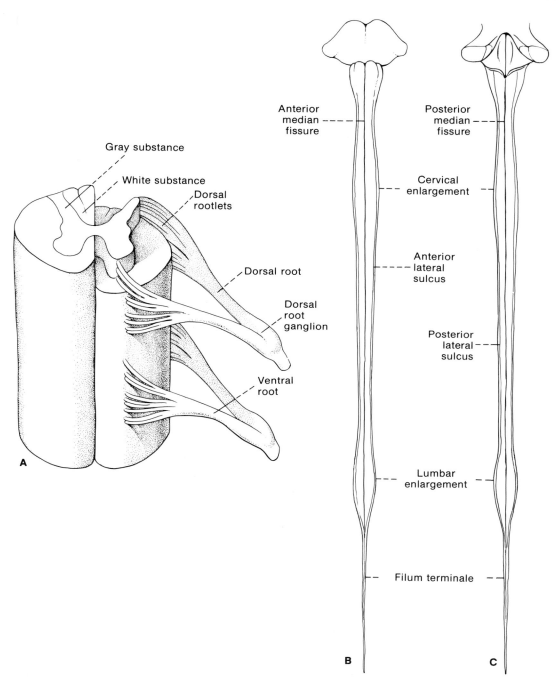

FIG. 46–1. The spinal cord. **A.** Section of the spinal cord with anterior and posterior nerve roots attached. **B.** Anterior view of the spinal cord. **C.** Posterior view of spinal cord.

thalamic tracts, both of which carry crossed exteroceptive impulses, together with the dorsal and ventral spinocerebellar, spinoolivary, spinotectal, and spinovestibular tracts. Descending pathways are the lateral corticospinal (crossed pyramidal), ventral corticospinal (uncrossed pyramidal), rubrospinal, olivospinal, tectospinal, vestibulospinal, and reticulospinal tracts. There are other less well defined tracts that may be important avenues of conduction, as well as

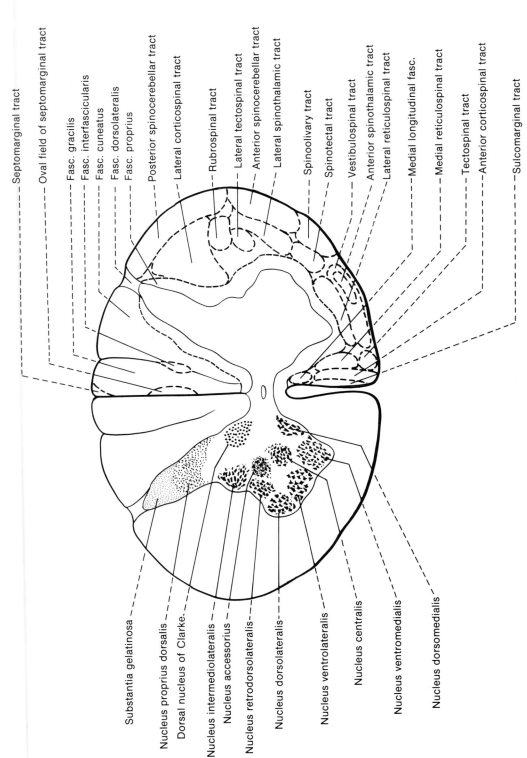

Septomarginal tract

Oval field of septomarginal tract

Fasc. gracilis

Fasc. interfascicularis

Fasc. cuneatus

Fasc. dorsolateralis

Fasc. proprius

Posterior spinocerebellar tract

Lateral corticospinal tract

Rubrospinal tract

Lateral tectospinal tract

Anterior spinocerebellar tract

Lateral spinothalamic tract

Spinoolivary tract

Spinotectal tract

Vestibulospinal tract

Anterior spinothalamic tract

Lateral reticulospinal tract

Medial longitudinal fasc.

Medial reticulospinal tract

Tectospinal tract

Anterior corticospinal tract

Sulcomarginal tract

Substantia gelatinosa

Nucleus proprius dorsalis

Dorsal nucleus of Clarke

Nucleus intermediolateralis

Nucleus accessorius

Nucleus retrodorsolateralis

Nucleus dorsolateralis

Nucleus ventrolateralis

Nucleus centralis

Nucleus ventromedialis

Nucleus dorsomedialis

FIG. 46–2. Cross section of the spinal cord showing the arrangement of cellular groups in the gray matter and fiber pathways in the white matter.

intersegmental, intrasegmental, and association pathways. There is a certain amount of intermingling of fibers within the various tracts, and it is not possible to outline or delineate the individual pathways as distinctly as diagrams would indicate.

The spinal cord extends from the foramen magnum, or the level of the upper border of the atlas, to the level between the first and second lumbar vertebrae. It is surrounded by pia mater, arachnoid, and dura mater. The pia mater is a delicate membrane that closely invests the spinal cord. The arachnoid is a transparent membrane that is close to the inner surface of the dura, but fine strands extend to the pia. The dura mater is a strong, fibrous membrane, penetrated by the nerve roots, which forms a firm, tubular sheath. It is separated from the wall of the vertebral canal by the epidural space, which contains areolar tissue and a plexus of veins. The subdural space is a potential space containing a small amount of fluid. The subarachnoid space, which extends to about the level of the second sacral vertebra, is a well-defined cavity containing cerebrospinal fluid. The dentate ligaments extend along the lateral surface of the spinal cord, between the anterior and posterior nerve roots, from the pia to the dura mater. They suspend the spinal cord in the vertebral canal. The spinal nerves, with their dorsal and ventral roots, are segmentally arranged in 31 pairs. There are 8 pairs of cervical nerves, 12 thoracic, 5 lumbar, 5 sacral, and 1 coccygeal. Situated on each dorsal root is the dorsal root ganglion. The spinal cord is greater in width and diameter in the cervical and lumbosacral regions, the site of nuclear centers that supply the extremities.

During the process of maturation the vertebral column elongates more than the spinal cord, and in the adult the spinal cord is shorter than the vertebral column and the spinal nerves course downward before making their exit through the intervertebral foramina. Those that originate in the lower part of the spinal cord become more and more oblique in their downward descent. The lumbar and sacral nerves descend almost vertically to reach their points of exit; these are designated the **cauda equina.** Consequent to this developmental change, there is a discrepancy between the segments of the spinal cord and the level of the spinous processes of the vertebrae. In the upper cervical area the cord level is about one segment higher than the corresponding spinous process; in the lower cervical and thoracic areas there is a difference of about two segments, whereas in the lumbar region there is a difference of almost three segments (see Fig. 5-11).

BLOOD SUPPLY

There is some individual variation in the blood supply of the spinal cord (Fig. 46-3). The anterior spinal (or anterior median spinal) artery is formed by the union of the arterial branches that pass caudally from each vertebral artery and unite in the midline near the foramen magnum. It descends the entire length of the spinal cord, taking a somewhat undulating course, and lies in or near the anterior median fissure. Below the fourth or fifth cervical segment the anterior spinal artery is fed or reinforced by unpaired anterior medullary arteries that arise from the lateral spinal arteries. These latter vessels enter the vertebral canal through the intervertebral foramina, and in the cervical region are branches of the ascending cervical artery; in the thorax, of the intercostals; in the abdomen, of the lumbar, iliolumbar, and lateral sacral arteries. They pierce the dural sheaths of the spinal roots and split into anterior and posterior radicular branches. The radicular arteries are asymmetric and sometimes absent. The largest medullary artery, often called the great radicular, or anterior medullary, artery of Adamkiewicz, supplies the lumbar enlargement, usually on the left side. The blood supply to any given level of the spinal cord is proportional to its cross-sectional area of gray matter, and the caliber of the anterior spinal artery is largest at the level of the lumbar and cervical enlargements.

The so-called posterior spinal arteries are really plexiform channels rather than distinct single vessels. They lie near the posterolateral sulci and the entrance of the rootlets of the posterior nerves. They also arise from the vertebral arteries, and posterior medullary arteries join them at irregular intervals. Central arteries, branches of the anterior spinal, being given off alternately to the right and left halves of the spinal cord at different levels, supply the anterior and central portions of the cord, and branches of the anterior and posterior spinal arteries form a peripheral anastomosis, the arterial vasocorona, which supplies the periphery of the cord, including the lateral and ventral funiculi. This anastomosis is least efficient in the region of the lateral columns. Within the substance of the cord the posterior spinal arteries supply the posterior horns and most of the dorsal funiculi, whereas the anterior spinal artery supplies most of the re-

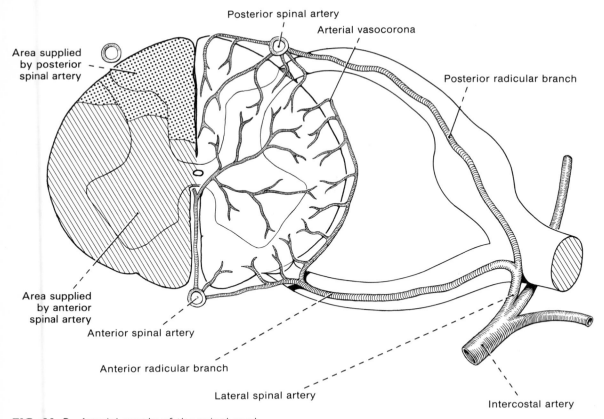

FIG. 46–3. Arterial supply of the spinal cord.

mainder of the cord. Certain boundary zones between ascending and descending sources of the blood supply are sites of least adequate circulation in the spinal cord. The fourth thoracic segment is one such site, and this is especially vulnerable to vascular occlusion and ischemic necrosis.

The venous drainage of the spinal cord courses from the capillary plexuses to peripheral venous plexuses that correspond somewhat to the arterial supply. The major portion of the venous drainage takes place through the intervertebral foramina into veins in the thoracic, abdominal, and pelvic cavities, but the spinovertebral venous plexus also continues upward into the intracranial cavity and venous sinuses; this may be a means of transport of tumor cells and other emboli to the brain.

PHYSIOLOGY AND PATHOPHYSIOLOGY

The spinal cord is essential to the regulation and administration of various motor, sensory, and autonomic activities of the body. By means of its segmentally arranged spinal nerves and its nuclear centers, it receives impulses at various levels and carries them to motor cells in the same or adjoining segments for distribution to appropriate muscles. Thus it provides for reflex action and governs motor activity. By means of its descending pathways from higher centers, it regulates and inhibits spinal cord reflexes and motor activity. Through its ascending pathways, it conducts impulses from the extremities, trunk, and neck to higher centers and to consciousness. It also has a regulatory and administrative action over various visceral activities. In disease of the spinal cord any or all of these functions may be affected, and one may often localize spinal cord lesions in both the transverse and the longitudinal planes by the neurologic examination.

Lesions of the spinal cord are characterized by sensory, motor, and autonomic changes. The resulting symptoms depend upon the location and extent of damage to various functional elements, and often upon the type of damage and the rapidity with which the lesion develops. If there is involvement of the posterior roots or of the sensory cells in the posterior horns of the gray matter, there are segmental sensory changes; there may be either a loss of certain or all varieties of sensation in the dermatomes supplied by the involved segments, or irritative phenomena such as pain and paresthesias. If there is involvement of the ascending pathways, loss of sensation, principally of the pain, temperature, and proprioceptive modalities, develops below the lesion. There is often a dissociation of sensation, with loss of some varieties but sparing of others. If there is involvement of the anterior horn cells or of the anterior roots, there is a lower motor neuron paralysis in the myotomes supplied by the involved segments, occasionally with either fasciculations or muscle spasm. If there is involvement of the descending motor pathways, either corticospinal, extrapyramidal, or vestibulospinal, there are changes in motor power and tone below the level of the lesion. If there is involvement of the intermediolateral cell group of the gray matter, the neuraxes of these cells, or the descending autonomic pathways, there are changes in autonomic function. Alterations of the reflexes, ataxia, disturbances of gait, dysfunction of the sphincters, and other abnormalities of function are all secondary to either isolated or combined motor, sensory, or autonomic involvement.

In order to localize spinal cord disease in the transverse plane, one must be familiar with the anatomy and function of the cell groups within the gray matter, the dorsal and ventral roots, and the peripheral afferent and efferent paths in the dorsal, lateral, and ventral columns. In order to localize disease in the vertical, or longitudinal, direction, one must be familiar with the segmental sensory, motor, reflex, and autonomic supply, and the relationship between the spinal cord segments and the vertebral bodies and spinous processes.

Motor Deficits. The motor deficits resulting from spinal cord diseases depend upon the site and extent of the lesion. There is usually a flaccid paralysis of those muscles supplied by the affected segment, and a flaccid paresis that later becomes spastic below the level of the lesion. The first through the fourth cervical segments innervate muscles that control movements of the head and neck. A lesion of the upper two or three cervical segments is usually rapidly fatal, owing to proximity to the important vasomotor and respiratory centers in the medulla; there may be hyperpyrexia. Involvement above the fourth cervical segment causes respiratory difficulty due to diaphragmatic paralysis; the patient is able to breathe only with the accessory mus-

cles of respiration. With a lesion at the fourth cervical segment respiration is possible through the function of the diaphragm and the accessory muscles of respiration, but there is paralysis of all four extremities.

The fourth or fifth cervical through the first or second thoracic segments control movements of the upper extremities. Involvement of the fifth or fifth and sixth cervical segments causes a syndrome resembling the upper arm type of brachial plexus palsy; there is paralysis of the rhomboid, supraspinatus, infraspinatus, teres major and minor, deltoid, biceps, and brachioradialis muscles, with loss of the biceps and brachioradialis reflexes and sometimes inversion of the radial reflex. The arms are adducted and may be in a position of internal rotation. With a lesion of the sixth cervical segment the biceps is predominantly affected, and the deltoid and triceps may both be intact. A lesion of the seventh cervical segment causes paralysis of the triceps and the extensors of the wrist and fingers; there is either loss of the triceps reflex or a paradoxic reflex with flexion instead of extension of the forearm. The patient holds his upper arm in abduction and his forearm in flexion, and there is usually flexion of the wrist and fingers. This position, if unilateral, is referred to as **Jolly's sign**; if bilateral, it is spoken of as either **Bradborn's** or **Thorborn's sign.** Involvement of the eighth cervical and first thoracic segments causes a syndrome that resembles the lower arm type of brachial plexus palsy; there may be an atrophic paralysis of the flexors of the wrist and fingers and the small muscles of the hand; the arm reflexes are preserved, but the wrist and finger flexion reflexes are affected.

The thoracic segments control movements of the trunk, thorax, and abdomen. Involvement of the midthoracic segments causes atrophic paralysis of the intercostal muscles; the abdominal reflexes are affected, and Beevor's sign may be present (Ch. 27). The segments from the first lumbar through the third sacral control movements of the lower extremities. A lesion of the first two or three lumbar segments causes paralysis of flexion and adduction of the thigh and of extension of the leg; the patellar reflex is lost. With a lesion of the fifth lumbar and first sacral segments there is loss of extension of the hip, with paralysis of plantar flexion and dorsiflexion of the foot, paralysis of flexion of the knee, and loss of the plantar and Achilles reflexes. Involvement of the second sacral segment causes paralysis of the small muscles of the foot. The lower sacral segments innervate the bladder, rectum, anus, and genitalia. A lesion of the third and fourth sacral segments causes paralysis of the rectum and bladder, impairment of erection, and loss of the anal and bulbocavernosus reflexes.

In all of these motor syndromes, a focal lesion that involves only the anterior horn cells will cause a flaccid loss of power, with consequent atrophy, that is limited to the involved myotomes. A lesion that involves the descending motor pathways will cause either a corticospinal or an extrapyramidal paralysis below the level of the lesion. If both the anterior horn cells and the descending tracts are affected, there will be a segmental flaccid paralysis, together with an upper motor neuron paresis below the level of the lesion.

Sensory Changes. The sensory changes associated with spinal cord lesions are usually segmental, or dermatomal, in distribution (see Fig. 5-10). There may be either loss or diminution of one or more modality, or perversions taking the form of either pain or paresthesias. The areas of diminution or loss, and the paresthesias as well, may involve the entire body below the level of the lesion, whereas the pain is usually segmental and affects only the dermatome supplied by the level of the lesion. The sensory loss is usually of the dissociated variety, with impairment of certain modalities and sparing of others. Pain, temperature, and proprioceptive sensations are predominantly affected. There may be hyperesthesia at the level of the lesion, with increased irritability even though the threshold may be raised. The level for pain and temperature sensations is most specific, and it may be difficult to delineate a definite level for either tactile or proprioceptive sensations. With cervical lesions, however, there may be marked proprioceptive loss as well as stereoanesthesia of the upper extremities (Ch. 8). **Lhermitte's sign,** the development of sudden, electriclike shocks spreading down the body on flexion of the neck, occurs in focal traumatic and neoplastic lesions at the cervical level, but is also seen in multiple sclerosis and spinal cord degenerations.

Autonomic Changes. The autonomic nervous system changes may vary. A lesion at the eighth cervical and first thoracic segments may cause a Horner's syndrome, but a Horner's syndrome may also follow a lesion of the descending autonomic pathways above this level. Transverse spinal lesions are followed, early in their course, by loss of sweating, vasodilation, loss of piloerection, increase in skin resistance, and increase in skin temperature below the level of the lesion. Later there is vasoconstriction with decrease in skin temperature, and there may be an increase in sweating and piloerection. Interruption of the descending pathways causes disturbances of bladder, rectal, and sexual functions. A lesion at the eighth cervical or first thoracic segment, above the thoracolumbar outflow, may cause a disturbance of the sympathetic innervation of the entire body. A lesion of the thoracic or upper lumbar portions of the spinal cord will cause a loss of sympathetic function that corresponds roughly to the levels of motor and sensory changes. A lesion below the third lumbar segment causes no disturbance in sympathetic function. A focal lesion at the first through the third lumbar segments causes impairment of ejaculation; a lesion of the third and fourth sacral segments causes an autonomous bladder and loss of erection.

Diagnostic Procedures. Special diagnostic tests may aid in the evaluation of disease of the spinal cord. The presence of either local tenderness or muscular rigidity may signify the level of the pathologic process. Electromyography assists in the localization of lesions if either the anterior horn cells or motor roots are involved. Tests of autonomic function may also aid in localization. Imaging procedures such as computed tomography and magnetic resonance with or without contrast enhancing substances are necessary for the accurate diagnosis and specific localization of spinal cord lesions. Plain radiographs of the spine are of some help but are less precise than the other imaging procedures. Myelography is less often needed when the imaging procedures are available, but still has use in supplementing them preoperatively with mass and structural lesions. Diskography is now rarely used. Spinal arteriography and venography have limited applications and are being replaced with magnetic imaging. However, if these diagnostic procedures are to be used, it is advisable to study not only the areas clinically suspected as the site of the pathology, but rather to search adjacent areas as well, if not the entire extent of the spinal cord, as clinical localizations may be deceptive, especially when mainly upper motor neuron signs are present. Lesions are often missed in the cervicomedullary region when the physician erroneously suspects thoracic or even lumbosacral lesions because of certain sensory or motor findings. Lumbar puncture and study of the cerebrospinal fluid may aid in the diagnosis of infectious myelopathies or subarachnoid hemorrhage.

LESIONS OF THE SPINAL CORD

There are many varieties of spinal cord lesions. Transverse syndromes are characterized by complete interruption of the continuity of the spinal cord; there is loss of all motor, sensory, and autonomic function below the level of involvement. Incomplete transverse lesions are followed by loss of function of certain portions of the cord; there may be dysfunction of one-half, one-quarter, or a certain portion or segment of the cord. Syndromes of the gray matter show segmental loss of function of certain cell groups. Disease of the ventral gray matter is followed by a segmental flaccid paralysis (anterior poliomyelitis, progressive spinal muscular atrophy); disease of the dorsal gray matter, by segmental sensory changes; disease of the gray commissure, by dissociation of sensation (syringomyelia). Syndromes of the white matter cause interference with the ascending and descending pathways. In disease of the dorsal funiculi there is interference with the ascending proprioceptive or related impulses, and in disease of the lateral columns, the lateral corticospinal, lateral spinothalamic, or other tracts may be affected. System disease is characterized by dysfunction of anatomically and functionally related systems of cells or fibers (spinocerebellar degenerations, posterolateral sclerosis, amyotrophic lateral sclerosis). Disseminated disease is manifested by patchy involvement, with many lesions of a focal nature (multiple sclerosis). Diffuse disease shows widespread involvement but some cells or fibers may be affected more than others.

A detailed history will usually give much information that is necessary to determine the etiology of spinal cord disease. Traumatic lesions are usually abrupt in onset. Compression of the spinal cord by extradural neoplasms, degenerative changes within the vertebral column, and focal infections of the meninges may cause a gradual onset of symptoms. Most intradural neoplasms are characterized by a progressive increase in manifestations of dysfunction, but occasionally the first symptoms come on precipitously. Vascular lesions, except for those associated with disseminated and diffuse involvement, and inflammatory myelitides appear abruptly. Most degenerative conditions are manifested by a slow and gradual progression of symptoms, although in some conditions, such as multiple sclerosis, there may be periods of remission and exacerbations.

Complete Transection

Complete transection of the spinal cord, whether of traumatic, neoplastic, vascular, or other origin, causes isolation of the segments below the level of the lesion. The upper portions of the cerebrospinal axis function normally, but motor, sensory, and autonomic functions are lost distal to the lesion. The term **transverse myelitis** is often used for syndromes that result in complete transection, even though the process may not be inflammatory in origin; in most cases the term *transverse myelopathy* is more appropriate.

If a transverse lesion is abrupt in onset, the state of spinal shock or diaschisis occurs. There is flaccid paralysis together with loss of all types of sensation, absence of autonomic function, and areflexia below the level of the lesion. Spinal shock usually lasts for about 3 or 4 weeks, after which the reflexes gradually return and become exaggerated, pathologic reflexes appear, muscle tone becomes increased, and the nature of the bladder and rectal dysfunction becomes altered. If infection supervenes, however, in the form of a severe urinary tract involvement or infected decubiti, the period of spinal shock is prolonged.

In transverse myelopathy there is a general loss of all types of sensation below the uppermost level of the lesion, and the lowest level of preserved sensation corresponds to the dermatome supplied by the lowest intact segment. This is most apparent and most clearly delineated with the exteroceptive sensations, especially the superficial pain and temperature modalities. There is loss of these sensations below the level of the lesion, or within one or two segments of the level of the lesion. It must be borne in mind, however, that there is some discrepancy between the spinal cord segments and the corresponding vertebral spinous processes. There may be hyperesthesia at the level of the lesion. The level for tactile sensation is seldom clearly delineated; proprioceptive sensations are also lost, but it is difficult to demonstrate a specific level for these.

After the initial period of flaccidity, the musculature below the level of the lesion becomes spastic, or sometimes spastic and rigid. There is increased tone, with increased resistance to passive movement. The muscle stretch reflexes return and then become hyperactive. The superficial reflexes do not return. Corticospinal tract responses may appear, but they do not do so as characteristically in complete as in incomplete transverse syndromes. There may be an exaggeration of sweating and piloerection below the level of the lesion, with changes in skin temperature and cutaneous vascular function. The bladder, first atonic and distended, with retention and overflow incontinence, becomes small and contracted; the patient develops a reflex type of neurogenic dysfunction. There may be priapism. With the development of these changes, reflexes of spinal automatism appear. These may be elicited by nociceptive stimuli up to the level of the lesion. They are usually of the uniphasic, or flexor, variety, and frequently are accompanied by the mass response with urination, defecation, and sweating below the level of the lesion.

The characteristic position in complete transverse lesions is one of flexion of the lower extremities. The paralysis and sensory loss are symmetric and total; voluntary power does not return; vasomotor and sphincter disturbances are evident; corticospinal tract responses are usually minimal, but defense responses are definite; there is a marked tendency toward the development of decubiti. Inasmuch as the response is mainly one of flexion, the extensor reflexes may be difficult to elicit. With transverse lesions of long duration there may be metabolic alterations, including increased excretion of proteins, fall in serum protein, increase of potassium and decrease of sodium and chlorides in the blood and tissue fluids, hypercalciuria, osteoporosis, testicular atrophy, gynecomastia, altered urinary excretion of 17-ketosteroids, and orthostatic hypotension. The hypertonicity of transverse spinal lesions is sometimes relieved by selective anterior rhizotomy, peripheral nerve section (obturator and others), posterior root section, selective cordectomy or myelotomy, or injection of alcohol or other substances into the subarachnoid space. Regeneration resulting from growth of neural elements within the spinal cord has been reported in experimental animals, but no functional regeneration has been observed in man following complete transverse lesions. With incomplete transection, however, or gradual compression of the cord, there may be recovery of function.

Incomplete Transection

If the spinal cord is only partially divided, the resulting signs and symptoms will depend upon the pathways and cellular structures involved. If there is a sudden onset, there may also be a period of spinal shock, but after recovery from this there is evidence that some portions of the cord have retained their function. The disturbance of superficial pain and temperature sensations depends upon the extent of the damage to the lateral spinothalamic tracts. Inasmuch as the impulses from the lower portions of the body are in the dorsolateral aspects of these tracts, and those from the upper portions of the body are ventral and medial, the sensory level depends upon the site of damage in the transverse plane. If only the lateral portion of one tract is affected, the level for loss of these sensations may be some distance distal to the lesion; it is always contralateral to the side of the cord involvement. Because tactile impulses are conducted to consciousness through both ipsilateral and contralateral pathways, there may be no demonstrable level for loss of such sensations. Proprioceptive sensations are lost on the side of the lesion; those from the lower portion of the body are medial, and an interruption of the lateral part of the tract may not affect them. The extent of motor change, autonomic nervous system dysfunction, and reflex disturbance depends upon the site and extent of the damage. In a partial lesion the motor changes are usually asymmetric and incomplete, and there is some return of voluntary power. The lower extremities may be in a position of extension if the vestibulospinal tracts are intact. The vasomotor changes are variable, but there is a lesser tendency toward the development of decubiti than in complete lesions. The bladder may be overactive, with a reduced capacity and precipitate micturition. There may be spinal defense reflexes, or reflexes of spinal automatism, but these are usually of the biphasic type with flexion followed by extension, or there may be a crossed extensor reflex or an extensor thrust. The muscle stretch reflexes are markedly hyperactive, especially the extensor responses. Babinski reflexes and other abnormal corticospinal tract responses are obtained. Sensory evoked potential studies may aid in differentiating complete from incomplete transections.

Hemisection of the spinal cord causes the **Brown – Séquard syndrome.** The essential findings, below the level of the lesion, are as follows: ipsilateral spastic paresis with increased reflexes and corticospinal tract responses; ipsilateral loss of proprioceptive sensation with sensory ataxia; contralateral loss of pain and temperature sensations extending to one or two segments below the level of the lesion. There may be little or no objective evidence of change in tactile sensation. The following additional neurologic changes may also be present: ipsilateral vasomotor paralysis below the level of the lesion; ipsilateral segmental flaccid paralysis in the myotome supplied by the level of the lesion; ipsilateral segmental loss of all sensation with vasomotor paralysis in the dermatome supplied by the level of the lesion; a zone of hyperesthesia above the anesthetic area, both ipsilaterally and contralaterally; bilateral anesthesia, hyperesthesia, or radicular pain in the distribution of the affected segments. A quadrantic lesion of the spinal cord that involves the dorsal quadrant causes ipsilateral loss of proprioceptive sensation and corticospinal paresis below the level of the lesion. Involvement of the ventral quadrant causes an ipsilateral segmental flaccid paralysis, due to involvement of the anterior horn cells, together with a contralateral loss of pain and temperature sensations below the level of the lesion. Pure hemisection or quadrantic lesions of the cord are rare; incomplete or partially bilateral involvements are more common.

Traumatic Lesions

Traumatic lesions of the spinal cord are usually abrupt in onset. They are most frequently associated with vertebral injuries such as fractures or dislocations of the vertebral column, or with gunshot, stab, or perforating wounds. The violence may be either direct or indirect. The regions of greatest mobility are most susceptible to trauma, and the fifth through seventh cervical, twelfth thoracic, and first lumbar levels are most often affected. Either physiologic interruption, usually temporary, or anatomic interruption of the cord, usually permanent, can occur without bony lesions. Birth injuries of the spinal cord usually follow difficult breech deliveries. The impairment of spinal cord function following trauma may be caused by actual damage to the cord, compression or mechanical blockage, interference with blood supply, herniation of intervertebral disks, extramedullary or intramedullary hemorrhages, or combinations of these. Anterior, posterior, or central injuries may occur. Spinal shock appears immediately if the lesion is

a severe or extensive one. Imaging studies may aid in diagnosis and localization.

Syndromes of spinal cord concussion, contusion, laceration, and compression have been described. **Concussion** of the spinal cord is said to follow indirect violence to the cord without fracture or dislocation. There is an immediate but transitory loss of sensory and motor function. It is said that there are no structural alterations, but there may be edema and mild intracellular and fiber changes of a reversible nature. Traction and compression of the peripheral nerves and nerve roots may cause some of the symptoms. If paralysis lasts more than 10–14 days, it is believed that the damage is more serious in type. In **contusion** of the spinal cord there are petechial hemorrhages into the cord, especially the gray matter, which cause focal disturbances of function. Recovery of function may or may not be complete. **Lacerations** of the spinal cord cause more severe disturbances of function than contusions. In actual **compression** of the spinal cord there is pressure on the structure with either partial or complete loss of function. The symptoms in all of these syndromes depend upon the location and the severity of the damage to the spinal cord. There may be manifestations of either complete or incomplete transection. Radicular pain, rigidity of the muscles supplied by the affected nerve roots, localized tenderness and rigidity of the spine, and motor, sensory, and autonomic nervous system changes may be found.

The syndrome of **acute central cervical spinal cord injury** usually follows severe hyperextension of the neck. There may be a dislocation of the vertebral bodies at the fifth and sixth cervical levels. There is more impairment of motor power in the upper than in the lower extremities, with varying degrees of sensory loss, and with recovery sensation and motor power return first in the legs, then in the upper arms, and finally in the hands. The central involvement of the cord may be mechanical or a result of vascular insufficiency. With **acute anterior spinal cord injuries** the clinical picture resembles that of thrombosis of the anterior spinal artery, and either lacerations of the cord or interruption of the blood supply, or both, may be responsible.

In the more common so-called **whiplash** or **flexion–extension injury** of the neck the pain and other symptoms are more often the result of damage to the soft tissues (muscles and ligaments) and stretching of nerves and nerve roots, than of actual trauma to the spinal cord itself. The symptoms and disability, however, do depend, at least in part, upon the type and severity of the injury, and there may be structural damage to the vertebral column with foraminal encroachment, compression of the vertebral artery, intervertebral disk herniation, and even spinal cord involvement in some cases.

Neoplasms

Neoplasms within the spinal canal may be either extradural or intradural. Intradural tumors may be either extramedullary or intramedullary. Tumors may be classified further according to their horizontal location and vertical level within the spinal canal. The onset of symptoms and signs in spinal cord neoplasms is usually a slow and progressive one, but on occasion the first manifestations appear precipitously. Pain and paresthesias are often symptoms of consequence, but motor, reflex, and vegetative changes are also important.

Extradural tumors may be either primary or metastatic in origin. There may be involvement of the vertebral bodies or extradural space by such neoplasms as carcinoma, sarcoma, lymphosarcoma, and multiple myeloma, with pressure on the spinal cord. **Intradural but extramedullary neoplasms** usually arise from the meninges, nerve roots, connective tissue, and blood vessels. These include meningiomas, neurofibromas, lipomas, dermoids, hemangiomas, and, commonly, metastatic tumors. In both groups the early manifestations are caused by compression, and later there is interference with blood supply. The essential symptoms and signs are listed in Table 46-1. Spontaneous pain is an early and prominent symptom; it may be radicular in distribution, and sharp and lancinating in character. It is often increased by movement and by increasing either the intracranial or intraspinal pressure. A history of prodromal root pains is sometimes obtained. The motor and sensory changes may be slow in onset because of a progressive loss of function of ascending and descending pathways. They often assume a Brown–Séquard distribution, with segmental alterations at the level of the tumor. There is contralateral loss of pain and temperature modalities, with ipsilateral loss of proprioceptive sensations. Inasmuch as the lateral portions of the lateral spinothalamic tract are primarily involved, the sensory loss may be more profound in the distal portions of the body; the defect in pain and temperature sensations may be prominent in the sacral areas. If there is anteroposterior pressure on the spinal cord, the proprioceptive sensations are severely affected.

TABLE 46-1. SIGNS AND SYMPTOMS DIFFERENTIATING BETWEEN EXTRAMEDULLARY AND INTRAMEDULLARY TUMORS OF THE SPINAL CORD

	Extramedullary Tumors	**Intramedullary Tumors**
Spontaneous pain	Radicular in type and distribution; an early and important symptom	Burning in type; poorly localized
Sensory deficit	Contralateral loss of pain and temperature; ipsilateral loss of proprioception	Dissociation of sensation; "spotty" changes
Changes in pain and temperature sensations in saddle area	More marked than at level of lesion	Less marked than at level of lesion
Lower motor neuron involvement	Segmental	Marked, widespread, atrophy, fasciculations
Upper motor neuron involvement	Prominent; early	Late, minimal
Muscle stretch reflexes	Increased early, markedly	Late, minimal changes
Corticospinal tract signs	Early	Late
Trophic changes	Usually not marked	Marked
Spinal subarachnoid block and changes in spinal fluid	Early, marked	Late, less marked

The motor changes are usually of a spastic type with little atrophy, but there may be segmental lower motor neuron involvement at the level of the lesion. There may be irritative motor phenomena, with spasm and defense reflexes. Hyperactive muscle stretch reflexes and corticospinal tract responses occur early. Trophic changes are not marked unless there is extensive spinal cord involvement. Changes in the content and pressure relationships of the spinal fluid occur early.

Intramedullary neoplasms (Fig. 46-4) are usually glial, ependymal cell, or vascular in origin. They frequently start in the gray matter of the cord in the vicinity of the central canal, and extend into the white matter (see Table 46-1). Spontaneous pain, if it occurs, is burning in type and poorly localized. Radicular pain is rare. The sensory changes are dissociated in type; there is segmental loss of pain and temperature sensations with little involvement of tactile or proprioceptive modalities. If the process extends to involve the lateral spinothalamic tract, it affects first the inner fibers, or those that have come from dermatomes just slightly below the level of the lesion. There may be spotty changes in sensation. The motor signs are those of lower motor neuron involvement, and there may be focal but often widespread paralysis, with atrophy and fasciculations. Paresis of the upper motor neuron type, an increase in the muscle stretch reflexes, and abnormal coticospinal tract signs appear late. Trophic changes may be marked. Alterations in the content and the pressure relationships of the spinal fluid occur later than in extramedullary neoplasms, and are less definite. The symptoms and signs of an intramedullary tumor may closely resemble those of syringomyelia.

The diagnosis and localization of spinal cord neoplasms can usually be confirmed by imaging studies such as magnetic resonance with or without contrast enhancement, computed tomography, and myelography. These studies demonstrate the mass lesion itself or outline displacements or obliteration of normal structures or spaces in the vicinity of the spinal cord. Plain roentgenograms are of limited value; they may show evidence of erosion of the vertebral processes, narrowing or separation of the pedicles, or even collapse of the bodies.

With space-occupying lesions within the vertebral canal, the flow of cerebrospinal fluid is often partially or completely blocked. The protein in the fluid may be elevated, sometimes assuming a yellowish discoloration. Neoplastic cells may be present in the fluid with some types of neoplasms, aiding in their identification and pathologic classification. The clinical manifestations associated with the tumor are sometimes increased following lumbar puncture, especially if there is a partial or total block and the hydrodynamics are altered by removal of some of the fluid. Thus, lumbar puncture and myelography must at times be postponed until the patient is ready for immediate decompressive surgery, should it be needed. Spinal fluid changes and changes on plain roentgenograms are more marked in extradural and extramedullary than in intramedullary tumors.

Herniated intervertebral disks that press on the spinal cord, nerve roots, or nerve fibers may give the symptoms of an extramedullary tumor. This is especially true when they occur in the cervical or thoracic regions of the cord. The more commonly encountered ruptured intervertebral disks in the lumbar and lumbosacral regions are considered with the syndromes of low back pain (Ch. 47).

Conus Medullaris and Cauda Equina Lesions. Neoplasms and lesions of other types in the region of the conus medullaris and the cauda equina may present some diagnostic difficulties. In lesions of the conus there is symmetric involvement, suggestive of an intramedullary lesion. In lesions of the cauda equina the manifestations are more asymmetric and are suggestive of nerve root involvement (Table 46-2).

Vascular Lesions

Vascular lesions affect the spinal cord less frequently than the brain or brain stem. However, thrombosis, embolism, hemorrhage, and atherosclerotic changes may occur.

Thrombosis of the anterior spinal artery causes ischemic necrosis and myelomalacia in the area of distribution of this vessel. It may occur at any level, but is most common in the boundary zones between ascending and descending sources of the blood supply, especially in the midthoracic areas. The onset is usually abrupt, with or without pain. There is a partial transverse myelopathy affecting predominantly the anterior horns and the ventral and lateral funiculi, with a flaccid paralysis at the level of the lesion and a spastic paresis below. Bowel and bladder functions are usually lost, but proprioceptive sensations are spared. The thrombosis is usually secondary to atherosclerosis of the ante-

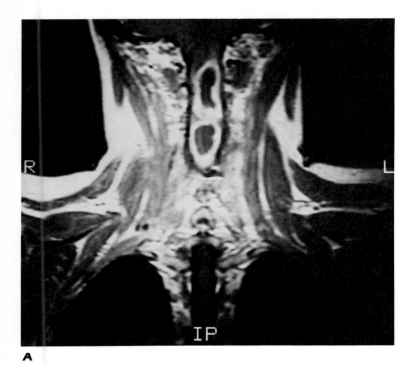

A

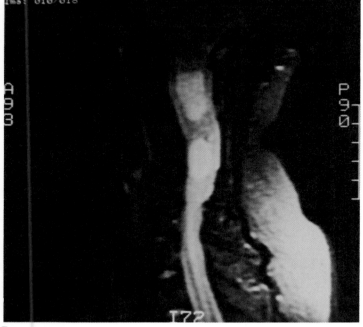

B

FIG. 46–4. Magnetic resonance images of a cervical glioma (TR 600, TE 20). **A.** Anteroposterior view. Lesion is the bilobed cystic area in top center. **B.** Lateral view.

TABLE 46-2. SIGNS AND SYMPTOMS DIFFERENTIATING BETWEEN LESIONS OF THE CONUS MEDULLARIS AND CAUDA EQUINA

	Conus Medullaris	**Cauda Equina**
Spontaneous pain	Not common or severe; bilateral and symmetric; in perineum or thighs	May be most prominent symptom; severe; radicular in type; unilateral or asymmetric; in perineum, thighs, and legs, back, or bladder; distribution of sacral nerves
Sensory deficit	Saddle distribution; bilateral, usually symmetric; dissociation of sensation	Saddle distribution; may be unilateral and asymmetric; all forms affected; no dissociation of sensation
Motor loss	Symmetric; not marked; fasciculations may be present	Asymmetric; more marked; atrophy may occur; usually no fasciculations
Reflex loss	Only Achilles reflex absent	Patellar and Achilles reflexes may be absent
Bladder and rectal symptoms	Early and marked	Late and less marked
Trophic changes	Decubiti common	Decubiti less marked
Sexual functions	Erection and ejaculation impaired	Less marked impairment
Onset	Sudden and bilateral	Gradual and unilateral

rior spinal artery, but it may also develop in association with either a dissecting aneurysm of the aorta or thrombosis of an aortic aneurysm, and it has been reported following aortography and operative procedures in the vicinity of the aorta. The cord dysfunction caused by neoplasms, herniated disks, and inflammatory involvement of the meninges may be the result of compression of the anterior spinal artery. Infarcts of the spinal cord are not common but may occur in association with atherosclerosis.

Meningeal hemorrhage, if subarachnoid, gives symptoms of subarachnoid hemorrhage (Ch. 53); if either subdural or extradural, it may cause focal manifestations. The term *hematorrhachia* is used for any hemorrhage into the spinal canal; it is usually traumatic in origin. Intraspinal hemorrhage and epidural hematoma produce focal manifestations. Hematomyelia may follow trauma to the spinal column or acute inflammation of the spinal cord; it may be associated with purpura or hemophilia. The lesion is usually in the vicinity of the spinal canal, and the symptoms are similar to those of syringomyelia. However, involvement may be either of the cord itself or secondary to pressure on it from inside or out-

side, causing a variety of symptoms and deficits. Angiomas, hemangiomas, arteriovenous malformations, varices of the meninges and spinal cord, and blood dyscrasias may cause focal symptoms that come on either abruptly or gradually, but there are also recurrent episodes of meningeal bleeding. Atherosclerotic changes, anemia, and hyperemia may cause focal, disseminated, or diffuse involvement. Progressive degenerative changes of the spinal cord with symptoms suggestive of posterolateral sclerosis may have an atherosclerotic basis. Symptoms similar to those of vascular occlusion may occur in decompression sickness, sometimes causing a transverse myelitis. In addition there are muscular cramps, paresthesias, vertigo, staggering, and nausea.

Inflammatory Lesions

The term **myelitis** is used to indicate inflammatory disease of the spinal cord. It is also used, however, for lesions that are not obviously inflammatory or are of unknown etiology; for these the term **myelopathy** would be more appropriate. Inflammatory transverse myelitis may be suppurative in type, secondary to meningitis, adjacent infections (such as osteomyelitis or tuberculosis of the vertebrae), or infections elsewhere in the body (pneumonia or septicemia), or it may be of viral or suspected viral origin. Myelitis is known to occur with specific viral infections, notably poliomyelitis, coxsackie and echoviruses, herpes zoster, rabies, human T-cell lymphotropic virus type I (tropical spastic paraparesis), and human immunodeficiency virus, as well as infections secondary to its immune suppressed state. Tuberculous, syphylitic, rickettsial, mycotic, and parasitic forms of myelitis also occur. Occasionally there is a sudden onset of transverse involvement, which may or may not follow symptoms of systemic infection and may or may not be accompanied by a pleocytosis in the cerebrospinal fluid. The source of the infection may not be determined, and the prognosis is unpredictable at the onset. Myelitis may develop on the basis of demyelination, as in certain cases of multiple sclerosis, in neuromyelitis optica, and in postvaccinal and postinfectious myelopathies. It may also occur with collagen disease and the use of intrathecal anesthetics or drugs, following radiation (both transiently and permanently), and electrical injuries, as a remote effect in association with visceral carcinoma, and as the so-called acute or subacute necrotic myelopathy, which may be of vascular etiology.

In **Landry's paralysis,** or **acute ascending paralysis,** there is an ascending motor deficit, usually with sensory changes that are less marked. This syndrome may be caused by an actual inflammatory disease of the spinal cord, predominantly in the anterior horn regions, or it may be associated with a polyradiculoneuritis (Landry – Guillain – Barré syndrome). In **anterior poliomyelitis** the inflammatory process is limited largely to the anterior horn cells, and there is a focal flaccid paralysis, segmental in distribution, with resulting atrophy. There is loss of both motor power and reflex action in the segments involved by the area of inflammation, often with associated vasomotor involvement, but no sensory changes. A meningeal reaction, with a pleocytosis in the cerebrospinal fluid, accompanies the process.

Meningeal inflammation may be accompanied by spinal cord involvement in the absence of transverse myelitis; adhesive spinal arachnoiditis usually causes both localized and disseminated changes. Cervical hypertrophic pachymeningitis produces focal manifestations suggestive of an extradural neoplasm; there may be associated pain and muscle spasm, sensory changes, and spinal subarachnoid block. A spinal epidural abscess may present symptoms of a focal, space-occupying, extramedullary lesion; there are usually associated signs of infection, along with tenderness to palpation over the area of the lesion in the back. While Pott's disease may cause cord symptoms, they are more often those of compression than of infection. Infections of the intervertebral disks cause pain and signs of systemic infection, but rarely cause spinal cord involvement. With all these extramedullary inflammations, signs of spinal cord disease, if they occur, may be the result of an interference with the blood supply rather than of an extension of the infectious process.

Degenerative Processes and System Diseases

So-called degenerative processes and system diseases of the spinal cord of unknown etiology may take various forms. The manifestations may be diffuse or disseminated, or may affect only certain cells and fiber systems.

In **progressive spinal muscular atrophy,** once known as chronic anterior poliomyelitis, there is atrophy with paresis and fasciculations secondary to degenerative changes in the anterior horn cells. In **amyotrophic lateral sclerosis** there are similar changes, together with evidence of corticospinal tract and bulbar involvement.

In **tabes dorsalis** the principal manifestations are loss of proprioceptive sensations and sensory ataxia secondary to involvement of the posterior funiculus. Associated involvement of the dorsal roots and dorsal root ganglia causes radicular pain, girdle sensations, decreased reflexes, loss of deep pain, and a delayed pain reaction. It may be that the pathologic process starts in the dorsal roots and progresses to the posterior funiculi. Other important changes include bladder dysfunction of an atonic type, rectal incontinence, impotence, and trophic disturbances in the form of penetrating ulcers and a Charcot type of arthropathy.

Primary lateral sclerosis has been described as a disease entity, but it may be the earliest manifestation of amyotrophic lateral sclerosis, posterolateral sclerosis, or multiple sclerosis, among others. In lateral sclerosis there is bilateral weakness with hyperreflexia, abnormal corticospinal tract signs, and loss of superficial reflexes, but no sensory disturbances. The syndrome of primary lateral sclerosis may also be associated with anterior spinal cord compression; the larger fibers, which mediate motor impulses, are affected earlier by pressure than the smaller fibers, which transmit pain and temperature sensations. A hereditary form of "primary lateral sclerosis" is not uncommon; with this tone is increased to a marked degree but the weakness is mild. This condition is termed familial spastic paraparesis. Usually the legs are more involved than the arms. Sensory impairment is absent, and bladder disturbances rare.

Posterolateral sclerosis is characterized by pathologic changes that involve predominantly the lateral column (corticospinal pathway) and the posterior funiculus. The clinical manifestations include weakness with hyperreflexia and abnormal corticospinal tract signs, loss of proprioceptive sensation with sensory ataxia, and autonomic manifestations with bladder and rectal involvement and impotence. Posterolateral sclerosis is most frequently associated with pernicious anemia, but it may appear in certain deficiency states, pellagra, diabetes mellitus, multiple sclerosis, and may occur as a disease *sui generis*. In **Friedreich's ataxia** there is involvement of the posterior columns and the spinocerebellar tracts; the lateral columns and the cerebellum are often affected. The ataxia is both spinal and cerebellar in type. Nystagmus is marked. The muscle stretch reflexes are absent owing to interruption of the sensory portion of the reflex arc. The Babinski sign is present.

These findings can be detected in other forms of hereditary spinocerebellar degenerations but in them the reflexes are usually exaggerated.

Syringomyelia (Fig. 46-5) is a disease in which the pathologic changes consist of gliosis, fibrosis, necrosis, and cavitation of the central portion of the spinal cord; the process often extends into the medulla as well (**syringobulbia**). Many etiologies have been suggested, but the condition is probably of developmental origin. Anomalies of or interference with the intramedullary blood supply lead to vascular insufficiency of the affected areas. The patients often have other malformations and disturbances of development. On occasion a syrinx may be associated with an intramedullary neoplasm, and, rarely, an intramedullary abscess or cyst may mimic it. Focal or noncommunicating syrinxes may occur with spinal multiple sclerosis. Those cases in which localized cavitation of the spinal cord develops secondary to trauma, compression, extramedullary vascular lesions, or meningeal inflammation and other causes can usually be differentiated pathologically from true syringomyelia. The degeneration usually occurs in the cervical enlargement; it starts in the region of the central canal and extends peripherally in an irregular fashion. The canal itself is not always involved in the process. Owing to interference with the decussating sensory fibers, the first manifestation is often a loss of pain and temperature sensations in the dermatomes sup-

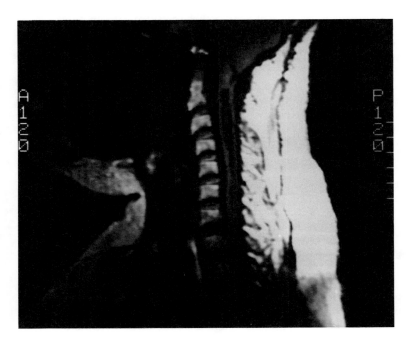

FIG. 46–5. Lateral magnetic resonance image of cervical syringomyelia (TR 600, TE 20), from a patient postoperative for Arnold–Chiari malformation. Syrinx is the tubular, dark central area throughout most of the length of the visualized spinal cord, to the right of the vertebrae.

plied by the involved segments, with relative sparing of tactile sensations. As the process extends there is involvement of the anterior horn cells, with focal paresis, atrophy, and fasciculations, and involvement of the cells of the intermediolateral column, with focal autonomic changes. Later there is pressure on the fiber pathways, with an upper motor neuron paresis and interruption of the ascending lateral spinothalamic tract. There may be extensive trophic changes in the skin and subcutaneous tissues, with indolent ulcers and infected whitlows. There may be painless ulcerations of the fingers (**Morvan's disease**) and edema and lividity of the hands (**main succulente**), as well as Charcot joints. The manifestations of syringomyelia resemble those of hematomyelia and intramedullary neoplasms. In syringomyelia, however, spontaneous pain and evidence of spinal fluid block are rarely encountered. The cavitary lesions of the spinal cord, including syringomyelia and others, are well demonstrated by magnetic resonance imaging.

Multiple sclerosis is characterized by disseminated lesions of the central nervous system. These are found in the spinal cord, where they affect largely the white matter, and also in the brain stem, cerebellum, cerebrum, and optic nerves. There may be fluctuation of symptoms, with remissions and exacerbations. Spinal cord involvement frequently causes a spastic paresis, hyperactive muscle stretch reflexes, loss of superficial reflexes, abnormal corticospinal tract signs, interference with proprioceptive sensations, and sensory ataxia. Disturbances of exteroceptive sensation are not common. In **neuromyelitis optica** there is, in addition to an acute optic neuritis, a rapidly progressive myelopathy, often with pain and paresthesias; it is felt to be a variety of multiple sclerosis.

Certain alterations of the spinal cord take place with the aging process. There is gliosis with demyelination of the fasciculus gracilis as well as atrophy of ganglion cells. These changes, along with ischemia secondary to atherosclerosis, may cause proprioceptive defects and progressive weakness of the lower extremities, but these are usually mild.

Developmental Disturbances and Congenital Defects

Developmental disturbances of various types may cause abnormalities of spinal cord function. These include, among others, heterotopias, spina bifida, agenesis, meningocele, myelocele, myelomeningocele, and myelodysplasias of various types and in various sites. Spina bifida, which is most frequent in the lumbosacral area, may cause a cauda equina syndrome with a flaccid paralysis of the lower extremities, sensory changes in the saddle area or perianal area, loss of bowel or bladder control, and trophic involvement. Developmental disturbances in the region of the atlas and axis are discussed in Chapter 18.

Other Causes of Spinal Cord Disease

Structural and other abnormalities of the vertebral column, especially those in the cervical region, may cause spinal cord and nerve root compression and thus bring about alterations of function. Osteomyelitis, syphilitic osteitis, rheumatoid arthritis, Paget's disease, Pott's disease, neoplasms, and severe osteoporosis may result in vertebral compression with consequent pressure on the spinal cord. There may be erosion of the vertebral bodies by a dissecting aortic aneurysm. Compression fractures of the vertebrae (sometimes occurring spontaneously), with resulting spinal cord and nerve root compression, may develop in patients with extensive osteoporosis or severe rheumatoid arthritis. Scoliosis of various etiologies may cause spinal cord symptoms. Absence of one or more of the cervical vertebrae (Klippel-Feil syndrome) may cause disturbances of function; this may be associated with the Sprengel deformity (congenital elevation of the scapula), and the wasting of the shoulder girdle muscles may simulate poliomyelitis. Rupture and protrusion of intervertebral disks at various levels may cause spinal cord symptoms, as may spondylosis and spondylitis of various etiologies. This is especially true in the cervical region, where spondylitis, usually either posttraumatic or degenerative, causes pressure on the emerging nerve roots as well as on the spinal cord, with resulting pain, weakness, and sensory changes in the radicular distribution and a significant and progressive myelopathy. Occasionally pressure on the vertebral arteries causes symptoms of vertebrobasilar insufficiency with transient attacks of vertigo and weakness. Myelopathy may develop as a result of nutritional deficiency and secondary to metabolic disturbances, such as hepatic disease.

The injection of foreign substances into the subarachnoid space, which may be done for either diagnostic or therapeutic purposes, may on occasion cause dysfunction of nerve roots, an aseptic meningitis that may be followed by a progressive or constricting arachnoiditis, or an actual myelitis. Fortunately these complications are rare, but the fact that they may occur should be a deterrent to the use of intrathecal injections except when specifically indicated. Excessive doses of radiation over the spinal cord may cause a radiation myelopathy, with necrosis of the parenchyma in the affected areas and thickening and proliferation of blood vessels; the damage to the nervous tissue may not become evident until 6 months or more after the therapy. A minor, transient form of myelopathy may occur earlier, even with smaller doses of radiation.

BIBLIOGRAPHY

Adams RD, Victor M. Principles of Neurology, 4th ed. New York, McGraw – Hill, 1989

Austin G (ed). The Spinal Cord: Basic Aspects and Surgical Considerations. Springfield, IL, Charles C Thomas, 1961

Brain R, Wilkinson M. Cervical Spondylosis and Other Disorders of the Cervical Spine. Philadelphia, WB Saunders, 1967

Di Chiro G, Wener L. Angiography of the spinal cord: A review of contemporary techniques and applications. J Neurosurg 1973;39:1

Feiring EH. Brock's Injuries of the Brain and Spinal Cord and Their Coverings, 5th ed. New York, Springer, 1974

Garland H, Greenberg J, Harriman DGF. Infarction of the spinal cord. Brain 1966;89:645

Gillilan LA. The arterial blood supply of the human spinal cord. J Comp Neurol 1958;110:75

Grieve S, Jacobson S, Proctor NSF. A nutritional myelopathy occurring in the Bantu on the Witwatersrand. Neurology 1957;12:1205

Henson RA, Parsons M. Ischaemic lesions of the spinal cord: An illustrated review. Q J Med 1967;36:205

Hughes JT. Pathology of the Spinal Cord. Chicago, Year Book Medical Pub, 1966

Jellinger K. Spinal cord arteriosclerosis and progressive vascular myelopathy. J Neurol Neurosurg Psychiatry 1967;30:195

Kahn EA. Role of the dentate ligament in spinal cord compression and the syndrome of lateral sclerosis. J Neurosurg 1947;4:191

Kincaid JC. Myelitis and myelopathy. In Joynt RJ (ed). Clinical Neurology. Philadelphia, JB Lippincott, 1989

Netsky MG. Syringomyelia: A clinicopathologic study. Arch Neurol Psychiatry 1953;70:741

Rosenblum ML, Levy RM, Bredesen DE (eds). AIDS and the Nervous System. New York, Raven Press, 1988

Schneider RC. The syndrome of acute anterior spinal cord injury. J Neurosurg 1955;12:95

Steegmann AT. Syndrome of the anterior spinal artery. Neurology 1952;2:15

Suh TH, Alexander L. Vascular system of the human spinal cord. Arch Neurol Psychiatry 1939;41:659

Tarlov IM. Spinal Cord Compression: Mechanism of Paralysis and Treatment. Springfield, IL, Charles C Thomas, 1957

Chapter 47

LESIONS CAUSING LOW BACK PAIN WITH LUMBOSACRAL RADIATION

The diagnosis of lesions that cause low back pain, pain of lumbosacral radiation, or both is one of the distressing problems of neurology and medicine in general. Such pain must always be regarded as a symptom, not a disease, and every attempt should be made to determine its etiology. Possible causes to be considered include the following: involvement of skeletal, muscular, and related structures; pelvic or abdominal disease; postural abnormalities; psychogenic factors. Among the frequent and important causes of such pain, however, are the neurogenic ones, and they must be carefully diagnosed before adequate treatment can be undertaken. The character and localization of the pain must be determined, and the examiner must decide whether the neurogenic difficulties are primary, or whether they are secondary to skeletal, muscular, or other disease.

The history is extremely important, especially if there is a relationship to trauma or infection, or if there have been previous episodes or recurrent manifestations. One must take into consideration the character of the pain and its exact distribution and areas of radiation, the presence of paresthesias and other subjective sensory changes, and the history of motor disturbances such as weakness and atrophy. Associated symptoms, such as bowel and bladder disturbances or rectal or genital anesthesia, may be important. The relationship of the pain to position and exercise may give relevant information. The pain of a ruptured intervertebral disk, for instance, may be more severe when the patient is seated than when he is standing, but it is usually increased by activity and by bending or stoop-

ing, especially when the legs are extended at the knees; it is characteristically intensified by coughing, straining, and sneezing. The pain of a spinal cord tumor may also be aggravated by increasing the intracranial or intraspinal pressure, but it is often more severe when the patient is lying down than when he is seated.

A complete examination of the back is essential. Abnormalities of posture, deformities, tenderness, and muscle spasm are important. With pain of sciatic or lumbosacral radiation there may be loss of the normal lumbar lordosis because of involuntary spasm of the back muscles. In addition there often is a lumbar scoliosis, with a compensatory thoracic scoliosis. Most commonly the list of the body is away from the painful side, and the pelvis is tilted so that the affected hip is prominent and elevated. The patient attempts to keep his weight on the sound limb. The list and scoliosis may, however, alternate, or be toward the painful side, and the patient's body may be bent forward and toward that side to avoid stretching the involved nerve. With very severe sciatic pain the patient will avoid complete extension at the knee, and may place only the toes on the floor, since dorsiflexion of the foot aggravates the pain by stretching the nerve. He may walk with small steps and keep his leg semiflexed at the knee. In bending forward he flexes his knee to avoid stretching the sciatic nerve (**Neri's sign**). In sitting he keeps the affected leg flexed at the knee and rests his weight on the opposite buttock. He may rise from a seated position by supporting himself on the unaffected side and placing one hand on his back while he bends the affected leg (**Minor's sign**).

Areas of maximal tenderness in the lumbosacral region should be determined, especially in those instances in which either manipulation or percussion of the spinous processes or pressure just lateral to them reproduces or accentuates the pain. A sharp blow with a percussion hammer, on or just lateral to the spinous processes while the patient is bending forward, may bring out the pain. The distribution of the muscle spasm may give objective information about the radiation of the pain, and not only the back muscles, but also the hamstrings and gastrocnemius may be in spasm. Flexion, extension, and lateral deviation of the spine are limited; the pain is usually accentuated on passive rotary extension of the lumbar spine toward the affected side while the patient is standing erect. Manipulation of the spine may be painful, and there may be localized tenderness at the sciatic notch and along the course of the sciatic nerve.

The neurologic examination must be carefully executed. Sensory changes are important and should be thoroughly evaluated. Either hypesthesia or hyperesthesia and hyperalgesia may be present. One should differentiate peripheral nerve and segmental changes. The exact localization of a ruptured intervertebral disk may depend upon the delineation of segmental changes in sensation. The motor examination should be complete, and one should carefully test motor power in the individual muscles and look for atrophy and fasciculations as well as muscle spasm. Reflex alterations are also important diagnostic criteria. Dysfunction of the sacral portion of the parasympathetic division may cause a neurogenic bladder and impotence.

Pelvic and rectal examinations must be performed to rule out neoplasms and infections originating outside the spine. Roentgenologic examinations, computed tomography, or magnetic resonance imaging and myelography are usually necessary. Diskography is now rarely needed. Electromyography helps to establish the presence of nerve and muscle involvement and aids in localization. Thermography has been advocated by some as an aid in localization of lumbosacral nerve root disorders, but its value is controversial.

SPECIAL DIAGNOSTIC PROCEDURES

A number of special diagnostic procedures should be performed during the examination of the patient who is suffering from pain in the low back with lumbosacral radiation. Some of these are of special interest to the orthopedist, but those that are essential to the neurologist are listed.

Lasègue's Sign. Flexion of the thigh at the hip while the leg is extended at the knee causes stretching of the sciatic nerve. Such stretching may be done as an active process if the patient bends over while his legs are extended at the knees, but it is done as a diagnostic neurologic test by passively flexing the hip of the supine patient while holding the leg in extension at the knee (Fig. 47-1). This maneuver may be carried out with the patient experiencing radiating pain if there is disease of the hip joint, but with either disease or irritation of the sciatic nerve, or of the nerve roots that enter into it, there is pain in the sciatic notch accompanied by pain and hypersensitivity along the course of the sciatic nerve. This is Lasègue's sign. The procedure, often called the **straight-leg-raising-test,** is similar to that used in eliciting Kernig's sign, but in the latter the thigh is flexed at the hip, and then an attempt is made to extend the leg at the knee. Both, when positive, indicate the presence of irritation of the meninges or of the lower lumbosacral nerve roots. In testing for Lasègue's sign, the examiner should note both the angle of hip flexion at which pain occurs and the amount and site of the pain experienced by the patient. The pain may be felt as a tight sensation or ac-

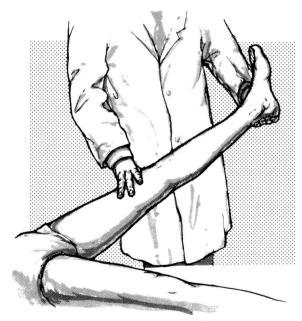

FIG. 47–1. *Method of eliciting Lasègue's sign.*

tual pain in the lumbar or sacral region, gluteal region, posterior aspect of the thigh, or the popliteal space, or sometimes in the opposite limb. There may even be numbness and paresthesias in the distribution of the affected nerve roots. The test is most positive if the maneuver reproduces the patient's subjective pain. Pain produced by flexion of less than 40° is indicative of movement of an affected nerve root against a protruded disk; if pain does not occur until flexion has been carried to 70° or 80°, one may assume that there is an abnormally sensitive nerve root, but not necessarily a demonstrable lesion of the root or protruded disk. Evidence of sciatic nerve or nerve root irritation can also be elicited by examining the patient while he is seated, with thighs at a right angle with the hips. The leg is then passively extended at the knee until pain is produced. It is generally believed, however, that the supine is preferable to the seated position for carrying out these maneuvers.

To test for the **buckling sign** the straight-leg test is carried out as previously described, by passively flexing the hip while the knee is extended, until the knee begins to flex or buckle. This is an involuntary reaction that signifies a release from the sciatic nerve tension that is producing the pain.

Various modifications of Lasègue's sign give additional information. The pain may be more severe, or elicited sooner, if the test is carried out with the thigh and leg in a position of adduction and internal rotation (**Bonnet's phenomenon**). Dorsiflexion of the foot (**Bragard's sign**) or of the great toe (**Sicard's sign**) while performing the examination increases the stretching of the tibial portion of the sciatic nerve and aggravates the pain (Fig. 47-2). The examiner may flex the hip until the first manifestations of pain are noted, and then flex either the toe or foot. In mild cases, no pain may be present with the usual Lasègue's test, but dorsiflexion of the foot or toe, after the hip is completely flexed, may cause pain. Sometimes the pain is brought on, while the patient is supine with his thighs and legs extended, merely by dorsiflexion of the foot or great toe. All the modifications of Lasègue's sign in which either the foot or great toe is dorsiflexed may be called nerve stretching tests; the term **Spurling's sign** is also used. A similar modification may be carried out by flexing the thigh to an angle just short of that necessary to cause pain, following which the neck is flexed; this may produce the same exacerbation of pain that would be brought about by further flexion of the hip. Occasionally the pain may be brought

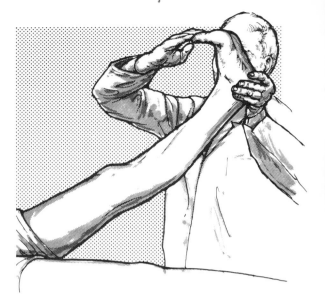

FIG. 47–2. Accentuation of Lasègue's sign by dorsiflexion of either the foot or the great toe.

on merely by passive flexion of the neck when the patient is recumbent with both the hips and knees extended.

In some patients with low back pain and lumbosacral radiation, flexion of the nonpainful thigh while the knee is extended causes an exacerbation of pain on the affected side. This has been called the **crossed straight-leg-raising test,** and some observers express the belief that it is pathognomonic of disk herniation.

In persons with upper lumbar root lesions, the pain pattern may be reproduced even in the absence of Lasègue's sign by the **bent knee pulling test.** The half-prone patient's bent knee is pulled backward by the examiner while he puts forward pressure on the buttock.

Nerve Pressure Signs. Tension on the sciatic nerve is increased when the tibial nerve is pressed in the popliteal space. The test for Lasègue's sign is carried out to the angle where pain is first noted, and then the knee is flexed about 20°. Following this the hip is further flexed to a degree just short of that causing pain, and firm pressure is applied in the popliteal space over the tibial nerve. When the test is positive, this causes sharp pain in the lumbar region, in the affected buttock, or along the course of the sciatic nerve. This test may also be carried out with the patient seated on a table. The affected leg is extended passively at the knee to the point at which pain is reproduced. It is then flexed slightly, and pressure is applied in the popliteal space, which, in cases of sciatic nerve or nerve root irritation, will cause pain.

O'Connell's Test. In carrying out this test, Lasègue's test is first carried out on the sound limb, and the angle of flexion and site of pain are recorded; the pain may be on the opposite side (**Fajersztajn's sign**). Then this test is carried out on the affected limb, and the angle and site of pain again noted. Then both thighs are flexed simultaneously while extension is maintained at the knee. The angle of flexion permitted may be greater than that allowed when either the affected limb or the sound limb is flexed alone. Finally, both thighs having been flexed to an angle just short of that which produces pain, the sound limb is lowered to the bed; this may result in a marked exacerbation of pain, sometimes associated with paresthesias.

Reverse Straight-Leg-Raising Test. With the patient lying prone, the knee is flexed to its maximum. The normal individual should complain of quadriceps tightness. With disk disease there is pain in the back or in the sciatic nerve distribution on the side of the lesion.

Viets' and Naffziger's Tests. Increase of the intracranial or intraspinal pressure causes exaggeration of radicular pain in patients with space-occupying lesions that press on the nerve roots. The pressure may be increased temporarily by coughing, sneezing, and straining, and by digital compression of the jugular veins. Pressure should be maintained until the patient complains of a fullness in the head, and the test should not be considered negative until venous return has been impeded for at least 2 min. Jugular compression can also be carried out with a sphygmomanometer cuff, maintaining a pressure of 40 mm Hg for 10 min (Naffziger's test). The patient may be in either the recumbent or upright position. In a patient with a ruptured intervertebral disk there will be radicular pain in the distribution of the affected nerve roots following jugular compression. The pain is similar to that which follows coughing and straining, and Viets' and Naffziger's tests are rarely positive in patients who do not have aggravation of pain when coughing and straining. Occasionally the pain may be noticed on the release of the pressure. A similar aggravation of the pain may sometimes be brought about merely by having the patient perform the Valsalva maneuver.

Patrick's Sign. This sign consists of pain in the hip when the heel or the external malleolus of the painful extremity is placed upon the opposite knee and the thigh is pressed downward. The pain thus occurs on simultaneous flexion, abduction, external rotation, and extension of the involved hip. When the maneuver is carried out it may be noted that the knee on the affected side is kept elevated and cannot be pressed toward the bed. Patrick's sign is positive in hip joint disease, but is usually absent in sciatic nerve involvement.

CAUSES OF LOW BACK PAIN WITH LUMBOSACRAL RADIATION

Low back pain with lumbosacral radiation may be due to many causes, and these should all be considered in arriving at a diagnosis. Involvement of the skeletal, muscular, and related structures that may cause pressure on and irritation of the lumbosacral plexus or its branches include the following: acute trauma with fractures or subluxations of the spine, fractures of the hip or pelvis, ligamentous or tendinous tears or strains, repeated mechanical strain, acute or chronic arthritis, congenital anomalies of the spine, spondylolisthesis, spondylolysis, sacralization of the fifth lumbar vertebra, bony spurs (osteosclerosis) of the lumbar spine, reduction of the lumbosacral joint space, disease of the sacroiliac area, diseases of the hip joint, narrowing of the intervertebral foramina, osteitis deformans, osteomyelitis, myositis, fibrositis, bursitis, irritation of the piriformis muscle, abnormally increased tension of the fascia lata, chronic postural anomalies, and hypertrophy of the ligamentum flavum. Intrapelvic and intraabdominal causes include neoplastic or inflammatory involvement of the pelvic and abdominal viscera, endometriosis, aortic obstruction or aneurysm, and fetal malposition during pregnancy. Spinal conditions include tumors of the vertebrae or spinal cord, tumors and inflammations of the cauda equina, meningitis, pachymeningitis, arachnoiditis, hemangiomas, arachnoid and extradural cysts, nerve root cysts and ruptured intervertebral disks. The sciatic nerve or its root may be affected by a primary neuritis, perineuritis, radiculitis, or the presence of a neuroma or neurinoma, or by trauma to the nerve itself or injection into it. Psychogenic etiologies must also be considered, especially in the presence of camptocormia or coccygodynia, or if the case is attributed to trauma for which compensation is being sought.

Intermittent pain in one leg or both that comes on after activity and is relieved by rest may be caused by a narrowed spinal canal — **lumbar spinal stenosis.** The underlying mechanism is probably intermittent ischemia of the cauda equina, and the syndrome has been referred to as intermittent claudication of the cauda equina. Widening of the spinal canal surgically may bring about relief. The syndrome occasionally occurs in patients with rheumatoid arthritis and Paget's disease.

The most common cause of low back pain with lumbosacral radiation is ruptured intervertebral disk. There may be either extrusion of a portion of the annulus fibrosus or rupture of the annulus with herniation of the nucleus pulposus. The protrusion may be either posterolateral or midline. In most cases there is a history of trauma that was followed by the onset of low back pain with radiation down one leg. The herniated, or protruded, nucleus pulposus presses upon the roots of the lumbosacral plexus and causes the symptoms. The radiation of the pain and the localization of the symptoms is dependent upon the degree and site of the herniation. Such herniation is most apt to occur in the lumbar region (Fig. 47-3), although it may occur in the cervical and thoracic areas also. In the lumbar spine the herniation most frequently occurs between the fourth and fifth lumbar vertebrae, with pressure on the fifth lumbar nerve root, or between the fifth lumbar and first sacral

bodies, with pressure on the first sacral root (Table 47-1).

Pain in the back with radiation down the posterior aspect of the thigh and the posterior or lateral aspect of the leg, to the heel or foot, is the most common symptom of a ruptured intervertebral disk. The pain is aggravated by coughing and straining and by bending either forward or to the affected side; it may be relieved by standing upright. Associated with the pain may be paresthesias, together with motor changes. In order to make an unequivocal clinical diagnosis of a ruptured intervertebral disk, certain objective sensory, motor, and reflex changes should be present. The sensory disturbances consist of either hypesthesia or hyperesthesia and hyperalgesia, most frequently in the distribution of the fifth lumbar or first sacral segments. Occasionally there are more diffuse sensory changes, even saddle anesthesia. Alterations in vibratory sensation are sometimes found. There may be referred hyperalgesia and muscle spasm when the skin of the back or loin on the affected side is stimulated.

The motor abnormalities may not be marked if only one nerve root is affected, since most muscles are supplied by more than one such root. There may, however, be weakness of the extensor hallucis longus, extensor digitorum brevis, tibialis anterior, or gastrocnemius muscles. The two sides should always be compared. In addition to weakness there may be atrophy, fascic-

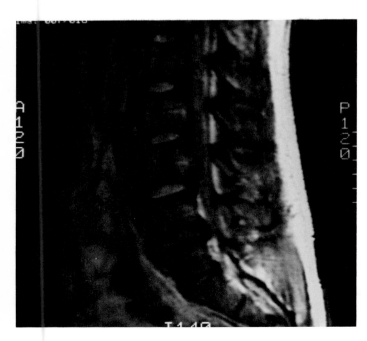

FIG. 47–3. Lateral lumbosacral magnetic resonance image (TR 800, TE 20), showing a disk herniation at the L5–S1 interspace.

TABLE 47-1. DIFFERENTIATION BETWEEN FOURTH LUMBAR AND FIFTH LUMBAR HERNIATIONS

	Fourth Lumbar Herniation	Fifth Lumbar Herniation
Site of lesion	Between fourth and fifth lumbar bodies	Between fifth lumbar and first sacral bodies
Nerve root affected	Fifth lumbar	First sacral
Radiation of pain and paresthesias (including site of pain in Lasègue's sign)	Lateral aspect of thigh, anterolateral aspect of leg, dorsal aspect of foot, occasionally affecting great toe	Posterior aspect of thigh, posterolateral aspect of leg, and lateral aspect of foot, including the heel and one or two outer toes
Superficial sensory changes	Hypesthesia or anesthesia, occasionally hyperesthesia, in the above-mentioned distribution, especially distally (fifth lumbar dermatome)	Hypesthesia or anesthesia, occasionally hyperesthesia, in the above-mentioned distribution, especially distally (first sacral dermatome)
Vibratory sensory changes	Occasionally loss or impairment over medial malleolus and medial aspect of foot and toes	Occasionally loss or impairment over lateral malleolus and lateral aspect of foot and toes
Motor changes	Paresis of extensor hallucis longus and occasionally of extensor digitorum brevis and tibialis anterior; atrophy of anterior calf muscles	Paresis of plantar flexors of foot (triceps surae); atrophy of posterior calf muscles
Reflex change	Tibialis posterior reflex may be absent	Diminished or absent Achilles reflex
Accentuation of pain	Pressure or percussion at the fourth lumbar interspace causes radiation of pain	Pressure or percussion at the lumbosacral interspace causes radiation of pain

ulations, or both. The most common reflex change is the loss of the Achilles response, but occasionally the tibialis posterior reflex is absent. Autonomic nervous system disturbances such as bladder and bowel dysfunction are less common. Bilateral involvement is not encountered unless there are bilateral herniations or a large ruptured disk in the midline. Under such circumstances the first through the lower sacral roots may be affected, and the clinical picture resembles that found with a lesion of the cauda equina. The sensory changes include the saddle and genital areas as well as the posterior aspects of the thighs and legs; there may be weakness of the triceps surae muscles bilaterally, one or both Achilles reflexes may be absent, and there may be sphincter disturbances and impotence.

In most patients with low back pain and lumbosacral radiation due to ruptured intervertebral disks, Lasègue's sign and associated signs of sciatic and nerve root irritation are positive. Roentgenograms often show evidence of reduction of the joint space between the fourth and fifth lumbar vertebral bodies or at the lumbosacral level, or other abnormalities. There may be electromyographic changes in those muscles supplied by the affected nerve roots. Computed tomography, magnetic resonance imaging, and at times myelography alone or in combination with the other imaging studies will identify the lesion and differentiate it from neoplasms and other conditions.

BIBLIOGRAPHY

Adams RD, Victor M. Principles of Neurology, 4th ed. New York, McGraw–Hill, 1989

Aird RB, Naffziger HC. Prolonged jugular compression: A new diagnostic test of neurological value. Trans Am Neurol Assoc 1940;66:45

Bradford FK, Spurling RG. The Intervertebral Disc: With

Special Reference to Rupture of the Annulus Fibrosus With Herniation of the Nucleus Pulposus, 2nd ed. Springfield, IL, Charles C Thomas, 1945

Brish A, Lerner MA, Braham J. Intermittent claudication from compression of cauda equina by a narrowed spinal canal. J Neurosurg 1964;21:207

Charnley J. Orthopaedic signs in the diagnosis of disc protrusion. Lancet 1951;1:186

Dimitrijevic DT. Lasègue sign. Neurology 1952;2:453

Falconer MA, Glasgow GL, Cole DS. Sensory disturbances occurring in sciatica due to intervertebral disc protrusions: some observations on the fifth lumbar and first sacral dermatomes. J Neurol Neurosurg Psychiatry 1947;10:72

Gardner RC. New test for intervertebral disk disease. An Intern Med 1971;75:480

Jabre JF, Bryan RW. Bent-knee pulling in the diagnosis of upper lumbar root lesions. Arch Neurol 1982;39:669

Keegan JJ. Diagnosis of herniation of lumbar intervertebral disks by neurologic signs. JAMA 1944;126:868

Love JG. The differential diagnosis of intraspinal tumors and protruded intervertebral disks and their surgical treatment. J Neurosurg 1944;1:275

Mixter WJ, Barr JS. Rupture of the intervertebral disk with involvement of the spinal cord. N Engl J Med 1934;211:210

O'Connell JEA. Sciatica and the mechanism of the production of the clinical syndrome in protrusions of the lumbar intervertebral discs. Br J Surg 1943;30:315

So YT, Aminoff MJ, Olney RK. The role of thermography in the evaluation of lumbosacral radiculopathy. Neurology 1989;39:1154

Viets HR. Two new signs suggestive of cauda equina tumor: root pain on jugular compression and the shifting of the lipiodol shadow on change of posture. N Engl J Med 1928;198:671

Wartenberg R. Lasègue sign and Kernig sign. Arch Neurol Psychiatry 1951;66:58

Woodhall B, Hayes G. The well-leg raising test of Fajerztajn in the diagnosis of ruptured lumbar intervertebral disc. J Bone Joint Surg 1950;32:786

PART H

Diagnosis and Localization of Intracranial Disease

The recognition and accurate localization of intracranial disease is one of the most important, and at the same time one of the most difficult, problems in neurologic diagnosis. It is essential not only to establish the presence of a lesion, but also to localize it accurately and to determine its nature and etiology. It is only after one accumulates all of the pertinent information that the treatment and prognosis can be considered.

A number of imaging and other specialized technics are now at our disposal to help in localizing structural intracranial disease, especially infarcts, masses, hemorrhages, demyelinative lesions, and others. These studies include computed tomography, magnetic resonance imaging, single photon computed tomography, radioactive brain scanning, positron emission tomography, and certain others. Such studies help to identify enlargement, distortions, or atrophy of structures, as well as the presence of abnormal structures and abnormally functioning structures. However, these studies often cannot positively identify the etiology of the abnormalities. They can differentiate between certain lesions, for example, hemorrhagic as opposed to occlusive vascular disorders. These studies, however, do not show abnormalities useful in day-to-day diagnosis in certain neurologic disorders, such as epilepsy, narcolepsy, migraine, and the like. The studies may also give misleading information, for example, demonstrating the presence of clinically silent cerebral infarcts or areas of altered attenuation on computed tomography or magnetic imaging that have no clinical correlations. With minor exceptions, the studies do not outline the extent of the actual neurologic dysfunction. Other tests, such as electroencephalography and evoked potential studies, yield information about disturbed function but are not precise in localization. This volume cannot describe the technical details of these tests. Excellent texts are devoted to each of these tests. The history, the general medical examination, and the neurologic examination are still of paramount importance in the diagnosis of intracranial disorders and will be dealt with in the present section.

The history is of utmost consequence (Ch. 2). In some diseases causing neurologic symptoms there may be no objective manifestations at any time, and in others, such as those causing periodic convulsions, there may be none between the attacks. In these, the diagnosis may have to be made on the basis of the history alone. Furthermore, the mode of onset, duration of symptoms, progression or regression of manifestations, and response to therapy may give pertinent clues to diagnosis. Vascular lesions are usually abrupt in onset, although occasionally intermittent or progressive. The onset of symptoms in intracranial neoplasms is usually progressive, and sometimes insidious; occasionally, however, the first manifestations appear precipitously. Degenerative diseases are usually slowly and gradually progressive, but in some, such as multiple sclerosis, there may be intermittent and remittent features. In posttraumatic states the history is usually self-revealing; in disturbances of development and hereditary affections the manifestations can often be traced back to birth or the postnatal period. In infections and toxic conditions one should be able to elicit a history of systemic as well as nervous system changes; and in occupational and nutritional disorders, one should be able to elicit a history of exposure to a toxic substance, physical or mental strain, or inadequate diet.

In cerebral disease even more than in involvement of other portions of the nervous system one must evaluate meticulously the often conflicting information that may be presented by those symptoms and signs that are the result, variously, of destruction, release, irritation, and partial assumption of function by healthy tissues. There may be either **neural shock,** or **diaschisis,** a temporary more or less complete cessation of function of nervous structures following an acute, catastrophic lesion, or a transient decrease of function in the areas surrounding a contusion, hemorrhage, or infarct owing to reversible ischemia, edema, or compression by the injured tissues. Furthermore, one must differentiate between the following: (1) positive symptoms, which may be due to either release or irritation; (2) negative symptoms, which follow loss of function of certain parts; (3) primary symptoms, correlated directly with either focal structural disease or local disorders of function; (4) secondary (indirect) manifestations, which occur as a result of overactivity of certain nervous mechanisms, owing to (a) release from the inhibition that is normally executed by the injured areas, (b) a functional alteration of the physiologic mechanisms of the parts damaged, or (c) reorganization of function of uninjured structures. There may be symptoms of both irritation and destruction, such as recurrent jacksonian attacks that are followed by a transitory localized paralysis (Todd's paralysis). In addition, edema, pressure from tumors and other expanding lesions, and interference with the circulation of the blood or with the flow of cerebrospinal fluid may cause dysfunction of distant parts of the brain or brain stem, producing symptoms and signs, known as false localizing signs, that suggest involvement of the opposite hemisphere or of other areas of the nervous system not affected by the primary process.

Localized lesions are limited to one region, and may affect all of the tissues regardless of their structures and functions. In diffuse disease the damage to the functional elements is usually incomplete, and certain structures suffer more than others. In system disease only anatomically and functionally related systems of cells or fibers are involved. When a lesion develops rapidly, negative symptoms are always greater and more widespread immediately after the onset; there may be recovery of function. Slowly progressive lesions, on the other hand, cause less severe disturbances of function in relation to their extent and severity. In all diseases of the nervous system, but especially in cerebral disorders, the most recently acquired, highly specialized, and most complex functions are the first to be affected, and the last and least complete to return during the recovery process.

The localization and diagnosis of disease of certain intracranial constituents are discussed elsewhere: The infratentorial structures (those below the tentorium cerebelli) are the cerebellum, midbrain, pons, and medulla. The functions of the cerebellum and the disturbances of function that result from disease are discussed in Part D, "The Motor System." Localization of disease of the midbrain, pons, and medulla is dependent upon a knowledge of the functions and distributions of the third through the twelfth cranial nerves as well as of the motor and sensory pathways that traverse these structures. The most important clinical conditions that may affect the midbrain and pons are discussed with the individual cranial nerves that have their nuclei of origin and termination within these structures; clinical involvement of the medulla is discussed in Chapter 18. The functions and disorders of some of the supratentorial structures are also discussed individually. The basal ganglia are dealt with in Chapter 22, and the hypothalamus in Part F, "The Autonomic Nervous System." In the present section clinical cerebral localization will be considered with respect to the cerebral cortex and certain noncortical areas of the cerebrum, namely, the thalamus, corpus callosum, and internal capsule.

Chapter 48
GROSS AND MICROSCOPIC ANATOMY OF THE CEREBRAL HEMISPHERES

For the diagnosis and localization of intracranial lesions it is necessary to have a general knowledge of cerebral anatomy and function. The brain, the seat of the higher sensory, motor, and intellectual functions, is composed of two hemispheres that are incompletely separated from each other by the median longitudinal fissure (Figs. 48-1, 48-2, and 48-3). At the bottom of this fissure lies a broad band of commissural fibers, the corpus callosum, which forms the chief bond of union between the hemispheres. Areas within the individual hemispheres communicate by means of association fibers, and the cerebrum is connected with lower centers by means of projection pathways. The brain is covered by a layer of gray matter, the cerebral cortex. Underneath is the white matter, which consists of the association, commissural, and projection fibers. At the base of each hemisphere are several gray masses, or nuclei, including the basal ganglia and the diencephalon, which consists of the thalamus, metathalamus, epithalamus, subthalamus, and hypothalamus. The cortex of the cerebrum with its underlying white matter is known as the pallium, or cerebral mantle; in the human this is tremendously expanded and forms by far the larger part of the hemispheres. The more primitive portions of the pallium are the paleopallium in the pyriform lobe area and the archipallium in the hippocampal formation; these constitute the rhinencephalon (allocortex), which is connected structurally and functionally with the limbic lobe. The phylogenetically more recent neopallium (isocortex) is highly developed only in mammals, and in humans constitutes the major portion of the cerebrum.

Each cerebral hemisphere is traversed by fissures and sulci (Figs. 48-4 and 48-5). The more important fissures divide the hemispheres into lobes, and these in turn are subdivided by the sulci into gyri, or convolutions. This separation of the parts of the brain has practical significance for anatomical purposes, but the divisions are arbitrary morphologic ones, and the individual lobes are not necessarily functional units. The classification of the various areas of the brain by physiologic and histologic criteria is discussed later.

On the lateral surface of the brain are two large fissures, the **lateral** or **sylvian,** and the **central,** or **rolandic.** The former begins on the basal surface of the brain and extends lateralward, posteriorly, and superiorly. The latter runs obliquely, nearly reaching the sylvian fissure; it makes an angle of 70% with the dorsal surface of the brain, and its peak is just behind the middle of the dorsal surface of the hemisphere.

The **frontal lobe,** which constitutes the anterior one-third of each hemisphere in man, extends, on the lateral surface of the brain, from the frontal pole to the rolandic fissure, and lies above, or rostral to, the sylvian fissure. On the medial surface of the brain it extends to the sulcus cinguli. It is made up of four principal gyri. The precentral gyrus, also known as the anterior central, or the posterior frontal, gyrus, is situated between the central and precentral fissures. The superior frontal gyrus is located rostral to the superior frontal sulcus; the middle frontal gyrus, between the superior and the inferior frontal sulci; the inferior frontal gyrus, beneath the inferior frontal sulcus. The middle

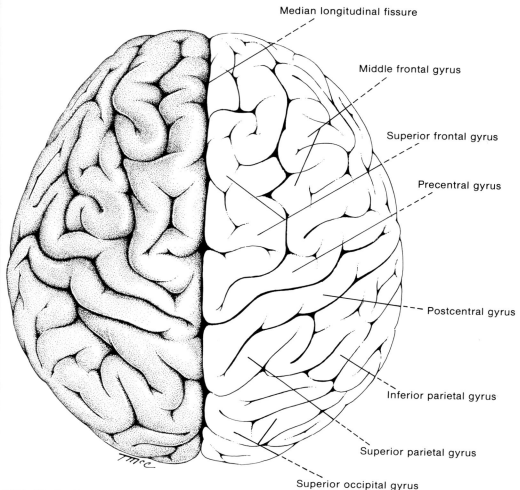

FIG. 48–1. *Gross structure of the cerebral hemispheres as seen from above.*

frontal sulcus runs through the middle frontal gyrus. The portion of the precentral gyrus that lies on the medial aspect of the brain above the sulcus cinguli is known as the paracentral lobule. Two divisions of the sylvian fissure, the anterior horizontal ramus, which runs anteriorly, and the anterior ascending ramus, which extends dorsally, divide the inferior frontal gyrus into the pars orbitalis, which lies below the anterior horizontal ramus, the pars triangularis, which is between the two rami, and the pars opercularis, which lies between the anterior ascending ramus and the rolandic fissure.

The **parietal lobe** extends from the central sulcus to an imaginary line drawn between the parietooccipital fissure and the preoccipital notch, and lies above the lateral fissure and an imaginary line connecting that fissure with the middle of the preceding line. It consists of five principal gyri. The superior parietal lobule lies above the interparietal sulcus; the postcentral (posterior central or anterior parietal) gyrus lies between the rolandic fissure and the postcentral sulcus; the inferior parietal lobule is situated beneath the interparietal sulcus; the supramarginal gyrus curves around the upturned end of the sylvian fissure; the angular gyrus is similarly related to the terminal ascending portion of the superior temporal sulcus.

The **temporal lobe** lies beneath the sylvian fissure and extends to the arbitrary limits of the parietal and occipital lobes; the tongue-shaped anterior projection terminates in the temporal pole, and the ventral surface lies on the floor of the middle cranial fossa. It contains three definite sulci, the superior, middle, and inferior tem-

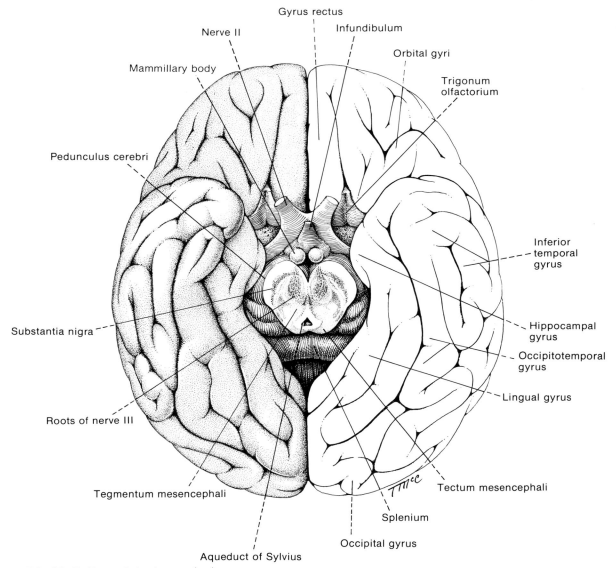

FIG. 48–2. Base of the human brain.

poral, dorsal to each of which is a gyrus bearing a similar name. The superior temporal gyrus, bordering on the lateral fissure, is marked in its posterior aspect by the presence of horizontal convolutions, the transverse temporal gyri, sometimes known as Heschl's convolutions. The inferior temporal sulcus is located on the basal portion of the lobe, and between it and the collateral fissure lies the fusiform gyrus. The **insula,** or island of Reil, may be considered as a lobe that lies buried at the depth of the lateral fissure. It is surrounded by the limiting, or circular, sulcus. Those portions of the frontal, parietal, and temporal lobes that overlie the insula are known as the frontal, parietal, and temporal opercula.

The **occipital lobe** occupies only a small part of the dorsolateral surface of the hemisphere, that area lying behind the line drawn between the parietooccipital fissure and the preoccipital notch, but it occupies a large triangular field between the parietal and temporal lobes on the medial aspect of the brain. The medial surface is traversed by the calcarine fissure, and the portion of the occipital lobe above this fissure is the cuneus, whereas that below is the lingual gyrus.

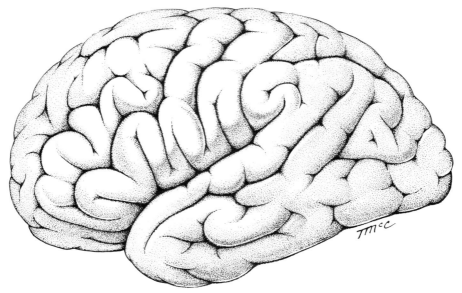

FIG. 48–3. Lateral view of the left cerebral hemisphere.

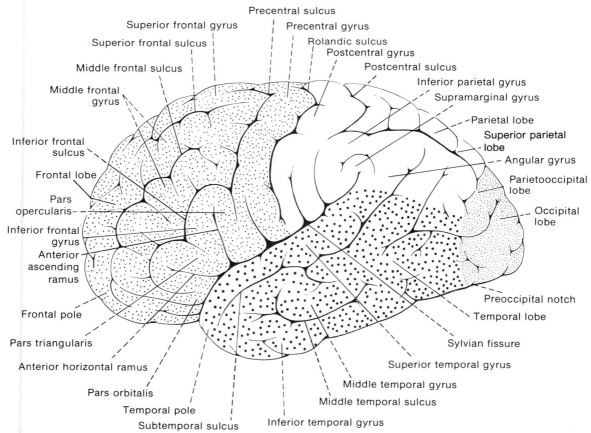

FIG. 48–4. Lobes, sulci, and gyri of the lateral aspect of the cerebral hemisphere.

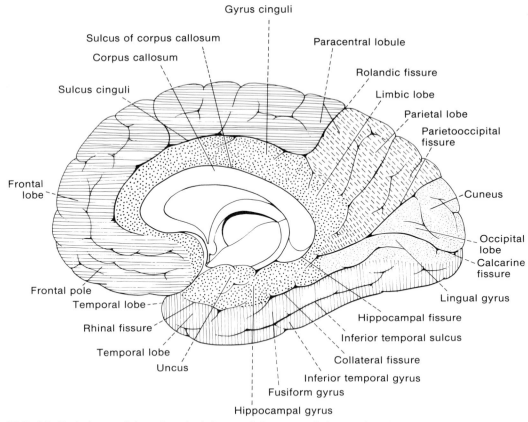

FIG. 48–5. Lobes, sulci, and gyri of the medial aspect of the cerebral hemisphere.

On the medial surface of the brain are the sulcus of the corpus callosum and the sulcus cinguli, between which lies the gyrus cinguli. The hippocampal gyrus is situated between the hippocampal fissure and the collateral fissure with its anterior projection, the rhinal fissure; its rostral extremity bends around the hippocampal fissure to form the uncus. It is connected with the gyrus cinguli by the isthmus, and the term gyrus fornicatus, or **limbic lobe,** is used to include the gyrus cinguli, isthmus, hippocampal gyrus, and certain subcortical structures including the amygdala and septal nuclei. These are usually considered parts of the rhinencephalon, but from a clinical point of view the hippocampal gyrus and uncus are sometimes assigned to the temporal lobe and the gyrus cinguli is divided between the parietal and frontal lobes.

The cerebral cortex is a laminated structure composed largely of cellular matter that dips into the fissures and sulci and covers the gyri and convolutions. About one third of the cortex is on the exposed surfaces of the brain and the remaining two thirds dips into the fissures and sulci. Von Economo has estimated that in addition to nerve fibers, neuroglia, and blood vessels, there are cell bodies of nearly 14 billion neurons in the cortex. The structure varies in thickness from 4.5 mm in the precentral gyrus to 1.25 mm near the occipital pole. The sizes and types of cells found in the cortex vary at different depths from the surface and in different portions of the brain, but in general they are arranged in fairly definite layers (Fig. 48-6), separated by myelinated bands. Ramón y Cajal described eight layers, but the usually accepted classification of the lamination is that of Brodmann, which is as follows:

    I. Lamina zonalis, or the molecular or plexiform layer, is the most superficial. It is covered by the pia and forms a dense tangential fiber network composed of the terminal dendrites of the deeper cells. The ganglion cells are small and few in number.

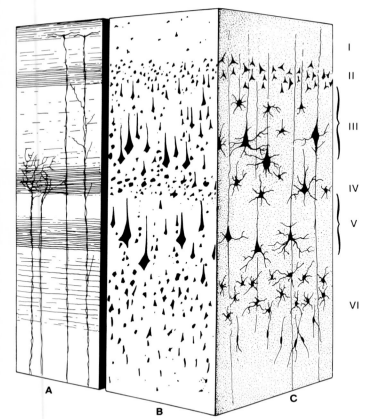

FIG. 48–6. Cell layers and fiber arrangement of the cerebral cortex. **A.** Weigert stain. **B.** Nissl stain. **C.** Golgi stain. Layers: **I.** Lamina zonalis. **II.** Lamina granularis externa. **III.** Lamina pyramidalis. **IV.** Lamina granularis interna. **V.** Lamina ganglionaris. **VI.** Lamina multiformis.

II. Lamina granularis externa, or the layer of small pyramidal cells, consists of many small, closely packed pyramidal cells.

III. Lamina pyramidalis, or the superficial layer of medium-sized and large pyramidal cells, may be divided into two substrata, the more superficial containing the medium-sized and the deeper one the large pyramidal cells.

IV. Lamina granularis interna, or the layer of small stellate cells, is characterized by the presence of a large number of small multipolar cells with short axons, among which are some small pyramidal cells.

V. Lamina ganglionaris, or the deep layer of medium-sized and large pyramidal cells, contains the largest cells of the cortex. In the motor region these are known as the giant pyramidal cells of Betz, and these, along with other neurons, give origin to the fibers of the corticospinal tract.

VI. Lamina multiformis, or the layer of polymorphic cells, contains irregular fusiform and angular cells, the axons of which enter the subjacent white matter.

Although the cortex of the entire brain can be divided into these six laminae, the histologic features vary from place to place, and this variation is probably responsible for differences in function. Individual areas present their characteristic appearances in thickness of the cortex as a whole, thickness and arrangement of specific cellular layers, cell structure, number of afferent and efferent myelinated fibers, and number and position of white striae. The differences in cellular structure have been spoken of as the cytoarchitectonic, and those of the fibrillary structures as the myeloarchitectonic, features of the cortex.

Histologic surveys based on the differences in the arrangements and the types of cells and the pattern of myelinated fibers have furnished several fundamentally similar cortical maps in which a number of cortical areas of slightly different structure have been described. These individual segments, the total of which has been variously estimated, have been grouped into regions that compare roughly to the boundaries imposed by the fissures and sulci. Flechsig, in 1876, outlined 36 areas of the cortex on the basis of the differences in the time of myelination of the nerve fibers. Campbell's publication, in 1905, based on work done in 1903, divided the human cortex into some 20 regions and described the cellular and fibrillary lamination of each. Elliot Smith, in 1907, identified 28 – 30 areas on the basis of gross examination; he noted the relative thickness of the gray and white matter, the texture, and the color in each region. Brodmann, in 1909, carried out more detailed observations and differentiated 47 separate fields by means of a histologic survey of the cortex using the Nissl method (see Fig. 23-1). His map of the cortex is commonly used in modern texts. C. and O. Vogt, in 1919, described over 200 areas; their work was based on the differences in the patterns of the myelinated fibers. In 1925 von Economo and Koskinas reduced all cortical variations to 5 fundamental types, but divided the cortex as a whole into 107 different areas; their work was based fundamentally on the work of Brodmann.

The classification of the brain into areas on the basis of histologic structure has attained greater value in functional localization than the division base on lobes and fissures. The granular cells, which make up the bulk of the second and fourth layers, are concerned with the reception of impulses, and hence these layers are the largest in the sensory areas. The pyramidal cells, on the other hand, are efferent in function, and are largest and most numerous in the motor areas, which regions also possess the thickest cortex. It has become obvious, however, that although the classifications described here are important from a topographic point of view, they cannot be correlated completely with the intrinsic functions of the individual regions. In their neurophysiologic research and functional localization, Dusser de Barenne, McCulloch, Bailey, von Bonin, and others, have used strychninization and observation of electrical activity (physiologic neuronography) to investigate the arrangement of associated and commissural systems within the hemispheres. They have shown that the histologic areas must be considered as somewhat arbitrary and artificial from a functional point of view. Furthermore, there are gradations of function, and limits between various zones cannot always be outlined specifically. Functional areas are gradually being defined by isotope studies including positron emission tomography and others. In spite of the fact, however, that many areas of the cortex cannot be distinguished from each other by histologic examination, the major zones described by the various anatomists are probably correct with respect to extent and boundaries, bearing in mind individual variations. Consequently, for both descriptive purposes and classification the numerical designations of Brodmann or modifications of them are most commonly used.

BIBLIOGRAPHY

Bailey P, von Bonin G. The Isocortex of Man. Urbana, IL, University of Illinois Press, 1951

Brodal A. Neurological Anatomy in Relation to Clinical Medicine, 3rd ed. New York, Oxford University Press, 1981

Brodmann K. Vergleichende Lokalisationslehre der Grosshirnrinde in ihren Prinzipien dargestellt auf Grund des Zellenbaues. Leipzig, JA Barth, 1909

Dusser de Barenne JG. Experimental researches on sensory localization in the sensory cortex of the monkey (Macacus). Proc R Soc Lond (Biol) 1924;96:272

McCulloch W. The functional organization of the cerebral cortex. Physiol Rev 1944;24:390

Penfield W, Rasmussen T. The Cerebral Cortex of Man: A Clinical Study of Localization of Function. New York, Macmillan, 1950

Poynter FNL (ed). The History and Philosophy of Knowledge of the Brain and its Functions. Springfield, IL, Charles C Thomas, 1958

Ramon y Cajal S. Studies on the Cerebral Cortex (Limbic Structures). Kraft LM (trans). Chicago, Year Book Medical Pub, 1955

Von Bonin G. Essay on the Cerebral Cortex. Springfield, IL, Charles C Thomas, 1950

Von Bonin G (ed). Some Papers on the Cerebral Cortex. Springfield, IL, Charles C Thomas, 1960

Von Economo C, Koskinas GN. Die Cytoarchitektonik der Hirnrinde des erwachsenen Menschen. Berlin, J Springer, 1925

Chapter 49

FUNCTIONS AND DISORDERS OF FUNCTION OF THE CEREBRAL CORTEX

The first concepts of the localization of cerebral functions were introduced by Gall and Spurzheim between 1800 and 1825; they also, however, attempted to correlate variations in function with the shape of the brain and skull, and thus introduced the pseudoscience of phrenology. Flourens (1823) found that large areas of the brain could be destroyed without causing symptoms and expressed the belief that the cerebrum functions as a single unit, denying the existence of localized action. Broca (1861) demonstrated that destruction of the left third frontal gyrus resulted in the loss of the ability to speak, and Fritsch and Hitzig (1870) showed that galvanic stimulation in the region of the central sulcus of the exposed brain of a dog was followed by movements of the opposite side of the body. Three years later Ferrier, using a faradic stimulus, described constant focal responses in the contralateral extremities on stimulating fixed points of the brain in cats, dogs, rabbits, and other animals, and the next year he carried out similar studies outlining in great detail the motor cortex of monkeys; he also produced paralysis by ablation of the excitable region. His work was followed by that of Horsley, Sherrington, and others. It is of interest that Jackson's prediction of the presence of an area in the cerebral cortex that governs isolated movements was made during the period 1864–1870 on the basis of his study of focal epilepsy, and that it preceded the experimental demonstrations just mentioned. In fact, Jackson was the first to point out that there is a motor cortex. The human cortex was first stimulated by Bartholow in Cincinnati in 1874,

in a 30-year-old patient whose skull was eroded by an epithelioma of the scalp. Needle electrodes plunged through the dura and into the cortex were stimulated by a faradic current, and motor and sensory responses were observed in the arms and legs.

These observations, confirmed and amplified by many experiments, have proved definitely that certain areas of the cerebral cortex possess specific functions. Physiologic studies on both animals and man, pathologic observations on the operating and autopsy tables, and careful clinical observations on patients with focal lesions have all shown that certain areas of the cortex influence the activity of subcortical, brain stem, and spinal centers. It is possible by careful histologic study to correlate these areas with regions that have characteristic cell and fiber lamination. Clinical manifestations of disorders in specific areas, however, can express themselves in widely differing manners.

Irritation, or excitation, of a center of brain function causes an overresponse of this focus; the symptoms are those of stimulation of the area. Destruction of a center causes either a reduction or a loss of function of the center, with resulting paralytic manifestations. Symptoms of release appear when the inhibiting effect of a higher center is removed. Signs of compensation are manifested when other structures or areas assume the activity of the diseased parts.

It must be recalled, when considering localization in the brain, that a "center" is not necessarily the focus that has sole control of a specific activity or one that has only one function, and that it can never function as an isolated unit. A center is merely the seat of greatest intensity of a function, and other contiguous and even far distant foci may control the same action to a certain extent. The center under consideration may also influence the function of distant areas as well as govern its own specific activity. In addition, there are many regions of the brain that do not respond to stimulation, and disease of such regions has been thought to cause no symptoms or signs. These are spoken of as "silent areas," but detailed clinical and physiologic studies have demonstrated the functional significance of most of these regions.

The concept of **cerebral dominance** in the diagnosis of lesions of the cerebral cortex must be considered. In lower animals both hemispheres seem to have equal influence. A particular attribute of the human brain, however, is the dominance of one hemisphere over the other in the control of certain functions, especially language, gnosis (the interpretation of sensory stimuli), and praxis (the performance of complex motor acts). The dominant hemisphere is the left one in at least 99% of right-handed individuals. It is the hemisphere that is contralateral to the hand, the foot, and the eye that the person uses by preference. Minor but definite anatomic differences between the cerebral hemispheres both in size and degree of development of certain structures have been observed by postmortem inspection and also by the newer imaging procedures *in vivo*. The situation is more complex in left-handed individuals. Many authors suggest that the left hemisphere is also dominant in 50% or more of left-handers, but some studies suggest that many left-handed individuals have language function in both hemispheres. Handedness and dominance are believed to be inherited. The nondominant hemisphere also has functions that it appears to control preferentially; for example, the conceptualization of space. These will be described below.

Some studies continue to deny the concept of localization in the cerebral cortex, and it has been stated that those functions believed to originate from particular parts of the brain depend upon the changing state of the entire nervous system. Both clinically and psychologically, however, there is definite evidence for cortical localization, and those areas of the brain whose functions have been verified are discussed in the following section. The physiology of the projection areas has been studied more than that of the association areas.

THE FRONTAL LOBES

The Motor Area

The posterior portion of the frontal lobe is designated the motor projection area, or the true motor area. This region coincides with the area gigantopyramidalis, or area 4 of Brodmann (see Fig. 23-1), and contains the giant pyramidal cells of Betz in layer V; at this site the gray matter is of maximum thickness. The cortex is agranular in type, with prominent pyramidal cells but no internal granular layer and a thin external granular layer. The Betz cells are extremely large, and those in the leg area may measure $60 \times 25 \mu$. Bucy, von Bonin, and others distinguish between area 4γ, the gigantopyramidal cortex, and area 4α, which is similar in structure but lacks the Betz cells (Fig. 49-1). This latter area covers most of the exposed surface of the precentral convolution at the level of the middle and inferior frontal gyri; it is similar in structure to area 6 (see "The Premotor Area") and is found only in the human brain. Area 4γ is situated mainly within the central fissure and is the only constituent of the motor cortex that extends to the medial surface of the brain. In man the motor area starts in the depths of the central sulcus and occupies the anterior wall of the sulcus and the adjacent part of the precentral, or posterior frontal, gyrus, together with that part of the paracentral lobule that lies rostral to the continuation of the central sulcus on the medial aspect of the hemisphere. It is narrow at its lower extremity, almost coming to a point just above the sylvian fissure, and is much wider rostrally.

The motor area gives rise to impulses that initiate volitional movements on the opposite side of the body (Fig. 49-2). It is subdivided into centers; each of these preferentially controls muscles that govern movements of individual parts of the opposite half of the body. These are represented in inverted order (see Figs. 23-3 and 23-4). The center for the pharynx and larynx is lowest, just above the sylvian fissure, and above that, in ascending order, those for the palate, mandible, tongue, lips, mouth, face, eyelids, forehead, neck, thumb, individual fingers, hand, wrist, forearm, arm, shoulder, upper thorax, diaphragm, lower thorax, abdominal muscles, thigh, leg, foot, toes, bladder, rectum, and genitalia. In the human the centers for the lower extremities as well as for those organs innervated by sacral nerves are situated on the medial aspect of the hemisphere. The areas for the

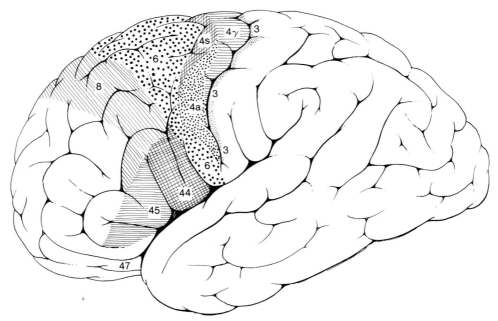

FIG. 49–1. Motor and premotor cortex of man. (Modified from Bucy PC (ed): The Precentral Motor Cortex. Illinois Monographs in the Medical Sciences. Urbana, IL, University of Illinois Press, 1944)

tongue, face, and digits are especially large, and each finger is represented individually. This is probably the result not of the size of the part, but of the number and complexity of movements executed by it. It must again be stressed that there is a certain amount of overlapping of the various areas, and that although the center that governs the movements of an individual portion of the body is predominantly located at one site, impulses from adjoining areas may also affect such movements. This multiplicity and wide extent of representation, as well as the existence of supplementary and secondary motor areas, may account for recovery of the function of individual parts of the body following focal lesions.

The motor area gives rise to the corticobulbar and corticospinal pathways, and the axons of the pyramidal cells, together with axons of other cells from this area, the premotor area, and parts of the parietal lobe, constitute the pyramidal, or corticospinal and corticobulbar, tracts that descend through the corona radiata, the genu and the anterior two-thirds of the posterior limb of the internal capsule, and the cerebral peduncle. The corticobulbar fibers terminate in the pons and medulla, but the corticospinal fibers continue their descent. At the pyramidal decussation, in the lower medulla, the majority of them (80% – 90%) cross and descend in the lateral

corticospinal pathways, while a few descend uncrossed in the ventral corticospinal pathways (see Fig. 23-6). The cells of the motor area undergo chromatolysis when the corticospinal tracts are sectioned, and the tracts degenerate when the motor cortex is destroyed.

The Premotor Area

Situated just anterior to the motor area, principally in its rostral portions, is the premotor area (see Fig. 49-1). This corresponds to area 6 of Brodmann (see Fig. 23-1) and is similar to area 4γ except for the absence of the giant pyramidal cells in layer V. The cells of layer V are, however, pyramidal in shape and obviously motor in type. Those in both layers III and V are arranged in a columnar pattern. The boundaries of the premotor area are less definite and distinct than those of the motor area, but roughly parallel the latter. The premotor area also exerts motor control over the opposite half of the body, and the localization within it parallels that in the motor region.

The portion of transitional cortex between areas 4 and 6 has been termed area 4s (Fig. 49-1). Some investigators have stated that stimulation of this region causes suppression of the

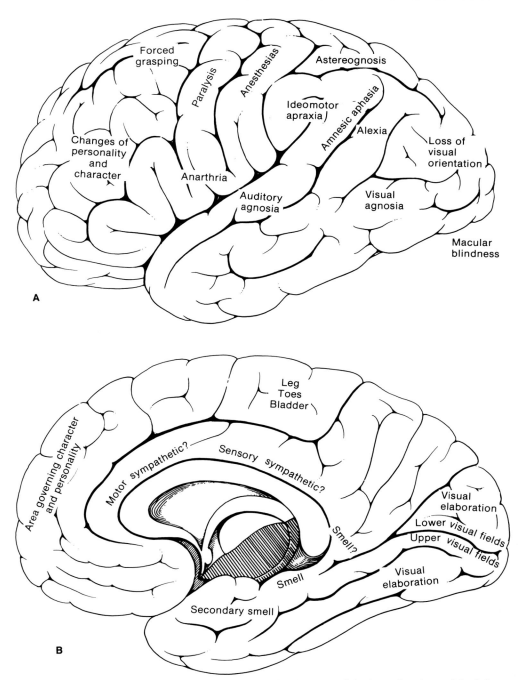

FIG. 49–2. Scheme of the cerebral hemispheres. **A.** Diagram of the lateral surface of the left hemisphere indicating the various symptoms that result from injury to certain areas. **B.** Medial surface of the right hemisphere showing symptoms following injury to various regions. (Modified from Bailey P. Intracranial Tumors, 2nd ed. Springfield, IL, Charles C Thomas, 1948)

activity of other cortical centers, especially area 4, with resulting muscular relaxation and loss of motor function, whereas ablation is followed by spasticity, hyperreflexia, and loss of fine movements. Other investigators, however, have questioned both the anatomic and physiologic existence of such a suppression area.

Lesions of the Motor and Premotor Areas

The details of the function of the motor and premotor areas, including the results of stimulation and ablation and the various concepts of corticospinal function and its disorders, are discussed in Chapter 23. The principal manifestation of a destructive lesion is paresis or paralysis of the opposite side of the body (see Fig. 23-8). This paralysis affects predominantly the distal portions of the extremities, and fine, skilled volitional movements are entirely abolished. Because the larynx, pharynx, palate, upper face, trunk muscles, diaphragm, rectum, and bladder are bilaterally innervated, the functions of these structures are little affected with unilateral lesions. It has generally been accepted by clinicians that the paresis or paralysis that follows lesions of the motor (and/or premotor) neurons or their neuraxes is of the spastic type (although it may be flaccid at the onset), and is accompanied by exaggeration of the muscle stretch reflexes as well as by pathologic reflex responses (Ch. 23). Irritation of the motor (and/or premotor) cortex causes motor responses of the corresponding contralateral portion of the body. Such irritation caused by a neoplasm or scar may result in focal or jacksonian convulsions. Stimulation experimentally or preceding surgical excision of epileptogenic foci causes discrete motor responses.

The motor and premotor areas also have connections with other important areas of the central nervous system. Frontopontine fibers, which make up an important part of the corticopontocerebellar tract, arise from the middle frontal convolution, anterior to areas 6 and 8. The impulses are carried to the pons, and after a synapse are relayed through the middle cerebellar peduncle (brachium pontis) to the contralateral cerebellar hemisphere. Loss of function of these fibers causes ataxia. At times it is difficult to differentiate between ataxia due to frontal lesions and that resulting from cerebellar involvement, but lesions of the frontal cortex or of the frontopontine fibers result in contralateral ataxia,

while a lesion of the cerebellar hemisphere causes ipsilateral ataxia. The premotor and motor areas have close connections with the basal ganglia. Focal epilepsy is sometimes alleviated by surgical excision of either meningocerebral cicatrices or foci of circumscribed atrophy in area 6, area 4, or both.

The Frontal Motor Eye Field

Area 8, which lies just anterior to area 6, is called the frontal motor eye field. It is the center for volitional control of conjugate ocular movements. Stimulation of this region, especially of area 8-alpha, beta, gamma of Vogt, causes strong, rapid conjugate deviation of the eyes to the opposite side, which may be accompanied by conjugate movement of the head and rotation of the trunk. If the lower portion of this area is stimulated, the eyes are deviated upward and laterally, and if the upper portion is irritated, they are moved downward and laterally. There may be associated opening of the eyelids and dilation of the pupils. Ablation of this area is followed by paresis of conjugate gaze to the opposite side and transient visual hemiagnosia; the eyes are turned toward the injured side, at least temporarily. This type of conjugate deviation is present for a few days after the occurrence of many infarcts of the middle cerebral artery territory. Area 8 (or 8s) also functions as a suppressor region with many of the same functions as area 4s. According to many anatomists, the frontal eye field extends into both area 6 and area 9.

The Motor Speech Areas

The lower portion of the motor and premotor region is known as Broca's area, or the motor speech area. The limits of this center are still being debated, but it is probably located in the region about the base of the precentral sulcus in the inferior frontal gyrus, and is situated in the left cerebral hemisphere in right-handed individuals and in either the right or left hemispheres (or in both) in left-handed persons. Area 44 of Brodmann is the principal site; this corresponds to the pars opercularis of the inferior frontal gyrus, but area 45 (in the pars triangularis), area 47 (in the pars orbitalis), and area 46 (above area 45) are also important. Possibly this region does not have the specific and localized functional characteristics that have been ascribed to it, and it may act only in association with the contiguous portions of the temporal and parietal lobes and the underlying insula. Stimulation of this region, however, has been followed by outbursts of logorrhea, or occasionally by slowed speech, and destructive lesions produce an oral expressive type of aphasia.

The Frontal Association Areas

The portions of the frontal lobe that lie anterior to area 6, area 8, and the motor speech centers are areas 9, 10, 11, 12, 32, and others. They are connected with the somesthetic, visual, auditory, and other sensory areas by association fibers, and with the thalamus and hypothalamus by projection fibers. They are often called the prefrontal areas, but inasmuch as they are frontal and not actually prefrontal, the term frontal association areas is a better one to use. From the point of view of cellular structure this region is strikingly different from areas 4 and 6. The cortex is thin and is particularly rich in granular cells, and the pyramidal cells in layer V are reduced in both size and number. These areas of the brain are the most conspicuously developed in man, and they have long been considered the seat of the higher intellectual functions, including memory, judgment, reasoning power, and the various perceptual, associative, and executive functions of the mind. Experimental studies, however, have given little information regarding their functions. Unilateral ablation in animals causes no obvious disturbance. Bilateral removal in humans is followed by restlessness, distractibility, failure of recent memory, and loss of ability to utilize past experiences. Much information concerning the functions of the frontal association areas has come from clinical observation of patients with degeneration, injuries, or tumors of the frontal lobes, and from examinations performed on those who have had these regions surgically removed.

The "case of the crowbar skull" is the first reported instance of an injury to the frontal lobes that was followed by personality changes. A man, aged 25 years, was injured in a powder explosion in 1848, and a crowbar was forced into the left frontal pole of the brain, making its exit from the skull just to the right of the coronal suture. He died 13 years later after having traveled extensively and having been, for a period of time, in Barnum's exhibit. He was said to have been irreverent, profane, impatient of restraint, and unable to hold a job. He was "a child in his

intellectual capacities, with the general passions of a strong man." Rylander in 1948 described 32 patients in whom part of one frontal lobe was removed in the treatment of either tumor or abscess. In the majority of cases about two thirds of the lobe was removed. In about one half of the patients there was bilateral involvement. The outstanding symptoms were diminished inhibition of affective response, euphoria, restlessness, loss of initiative, and disturbances of intellectual faculties characterized by loss of attention, slowing of intellectual processes, loss of memory for details, and difficulty with associations. About one fifth of the patients showed significant personality changes along with a marked increase in appetite and weight. In most instances the mental symptoms and alterations in personality did not affect the patient's ability to lead a normal social existence, but they did interfere with intellectual work. Many cases of unilateral frontal lobectomy have been reported in which no discernible alterations in mental functions were present. On the other hand, slight changes in personality and minimal loss of initiative and impairment of abstract thinking have been described. These symptoms are more marked if the left frontal lobe is removed in a right-handed individual.

Some studies have been described of patients who have had both frontal lobes removed in the excision of large tumors. Brickner reported the history of a 40-year-old stock broker who underwent a bilateral frontal lobectomy for the removal of a meningioma. The excision was carried back as far as the premotor regions, and areas 9, 10, 11, 12, 45, 46, 47, and parts of 8, 32, and 44 were extirpated, slightly more on the right than on the left. Psychologic observations, reported 6 and 8 years after the operation, revealed the following problems: Slowing and stereotype of mental activity; limitation in the capacity to associate and synthesize, with distractibility and impairment of selection, retention, and learning; loss of judgment, initiative, and the ability to reason abstractly; and defective emotional restraint, with euphoria, boasting, hostility, temper outbursts, and lack of sexual inhibitions. On the Stanford–Binet test his intelligence quotient was 94, although his mental age was only 9 years on the Pintner–Paterson scale. He lacked appreciation of the gravity of his situation and had learned nothing since the operation. In contrast to this report, Ackerly found only moderate emotional changes and no permanent defect in intellectual status of a patient whose entire right prefrontal area was removed, even though there had been a previous partial destruction of the left prefrontal area.

The functions of the frontal association areas may be indicated by a review of the alterations of these functions that take place in the various degenerative and atrophic lesions of the frontal lobe. In dementia paralytica, Alzheimer's disease, Pick's disease, and dementias associated with infectious and nutritional disorders, the earliest change is often a loss of memory, especially of recent memory or of retention and immediate recall. This may be followed by an impairment of judgment, especially in social and ethical situations. Absence of the restraint imposed by the inhibitions that have been acquired through training may lead to an increase in natural appetites and carelessness in habits of dress and personal hygiene. Sexual promiscuity may develop. Loss of ability to carry out business affairs results. The ability to perceive abstract relationships is impaired early. The patient may be able to carry out simple, well-organized actions, but is incapable of dealing with new problems, although they may be within the scope and range usually handled by a person of similar age and education. Attempted tasks are solved in a roundabout manner, and those requiring a deviation from established mental habits and an adaptation to unfamiliar situations are the most difficult to perform. The power of attention is lessened, and distractibility may be marked. There is difficulty in comprehension and loss of ability to make associations, especially in acquiring and synthesizing new material. The time needed for solving intellectual problems is prolonged, and the patient fatigues rapidly. Emotional lability may be outstanding, with vacillating moods and outbursts of crying, rage, or laughter, even though the patient had formerly shown an even temperament and steady habits. There may be marked irritability. The mood is often one of euphoria with an increased sense of well-being, and with facetiousness, levity, and senseless joking and punning (**witzelsucht**). Apathy and indifference may be present. The patient may fail to link immediate impressions with past experience, and this can lead to confusion and disorientation. There is progressive dementia as the deterioration increases.

Similar symptoms may be encountered in patients with neoplasms of the frontal lobe. In neoplasms, however, either *witzelsucht* and euphoria or indifference and apathy are early manifestations, and may be evident before memory loss and difficulties with judgment become apparent. Often, however, there are other signs of intracranial disease. Pressure on the motor areas may cause pareses, focal or generalized convulsive manifestations, frontal ataxia, or forced grasping, pressure on either the olfactory or visual pathways may produce either anosmia or visual defects; increase in intracranial pressure may be evident by the presence of headaches, papilledema, and a slow pulse.

Although it is known that extensive impairment of function occurs with lesions of the anterior portion of the frontal lobes, further localization is not possible from the examination alone. There is no definite focus whose removal leads to dementia, and massive lesions of the frontal lobes, especially when unilateral, may cause few symptoms, particularly if the lesion is in the non-dominant hemisphere. Some psychologic studies have indicated that disturbance of such functions as retention and learning are dependent upon the size of a lesion, whereas impairment of intellectual ability is more dependent upon the site of the lesion, and is more marked with left-sided involvement.

The original concept of Hughlings Jackson that the brain functions as a whole intellectually and emotionally may account for the fact that extensive lesions in the frontal lobes may be necessary before impairment is obvious. This theory is stressed by those who state that there is no representation of function in the cerebrum, and express the belief that the cortex merely selects, abstracts, and integrates patterns of nervous activity, and that differences in intellectual ability are dependent upon the amount of activity of the brain rather than the function of individual cellular components. It is generally accepted, however, that the disturbances of the mental, intellectual, and emotional processes just described are symptoms of dysfunction of the association areas, not only frontal, but, when severe, including also the parietal, temporal, and limbic lobes. It is not possible to state whether they are the result of irritation, destruction, or both, but they are probably caused by both. In cases of brain tumor, however, where there may be marked changes in personality and memory, the removal of an entire frontal lobe may to all appearance return the patient to normal; in such instances the symptoms are probably those of irritation, or related to pressure and edema. Following hemispherectomies performed in patients with infantile hemiplegia and convulsions, behavioral and mental symptoms have improved without an increase in the motor deficit. In the progressive dementias, however, and in observations such as those of Brickner, identical symptoms are the result of destruction of brain tissue.

The observation that lesions of the frontal lobes may decrease emotional and affective responses and relieve anxiety, apprehension, and nervous tension led to the operation of prefrontal leukotomy, or lobotomy, for the relief of mental symptoms. This procedure, first performed in Portugal by Moniz in 1936, was done extensively over a period of years in the treatment of patients with manic-depressive psychosis, involutional depressions, schizophrenia, and obsessive-compulsive states, and to decrease the reaction to intractable pain of organic disease. It has been discontinued for the most part. The operation consisted of cutting the white matter in the plane of the coronal suture in each frontal lobe; the association fibers that connect the prefrontal areas with the subcortical gray masses, especially the thalamus and hypothalamus, were also usually sectioned. Several modifications of the technic existed, some with thalamotomy included. Undesirable reactions were often more prominent than relief of symptoms following these procedures, and for this reason as well as their unpredictability, and because of questions raised about their moral justification, they have been largely abandoned. Pharmacotherapy has replaced them.

THE PARIETAL LOBES

The postcentral region is composed of areas 3, 1, and 2; it occupies all but the lowest part of the postcentral gyrus and is continued over the superomedial border into the adjoining part of the paracentral lobule. In the depth of the central fissure area 3 joins area 4. In the postcentral area there is the typical sensory cortex with all six layers well developed. The anterior parts are very thin. They are characterized by the density of the granular layer and the presence of granular cells that have replaced other nuclei in the outer pyramidal layer. The largest nuclei are found in the inner layer of the large pyramidal cells. They are smaller than the giant cells of Betz and occur discretely rather than in clusters. In the posterior parts the large pyramidal cells are reduced both in size and number, and the granular layer is wider but is not so densely packed with cells.

Area 5a, or the preparietal area, is situated in the upper part of the parietal lobe, just posterior to area 2. It contains large, deep pyramidal cells, some as great as the smaller Betz cells in area 4.

Area 5b, the superior parietal area, occupies a large part of the superior parietal lobule in man and extends over the medial surface of the hemisphere to include the precuneus. Area 7, the inferior parietal area, constitutes the major portion of the inferior parietal lobule; it includes the supramarginal and angular gyri, which are sometimes separately designated as areas 40 and 39, respectively. In areas 5b, 7, 39, and 40 there are no large pyramidal cells in layer V; the granular layers are of great depth and density.

The postcentral region is the somesthetic sensory, or sensory receptive, area. It receives enormous projections from the nuclei ventralis posterolateralis and posteromedialis of the lateral nuclear mass of the thalamus. These relay impulses from the spinothalamic tracts, medial lemnisci, and secondary trigeminal tracts, and traverse the posterior limb of the internal capsule. The various regions of the body are preferentially represented in specific portions of the postcentral gyrus, and the pattern roughly parallels the motor localization on the opposite lip of the central fissure, although it is not as definite or as well defined (see Figs. 5-4 and 49-2). The distal portions of the extremities are widely represented. Cutaneous sensations for the face and body may have bilateral representation, but those for the extremities, as well as deep sensations, have only contralateral representation. The somesthetic area may extend posteriorly into areas 5 and 7, and even rostrally into the precentral gyrus (areas 4 and 6). The receptive fields differ somewhat for the various sensory modalities. Secondary and supplementary sensory areas have been described adjacent to the ends of the primary area.

The superior and inferior parietal lobules (areas 5 and 7) constitute the psychosensory or sensory association area. This has connections with the postcentral gyrus by means of association pathways, and receives fibers from the nuclei lateralis dorsalis and posterior of the thalamus. No localization of function has been determined in the parietal lobe posterior to the postcentral gyrus, although localization is somewhat more definite near to this gyrus than distant from it.

The functions of the parietal lobe are essentially those of reception, correlation, analysis, synthesis, integration, interpretation, and elaboration of the primary sensory impulses that are received from the thalamus. The somesthetic area is the initial reception center for afferent impulses, especially for tactile, pressure, and position sensations. It is necessary for the discrimination of the finer, more critical grades of sensation and for the recognition of intensity. Stimulation of this area by either artificial excitation or disease processes produces paresthesias on the opposite side of the body. There are tactile and pressure sensations, with numbness, tingling, sensations of constriction and movement, and occasional thermal sensations, but rarely pain. Such sensations may precede jacksonian convulsions as an aura of the seizure, or may accompany the convulsion, and the spread of the stimulus follows the same general pattern as in the motor area. On stimulation of the postcentral gyrus in animals there is evidence of bilateral paresthesias. Destructive lesions are followed by a raising of the sensory threshold on the opposite side of the body, but both exteroceptive and proprioceptive sensations are perceived and complete anesthesia is not present.

The sensory association areas are essential for the synthesis and interpretation of impulses, appreciation of similarities and differences, interpretation of spatial relationships and two-dimensional qualities, evaluations of variations in form and weight, and localization of sensation. Irritation of these areas is followed by minimal symptoms such as vague paresthesias or hyperesthesias on the opposite side of the body. Destructive lesions produce a complex of symptoms affecting mainly the gnostic aspects of sensation. Simple appreciation of the stimulation of primary sensory endings remains, but perceptual functions are lost. There is impairment of those aspects of sensation that involve interpretation of stimuli, analysis and synthesis of individual modalities, correlation and elaboration of impulses, integration into concrete concepts, and calling out of engrams to aid in association and identification. Attempts have been made to associate these various functions with individual portions of the parietal lobe, but such localization has yet to be confirmed.

The clinical manifestations of parietal lobe lesions are described in Chapter 8. The extremities, especially their distal parts, are more affected than the trunk and face, and the midline is spared on the latter areas. The threshold for superficial pain may be raised slightly, and the pain of a phantom limb has been relieved by removal of the area of cortical representation of the limb. There is loss of temperature discrimination, especially in the intermediate ranges; light touch is little disturbed, but tactile discrimination and localization may be profoundly affected. Recognition of joint position, awareness of passive movement, and spa-

tial orientation are impaired, and as a result there may be sensory ataxia and pseudoathetoid movements. Stereognostic sense, the appreciation of similarities and differences in size and weight, localization of stimulation, recognition of textures, identification of figures written on the skin, and two-point discrimination are all lost. The time required for sensory adaptation is prolonged. **Sensory inattention,** or **extinction,** on the affected side of the body is often an early and important finding: with simultaneous stimulation of identical areas on the two sides of the body, the stimulus is not perceived on the side opposite the affected parietal lobe, although sensation on that side may be normal to routine testing.

Lesions of the parietal lobe, predominantly the subordinate one, may also cause defects in orientation of the opposite side of the body in space, in identification of portions of the body, and in awareness of disease. Unilateral neglect, usually of the left side of the body, is often the result of non-dominant parietal lobe lesions; also, functions dealing with spatial synthesis and orientation are impaired with non-dominant lesions, causing the phenomena of constructional apraxia and other disturbances. **Autotopagnosia** or **somatotopagnosia** is the loss of power to orient the body or the relation of its individual parts; there may be loss of identification of one limb or one part of the body. **Amorphosynthesis** is the lack of recognition of the opposite side of the body and of space. **Anosognosia,** the ignorance of the existence of disease, is used specifically to imply the lack of awareness of hemiplegia, or a feeling of depersonalization toward paralyzed parts of the body or a loss of perception of them. The patient may deny the existence of paresis and believe that he is able to use the affected extremities in a normal manner. Along with this there may be unilateral neglect of the involved portion of the body.

The posterior and inferior portions of the parietal lobe, especially the angular and supramarginal gyri and the areas in close proximity to the occipital and temporal lobes, are associated in function with the visual and auditory systems. The optic radiations course through a portion of the parietal lobe to reach the visual cortex, and a deeply placed lesion of the lobe may cause either an inferior quadrantic or a hemianopic defect of the visual fields. Stimulation of the angular gyrus causes contralateral deviation of the eyes. The angular and supramarginal gyri of the dominant hemisphere are important in relation to language and related functions, and lesions in these areas may be responsible for various types of receptive aphasia, agnosia, and sensory apraxia; these are discussed in Chapter 52.

Occasionally parietal lesions have been reported to result in contralateral muscular atrophy, with flaccidity, either absence or increase of muscle stretch reflexes, and trophic changes that consist of smooth, shiny skin, decrease in skin temperature, dry, brittle hair and nails, and edema. Secondary to the sensory disturbances there may be hypotonia and slowness of movement of the opposite side of the body, especially of the proximal muscles, with ataxia and pseudoathetoid groping movements. Focal motor seizures and partial paralysis involving the contralateral portions of the body can occur with parietal lesions. These may be caused by an interruption of communication with areas 6 and 4, or may denote that the parietal lobe also possesses motor functions.

THE OCCIPITAL LOBES

The occipital lobe is more nearly a structural and functional entity than are any of the other cerebral lobes. All of its functions are concerned either directly or indirectly with vision. It is composed of areas 17, 18, and 19 of Brodmann.

The visual receptive area (area 17) is located on the lips of the calcarine fissure and adjacent portions of the cuneus and lingual gyrus, and extends around the occipital pole to occupy a portion of the lateral surface of the hemisphere. The cortex is granular in type. It is extremely thin, but layer IV is relatively thick and is subdivided by a light band into three sublayers. The middle sublayer is occupied by the greatly thickened outer band of Baillarger, here known as the band of Gennari, which is visible to the naked eye in sections of the fresh cortex and has given the region the name area striata. The optic radiations, or geniculocalcarine tract, pass from the lateral geniculate body to the striate cortex on the upper and lower lips of the calcarine fissure. These fibers convey impulses from the ipsilateral half of each retina. Those from the lower half terminate on the lower lip of the fissure, and those from the upper half, on the upper lip. The macular fibers occupy the posterior portion of the region, in a wedge-shaped area with its apex anterior, and have a wide cortical distribution. Impulses from the paracentral and peripheral retinal areas are represented more anteriorly in serial concentric zones (see Fig. 10-3). The striate area is the receiving center for visual impressions; color, size, form, motion, illumination, and transparency are perceived and determined there. The recognition and identification of objects, however, requires the associated function of the adjoining visuopsychic areas, discussed in the next paragraph. Stimulation, or irritation, of the calcarine cortex produces unformed visual hallucinations, such as scotomas and flashes of light, in the corresponding fields of vision. Destructive lesions result in defects in the visual fields supplied by the affected areas. Destruction of both striate regions causes total blindness.

The parastriate, or parareceptive, region, area 18, receives and interprets impulses from area 17; it is essential for the recognition and identification of objects. It is said that memories of inanimate objects are "stored" in the lateral and inferior part, and those for animate objects and for the body itself in the upper part. The peristriate (perireceptive or preoccipital) region, area 19, has connections with areas 17 and 18 and with other portions of the cortex. It functions in more complex visual recognition and perception, revisualization, visual association, and spatial orientation. These regions are classed together as the visuopsychic areas; the cortex is thicker than in the striate region, and there is an increase in the size and number of cells in layer III, but almost complete absence of large cells in layer V. Stimulation of these regions causes formed visual hallucinations, and destruction is followed by difficulty with fixation and with maintaining visual attention, loss of stereoscopic vision, impairment of visual memory, difficulty with accurate localization and discernment of objects, and disturbances in the spatial orientation of the visual image, especially for distance, in the homonymous field. There is loss of ability to discriminate with respect to size, shape, and color. There may be errors in the patient's ability to localize either himself or stationary or moving objects in space, with a loss of visual perception of spatial relationships. There may be distortion of objects, or metamorphopsia. In bilateral lesions there may be marked loss of visual orientation with anosognosia, or denial of blindness (**Anton's syndrome**), due to interruption of the pathways between the striate cortex and other centers. Visual aphasias are discussed in Chapter 52.

Areas 18 and 19, especially the latter, also contain the cortical centers for optically induced eye movements and optic fixation reflexes, in contrast to the volitional center in the frontal lobe. Corticofugal fibers pass through the optic radiations to the superior colliculus and tegmentum of the midbrain and then, partly by way of the paramedian pontine reticular formation, through the medial longitudinal fasciculus and other tracts to the nuclei of the ocular nerves. There are also association pathways from the occipital to the frontal cortical areas, with radiation of impulses to the frontal cortex before they descend in the internal capsule. Stimulation causes a slow, forced, conjugate deviation of the eyes to the opposite side and pupillary constriction; ablation is followed by loss of following and reflex ocular movements and of optic fixation reflexes. Although voluntary control is maintained, there may be difficulty in focusing the eyes.

THE TEMPORAL LOBES

The auditory receptive region (areas 41 and 42) is located in the transverse temporal gyri (Heschl's convolutions), which lie on the dorsal surface of the posterior part of the superior temporal convolution, partly buried in the floor of the lateral sulcus. Area 41 occupies the middle of the anterior transverse gyrus and is surrounded by area 42, which extends on the lateral surface of the middle region of the superior temporal gyrus. Area 41 is composed of granular cortex similar to that in the parietal and occipital receptive regions; area 42 has a number of large pyramidal cells in layer III. The auditory radiations pass from the medial geniculate body to the auditory receptive region. Hearing is bilaterally represented in the temporal lobes, although a greater number of impulses may be received from the contralateral ear. There is some localization of the various auditory impulses in the temporal lobe; it has been suggested that high-pitched tones are received in the more medial and posterior portions, whereas low tones are received more laterally and anteriorly. From the cortical centers, connections are made with adjacent areas in the superior temporal convolution where sound, word, and memory patterns are stored. In this region auditory impressions are differentiated and interpreted as words. It is believed that the superior temporal convolution may also receive vestibular impulses, but the exact localization of cortical centers for these impulses is not known.

Stimulation of the superior temporal gyrus produces vague auditory hallucinations in the form of tinnitus and sensations of roaring and buzzing, and stimulation of adjacent areas causes vertigo and a sensation of unsteadiness.

Unilateral destruction of the transverse temporal gyri does not cause deafness (because there is bilateral representation of hearing) although there may be an impairment of the localization of sounds on the opposite side, especially in regard to the distance from which the sounds are coming. Furthermore, there may be a bilateral dulling of auditory acuity with a perceptible difference in the intensity of sounds and impairment in the recognition of musical notes. Unilateral destructive lesions of the superior temporal convolution may, in addition, cause difficulty with equilibrium and a sensation of unsteadiness and falling to the opposite side. Bilateral destruction of the temporal lobes may cause deafness. A destructive lesion in the region of the anterior transverse temporal gyrus or the adjacent posterior and lateral portion of the superior temporal convolution (Wernicke's area) on the left in right-handed persons will cause a loss of ability to comprehend spoken words. The auditory receptive aphasias are discussed in Chapter 52.

The functions of the remainder of the temporal lobes have been less specifically defined in the past, and those areas other than the ones dealing with the auditory and vestibular systems have often been referred to as "silent" ones. Experimental and clinical studies, however, have demonstrated some important functions and have shown the relationship of the temporal lobes to various clinical syndromes and disease processes. Certain regions are related to the visual system, and stimulation of the middle temporal gyrus (area 21) causes contralateral deviation of the eyes, often accompanied by similar deviation of the trunk and adversive and synergic movements of the opposite arm and leg. The optic radiations pass through the temporal lobe and curve around the descending horn of the lateral ventricle; encroachment on them may cause either a superior quadrantic or hemianopic defect in the visual fields. Irritation of these fibers or of certain portions of the temporal cortex may cause visual hallucinations that are better formed and organized than the hallucinations associated with occipital lobe lesions.

The posterior portions of the middle and inferior temporal convolutions communicate with the cerebellum through the temporopontocerebellar pathways, and unilateral destruction of these regions may cause contralateral ataxia. Ablation of major portions of one temporal lobe, especially the anterior region, causes few or no symptoms in experimental animals, but bilateral ablation produces a characteristic set of symptoms (**Klüver – Bucy syndrome**). This consists of psychic blindness or visual agnosia, loss of fear and rage reactions, increased sexual activity, bulimia, hypermetamorphosis (excessive tendency to attend and react to every visual stimulus), and a severe memory defect. These manifestations occur only if the uncus and hippocampus are included in the ablation. From an anatomic and physiologic point of view these latter regions on the medial aspect of the lobe, along with the amygdaloid complex, belong to the limbic lobe, but they are considered parts of the temporal lobe by most clinicians.

Penfield and his associates have demonstrated that stimulation of the temporal lobe cortex in epileptic patients gives rise to illusions of perception, hallucinations, and automatisms. Furthermore, they were able to elicit psychic responses on stimulation of the lateral and superior surfaces, and to produce "memories," or instances in which the patient would relive earlier experiences. Consequently Penfield stated that the temporal lobe is used in the interpretation of current experiences and in recall of memories. On the basis of these observations, as well as electroencephalographic, anatomic, and pathologic studies and experimental investigation, the relationship of the temporal lobe and contiguous structures to a specific type of epileptic syndrome is well accepted. Jackson, in 1873 and subsequent years, described seizures characterized by olfactory and visual hallucinations, dreamy states and reminiscences, automatisms, and gastric and autonomic symptoms, and observed that they were associated with lesions of the medial aspect of the temporal lobe. He referred to these as the "uncinate group of fits," but clinicians in general have used the term uncinate only for those with olfactory hallucinations.

The terms psychomotor and temporal lobe seizures were often used synonymously for these attacks. The preferred term is now **complex partial seizures.** They include some or all of the following: automatisms consisting of brief or prolonged inappropriate but seemingly purposeful automatic movements; disordered consciousness, usually with amnesia for the period of abnormal behavior; perceptual illusions and hallucinations that may be visual, auditory, olfactory, or gustatory; motor accompaniments of the olfactory and gustatory hallucinations (chewing, tasting, and swallowing movements), pilomotor ("gooseflesh") phenomena; disorders of recognition and recall, often with reminiscences, dreamy states, and phenomena such as *déjà vu* and *déjà pensé* in which the patient expe-

riences either visual manifestations or thoughts that seem strangely familiar to him and that he feels he has lived through or observed previously; psychic manifestations such as anxiety, fear, rage, obsessive thoughts, compulsive speech or actions, or feelings of unreality. These phenomena have been found to be associated with abnormal discharges or pathologic lesions of the anterior and medial portions of the temporal lobes, including the hippocampal gyrus, uncus, amygdaloid complex, and hippocampus, or the subcortical connections of these structures, many of which actually belong to the limbic system. Relay of impulses to the hypothalamus, thalamus, or mesencephalic reticular formation may also be of importance. In certain cases of such complex partial seizures there may be associated involvement of the insula, posterior orbital surface of the frontal lobe, basal ganglia, frontal association areas, or contiguous structures. It has been demonstrated that removal of a portion of the abnormally discharging temporal lobe has been an effective therapy in certain cases of such seizures, when medication fails to alleviate them adequately. In rare instances bilateral lobectomy has been attempted, but a syndrome similar to that described by Klüver and Bucy in animals has been reported in humans subjected to such bilateral ablations.

Foci of abnormal tissue, neoplastic or other, in the temporal lobe of certain persons with complex partial seizures can be visualized by magnetic resonance imaging. Abnormal metabolism and blood flow may be demonstrated in some by positron emission tomography or other radioisotope studies, and cortical or intracortical electroencephalographic recordings can help localize abnormal foci or paroxysmal discharges prior to temporal lobe resection.

Disease of the temporal lobes may also be manifested by symptoms other than the phenomena described. Major convulsions occur frequently with neoplasms and similar lesions. A tumor of the superior aspect of the temporal lobe may press upon the lower frontal and parietal areas and cause either motor and sensory changes in the face and arm or focal convulsions before evidence of primary localization to the temporal lobe is apparent. Neoplasms of the temporal lobes are second only to those of the frontal lobes in the frequency with which they are accompanied by mental symptoms, among which are the following: psychic manifestations varying from vague personality changes to frank behavioral disturbances; emotional abnormalities such as anxiety, depression, fear, and anger;

paranoia; memory defects; learning and cognitive disabilities; slowing of cerebration, and apathy. These are most apt to occur with diffuse and rapidly growing lesions, especially if the dominant hemisphere is affected. A neoplasm of the medial aspect may press on the midbrain and cause dilation of the ipsilateral pupil, a third nerve palsy, or even decerebrate motor activity.

THE LIMBIC LOBES

The hippocampal gyrus, uncus, isthmus, and gyrus cinguli are usually grouped together as the limbic lobe or system. Closely related are the subcallosal and retrosplenial gyri, pyriform area, hippocampus, and various subcortical structures including the amygdala and septal nuclei. Certain of these are often included in the temporal lobe, but anatomically and physiologically they are placed in the limbic system, or "visceral brain." The insula and the medial and posterior orbital gyri of the frontal lobe are closely allied, although not actually a part of the limbic system. Phylogenetically the majority of these structures are a part of the rhinencephalon, the major portion of the cerebral hemisphere in lower forms, and are related to the olfactory and gustatory systems, which are so important in these forms. In the human, however, the development of the neopallium overshadows the olfactory and gustatory portions of the brain, the connections of which are primarily subcortical and relate to thalamic and hypothalamic centers. The cingulate gyrus may be more closely related in function to the frontal and parietal lobes, but the hippocampal gyrus and uncus, even though allied anatomically to the temporal lobe, are undoubtedly in part olfactory and gustatory in function, and the fibers of the lateral olfactory stria terminate in them. Irritation, or stimulation, of these produces either olfactory or gustatory hallucinations. These are often very disagreeable and are described with difficulty. For example, the patient may describe the taste of blood, the odor of burning rubber, or of decaying material. The hallucinations may be accompanied by smacking or licking of the lips, tasting movements of the tongue, swallowing, and salivation, and constitute an important part of the complex partial seizure. Destruction of these areas is not followed by loss of smell or taste because of their bilateral connections.

It is generally conceded by anatomists and physiologists that smell and taste are functionally related, and that the central connections dealing with gustatory sensations are correlated with those for olfactory sensations, not only in the uncus and hippocampal gyrus, but also in the thalamus and hypothalamus. It has been stated that area 43, or the pararolandic operculum, which overlies the lower aspects of the parietal and frontal lobes, has both sensory and motor functions concerned with taste. The posterior portion of this area, which overlies the locus for somatic sensation from the tongue, may be the cortical center for gustatory sensation, and the anterior portion has been called the site for the control of movements necessary for tasting and swallowing. Stimulation of area 43 may be followed by smacking, tasting, and swallowing movements, and by gustatory hallucinations.

The limbic lobe and related structures have rich connections with the hypothalamus and thalamus, and play an important part in the central regulation of the autonomic nervous system (Ch. 40) as well as of visceral and sexual functions and the autonomic aspects involved in emotional expression. In addition to the oral and alimentary reactions just mentioned, stimulation of certain of the areas may cause genital and sexual responses, and manifestations of rage, fear, and defense. Abnormal affective and emotional responses, fear, and aggressive behavior may be lessened by interruption of the connections between these cortical areas and the thalamus and hypothalamus. Bilateral or even unilateral lesions or resection of the hippocampus and hippocampal gyrus are followed by marked impairment of recent memory. Bilateral lesions of the cingulate gyrus (area 24) cause apathy, akinesia, and mutism. It is probable that many of the manifestations of complex partial seizures are the result of involvement of the limbic lobe rather than the temporal lobe. The relationship of the various structures included in the "visceral brain" to emotional and mental disease is assuming increasing importance (Ch. 42).

OTHER CORTICAL AREAS

Only those regions of the cerebral cortex whose functions have been either demonstrated experimentally or observed clinically have been discussed; these are principally the projection areas. Cytoarchitectural studies show that there are many other distinct regions that may be significant clinically, but the functions of these areas are either less well defined or as yet unknown. In view of the lack of definite knowledge of their functions, they cannot at this time be considered from a clinical point of view.

BIBLIOGRAPHY

Ackerly S. Instinctive, emotional and mental changes following prefrontal lobe extirpation. Am J Psychiatry 1935;92:717

Bartholow R. Experimental investigation into the functions of the human brain. Am J Med Sci 1874;67:305

Brickner RM. The Intellectual Functions of the Frontal Lobes: A Study Based Upon Observation of a Man With Partial Bilateral Frontal Lobectomy. New York, Macmillan, 1963

Brodal A. Neurological Anatomy in Relation to Clinical Medicine, 3rd ed. New York, Oxford University Press, 1981

Brodal A. The hippocampus and the sense of smell: A review. Brain 1947;70:179

Bucy PC (ed). The Precentral Motor Cortex. Illinois Monographs in the Medical Sciences. Urbana, IL, University of Illinois Press, 1944

Critchley M. The Parietal Lobes. London, Edward Arnold & Co, 1953

Dejong RN. "Psychomotor" or "temporal lobe epilepsy": A review of the development of our present concepts. Neurology 1957;7:1

Dejong RN. The hippocampus and its role in memory: Clinical manifestations and theoretical considerations. J Neurol Sci 1973;19:73

Ferrier D. The Function of the Brain. New York, GP Putnam's Sons, 1886

Fisher CM. Disorientation for place. Arch Neurol 1982;39:33

Foerster O. The motor cortex in man in the light of Hughlings Jackson's doctrines. Brain 1936;59:135

Fritsch G, Hitzig E. Ueber die Elektrische Erregbarkeit des Grosshirns. Arch Anat Physiol Wissensch Med 1870;37:300

Fulton JF. Functional Localization in Relation to Frontal Lobotomy. New York, Oxford University Press, 1949

Gibbs EL, Gibbs FA, Fuster B. Psychomotor epilepsy. Arch Neurol Psychiatry 1948;60:331

Goody W. Cerebral representation. Brain 1956;79:167

Green JB. Pilomotor seizures. Neurology 1984;34:837

Halstead WB. Brain and Intelligence: A Quantitative Study of the Frontal Lobes. Chicago, University of Chicago Press, 1947

Harlow JM. Passage of an iron rod through the head. Boston Med Surg 1848;39:389

Jacobs L, Gossman MD. Three primitive reflexes in normal adults. Neurology 1980;30:184

Kimura D. Speech representation in an unbiased sample of left-handers. Hum Neurobiol 1983;2:147

Klüver H, Bucy PC. "Psychic blindness" and other symptoms following bilateral temporal lobectomy in rhesus monkeys. Am J Physiol 1937;119:352

Krynauw RA. Infantile hemiplegia treated by removing one cerebral hemisphere. J Neurol Neurosurg Psychiatry 1950;13:243

McGlone J, Young B. Cerebral localization. In Joynt RJ (ed). Clinical Neurology. Philadelphia, JB Lippincott, 1989

Mettler PA, Pool JL, Landis C et al. Selective Partial Ablation of the Frontal Cortex. New York, PB Hoeber, 1949

Meyer E, Beck E, Mclardy T. Prefrontal leucotomy: A neuroanatomical report. Brain 1947;70:18

Moniz E. Tentatives Operatoires dans le Traitment de Certaines Psychoses. Paris, Mason & Cie, 1936

Penfield W, Jasper H. Epilepsy and the Functional Anatomy of the Human Brain. Boston, Little, Brown & Co, 1954

Ropper AH. Self-grasping: A focal neurological sign. Ann Neurol 1982;12:575.

Rylander G. Personality analysis before and after frontal lobotomy. Ass Res Nerv Dis Proc 1948;27:691

Taylor J (ed). Selected Writings of J. Hughlings Jackson. London, Hodder & Stoughton, 1931

Terzian H, Ore GD. Syndrome of Klüver and Bucy reproduced in man by bilateral removal of the temporal lobes. Neurology 1955;5:373

Tweedy J, Reding M, Garcia C et al. Significance of cortical disinhibition signs. Neurology 1982;32:169

Von Monakow C. Die Lokalisation im Grosshirn und der Abbau der Function der korticalen Herde. Wiesbaden, JF Bergmann, 1914

Williams D. Man's temporal lobe. Brain 1968;91:639

Chapter 50

FUNCTIONS AND DISORDERS OF FUNCTION OF CERTAIN NONCORTICAL AREAS OF THE CEREBRUM

The diagnosis and localization of intracranial disease are dependent to a large extent upon evidence of disturbances of function of the cerebral cortex and the white matter underlying it. There are structures deeper in the cerebrum, however, whose functions are also of clinical importance. Some of these, such as the basal ganglia and related nuclear centers, are discussed elsewhere (Ch. 22) and will not be dealt with here. Others lack known clinical significance. Evidence of involvement of the following structures and complexes, however, may give important diagnostic and localizing information.

THE THALAMUS

The thalamus (Fig. 50-1) is one of the major constituents of the diencephalon. It is a large ovoid structure that is placed medially in the cerebrum. Its dorsal aspect forms the floor of the lateral ventricle, and it is bounded medially by the third ventricle and laterally by the internal capsule and basal ganglia; ventrally it is continuous with the subthalamus. Its nuclear centers have been classified and named variously, but in general the terminology of Walker is used. The nuclei of the thalamus are classed morphologically into specific groups.

The anterior nuclear group occupies the anterior part of the thalamus and projects into the lateral ventricle. It consists of the nuclei anterodorsalis, anteroventralis, and anteromedialis, whose connections are largely with the cingulate cortex and the hypothalamus. The nuclei of the midline are clusters of cells that lie close to the wall of the third ventricle and in the massa intermedia. They are connected chiefly with the hypothalamus, for visceral functions, but are poorly developed in man. The medial nuclei lie between the nuclei of the midline and the internal medullary lamina. Their most important representative is the nucleus medialis dorsalis, or the dorsomedial nucleus, which has connections with other thalamic nuclei, the preoptic and hypothalamic regions, the parolfactory area, the corpus striatum and globus pallidus, the amygdaloid complex, areas 8, 9, 10, 11, 12, 44, 45, 46, and 47 of the frontal cortex, and possibly areas 40 and 42 on the temporal operculum. The anterior, midline, and medial nuclei are centers for the correlation of interoceptive impulses, including olfactovisceral, general visceral, and probably gustatory impulses, with exteroceptive and equilibratory sensations. They are closely related to the hypothalamus and periventricular gray matter. The connections of the medial nuclei with the frontal cortex are of significance in the anatomic basis for behavior and personality.

The major component of the group of intralaminar nuclei is the nucleus centromedianus, which has connections with the caudate, putamen, and globus pallidus. The nucleus reticularis has been regarded as one of the regions of termination for ascending multisynaptic pathways and as a relay center in an activating system to the cortex.

The ventral nuclear group lies between the internal medullary lamina and the internal capsule, anterior to the pulvinar. Its most rostral portion is the nucleus ventralis anterior, which receives fibers from the globus pallidus and the

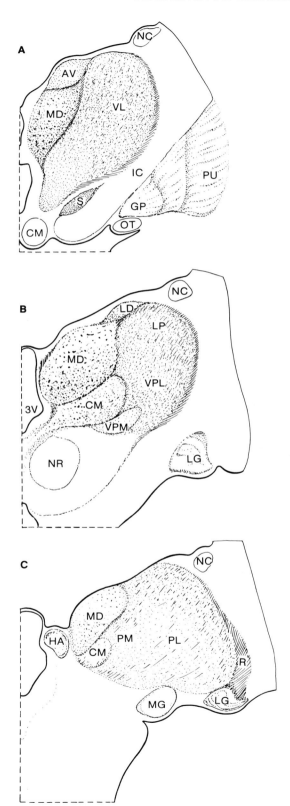

caudate nucleus and sends other fibers to the globus pallidus, caudate, and putamen, and possibly to the premotor cortex. Behind it lies the nucleus ventralis lateralis, which receives dentatothalamic and rubrothalamic fibers from the brachium conjunctivum and red nucleus, as well as fibers from the frontal cortex; it sends impulses to the motor and premotor cortex of the frontal lobe. It is a relay station from the cerebellum and red nucleus to the cerebral motor centers. The posterior part of the ventral division is the nucleus ventralis posterior, the largest cell mass in the ventral nuclear group. It is divided into four parts, the nuclei ventralis posteromedialis, posterolateralis, posteroinferior, and intermedius, but the first two are the most important. Within the nucleus ventralis posteromedialis terminate the fibers of the secondary trigeminal tracts, and within the nucleus ventralis posterolateralis the fibers of the spinothalamic tract and the medial lemniscus terminate. By means of thalamocortical fibers arising in these centers, impulses are relayed to the somesthetic sensory cortex in the postcentral gyrus.

Within the thalamus the receptive area for the face is located medially and caudally, that for the leg laterally and rostrally, and that for the arm in an intermediate position. These respective areas are connected with corresponding regions of the sensory cortex by specific portions of the thalamic radiations. Impulses from the upper areas of the body (medial part of the thalamus) travel to the inferior portions of the postcentral gyrus; those from the lower regions of the body (lateral part of the thalamus), to the superior sensory centers; those from the intermediate regions of the body and parts of the thalamus, to the middle portion of the sensory cortex.

FIG. 50–1. Cross section of the human thalamus showing the principal nuclear masses at three levels. **A.** Anterior thalamus. **B.** Midthalamus. **C.** Posterior thalamus. (*AV,* Nucleus anteroventralis. *CM,* Nucleus centrum medianum. *GP,* Globus pallidus. *HA,* Habenula. *IC,* Internal capsule. *LD,* Nucleus lateralis dorsalis. *LG,* Lateral geniculate body. *LP,* Nucleus lateralis posterior. *MD,* Nucleus medialis dorsalis. *MG,* Medial geniculate body. *NC,* Caudate nucleus. *NR,* Red nucleus. *OT,* Optic tract. *PM,* Medial nuclear group of pulvinar. *PU,* Putamen. *S,* Subthalamic nucleus. *VL,* Nucleus ventralis lateralis. *VPL,* Nucleus ventralis posterolateralis. *VPM,* Nucleus ventralis posteromedialis. *3V,* Third ventricle. *PL,* Lateral nuclear group of pulvinar. *R,* Nucleus reticularis)

The lateral nuclear group consists of the pulvinar and the nuclei lateralis dorsalis and posterior. The latter two receive fibers from other thalamic nuclei and communicate with the cortex of the posterior parts of the parietal lobe. The pulvinar is a large mass that forms the caudal extremity of the thalamus. Fibers project to it from other thalamic nuclei and possibly from the geniculate bodies, and it has connections with the peristriate area and the posterior parts of the parietal lobes. These nuclei are closely interrelated with the cerebral cortex, particularly with the parietal area, and are believed to integrate and reinforce cortical discharges.

The lateral and medial geniculate bodies are thalamic nuclei that have been displaced downward so that they lie lateral to the upper end of the mesencephalon under cover of the pulvinar. The portion of the thalamus in which they are situated is sometimes referred to as the metathalamus. The lateral geniculate bodies receive the fibers of the optic tracts, and after a synapse relay the impulses to the striate cortex through the geniculocalcarine pathways. There is a specific anatomic relationship between the various portions of the retinas, localization in the geniculate bodies, and the site of termination of the impulses in the occipital cortex (see Fig. 10-3). The medial geniculate bodies receive impulses from the cochlear nuclei by way of the lateral lemnisci and send them via the thalamotemporal radiations to the auditory areas in the superior temporal convolutions (see Fig. 14-2).

The thalamus may also be subdivided into the dorsal thalamus and the ventral thalamus. The former, which includes the constituents already described, is a receptive center for impulses, in most cases after synapse in lower regions, and transmits them to the corpus striatum and the cerebral cortex. The ventral thalamus, or subthalamus, is on the efferent side of the arc; it conducts impulses received from the dorsal thalamus, the motor cortex, and the lenticular nucleus to the lower efferent centers in the midbrain, pons, medulla, and spinal cord. It is an upward prolongation of the tegmental region of the midbrain and forms a zone of transition between the tegmentum and the thalamus. It occupies a triangular area between the dorsal thalamus above, the internal capsule and cerebral peduncle laterally, and the hypothalamus medially. The epithalamus, above the thalamus, includes the habenular nuclei and their connections, and the stria medullaris, epiphysis, and posterior commissure; it is an olfactosomatic correlation center for conscious and reflex response to olfactory stimulation, and also has endocrine functions. The hypothalamus, below the thalamus, is discussed in Part F, "The Autonomic Nervous System."

The thalamus is connected with the cerebral cortex by the thalamic peduncles. The anterior thalamic peduncle consists of frontothalamic, thalamofrontal, striothalamic, and thalamostriatal fibers that run in the anterior limb of the internal capsule. The thalamocortical fibers are believed to allow certain emotional impulses or "feeling tones" to reach the cortex. The superior thalamic peduncle consists of thalamoparietal fibers that transmit sensation from the thalamus to the cortex; these fibers run in the posterior limb of the internal capsule. The posterior thalamic peduncle contains the optic radiations from the lateral geniculate body to the occipital cortex, and the inferior thalamic peduncle carries auditory radiations from the medial geniculate body to the temporal cortex.

The thalamus has various functions. It is the principal relay center in the forebrain. It receives pain and temperature impulses from the spinothalamic and dorsal secondary ascending trigeminal pathways, tactile and proprioceptive sensations from the medial lemniscus and ventral secondary ascending trigeminal tract, cerebellar projections from the brachium conjunctivum, afferent fibers from the optic and auditory systems, and also olfactory and gustatory impulses. After an interruption these are forwarded to cortical levels. It is also a complex integrating nuclear mass. Impulses are not passed through it without changes, but are associated and synthesized. The thalamus is connected with the cerebral association areas and not only projects to the cortex but also receives fibers from it. The thalamus is principally a relay station for sensory impulses, but when the impulses reach the thalamus the person may have a vague awareness of the presence of the stimulus, with a crude, uncritical consciousness of it. The thalamus may also be the end-station in the quantitative appreciation of pain, heat, cold, and heavy contact. It is more important, however, in the affective than in the discriminative aspects of sensation.

Lesions of the thalamus may be followed by a definite complex of symptoms. The **thalamic syndrome** of Dejerine and Roussy results from damage that predominates in the nuclei ventralis posterolateralis and posteromedialis, and also from interruption of pathways going from the thalamus to the cortex. It is usually caused by a vascular lesion, most frequently either rupture or occlusion of one of the thalamogeniculate branches of the posterior cerebral artery. A characteristic group of symptoms develops. There is diminution of sensation on the opposite half of the body without complete anesthesia. The limbs and trunk are usually affected more than the face, which may be spared. There is usually a disturbance of deep sensibility — postural sense, and appreciation of passive movement, heavy contact, and deep pressure. The defect may range from slight to profound. Cutaneous sensations are also impaired, but the change may be transient. The threshold for tactile, pain, and temperature sensations is raised, but pain sense exhibits a specific alteration. All stimuli, when effective, excite unpleasant sensations, and even the lightest stimulus may evoke a disagreeable, burning, agonizing type of pain response in the affected part of the body. Light touch, extremes of hot and cold, roughness, tickling, and even the pressure of clothing or bedclothes may excite marked discomfort. Various visceral and affective states as well as auditory and visual impulses may also cause the response. As a result the patient may complain of intractable pain not relieved by ordinary analgesics. Owing to the presence of this hyperpathia, or hyperaffectivity, in spite of the raised sensory threshold, the term **anesthesia dolorosa** has been associated with this symptom complex. The thalamic overaction is the result of either irritation of the thalamus or release from higher cortical control. Every stimulus acting on the thalamus produces an excessive effect on the contralateral half of the body, especially as far as the affective element, the pleasant or unpleasant character in its appreciation, is concerned. Occasionally, pleasurable stimulation, such as that produced when a warm hand is applied to the skin on the affected side, may be markedly accentuated.

In addition to the sensory changes, the thalamic syndrome may include also, on the opposite side of the body, a transient or permanent hemiparesis resulting from damage to the adjacent corticospinal tract in the internal capsule, a hemiataxia with choreiform or choreoathetoid movements resulting from involvement of the cerebellorubrothalamic connections, a mimetic type of facial paresis with weakness present on emotional but not on voluntary contraction, and a quadrantic or hemianopic visual field defect. Increased emotional lability, with easily precipitated laughter and crying, may also be present.

Prolonged psychic disturbances, including confusion, amnesia, and confabulation, have been reported following surgical procedures performed on regions of the thalamus for the treatment of hyperkinetic and other disorders. Pathologic alterations of thalamic functions have been described in association with some psychiatric illnesses. Penfield and his associates have included the thalamus, especially the intralaminar and reticular nuclei, along with the reticular formation of the midbrain and brain stem, the tegmentum of the midbrain, and the basal diencephalic area, in the so-called centrencephalic integrating system in which certain "deep level" epileptic seizures, including absence and some other generalized attacks, originate. Epileptic discharges arising in this complex appear simultaneously in both cerebral hemispheres, and the electroencephalographic abnormality that accompanies them is bilaterally synchronous. If such a system does exist, however, it is probably caudally placed, mainly in the reticular formation (discussed later in this chapter), and epilepsy may not arise in the diencephalon, although this portion of the brain may be involved in the propagation of generalized seizures. On the other hand, "diencephalic seizures" have been described by some.

Aphasias have been reported to occur, although rarely, from unilateral vascular lesions of the thalamus alone. The vascular insult may have been occlusive or hemorrhagic.

The clinical manifestation of lesions in other portions of the thalamus are poorly understood. Involvement of the anterior part causes few sensory changes. Unmotivated laughter and crying, occurring without associated affective changes, are thought to be caused by lesions of the anterior thalamic peduncle. However, such unmotivated manifestations, also termed **emotional incontinence,** have also been described with lesions, usually bilateral, of many cortical and subcortical hemispheric areas.

Both severe dementia and choreoathetoid movements have been reported with symmetric degeneration of the thalamus affecting principally the anterior, medial, and lateral nuclei, and it has been suggested that an affection of the thalamus may be a major feature of some psychoses and degenerative diseases. The relief of mental and emotional symptoms that followed frontal lobotomy may have been the result of interruption of the pathways between the frontal regions and the thalamus; similar relief of symptoms and also amelioration of hyperkinetic disorders have been reported following the placing of circumscribed lesions or stimulators in the thalamus. The dorsomedial nucleus has been destroyed by stereotaxic surgery in the treatment of psychotic states and personality disorders; lesions or stimulators have also been placed in this nucleus and in the nuclei ventralis posteromedialis and posterolateralis for the control of intractable pain; destructive lesions have been made in the nucleus ventralis lateralis and other thalamic nuclei for the relief of the tremor and rigidity of Parkinson's disease and in the treatment of other dyskinetic states.

THE CORPUS CALLOSUM

The corpus callosum is the largest of the commissural systems of the brain. It consists of a broad band of white fibers located at the bottom of the medial longitudinal fissure, and connects the neopallium of the two hemispheres. It is composed of a major portion, or body, an anterior genu ending in the rostrum, and a thickened posterior termination, or splenium. Fibers connecting the anterior portions of the frontal lobes, including the speech areas, course through the anterior third; the body carries fibers from the posterior portions of the frontal lobes and from the parietal lobes; the splenium contains fibers from the temporal and occipital lobes.

The corpus callosum facilitates the cooperation of the two cerebral hemispheres, especially in man, in whom each hemisphere is dominant for some functions. The clinical significance of the corpus callosum, however, is not well understood, for its absence may cause no symptoms. Furthermore, it may be difficult to differentiate between signs caused by disease of the corpus callosum and those resulting from disease of contiguous parts. The statement has been made many times that lesions of the middle third of this structure cause apraxia, or the inability to carry out skilled movements, and that involvement of the anterior third causes both apraxia and aphasia (Ch. 52). With acute lesions there may be emotional excitement, confusion, and irritability, followed by apathy, drowsiness, and personality changes, and later by stupor and coma. While certain of these symptoms may result from disease of the corpus callosum itself, others are due to involvement of neighboring areas, including the corona radiata and the cingulate gyri. The corpus callosum has been sectioned in an attempt to relieve convulsive attacks, principally to stop the spread of the epileptogenic discharge from one hemisphere to the other. The results have been encouraging in well-selected cases.

Various clinical syndromes of involvement of the corpus callosum have been described. Agenesis is most frequently discovered only by autopsy, computed tomography, or magnetic resonance imaging. There may be mental deficiency and convulsions, and there may be hemiplegia and paraplegia resulting from lesions affecting contiguous structures. These symptoms are usually associated with additional congenital malformations of the brain. Primary degeneration of the corpus callosum, **Marchiafava – Bignami disease,** is a rare condition probably related to chronic alcoholism and undernutrition. Animal and some human studies indicate that section of the corpus callosum and anterior commissures results in impairment in the transfer of information from one hemisphere to the other. Events and stimuli that have been learned by one half of the body fail to evoke evidence that they are understood when they are presented to the other side. With tumors of the corpus callosum mental symptoms are prominent; they consist of apathy, drowsiness, loss of memory, difficulty in concentration, personality changes, and other manifestations suggestive of frontal lobe involvement. Apraxia is present in only some patients. Thrombosis of the anterior cerebral artery causes softening of a large portion of the commissure. It has been said that there is always motor apraxia on the left, regardless of the side of the lesion, but observations have shown that this is not always the case. In all of these conditions, the clinical diagnosis of involvement of the corpus callosum is dependent upon the presence of signs referable to disease of neighboring parts of the brain, or on imaging studies.

THE INTERNAL CAPSULE

The cerebral hemisphere is connected with the brain stem and spinal cord by an extensive system of projection fibers, some of which are efferent, others afferent. These fibers either arise from or terminate in the entire extent of the cortex, and within the white substance of the hemisphere they appear as a radiating structure, the corona radiata. They converge into a broad band, the internal capsule, which continues to the underlying structures (see Fig. 23-5). This tract is composed of all of the fibers, both efferent and afferent, which communicate with the cerebral cortex. A large part of the internal capsule is composed of the thalamic radiations, and the rest consists of efferent fibers to lower structures. Below the level of the thalamus the descending systems make up the cerebral peduncle of the midbrain.

The internal capsule separates the lentiform nucleus, which is lateral to it, from the caudate nucleus anteromedially and the thalamus posteromedially. Between the caudate and the thalamus it bends sharply at the genu. In horizontal section the internal capsule is seen to be composed of three parts. The frontal portion is the shorter anterior limb, or lenticulocaudate division, which extends rostrally and laterally between the lentiform and caudate nuclei. The junctional zone is the genu, or geniculate portion, which forms an obtuse angle between the two limbs. The longer posterior limb, or lenticulothalamic division, extends laterally and posteriorly between the lentiform nucleus and the thalamus; its caudal extremity is divided into a retrolenticular portion, which projects behind the lentiform nucleus to reach the occipital cortex, and a sublenticular portion, which passes below the posterior part of this nucleus to reach the temporal lobe.

The anterior limb of the internal capsule is composed of the frontopontine tract and the anterior thalamic radiations. The former, which carries the corticopontocerebellar impulses from the frontal region, conveys fibers that arise in the premotor region of the frontal cortex, probably from the middle frontal convolution anterior to areas 6 and 8, to the homolateral pontine nuclei. After a synapse, the impulse is transmitted through the brachium pontis to the opposite cerebellar hemisphere. The anterior thalamic radiations, or anterior thalamic peduncle, carry the following: 1) thalamofrontal fibers from the nucleus ventralis lateralis to the motor and premotor cortex, from the anterior nuclear group of the thalamus to the cingulate gyrus and inferior region of the frontal cortex, and from the nucleus medialis dorsalis to the frontal association areas; 2) frontothalamic fibers from the motor and premotor regions to the lateral nuclear mass, especially the nucleus ventralis lateralis, as well as from the frontal association areas to the nucleus medialis dorsalis; and 3) thalamostriate and striothalamic fibers. Projections from areas 4s, 8, 9, and possibly other regions of the frontal cortex to the caudate nucleus may also be carried through the anterior limb.

The corticobulbar tracts are situated at the genu of the internal capsule; they carry impulses from the lower portion of the precentral (and premotor) cortex to the motor nuclei of the cranial nerves. The fibers to the eye muscles and face are placed most anteriorly, and those to the mouth and tongue extend a short distance into the posterior limb. The corticobulbar impulses pass largely but not entirely to contralateral nuclei.

The posterior limb of the internal capsule has many important constituents. The corticospinal and corticorubral tracts are situated in the anterior half or two thirds of the lenticulothalamic portion. The corticospinal pathway carries impulses from the upper portion and the paracentral region of the precentral (and premotor) cortex to the nuclei of the spinal cord, predominantly on the opposite side. The fibers destined for the arm are more anterior than those for the leg. It is important from both anatomic and clinical points of view that the pyramidal pathway, which includes both the corticobulbar and corticospinal tracts, is situated in a small area of the internal capsule, occupying the genu, the anterior portion of the posterior limb, and perhaps a very small portion of the anterior limb. The arrangement of the fibers differs somewhat from the order of cortical representation (see Fig. 23-3): in the internal capsule the fibers to the eyes and face are placed most anteriorly, followed, in a backward direction, by those to the mouth, tongue, shoulder, arm, forearm, hand, fingers, thumb, trunk, hip, leg, ankle, and toes. The corticorubral tract, which is lateral to the corticospinal pathway, carries impulses from the frontal cortex, probably mainly area 4, to the ipsilateral red nucleus, as well as rubrocortical fibers from the red nucleus to the cortex. Corticonigral and corticosubthalamic impulses may accompany the corticorubral tract. Fibers from the frontal cortex, areas 4 and 6, to the caudate nucleus, putamen, and globus pallidus are carried as collaterals of the corticospinal neurons.

The thalamic radiations that compose the superior thalamic peduncle make up a large portion of the posterior limb of the internal capsule. These consist of the thalamocortical fibers from the nuclei ventralis posteromedialis and posterolateralis to the somesthetic sensory cortex in the postcentral gyrus, as well as those from the nuclei lateralis dorsalis and posterior to the posterior parts of the parietal lobe. It may be that some thalamofrontal fibers from the nucleus ventralis lateralis to the motor and premotor cortex are also carried with these thalamic radiations, as well as thalamolenticular, lenticulothalamic, and striothalamic impulses. The temporopontine and occipitopontine fibers that carry corticopontocerebellar impulses from association areas in the middle and inferior temporal convolutions and also from the anterior portion of the occipital lobe (or lower parietal region) to the homolateral pontine nuclei, and thence to the contralateral cerebellar hemisphere, also course through the posterior limb of the internal capsule, as do the optic and auditory radiations.

The optic radiations, or the posterior thalamic peduncle, make up most of the retrolenticular portion of the posterior limb. They constitute the geniculocalcarine tract and carry impulses from the lateral geniculate body, and possibly the pulvinar, to the striate cortex. Corticofugal fibers from areas 18 and 19, especially the latter, to the superior colliculus (anterior quadrigeminal body) and its surrounding areas, and then through the medial longitudinal fasciculus to the nuclei of the ocular nerves, pass with the optic radiations, as do communications between the pulvinar and the peristriate area. The occipitopontine fibers are also in the retrolenticular division.

The auditory radiations, or the inferior thalamic peduncle, constitute the major portion of the sublenticular division of the posterior limb. They carry impulses from the medial geniculate body to the auditory areas in the transverse temporal convolutions, through the thalamotemporal radiations. There may also be some impulses that pass in the opposite direction. The temporopontine fibers are also in the sublenticular division, as are some of the thalamostriatal, striothalamic, thalamopallidal, and pallidothalamic fibers.

The internal capsule is of major clinical importance. As can be seen from the previous description, fiber pathways that communicate with various areas of the brain converge here and are concentrated in a small area. The blood supply of the region is such that hemorrhages and vascular occlusions frequently affect the structure. Owing to the close crowding of the fibers in the internal capsule, a small lesion may cause a profound contralateral hemiplegia; this is especially true of involvement at or just posterior to the genu. Posterior lesions are accompanied by sensory changes and hemianopic defects. Involvement of the anterior limb of the internal capsule may cause symptoms of thalamic release with unmotivated laughter and crying. Owing to the proximity of the internal capsule to the basal ganglia and the thalamus, lesions of the capsule may also affect these structures.

THE RETICULAR FORMATION

Groups of cells situated in the reticular formation of the midbrain, pons, and medulla and in the thalamus (especially the intralaminar and reticular nuclei) and contiguous areas perform many functions that are widespread in their pattern of effects. Collectively, these are known as the reticular formation, the reticular activating system, or the ascending and descending multisynaptic projection system. Into this complex come collaterals of the long ascending paths as well as motor collaterals from the descending corticospinal, extrapyramidal, and other pathways. In addition there are connections with the cerebellum and the various cranial nerve nuclei. Intimate synaptic relations connect all these fiber systems, and projections are sent out in both rostral and caudal directions. The actions of this complex include the facilitation or suppression of motor activity, reflex response, and movement. It has similar influences on sensory conduction, which it may either inhibit or enhance.

The reticular activating system also plays an important part in regulating awareness to sensation, arousal to wakefulness, and alerting to attention, as well as in the control of neuroendocrine functions. It participates in determining not only the level but also the content of consciousness. Consequently it may have an influence in the control of emotional states and behavior. It may correspond closely to the so-called centrencephalic integrating system in which certain "deep-level" epileptic seizures are said to originate. The syndrome of akinetic mutism (Ch. 54) may result from involvement of the reticular activating system. Many of the drugs that inhibit or enhance motor or sensory responses, affect consciousness and behavior, and control certain varieties of epileptic attacks, have their sites of action in this small area of the brain. Investigations on the reticular formation are demonstrating the widespread influence it has in the activation and regulation of nervous system function.

BIBLIOGRAPHY

Adams RD, Victor M. Principles of Neurology, 4th ed. New York, McGraw–Hill, 1989

Akelaitis AJE. Psychobiological studies following section of the corpus callosum. Am J Psychiatry 1941;97:1147

Bruyn RP. Thalamic aphasia. J Neurol 1989;236:21

Cooper IS. Clinical and physiological implications of thalamic surgery for disorders of sensory communication. J Neurol Sci 1965;2:493

Dejerine R, Roussy G. La syndrome thalamique. Rev Neurol 1906;14:521

Ettlinger EG (ed). Functions of the Corpus Callosum. Ciba

Foundation Study Group No. 20. Boston, Little, Brown & Co, 1965

French JD. The reticular formation. J Neurosurg 1958;15:97

Gazzaniga MS, Riese GL, Springer SP et al. Psychologic and neurologic consequences of sectioning the cerebral commissures in man. Neurology 1975;25:10

Goldstein MN, Joynt RJ. Long-term follow-up of a callosal-sectioned patient. Arch Neurol 1969;20L:96

Jasper AH, Proctor LD, Knighton RS, Noshay WC et al. The Reticular Formation of the Brain. Boston, Little, Brown & Co, 1958

Loeser JD, Alvord EC Jr. Agenesis of the corpus callosum. Brain 1968;91:553

Magoun HW. The ascending reticular activating system. Assoc Res Nerv Dis Proc 1950;30:480

Penfield W, Jasper H. Epilepsy and the Functional Anatomy of the Human Brain. Boston, Little, Brown & Co, 1954

Walker AE. The Primate Thalamus. Chicago, University of Chicago Press, 1938

Watkins ES, Oppenheimer DR. Mental disturbances after thalamolysis. J Neurol Neurosurg Psychiatry 1962; 25:243

Williams D. The thalamus and epilepsy. Brain 1965; 88:530

Wilson DH, Reeves A, Gazzaniga M et al. Cerebral commissurotomy for control of intractable seizures. Neurology 1977;27:708

Chapter 51

THE BLOOD SUPPLY OF THE BRAIN, AND THE VASCULAR SYNDROMES

THE CEREBRAL ARTERIES

The brain receives its blood supply from the vertebral and the internal carotid arteries. Although these vessels communicate with each other, in general branches derived from the vertebral arteries supply the caudal half of the brain, including the brain stem, midbrain, occipital lobes, inferior portion of the temporal lobes, and most of the thalamus, while branches of the internal carotid arteries supply the basal ganglia, frontal and parietal lobes, the lateral portion of the temporal lobes, and most of the internal capsule. Branches of these arteries and communications between them make up the arterial circle of Willis at the base of the brain (see Fig. 18-1). The central arteries arise from the circle of Willis and the proximal portions of the principal cerebral arteries, and dip perpendicularly into the brain substance. They are terminal branches and do not anastomose with each other, and thus occlusion of one of these vessels produces infarction of the area deprived of its blood supply. Cortical branches arise from distal portions of the arteries and enter the pia mater where they form a superficial plexus of anastomosing vessels; from these plexuses smaller terminal branches enter the brain substance at right angles. Owing to the anastomosis of the larger cortical arteries, occlusion of one of them may be compensated to a variable extent by the blood supply from neighboring branches.

The two vertebral arteries enter the cranial cavity through the foramen magnum and run rostrally along the ventral surface of the medulla. They unite at the lower border of the pons to form the basilar artery. The basilar artery ends at the upper border of the pons by dividing into the two posterior cerebral arteries. Two important branches of the vertebral artery are the posterior inferior cerebellar artery, which winds around the medulla to the inferior surface of the cerebellum, and the anterior spinal artery. The posterior spinal and the medullary arteries are smaller branches. Branches of the basilar artery are the two anterior inferior cerebellar arteries, the two internal auditory arteries, several pontine branches, and the two superior cerebellar arteries. There is some variation in the presence and distribution of these branch vessels; also, one of the vertebral arteries is often hypoplastic.

The posterior cerebral arteries are formed by the bifurcation of the basilar artery. Each one extends backward and laterally around the cerebral peduncle, where it is close to the upper border of the pons, parallel to the superior cerebellar artery, and in front of the oculomotor nerve. After receiving the posterior communicating branch from the internal carotid artery, the posterior cerebral artery continues along the medial surface of the corresponding cerebral hemisphere, beneath the splenium of the corpus callosum, to reach the medial and inferior surfaces of the temporal lobe and the medial surface of the occipital lobe (Fig. 51-1), where it divides into its four cortical branches: 1) the anterior temporal artery supplies the uncus and the anterior parts of the inferior temporal, fusiform, and hippocampal gyri, exclusive of the temporal pole, which is supplied by the middle cerebral artery; 2) the posterior temporal artery supplies the rest of the fusiform and inferior temporal

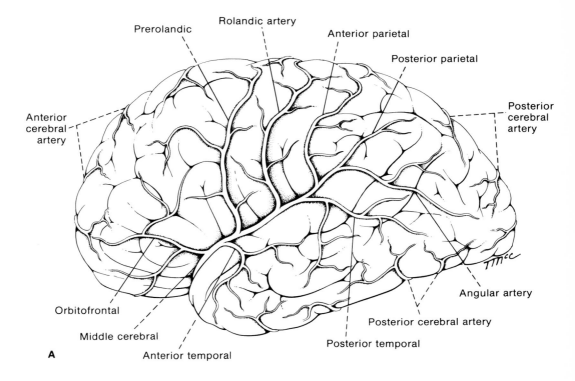

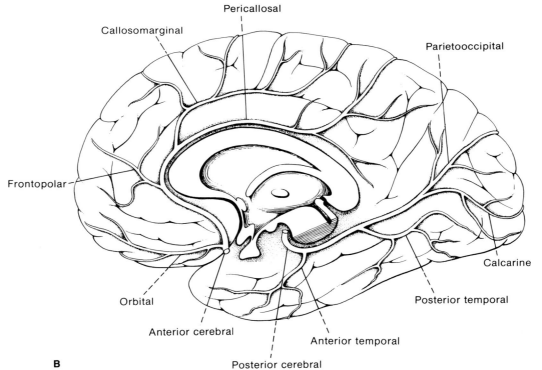

FIG. 51–1. Blood supply of the cerebral cortex. **A.** Lateral surface of the brain. **B.** Medial surface of the brain.

gyri; 3) the calcarine artery supplies the lingual gyrus and the inferior half of the cuneus; 4) the parietooccipital, or posterior occipital, artery supplies the upper part of the cuneus, with branches to the splenium of the corpus callosum. Thus the cortical branches of the posterior cerebral artery provide blood to the medial surface of the occipital lobe, including all of the visual receptive area, the medial and inferior surfaces of the temporal lobe, and the splenium of the corpus callosum. Their terminal branches wind around the borders of the hemisphere and supply a portion of the lateral surfaces of the temporal and occipital lobes and a small part of the superior parietal lobule. They anastomose with branches of the middle and anterior cerebral arteries.

The deep branches of the posterior cerebral artery are the following: the posterior choroidal arteries, of which there usually are two, encircle the cerebral peduncle and give off branches to the midbrain, the tela choroidea and choroid plexus of the third ventricle, and the superomedial surface of the thalamus; the posteromedial arteries, derived from the posterior communicating artery as well as the posterior cerebral, supply the hypophysis, infundibulum, tuberal and mammillary regions of the hypothalamus, walls of the third ventricle, medial and anteromedial portions of the thalamus, subthalamic structures, tegmentum of the midbrain, red nucleus, and medial portion of the cerebral peduncle; the posterolateral, or thalamogeniculate, arteries supply the caudal half of the thalamus, the posterior portion of the internal capsule, the superior cerebellar peduncle, the superior colliculus, and the geniculate bodies.

Each internal carotid artery arises in the neck as one of the terminal branches of the common carotid artery. It passes through the carotid canal in the petrous portion of the temporal bone and enters the cranial cavity through the foramen lacerum. It makes a series of turns within the cavernous sinus, and just before leaving this structure gives off the ophthalmic artery. It reaches the brain lateral to the optic chiasm and near the medial side of the temporal pole and the medial and lower extremity of the lateral cerebral fissure. It then divides into two terminal branches, the anterior and middle cerebral arteries. Before dividing, however, it gives off the posterior communicating artery, which connects the internal carotid and posterior cerebral arteries, and the anterior choroidal artery, which runs backward to reach the choroid plexus of the lateral ventricle.

The anterior cerebral artery, normally the smaller of the two terminal branches of the internal carotid artery, crosses the anterior perforated space above the optic nerve and runs forward and medially to the medial longitudinal fissure; just in front of the optic chiasm it is joined with the opposite anterior cerebral artery by the anterior communicating artery. It then travels forward and rostrally within the interhemispheric fissure, where it lies on the medial surface of the hemisphere close to the corpus callosum (see Fig. 51-1). It curves around the genu of this body and then backward, and continues along the upper surface of the corpus callosum to the posterior parietal region. Along this course the artery gives off four cortical branches: (1) the orbital artery arises where the main trunk turns upward, and it spreads out over the orbital surface of the frontal lobe, supplying the olfactory lobe, gyrus rectus, and medial and inferior portions of the orbital gyri; (2) the frontopolar artery supplies the medial surface of the prefrontal region as far forward as the frontal pole; (3) the callosomarginal artery arises opposite the genu of the corpus callosum and courses backward in the cingulate sulcus; it gives off the anterior internal frontal branch about the middle of the superior frontal gyrus, the middle internal frontal branch at the posterior extremity of the superior frontal gyrus, and the terminal posterior internal frontal branch in the region of the paracentral lobule; (4) the pericallosal artery continues backward over the body and posterior part of the corpus callosum to anastomose with branches of the posterior cerebral artery. Numerous small branches of both the anterior cerebral and pericallosal arteries penetrate the corpus callosum. Thus the cortical branches of the anterior cerebral artery supply the medial and orbital surfaces of the frontal lobe, the medial surface of the parietal lobe as far as the parietooccipital fissure, the cingulate gyrus, and the genu and anterior four fifths of the corpus callosum; these areas include the motor and somesthetic centers in the paracentral lobule. Their terminal branches, like those of the posterior cerebral artery, wind around the border of the hemisphere to supply a small portion of the lateral surface, in this case, of the frontal and parietal lobes.

The largest of the deep, or central, branches of the anterior cerebral artery is the recurrent artery of Heubner, or the medial striate artery. It takes a recurrent course, and after giving a few branches to the orbital cortex, passes through the anterior perforated space to join the deep branches of the middle cerebral artery. It supplies the lower part of the head of the caudate nucleus, the lower part of the frontal pole of the putamen, the frontal pole of the globus pallidus, the adjacent frontal half of the anterior limb of the internal capsule, and the anterior portions of the external capsule and lateral ventricle. The anteromedial group of central arteries arises from the anterior cerebral and anterior communicating arteries and supplies the anterior hypothalamus, including the preoptic and suprachiasmatic regions, the genu of the corpus callosum, the septum pellucidum, the anterior pillars of the fornix, and part of the anterior commissure.

The middle cerebral artery is the largest of the cerebral arteries (see Fig. 51-1). It travels first laterally and then laterally, posteriorly, and upward in the sylvian, or lateral, fissure, over the surface of the insula and between the frontal and temporal lobes. It gives off many cortical branches that supply the lateral surface of the brain. The anterior temporal artery curves out of the lateral fissure and runs backward over the temporal lobe; it supplies the temporal pole and the anterior third of the superior and middle temporal gyri. The orbitofrontal artery supplies the lateral part of the orbital surface of the frontal lobe, the lateral surface of the orbital gyri, and the lateral surface of the inferior frontal convolution. The prerolandic artery runs for a short distance in the central fissure and then curves over the precentral gyrus to enter the precentral fissure, supplying the lower and anterior portions of the precentral gyrus and the posterior portions of the middle and inferior frontal convolutions.

The rolandic artery runs over the opercular part of the postcentral gyrus and then enters the central fissure; it supplies the posterior portion of the precentral gyrus and the anterior portion of the postcentral gyrus. The anterior parietal artery curves over the opercular portion of the parietal lobe and extends to the interparietal fissure, supplying the posterior border of the postcentral gyrus and the anterior parts of the other parietal convolutions. The posterior temporal artery descends from the lateral fissure and supplies the posterior two thirds of the superior and middle temporal convolutions. The posterior parietal (supramarginal) artery arises near the end of the lateral fissure and supplies the supramarginal gyrus and the posterior part of the inferior parietal lobule. The middle cerebral artery terminates as the angular artery, which supplies the angular gyrus and the adjoining parts of the parietal lobe.

These branches anastomose with branches of the anterior and posterior cerebral arteries that project onto the lateral surface of the hemispheres. Thus the cortical branches of the middle cerebral artery supply the lateral surfaces of the frontal and parietal lobes, and the lateral and upper surface of the temporal lobe, the insula, and the lateral part of the orbital gyri. These areas include the middle and inferior frontal convolutions, the lateral parts of the premotor and precentral regions, the postcentral gyrus, the superior and inferior parietal lobules, the angular and supramarginal gyri, the superior and middle temporal convolutions including the temporal pole, and the preoccipital region. Situated in these areas are the language centers, the auditory receptive area, and the major portion of the motor and somesthetic cortex.

The deep, or central, branches of the middle cerebral artery arise from the proximal part of the vessel. They constitute the anterolateral group, or lateral and medial striate arteries, which pierce the anterior perforated substance and supply the whole of the putamen except for its anterior pole, the upper part of the head of the caudate nucleus, and the whole of its body, the lateral part of the globus pallidus, and the posterior part of the anterior limb, the genu, and the anterior third of the posterior limb of the internal capsule. Under most circumstances it is not possible to distinguish among the striate arteries any individual branch such as the lenticulostriate artery, although Charcot and others expressed the belief that there was such a vessel, the largest of the group, which they termed the "artery of cerebral hemorrhage" because they believed that it was frequently the site of such hemorrhage.

The anterior choroidal artery arises from the internal carotid artery just before its bifurcation. It passes backward along the optic tract and around the cerebral peduncle as far as the lateral geniculate body, where its main branches turn to enter the inferior horn of the lateral ventricle; it supplies the choroid plexus of the lateral ventricle. During its course it gives branches to the optic tract, hippocampus, tail of the caudate nucleus, medial and intermediate portions of the globus pallidus, posterior two-thirds of the posterior limb of the internal capsule, middle third of the cerebral peduncle, and outer part of the lateral geniculate body. The retrolenticular and sublenticular portions of the internal capsule are also supplied by this artery. Branches of the posterior communicating artery enter the base of the brain between the infundibulum and the optic tract, and supply the genu and anterior one third of the posterior limb of the internal capsule, the anterior one third of the thalamus, and the walls of the third ventricle.

Studies of the circle of Wills have shown that it is subject to wide variations in configuration and that anomalous formations are frequent. There may be hypoplasia of one or more components, which may have a string-like caliber, or there may be duplication or triplication of vessels, absent vessels, or persisting embryonic origin of certain of the constituents (Fig. 51-2). The circle is actually normal in only about one half of individuals without evidence of nervous system disease. Anomalies occur in about 80% of patients with neural dysfunction.

Clinical and investigative studies have provided insights regarding the cerebral circulation. Angiography has given much important information about the distribution of the major cerebral arteries and their communications, and has demonstrated the effects on cerebral circula-

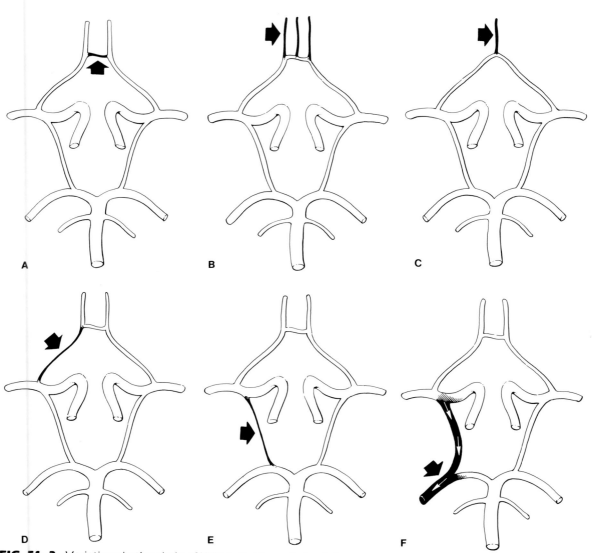

FIG. 51–2. Variations in the circle of Willis. **A.** Hypoplasia of the anterior communicating artery. **B.** Anomalous anterior cerebral arteries. **C.** Fusion of the anterior cerebral arteries. **D** and **E.** Hypoplasia of branches of the internal carotid artery. **F.** Posterior cerebral artery from the internal carotid artery. (Modified from Alpers BJ, Berry RG, Paddison RM. Arch Neurol Psychiatry 1959; 81:409–418)

tion of their obstruction. Investigations of cerebral blood flow and metabolism by means of various physiologic technics have revealed the relationship of the cerebral circulation to such factors as arterial blood pressure, venous pressure, cerebrovascular resistance, oxygen and carbon dioxide tension, and intracranial cerebrospinal fluid pressure. Such technics also show the effects on cerebral circulation and oxygen consumption of autonomic nervous system stimulation and depression, various drugs and metabolites, and disease processes of either the vessels or the blood itself.

Cerebral blood flow is studied with a variety of technics. The least invasive ones include single photon emission computed tomography, xenon clearance studies, and positron emission tomography. Both total and regional cerebral blood flow may be evaluated. The intactness of the vessels themselves can be examined by conventional angiography or by digital subtraction technics employing arterial or venous routes. Doppler and other ultrasonic tests detect the presence of occlusions or stenoses in the large neck vessels in a noninvasive manner, and transcranial Doppler studies promise help with evaluation of flow in the intracranial vessels. Magnetic resonance imaging also displays stenoses or other focal abnormalities of certain intracranial vessels. These magnetic images, as well as computed tomography and conventional angiography admirably define intracranial vascular lesions such as aneurysms, angiomas, and malformations. Computed tomography identifies intracranial hemorrhagic lesions reliably and often provides, as does magnetic imaging, evidence of cerebral infarction in various vascular territories.

THE CEREBRAL VEINS AND THE VENOUS SINUSES

The cerebral veins do not parallel the cerebral arteries; they possess no valves, and their walls, owing to the absence of muscular tissue, are extremely thin. They may be divided into an external, superficial, or cortical group, and an internal, deep, or central group (Fig. 51-3). Studies of the venous phase of angiography as well as injection of contrast material into the venous sinuses have both aided in diagnosis of intracranial disease and broadened our knowledge of the distribution of venous channels.

The external veins arise from the cortex and medullary substance of the hemisphere. They anastomose freely and form a network of large trunks in the pia mater. The superior cerebral veins, 8 – 12 in number, drain the superior, lateral, and medial surfaces of the hemispheres above the sylvian and callosomarginal fissures. Most of them are lodged in the sulci between the gyri, although some of the larger trunks run across the convexity of the gyri. They pierce the arachnoid membrane and the inner layer of the dura mater, and after a short intradural course terminate in the superior sagittal sinus or its venous lacunae. The arrangement on the two sides is asymmetric, and a separation into anterior and posterior groups is usually evident. The anterior veins drain the upper parts of the frontal lobe and enter the sinus at right angles to its lateral wall. The larger posterior veins drain the parietal region and are directed forward before entering the sinus; some from the convex surface of the occipital lobe may terminate in the transverse sinus.

The inferior cerebral veins are small and drain the basal surfaces of the hemispheres and the lower portion of the lateral surfaces. Those on the orbital surface of the hemisphere enter the superior veins and thus reach the superior longitudinal sinus. Those of the temporal lobes anastomose with the middle cerebral veins and enter the cavernous, sphenoparietal, transverse, and superior petrosal sinuses. The middle cerebral vein traverses the lateral fissure and drains the insula and the opercular region. It terminates in either the cavernous or sphenoparietal sinus, or occasionally in the transverse or superior petrosal sinus. It is connected with the superior sagittal sinus by the great anastomotic vein of Trolard, and with the transverse sinus by the small, or posterior, anastomotic vein of Labbé.

The deep cerebral veins drain the interior of the hemispheres. The choroidal vein runs the entire length of the choroid plexus and receives branches from the hippocampus, fornix, and corpus callosum. The terminal vein commences in the groove between the caudate nucleus and thalamus and receives many tributaries from these structures as well as from the internal capsule. Near the interventricular foramen the terminal and choroidal veins fuse to form the internal cerebral vein. The basal vein (of Rosenthal) is formed at the anterior perforated space by the union of a small anterior vein that accompanies the anterior cerebral artery, the deep middle cerebral vein, and the inferior striate vein; it passes backward around the cerebral peduncle to end in the internal cerebral vein, and receives tributaries from the cingulate gyrus,

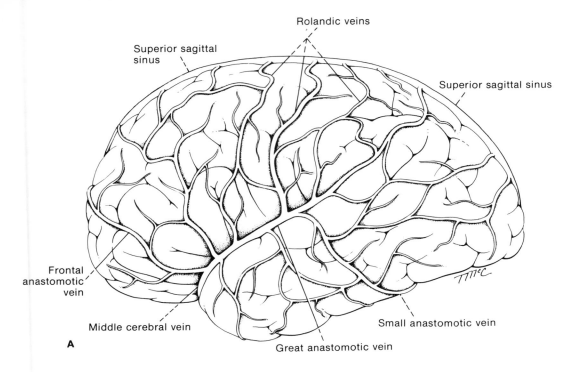

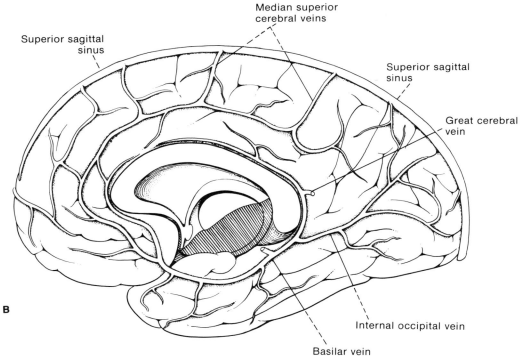

FIG. 51–3. Venous drainage of the cerebral cortex. **A.** Lateral surface. **B.** Medial surface.

anterior part of the corpus callosum, orbital surface of the frontal lobe, olfactory groove, optic chiasm, hypophysis, cerebral peduncle, interpeduncular fossa, inferior horn of the lateral ventricle, hippocampal gyrus, and midbrain. The internal occipital vein also enters the internal cerebral vein.

The great cerebral vein of Galen is formed just behind the pineal body by the union of the two internal cerebral veins. It is a short median trunk that curves backward and upward around the splenium of the corpus callosum and ends in the anterior extremity of the straight sinus.

The venous sinuses of the dura mater are channels that are situated between the two layers of the dura; the cerebral veins terminate in them (Fig. 51-4). The superior sagittal (or longitudinal) sinus occupies the convex, or attached, margin of the falx cerebri from the foramen cae-

cum to the region of the internal occipital protuberance, where it is continued as one of the transverse sinuses. In its middle portion it gives off a number of lateral diverticula, or venous lacunae, into which protrude the arachnoid granulations, or pacchionian bodies. It receives the superior cerebral veins, veins from the diploë and dura mater, and, in the parietal region, emissary veins from the pericranium. In early childhood it receives branches from the nasal veins. The inferior sagittal (or longitudinal) sinus is situated in the posterior half or two thirds of the free margin of the falx cerebri and receives veins from the falx and from the medial surfaces of the hemispheres. It terminates in the straight sinus, which is situated at the junction of the falx cerebri and tentorium cerebelli and runs backward to end in the transverse sinus opposite the one in which the superior sagittal sinus ends. It

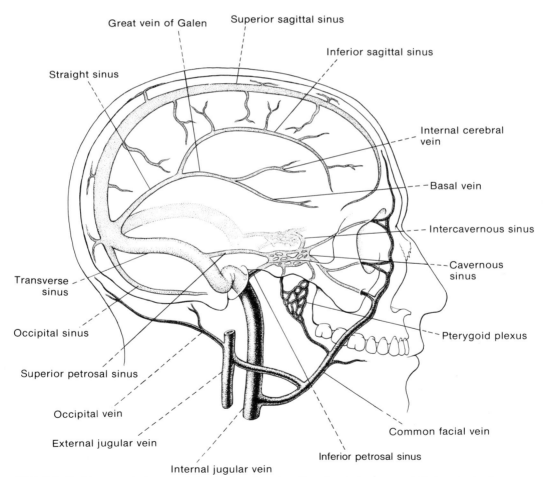

FIG. 51–4. Venous drainage of the brain, showing the dural sinuses and their principal connections with extracranial veins.

receives, in addition to the inferior sagittal sinus, the great cerebral vein of Galen and the superior cerebellar veins.

The transverse (lateral) sinuses begin in the region of the internal occipital protuberance as continuations of the superior sagittal and straight sinuses, and pass laterally and forward in the attached margin of the tentorium cerebelli to the petrous portion of the temporal bone. They then pass downward and medially to reach the internal jugular foramen where they end in the internal jugular veins. Those portions that occupy the groove on the mastoid part of the temporal bone are sometimes called sigmoid sinuses. The transverse sinuses receive blood from the superior petrosal sinuses, inferior cerebral and inferior cerebellar veins, and emissary and diploic veins. The occipital sinus begins at the margin of the foramen magnum and courses through the lower attached margin of the falx cerebri to the transverse sinus. The place of union of the superior sagittal, straight, transverse, and occipital sinuses is the confluence of sinuses, or torcular Herophili.

The cavernous sinuses are placed on each side of the body of the sphenoid bone, lateral to the sella turcica, and extend from the superior orbital fissure to the petrous portion of the temporal bone. They open behind into the petrosal sinuses. The internal carotid artery and the carotid plexus are on the medial wall of the sinus, and lateral to them are the abducens, oculomotor, and trochlear nerves, and the ophthalmic and maxillary divisions of the trigeminal nerve (see Fig. 11-2). The cavernous sinuses receive the ophthalmic veins, some of the cerebral veins, and the small sphenoparietal sinus that courses under the surface of the small wing of the sphenoid bone. The two sinuses communicate with each other by the anterior and posterior intercavernous sinuses.

The superior petrosal sinus connects the cavernous with the transverse sinus and receives cerebellar and inferior cerebral veins and veins from the tympanic cavity. The inferior petrosal sinus connects the cavernous sinus with the internal jugular vein and receives the internal auditory veins and veins from the cerebellum and medulla. The basilar plexus consists of several interlacing venous channels between the layers of the dura mater on the basilar part of the occipital bone; it connects the two inferior petrosal sinuses and communicates with the vertebral venous plexuses. Emissary veins pass through apertures in the cranial wall and establish communications between the sinuses inside the skull

and veins external to it. Diploic veins occupy channels in the diploë of the cranial bones and communicate with the sinuses of the dura mater, veins of the pericranium, and meningeal veins.

SYNDROMES OF CEREBROVASCULAR DISEASE

A large body of knowledge has accumulated concerning cerebrovascular disease and is covered in appropriate texts on this subject. Some of the clinical symptoms and features of the examination of persons with cerebrovascular disease are covered in Chapter 53. Only brief mention of the scope of cerebrovascular disease and its general outline can be made here, to be followed by a description of certain intracranial and extracranial vascular syndromes that have not already been covered with the discussions of the basilar and vertebral vessels.

Stroke continues to be the third leading cause of death in the United States. Well-known risk factors include hypertension, heart disease, smoking, diabetes mellitus, elevated blood lipids, and advancing age. Strokes affect populations differently. In some Asiatics intracranial hemorrhages are more common than in Caucasians; blacks have more occlusive cerebrovascular disease than do whites in the United States; older white males are especially prone to extracranial disease of the vessels to the brain, whereas in blacks there is a predominance of intracranial stenoses and occlusions. Thus, the patient's background, age, and sex help to determine the probabilities of what type of stroke may have occurred in a given person.

Generally, cerebrovascular disease has been divided into occlusive and hemorrhagic types. Recent compilations have established that some two thirds of initial strokes are atherothrombotic infarctions, 16% are embolic, 4% intracerebral hemorrhages, 10% subarachnoid hemorrhages, and 3% other types. The distributions, however, vary somewhat between populations, as already mentioned. Occlusive cerebrovascular disorders can be further subdivided into those due to thrombotic occlusion of a vessel, those due to embolic occlusion from distant sources such as the heart or the great vessels in the neck and chest, watershed infarcts occurring at border zones of perfusion when there is a general decrease in cerebral perfusion, lacunar infarcts (less than 2 cm in diameter and usually deep, the result of occlusion of perforating "end" arteries), transient ischemic attacks, and reversible ischemic neurologic deficits or "transient strokes." Transient ischemic attacks and reversible ischemic neurologic deficits initially present as do other cerebrovascular occlusive syndromes, but resolve after variable times to leave no detectable clinical deficits. Commonly, transient ischemic attacks last 10 – 15 minutes or a little longer and resolve completely no later than 24 hours after their onset. Reversible ischemic neurologic deficits may persist for up to one or two weeks. Authorities disagree as to the definitions of transient ischemic attacks and reversible deficits; some lump them together as simply representing small strokes. Debate also continues concerning the etiology and pathogenesis of transient ischemic attacks, whether they are mainly embolic or other phenomena. Some define reversible occlusive syndromes as those leaving no detectable clinical residual and also no residual abnormalities on imaging studies.

Either stenosis or occlusion of extracerebral and even extracranial arteries may be responsible for a large portion of cerebrovascular disease. The affected vessels may be in the neck or chest and include the common and internal carotids, the vertebrals, and the arch of the aorta.

Most instances of vascular occlusive disease are secondary to atherosclerotic involvement of the affected arteries. Thickening of the intima of the large arteries is accompanied by accumulation of lipids, formation of atherosclerotic plaques and at times ulcers, and eventually a decrease in the caliber of the vessels, especially at the site of bifurcations, branchings, and curves (Fig. 51-5). With thickening of the atherosclerotic plaque the lumen of the vessel narrows and blood flow diminishes. With a sudden drop of systemic blood pressure the vessel may be temporarily occluded, symptoms occurring due to decrease in blood supply to the terminal branches of the affected artery. More serious in consequence is formation of a thrombus at the site of a plaque with resulting complete occlusion of the vessel.

Other causes of vascular occlusion and consequent cerebrovascular syndromes include vascular inflammatory disease, trauma to the vessels, mechanical obstruction, dissection of the vessel walls, fibromuscular dysplasia, arteriopathies such as Takayasu's arteritis, Moyamoya disease, and others.

The nerve cells of the brain are highly sensitive to variations in the blood, oxygen, and glucose supply. The cerebral circulation, through the communications of the circle of Willis and the anastomoses of the cortical branches, aids in maintaining as constant a supply of both oxygen and blood as possible, and in providing adequate collateral circulation in case of local damage. The lack of anastomosis of the central branches makes the deep parts of the brain more vulnerable to vascular disease. Intermittent cerebrovascular insufficiency often relates to involvement of the extracerebral vessels and may cause transient ischemic attacks with symptoms referable to the areas supplied by the terminal branches of the affected arteries. Such attacks may progress in severity, with a decreasing return of function after each episode. Complete ischemia is followed in a relatively short period of time by irreversible changes that lead to necrosis and scarring. Focal cerebral damage of vascular origin is in most cases the result of either infarct formation or hemorrhage. Hemorrhage results from rupture of one of the intracerebral vessels, and may be secondary to hypertension, aneurysmal dilation, vascular anomaly, blood dyscrasia, or other causes. An infarct results from interruption of the blood supply; this may be due to either thrombus formation, with obliteration of the vessel lumen, or embolism, with obstruction by lodging of a foreign particle in a vessel that is too small to permit its passage. The onset of symptoms with all of these is usually abrupt — the so-called stroke — although the symptoms of thrombosis occasionally appear more gradually than those of either hemorrhage or embolism. The possible development of unilateral cerebral edema in association with vascular occlusion may suggest the presence of a neoplasm. Cerebral arteries are occasionally compressed by neoplasms or by a sudden increase in intracranial pressure.

Because specific areas of the brain are supplied by individual arteries, occlusion or rupture of such vessels produces disturbances of function of these regions with characteristic signs and symptoms of disease. By appraisal of these signs and symptoms the disease process can usually be clinically localized and the affected blood vessel identified. It must be remembered, however, that there is variability in the vascular supply to the brain, and that anomalies of the cerebral vessels are frequently encountered. Furthermore, the symptoms of vascular disease may be influenced by the richness of anastomosis of cerebral vessels, the ability of healthy parts of the brain to assume the functions of destroyed areas, and the dominance of certain cerebral centers over others. In some patients who have extensive vascular disease, especially of the extracranial arteries, but who have been without

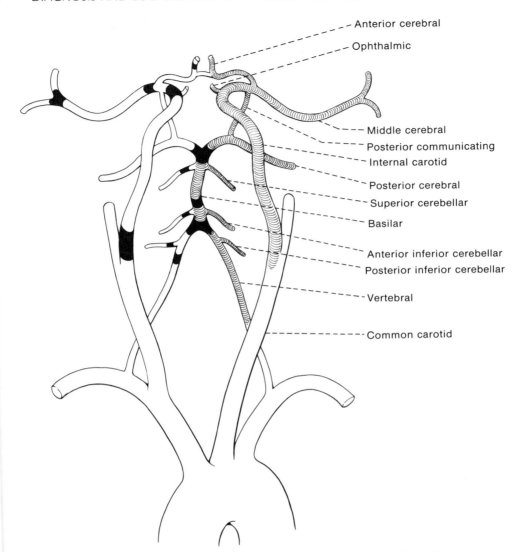

FIG. 51–5. Diagram of the cerebral circulation showing sites of predilection for atherosclerosis and occlusion at bifurcations, branchings, and curves. (Modified from Alpers BJ, Berry RG, Paddison RM. Arch Neurol Psychiatry 1959; 81:409–418)

symptoms because the blood supply to the brain is still adequate, the occlusion of a vessel may result in symptoms and signs referable not only to the distribution of the recently thrombosed artery but also to areas whose circulation had previously been impaired.

A discussion of the vascular supply to the various areas of the brain and of the common syndromes of occlusion and rupture of the more important arteries is given here. Syndromes of insufficiency, occlusion, and rupture of the vertebral and basilar arteries and their branches are described in Chapter 18, as well as in the discussion of the ocular, trigeminal, and facial nerves.

The areas of distribution of each of the cerebral arteries have been described in detail. To aid in visualization of vascular disease, however, the various areas of the brain and the arteries that supply them are listed. The cerebral cortex receives blood from the anterior, middle, and posterior cerebral arteries. The anterior cerebral artery supplies the medial surfaces and upper portions of the convexities of the frontal and parietal lobes, and the cortex of the cingulate gyrus including the motor and somesthetic cortex for the lower extremity. The middle cerebral artery supplies the cortex of most of the convexity of the brain — the lateral aspects of the frontal and parietal lobes, the upper portion of the temporal lobe including the temporal pole, and the insula; it is distributed to the motor and somesthetic areas for the face and upper extremity, the motor speech area, the auditory receptive region, and important association foci. The posterior cerebral artery supplies the medial and inferior parts of the temporal lobe, exclusive of the temporal pole, and the medial aspect of the occipital lobe, including the visual receptive area.

The caudate and putamen are supplied primarily by striate branches of the middle cerebral arteries, but their anterior extremities receive blood from the anterior cerebral artery. The medial and intermediate segments of the globus pallidus are supplied by the anterior choroidal artery, but the lateral segment receives blood from both the striate branches of the middle cerebral and anterior choroidal artery. The thalamus is supplied by the deep branches of the posterior cerebral and posterior communicating arteries, and by the anterior choroidal artery. The anterior hypothalamus is supplied by the branches of the anterior cerebral artery, and the posterior hypothalamus and subthalamus by branches of the posterior communicating and posterior cerebral arteries. The anterior part of the anterior limb of the internal capsule is supplied by the anterior cerebral artery; the posterior part of the anterior limb, the genu, and the anterior part of the posterior limb receive their blood supply from the middle cerebral and posterior communicating arteries; the posterior portion of the posterior limb is supplied by the anterior choroidal artery and the deep branches of the posterior cerebral artery. The genu may receive a few small filaments directly from the internal carotid artery.

Lacunar infarcts are often silent and discovered incidentally on imaging studies. When symptomatic they usually produce incomplete pictures of the syndromes of the major vessels to be described below, often pure hemiparesis without sensory loss, and similar deficits.

Occlusion or rupture of the anterior cerebral artery is much less common than involvement of the middle cerebral and its branches. If it occludes before the origin of the recurrent branch, contralateral spastic hemiplegia results, the leg being affected more than the arm or face. There may be mental symptoms in the nature of memory loss, sluggishness, emotional lability, confu-

sion, and disorientation, and at times actual dementia. If the lesion is left-sided, there is some expressive aphasia, which may be temporary, and there is apraxia on the right, which may be masked by the paresis. If the lesion is right-sided, there is left-sided apraxia that, again, may be masked. It is stated that there may be a left-sided apraxia with a right-sided hemiplegia in lesions of the left anterior cerebral artery. There often is sensory impairment of the lower extremity. There may be peculiar sucking and chewing movements and snout and sucking reflexes, with grasping and groping reflexes on the affected side. There is often transient urinary incontinence.

If the anterior cerebral artery is occluded after the origin of the recurrent artery, the hemiplegia will predominate in the leg, which is often flaccid. There will be sensory changes, as previously mentioned, and the apraxia may be present in the left arm, regardless of the side affected by the paralysis. The mental changes, aphasia, and forced grasping are as mentioned before. If only the artery of Heubner is occluded, there will be paresis of the face, tongue, and shoulder on the opposite side, owing to infarction of the anterior part of the internal capsule, and there may be rigidity and hyperkinesias, resulting from striatal involvement. Some doubt that such a constellation has been conclusively demonstrated, however. If only the callosal branches are involved, there may be apraxia and mental changes without paresis. If only the paracentral lobule is affected, there may be paralysis and sensory changes in the leg with sparing of the arm. Bilateral involvement of the anterior cerebral arteries may cause the syndrome of pseudobulbar palsy. Rupture of the anterior communicating artery causes symptoms of subarachnoid hemorrhage, with or without features of anterior cerebral artery infarction unilaterally or bilaterally, resulting from spasm related to the bleeding.

Symptoms resulting from occlusion or rupture of the posterior cerebral artery (Fig. 51-6) include hemiplegia, hemianesthesia, homonymous hemianopia, receptive aphasia with alexia predominating, hyperkinetic phenomena, asynergia, and third nerve paralysis; there may be temporary bilateral blindness. Due to abundant anastomoses, however, involvement of the entire area is rare, and the peduncular region in particular escapes. Occlusion near the origin of the artery causes a hemianesthesia of the thalamic type, and the hemiparesis is mild but is accompanied by some asynergy owing to involvement of the superior cerebellar peduncle. The

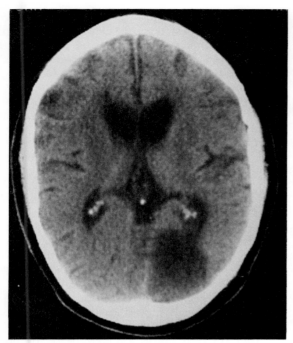

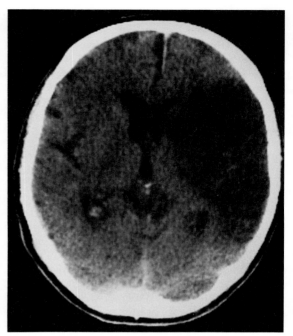

FIG. 51–6. Computed tomogram of a patient with multiple cerebral infarcts, the most prominent being in the territory of the left posterior cerebral artery (dark area in bottom right of figure).

FIG. 51–7. Computed tomogram showing a large infarct (dark area on right of figure) in the territory of the left middle cerebral artery. The frontal horn of the left lateral ventricle is distorted and partly obliterated.

most common syndrome of the posterior cerebral artery is one involving the cortical branches, the calcarine is most often affected; there is resulting hemianopia, with or without alexia, depending on the hemisphere affected.

Occlusion or rupture affecting the entire middle cerebral artery (Fig. 51-7) produces such widespread softening of one hemisphere that profound coma takes place at once, with complete hemiplegia, hemianesthesia, and hemianopia, and with aphasia if the lesion is in the dominant hemisphere (and the patient is alert enough to be tested for it); death usually follows. If the perforating branches alone are involved, the syndrome of capsular hemiplegia occurs, with hemiparesis affecting especially the face and upper extremity, often accompanied by sensory loss. Extreme rigidity and contractures may develop. If the trunk of the artery is affected after the origin of the perforating branches, or if the cortical branches are involved, there may be localized pareses and sensory changes, aphasia of varying types, astereognosis, apraxia, or a hemianopic defect, depending on the site of the occlusion and the collateral. Involvement of the orbitofrontal artery on the left causes expressive

aphasia; of the prerolandic artery, paresis of the opposite side of the face and tongue; of the rolandic artery, both paresis and hypesthesia of the opposite face and arm; of the anterior parietal artery, contralateral astereognosis; of the posterior temporal artery on the left, auditory receptive aphasia; of the supramarginal and angular arteries, hemianopia or, if on the left, visual receptive aphasia and apraxia. Two or more branches may be occluded simultaneously. Because of its large distribution and its flow pattern, the middle cerebral artery and its branches are most often involved in cerebrovascular occlusive disease, both thrombotic and embolic.

Occlusion of the internal carotid artery, if it occurs suddenly, is followed in most instances by a severe contralateral hemiplegia and hemianesthesia, often with ipsilateral blindness due to occlusion of the ophthalmic artery. If the dominant hemisphere is affected, there is complete aphasia. Pathologically there is infarction of the entire hemisphere with the exception of the thalamus, inferior portion of the temporal lobe, and medial portion of the occipital lobe. Convulsions may occur at the onset. If the occlusion takes place gradually, and if the circulation of the circle of Willis is adequate, there may be very few symptoms. Since the introduction of vascular studies it has become apparent that occlusion of the internal carotid artery occurs much more frequently than was realized in the past, and usually takes place in the neck just above the bifurcation of the common carotid or at the level of the carotid sinus. With atherosclerotic involvement of this vessel there may be transient, recurring symptoms of cerebrovascular insufficiency, or if the occlusion is gradual in onset there may be premonitory manifestations consisting of contralateral hemiparesis or monoplegia, paresthesias, or visual field defects, along with aphasia and ipsilateral monocular blindness owing to impairment of circulation through the ophthalmic artery. There may be secondary embolic phenomena. Occasionally it is necessary to occlude the internal carotid artery surgically to stop hemorrhage. If the vessel can be occluded gradually there may be no untoward symptoms. Atherosclerosis, stenosis, and near-occlusion of the internal carotid in the neck or of its origin in the mediastinum may be treated surgically by thrombendarterectomy and reconstruction of the vessel wall but there is little or no evidence that the procedure results in improvement in neurologic function after a completed stroke, and its prophylactic value is still debated.

Occlusion or rupture of the anterior choroidal artery is followed by hemiplegia and sensory defects, affecting principally the leg, and either a quadrantic or hemianopic field defect opposite to the side of the lesion, together with added signs resulting from involvement of the basal ganglia, hippocampus, thalamus, and mesencephalon.

Aneurysms of the intracranial vessels develop preferentially at bifurcations and in the circle of Willis. Common sites are the anterior communicating artery, the tip of the basilar artery, and the takeoff of the posterior communicating vessels. Aneurysms may cause localized compression of cranial nerves. The third nerves and the visual pathways (optic nerve, chiasm, or tract) are affected most frequently. When the aneurysm is located on that portion of the internal carotid artery that lies within the cavernous sinus, the third, fourth, and sixth nerves and the ophthalmic division of the fifth may be involved. Rupture of aneurysms of the circle of Willis or more distal portions of the arteries at the base of the brain causes sudden spontaneous subarachnoid hemorrhage. There may be loss of consciousness and generalized convulsions at the outset. The symptoms are largely those of meningeal irritation with intense nuchal or occipital headache, stiff neck, and photophobia, but there may also be manifestations of focal nervous system dysfunction and signs of increased intracranial pressure. The spinal fluid is under increased pressure and contains blood; within a short time the supernatant fluid becomes xanthochromic. Arteriovenous aneurysms within the cavernous sinus may cause proptosis, chemosis, dilation of the conjunctival vessels, engorgement of the retinal veins, papilledema, and cranial nerve involvement, together with a pulsating exophthalmos. A bruit can often be heard over the eye or forehead. The pulsation of the eye can be abolished by compression of the ipsilateral common carotid artery. Imaging studies and angiograms define aneurysms and can demonstrate the hemorrhage.

Intracranial hemorrhage may be the result of rupture of vascular malformations; the signs and symptoms depend on the location of the malformation, which is readily demonstrated by imaging studies.

Intracerebral hemorrhage (Fig. 51-8) most often takes place in the basal ganglia from rupture of the perforating branches of the vessels to this region. Hemorrhage in other locations may

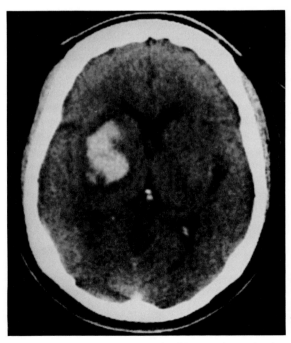

FIG. 51–8. Typical intracerebral hemorrhage in the right basal ganglia (white area to left of center of figure) as demonstrated on computed tomogram.

relate to blood dyscrasias, microaneurysms, amyloid degeneration, or conversion of an embolic infarction into a hemorrhagic infarction. Hemorrhages are easily demonstrated by computed tomography; their signs and symptoms depend on the extent and location of the bleeding.

SYNDROMES OF OCCLUSION OF THE CEREBRAL VEINS AND VENOUS SINUSES

Syndromes of occlusion of the cerebral veins and of the venous sinuses occur less frequently than those of the cerebral arteries; the sinuses are affected more often than the veins. Thrombosis of the cerebral veins or venous sinuses is usually secondary to trauma, infection, cachexia, or blood dyscrasia, and occurs most often in infants and children. Cerebral venous occlusion has also been attributed to the use of oral contraceptives, and it may occur in the puerperium.

Occlusion of the superior cerebral veins may cause either motor or sensory changes on the opposite side of the body, depending upon whether the anterior or posterior group is affected. Occlusion of either the middle cerebral or small anastomotic vein may cause weakness of the facial muscles; if the occlusion is on the left, there may be aphasia. Obliteration of the internal occipital vein produces hemianopia. Occlusion of the great cerebral vein of Galen may cause coma, hyperpyrexia, tachycardia, contraction of the pupils, either convulsions or tonic fits, decerebrate rigidity, and papilledema.

Occlusion of the superior sagittal sinus in young children is followed by generalized convulsions, spastic paralysis, and distention of the veins of the scalp and nose. In adults disease of this sinus is followed by spastic paralysis and cortical sensory changes, with more marked involvement of the lower than the upper extremities. There may be jacksonian convulsions, loss of sphincter control, nausea and vomiting, delirium, apathy, stupor, papilledema, and edema and dilation of the veins of the scalp, eyelids, and forehead. Thrombosis of the straight sinus causes decerebrate rigidity and other manifestations similar to those of occlusion of the great vein of Galen.

The transverse sinus may be occluded or may be subject to thrombosis in disease of the middle ear or mastoid; the thrombus extends into the jugular bulb and vein. In addition to symptoms of septicemia, there may be headache, nausea and vomiting, tenderness and induration of the jugular vein on the involved side, edema and distention of the veins of the neck and mastoid area, meningeal signs, and papilledema that is most marked ipsilaterally, together with auditory and vestibular involvement, and sometimes dyspnea, dysphagia, and bradycardia owing to vagus involvement. The Queckenstedt maneuver on the affected side fails to cause a rise in spinal fluid pressure (Ch. 57).

Thrombosis of the cavernous sinus may complicate infections of the orbit, nose, paranasal sinuses, or contiguous areas of the face on the involved side. In addition to manifestations of septicemia there is pain in the eyes and forehead, with ipsilateral proptosis, chemosis, edema of the eyelid and conjunctiva, papilledema, dilation of the retinal veins, retinal hemorrhages, and involvement of the third, fourth, and sixth nerves and the ophthalmic division of the trigeminal nerve. The process may extend to the opposite side.

Thrombosis of the dural sinuses may be one of several causes of brain swelling of "unknown" etiology, or so-called pseudotumor cerebri. The process may have its origin in the transverse sinus of one side and may extend to either the superior sagittal or straight sinus and cause intracranial hypertension through interference with absorption of cerebrospinal fluid.

BIBLIOGRAPHY

Alpers BJ, Berry RG, Paddison RM. Anatomic studies of the circle of Willis in normal brain. Arch Neurol Psychiatry 1959;81:409

Carpenter MB, Noback CB, Moss ML. The anterior choroidal artery: its origin, course, distribution, and variations. Arch Neurol Psychiatry 1954;71:714

Corday E, Rothenberg SF, Putnam TJ. Cerebral vascular insufficiency: An explanation of some types of localized cerebral encephalopathy. Arch Neurol Psychiatry 1953; 69:551

Dandy WE. Intracranial Arterial Aneurysms. Ithaca, Comstock, 1944.

Field WS (ed). Pathogenesis and Treatment of Cerebrovascular disease. Springfield, IL, Charles C Thomas, 1961

Fisher M. Occlusion of the internal carotid artery. Arch Neurol Psychiatry 1951;65:346

Gillilan LA. The arterial and venous blood supplies to the forebrain (including the internal capsule) of primates. Neurology 1968;18:653

Kaplan HA, Ford DH. The Brain Vascular System. Amsterdam, Elsevier, 1966

Kety SS. Circulation and metabolism of the human brain in health and disease. Am J Med 1950;8:205

Klonoff DC, Andrews BT, Obana WG. Stroke associated with cocaine use. Arch Neurol 1989;46:939

Marshall J. The Management of Cerebrovascular Disease. Boston, Little, Brown & Co, 1965

Meyer JS, Denny – Brown D. The cerebral collateral circulation. Neurology 1957;7:447

Millikan CH, McDowell F, Easton JD. Stroke. Philadelphia, Lea & Febiger, 1987

Murphy JP. Cerebrovascular Disease. Chicago, Year Book Medical Pub, 1954

Riggs HE, Rupp C. Variation in form of circle of Willis. Arch Neurol 1963;8:8

Robinson MK, Toole JF. Ischemic cerebrovascular disease. In Joynt RJ (ed). Clinical Neurology. Philadelphia, JB Lippincott, 1989

Ross JS, Masaryk TJ, Modie MT, Harik SI et al. Magnetic resonance angiography of the extracranial carotid arteries and intracranial vessels: a review. Neurology 1989; 39:369

Schmidt CF. The Cerebral Circulation in Health and Disease. Springfield, IL, Charles C Thomas, 1950

Schoenberg BS, Anderson DW, Haerer AF. Racial differentials in the prevalence of stroke: Copiah County, Mississippi. Arch Neurol 1986;43:565

Vander Eecken HM, Fisher M, Adams RD. The arterial anastomoses of the human brain and their importance in the delimitation of human brain infarction. J Neuropathol Exp Neurol 1952;11:91

Vinken PJ, Bruyn GW (eds). Vascular diseases of the nervous system. In Handbook of Neurology. Amsterdam, North Holland, 1972

WHO Task Force on Stroke and Other Cerebrovascular Disorders. Stroke-1989. Recommendations on stroke prevention, diagnosis, and therapy. Stroke 1989;20:1407

Wright IS, Luckey EH (eds). Cerebral Vascular Diseases. New York, Grune & Stratton, 1955

Chapter 52

APHASIA, AGNOSIA, AND APRAXIA: EXAMINATION OF LANGUAGE AND RELATED FUNCTIONS

Language is defined as audible, articulate human speech that is produced by the action of the tongue and vocal cords, and **speech** as utterance of vocal sounds that convey ideas, or the faculty of expressing thoughts by words (articulate sounds that symbolize and communicate ideas). Speech is more than a motor activity; it is the mechanism by which one gives external expression to internal symbolization, or thinking. Language and speech are considered to be attributes of the human race. Thoughts and ideas, however, are not only expressed in speech, by auditory symbols, but also in writing, by graphic symbols, and in gestures and pantomime, by motor symbols. Consequently language may be regarded as any means of expressing or communicating feeling or thought, usually by spoken words, but also by writing and gestures. Furthermore, such expression, to be accurate and comprehensible, requires not only the motor acts necessary for execution, but also the reception and interpretation of these acts when they are carried out by others, along with the retention, recall, and visualization of the symbols. Speech is as dependent upon the interpretation of the auditory and visual images that reach consciousness and the association of these images with the motor centers that control expression as upon the motor elements of such expression.

An important part of cerebral, or cortical, function is concerned with the ability of the individual to express himself by speech, writing, and gestures; to comprehend spoken and written words and gestures; to recognize the significance of various sensory stimuli; and to carry out purposive or complex movements. A de-

tailed discussion of these subjects would of necessity be too comprehensive for this book, and indeed would merit a complete monograph. The importance of these functions in neurologic diagnosis, however, warrants a general review, together with an outline of an examination of language and related functions.

The word **aphasia** has been used as a general term to include all disturbances of language that are caused by lesions of the brain but are not the result of faulty innervation of the speech muscles, involvement of the organs of articulation themselves, or general mental or intellectual deficiency. It may include those varieties of **agnosia,** or failure to recognize the importance of sensory stimuli, and of **apraxia,** or loss of ability to carry out purposive acts, which have to do with language. Furthermore, because of the close association of language with other forms of symbolic interpretation and expression, it is pertinent to discuss all varieties of agnosia and apraxia along with a consideration of aphasia.

Gall, along with his associate Spurzheim, is credited with one of the earliest descriptions of disturbances of language function and early in the nineteenth century suggested that speech functions were localized to the frontal lobes. Lordat (1823) expressed the opinion that "alalia" was due to asynergy of the muscles used for speech. Bouillaud (1825) first noted that the ability to form words could be lost even though the words were retained in memory and the motor functions for carrying out speech were intact; he believed that the faculty of language was situated in the frontal lobes. Dax (1836) made a statement that word memory is a function of the left cerebral hemisphere. Broca (1861) noted loss of speech associated with a lesion of the inferior frontal convolution on the left. Because the loss of speech was not the result of paralysis of the speech organs, the defect was called aphemia. Trousseau (1862) first used the term aphasia. Wyllie (1866) and Bastian (1869) observed that patients with motor aphasia might have difficulty in the comprehension of spoken words, and Wernicke (1874) described sensory aphasia, or loss of comprehension of words, due to abolition of sound images (**word deafness**), with a lesion of the left superior temporal gyrus. Later he reported that a lesion somewhat posterior to the superior temporal gyrus, in the region of the angular gyrus, was followed by inability to comprehend written words (**alexia,** or **word blindness**).

The development of the concepts of speech functions has a complex history. On the basis of the aforementioned observations Bastian, Broadbent, Wernicke, and others attempted to establish an anatomic classification of the aphasias and to map out the various language centers and their connections. Aphasias were classified as motor, with lesions in the lower precentral region, and sensory, with lesions in the superior temporal, angular, or supramarginal gyri, and were subdivided into cortical, subcortical, and transcortical groups. In the first only specific centers were affected; in the subcortical groups, the deeper structures below the center; in the transcortical group, the association pathways between the various centers.

Other investigators, however, made functional, or physiologic, classifications. Hughlings Jackson stressed the complexity of language disorders. Starr (1889) stated that he had failed to find any cases that substantiated Broca's viewpoint. Marie (1906) expressed the belief that every true aphasia involves defects in general intelligence as well as in special language functions, and in the comprehension of spoken words as well as in speech. He examined the brains of Broca's first two patients and stated that his observations did not afford support for Broca's conclusions; he expressed the belief that the third frontal convolution plays no special role in speech. Since Marie's times the investigators of aphasia have fallen into two general groups: those who continue to stress an anatomic basis and those who use a psychologic approach. The latter believe that language must be considered as a coherent whole and that one must analyze not only the speech disturbance but also the psychologic changes that appear

with cerebral lesions. Head considered aphasia to be a disorder of symbolic formulation and expression or a complexity of language disintegration. On the basis of his analysis of cases he described the following four varieties: **Verbal aphasia** consists of a difficulty in the formulation of words, with, as a result, a restricted vocabulary. **Syntactical aphasia** is characterized by loss of the ability to arrange syllables or words in proper sequence (**jargon aphasia**). **Nominal aphasia** is loss of the memory for words, or inability to name objects, colors, etc. **Semantic aphasia** is characterized by the lack of recognition of the full symbolic significance of words and phrases.

It is still not possible to separate definitely the anatomic and the physiologic substrata of aphasia. It may be, as Freud suggested, that the so-called speech centers are only cornerstones of a larger cortical area in the dominant hemisphere concerned with speech, or as Symonds has postulated, that circuits are affected more than centers. Later investigators, including Wilson, Bay, Brain, Critchley, and Geschwind, have correlated and combined the anatomic, physiologic, and psychologic features of language disorders, and have emphasized the interdependence of speech, language, thought, memory, gestures, and behavior.

Aphasia has been defined variously. A simple definition states that it is a disorder of previously intact language abilities secondary to brain damage. A broader and more comprehensive definition considers it a defect in (dysphasia) or loss of (aphasia) the power of expression by speech, writing, or gestures or a defect or loss in the ability to comprehend spoken or written language or to interpret gestures, secondary to brain damage. If the term aphasia is used, it is implied that there is no paralysis or disability of the organs of speech or of muscles governing other forms of expression, and no loss of hearing or vision. Most aphasias are complex phenomena, and varying combinations of expressive and receptive difficulty may be present. Furthermore, it is often helpful to differentiate between fluent and nonfluent disorders of expression, and between those with and without repetition difficulty (Geschwind).

Before considering the examination of the aphasic patient, it is well to recall that there are three cortical levels as far as reception of impulses is concerned. The first is the level of "arrival," a function of the primary cortical reception areas; at this level one perceives, or sees and hears, without further differentiation of the impulses. The second level is that of "knowing," or gnostic function, concerned with the recognition of impulses, formulation of engrams for recall of stimuli, and revisualization. The third level, the one of greatest importance in aphasia, is that which has to do with recognition of symbols in the form of words, or the higher elaboration and association of learned symbols as a function of language. There are also three levels of speech function, and in aphasic defects the most automatic of these is least frequently affected, and the least automatic most often involved. The most automatic is the emotional level, and the patient may be able to respond to a painful or emotional stimulus with the word "ouch," or perhaps can give vent to an expletive, even though the other functions of speech are entirely absent. The next is the propositional level, or that concerned with casual, automatic speech; the patient may be able to answer questions with words such as "yes" and "no" even though other elements of speech are severely impaired. The highest level is the volitional, or intellectualized, which is the first to be affected and the last to return. The patient is unable to repeat words said by the examiner or to make statements that require thought and concentration. It is of interest that in the return of speech during recovery from aphasia, those languages that were learned earliest in life or learned most thoroughly may be the first to come into use. Multilinguals appear to have several centers for speech in somewhat discrete but overlapping cortical areas. Modern imaging technics and blood flow or cerebral metabolism studies are gradually adding to our knowledge of the regions of the brain involved in the various speech-related processes.

THE EXAMINATION OF THE PATIENT WITH APHASIA, AGNOSIA, AND APRAXIA

The detailed testing of language and related functions in the patient who shows evidence of aphasia, agnosia, or apraxia may be carried out after the rest of the neurologic examination has been completed. Appraisal, however, during the taking of the history as well as throughout the routine examination, may provide valuable information regarding both expressive and receptive defects.

The history is extremely important in the evaluation of the aphasic patient. It should include not only information about the patient's present and past illnesses (Ch. 2), but also data relative to cultural background, education, and training. The examiner should determine the patient's native tongue, the order in which he has learned other languages, and his fluency in all languages he has known. School achievements, the last grade reached, and age at completion of formal education should be ascertained. Other important elements in the history include the patient's linguistic and reading habits, speech defects and handicaps, mathematical ability, and occupational pursuits. It is important to know not only the patient's dominance of hand, eye, and foot in writing and other acts, but also whether this dominance (especially handedness) is native to him or is the result of training. A family history of either left-handedness or ambidexterity as well as of speech handicaps may be relevant.

Before attempting to evaluate disturbances in language function, the examiner must appraise the patient's vocabulary, intellectual capacity, emotional state, sensorium, orientation, attention, memory, retention, and recall (Ch. 4). Obviously, it is not possible to evaluate disturbances of language function in patients who are confused, semistuporous, or markedly agitated or depressed. Furthermore, fright and other emotional states as well as the conversion mechanisms of hysteria may produce defects in both expression and reception that may simulate those of organic disease. The remainder of the neurologic examination, of course, contributes essential information.

All tests should be carried out in a quiet environment with minimal distractions; fatigue and irritation should be avoided. If fatigue is apparent, or if the findings are equivocal, it may be necessary to repeat the examination at another time. It is not possible, in testing aphasia, agnosia, and apraxia, to separate expressive and receptive factors completely; it is necessary for the patient to comprehend visual and auditory impulses if commands are to be understood, but responses to such commands are performed by expressive faculties. However, the examiner should attempt to evaluate the various components of language individually, and then record the results. At the completion of the examination the findings and patient's performance as a whole can be synthesized. The listing that follows contains the essential points to be evaluated.

Speech

When testing speech, or the formulation and expression of ideas and feelings by means of spoken words, phrases, or more complex statements, one must consider spontaneous, automatic, emotional, propositional, and volitional varieties as well as abstract speech.

Spontaneous Speech. The patient's use of words in giving the history and in relating symptoms should be evaluated. Appraisal of spontaneous narration may be an important part of the speech investigation, and it is often valuable to make verbatim recordings. The examiner should note pronunciation, enunciation, formation not only of words but also of sentences, fluency, cadence, rhythm, prosody, elision of syllables or words, omission or transposition of words, misuse of words, circumlocutions, repetition, perseveration, paraphasic defects, jargon, and the use of neologisms. The patient's ability to talk, form simple words, and utter less familiar words and those of several syllables should be detected, as well as the extent of the patient's vocabulary and his ability to formulate grammatical sentences and to express himself and his ideas accurately in speech. Any deviation from the normal should be appraised. Among the abnormalities in spontaneous speech, the following clues suggest a defect and have diagnostic significance: slight errors in word formation with omission or substitution of letters, such as the use of "inconscious" for "unconscious," "thumbness" for "numbness;" misplacement not only of letters, but also of syllables and words; the use of unusual synonyms or circumlocutions in order to avoid the use of a word that cannot be recalled; discrepancies in the implication of words; omissions of words; hesitations and inappropriate pauses; perseveration; verbal stereotype; neologisms; agrammatism; jargon or gibberish; the use of pantomime or gesture to compensate for defects in oral expression. In severe aphasia the patient may be unable to utter a single word; in other cases there may be recurring utterance of syllables, a specific word, "yes" or "no" or both, a phrase, or a fragment of meaningless jargon.

Automatic Speech. Word series that were well learned in early life may be retained even when spontaneous speech is lost; these may be considered a part of automatic speech. The patient is asked to state his name, repeat the alphabet, count, list the days of the week or months of the year, spell simple words, and repeat simple poems and nursery rhymes.

Emotional Speech. Emotional speech is important, and the patient may be unable to speak consecutively while retaining the ability to express himself by the use of expletives, swearing, or other emotional responses.

Volitional Speech. Volitional, or intellectualized, speech, is apparent in the patient's spontaneous utterances, but some of these may be reflex or semiautomatic. Volitional speech is further tested by having the patient speak from dictation and repeat simple sounds, words, short phrases, and sentences spoken by the examiner. These should contain most English sounds and should include digit and letter sequences, nonsense syllables, disconnected words, short phrases and sentences, and short stories.

Functional and Abstract Speech. Functional speech is tested by having the patient spell complex words and define simple words and objects. Abstract language is evaluated by noting the patient's ability to define or interpret proverbs.

Singing. Musical speech or singing can be tested. The patient may retain his ability to sing, even though he is unable to talk. Retention of a melody may aid in the recall of words that the patient associates with it.

Recall of Words and Naming of Objects. The patient should be asked to recall words and use them as names. He may first be asked to name colors and simple objects such as a key, pencil, coin, book, watch, or parts of the body. He may then be asked to name more complex and less common objects, such as the parts of a watch (stem, hands, crystal, etc.) or the individual structures of the eye. Finally he may be asked to name and describe what he sees in pictures. If the patient is unable to recall words or names, he may be asked to select the correct name out of a group of words suggested to him (reinforcing expression by either auditory or visual symbols), or to tell the number of letters or syllables in the word he wishes to speak. Writing as well as speech should be considered in the evaluation of the patient's ability to formulate ideas and express himself.

Spontaneous Writing. Spontaneous writing may be evaluated by having the patient write, in both print and script, whatever he desires; this may include name and address or short sentences. A letter recently written by the patient, if available, may give pertinent information about the ability to express thoughts in writing. As in the evaluation of spontaneous speech, errors such as the omission or substitution of letters, misspelling, or elision of syllables or words should be noted. The presence of mirror writing may also give diagnostic information, since it may be a symptom of a disturbance of cerebral dominance.

Automatic or Semiautomatic Writing. The patient is asked specifically to write his name and address, spell simple words, and write the days of the week or the months of the year.

Volitional Writing. Volitional writing is tested in a variety of ways. The patient may be asked to write, in both print and script, letters, words, and sentences that are dictated to him. This involves not only volitional writing, but also the ability of the patient to translate auditory symbols into visual ones and is possible only when comprehension of speech is not seriously defective. The patient may be asked to copy, in both print and script, printed and written material. This tests not only volitional writing, but, in addition, the ability to comprehend visual symbols and to translate one visual symbol into another, and is possible only when visual receptive functions are intact.

Recall of Words and Naming of Objects. As with the evaluation of speech, the patient is asked to recall words and to name objects by having him write down names and colors of simple and complex objects.

Comprehension of Spoken Language

The patient's responses to verbal requests and commands and to everyday questions and comments give information about his ability to understand articulate speech, or spoken language, but for an adequate evaluation specific tests may be given, arranged in order of increasing complexity. It should be noted whether the patient has more difficulty with polysyllabic words and long sentences than with simple words and short sentences, and whether concepts as well as words are recognized. He is first asked to point to objects that have been named for him. Simple requests are then given in the form of short sentences, such as "Place your finger on your nose," "Close your eyes," "Show your teeth," "Turn out the light," and "Open the door." These requests are then made somewhat more complex: "Place your right hand on top of your head," "Put your left index finger on your right ear," "Turn to page 87 in this book." Compound sentences and double or complex commands may finally be em-

ployed: "Put out your hands and close your eyes," "Place one hand on your head, turn around, and sit down," "Take that coin from the table and give it to me," "Place one coin on the table, give me the second, and keep the third in your hand." In Marie's paper test the patient is told, "Here is a piece of paper; tear it in four parts and place one on the table, give one to me, and keep two for yourself." A group of coins of different denominations can be presented. The patient is asked to pick out individual ones and rearrange them in patterns of increasing value. Auditory comprehension also can be evaluated by making definite statements that are either true or false, and asking the patient to indicate the answer by saying "yes" or "no" or by making the appropriate gesture. Both comprehension and retention are evaluated by telling a short story and then asking questions about it that can be answered similarly.

Comprehension of Written Language

The patient's ability to understand written language is evaluated by having him demonstrate his skill in reading. The tests are arranged in order of increasing difficulty, beginning with numbers and letters, then passing to words, both short and complex, and proceeding to phrases and simple and complicated sentences. The ability to read both printed material and script should be noted. The patient may first be given cards bearing the names of simple objects, such as a key or a pencil, which are placed on a table before him, and he should point to the objects when he reads their names. Then the examiner should verbally recite the names of the objects, and the patient should be asked to point to the card bearing the appropriate name. Simple written commands, and finally more complex commands, such as "Place your hand on your head," then "Place your right index finger on your left eye," should be presented in block letters or legible script. Later he is asked to read, both aloud and silently, simple printed material and then sentences of increasing complexity, and to explain the meaning. One notes the ability to recognize and comprehend the meaning of letters and syllables and the significance of simple sentences, either true or false, and then more complex written material. If the patient is unable to express what has been read, questions should be asked that can be answered by "yes" or "no," or by gestures. When the patient reads aloud and then explains what has been read, oral expression is tested as well as reading. The patient may be able to understand what he has read silently, although the ability to read aloud or translate visual symbols into oral ones is lost. It is also important to determine whether the patient is able to read his own writing.

Expression by Gestures and the Comprehension of Symbols and Gestures

Expression and comprehension of symbols may be examined specifically by having the patient write mathematical figures and musical symbols, and having him state the significance of each, as well as of letters, symbols such as the Red Cross and abbreviations such as YMCA. He may also be asked to interpret the meaning and significance of pictures, such as a child preparing to hand a happy-looking puppy his food.

When patients are unable to express themselves by either speech or writing, it is important to note their ability to express themselves by gestures, and, likewise, with those unable to comprehend spoken or written language, to note their comprehension of pantomime, gestures, and symbols. A patient who is unable to make his desires known in other ways may indicate responses and desires by shaking or nodding the head, shrugging the shoulders, or demonstrating visible emotional reactions. Although incapable of expression through spoken or written words, the patient may recognize symbolic gestures. A patient who is unable to understand either oral or written commands may imitate the actions of the examiner in placing a finger to the nose or putting out the tongue.

Drawing

The patient's ability to express himself in drawing is tested by having him first draw simple objects such as a square, circle, triangle, or cross, and then more complex pictures such as a cube, man, house, or daisy. He should also be asked to trace or copy figures, or reproduce them immediately after presentation, and to draw from a model.

Calculation

The patient's arithmetical ability is examined first by having him do simple computations involving addition, subtraction, multiplication, and division, and then by having him solve sim-

ple and more complex problems, both orally and on paper.

Gnostic Functions

The recognition of sensory stimuli other than those specifically involved in language functions should also be noted. When testing vision, this includes the appreciation of color, form, and direction, perception of space, identification of geometric figures and pictures, recognition of fingers and parts of the body, comprehension of laterality, and identification of both inanimate and animate objects. It is important to determine whether the patient recognizes objects even if unable to name them. The patient may recall the name on hearing it said although he cannot state it spontaneously. The patient should be asked not only to name colors (an expressive function), but also to match them (a gnostic process). In the auditory field one notes the patient's ability to recognize inarticulate sounds, tone, and music. Identification of such sounds as the ringing of a bell, clinking of coins, jingling of keys, and crumpling of paper, and recognition of simple musical melodies, should be evaluated. In the tactile field one notes the patient's recognition of objects by feeling them, his comprehension of letters and figures made of wood or plastic, and the identification of parts of the body from tactile stimulation. The routine tests for cortical sensory functions are described in Part B, "The Sensory System." In testing for the syndrome of finger agnosia the patient should be asked to point to individual fingers and parts of his body when his eyes are both open and closed, and to name and select fingers and parts of the body, both his own and the examiner's, when looking at them, when the examiner points to them, and (with eyes both open and closed) when they are touched. The patient should also be asked to indicate laterality, both on his own and the examiner's body.

Performance of Purposive Acts

Eupractic functions and their disturbances may be tested by having the patient carry out various purposive acts. Muscular weakness and incoordination resulting from either muscular or cerebellar dysfunction or loss of proprioceptive sense must be differentiated from loss of the ability to formulate motor plans and perform skilled movements; and spontaneous, more or less reflex or automatic acts must be distinguished from volitional ones. It is important to determine whether the patient recognizes the nature of common objects and understands their use and function. The execution of spontaneous, requested, and imitative (mimicking the examiner) movements is observed, and the ability to perform movements with each hand individually and both hands together is noted.

The patient may first be asked to stand, walk, sit, protrude the tongue, and carry out simple acts with hands and feet, such as making a fist, separating fingers, and stamping the foot; then to perform movements directed to parts of the body, such as placing one hand on top of the head, touching the nose with the index finger, and placing one heel on the opposite knee. It must be determined whether weakness or ataxia is present and if the movements are performed skillfully, or in a crude manner. Dexterity for fine movements is important. The patient is then asked to do various symbolic actions involving pantomime and gesture, such as throwing a kiss, waving good-bye, shaking hands, greeting a friend, beckoning, threatening, or pretending to play the piano. Then he is asked to demonstrate the use of simple objects, such as a key, comb, pen, scissors, hammer, screw, and toothbrush, both by pantomime and with the use of the available objects. He may be asked to wind a watch, dress himself, button his clothes, strike a match, stamp a letter, tie a knot, or drink a glass of water. To test for constructional apraxia the patient is requested to draw figures and pictures, and to copy designs made by the examiner; then to form geometric figures with matches and toothpicks, and more complex three-dimensional structures with blocks, and again to copy designs made by the examiner.

Simultaneous Testing of Gnostic and Eupractic Functions

In many of the tests just described both receptive and expressive elements and gnostic and eupractic functions are evaluated simultaneously. Combined functions may be evaluated in other ways. One may determine whether the patient is able not only to recognize objects, but also to name them, tell their use, and then use them, and whether he is able to understand what he has said and written. If a patient is asked to set a clock both on command and by duplication of the setting of another clock, auditory and visual receptive functions as well as the ability to perform purposive acts are evaluated,

and if he is asked to tell the time and to write it down, expression by both speech and writing are tested. The use of simple games and puzzles may provide information. The patient may be able to play some games more or less automatically, yet be unable to explain what he is doing or to follow commands.

Chesher outlined a simple and brief routine that may be used in the examination of an aphasic patient wherein both receptive and expressive functions are tested together. The patient is given a few simple objects, such as a key, pencil, penny, matchbox, pair of scissors, and comb. The following requests are then made: (1) Name the objects. (2) Say the names after the examiner (repetition of single words). (3) Point to the objects as their names are called (comprehension of spoken words). (4) Read printed words giving the names of the objects. (5) Point to the object on reading its name (comprehension of printed words). (6) Write the names of the objects. (7) Write the names from dictation. (8) Copy the names. (9) Spell the names aloud. To this may be added tests for gnostic and eupractic functions by asking the patient to identify the objects by feeling them and by having him demonstrate their use. Another simultaneous test for both auditory and visual comprehension and motor execution may be carried out by giving the patient four coins of different denominations and four numbered plates, then requesting that the coins be placed on the respective plates in accordance with both oral and written commands.

Revisualization

The patient's ability to revisualize may be appraised by having him tell the color of various familiar objects, describe the physical characteristics of friends, and both describe and draw the plan of his home. Recall of auditory stimuli is tested by asking the patient to recite simple poems or sing songs, and recall of both auditory and visual stimuli by having him spell aloud words given by the examiner.

Additional Methods of Testing

Intelligence tests, both of the language and non-language varieties, vocabulary tests, word association tests, performance tests, sentence completion tests, form boards, imitation and sorting tests, digit-symbol substitution tests, drawing and picture completion, and other special methods of examination, including the Bender visual-motor gestalt test, the Kohs block design exercises, and examination with the use of the tachistoscope, have paramount value in the final evaluation of the asphasic patient. Many of these tests are mentioned in Chapter 4. Technics using test boards, cards, and specialized equipment, such as the Halstead-Wepman aphasia screening test and Reitan's modification of it, the Wepman-Jones test, Eisenson's test, the Minnesota test for the differential diagnosis of aphasia, and Schuell's short examination for aphasia, are used by many clinicians and speech pathologists.

CLASSIFICATION OF THE APHASIAS, AGNOSIAS, AND APRAXIAS, AND THEIR VALUE IN CEREBRAL LOCALIZATION

The diagnosis and classification of the aphasias and related disorders are complex problems. These disorders occur in varying degrees of severity and are frequently mixed in type. There have been many attempts at classification, from anatomic, physiologic, and psychologic points of view. A strictly anatomic classification does not apply in all instances, for a small lesion may be followed by severe impairment of both expression and comprehension, whereas an extensive lesion sometimes causes an isolated defect. Lesions that appear similar in size and location on imaging studies may be associated with somewhat variable aphasic syndromes even in persons with identical cerebral dominance for speech, and lesions appearing in different locations or being of variable sizes may produce similar aphasic syndromes. Nevertheless, some general relationships exist between anatomic sites and aphasic types.

On the other hand, a classification stressing only function also may be unsatisfactory, for every motor act has a sensory element, and sensory function often can be revealed only by motor expression. The classification used herein is essentially a functional one but is also practical, especially if the examiner correlates function with anatomic knowledge. In this classification the aphasias are designated as predominantly expressive, predominantly receptive, expressive-receptive, and amnesic varieties. Expressive aphasia is closely related to or perhaps identical with apraxia of the muscles of speech or writing. Receptive aphasias and visual and auditory agnosias clinically seem similar. All agnosias in-

volve failure to interpret stimuli and are disabilities in the receptive fields. Most disorders of speech are complex and involve both reception and expression, although one is usually affected more than the other.

Another widely used classification of aphasia is that proposed by Benson, Geschwind, and their associates at the Boston Veterans Administration Research Unit. They divide aphasias into syndromes with repetition disturbance (Broca, Wernicke, conduction, pure word deafness, aphemia, and global types), and syndromes without repetition disturbance (transcortical types, anomic, and subcortical types). The investigators stress the fact, however, that few patients conform to any one type, but most have a symptom picture that resembles one of the listed types more than the others. Also, in classifying patients with aphasia, it must be remembered that the clinical picture may vary during the development and resolution, if any, of the disorder.

Despite statements by Head and others that language must be considered a coherent whole and a function of the entire brain, clinical studies and surgical and autopsy confirmations have shown that the aphasias and related disorders have some localizing significance. Furthermore, although a functional classification is used, disturbance of physiology can often be correlated with anatomic localization. In most instances the lesion that causes an aphasia, and some of the agnosias and apraxias as well, is located in the dominant hemisphere. This is especially true of right-handed persons, in 99% or more of whom the lesion causing an aphasia is in the left hemisphere. Cerebral dominance for language is not so definite in left-handed individuals, who make up from 5% to 10% of the population. Some of these may have bilateral speech representation, but it is usually unilateral. In about 60% of left-handed people the lesion that causes an aphasia is in the left hemisphere; the speech defect that follows a lesion of the right hemisphere is often less severe and more transient.

Apparent inconsistencies between handedness and the side of the lesion responsible for an aphasia may result from several factors. Handedness is usually inherited, but many native sinistrals have been trained to use only the right hand; left-handedness occasionally is the result of disease of the motor areas of the left hemisphere in early life; injuries and amputations in childhood may bring about a change in handedness and possibly also in dominance for speech. It is generally believed that dominance for language localizes to the left hemisphere by the age of 8. Many ambidextrous persons are shifted left-handed people. The presence of an aphasia may not only lateralize a lesion, but may also further localize it. Aphasias of the expressive type, in most instances, result from a lesion anterior to the rolandic fissure, and those of the receptive variety are usually caused by disturbances posterior to this fissure, in the temporal and parietal regions (Fig. 52-1). Some authors emphasize that speech disturbances can arise from the entire perisylvian area and structures deep to it, with more motor abnormalities from anterior lesions and more sensory (receptive) deficits from posterior lesions.

Aphasias may be the result of a wide variety of cerebral lesions. A vascular origin constitutes the most common cause, followed by trauma and neoplasms. Congenital aphasia does occur, but is extremely rare. The prognosis for recovery is good with acquired aphasia that develops in childhood, although there may be some impairment of intellectual development owing to involvement of the dominant hemisphere. The prognosis for recovery is usually also good with aphasia in ambidextrous persons and in left-handed individuals, regardless of whether the responsible lesion is in the left or right hemi-sphere. The relationship between aphasia and intelligence is a controversial subject, inasmuch as psychomotor testing is difficult if either the expressive or receptive aspects of language function are much impaired. In testing dysphasic or mildly aphasic individuals, however, and those with lesions of the left cerebral hemisphere without clinical evidence of speech impairment, there is often some evidence of difficulty with verbal tests and conceptual thinking, whereas in persons with lesions of the right hemisphere there is difficulty with the performance tests and especially with visuospatial functions.

EXPRESSIVE APHASIA

The predominantly expressive, or motor, aphasias are characterized by a defect or loss in the power of expression by speech, writing, or gestures.

Oral expressive aphasia corresponds to the motor aphasia of Broca and the verbal aphasia of Head. Although there is no loss of function of the organs of articulation, the patient is unable to form words or to combine or integrate the movements of the organs of articulation that are

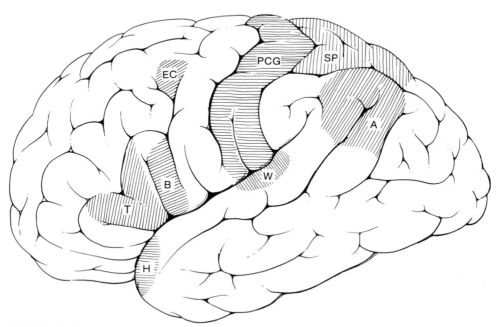

FIG. 52–1. Centers important in language. **A.** Angular gyrus. **B.** Broca's area. **EC.** Exner's writing center. **H.** Henschen's music center. **SP.** Superior parietal lobule, which with **PCG** (postcentral gyrus) is important in tactile recognition. **T.** Pars triangularis. **W.** Wernicke's area. (Modified from Nielson JM. Agnosia, Apraxia, Aphasia: Their Value in Cerebral Localization, 2nd ed. New York, Paul B Hoeber, 1946)

necessary for speech. He knows what he wishes to say, but is unable to say it, or to say it correctly. He may be unable to talk spontaneously, repeat, or read aloud. He is able to hear and understand spoken language and to read and comprehend written language but is unable to repeat what he hears and reads. He can identify objects but not name them. He may be able to write and draw, although under most circumstances the lesion causing the aphasia also causes paralysis of the right hand. There may be loss of expression of recently acquired languages or those not thoroughly learned, with preservation of those learned early in life or most thoroughly learned. There may be loss of volitional and propositional speech, but preservation of automatic and emotional speech. Singing may be retained even though speech is lost. Occasionally speech is limited to the repetitive utterance of a single word or phrase. In mild cases (dysphasia) there may be only slight errors in word formation, occasional circumlocutions, or reduction of vocabulary, often brought out only by stressing the patient through requesting specific information in a rapid-fire manner. In others perseveration or **palilalia** (recurring utterance of syllables, words, or phrases) may be evident. Dysarthria is sometimes present in aphasic patients, either due to coincidental lesions affecting the articulatory apparatus at a lower level or as the result of apraxia of the muscles of articulation.

It is important to differentiate between expressive aphasia (**aphemia,** or loss of speech) and the various disorders of articulation. **Dysarthria** is the imperfect utterance of sounds or words; symbolic formulation of words is normal and phonation is preserved, but disease of the nerves to the organs of articulation or of the central regulation of the nerves interferes with clear enunciation. **Anarthria** is the total loss of ability to articulate; it is caused by more extensive dysfunction of the nerves or their regulatory centers. **Dysphonia** and **aphonia** are disorders of function of the larynx in which phonation is lost even though articulation may be preserved; the dysfunction may be caused by either disease of the larynx or hysteria. **Dyslalia** is a disturbance of utterance in which there is no organic neurologic defect, but there is structural damage to the articulatory system.

Although it has been stated that oral expressive aphasia is usually caused by a lesion in the lower motor region of the dominant hemisphere, principally about the base of the precentral sulcus in the posterior part of the inferior frontal convolution (Broca's area) and the adjoining gyri

(areas 44, 45, 46, and 47 of Brodmann), such accurate localization is seldom possible. Lesions in many widespread areas in front of or along the rolandic fissure may cause motor aphasia (see Fig. 52-1). Penfield and Roberts state that Broca's area, or the frontal cortex in its immediate vicinity, is important in speech and should be avoided during surgery, but comment that most persisting aphasias follow extensive lesions of the left hemisphere, including, in most cases, the posterior temporoparietal region. They produced transient dysphasia with limited excisions of many areas in the dominant hemisphere. Probably the aphasia following a lesion of a specific cortical area may not be the result of specific loss of function of this region, but rather a disturbance of the connections between this region and other portions of the brain, particularly those relating to recognition and interpretation of spoken and written words. Arguments concerning the function and limits of Broca's area continue.

Loss of expression by writing is usually called **agraphia;** it is characterized by inability to formulate words in either script or printing in the absence of paralysis of the arm or hand. It usually is associated with oral expressive aphasias and apraxias, and may indicate the presence of a somewhat larger lesion that also involves the hand area ("Exner's writing center" in the middle frontal convolution, Fig. 52-1). There may, however, be loss of the ability to write although speech is retained. The defect is essentially an apraxia of the right hand. In place of agraphia there may be contraction of words, elision of letters or syllables, transposition of words, or mirror writing. In dissociated dysgraphia there may be difficulty in writing spontaneously or to dictation, but retention of the ability to copy written or printed material. Agraphia may also follow a lesion posterior to the rolandic fissure and may accompany the Gerstmann syndrome (see under "Agnosia").

Loss of expression by gestures may be a significant part of an aphasic defect. Speech and writing are both means of self-expression by use of symbols, one by spoken words, the other by writing. There are, however, additional types of expression that involve different symbols, such as gestures, mimicry, and pantomime. In a severe, or global, aphasia the patient may be unable to nod his head to signify "yes" or to shake his head to indicate "no." The ability to use his hands in talking, shrug his shoulders, and express himself by other gestures and movements may be lost. The term **asymbolia** is sometimes used for the inability of expression by symbols, and **amimia** for defects in expression by gestures and mimicry.

Motor, or **kinetic, apraxia** is loss of the ability to carry out purposeful acts in the absence of paralysis. Most of the expressive aphasias that have been mentioned are actually varieties of motor apraxia, and in reality all motor acts are means by which the individual expresses himself, although eupraxia is not a function of language. The apraxias are discussed later in this chapter.

RECEPTIVE APHASIA

The predominantly receptive aphasias are characterized by a defect or loss of ability to comprehend spoken or written language or to interpret gesture.

Visual receptive aphasia is also known as visual sensory aphasia. In its pure form it is characterized by loss of the ability to comprehend the meaning or significance of printed or written words in the absence of actual loss of vision: this is known as **alexia,** or **word blindness.** Actually, however, there are many varieties of disturbances of visual reception in addition to true word blindness.

Area 17 of Brodmann, or the striate cortex, is the site of the primary reception, or arrival, of the visual impulses. A lesion here causes loss of perception, or blindness, which is restricted in extent to the visual field affected. Area 18 is concerned with gnostic functions, or the recognition of the stimulus. A lesion in this area causes a visual agnosia for objects: the patient sees the objects but cannot identify them and reacts to them as a blind person would. He may retain the ability to distinguish them in other ways, as by touch. This syndrome is designated **psychic blindness,** or **mind blindness.** There may be either loss of recognition of the object with retention of color vision, or loss of color perception (**color agnosia,** or **achromatopsia**); interpretation of form and shape is also impaired. Occasionally visual agnosia is limited to nonidentification of the human face (**prosopagnosia**); another type is characterized by loss of the ability to interpret pictures and gestures.

Area 19 is important in revisualization, activation of engrams, and space perception. Lesions in this region cause a visual agnosia that is characterized by loss of the ability to revisualize, or to describe an object after it has been seen, although the object may be identified when the patient sees it; there is loss of memory for objects and persons. There is also loss of the ability to localize and to perceive distance, space relationships, and motion (**visual spatial agnosia**); there may be disorganization of spatial judgment and visual disorientation in which the patient cannot find his way in familiar surroundings. The patient may be able to perceive parts but not the whole of a pattern, and may have difficulty with constructional tasks, copying, and drawing. In the **Charcot – Wilbrand syndrome** there is visual agnosia together with loss of revisualization; the patient cannot draw from memory.

The region of the angular gyrus (area 39 of Brodmann) and the adjacent cortex in the dominant hemisphere (see Fig. 52-1) have been said to be essential for the recognition and interpretation of symbols in the form of letters and words, and the association of learned symbols as a function of language. A lesion of this region, or of the connections between it and the striate cortex, causes alexia, or word blindness. There is loss of the powers of recognition, interpretation, and recall of the visual symbols of language; written and printed words have no meaning, although the patient may talk without difficulty and understand what is said to him. The recognition of letters and syllables as well as of words may be impaired. Occasionally the patient with alexia may be able to read by kinesthetic sense, and can recognize embossed letters by feeling them even though he cannot identify them when he sees them. In congenital or developmental dyslexia there may be a severe reading disability, often with difficulty in writing as well. This occurs most often in boys and may be inherited.

Impulses from the striate cortex go to both angular gyri, but they go only to the dominant hemisphere for recognition of language symbols. Consequently a unilateral lesion of either area 18 or 19 may cause agnosia for objects, color, form, space perception, or motion, or loss of revisualization in the opposite visual field, whereas a lesion of the major angular gyrus causes alexia. In bilateral lesions there may be **anosognosia,** or denial of blindness, owing either to involvement of the striate cortex itself or to interruption of fibers from it to other cortical areas.

Auditory receptive aphasia is also known as auditory sensory aphasia, auditory agnosia, and **Wernicke's aphasia.** In its pure form it is characterized by loss of the ability to comprehend the significance of spoken words in the absence of deafness (**word deafness**).

The three cortical levels for the reception and interpretation of the auditory impulses are not as clearly defined as those for the reception and interpretation of visual impulses. Areas 41 and 42, located in the transverse temporal gyri (Heschl's convolutions) on the dorsal surface of the posterior portion of the superior temporal convolution, are probably the centers for both primary reception and recognition of auditory impulses. Certain authorities, however, designate the medial geniculate bodies as the primary receptive areas, and Heschl's convolutions as the centers for recognition; others state that areas 41 and 42 are the receptive regions, and that the adjacent paratransverse portions of the superior temporal convolutions function in the recognition of sounds. Lesions of areas 41 and 42, or the regions immediately surrounding them, may cause a general auditory agnosia in which the patient loses his ability to recognize or interpret ordinary sounds, such as the ringing of a bell, and also his memory for them. This is **psychic deafness;** there may also be loss of "reauditorization" of sounds. Owing to the fact that auditory impulses pass to both temporal lobes and there is little unilateral cerebral dominance for ordinary sounds, there is never any marked disability, either deafness or complete auditory agnosia, with unilateral temporal lobe lesions.

Wenicke's area, which occupies a crescentic zone in the posterior third of the superior temporal convolution of the dominant hemisphere, just lateral to the transverse temporal gyrus of Heschl, has been called the center for the recognition, interpretation, and recall of word symbols and their association as a function of language (see Fig. 52-1). A lesion at this site may cause an auditory receptive aphasia, auditory verbal agnosia, or word deafness. There is loss of ability to comprehend the significance of spoken words or recall their meaning: the patient can still hear and can recognize voices, but not the words that they utter, and he cannot repeat what he hears. He can read without difficulty, and may be able to speak normally, but the loss of ability to comprehend the significance of spoken words includes those spoken by the patient himself as well as by others, so that there is usually a syntactical defect, or inability to arrange words in proper sequence, accompanied by the employment of incorrect or unintelligible words, unconventional and gibberish sounds, and senseless combinations. The patient is not aware of his errors in speaking. The resulting misuse of words and defect of sequence is termed **agrammatism, paraphasia,** or **jargon aphasia.** He may be able to repeat what others have said even though he does not understand the meaning. Word deafness occasionally is congenital.

Other Sensory Aphasias. Conduction **aphasia** is a term used by some to connote a sensory aphasia characterized by paraphasic output, fairly good comprehension of spoken language, but very poor repetition. Lesions of the arcuate fasciculus have been proposed as a cause, but disagreements continue about the localization of this disorder.

Receptive aphasia for gestures is usually a part of an extensive aphasic or agnostic defect. It may be referred to as either **asymbolia** or **amimia,** the inability to comprehend the meaning of acts, symbols, gestures, or pantomime. Ideational, or sensory, apraxia is discussed with the apraxias.

EXPRESSIVE – RECEPTIVE APHASIA

Although many patients with aphasia show predominantly receptive or predominantly expressive difficulties, combinations of the two are most frequently encountered in clinical practice. It is occasionally difficult or impossible to distinguish between the defects or to determine whether the receptive or expressive component is affected most seriously. For this reason specific localization of the lesions that cause aphasia cannot always be made clinically by neurologic examination alone. Oral expressive aphasia occurs with a lesion of the frontal lobe, but on the other hand the paraphasia that occurs with a receptive defect in the temporal region may cause similar changes in speech. Agraphia is usually caused by frontal involvement, but it may also be associated with posterior lesions. Alexia is most frequently caused by either defects in the connections between the occipital cortex and the lower parietal regions or by involvement of the angular gyrus, but it may also occur with frontal lesions. Expressive-receptive aphasias may, like the other types, vary in degree of involvement, just as they may vary in the extent to which the individual language functions are affected. The mixed defect in which there is complete or almost complete loss of both expression and perception of language is termed a **global** or **total aphasia,** or sometimes **central aphasia.**

Attempts have been made to correlate both mixed and global aphasias with isolated lesions of the brain, although under most circumstances defects in both the expressive and receptive fields are the result of either extensive cortical lesions or subcortical damage with interruption of the association pathways. Involvement in the region of the so-called quadrilateral space of Marie, which is situated between the cortex externally and the internal capsule medially and within the limits of the insula anteriorly and posteriorly, may cause interruption of the association fibers that course through the external capsule to connect Broca's area with the other language centers; there may be a mixed aphasia characterized by agraphia and paraphasia or by alexia and oral expressive aphasia. The so-called **transcortical aphasias** may have motor, sensory, or mixed varieties. Repetition is spared. Interruptions of cortical connections, or isolation of speech centers are held responsible for these aphasias. Echolalia occurs with mixed transcortical aphasia, and various motor or sensory speech deficits with preserved ability to repeat words occur in the other types.

Mixed aphasia, often temporary, may also occur in lesions of the internal capsule as a result of interruption of the association bundles that pass just above and below the lentiform nucleus and connect the frontal, temporal, and parietal regions.

Idiokinetic apraxia results from interruption of the impulses between the site of comprehension and that of execution of the act. Amimia and asymbolia may be either expressive (loss of ability to perform gestures or pantomime), or receptive (loss of comprehension of such acts).

Mixed aphasias often evolve over time, with different degrees of regression of certain features from those of the others.

AMNESIC APHASIA

Amnesic aphasia has been defined as a difficulty in evoking the names for objects, conditions, or qualities, with serious limitations in speaking and writing. This type of aphasia corresponds to the nominal variety of Head, or anomia. The disability is said to be different from that of the typical expressive disorder; speech is correctly articulated, but is hesitant and fragmentary owing to difficulty in the recall of certain names and words. Comprehension of spoken and written language is relatively satisfactory, but non-language performances are generally superior to language performances. The patient, however, has a fairly accurate understanding of a concept even when he cannot produce the name as a

symbol for it, and he can almost always recognize the correct word and select it from a number of terms suggested to him.

Amnesic aphasia is relatively rare. Nielsen and others have postulated the presence of a language formulation center in the posterior temporal region between Wernicke's area and the angular gyrus (the upper parts of areas 22 and 37), where engrams are stored for both visual and auditory memory of words, and have expressed the belief that a lesion here, or interruption of the association pathways, causes amnesic aphasia. This variety of aphasia, however, is extremely difficult to differentiate from the oral expressive type, and it must be concluded that amnesic aphasia, if it does exist as an entity, is probably caused by a diffuse rather than a focal lesion. **Semantic aphasia,** in which there is a quantitative reduction in the capacity for comprehension of speech, with lack of recognition of the full significance of words and phrases, may be related to amnesic aphasia. It is rarely associated with focal lesions, and is found in toxic, degenerative, and fatigue states.

AMUSIA

The loss of the ability to appreciate music may also occur in patients with aphasia or agnosia. Both receptive and expressive amusias have been described. There has been speculation as to the site of the lesion producing amusia, and the evaluation of it is hindered by the fact that the patient must not have any significant other type of dysphasia that hinders evaluation, and must have had a premorbid appreciation of music. Also, the examiner must have some degree of appreciation of music to assess the patient. Wertheim describes a comprehensive test for the evaluation of amusia. Different features of musical ability appear to be distributed between the two hemispheres; thus, elements of amusia may develop from lesions of either.

AGNOSIA

Agnosias of all types are characterized by loss of the ability to comprehend the meaning or to recognize the importance of various types of stimulation; these are actually receptive defects. Gnosis is the higher synthesis of sensory impulses, with resulting appreciation and perception of stimuli. Auditory and visual agnosias in which there is loss of recognition of symbols that have to do with language are essentially aphasias, but other receptive defects in the nonlanguage field also have diagnostic importance.

There are varieties of agnosia in which the receptive defect involves the inability to identify stimuli, even though they are perceived. Such stimuli may be cutaneous or postural. **Astereognosis,** or **tactile agnosia,** is the loss of power to perceive the shape and nature of superficial contact alone, in the absence of any demonstrable sensory defect. Although the term tactile agnosia is used, there is a defect in the higher correlation of proprioceptive sensations as well. Astereognosis follows lesions of the parietal lobe, principally in the cortex of the posterior portions and the superior parietal lobule, although occasionally in the thalamic radiations. There is no cerebral dominance in the interpretation of cutaneous and proprioceptive stimuli, and the defect is always contralateral to the lesion. Some observers use the term astereognosis for minor defects in which the patient is unable to recognize form, and tactile agnosia for more profound difficulties, which are characterized by loss of the ability to identify objects.

Anosognosia is defined as the ignorance of the existence of disease, and the term has been used specifically to imply the imperception of hemiplegia, or a feeling of depersonalization toward or loss of perception of paralyzed parts of the body. It may vary from a mere imperception of weakness, in which the patient may believe that he can move his paretic limbs in a normal manner, to a lack of concern for the hemiparesis or even denial of its existence. The defect usually follows a lesion of the inferior parietal region in the vicinity of the supramarginal gyrus in the hemisphere that is contralateral to the paralysis, and it usually occurs with a lesion of the nondominant hemisphere, although there have been reports of similar disturbances with involvement of the dominant half of the brain. A lesion of the thalamic radiations may possibly cause the same syndrome. Associated with anosognosia there may be loss of awareness of one half of the body, a feeling of absence of the paralyzed extremities, or unilateral neglect (motor, sensory, and visual) of one side of the body. There may also be anosognosia for blindness and deafness. The term anosognosia has also been used to indicate denial of illness in general and of events in the patient's recent experience, often with associated disorientation and confabulation; this has usually been reported with diffuse cerebral disease (Weinstein and Kahn).

In **autotopagnosia,** or **somatotopagnosia,** there is loss of the power to identify or orient the body or the relation of its individual parts — a defect in body awareness. The patient may have complete loss of personal identification of and amnesia for one limb or one half of the body. He may drop his hand from a table onto his lap and believe that some object has fallen, or he may feel an arm next to his body and be unaware that it is his own. He may be unable to point out the paretic extremities or to distinguish laterality. Lack of awareness of one half of the body has been referred to as agnosia of the body half. Autotopagnosia occurs with lesions of either the thalamoparietal pathways or the cortex bordering on the interparietal sulcus, especially near the angular gyrus. Like anosognosia, it usually occurs with lesions of the nondominant hemisphere, but has been reported also with involvement of the left parietal lobe. Denny-Brown and Banker have reported what they term **amorphosynthesis,** a disorder of recognition of the opposite side of the body and of spatial relationships, with a lesion of the left parietal lobe. Most disturbances with visuospatial relations, however, including visuospatial neglect, occur with right hemisphere lesions.

In the syndrome of **finger agnosia of Gerstmann** there is loss or impairment of the ability to recognize, name, or select individual fingers, either when the patient is looking at them or when the examiner points to them. This may apply to both the patient's and the examiner's fingers. Associated with this are disorientation of right and left (confusion of laterality), agraphia, and acalculia. It has been reported to result from a lesion of the angular gyrus, or of that portion of the parietal lobe between the angular gyrus and the occipital region, in the dominant hemisphere. Partial syndromes, however, and various combinations of its component parts, may occur with focal lesions of other areas in the dominant hemisphere or even with diffuse cerebral disease.

Prosopagnosia, or agnosia for faces, is a perceptual defect of specific nature and may be detected following a lesion of the posterior portion of the minor hemisphere, although usually there are bilateral lesions. There may be associated phenomena, including defects in the contralateral visual field, constructional apraxia, visuospatial defects, and disturbances of the body scheme. Apractic agnosia, usually associated with involvement of the parietooccipital region of the nondominant hemisphere, is a combination of agnostic and apractic defects. In addition to body scheme disturbances of the anosognostic type, there are constructional disabilities, apraxia for dressing, and difficulties with spatial orientation. Those agnosias that are largely visual are discussed under "Receptive Aphasia" and in Chapter 10.

APRAXIA

Apraxia is a defect in the ability to carry out purposive, useful, or skilled acts, especially if complicated; there is loss of the capacity to use objects correctly. Apraxia may be defined as the inability to move a certain part of the body in accordance with a proposed purpose, the motility of the part being otherwise preserved. Sometimes the term **mind blindness** is used as a synonym. Purposive acts are built up by the synthesis of simple individual movements. The performance of complex and skilled motor activity requires intact motor strength and power, normal coordination, and adequate tonus and sensation. In addition, however, the psychic elaboration of an ideational plan must be present before any skilled act can be carried out. The perfect performance of motor activity is known as **eupraxia,** and loss of such performance is **apraxia,** which, of course, cannot be diagnosed if there is paresis or paralysis, ataxia, rigidity, akinesia, hyperkinesia, or sensory loss. One must also exclude, in the diagnosis of apraxia, difficulties due to loss of comprehension, dementia, and auditory and visual defects. Oral expressive aphasia and other varieties of expressive aphasia are probably apractic defects.

Kinetic, or motor, apraxia is the simplest of the apraxias. It usually affects only one limb, principally an upper extremity, although it may be more extensive and include the throat and head region, and it may be bilateral. There is no motor weakness and the extremity can be used for unconscious and associated movements, but not for deliberate, purposeful acts. The patient may be able to carry out activities in which he uses the limb as a whole, but he cannot execute fine motor acts with the individual fingers. He cannot perform movements that he has learned, acquired, and brought to perfection. There is a loss of dexterity that resembles ataxia, and all skilled movements, even those of a simple pattern, are carried out in crude, garbled, unsteady manner; learned acts are performed clumsily, as though for the first time. The difficulty is equally pronounced whether the act is spontaneous, requested, or imitative. The patient is unable to employ objects whose use he understands, even though he can see and recognize the objects, name them, and tell their use.

Kinetic apraxia may be interpreted as an expressive defect. It is in most instances caused by a lesion of the cell groups in the precentral or premotor cortex (areas 4 or 6) that are essential for executing the movement, or of their descending neuraxes. The apraxia is usually contralateral to the lesion; in cases of outstanding cerebral dominance, it may be bilateral. There may be apraxia of the left upper extremity in right-handed persons in association with a cortical lesion that causes paralysis of the right upper extremity, although in many instances damage to both hemispheres is necessary for bilateral apraxia. Kinetic apraxia also has been reported with lesions of the anterior portion of the corpus callosum (Ch. 50). It occurs on the left in right-handed persons with pronounced dominance of the left hemisphere, and is said to result from interruption of the commisural fibers that convey the dominating influence to the right side of the brain. Section of the corpus callosum has been carried out in humans, however, without causing apraxia but causing disturbances in the transfer of information learned by one side of the body to the other. This absence of apraxia has been explained on the basis of either representation of eupractic functions in both hemispheres or ability to use other subcortical pathways. Apraxia of gait (Ch. 32) is probably a kinetic apraxia. There is loss of the ability to use the lower limbs properly in walking, although there is no demonstrable motor weakness or sensory impairment. In addition there often are perseveration, hypokinesia, rigidity, and *gegenhalten*. This occurs with extensive cerebral lesions, usually of the frontal lobes.

Ideokinetic (ideomotor or "classic") apraxia is caused by an interruption of the pathways between the center for formulation of an act and that for execution of the act: there is a break in the continuity of the association fibers between the site where the ideational plan is elaborated and the center that governs the motor mechanism. The idea is correctly formulated, but the plan fails to reach motor expression. The patient can carry out simple movements and spontaneous and automatic acts, but he cannot execute complex movements, either voluntary or imitative, if they require a sequence of muscular activities, or if he has to plan the act before performing it. The patient may be able to perform the constituent parts of an act, but he is unable to synthesize the correct combination of single muscular responses necessary for the execution of a complex movement. He may know what he wishes to do and be able to describe the act, but he is unable to execute the act when he wants to or on command. The patient may button his clothes or comb his hair normally when such acts are carried out automatically, yet he is unable to do these things on request. When asked to throw a kiss he may place the back of his hand to his mouth and may perform sucking rather than kissing movements with his lips. He may be unable to manipulate objects such as a hammer or screwdriver, although he can explain their use. The movements in idiokinetic apraxia, like those of kinetic apraxia, may be crude and incoordinated, and may resemble the motor responses in ataxia and athetosis. The predominance of an apractic element in certain cases of oral expressive aphasia may be demonstrated by noting the patient's inability to protrude his tongue or wet his lips on command, although he can carry out these acts unconsciously and can use these portions of the speech apparatus normally for other purposes and in forming those words that he is able to utter. Loss of ability to sing or to play musical instruments may constitute a musical apraxia.

Idiokinetic apraxia is often bilateral and affects the extremities of both sides equally. It has been ascribed to lesions of the supramarginal gyrus (area 40), the arcuate fasciculus, the motor and premotor areas, and the body of the corpus callosum. The first-named site is probably the most important, and frontal lesions are believed to produce predominantly kinetic varieties of apraxia. A cortical or subcortical lesion of the right supramarginal gyrus may cause idiokinetic apraxia limited to the left side, but a cortical or subcortical lesion of the left supramarginal gyrus produces bilateral apraxia. A lesion of the corpus callosum may cause apraxia on the left in right-handed individuals, owing to interruption of the commissural pathways. Even lesions confined to the basal ganglia and thalamus may cause apractic phenomena.

Ideational, or sensory, apraxia is characterized by loss of the ability to formulate the ideational plan that is necessary for executing the several components of a complex act. It is true mind blindness. Kinesthetic memory and the appreciation of the nature of the act are defective, and as a result the motor mechanism that is essential for its execution cannot be produced. The general conception of the act is incorrect or imperfect. Simple and isolated movements are normal, and the component parts may be executed properly, but they cannot be synthesized into a purposeful plan, and may be performed in the wrong order or in faulty combinations. Consequently, there is a distortion of the entire performance, with incorrect adjustment in space and time of the individual elements. The confusion and disturbance of motor activity resemble those seen in extreme absent-mindedness. In attempting to light a cigarette the patient may strike the match on the wrong side of the box, or he may place the match in his mouth and attempt to strike the cigarette.

Ideational apraxia is actually a variety of agnosia, and it is almost always bilateral. It has been ascribed to focal lesions of the posterior part of the left parietal lobe, the left supramarginal gyrus, and the corpus callosum, but in most instances it is the result of diffuse or bilateral rather than localized cerebral involvement. It occurs most frequently in toxic states and in diffuse cerebral degenerations such as dementia paralytica, multi-infarct dementia, Alzheimer's disease, and others. Symptoms resembling it are sometimes found in neuroses, functional psychoses, fatigue states, and extreme absent-mindedness. If the manifestations are unilateral they are probably symptoms of tactile agnosia rather than ideational apraxia.

The constructional apraxia of Kleist is characterized by loss of visual guidance, impairment of the visual image, and disturbance of revisualization. The patient is unable to guide his movements by vision or by visual memory. He cannot write when his eyes are open, but may be able to write either automatically or by kinesthetic memory when his eyes are closed. He cannot guide his hand in constructing small geometric figures and in building forms with blocks. In drawing the figure of a man he may place the eyes outside of the head. This variety of apraxia is probably caused by interruption of the pathways between the occipital and parietal regions of the brain, usually in the vicinity of the angular gyrus. It may occur with lesions in several locations of either hemisphere, but is more frequent and more severe if they are right-sided.

Apraxia for dressing may also be a specific type of loss of purposive movement, although it is probably a blend of apraxia and agnosia. The lesion responsible is in the parietooccipital region, usually on the right side. This is combined with constructional, anosognostic, and visual difficulties in the syndrome of apractic agnosia.

SUMMARY

Aphasia, agnosia, and apraxia are important in the diagnosis and localization of intracranial disease, although it is not always possible to localize a lesion clinically by the presence of these difficulties alone. There is still a difference of opinion regarding anatomic features, pathologic physiology, and classification into definite categories. Furthermore, it is not always possible to differentiate the individual types, distinguish between expressive and receptive defects, separate apractic and agnostic elements, and localize specifically the lesion that is causing the difficulty from the neurologic examination alone. Aphasia, agnosia, and apraxia must be regarded as general terms, but individual varieties may indicate the presence of focal involvement of the nervous system. Certain conclusions that aid in diagnosis may be drawn from the following paragraphs.

As was stated, in a large majority of cases aphasia is situated in the dominant, or major, cerebral hemisphere. Unilateral dominance is more marked for language than for nonlanguage functions, and it does not play as great a part in the agnosias and apraxias that are not related to language disabilities. The minor hemisphere is thought to assume some of the functions of the dominant one in the control of speech, but this occurs to a variable degree in different individuals. It does so with great facility in some instances, with difficulty in others, and not at all in some. This bilaterality of speech functions, or compensatory action of the opposite hemisphere, is important both in the development of and in the recovery from aphasia.

Various centers have been described that are important in the regulation of language function. These are widely separated in the cortex of the dominant cerebral hemisphere (see Fig. 52-1). These centers are not areas that have an isolated function, but they are regions that are more important than the surrounding portions of the cortex in the performance of certain activities. Furthermore, they can never function alone, but only in cooperation with each other and with other parts of the brain. It is not possible, in most instances, from clinical examination alone, to state whether the process that causes an aphasic defect is cortical, subcortical, or transcortical. A small, localized lesion may on occasion result in

a widespread loss of the various elements of speech function, whereas destruction of a large area may cause impairment of only one phase of either expression or interpretation. Even though there may be complete loss of volitional and propositional speech, due to a lesion of the dominant hemisphere, emotional speech may be retained, possibly as a function of the opposite hemisphere.

The centers that govern motor activity and the expressive elements of language are situated in the motor region of the brain, anterior to the rolandic fissure. Many cases of purely oral aphasia have been observed in which the lesion was localized to Broca's area, and cases of expressive aphasia involving writing and drawing in which the lesions were situated just above this site. Similar disabilities, however, have been found occasionally in patients with lesions in the temporal and parietal lobes. The centers that have to do with interpretation and with receptive elements of language are situated posterior to the rolandic fissure, in the temporal, parietal, and occipital lobes. Many cases of visual receptive aphasia have been studied in which the lesion was localized to the region of the angular gyrus, and of auditory receptive aphasia with the lesion restricted to the superior temporal convolution. Abnormalities of comprehension of written and spoken language, difficult to differentiate from visual and auditory receptive aphasia may, however, be caused by more anterior lesions.

The agnosias, other than those concerned with vision and audition, are somewhat less well localized; they are mainly the result of parietal lobe lesions, and the symptoms are contralateral to the side of cerebral involvement. Syndromes characterized by disturbance of the body scheme of an anosognostic type, however, are usually the result of lesions of the nondominant parietal area, although the syndrome of finger agnosia usually occurs with involvement of the parietooccipital region on the dominant side. The localization of the apraxias is not as specific as that of the aphasias, but it may be said that the motor apraxias are the result of lesions anterior to the rolandic fissure, whereas sensory apraxias follow involvement posterior to this fissure. Kinetic apraxia is usually associated with a lesion of the precentral gyrus, idiokinetic apraxia with a lesion of the parietal lobe, especially the supramarginal gyrus, and ideational apraxia with diffuse brain involvement, but variations may occur with all of these localizations. The relationship of the corpus callosum to the apraxias is still disputed, and there is a possibility that any one of the varieties may be caused by a callosal lesion. Cerebral dominance probably plays a major part only in idiokinetic apraxia, although kinetic apraxia of the left upper extremity has been reported in right-handed individuals with cortical lesions that cause paralysis of the right upper extremity. There is a possibility that some instances of ideational apraxia, which is essentially an agnosia, may follow lesions of the left parietal lobe, especially the supramarginal gyrus.

A careful and detailed examination is indicated whenever the presence of aphasia, agnosia, or apraxia is suspected. It is important to bear in mind that nonorganic causes may produce symptoms that resemble those of aphasia. Fatigue states, drug ingestion, and hysterical processes may cause language defects that simulate aphasia, and the disorganized speech that is apparent in many of the functional psychoses is often difficult to differentiate from a specific disability of language function. In diffuse organic brain disease, too, there may be difficulties with speech, and paraphasic defects that resemble those encountered in some aphasias may be seen. In both functional and organic psychoses, however, there usually are associated changes in behavior, orientation, and mood. On the other hand, a patient with either an expressive or receptive aphasia may be thought to be psychotic because of his irrelevant and disorganized speech. A definite diagnosis of aphasia, agnosia, or apraxia is not always possible in the presence of confusion, lowered consciousness, dementia, or amentia. On the whole, however, unless the involvement is extensive or there are multiple cerebral lesions, there need be no definite or permanent impairment of higher intellectual functions, memory, or judgment in the aphasic patient, even though a superficial appraisal may suggest the presence of marked intellectual deterioration. The apraxias, especially the ideational varieties which are usually the result of diffuse lesions, are often accompanied by intellectual impairment.

In the study of the aphasic, the apractic, and the agnostic patient, neurology meets psychiatry, physiology meets psychology, and clinical evaluation and judgment are extremely important.

BIBLIOGRAPHY

Adams RD, Victor M. Principles of Neurology, 4th ed. New York, McGraw – Hill, 1989

Akelaitis AJ. A study of gnosis, praxis and language following section of the corpus callosum and anterior commissure. J Neurosurg 1944;1:94

Alajouanine T. Verbal realization in aphasia. Brain 1956;79:1

Alajouanine T, Lhermitte F. Acquired aphasia in children. Brain 1965;88:653

Alexander MP, Naeser MA, Palumbo C. Broca's area aphasias: Aphasia after lesions including the frontal operculum. Neurology 1990;40:353

Bay E. Aphasia and non-verbal disorders of language. Brain 1962;85:411

Benson DF, Geschwind N. The aphasias and related disturbances. In Joynt RJ (ed). Clinical Neurology. Philadelphia, JB Lippincott, 1989

Benton AL. Right-left Discrimination and Finger Localization: Development and Pathology. New York, PB Hoeber, 1959

Brain R. Speech disorders: Aphasia, Apraxia, Agnosia. Washington, DC, Butterworth's, 1961

Brain R. The neurology of language. Brain 1961;84:145

Brown JR, Simonson J. A clinical study of 100 aphasic patients. I. Observations on lateralization and localization of lesions. Neurology 1957;7:777

Buchman AS, Garron DC, Trost – Cardamone JE, Wichter MD et al. Word deafness: One hundred years later. J Neurol Neurosurg Psychiatry 1986;49:489

Chesher EC. Aphasia. I. Technique of clinical examination. Bull Neurol Inst NY 1937;6:134

Critchley M. The Parietal Lobes. London, Edward Arnold & Co, 1953

Critchley M. Developmental Dyslexia. London, W Heinemann Medical Books, 1964

Denny – Brown D. The nature of apraxia. J Nerv Ment Dis 1958;126:9

Denny – Brown D, Banker BQ. Amorphosynthesis from left parietal lesion. Arch Neurol Psychiatry 1954;71:302

DeRenzi E, Faglioni P, Scarpa M, Crisi G. Limb apraxia in patients with damage confined to the left basal ganglia and thalamus. J Neurol Neurosurg Psychiatry 1986;49:1030

DeReuck AVS, O'Connor W (eds). Ciba Foundation Symposium. Disorders of Language. Boston, Little, Brown & Co, 1964

Eisenson J. Examining for Aphasia, 2nd ed. New York, Psychological Corp, 1954

Ettlinger G, Jackson CV, Zangwill OL. Cerebral dominance in sinistrals. Brain 1956;79:569

Freud S. On Aphasia: A Critical Study. New York, International Universities Press, 1953

Gall FJ, Spurzheim JC. Anatomie et Physiologie du Systeme Nerveux en General et du Cerveau en Particulier (4 vols). Paris, F Schoell, 1810 – 1819

Gerstmann J. Fingeragnosie: Eine Umschreibene Störung der Orientierung am Eigenen Körper. Klin Wochenschr 1924;37:1010

Gerstmann J. Some notes on the Gerstmann syndrome. Neurology 1957;7:866

Geschwind N. Disconnection syndromes in animals and man. Brain 1965;88:237, 585

Geschwind N. Aphasia. N Engl J Med 1971;284:654

Geschwind N, Sheremata WA, Bouchard R et al. Conduction

aphasia: A clinicopathological study. Arch Neurol 1973;28:339

Goldstein K. Language and Language Disturbances. New York, Grune & Stratton, 1948

Goodglass H, Quadfasel FA. Language laterality in left-handed aphasics. Brain 1954;77:521

Graff – Redford NR, Welsh K, Godersky J. Callosal apraxia. Neurology 1987;37:100

Granich L. Aphasia: A Guide to Retraining. New York, Grune & Stratton, 1947

Halstead WC, Wepman JM. The Halstead – Wepman aphasia screening test. J Speech Dis 1949;14:9

Head H. Aphasia and Kindred Disorders of Speech. Cambridge, MA,: The University Press, 1926

Hecaen H, De Ajuriaguerra J. Left Handedness: Manual Superiority and Cerebral Dominance. New York, Grune & Stratton, 1964

Hecaen H, Angelergues R. Agnosia for faces (prosopagnosia). Arch Neurol 1962;7:92

Heimburger RG, Reitan RM. Easily administered written test for lateralizing brain lesions. J Neurosurg 1961; 18:301

Kennedy F, Wolf A. The relationship of intellect to speech defect in aphasic patients, with illustrative cases. N Nerv Ment Dis 1936;84:125, 293

Kertesz A. Classification of aphasic phenomena. Can J Neurol Sci 1976;3:135

Lhermitte F, Gautier JC. Aphasia. In Vinken PJ, Bruyn GW, Critchley M et al (eds). Disorders of Speech, Perception, and Symbolic Behavior. Handbook of Clinical Neurology, vol 4. Amsterdam, North Holland, 1969

Monrad – Krohn GH. The prosodic quality of speech and its disorders. Acta Psychiatr Scand 1947;22:255

Mountcastle VB (ed). Interhemispheric Relations and Cerebral Dominance. Baltimore, Johns Hopkins Press, 1962

Nielsen JM. Agnosia, Apraxia, Aphasia: Their Value in Cerebral Localization, 3nd ed. New York, PB Hoeber, 1946

Penfield W, Roberts L. Speech and Brain Mechanisms. Princeton, Princeton University Press, 1959

Piercy M, Smyth VOG. Right hemisphere dominance for certain non-verbal skills. Brain 1962;85:775

Riese W. The early history of aphasia. Bull Hist Med 1947;21:322

Russell WR, Espir MEL. Traumatic Aphasia: A Study of Aphasia in War Wounds of the Brain. London, Oxford University Press, 1961

Schuell HM. Minnesota Test for Differential Diagnosis of Aphasia (research edition). Minneapolis, University of Minnesota Press, 1955

Schuell HM. A short examination for aphasia. Neurology 1957;7:625

Schuell HM, Jenkins JJ, Jimenez – Pabon E. Aphasia in Adults: Diagnosis, Prognosis, and Treatment. New York, Hoeber Medical Division, Harper & Row, 1964

Subirana A. The prognosis in aphasia in relation to cerebral dominance and handedness. Brain 1958;81:415

Symonds C. Aphasia. J Neurol Neurosurg Psychiatry 1953;16:16

Tanridag O, Kirshner HS. Aphasia and agraphia in lesions of the posterior internal capsule and putamen. Neurology 1985;35:1797

Watson RT, Heilman KM. Callosal apraxia. Brain 1983;106:391

Weinstein EA, Kahn RL. The syndrome of anosognosia. Arch Neurol Psychiatry 1950;64:772

Weisenburg TH, McBride KE. Aphasia: A Clinical and Psychological Study. New York, Commonwealth Fund, 1935

Wepman JM, Jones LV. Studies in Aphasia: An Approach to Testing. Chicago, Education – Industry Service, 1961

Wertheim M. The amusias. In Vinken PJ, Bruyn GW, Critchley M et al (eds). Disorders of Speech, Perception, and Symbolic Behavior. Handbook of Clinical Neurology, vol 4. Amsterdam, North Holland, 1969

Wilson SAK. Aphasia. London, K Paul, Trench, Trubner & Co, Ltd, 1926

Zangwill OL. Cerebral Dominance and Its Relation to Psychological Function. Springfield, IL, Charles C Thomas, 1960

Chapter 53
DIFFERENTIAL DIAGNOSIS OF INTRACRANIAL DISEASE

The differential diagnosis of intracranial disease depends upon a thorough knowledge of the anatomy and physiology of the cerebrum, including both the cortical and subcortical structures and the blood supply of each, together with a familiarity with the changes in function that may be brought about by various pathologic processes. Not only must the presence and localization of an intracranial lesion be established but also its nature and etiology must be determined before treatment can be suggested and prognosis can be evaluated.

Disease of the brain, like disease of other portions of the body, may be caused by neoplasms, vascular damage, infection, trauma, toxic substances, metabolic changes, degenerative processes, and developmental disturbances. These various pathologic processes may cause not only focal damage resulting in disturbed function of one or more areas, but also alteration of function of neighboring or adjacent areas by edema and pressure. Certain processes appear to involve wide areas of the cerebrum, causing diffuse dysfunction. In addition, certain types of intracranial disease may produce increased intracranial pressure; subjectively this may be manifested by the presence of headaches of increasing severity, nausea, vertigo, vomiting, visual loss, and drowsiness, and objectively by papilledema, ocular muscle palsies, and slowing of the pulse rate. If there is a marked increase in intracranial pressure there may be elevation (or in later stages decline) of the blood pressure, slowing of the respiratory rate, apathy, stupor, generalized convulsions, and coma. In children there may be a "cracked-pot" resonance (Mace-

wen's sign, a clear, drum-like sound when the head is percussed), enlargement of the head, or separation of the sutures. In infants, the fontanelles may bulge. Pressure by the edematous brain in the region of either the incisura of the tentorium cerebelli or the foramen magnum may cause signs of false localization.

The first procedures to be carried out in the differential diagnosis of intracranial disease are those which are essential to the diagnosis of any neurologic condition. The examiner should obtain a detailed history, and follow this by physical and mental examinations and a careful neurologic appraisal. The history may give significant information. With cerebrovascular disease there is often a sudden onset of symptoms that is followed by either complete or incomplete recovery or death; occasionally the symptoms are transitory, or there may be recurring small episodes with usually a gradual increase in severity. With trauma and acute infections, as with cerebrovascular disease, the onset is sudden, followed by variable degrees of recovery or by death; with some infections, however, there may be prodromata and a progressive course. With neoplasms and degenerative diseases the symptoms and signs are usually progressive in character, although occasionally the onset is abrupt. In multiple sclerosis there may be remissions followed by exacerbations of increasing severity. The importance of the history in the differential diagnosis in such conditions as headaches and convulsive disorders is stressed in Chapter 2.

Under most circumstances it is necessary to resort to ancillary diagnostic measures. Roentgenographic or imaging studies are essential in cases of trauma. Plain radiographs may show fractures or displacements of calcified structures; computed tomography or magnetic imaging may show bony lesions, hemorrhages, distortions of the ventricular spaces, edema, or other signs of focal damage. Increased intracranial pressure may be manifested on plain radiographs by increased convolutional markings and erosion of the clinoid processes or of the sella turcica. Magnetic imaging or computed tomography may disclose obliteration of normal cerebral convolutional markings, increased size of the ventricles, or differential blocks in the cerebrospinal fluid spaces. In children with increased intracranial pressure there may be enlargement of the head and separation of the sutures. Localized neoplasms may cause focal areas of erosion on plain radiographs, along with unusual vascular markings, areas of osseous proliferation or hyperostosis, or intrasellar erosion. Intracranial calcifications may be seen in oligodendrogliomas, astrocytomas (rarely), aneurysms, angiomas, hematomas, chronic abscesses, tuberculomas, craniopharyngiomas, and some parasitic diseases. Displacement, or shift, of the calcified pineal gland to one side, or in the anterior, posterior, upward, or downward direction is often the result of a focal mass lesion.

Magnetic imaging and computed tomography have largely replaced plain roentgenograms in the diagnosis of intracranial masses, be they neoplastic, infectious, or hemorrhagic. For most mass lesions, magnetic imaging produces a more precise demonstration than does computed tomography; however, intracerebral hemorrhage is exquisitely shown on computed tomographs. Radioactive brain scanning has been largely abandoned in the diagnosis of intracranial masses, but is helpful in the demonstration of differential blood flow and focal perfusion if used in the technic of single photon emitted computed tomography.

Pneumoencephalography, ventriculography, and echoencephalography are no longer in routine use for intracranial diagnosis. Examination of the cerebrospinal fluid is often essential in the diagnosis of intracranial disease but should usually be postponed until imaging procedures have ruled out the presence of a focal mass, and lumbar puncture should be performed only when there is a definite indication for this procedure.

Other ancillary diagnostic procedures often add information that is important to the understanding of the disease process and to diagnosis and differential diagnosis as well as to localiza-

tion. Electroencephalography helps with the evaluation of epilepsy or the presence of abnormal paroxysmal discharges, focal or generalized. It also aids in determining the presence of focal nonparoxysmal disturbances such as masses or infarcts, but its specificity is not great for these purposes. It helps to establish the presence of diffuse encephalopathy and its severity. It can also aid in the determination of brain death. Evoked potentials, discussed with the cranial nerves and sensory systems, have a limited role in the assessment of the integrity of the visual, auditory, and sensory pathways and in the determination of brain death.

Angiography gives relevant information in the interpretation of both extracranial and intracranial vascular disease, as well as in determining the presence or absence of aneurysms and the vascular changes associated with neoplastic disease.

Positron emission tomography is primarily a research tool for investigation of abnormalities, focal or diffuse, of cerebral blood flow and metabolism.

Doppler blood flow studies and related ultrasound studies help with the evaluation of the large vessels in the neck, and to a lesser extent of the intracranial ones, and magnetic imaging can demonstrate some intraluminal vascular lesions.

Cerebral biopsy may be used for the diagnosis of tumors and to distinguish various types of cerebral degenerations. It can also help diagnose herpes simplex encephalitis, and, rarely, other infectious processes. This technic is used infrequently, and only when it is believed that information essential to therapy may be obtained.

The differential diagnosis of the various causes of headaches alone constitutes one of the most important problems in the identification of intracranial disease. A headache, it must be recognized, is a symptom and not a disease, and it is always essential to determine the cause of the symptom. Individuals react differently to headaches, and some have a special susceptibility to them. Migraine, for example, affects 10% – 20% of the population to some degree, and may be familial. Many etiologies and mechanisms of headaches have to be considered, some of the more important of which are distention or dilation of extracranial or intracranial arteries, contraction or irritation of the muscles and fasciae in the cervical and suboccipital regions, irritation of the pain-afferent cervical and cranial nerves or neuralgias of these nerves, inflammation or irritation of the basal meninges, focal intracranial disease, disease of other structures in the region of the head and neck (eyes, ears, nose, paranasal sinuses, throat, teeth, cervical spine), systemic disease (infections, allergy, anemia or polycythemia, endogenous or exogenous toxins), and psychogenic or conversion mechanisms. For the accurate diagnosis of the cause of a headache, especially if it is of a chronic or recurring type, not only a detailed history and thorough physical and neurologic examination are necessary, but also, in some cases, examination of the eyes, ears, paranasal sinuses, and teeth, tests for allergies, psychologic studies, cerebral imaging procedures, cerebrospinal fluid examination, and, on occasion, certain of the other ancillary procedures previously listed.

INTRACRANIAL NEOPLASMS

The term intracranial neoplasm is used to designate all tumors that involve the structures within the skull; it includes intrinsic neoplasms of the brain substance, meninges, cranial nerves, and pituitary and pineal glands, as well as metastatic tumors that affect these structures and neoplasms of the skull that invade the intracranial space. The symptoms and signs of such tumors depend upon their location, expansile nature, and pathologic peculiarities, as well as upon their tendency to cause an increase in intracranial pressure. Their prognosis depends upon their pathologic characteristics, location, accessibility to surgery, response to radiation and chemotherapy, as well as upon the extent of involvement of important intracranial structures and the stage at which the diagnosis is made; early diagnosis is, of course, important. Their onset is usually insidious but occasionally, as in the case of the glioblastoma multiforme, is abrupt.

Focal manifestations of intracranial tumors include irritative phenomena such as jacksonian or generalized convulsive seizures, and symptoms of destruction such as progressive paralysis. They may cause motor, sensory, auditory, visual, olfactory, gustatory, mental, endocrine, or hypothalamic disturbances, as well as cranial nerve dysfunctions. Tumors arising in "silent areas" may reach considerable size before they become apparent. The majority of the intracranial tumors in adults (except for acoustic neurinomas) arise above the tentorium cerebelli, whereas the majority of tumors in children (except for craniopharyngiomas) arise below the tentorium. The expansile nature of neoplasms, as well as their tendency to block the circulation of the cerebro-

spinal fluid and interfere with its absorption, causes symptoms and signs of increased intracranial pressure.

Important early symptoms and signs of intracranial neoplasms include the following: enlargement of the head, spreading of the sutures, bulging fontanelles, and Macewen's sign in infancy and early childhood; vomiting without apparent cause in childhood; headaches, progressive paralysis, and either focal or generalized convulsions that have their onset in adult life; failing vision in all age groups; mental and personality changes. Headaches, when present, need not necessarily be severe, and may be either focal or diffuse. The presence of minimal but early neurologic signs is important in diagnosis. These include slight alterations in the visual fields, reflex inequality, minor cranial nerve dysfunction, and early manifestations of papilledema. The later signs of marked increase of intracranial pressure are listed earlier in this chapter.

Approximately 50% of all intracranial neoplasms belong to the glioma group (Fig. 53-1). These neoplasms, which are primary tumors of the brain substance, have been subdivided variously by neuropathologists and neurosurgeons, and their nomenclature is still disputed. They arise in various regions of the brain and are composed of cells of neuroectodermal origin, some of which are glial, others neuronal. The individual tumors of this group are characterized by excessive proliferation of either embryonic cells or adult supporting or neuronal cells, or a mixture of the two. All are malignant, but some more so than others. They are usually classified according to their histogenesis, which gives some information regarding both growth history and degree of malignancy. Correlation of the histopathology, clinical manifestations, and usual localization of each has made it possible to learn much about their course and prognosis.

The astrocytoma is the most common primary intracerebral neoplasm, and constitutes about one third of the gliomas. It is intermediate in rapidity of growth and degree of malignancy. Astrocytomas have been classified microscopically as fibrillary and protoplasmic; they are found predominantly in the cerebral hemispheres of adults and the cerebellar hemispheres of children. Astroblastomas are composed of relatively primitive and rapidly growing cells, and consequently are more malignant; they occur principally in the cerebral hemispheres. The glioblastoma multiforme (astrocytoma grade IV) is one of the most malignant neoplasms of the

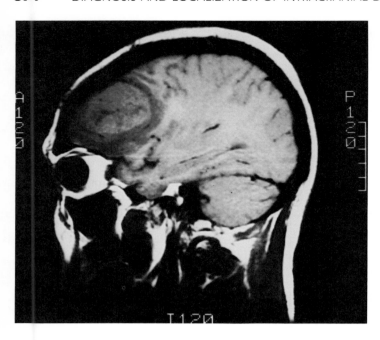

FIG. 53–1. Parasagittal cerebral magnetic resonance image (TR 700, TE 20) of a patient with a large frontal lobe glioma (top left) with necrotic and cystic (dark) components.

brain; it also is a common glioma. Tumors of this type are composed of primitive, rapidly growing cells; they often have a dramatic and sudden onset within the white matter of the cerebral hemispheres and usually progress rapidly to a fatal termination.

Oligodendrogliomas grow fairly slowly and are of low malignancy. These tumors often contain areas of calcification; they can sometimes be diagnosed or suspected and localized by plain roentgenograms of the skull. Spongioblastoma polare is of intermediate malignancy, but, as it usually occurs in portions of the nervous system that are relatively inaccessible to surgery, prognosis is poor. In children these tumors are frequently present in the region of the optic nerves and chiasm and are often referred to as optic nerve gliomas; in adults they occur in the region of the brain stem, the corpus callosum, and the undersurface of the cerebral hemispheres. Medulloblastomas are very malignant tumors that show a predilection for the region of the roof plate of the fourth ventricle in children, and cause the midline cerebellar syndrome (Ch. 24). They sometimes metastasize, especially to the spinal cord and nerve roots. Medulloblastomas comprise about 15% of the gliomas.

Other tumors of the glioma group include ependymomas, pinealomas, ganglioneuromas, neuroblastomas, medulloepitheliomas, neuroepitheliomas, and papillomas of the choroid plexus. Ependymomas, like medulloblastomas,

have a predilection for the roof plate of the fourth ventricle and may cause midline cerebellar syndromes, although they also originate in the cerebrum, brain stem, and spinal cord. They may seed along the neuraxis. Pinealomas, which usually arise in the region of the pineal gland, are often classed with the gliomas; they are relatively rare, usually occur in males between the ages of 15 and 25 years, and often press upon the superior colliculi and give rise to the pineal, or Parinaud's, syndrome, with paresis of upward gaze and disturbances of pupillary responses. Pinealomas also cause autonomic symptoms because of pressure on the hypothalamus, and signs of rapidly increasing intracranial pressure owing to early obstruction of the sylvian aqueduct. Pubertas praecox, which has often been described in association with pinealomas, is probably the result of pressure on the ventromedial and lateral tuberal nuclei of the hypothalamus and on the mammillary bodies.

The meningiomas are relatively benign tumors that make up about 16% of all intracranial neoplasms. They produce symptoms and signs by pressure on the brain and only rarely turn malignant and actually infiltrate it. Accordingly, their prognosis is better than that for tumors of the glioma group, although the technical aspects of surgical removal may be difficult because of their vascularity, great size, and tendency to involve the major dural sinuses. The clinical course is usually long so that the tumor may have attained great size before it is recognized, although computed tomography and magnetic resonance imaging have permitted earlier diagnosis in many instances. Meningiomas usually arise from the arachnoid granulations. The bones of the skull in juxtaposition to them may show either erosion or thickening with localized hyperostosis on plain roentgenograms. There may be tenderness to pressure or percussion of the skull over their location. Irrespective of their exact histologic origin, architecture, and cell type they produce characteristic syndromes that are dependent upon the sites of development and that may be classified regionally. They are usually supratentorial.

Olfactory groove meningiomas arise from the cribriform plate area of the ethmoid bone and produce a clinical syndrome that is characterized by bilateral anosmia, often with optic atrophy on one side and papilledema on the other (the Foster–Kennedy syndrome, Ch. 9). Sphenoidal ridge meningiomas may grow either forward under the frontal lobe to the orbital plate or backward into the middle fossa; they produce unilateral proptosis, papilledema, and anosmia, and often cause temporal lobe manifestations with a hemianopic visual field defect and uncinate attacks. Parasagittal meningiomas arise from the wall of the superior longitudinal sinus and may be attached to the falx cerebri as well; they are manifested clinically by a progressive

spastic paresis of one or both lower extremities, with, in addition, jacksonian convulsive seizures that originate in one or both feet, and problems with bladder control. Meningiomas that arise in the foramina of the individual cranial nerves affect most frequently the eighth, second, and fifth nerves. A meningioma in the region of the eighth cranial nerve may cause a clinical syndrome that cannot be distinguished from that of the acoustic neurinoma (Fig. 53-2). Tumors that arise from the arachnoid sheath of the optic nerve, even in the orbit itself, produce a unilateral, painless exophthalmos with primary optic atrophy. Such lesions are easily visualized by imaging studies. Meningiomas that arise in association with the trigeminal nerve may involve the gasserian ganglion and cause pain and sensory change in the distribution of the individual divisions of the nerve, and often motor changes as well. Meningiomas of the tuberculum sellae may cause a syndrome that simulates that of either a pituitary adenoma or a craniopharyngeal duct tumor, with bitemporal hemianopia, bilateral optic atrophy, and endocrine changes. Meningiomas en plaque consist of sheetlike proliferations that are usually found at the base of the brain.

Acoustic neurinomas constitute from 5% to 10% of all intracranial tumors. They arise from the perineurium of the eighth cranial nerve near to or within the internal acoustic meatus and

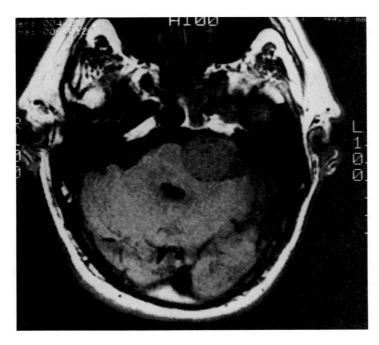

FIG. 53–2. Magnetic resonance image (TR 600, TE 20) of the posterior fossa of a patient with a large left cerebellopontine angle tumor, likely an acoustic neurinoma or meningioma. Lesion is just to the right of center of the figure.

cause the characteristic cerebellopontine angle syndrome. Tinnitus and progressive deafness are usually the first symptoms, and may be present for a long period before other manifestations are noted. Other symptoms include numbness and/or pain of the ipsilateral side of the face (trigeminal nerve involvement), a peripheral facial palsy (seventh nerve), attacks of vertigo (vestibular portion of the acoustic nerve), ipsilateral cerebellar signs (involvement of either the cerebellum or the cerebellar peduncles), and an ipsilateral sixth nerve palsy. There may be dysphagia and dysarthria (affection of the bulbar nerves). Following these manifestations there are signs of increased intracranial pressure with headaches, papilledema, and vomiting. The fully developed syndrome consists of the following objective manifestations: nerve deafness with absence of the labyrinthine response; facial weakness; cerebellar signs; loss of the corneal reflex. The lesion may be demonstrated in the internal acoustic foramen by imaging technics. The tumor has been variously described as a neuroma, neurinoma, neurofibroma, perineural fibroblastoma, and Schwannoma. It may be a manifestation of von Recklinghausen's disease, or neurofibromatosis (type II), a familial disorder; sometimes there may be bilateral such neoplasms in persons with this disease. These tumors of the cerebellopontine angle are usually encapsulated and are relatively benign. The prognosis is good if the diagnosis is established early, but surgical removal is difficult in late stages.

Blood vessel tumors include angiomas, hemangiomas, and hemangioblastomas. Angiomas of the cerebral hemispheres may be accompanied by unilateral facial nevi in the distribution of the ophthalmic nerve or in the distribution of the maxillary branch of the trigeminal nerve (Sturge – Weber syndrome, Weber – Dimitri disease, or encephalotrigeminal angiomatosis). Angiomas of the retina (von Hippel's disease) may be accompanied by hemangioblastomas of the cerebellum (von Hippel – Lindau disease). Angiomas present fairly typical characteristics on imaging studies. On plain roentgenograms in Sturge – Weber syndrome there are calcium deposits within the cerebral cortex.

Tumors of the hypophysis may be of various types. They frequently impinge on the optic chiasm and cause bi-temporal hemianopia and bilateral optic atrophy as well as signs of endocrine dysfunction. Adenomas commonly affect the anterior lobe. With chromophobe adenomas, which are the most frequent, there are signs of

hypopituitarism, with amenorrhea in the female and loss of potency and libido in the male; in both sexes there are other endocrine changes, with loss of body hair, alterations in the skin, and obesity. Acidophilic (eosinophilic) adenomas produce the syndrome of acromegaly, with increase in the size of the skull, jaw, and hands, and a generalized osseous overgrowth that results in gigantism; these changes are also accompanied by amenorrhea and loss of potency. With basophilic adenomas there are manifestations of Cushing's syndrome, with obesity, hypertension, cyanosis, hypertrichosis, and abdominal striae. Both the chromophobe and acidophilic adenomas are characterized by a cellular proliferation and an increase in the size of the gland. Since the hypophysis is confined by a capsule of dura mater and the bony structure of the sella turcica, these tumors immediately meet with resistance to their growth. The walls of the sella turcica become eroded and thinned by constant pressure, and the sella becomes greatly enlarged. The capsule of dura mater becomes greatly distended, and as the tumor bulges upward it produces pressure on the optic chiasm, at first from below and behind, so that the characteristic bitemporal, upper quadrantic visual field defect is produced. Later, there is a bitemporal hemianopia, and finally, complete blindness, often with optic atrophy; occasionally there are homonymous defects. The intrasellar erosion may be diagnosed by imaging procedures or even plain roentgenograms of the skull, but often the lesion can be identified before it reaches great size because of its endocrine and neurologic manifestations and the abnormalities of blood and other endocrine tests secondary to it.

Craniopharyngiomas include those tumors that have also been known as hypophyseal duct tumors, suprasellar or epithelial cysts, Rathke's pouch neoplasms, and adamantinomas. They are of congenital origin and arise from cell rests in the region of the sella turcica; they become manifest most frequently in childhood or young adult life. There are signs of hypophyseal dysfunction, often with a Fröhlich's syndrome (adiposogenital dystrophy), together with signs of pressure on the optic nerves or chiasm, stimulation or paralysis of important hypothalamic structures, and hydrocephalus due to obstruction of the foramen of Monro. These lesions often have elements of calcification and cyst formation. They are easily visible on imaging procedures (Fig. 53-3), preferably with coronal views. Other congenital tumors include dermoid

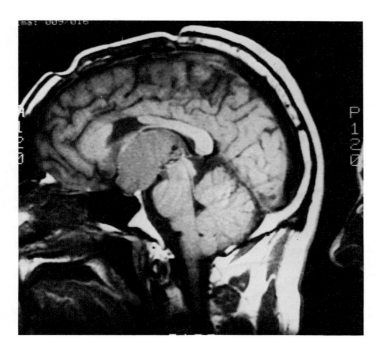

FIG. 53–3. Sagittal cerebral magnetic resonance image (TR 600, TE 20) of a patient after operative attempts to remove a large craniopharyngioma. The large uniform mass in the center of the figure, above the pons and below the corpus callosum, is residual tumor.

cysts, colloid cysts, teratomas, cholesteatomas, chordomas, chondromas, and hamartomas. These may be intracerebral, subpial, or intradural in location and may arise in any of the cranial fossae.

Metastatic tumors, which once constituted about 10% – 20% of all intracranial tumors, are encountered with increasing frequency, presumably because of longer lifespan and a resultant increase in the malignancy rate and other factors, including environmental effects. They may be single or multiple. Primary bronchogenic carcinomas are especially likely to metastasize to the brain, but carcinomas of the breast, gastrointestinal tract, thyroid, prostate, or other organs, as well as hypernephromas and sarcomas, may also invade the brain. Melanosarcomas often cause diffuse meningeal and cerebral symptoms. Carcinoma of the nasopharynx or neck may invade the cranial cavity by direct extension and erosion; diffuse cranial nerve palsies may be the earliest symptoms. Meningeal carcinomatosis may give a clinical picture resembling a chronic meningitis. Neoplasms previously considered rare or unusual occur with greater frequency in the central nervous systems of persons with compromised immune systems, including those due to human immunodeficiency virus infections and iatrogenic immune suppression.

Granulomas of various types, including syphilitic gummas, tuberculomas, and granulomas associated with schistosomiasis, actinomycosis, cysticercosis, and echinococcosis may give manifestations of cerebral tumor. Tumors of the bones of the skull, such as osteomas and myelomas, as well as Paget's disease (osteitis deformans) may also affect intracranial structures.

VASCULAR DISEASE

Vascular disease of the brain accounts for much of the organic nervous system disease encountered in the general practice of medicine. The more common syndromes of cerebrovascular disease, both intracranial and extracranial, are discussed in Chapters 51 and 19.

Intracerebral hemorrhage was once regarded as the most common cerebrovascular syndrome, but it is now known to occur less frequently than cerebral infarction. It usually has an abrupt onset. It is often a disease of hypertensive individuals. It may begin during periods of unusual physical exertion or emotional stress; it most commonly affects the deep, or striate, branches of the middle cerebral artery. There may be premonitory symptoms characterized by occipital or nuchal headache, vertigo, syncope, epistaxis, or transient motor or sensory symptoms. There is then a sudden appearance of hemiplegia, and with the larger lesions often coma, shock, a drop in blood pressure, stertorous breathing, and feeble pulse. The prognosis depends on the size and location of the hemorrhage. Small lesions may produce only few symptoms and are being recognized mainly because the imaging procedures are very sensitive in their detection. Intracerebral hemorrhage may also occur in association with anomalies of the blood vessels, trauma (delayed posttraumatic intracerebral hemorrhage, or spät-apoplexie), and blood dyscrasias (leukemia, purpura, hemophilia, polycythemia, sickle cell disease, etc.).

Cerebral infarction may develop either secondary to cerebral thrombosis or to cerebral embolism. Cerebral thrombosis is usually secondary to atherosclerosis, although rare causes include giant cell, poly-, and syphilitic arteritis, ruptured saccular aneurysms, and hematologic disorders. Atherosclerotic plaques tend to form at bifurcations and other sites of narrowing of the arteries, and these may completely occlude the artery. Hypertension aggravates the atherosclerotic process and in addition is associated with special segmental degeneration resulting in involvement of smaller vessels. The onset of symptoms is often more gradual than it is with cerebral hemorrhage, but occasionally it is sudden. There is less apt to be coma or shock. Inasmuch as smaller or terminal vessels may be affected, the symptoms are often focal in character. Cerebral embolism is always secondary to disease elsewhere in the body. In most cases the embolic material consists of a fragment that has broken away from a thrombus within the heart, and there is usually a history of chronic, subacute, or acute cardiac disease. Emboli may also dislodge from atherosclerotic lesions in the neck vessels or even from intracranial proximal vessels. Emboli consisting of tumor cells, air, fat, or infectious material are rare. The embolus usually stops at a bifurcation or other site of arterial narrowing, and occlusion and resulting infarction follow.

Either stenosis or occlusion of the extracranial arteries is responsible for a large percentage of instances of so-called cerebrovascular disease. Brief periods of vascular insufficiency, in the distribution of either the carotid (Ch. 51) or vertebrobasilar (Ch. 19) system, cause episodes of transient cerebral ischemia without infarct formation. These transient ischemic episodes may crescendo and result in cerebral infarction in one third of the cases; they continue without worsening in another third, and they eventually stop in the remaining third. Diffuse cerebrovascular disease may cause a slowly progressive impairment of brain function. Cerebral athero-

sclerosis, hypertensive encephalopathy, progressive occlusion of the internal carotid arteries, systemic diseases such as diabetes mellitus that are accompanied by vascular changes, and the now rare syphilitic endarteritis may cause diffuse brain damage. Multiple focal areas of infarction with nerve cell degeneration, glial infiltration, and focal atrophy, scarring, and cystic degeneration are found at autopsy. Imaging studies or pathologic examination show multiple small (and some larger) infarcts, the so-called lacunes. The onset may be insidious, with transient intermittent or recurring apoplectic attacks of varying severity that are followed by partial recovery, but often the course progresses in a stepwise manner. There may be impairment of circulation in certain regions before the vessels are completely occluded. The most common syndrome, that of progressive mental and intellectual deterioration, is largely manifested by changes in frontal lobe function, the so-called **multi-infarct dementia.** There may also be vertigo, transient periods of loss of consciousness, temporary sensory and motor changes, convulsions, and, especially in hypertensive encephalopathy, headaches.

Hypertensive crisis has become much less common since the introduction of effective antihypertensive therapy. With such crisis, there may be premonitory signs of headache, irritability, fatigue, and lowered consciousness that are followed by the sudden onset of severe headache, drowsiness, vomiting, convulsions, and coma. There is marked edema of the brain, with focal areas of destruction, either miliary or extensive.

In Binswanger's disease, or progressive subcortical encephalopathy, there are multiple small areas of atherosclerotic infarction in the white matter of the brain, with sparing of the cortex. These changes are visible on computed tomography and magnetic resonance images but unfortunately they are not specific or diagnostic. Whether these changes are sufficiently distinctive to deserve a specific eponymic designation continues to be disputed.

Repeated cerebrovascular accidents, affecting first one hemisphere and then the other, may give rise to the syndrome of pseudobulbar palsy.

Syndromes of cerebral anemia and hyperemia have also been described. The former is characterized by vertigo and syncope; the latter, which may result from hypertension, venous obstruction, or polycythemia, is manifested by headache, severe dizziness, focal signs, convulsions, and coma. Leukemia, the lymphomas, and

Hodgkin's disease may also affect the nervous system.

Spontaneous subarachnoid hemorrhage is usually the result of rupture of an aneurysm of one of the branches of the arterial circle of Willis, although it may be caused by trauma, bleeding from a cerebral neoplasm (especially one impinging on the meninges or the ventricles), rupture of a vascular anomaly, blood dyscrasia, or intracerebral or intraventricular hemorrhage. The onset is usually precipitous. The patient develops a sudden, severe headache, often occipital or nuchal. He may state without prompting that the headache felt as if he had been hit on the back of the head by a baseball bat or a brick. The headache may be accompanied by convulsions, obtundation, or coma. Vertigo, vomiting, lethargy, and bradycardia are often present. The principal signs are those of meningeal irritation—stiff neck, Kernig's and Brudzinski's signs, and photophobia. Focal neurologic changes, ocular muscle palsies, papilledema, and retinal as well as subhyaloid hemorrhages may develop. The diagnosis is confirmed by finding blood or xanthochromia in the cerebrospinal fluid, and by imaging or angiography.

Intracerebral angiomas and arteriovenous anomalies may cause convulsions, localized headaches, and focal neurologic signs. They occasionally rupture and cause subarachnoid bleeding; they are a common cause of recurrent subarachnoid hemorrhage in children, adolescents, and young adults. In older adults ruptures of aneurysms are more common causes of subarachnoid hemorrhage than are ruptures of vascular malformations.

Subdural hematomas and hygromas are usually posttraumatic in origin although in many cases no history of trauma is obtained. They may occur immediately after injury or may be delayed. A symptom-free period between the time of injury and development of symptoms is common. Then signs of increased intracranial pressure develop along with signs of focal cerebral involvement. The diagnosis can usually be established by imaging procedures (Fig. 53-4); on occasion arteriography will help in delineating the lesion.

Extradural bleeding is also posttraumatic in origin; there is usually loss of consciousness followed by a brief lucid interval, and then deepening stupor accompanied by signs of increasing intracranial pressure. There is often a dilated pupil, which may not react either to light or in accommodation, on the side of the hemorrhage, with a contralateral hemiplegia. If the mass lesion compresses the opposite cerebral peduncle against the incisura, the hemiplegia may be ipsilateral— a false localizing sign. There may be a fracture line in the region of the middle meningeal artery. Imaging studies demonstrate the hemorrhage.

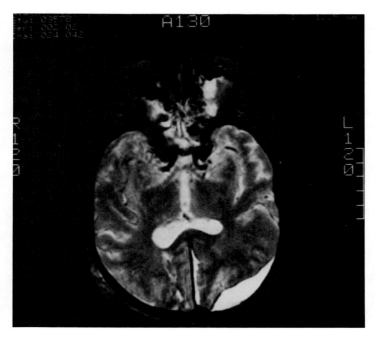

FIG. 53–4. Cerebral magnetic resonance image of a patient with a subacute left occipital subdural hematoma. The lesion is the crescent-shaped white area in the bottom right of the figure.

Diseases of the cerebral veins and venous sinuses are discussed in Chapter 51.

INTRACRANIAL INFECTIONS

Intracranial infections may cause either diffuse or focal involvement, and the infectious process may affect the meninges, the brain tissue, or both. The presentation may be acute, subacute, or chronic. The more severe clinical manifestations of meningitis are usually those of a meningoencephalitis, and some of the diagnostic criteria in the encephalitides are the result of associated meningeal involvement.

Meningitis

Infectious involvement of the pachymeninges is rare. It usually either follows osteomyelitis of the skull associated with disease of the paranasal sinuses or the mastoid air cells, or trauma with extension to the large dural sinuses. There is formation of purulent material in the extradural and subdural spaces, often with extension to the large dural sinuses. The process may spread through the arachnoid to produce a leptomeningitis. Signs of systemic infection (fever, leukocytosis, etc.) are present, together with signs of increased intracranial pressure, and there may be focal cerebral manifestations that appear as a result of thrombosis of the dural sinuses and interference with the venous drainage of the brain. The collections of purulent material may be seen on computed tomography or magnetic resonance imaging. The cerebrospinal fluid pressure may be increased and the fluid may show evidence of meningeal inflammation. Syphilitic pachymeningitis (cervical hypertrophic pachymeningitis) is now rare. It tends to affect the lower cervical spinal cord area, producing atrophy of the hand muscles, and resembles syringomyelia in its other clinical features.

Leptomeningitis is caused by a variety of pathogenic microorganisms. Purulent, or suppurative, meningitis is acute in onset, and is most frequently due to invasion of the meninges by an organism of the coccus group. The meningococcal, pneumococcal, streptococcal, staphylococcal, and Hemophilus varieties are the most important, although Neisseria gonorrheae may also cause a purulent meningitis. In children, Hemophilus influenzae infections predominate. In infants, common organisms include coliforms, streptococci, pseudomonas,

Listeria, and staphylococci. The organisms may gain access to the meninges by any of the following mechanisms: by continuity along the nerve sheaths and cerebrospinal fluid pathways to the subarachnoid space; by direct extension from the nasal passages through the cribriform plate of the ethmoid bone (rhinogenous meningitis); by contiguity from infections of the paranasal sinuses, mastoid cells, and bones of the skull, with production of localized external pachymeningitis, internal pachymeningitis, and then leptomeningitis (rhinogenous and otogenous meningitis); as a consequence of a penetrating injury or compound fracture of the skull (traumatic meningitis); through the blood stream by metastasis from infections elsewhere in the body; or as a result of systemic infections. The onset is sudden, with headache, stiff neck, signs of infection (fever and leukocytosis), and sometimes coma and/or convulsions. There may be irritability, restlessness, photophobia, ocular muscle palsies, and dissociation of extraocular movements, as well as objective manifestations of meningeal irritation with nuchal rigidity and Kernig's and Brudzinski's signs. If the patient is already deeply comatose, or if the process is present in a young infant, the signs of meningeal irritation may not be evident. The cerebrospinal fluid changes consist of marked polymorphonuclear pleocytosis, increase in protein, and decrease in glucose. Often the causative organism can be demonstrated by smear or culture. If, however, any antibiotic therapy has been given before the evaluation of the cerebrospinal fluid, it is usually impossible to demonstrate the organism. Furthermore, prior antibiotic or corticosteroid therapy may mask the typical cerebrospinal fluid findings of purulent meningitis and erroneously suggest a diagnosis of viral meningitis. Counterimmunoelectrophoresis can identify the causative organisms in some such circumstances, as may other serologic methods of antigen detection. Blood cultures may also be helpful at times.

The subacute (nonsuppurative) meningitides are somewhat more gradual in onset than the purulent types, but the clinical manifestations are similar. In tuberculous meningitis the pleocytosis is less marked than that seen in the acute varieties, and there are both lymphocytes and polymorphonuclear cells, but predominantly the former; the changes in the chemistry of the cerebrospinal fluid are similar. In a fairly large percentage of cases the causative organism cannot be demonstrated by direct stain, but in most instances it is detected by either culture or animal inoculation. In the meningitis caused by *Cryptococcus neoformans* (*Torula histolytica*), the most common form of fungal infection of the nervous system, the onset of symptoms is less abrupt than in tuberculous meningitis, but the cerebrospinal fluid picture is similar; the diagnosis is made by finding the organisms in the fluid, preferably by staining them with India ink, or by culturing them on Sabouraud's agar. Many patients have positive serum tests for cryptococcal antigen. Fungal infections, as well as a variety of bacterial, viral, and even parasitic infections of the meningeal spaces are common in immunosuppressed persons, especially those with human immunodeficiency virus infection.

There are many meningitides in which the cerebrospinal fluid response is predominantly a lymphocytic one, with 25 – 50 cells, or even 200 or more per cu mm. There are few other changes in the cerebrospinal fluid, and the course is often benign. These are often called instances of aseptic meningitis because no organism is found in the fluid on direct examination or by the usual culture methods. Many of them are, however, of viral origin, and in some of them the virus has been isolated from the fluid by special technics. In others the virus has been detected in the feces or in nasal and pharyngeal washings, or the diagnosis has been confirmed by rising antibody titers on sequential examinations of the serum. Among the most common causative viruses are the virus of lymphocytic choriomeningitis, the Coxsackie and ECHO viruses, and the viruses of mumps, herpes zoster, and herpes simplex. Poliomyelitis virus, now very rare, and those responsible for the arthropod-borne encephalitides may cause a similar meningeal response.

It is important to remember that signs of meningeal irritation, often with a definite meningitis, may occur in association with systemic diseases of various types. Brucellosis, typhoid fever, malaria, subacute bacterial endocarditis, and other systemic infections may be complicated by meningeal involvement and its signs, as well as by encephalitic manifestations, as discussed later. With brain abscesses, especially if near either the surface of the brain or the ventricles, definite meningeal signs and cerebrospinal fluid alterations may be present. There are moderate meningeal signs in dementia paralytica, and rarely an acute syphilitic meningitis develops with a marked lymphocytic pleocytosis and other signs of meningeal involvement.

Carcinomatous meningitis is being increasingly recognized. Also known as meningeal carcinomatosis, it may occasionally be part of some other disseminated neoplasms. Because of the lymphocytic reaction in the cerebrospinal fluid, along with an increase in the protein content and a decrease in glucose, the illness may be mistaken for a subacute infectious meningitis. With careful staining of the cells, however, and histologic study of the stained sediment, it may be found that some of the cells that were thought to be lymphocytes are, in reality, neoplastic cells. A similar meningeal reaction may occur in association with leukemia and lymphoma. A subacute meningeal reaction may occur in sarcoidosis; there may be associated cranial nerve dysfunction, optic neuritis, and encephalitic manifestations. Acute meningeal symptoms may also be present with infectious mononucleosis. In addition, encephalitic, myelitic, and neuritic involvement may develop. Recurring meningitis, usually bacterial, may be secondary to traumatic cerebrospinal fluid rhinorrhea. A benign recurrent meningitis for which no etiology has been found is known as **Mollaret's meningitis.** Recurring meningitis may be a feature of Behçet's syndrome, of unknown etiology, which also causes recurrent orogenital ulcerations. Lyme disease (borreliosis) may also cause recurring meningeal symptoms.

In both the aseptic meningitis and meningismus there may be objective manifestations that suggest invasion of the meninges. The former occurs when there is a pyogenic infection near the meninges that has not yet invaded them, or as a reaction on the part of the meninges to the introduction of drugs, air, contrast media, etc. There is an increase in the spinal fluid pressure and protein content, often with a marked pleocytosis, but no organisms are detected. The syndrome is probably the result of increased permeability of the perineural and perivenous lymph spaces. Occasionally it is the precursor or first stage of purulent meningitis. Meningismus is a reaction to a systemic infection or febrile illness, usually in children. The spinal fluid pressure is increased, but the fluid itself is normal.

Cystic, adhesive, or **optochiasmatic arachnoiditis** is a focal involvement of the meninges in the region of the optic chiasm; there may be papilledema, loss of vision, ocular muscle palsies, and exophthalmos.

In the syndrome referred to as pseudotumor cerebri (benign intracranial hypertension, brain swelling of unknown cause, or otitic hydrocephalus) there is brain edema leading to an increase in spinal fluid pressure and papilledema, but no pleocytosis. Pseudotumor cerebri is sometimes secondary to thrombosis of the dural sinuses, but other causes seem to be associated with generalized infections, trauma, or metabolic/toxic disturbances.

Encephalitis

Encephalitis, or inflammation of the brain, may be the result of the response of the cerebral tissues to a wide variety of infections, and sometimes to toxins or irritants as well. Some of these clinical and pathologic syndromes are more properly termed encephalopathies; the diagnosis of encephalitis is usually restricted to those diseases in which there is a diffuse, nonpurulent cerebral inflammation that affects principally the gray matter. Following the first World War a widespread epidemic of encephalitis lethargica, or von Economo's encephalitis, occurred. This was characterized in its acute stages by lethargy or other disturbances in the sleep cycle, ocular muscle paresis, fever, headache, confusion and disorientation, either stupor or hyperexcitability, and occasionally hyperkinetic phenomena. There were mild meningeal signs with a moderate pleocytosis in the cerebrospinal fluid. The disease had a high mortality, and many patients seemed to recover but later developed other signs of nervous system damage. In children these sequelae took the form of personality or behavior disorders, and in the adult, parkinsonian manifestations, oculogyric crises, blepharospasms, and other ocular disturbances and hypothalamic changes. The disease is rarely, if ever, diagnosed today. A viral etiology was suspected, but no causal agent was ever isolated.

Epidemic encephalitides that are somewhat similar to the von Economo variety, but are caused by specific viruses that have been identified, occur in all parts of the world. These include St. Louis encephalitis and eastern and western (equine) encephalitis in the United States, Russian spring–summer encephalitis, Japanese B encephalitis, Australian X disease, and many others, including similar diseases in domestic and other animals. The clinical picture varies, depending upon the specific virus involved, the part of the nervous system maximally affected, the age of the patient (the symptoms are more severe in infants and aged persons), and other factors. There may or may not be residuals and sequelae. In most of these encephalitides the neurotropic virus is arthropod-borne, and is transferred to man by mosquitoes and ticks, usually from a reservoir of infection in certain wild and domestic animals

and birds. The diagnosis can be confirmed (usually retrospectively) by complement fixation and neutralization tests. Poliomyelitis and rabies also cause an encephalitis that affects principally the gray matter; in the former, however, the involvement is predominantly in the anterior horn cells of the spinal cord, and in the latter, in the brain stem, rather than in the midbrain, basal ganglia, hypothalamus, or cortex.

Subacute sclerosing panencephalitis is a rare disease of childhood and adolescence characterized by increasing dementia, ataxia, and myoclonus. The course is slowly progressive and death may occur in weeks or months. There may be slight pleocytosis in the spinal fluid and elevated IgG although the total protein content may be normal. Measles antibodies have been demonstrated within nerve cells and inclusion bodies in the brain. High titers for measles antibodies are also present in the blood and spinal fluid. Measles virus is now considered the etiologic agent.

A demyelinating disorder called **progressive multifocal leukoencephalopathy** may develop, usually in debilitated patients with leukemia, lymphomas, and other chronic illnesses. The common denominator is that the patient has an impairment of immunologic responses. Viruses of the papova group have been incriminated. Rapidly progressive neurologic dysfunction with involvement of any portion of the central nervous system may occur. Imaging studies may suggest the diagnosis; there is no effective treatment.

Creutzfeldt – Jakob disease, or subacute spongiform encephalopathy, is a transmissible disease caused by a "slow virus" or subviral particle called prion. The clinical features include dementia with extrapyramidal, corticospinal, and cerebellar signs, myoclonic movements, and fasciculations. The course is progressive, with death usually occurring within one year.

Cytomegalus infection (cytomegalic inclusion body disease) may be a cause of stillbirth or neonatal death. It is a common superinfection of the human immunodeficiency virus syndrome. There is involvement of the brain and also of the kidneys, liver, and other organs. In the congenital variety, cytomegalic disease may cause hydrocephalus, microcephaly, and other developmental defects of the brain. In adults with the immunosuppressive syndromes, cytomegalic disease may present a picture of protean cerebral involvement. There are intranuclear and cytoplasmic inclusion bodies in the involved organs and also in the epithelium of the salivary and pancreatic ducts and elsewhere. The lesions resemble those caused by salivary gland viruses of various animals.

The term encephalitis may also be applied to those instances of cerebral involvement that occur in association with septicemia, inflammatory processes elsewhere in the body, subacute bacterial endocarditis, and pulmonary disease. Pathologically there may be either diffuse involvement or multiple miliary lesions. The now rare dementia paralytica, or syphilitic meningoencephalitis, is a widespread, parenchymatous affection caused by *Treponema pallidum*. Postinfectious and postvaccinial encephalomyelitis is characterized by a diffuse perivascular destruction of nervous tissue, especially the myelinized structures, and pathologically may resemble the demyelinating diseases more closely than the encephalitides. Such demyelinating changes may occur after certain types of vaccination, or in association with smallpox, chickenpox, measles, rubella, mumps, and certain types of pneumonia. They probably result from an immunologic reaction.

A clinical picture suggestive of either meningitis or encephalitis, frequently that of a meningoencephalitis or even a meningoencephalomyelitis, may occur as a complication or a secondary manifestation of many systemic diseases. Some of these may be listed as follows: virus infections such as herpes zoster, herpes simplex, dengue, yellow fever, mumps, Asian influenza, and infectious hepatitis; chlamydial infections such as psittacosis, cat-scratch disease, and lymphogranuloma venereum; spirochetal infections such as relapsing fever and Weil's disease as well as Lyme disease; rickettsial infections such as typhus, tsutsugamushi disease, tick-bite fever, and Rocky Mountain spotted fever; bacillary infections such as typhoid fever, anthrax, and tularemia, and secondary invasion by *Mycobacterium leprae, Proteus vulgaris, Pasteurella pestis, Escherichia coli*, and *Pseudomonas aeruginosa*; infections with fungi, yeasts, and molds such as *Mucor, Candida, Nocardia, Listeria, Blastomyces, Coccidioides, Aspergillus, Histoplasma, Leptothrix, Sporotrichum, Cryptococcus, Endomyces*, and *Actinomyces*; involvement by protozoa such as *Plasmodium* (malaria), *Endamoeba histolytica, Trypanosoma* (African sleeping sickness and Chagas' disease), and *Toxoplasma* (often in association with human immunodeficiency syndrome); invasion by parasites such as *Trichinella, Paragonimus, Toxocara, Echinococcus, Taenia*, and *Schistosoma*. Diseases such as rheumatic fever followed by Sydenham's cho-

rea, infectious mononucleosis, brucellosis, malaria, periarteritis nodosa, systemic lupus erythematosus, and sarcoidosis may cause widespread cerebral and meningeal involvement. Encephalomyelitic symptoms may be important manifestations of Behçet's syndrome (see above). A syndrome consisting of uveitis, retinal hemorrhage and detachment, alopecia, vitiligo, and deafness, often with associated nervous system signs, has been described by Harada, Vogt, Koyanagi, and others. Involvement of the meninges and/or the cerebral structures may occur as a complication of middle ear or mastoid disease, sinus infections, petrositis, thrombosis of the venous sinuses, osteomyelitis, and penetrating injuries or compound fractures of the skull.

Cerebral involvement frequently, if not routinely, occurs with human immunodeficiency virus infection. A dementia results from the virus itself, and a host of secondary cerebral and spinal-meningeal disorders arise from the immune-suppressed condition, including viral, bacterial, fungal, tuberculous, syphilitic, protozoal, and other parasitic infections, abscesses, and unusual neoplasms such as lymphoma and sarcoma.

Brain Abscess

A brain abscess is a focal area of encephalitis. One must be particularly alert to the possibility of this diagnosis. Once brain abscesses were common and borne in mind by all physicians. They have become relatively rare since the introduction of antibiotic therapy. In the beginning the abscess consists of a localized collection of purulent exudate with softening of the surrounding cerebral tissues (*cerebritis*). In most instances the abscess becomes encapsulated after a period of 2 – 6 weeks. The etiology of brain abscesses is varied, and many mechanisms may be responsible. They may develop either by contiguity or continuity from osteomyelitis of the skull, infections of the pachymeninges or leptomeninges, involvement of the mastoid cells and paranasal sinuses, infections of the face and orbit, and affection of the venous sinuses within the skull. They may originate by metastasis from systemic infections, involvement of the heart or lungs, or focal infectious processes (by the hematogenous route), and sometimes follow extraction of abscessed teeth. They may be produced by direct implantation from penetrating wounds or compound fractures of the skull. Otogenous abscesses (those that complicate infection of the middle ear, mastoid cells, or petrous pyramid) are usually in either the temporal lobe or the cerebellum; rhinogenous abscesses (those that follow infections of the nose and paranasal sinuses) are usually in the frontal lobes.

The clinical diagnosis of brain abscess is suspected on the basis of signs of systemic infection (fever, leukocytosis, etc.), manifestations of rapidly increasing intracranial pressure, and signs of focal nervous system involvement. Except for the signs of infection and the frequently rapid increase in symptoms, the clinical picture is quite similar to that encountered with cerebral neoplasms. It must be remembered that abscesses near either the surface of the brain or the ventricles may be accompanied by meningeal involvement, and that there may be definite signs of a meningitis. Computed tomography and magnetic imaging have revolutionized the diagnosis of brain abscesses; ring-shaped lesions with central "liquid cores" are characteristic (Fig. 53-5 and Fig. 53-6). A lumbar puncture in the presence of a brain abscess may cause either rupture of the abscess or dissemination of the meningeal infection; it may even cause herniation of the brain or brainstem due to the mass effect of the abscess.

Extradural abscess (pachymeningitis externa) is a collection of pus between the dura and the skull; *subdural abscess* (pachymeningitis interna) is a collection of purulent material between the dura and the arachnoid. Both of these conditions may be produced by the same processes that cause the development of brain abscesses, and the symptoms and diagnostic signs are similar. It is important, however, to make a correct differential diagnosis, since the prognosis and treatment vary. The imaging procedures usually differentiate these conditions.

CEREBRAL TRAUMA

In most instances traumatic involvement of the brain may be diagnosed from the history alone. It must be remembered, however, that trauma may occur consequent to acute alcoholic intoxication or epilepsy, and that no history of injury may be recalled or presented. Also, trauma may precipitate other pathologic changes, such as subarachnoid, extradural, subdural, or intracerebral hemorrhage. Furthermore, the late posttraumatic sequelae, especially if they are complicated by the presence of nonorganic manifestations, may be exceedingly difficult to appraise. The imaging studies, computed tomography and magnetic resonance, permit a comprehensive noninvasive appraisal of the intracranial extent of head trauma by showing areas of hemorrhage, edema, distortion of normal structures, presence of foreign bodies, etc.;

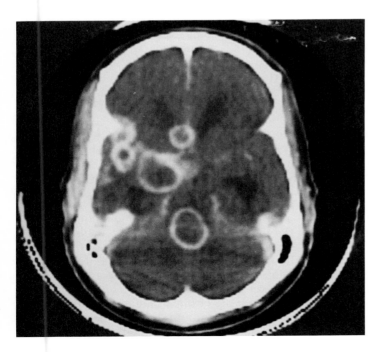

FIG. 53–5. Computed cerebral tomogram of a patient with multiple cerebral abscesses. At least five ring-shaped lesions are scattered through the brain.

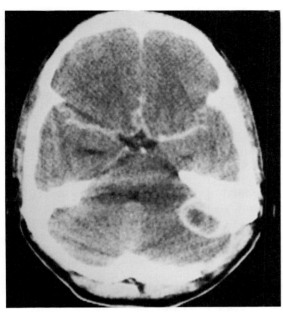

FIG. 53–6. Computed cerebral tomogram of a patient with a left cerebellar abscess. Lesion is the ring-shaped structure in the lower right of the figure.

they do not, however, outline all dysfunctional areas of the brain.

Acute head injuries are of two main types. Nonpenetrating, or "closed," head injuries are those in which there has been no exposure of the meninges or brain as a result of the trauma; the scalp alone is wounded, or if the skull has been injured, there is only a small linear fracture without displacement of the fragments, rupture of the dura, or penetration or exposure of the brain substance. Penetrating, or "open" head injuries are those that occur in association with either compound or depressed fractures or penetrating wounds. There is tearing of the dura with exposure of the brain substance and penetration of the brain by fragments of bone, metal, or other foreign bodies.

The general symptoms of head injury may occur with all forms of trauma, although all of these symptoms need not be present in every case. Headache is probably the most common manifestation; it may vary in location, type, severity, and duration. If the headache persists, one must consider the possibility that complications have developed, or in some instances, posttraumatic neurotic reactions. Dizziness, usually a light-headed sensation or imbalance when walking (ocasionally true vertigo), is probably second to headache in frequency; its persistence

has the same implications. Postural dizziness or vertigo secondary to head trauma are felt, however, to have at least a partially organic basis (Ch. 14). Disturbances of consciousness are commonly encountered. There may be either brief or prolonged coma after a head injury, or fluctuations in the level of consciousness. There may be no complete loss of consciousness, but a lowering of the patient's awareness of his surroundings, with confusion, disorientation, and delirium. The period of true unconsciousness may be relatively short, but the return to normal consciousness may be prolonged, with disorientation, confusion, irritability, and lethargy. Retrograde amnesia is almost always present if there has been a loss of consciousness and may cover a period that varies from a few seconds to minutes or even hours preceding the time of the injury. Posttraumatic (anterograde) amnesia may cover the period of confusion.

Changes in the body temperature, pulse, and respirations are common after head injuries. There may be a moderate hyperthermia, but occasionally there is hypothermia. The pulse may be rapid and feeble, especially if shock occurs; with increased intracranial pressure there is bradycardia. The respirations may be rapid, feeble, and shallow, or they may be depressed and irregular. Cheyne-Stokes respirations are sometimes observed. Signs of increasing intracranial pressure (slow pulse and respirations, papilledema, and vomiting) are of grave prognostic import.

The cerebrospinal fluid may be under increased pressure. Examination of the cerebrospinal fluid is not routinely necessary after head trauma, unless infection is suspected. Following a cerebral laceration or subarachnoid bleeding the fluid is bloody. Cerebrospinal fluid rhinorrhea is a complication of fractures in the frontal region and is caused by a fistula that forms a direct communication between the subarachnoid space and the nasal cavity, either through the cribriform plate or the frontal or ethmoid sinuses. This fistula is a direct pathway by which infections may enter the intracranial cavity, and its presence may lead to the development of meningitis, usually bacterial in type, and at times repeatedly.

The focal symptoms of head injury are dependent, of course, upon the site of the pathologic change. They may consist of sensory, motor, and other manifestations. Anisocoria and cranial nerve dysfunctions may or may not have localizing value. The cranial nerves most frequently affected are those to the muscles of ocular movement and the olfactory, facial, and acoustic nerves.

The term **concussion** has been applied to those cases of cerebral injury where there is no demonstrable pathologic alteration of tissue. There may be loss of consciousness lasting from a few seconds to hours, probably resulting from either transient hydrodynamic pressure changes or cerebral anemia; it is usually followed by amnesia for the actual moment of the accident. Concussion can be defined as the direct effect of violence on the nerve cells of the brain resulting in a temporary depression or cessation of function without immediate detectable evidence of structural changes in these cells. It has also been suggested that the loss of consciousness and other symptoms may be the result of a reduction of activity in the reticular formation at the midbrain level. If the loss of consciousness is prolonged, however, and there is retrograde amnesia with headache, vertigo, pupillary inequality, paresis of ocular muscles, vomiting, and impaired mentation, then cerebral edema with congestion and petechial hemorrhages has probably occurred, along with damage to the neurons and nerve fibers that may or may not be reversible. Imaging studies may demonstrate some of these changes. The electroencephalogram taken soon after such injury usually indicates a stage of excitation followed by depressed activity. Post-traumatic sequelae- headaches, convulsions, dizziness, emotional lability, irritability, and memory changes all suggest that cerebral damage has occurred.

If there has been either contusion or laceration of the brain, there are definite structural alterations that may produce focal signs of cerebral dysfunction, often with permanent residual effects. There may be associated hemorrhages into the subarachnoid space, diagnosed by imaging or lumbar puncture. With generalized cerebral contusions the brain is often swollen and edematous. There may be multiple, minute, punctate perivascular hemorrhages. The perivascular spaces are distended and there may be areas of focal necrosis. The predominant damage may be either at the site of the injury or on the opposite side of the brain (**contrecoup**). With lacerations there are tears of the affected tissues.

Serious complications of compound and depressed skull fractures and of severe contusions and lacerations include cerebral compression, intracerebral hematoma, extradural hemorrhage, subdural hematoma and hygroma, subarachnoid hemorrhage, posttraumatic meningitis and brain abscess, focal cerebral cicatrices, osteomyelitis of the skull, traumatic pneumocephalus, arteriovenous aneurysm, and posttraumatic epilepsy.

If there are prolonged posttraumatic manifestations, in the absence of definite focal changes such as those that follow contusions and lacerations, it is often difficult to differentiate between organic residuals and superimposed nonorganic changes. The most common symptoms, which include headaches, dizziness, fatigue, irritability, insomnia, personality changes, intolerance to alcohol, and tremors may occur in either posttraumatic encephalopathy or posttraumatic functional syndromes. The posttraumatic, or postconcussion, syndrome may be in part organic and in part psychogenic. This is particularly evident when the opportunity for secondary gain is present and litigation is underway. When objective signs are absent on examination it is difficult to differentiate between an organic postconcussion syndrome, a psychogenic reaction precipitated by the injury (at a subconscious level), and even frank malingering for possible financial or other secondary gain. The presence of focal signs, ocular muscle palsies, organic mental changes, imaging changes, focal cerebral abnormalities of perfusion and metabolism on special studies, electroencephalography, or evoked potential examinations, argue strongly in favor of persisting structural alterations. Even their presence, however, does not rule out nonorganic "overlay" along with organic deficits.

Repeated trauma, such as that suffered in boxing injuries, produces multiple petechial hemorrhages, often in the deeper parts of the cerebrum. This may result in traumatic dementia, or the "punch-drunk" syndrome, with deterioration of memory and intellect, and motor changes consisting of ataxia and evidence of both corticospinal and extrapyramidal disorders.

TOXIC INVOLVEMENT OF THE CENTRAL NERVOUS SYSTEM

The adjective *toxic* is often used loosely in referring to involvement of both the peripheral and the central nervous system. Many exogenous toxins, however, have a definite effect on nervous structures, central as well as peripheral, and toxins of endogenous origin may also cause neurologic manifestations. Certain toxic encephalopathies are difficult to differentiate clinically from encephalitides of viral origin. The possibility of either exposure to or ingestion of toxins must always be remembered when the clinician is confronted with a bizarre picture of cerebral dysfunction or evidence of diffuse brain damage. A toxin screen of blood, and at times of other body fluids or tissues is a necessary diagnostic aid in the assessment of persons with encephalopathies of uncertain cause.

Ethyl alcohol acts upon the central nervous system through various mechanisms. Acute intoxication is caused by its depressant action. Disorders of thought and conduct are commonly the first symptoms to appear, with lack of judgment from loss of normal inhibition. Later coordination is affected, with staggering, dysarthria, and diplopia. The state of consciousness is progressively lowered, and coma may result. Blood alcohol levels readily confirm the diagnosis. Abstinence, or withdrawal, symptoms include tremulousness, at times seizures, hallucinations, and delirium tremens. The so-called alcoholic polyneuropathy, Korsakoff's and Wernicke's syndromes and amblyopia are nutritional disorders, resulting from deficiency of the B complex vitamins, especially thiamine. The Marchiafava – Bignami syndrome and central pontine myelinolysis also occur in alcoholics. Chronic ingestion of alcohol in large amounts may lead to progressive cerebellar degeneration and mental disorientation. Methyl alcohol has a toxic effect on the optic nerves, often causing optic atrophy and blindness, but it may also cause an encephalopathy, sometimes fatal.

Almost any drug, especially if taken in excess, is a potential cause of encephalopathy. Bromides and barbiturates, both of which are sedatives and anticonvulsants, in large doses, on prolonged use, and in susceptible individuals, cause lethargy, confusion, delirium, and mental symptoms with a toxic psychosis that resembles organic delirium. Excessive amounts may cause coma and death. Other hypnotics may cause similar symptoms. The phenothiazine preparations and other tranquilizers such as reserpine, meprobamate, the benzodiazepines, and others, including some of the antihistamines, are also sedatives, especially when used in large doses, and may cause lethargy, depression, and even coma and death. Addiction may develop with the use of many of the above drugs, and on withdrawal there may be insomnia, delirium, and convulsions. Abuse of phencyclidine may cause intracerebral hemorrhage. The phenothiazines, butyrophenones, and reserpine may also cause extrapyramidal manifestations, including parkinsonism, dyskinesias, dystonic reactions, and akathisia at times with severe hyperpyrexia.

Phenytoin may also cause lethargy and confusion; in toxic doses it produces vertigo, ataxia, nystagmus, ocular palsies, and cerebellar manifestations. Other anticonvulsants, including carbamazepine, primidone, valproate, and others may produce some or all of the same effects.

Alkaloids of opium such as morphine, codeine, heroin, and their synthetic derivatives or related analgesics have a narcotic action on the central nervous system as well as a depressant action on vital centers that may lead to death; in certain susceptible individuals they may act as excitants and cause mania and even convulsions. The general anesthetics such as ether, chloroform, and nitrous oxide affect the central nervous system principally by their depressant action on the vital centers and the secondary production of anoxia. Cocaine, used as a local anesthetic or as a street drug may, in large doses or in susceptible individuals, cause symptoms of central nervous system stimulation that may lead to convulsions; stimulation may be followed by depression and death due to respiratory failure. Focal central nervous system deficits may also be the consequence of vascular occlusion or intracerebral hemorrhage from cocaine abuse.

Strychnine, a central nervous system stimulant, may be responsible for fatal convulsions. Other stimulants, such as picrotoxin, caffeine, amphetamine, and methylphenidate may also cause insomnia, tremors, excitement, and on occasion convulsions. Similar effects may also be seen from other psychotropic drugs, including the tricyclic compounds. The monoamine oxidase inhibitor group of drugs are also antidepressants. In some patients, and especially when used in combination with some other drugs, particularly the tricyclic group just mentioned, the monoamine oxidase inhibitor drugs can cause headache, hypertensive crises, and even cerebral hemorrhage. Convulsions may also result when the drugs are used in combination. Likewise, when monoamine oxidase inhibitors are used, aged cheese, wines, beer, and other foods containing tyramine should be avoided, as hypertensive crises may be precipitated by tyramine in patients using these drugs.

Among the heavy metals, lead is best known for its toxic action. In adults lead poisoning is usually manifested by a peripheral neuritis, motor in type, but in children there may be a lead encephalopathy with headache, tremors, convulsions, hemiplegia, and papilledema; the symptoms may resemble those of brain tumor. Pathologically there is evidence of severe damage to the brain, with edema and perivascular hemorrhages. Mercury causes a mixed peripheral neuropathy and may produce a toxic encephalopathy with irritability, tremors, ataxia, and mental symptoms. Inorganic arsenical compounds, especially arsenic trioxide (arsenous acid) and potassium arsenite (Fowler's solution), cause a mixed peripheral neuropathy, whereas organic arsenical compounds may produce an intense hemorrhagic encephalopathy with perivascular hemorrhages, pronounced cerebral damage, and optic atrophy. The accidental ingestion of soluble barium can cause paresthesias, tremor, and muscle weakness followed by paralysis. Bismuth intoxication is rare but can result in personality alterations, convulsions, and peripheral neuropathy. Zinc intoxication is also rare but tremors, personality changes, and profound weakness can occur after chronic exposure ("brass-founders' ague" or "metal fume fever"). Thallium produces not only a peripheral neuropathy but also retrobulbar neuritis, cranial nerve palsies, delirium, and convulsions; generalized alopecia accompanying the neurologic signs is characteristic. Chromium may cause central nervous system symptoms that resemble those of lead encephalopathy. Manganese seems to have a highly selective action on the basal ganglia, and poisoning by it causes a syndrome that closely resembles Parkinson's disease; there may also be disseminated involvement and psychiatric symptoms. Intoxication with gold salts, which can result from their use in the treatment of rheumatoid arthritis, causes either excitement, confusion, and hallucinations, or apathy and withdrawal.

Carbon monoxide, owing to its affinity for hemoglobin, causes symptoms of tissue anoxia. Neurologic symptoms of carbon monoxide poisoning consist of headache, weakness, vertigo, dimness of vision, lethargy, confusion, syncope, coma, and convulsions. If a patient survives acute carbon monoxide poisoning, there may be diffuse cerebral changes, often with an extrapyramidal syndrome due to basal ganglion involvement, probably the result of selective destruction of susceptible structures by the anoxia. Cyanide preparations also interfere with oxygenation of tissues, not, however, by decreasing the oxygen in the blood, but by rendering the tissues incapable of utilizing oxygen. Cyanide poisoning is usually fatal, and asphyxial convulsions precede death. Recovery from cyanide intoxication is rare, and the existence of chronic manifestations is questionable.

Certain organic solvents and noxious gases and vapors affect the nervous system largely through their effect on the myelin. In acute carbon tetrachloride poisoning there is vertigo with lethargy followed by convulsions and coma. Methyl bromide and methyl chloride cause headache, vertigo, ataxia, pareses, visual symptoms, delirium, convulsions, and coma. Various benzene derivatives, including some of the aniline dyes, cause neuritic manifestations, pseudomyasthenic symptoms, retrobulbar neuritis, ataxia, delirium, stupor, and coma. Some of the aniline, or coal tar, antipyretics, such as acetanilid, acetophenetidin, aminopyrine, and antipyrine, cause similar neurologic changes, and the former two also have a secondary effect on the nervous system through the production of methemoglobinemia. Carbon disulfide is highly toxic to the nervous system; it causes peripheral neuropathy, optic atrophy, headache, vertigo, delirium, dementia, and parkinsonian symptoms. Trichloroethylene poisoning is characterized by peripheral (particularly trigeminal) neuropathy, disturbances of consciousness, retrobulbar neuritis, and convulsions. Tetrachlorethylene may also cause delirious states. Triorthocresyl phosphate is known especially for its effects on the peripheral nerves, but it may cause diffuse central nervous system changes as well, among them spastic paraparesis from involvement of the spinal cord. The organic phosphate inhibitors of cholinesterase that are used as insecticides may have central as well as peripheral actions and can cause respiratory failure, convulsions, coma, and death.

Other pharmacologic preparations may also have toxic effects in large doses or in susceptible individuals. The salicylates in high doses may cause stimulation followed by depression; they also have a specific effect on the eighth nerve, as does quinine. The sulfonamides may affect the peripheral nerves, or they may cause vertigo, ataxia, confusion, nausea and vomiting, delirium, and convulsions. Among other substances that have a toxic effect on the nervous system are atropine and related cholinergic drugs, including those used for the treatment of Parkinson's disease; levodopa and related substances, the dopaminergic drugs, penicillin, streptomycin, and other antibiotics; cortisone, corticotropin, and allied steroid preparations; and the antihistamine drugs. Many less common drugs and chemicals are toxic to the nervous system, including phosphorus, nicotine, formaldehyde, nitrites, tetrachloroethane, nitrobenzene, trinitrobenzene, trinitrotoluene (TNT), bulbocapnine, apiol, and absinthe. *Cannabis sativa* (marijuana), D-lysergic acid diethylamide, mescaline, and other hallucinogens alter mental function to various degrees.

Organic poisons may have both central and peripheral actions. Curare acts principally at the myoneural junction. Diphtheria toxin has a predilection for peripheral nerves. Botulinus toxin affects the medullary centers, although it may also act on the myoneural junction and peripheral nerves. In botulism mild gastrointestinal symptoms are followed by diplopia, blurring of vision, dimness of vision, dysarthria, dysphonia, generalized muscular weakness, lethargy, and paralysis of muscles supplied by the midbrain and medullary nerves.

The convulsive seizures and intense reflex activity of tetanus probably result from the action of the toxin upon the central nervous system, although there may also be a direct action upon muscles and the end-plates of the motor nerve fibers.

The toxin of the poisonous mushrooms *Amanita muscaria* and *A. phalloides* produces nausea, vomiting, confusion, irritability, delirium, convulsions, and coma. The neurotoxin of the ticks *Dermacentor* and *Amblyomma* causes an ascending paralysis while the tick is engorging; this subsides after the tick has been removed. In ergotism pain and tingling of the extremities secondary to peripheral vasoconstriction are the most prominent symptoms, although there may be abdominal pain, psychotic symptoms, and convulsions. In lathyrism, which develops following the ingestion of certain leguminous plants, there is nausea with vomiting, and later spastic paralysis and mental symptoms. Poisoning by snake venoms causes paralysis of nerve endings and respiratory centers, with convulsions and respiratory paralysis; spider venoms cause pain, restlessness, anxiety, vomiting, cyanosis, and collapse. The encephalopathy with cerebral edema and vascular changes that may develop following stings by bees and other insects is probably an allergic response.

The term *toxic* is often applied to the cerebral changes that may occur with systemic infections and febrile states; most likely, however, metabolic alterations, inflammation, and other processes are also involved. The postinfectious and postvaccinial encephalitides are sometimes referred to as toxic processes; the demyelination that occurs in these, however, is probably the result of an immune reaction. Endogenous toxins, such as those associated with uremia and he-

patic disease, also cause nervous system dysfunction; these will be discussed with the metabolic disturbances.

Extensive burns are frequently associated with evidence of severe intoxication. Somnolence, apathy, and delirium are not uncommon; decerebrate rigidity may occur. Pathologically there may be vascular changes, perivascular infiltrations, and edema; thromboses of the venous sinuses may occur. Later there is degeneration of the ganglion cells of the brain, along with glial infiltrations, scarring, atrophy, and demyelination. Heat exhaustion, heat stroke, and sunstroke may cause headache, vertigo, lethargy, delirium, convulsions, and coma; impairment of the vital centers causes hyperpyrexia, anhidrosis, disorders of water and electrolyte metabolism, and shock. Pathologically there may be cerebral edema, congestion, and petechial hemorrhages, causing irreversible memory difficulties, loss of ability to concentrate, and irritability. Prolonged hypothermia may also cause brain damage, characterized by confusion, disorientation, amnesia, and disturbances of consciousness.

Lightning and electrical currents may cause death; with the former, symptoms of parasympathetic hyperactivity predominate; the latter cause generalized cytotoxicity that is often fatal. If the shock is not immediately fatal, there may be unconsciousness for a variable period of time, with or without convulsions. Generally, low-voltage shock causes ventricular fibrillation and high-voltage produces asystole and respiratory arrest, probably because of injury to centers in the medulla. Patients who recover may show visual disturbance, headache, convulsions, and spinal cord and peripheral nerve dysfunction. Pathologically there are petechial hemorrhages, necrosis of the neurons, and degenerative cortical changes.

The adult nervous system is relatively resistant to ionizing radiation, although excessive amounts of radiation therapy to the brain or spinal cord may cause delayed, progressive, irreparable damage to these structures, usually after six or more months have elapsed. The peripheral nerves, nerve roots, and plexuses may be similarly affected. Relatively small amounts of radiation to the developing brain, especially in the early stages of development of the fetus, may cause microcephaly, hydrocephalus, and other developmental anomalies.

Anoxia, whether due to lack of oxygen in the surrounding air, obstruction of the airway, paralysis of the muscles of respiration, impaired circulation of the blood to the brain, impaired utilization or transport of oxygen by the blood, cardiac failure or prolonged circulatory arrest, protracted anesthesia, neonatal asphyxia, carbon monoxide poisoning, high altitude flying, decompression, or blast injury, may cause either transient or irreversible manifestations. The gray matter is most susceptible to oxygen deprivation, and the most pronounced changes are in the cerebral cortex, basal ganglia, hypothalamus, brain stem nuclei, and cerebellum. There may be hemorrhagic changes as well. If the patient survives there may be permanent residuals, with paralyses, a clinical state resembling either decerebrate rigidity or parkinsonism, intellectual loss, and occasionally blindness. Delayed neurologic deterioration may develop following anoxia. Postanoxic action, or intention, myoclonus may develop. The symptoms of decompression sickness, namely pains, confusion, disturbances of consciousness, convulsions, and paralyses, are due to multiple small infarcts caused by nitrogen bubbles in the blood stream.

METABOLIC ALTERATIONS AFFECTING THE CENTRAL NERVOUS SYSTEM

The term metabolic alterations is used to include a wide variety of systemic disorders — endocrine, deficiency, hepatic, renal, and others — that may affect the nervous system either directly or indirectly. The brain and its functions are extremely sensitive to disturbances in the physiology of the body, and the first clinically apparent symptoms and signs of many systemic diseases may be due to their effect on the nervous system. Certain of these — vascular disease, infections, and toxic involvement — have already been discussed. A survey of the effects of some of the other disturbances of body function follows.

Diabetes mellitus most often affects the peripheral nervous system. There is usually a diffuse polyneuropathy, although there may be a mononeuritis, mononeuritis multiplex, cranial nerve involvement (especially the oculomotor and abducens nerves), and visceral changes secondary to the affection of the autonomic nerves. It has been postulated that both metabolic alterations and deficiency factors may be responsible for these. The cerebral changes that are often encountered in patients with long-standing diabetes and in older patients with the disease are usually of vascular origin, either focal or diffuse. It is known that there is a predilection for the development of atherosclerosis in patients with diabetes. Although diabetic myelopathy and encephalopathy are rare, both have been described pathologically. So-called diabetic amyotrophy is probably the result of a mononeuritis multiplex or a radiculopathy. In nonketotic hyperglycemic coma symptoms of cerebral dysfunction and (usually focal) convulsions precede the loss of consciousness.

Hypoglycemia also affects the nervous system through the production of autonomic symptoms, sensory changes, paresis, irritability, hyperkinesias, psychic manifestations, convulsions, and coma; there may be irreversible cerebral damage due to edema, perivascular infiltrations, extravasation of blood, swelling of axis cylinders, and degeneration of the ganglion cells. Hypoglycemia may result from excessive doses of insulin (especially regular, or crystalline, insulin), organic or functional hyperinsulinism, or the administration of insulin shock in the treatment of psychoses.

Endocrinopathies may have either primary or secondary effects on the nervous system. Disorders of the pituitary gland are discussed in Chapter 42.

Congenital deficiency of thyroid secretion causes cretinism, with retarded mental and physical development. Acquired deficiency causes myxedema, with lethargy, weakness, slowness of speech, fatigue, and, on occasion, coma. Myxedema may result in an elevation of the cerebrospinal fluid protein, and on examination of reflexes slowness of muscle contraction and relaxation is found. Hyperthyroidism causes weakness, nervousness, irritability, and tremors; there may be exophthalmos and ocular palsies. Thyrotoxic myopathy is discussed in Chapter 29. A form of periodic paralysis may be associated with hyperthyroidism.

Decrease of parathyroid function causes hypocalcemia, tetany (Ch. 28), convulsions, and occasionally psychotic manifestations. Hyperparathyroidism causes hypercalcemia, bone changes (osteitis fibrosa cystica), nephrolithiasis with resulting renal changes, muscle weakness, and occasionally psychotic episodes and organic mental changes.

Adrenal hypofunction causes Addison's disease, with hypotension and marked weakness, fatigability, and weight loss. There may be psychotic manifestations. Adrenal hyperfunction causes adrenal virilism and the adrenogenital syndrome. A tumor of the adrenal cortex can also cause primary aldosteronism, with hypertension, hypokalemia, hypernatremia, recurring attacks of severe muscular weakness, and occasionally tetany and diabetes mellitus. A chromaffin cell tumor of the adrenal medulla (pheochromocytoma) causes either sustained or intermittent hypertension. With the latter there are paroxysmal attacks of headache, palpitation, precordial pain, and other symptoms of hyperadrenalism; the hypertension may give rise to cerebral hemorrhage, pulmonary edema, or cardiac failure.

Paroxysmal attacks of flushing, usually unaccompanied by an increase in blood pressure, characteristically occur in the carcinoid syndrome.

Vitamin deficiencies may be responsible for a variety of neurologic disorders. Vitamin A deficiency in infants may cause mental retardation, hydrocephalus, and signs of increased intracranial pressure.

Deficiencies of many of the constituents of the vitamin B complex cause serious nervous system alterations. Thiamine deficiency affects both the peripheral nerves and the central nervous system. In beriberi, the result of prolonged thiamine deficiency, severe polyneuritis results. There may be retrobulbar neuropathy and cerebral changes as well. The polyneuropathy, Korsakoff's and Wernicke's syndromes, and amblyopia of chronic alcoholism are thought to be secondary to thiamine deficiency.

Severe and prolonged deficiency of niacin (nicotinic acid) causes pellagra, in which there are both spinal cord involvement and mental symptoms. Pyridoxine (B-6) deficiency in infants causes irritability, motor activity, and convulsions. In adults pyridoxine deficiency has been encountered in patients taking isoniazid, with resulting polyneuropathy and, on occasion, convulsions. Excessive use of pyridoxine for therapeutic reasons may also cause a neuropathy. Deficiency or failure of absorption of cyanocobalamin (B-12) is responsible for pernicious anemia, in which the primary neurologic changes are in the posterior and lateral columns of the spinal cord and the peripheral nerves, but the cerebrum and optic nerves may be affected as well.

Vitamin C deficiency causes scurvy, with symptoms of hyperirritability, generalized tenderness, and a tendency toward bleeding. Hemorrhagic lesions in the peripheral nerves and central nervous system may occur.

A deficiency of vitamin D causes a disturbance of calcium metabolism that, in some cases, may lead to the development of tetany.

Hepatic disorders of serious consequence may cause a constellation of neurologic alterations and symptoms. Among the underlying disease processes are cirrhosis, acute and chronic hepatitis, and disturbances of the portal or hepatic circulation, including portacaval anastomoses. There may be motor symptoms, including tremors, asterixis, and rigidity, and mental changes consisting of lethargy, irritability, depression, confusion, disorientation, delirium, and coma. A disturbance of nitrogen metabolism with an increase in the concentration of blood ammonia is thought to be responsible, at least in part, for the cerebral changes and resulting symptoms.

Uremia develops with renal failure. An accumulation of toxic substances in the body fluids may lead to the development of apathy, fatigue, headache, drowsiness, delirium, stupor, convulsions, and coma. Neuropathy is usually present with chronic renal failure. Convulsions, encephalopathy, and psychotic states may also occur in patients undergoing hemodialysis in the treatment of renal disease as part of the so-called dysequilibrium syndrome. Dialysis dementia, beginning with speech disturbances and myoclonus, has been described in persons on long-term hemodialysis; it was probably caused by aluminum toxicity. Following renal transplantation the uremic neuropathy may reverse, but there may be other neurologic symptoms. If the transplanted kidney immediately begins to function well, the sudden shift of electrolytes may cause a series of seizures. If there is rejection, there may be increasing hypertension and the symptoms of a toxic psychosis.

The encephalopathy that may accompany chronic pulmonary insufficiency or respiratory failure causes headaches, confusion, tremors, somnolence, stupor, and coma; there may be papilledema and others signs of an increase in intracranial pressure.

Disturbances of water and electrolytes may cause cerebral changes and neurologic symptoms. Dehydration results from either excessive loss of water via the kidneys, gastrointestinal tract, and skin, or decreased fluid intake. There may be fatigue, weakness, and irritability, and in late stages delirium, stupor, and coma. Water intoxication may have many etiologies, including excessive or inappropriate secretion of antidiuretic hormone, renal insufficiency, and sodium depletion. It is sometimes iatrogenic or self-induced. There is reduction of awareness and responsiveness, followed by convulsions and signs of increased intracranial pressure.

Disturbances of the electrolytes consist of alterations of the concentrations of anions (sodium, potassium, calcium, and magnesium) and cations (bicarbonate, chloride, phosphate, and sulfate) in both extracellular and intracellular fluids, as well as changes in the acid-base balance. There is seldom a simple, one-factor electrolyte change. Dehydration may be accompanied by hypernatremia, overhydration by hyponatremia. With prolonged vomiting, hypochloremic alkalosis is accompanied by hypokalemia. Metabolic acidosis may provoke hypokalemia. Hypernatremia may be accompanied by hypokalemia. A variation of either single or multiple factors may alter neurologic functions and cause non-specific symptoms consisting first of lassitude, lethargy, depression, and irritability, and then a confusional mental state progressing to delirium, collapse, and convulsions or coma. Occasional focal weakness or convulsions may result from general electrolyte or other metabolic derangements. Somewhat specific features that accompany altered concentrations of certain electrolytes are the following: With either an excess or a deficiency of potassium there may be flaccid muscular weakness or paralysis, including the muscles supplied by the cranial nerves, and myocardial and electrocardiographic changes. With either alkalosis or hypocalcemia there may be tetany. Magnesium in high concentrations may cause neuromuscular depression, and a deficiency may cause irritability, confusion, seizures, tremors, and choreic movements. Hypokalemic, hyperkalemic, and normokalemic varieties of periodic paralysis have been described (Ch. 21). With hypernatremic encephalopathy, vascular damage with hemorrhagic lesions within the brain may occur, as well as subarachnoid hemorrhages. Overly rapid attempts to correct sodium imbalances, especially hyponatremia, may precipitate the syndrome of central pontine myelinolysis, discussed earlier.

Many disturbances of neurologic function result from multiple underlying metabolic alterations, and may be among the causes of stupor, coma, and other disturbances of consciousness (Ch. 54). In general, those disorders affecting the nervous system that result from deprivation of oxygen or from metabolic cofactors, diseases of other organs, toxins, or acid–base disturbances have been referred to as secondary metabolic encephalopathies.

Biochemical investigations, chromosome studies, and other avenues of research have shown that there are many neurologic diseases in which the pathologic alterations and clinical manifestations are the result of an inborn error of metabolism. The proliferation of knowledge in this area has been so rapid that entire texts are devoted to it. Only a few of the many hundreds of described conditions can be mentioned here. Wilson's disease is a genetically determined disorder of copper metabolism; there is a decrease of ceruloplasm in the blood with accumulations of copper in the brain, liver, and other organs, and the pathologic alterations and symptoms are probably the result of copper toxicity (Ch. 22). Disorders of lipid metabolism include Gaucher's disease, Niemann – Pick disease, Fabry's disease, Farber's disease, Wolman's disease, Schüller – Christian disease, Tay – Sachs disease, and the late infantile and juvenile forms of lipidosis, the group of leukodystrophies (Krabbe's, metachromatic, adrenoleukodystrophy, and variants), and many others; the central nervous system may be affected either primarily or secondarily in these, and different lipid and other factors are involved in the various syndromes.

Porphyria is a biochemical disorder in which there is an excessive formation and excretion of porphobilinogen and its precursors in the urine and feces. There are several varieties of the disease. The most important one from a neurologic point of view is **acute intermittent porphyria,** which is inherited as a dominant trait. In this there are recurring symptoms consisting of abdominal pain, hypertension, polyneuritis, mental changes, convulsions, and the excretion of burgundy-red urine. Pathologically, patchy areas of demyelination in the central nervous system and degenerative changes in the dorsal root ganglia and anterior horn cells may be present.

Phenylketonuria is a common inherited defect in the hydroxylation of phenylalanine, with secondary alterations in the metabolism of other aromatic amino acids. Unless promptly treated with a low-phenylalanine diet it causes irreversible changes in the developing brain. There are many other diseases, most of which are inherited and cause both mental deficiency and gross neurologic changes, which are associated with biochemical abnormalities or result from a deficiency of enzyme activity; some of these include cystinuria, Hartnup disease, gargoylism (Hurler's disease), histidinemia, tyrosinemia, maple syrup urine disease, other aminoacidopathies, galactosemia, Leigh's disease (subacute necrotizing encephalomyelopathy), Lesch – Nyhan disease, pseudo-hypoparathyroidism, and the glycogen storage disorders.

DISTURBANCES OF DEVELOPMENT

The brain, as well as other parts of the body, may fail to develop normally during intrauterine life or may be either injured or deformed at the time of birth. Microcephaly, macrocephaly, cerebral dysplasia and dysgenesis, congenital absence of structures (*e.g.*, the corpus callosum), lissencephaly, and other abnormalities of the gyri and convolutions may result. Heterotopias, encephalocele, porencephalic cysts, hydranencephaly, and congenital hydrocephalus may also result from abnormalities of brain growth during the embryonic and fetal periods. In most instances these are manifested by mental deficiency, paralytic or dyskinetic phenomena, and convulsions. Congenital spastic paraplegia (Little's disease), cerebral diplegia, infantile hemiplegia, status marmoratus, congenital athetosis, dystonia, and ataxia may be the result of many factors, including abnormalities of development, prolonged or precipitate labor, perinatal anoxia, meningitis or encephalitis preceding or immediately following birth, injury or hemorrhage during delivery, kernicterus, and maternal infections such as toxoplasmosis, cytomegalic inclusion-body disease, acquired immune deficiency syndrome, and rubella. Malformations or abnormalities of development of the skull and cervical spine, including craniostenosis, craniofacial dysostosis (Crouzon's syndrome), hypertelorism, spina bifida, and cranium bifidum, also affect cerebral development and cause neurologic symptoms.

There are many causes for congenital mental retardation, including the inborn errors of metabolism just mentioned, but in many patients no etiology is determined. The following, however, are among the specifically classified syndromes, in some of which the mechanism is known: cretinism, or congenital thyroid deficiency, Down's syndrome, Prader–Willi syndrome, cri du chat syndrome, and other chromosomal aberrations; tuberous sclerosis (Bourneville's disease), neurofibromatosis (von Recklinghausen's disease), and other phakomatoses; Lowe's cerebrooculorenal syndrome, Heller's syndrome (dementia infantilis), Rett's syndrome, and the Cornelia de Lange syndrome, characterized by mental retardation, microcephaly, peculiar facies, and skeletal anomalies, especially of the extremities.

DEGENERATIVE PROCESSES AND MISCELLANEOUS DISORDERS

There are many diseases of the nervous system whose etiology and mode of production are not known. Some of these have been shown to be hereditary conditions, and others may yet prove to be hereditary. The majority, however, have no familial pattern, and their cause remains obscure. There are many theories regarding the etiology of this large group of conditions; they may be caused by some unknown infectious process, vascular diseases, an inherent disorder of metabolism or a deficiency or dysfunction of certain enzyme systems, unknown toxins, or autoimmune causes. For lack of better means of classification, the members of this large group of diseases are often called degenerative conditions, and most of them are characterized by progressive impairment of function. Onset is insidious and asymptomatic, and the course is chronic and increasingly deteriorating. Many degenerative diseases seem to be associated with the aging process. Many of the familial degenerative disorders are being recognized as associated with certain chromosomes and specific loci on them.

Disorders that are (under most circumstances) heredofamilial are Huntington's chorea, Wilson's disease, Hallervorden–Spatz disease, dystonia musculorum deformans, essential tremor, the lipidoses, myoclonus epilepsy (Unverricht's disease), the phakomatoses (including tuberous sclerosis, ataxia telangiectasia, von Hippel–Lindau disease, and neurofibromatosis), as well as other disorders of the nervous and neuromuscular systems which are not classified as cerebral disorders (the spinocerebellar degenerations, hereditary ataxia with muscular atrophy, parenchymatous cerebellar degeneration, olivopontocerebellar atrophy [Fig. 53-7], the muscular dystrophies, certain hereditary muscular atrophies, Charcot–Marie–Tooth disease, and the hereditary neuropathies).

Cerebral degenerative diseases that develop during the presenile and aging periods and that, under most circumstances, are not heredofamilial are Alzheimer's and Pick's diseases and normotensive hydrocephalus. Two other commonly encountered diseases of the nervous system whose etiologies remain obscure are multiple sclerosis (Fig. 53-8 and Fig. 53-9) and amyotrophic lateral sclerosis. Familial instances of each do occur, but these are rare. Environmental as opposed to hereditary influences in

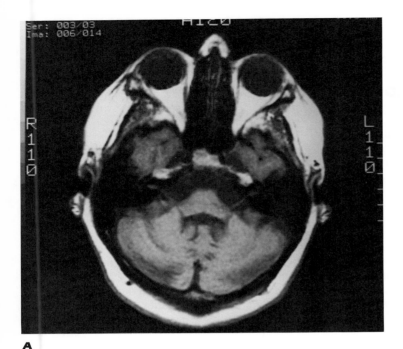

A

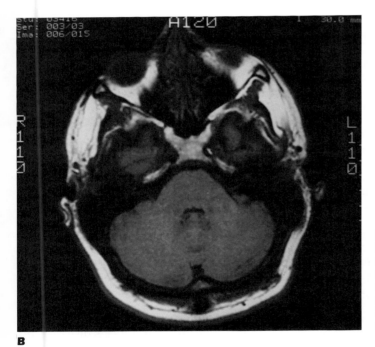

B

FIG. 53–7. A. Computed tomogram through the posterior fossa of a patient with olivopontocerebellar atrophy. Note enlarged fourth ventricle in lower third center of figure, with adjacent marked atrophy of the middle cerebellar peduncles. **B.** Similar tomogram of a normal person of same age for comparison with **A.**

the causation of these conditions continue to be debated. On the other hand, there is a familial form of Alzheimer's disease, occurring in up to 20% of the cases, and related to a specific chromosome. Huntington's chorea is a dominantly inherited disorder with chromosome 4 involve-

ment, but the mechanism for its development remains unknown. Biochemical alterations have been found in the brains of persons with this disorder, including reduced amounts of gamma-aminobutyric acid and the enzyme glutamic acid dehydroxylase, in the basal ganglia and degen-

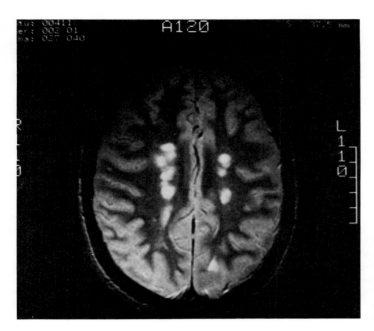

FIG. 53–8. Cerebral magnetic resonance image (TR 3200, TE 20) of a patient with multiple sclerosis, showing a number of bilateral irregular scattered bright white demyelinating lesions, mainly in subcortical and periventricular white matter.

eration of cholinergic striatal interneurons, but the relationship of these abnormalities to the disease has not been clarified. A variety of less specific biochemical changes has been described in the brains of persons dying from several of the other degenerative conditions just listed.

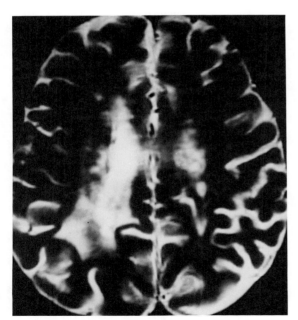

FIG. 53–9. Another patient with multiple sclerosis. Extensive and confluent irregular periventricular areas of demyelination are shown in bright white.

There are certain miscellaneous disorders that affect the nervous system. The collagen disorders (polyarteritis nodosa, disseminated lupus erythematosus, giant cell arteritis, scleroderma, and dermatomyositis) may involve the central or peripheral nervous system or the muscles. Sarcoidosis may cause a meningeal reaction, cranial nerve palsies, optic neuritis, and encephalitic symptoms. Primary amyloidosis may cause a peripheral neuritis, often with extensive autonomic changes; the spinal cord and brain are usually spared. Carcinoma may affect the nervous system through metastasis or direct extension, by pressure on nerves or nerve roots, or as a carcinomatous meningitis; in addition, however, neuromyopathies, cerebellar degeneration, and even myelopathies and encephalopathies have been reported in association with carcinomatosis. Immunologic factors have been tentatively identified in their causation. Neurologic manifestations of allergy, hypersensitivity, and anaphylaxis include angioneurotic edema, postvaccinial and postinfectious encephalomyelitis, serum neuropathy, and the reactions to some insect bites and drugs. Certain instances of vascular headaches may be due to hypersensitivity. Some disorders that secondarily involve the nervous system such as the collagen diseases, as well as specific neurologic conditions such as myasthenia gravis and Guillain-Barré syndrome have associated and probably causative immunologic disturbances.

BIBLIOGRAPHY

Adams RD, Fisher CM, Hakin S, Ojemann RG, Sweet WH. Symptomatic occult hydrocephalus with "normal" cerebrospinal-fluid pressure: a treatable syndrome. N Engl J Med 1965;273:117.

Adams RD, Victor M. Principles of Neurology, 4th ed. New York, McGraw – Hill, 1989

Aita J. Neurologic Manifestations of General Diseases. Springfield, IL, Charles C Thomas, 1964

Alexander E, Davis CH. Macewen's sign — "The cracked pot sound." Surg Neurol 1987;27:519

Allison RS. The Senile Brain: A Clinical Study. London, Edward Arnold, 1962

Bailey P. Intracranial Tumors, 2nd ed. Springfield, IL, Charles C Thomas, 1948

Bale JF, Perlman S. Viral Encephalitis. In Joynt RJ (ed). Clinical Neurology. Philadelphia, JB Lippincott, 1989

Bartter FC, Schwartz WH. The syndrome of inappropriate secretion of antidiuretic hormone. Am J Med 1967;42:790

Brain R, Norris FH Jr (eds). Remote Effects of Cancer on the Nervous System. New York, Grune & Stratton, 1965

Brock S (ed). Injuries of the Brain and Spinal Cord and Their Coverings, 4th ed. New York, Springer, 1960

Chiappa KH. Evoked potentials in clinical medicine. In Joynt RJ (ed). Clinical Neurology. Philadelpha, JB Lippincott, 1989

Courville CB. Commotio Cerebri. Los Angeles, San Lucas Press, 1953

Cumings JN, Kremer M (eds). Biochemical Aspects of Neurological Disorders. Springfield, IL, Charles C Thomas, 1959

Dalessio DJ (ed). Wolff's Headache and Other Head Pain, 5th ed. New York, Oxford University Press, 1987

DeJong RN, Magee KR. Treatment of the metabolic and toxic disorders of the nervous system. In Forster FM (ed). Modern Therapy in Neurology. St Louis, CV Mosby, 1957

DeJong RN. The neurologic manifestations of diabetes mellitus. In Vinken PJ, Bruyn GW, Klawans HL (eds). Handbook of Clinical Neurology, vol 27, Metabolic and Deficiency Diseases of the Nervous System, part I. Amsterdam, North Holland, 1976

Dodge PR, Swartz MN. Bacterial meningitis — a review of selected asp0ects. N Engl J Med 1965;272:954, 1003

Evans JP. Acute Head Injury. Springfield, IL, Charles C Thomas, 1950

Farmer TW, Wingfield MS, Lynch SA et al. Ataxia, chorea, seizures, and dementia. Pathologic features of a newly defined familial disorder. Arch Neurol 1989;46:774

Fields WS, Blattner RJ (eds). Viral Encephalitis. Springfield, IL, Charles C Thomas, 1958

Gajdusek DC, Gibbs CJ Jr, Alpers M. Experimental transmission of a kuru-like syndrome to chimpanzees. Nature 1966;209:794

Gibbs CJ Jr, Gajdusek DC, Asher DM et al. Creutzfeldt – Jakob disease (subacute spongiform encephalopathy): Transmission to the chimpanzee. Science 1967;161:388

Glaser GH. Metabolic encephalopathy in hepatic, renal and pulmonary disorders. Postgrad Med 1960;27:611

Haerer AF, Udelman HD. Acute brain syndrome due to tetrachlorethylene ingestion. Am J Psychiatry 1964;121:78

Hagberg B, Aicardi J, Dias K, Ramos O. A progressive syndrome of autism, dementia, ataxia, and loss of purposeful hand use in girls: Rett's syndrome: Report of 35 cases. Ann Neurol 1983;14:471

Halperin JJ, Luft BJ, Anand AK et al. Lyme neuroborreliosis: Central nervous system manifestations. Neurology 1989;39:753

Henson RA, Hoffman HL, Urich H. Encephalomyelitis with carcinoma. Brain 1965;88:449

Kinkel PR. Nuclear magnetic resonance imaging in clinical neurology. In Joynt RJ (ed). Clinical Neurology. Philadelphia, JB Lippincott, 1989

Klawans HL, Rubovits R. Central cholinergic-anticholinergic antagonism in Huntington's chorea. Neurology 1972;22:107

Menkes JH, Richardson F, Verplanck S. Program for detection of metabolic diseases. Arch Neurol 1962;6:462

Munro D. The Treatment of Injuries to the Nervous System. Philadelphia, WB Saunders, 1952

Perry TL, Hansen S, Kloster M. Huntington's chorea: Deficiency of gamma-amino butyric acid in brain. N Engl J Med 1973;288:311

Plum F. Metabolic encephalopathy. In Tower DB, Chase TN (eds). The Nervous System. Vol 2, The Clinical Neurosciences. New York, Raven Press, 1975

Plum F, Posner JB, Hain RF. Delayed neurological deterioration after anoxia. Arch Intern Med 1962;110:18

Prusiner SB. Creutzfeldt – Jakob disease and scrapie prions. Alzheimer Dis Assoc Disord 1989;3:52

Richardson JC, Chambers RA, Heywood PM. Encephalopathies of anoxia. Arch Neurol 1959;1:178

Rosenblum ML, Levy RM, Bredesen DE (eds). AIDS and the Nervous System. New York, Raven Press, 1988

Rowland LP (ed). Merritt's Textbook of Neurology, 8th ed. Philadelphia, Lea & Febiger, 1989

Sherlock S, Summerskill WHJ, White LP, Phear EA. Portalsystemic encephalopathy: Neurological complications of liver disease. Lancet 1954;2:453

Smadel JE, Bailey P, Baker AB. Sequelae of the arthropodborne encephalitides. Neurology 1958;8:873

Smith DW. Recognizable Patterns of Human Malformations. Philadelphia, WB Saunders, 1970

Stanbury JB, Wyngaarden JB, Fredrickson DS, Goldstein JL et al. The Metabolic Basis of Inherited Disease, 5th ed. New York, McGraw – Hill, 1983

Swartz MN, Dodge PR. Bacterial meningitis — a review of selected aspects. N Engl J Med 1965;725, 779, 842, 898

Symonds C. Concussion and its sequelae. Lancet 1962;1:1

Tobis JS, Lowenthal M. Evaluation and Management of the Brain-damaged Patient. Springfield, IL, Charles C Thomas, 1960

Tyler HR. Neurological complications of dialysis, transplantation, and other forms of treatment in chronic uremia. Neurology 1965;15:1081

Walton JN. Subarachnoid Hemorrhage. Edinburgh, E&S Livingstone Ltd, 1956

Ward AA Jr. Physiologic basis of concussion. J Neurosurg 1958;15:129

Youmans JR (ed). Neurological Surgery, 3rd ed. Philadelphia, WB Saunders, 1990

Zimmerman HM, Netsky MG, Davidoff LM. Atlas of Tumors of the Nervous System. Philadelphia, Lea & Febiger, 1956

PART I
Special Methods of Examination

Chapter 54

THE EXAMINATION IN COMA, IN OTHER STATES OF DISORDERED CONSCIOUSNESS, AND IN BRAIN DEATH

The **state of consciousness** is the level of the individual's awareness and the responsiveness of his mind to himself, the environment, and the impressions made by his senses. This level of awareness may be disturbed in various ways and degrees by alterations in cerebral function as well as by nonorganic factors. In coma, stupor, and hypersomnia there is lowering of consciousness; in confusion and delirium there is a clouding of consciousness; in amnesia there is a loss of memory that usually affects only a particular period of time or certain experiences; in the convulsive state there is either a paroxysmal decrease of consciousness or amnesia, usually accompanied by motor phenomena or disturbances in behavior.

Coma is defined as a state of complete loss of consciousness from which the patient cannot be aroused by ordinary stimuli. It is a state of complete unresponsiveness to the environment. The patient makes no voluntary movements. Reactions are limited to elemental reflexes, and even some of these may be impaired. In profound coma painful stimuli such as pressure on the eyeballs and pinching of the skin fail to arouse the patient. Corneal sensations and reflexes are absent. The pupils may be either dilated or contracted and do not react to light. The swallowing and cough reflexes are abolished and the patient is unable to swallow either liquids or solids. There is incontinence of sphincters. As consciousness diminishes, the muscle stretch reflexes may be exaggerated and extensor plantar responses are obtained. In deep coma, both superficial and deep reflexes are lost and no movement of the toes occurs on plantar stimulation.

Stupor is a state of partial or relative loss of response to the environment in which the patient's consciousness may be impaired in varying degrees. In stupor no significant defect of the elemental reflexes is present. The patient is difficult to arouse, and although brief stimulation may be possible, responses are slow and inadequate. The patient is otherwise oblivious to what is happening in the environment, and promptly falls back into the stuporous state. In stupor bordering on coma the patient may respond only to painful stimulation, but in lighter stages the patient may react to noises, calls by name, visual threats, and even verbal commands, and he may be able to execute simple acts such as shutting the eyes and protruding the tongue. The corneal and pupillary reflexes are sluggish or normal, and no consistent changes in the superficial and muscle stretch reflexes are detected. Pathologic reflexes may be obtained; swallowing, coughing, and sphincter control are preserved. The patient usually makes no spontaneous movements except when aroused.

Lethargy, hypersomnia, or **somnolence,** is a morbid drowsiness, or a continued or prolonged sleep; the patient can usually be aroused or awakened and then appears to be in complete possession of his senses, but may fall asleep as soon as the stimulation is removed.

Syncope is a transient, partial or complete suspension of consciousness that is usually accompanied by temporary respiratory and circulatory impairment, with a rapid, feeble pulse, rapid respirations, pallor, increased perspiration, and coldness of the skin.

Amnesia is a loss of memory that usually affects either a circumscribed period of time or certain experiences without loss of orientation for the immediate environment.

A **fugue state** is a disturbance of consciousness, often lasting hours or even days, in which the patient performs purposeful acts. Afterwards, the patient does not consciously remember actions carried out during the period. It may develop in association with various psychiatric disorders or, if brief, be an epileptic phenomenon.

Confusion is a state in which only a mild lowering of the level of consciousness develops and the elemental responses, simple mental functions, and reactions to ordinary commands are intact. The impairment of the patient's awareness is manifested by defects in the attention span and memory, and loss of normal appreciation for and perception of the environment. The chief symptoms may be in the field of orientation, with a defect in time sense and loss of identification of self and others. There is impaired capacity to think clearly and with customary rapidity, and to perceive, respond to, and remember questions or directions.

Delirium is characterized by confusion with disordered perception and loss of attention, but manifestations of motor and sensory irritability together with abnormal mental phenomena are also evident. Disorientation for time is more marked than that for either place or person, and there often are fluctuations in the level of attention, frequently with diurnal or nocturnal variations. Excitement is an outstanding symptom. The patient is restless and there may be hyperkinesias with marked motor activity and an increased response to all types of stimuli, many of which are interpreted incorrectly. Psychic symptoms include incoherence, illusions, hallucinations, and delusional ideation.

The **convulsive state** is a transient episode of uncontrollable motor activity, either focal or generalized, which usually is accompanied by clouding or loss of consciousness. The motor activity may alternate with either rigidity or atonia. In the postconvulsion period there may be coma, stupor, a desire to sleep, and confusion, disorientation, or other psychic manifestations. Other types of epilepsy include focal seizures in which the motor phenomena are confined to one extremity or one side of the body, with or without sensory manifestations or loss of consciousness; brief periods of altered or obtunded conscious-

ness; usually without motor accompaniments; automatisms with associated amnesia; disturbances of feeling or behavior, hallucinations, and signs of alterations in the function of the autonomic nervous system; myoclonic and akinetic seizures, and various combinations or abortive forms of seizures.

These varieties of disordered consciousness are usually indicative of organic disease of the central nervous system, although many of them may be similar to those encountered in hysteria or psychotic states. Coma, stupor, and delirium, as well as the convulsive and postconvulsive states, constitute emergency situations requiring evaluation with the least possible delay. Treatment must be instituted immediately; the mode of therapy varies depending upon the etiology. It is always important to determine the causative factors and to discriminate between organic and psychogenic etiologies. This latter differentiation is not always simple, however, and a detailed examination with prolonged observation or electrophysiologic monitoring is sometimes necessary. It is the general practitioner of medicine or the emergency room physician who is usually called upon to diagnose and treat states of acutely developing disorders of consciousness, often under circumstances rendering evaluation difficult. Inasmuch, however, as most such disturbances are fundamentally neurologic problems and are associated with altered function of higher nervous centers, the neurologist is often sought as a consultant, especially if the diagnosis is difficult to establish.

Coma, stupor, and allied states must always be distinguished from mutism, in which the patient is completely withdrawn from the environment and is unable or refuses to speak; and from negativism, in which, because of mental disease, the patient presents an abnormality of behavior characterized by either failure to perform acts that are commanded or suggested (passive negativism), or performs acts that are the opposite of those suggested (active negativism). In aphasia, as a result of focal rather than diffuse brain damage, there is a defect in either expression or interpretation of language functions; usually both are present.

The examination of the comatose, stuporous, or delirious patient, or of the individual exhibiting either a convulsive paroxysm or a postconvulsion state, often presents many difficulties and may require special methods of investigation. The general observation of the state of consciousness, including the alertness of the individual, attention span, reaction time, accessibility, and interest in the environment, are mentioned in Chapters 3 and 4. Occasionally, however, an alteration of consciousness is present to such a degree that the usual procedure of examination cannot be followed. Special details that must be considered under such circumstances are outlined.

THE EXAMINATION OF THE COMATOSE PATIENT

Unless the cause of the coma is immediately apparent, emergency measures must be instituted at once, even before a detailed history and examination are in order. Support of vital functions should be assured by providing airway, intravenous access, and oxygen. Emergency blood samples are drawn, and glucose and thiamine administered intravenously. Naloxone should be given parenterally if narcotic poisoning is suspected. Preparations for intubation, respiratory support, and use of pressor agents must be made, should they become necessary. It must always be assumed that a cervical spine fracture may be present; the neck should be immobilized or stabilized until a fracture can be ruled out.

The History

After the initial stabilization, the detailed examination should be preceded in every instance by a reliable history. In states of disordered consciousness it is usually impossible to obtain such a history from the patient, and it may be necessary to obtain the essential information from a friend, relative, observer, or the referring physician. It should include not only the mode of onset and manifestations of the present episode but also an account of the patient's past health, both physical and emotional. A history, for instance, of prior convulsive attacks, cerebrovascular symptoms, diabetes mellitus, or hypertension; of pulmonary, cardiac, hepatic, renal, or endocrine disorders; or of alcoholism, abuse of drugs or other substances, past depressions, or suicidal attempts may give important clues and aid the physician in initiating therapy without delay. Specific details that must be remembered in eliciting the history of what transpired immediately preceding the period of disordered consciousness are obtained separately.

If there is a history of trauma, one should determine the type, site, and severity of the injury, the time interval between the injury and loss of consciousness, and the degree and character of the loss of consciousness. With middle meningeal hemorrhage and consequent epidural hematoma there may have been coma that was followed by a lucid interval and then, in turn, by progressively deepening stupor. When a subdural hematoma develops the trauma may have been less recent. It is important to bear in mind that an epileptic convulsion may cause serious cerebral trauma, but that head injury may also cause immediate convulsions. It is also important to remember that alcoholism and trauma may occur together and that one may be a complication of the other.

Some information should always be obtained relative to the cardiovascular status, and a history of hypertension, diabetes, hyperlipidemia, and blood coagulation abnormalities may aid in the diagnosis of cerebrovascular insufficiency, cerebral thrombosis or hemorrhage, or subarachnoid hemorrhage. A history of cardiac disease such as acute, vegetative, or subacute bacterial endocarditis, atrial fibrillation, or prior cardiac surgery may contribute to the diagnosis of cerebral embolism. Pulmonary diseases, especially neoplasms, may lead to suspicion of metastatic disease; infections suggest brain abscess. Neoplasms of various other organs often disseminate to the brain and, of course, must be considered when obtaining the history. Fractures of the long bones may also suggest the presence of fat embolism to the brain. A history of infections, either generalized or focal, but especially infections around the head and face, may be important in the diagnosis of coma, delirium, and convulsions. Meningitis, encephalitis, and brain abscesses may complicate either systemic or localized infectious processes. A history of recurrent or persistent headaches, visual disturbances, convulsions or transient disturbances of consciousness, or personality changes may suggest the presence of brain tumor, brain abscess, subdural hematoma, encephalitis, or metabolic encephalopathies.

The past mental history is also pertinent in the evaluation of the comatose patient. The previous habits and mental reactions may be informative in the diagnosis of alcoholic intoxication, abuse of narcotics, or other substances, asphyxiation, and suicidal attempts. Furthermore, hysteria and functional psychoses may cause symptoms resembling those encountered in organically caused states of disordered consciousness.

The General Examination

If the patient is entirely uncommunicative and if no further informative history can be obtained from the relatives or observers, the physician has to rely entirely upon the examination in the diagnosis of stuporous, comatose, or delirious states. The investigation is limited to the objective findings, that is, to those signs elicited without the cooperation of the patient. The examination may be far from satisfactory, but every patient, no matter how stuporous, noncooperative, or even negativistic or entirely antagonistic, can be examined to some degree, and some helpful information can be obtained.

In the general observation the examiner should note the patient's apparent age, appearance, and behavior, neatness and cleanliness of clothes and person, signs of acute or chronic illness, and evidence of trauma or blood loss. In attempting to appraise the depth of impaired consciousness, one should note stertorous breathing and incontinence as well as responses to noises, verbal commands, visual stimuli, threats, and tactile and painful stimulation. Evidence of somatic disease may be manifested by the presence of fever, cyanosis, jaundice, pallor, and signs of dehydration and loss of weight. These signs of generalized disease are discussed in greater detail in Chapter 3.

The posture of the body and its parts, all spontaneous acts, and all voluntary and involuntary movements should be carefully appraised. The positions assumed by the body as a whole and by the limbs are significant. In meningitis there may be opisthotonos with retraction of the head but with marked flexion of the thighs and legs. In hysteria there may also be opisthotonos, but the lower extremities are in extension and the patient assumes the so-called *arc de cercle*. The tonus of the body and the extremities, abnormalities of posture, and the reaction of the parts of the body to painful and other stimuli and to being placed in awkward or uncomfortable positions may give some clue regarding obvious paralyses, not only of the limbs, but also of the face and trunk muscles. The general activity (immobile, underactive, retarded, restless, or hyperkinetic); tonus (limp, relaxed, rigid, or tense); and the presence of abnormal movements (tremors, twitches, tics, grimaces, and spasms) should

all be noted. **Carphology (floccilation)** is an involuntary tugging at the sheets and picking of imaginary objects from the bedclothes, and **jactitation** is a tossing to and fro on the bed; these may be seen in acute disease, high fevers, and exhaustion. Motor unrest and excessive activity are seen in both organic and psychogenic states. Stereotypy appears in psychoses, but also in organic delirium. If convulsions occur, the examiner should note the distribution of the convulsive movements, their spread, and associated manifestations, such as the degree of impairment of consciousness, frothing at the mouth, tongue-biting, and incontinence.

The behavior of the patient should be observed closely and as often as necessary until the diagnosis is established. One should note the patient's reactions to physicians, nurses, and relatives. Do the eyes follow people? Is some awareness present of what is happening in the immediate environment? The conduct may be constant or it may be variable from time to time and influenced by special occurrences. The patient, for instance, may appear to be completely unconscious and fail to respond to any type of stimulation while the observer is in the room, yet when not aware of being watched, he may open his eyes, make furtive glances, and move around. Both spontaneous acts and defense movements are important. The former may, on occasion, signify playfulness, mischievousness, or assaultiveness. It should be determined whether or not the patient, regardless of the degree of loss of consciousness, appears comfortable and natural, or assumes unnatural postures and manners.

The ability to eat voluntarily, refusal of food, the need for assistance while eating, and actions while eating or being fed should be observed. Ability to perform routine toilet needs should be recorded. In testing social reactions and responses to stimulation of various types the physician should note the degree of reaction and whether the movements are slow, abrupt, or natural. It should be noted whether slow actions show only initial retardation or consistent slowing throughout their duration. The patient may be given simple commands such as to protrude the tongue, move the extremities, and make a fist. The type of motor response is noted. There may be compliance and automatic obedience to verbal commands, failure to reply, or negativistic responses. The primitive response of forced grasping seen in patients with disturbed states of consciousness and organic mental syndromes must be differentiated from automatic obedience to commands. The former is a reflex and occurs after stimulating the palm without any requests to the patient. It should be noticed whether either distraction or commands influence the reaction to various stimuli.

The facies may afford valuable clues in diagnosis. The facial expression may be alert, attentive, smiling, placid, masklike, apathetic, frowning, sulky, scowling, perplexed, bewildered, fearful, distressed, tearful, fixed, tense, angry, changeable, depressed, ecstatic, dramatic, grimacing, or vacant. It may be either constant or variable; if the latter, the precipitating stimuli should be noted. The facial expression may afford information regarding emotional responsiveness, but a display of emotional responses by acceleration of the pulse and respirations, changes in the color of the face, perspiration, tears, and smiling should also be noted. One should note the presence of spontaneous emotional display, whether affective responses appear when reference is made to members of the family and certain personal facts or when visitors appear, and whether jokes or sad news elicit any change in facial expression or other responses. The effect of unexpected stimuli, such as clapping of the hands and flashes of light, on the emotional reaction should also be observed.

Evidence of communicativeness and expression by speech, writing, and gesture should be carefully evaluated. Does the patient take the initiative in speech, and answer when addressed or stimulated? Although unable to talk, apparent efforts to speak may be observed by lip movements, whispers, or nodding or shaking of the head. The patient may be consistently mute or may have periods of speech, either emotionally precipitated or spontaneous. The exact utterances, with the accompanying emotional reactions, should be noted. Occasionally a patient who fails to talk may be able to write or to express feelings by means of gestures or pantomime. Perseveration (persistence of one reply or one idea in response to questions), palilalia (continued repetition of a word or phrase), echolalia (imitation of the speech of others), and echopraxia (imitation of the actions of others) are found in both organic and psychogenic states.

The Glasgow coma scale of Teasdale and Jennett has gained wide acceptance in the repeated evaluations of persons with impaired consciousness, especially if due to head trauma. This scale can be used by paramedical personnel as well as physicians. Scores are obtained for ocular, verbal, and motor functions, and the three scores totaled. In regard to eye opening, a score

of 4 is given if eyes open spontaneously, 3 if they open only to verbal stimuli, 2 if only to pain, and 1 if they never open. For best verbal response, 5 points are given if the patient is oriented and converses, 4 if disoriented yet converses, 3 if he uses inappropriate words, 2 if he makes incomprehensible sounds, and 1 if he makes no verbal response. For best motor response, 6 points are given if the patient obeys motor commands, 5 if he localizes pain, 4 if he exhibits flexion withdrawal, 3 for decorticate rigidity, 2 for decerebrate rigidity, and 1 for no motor response. An alert person with normal eye and motor responses would thus rate a total of 15 points, whereas one in profound coma would rate 3 points.

The Physical Examination

The physical examination should be carried out in detail, usually preceding the neurologic examination. The general appearance of the patient may give evidence of either chronic or acute illness. Signs of dehydration, emaciation, cachexia, or fever may be evident. The body habitus and general build of the patient may give some clue regarding susceptibility to disease. The color of the skin is significant. Pallor may indicate recent hemorrhage, anemia, vasomotor syncope, or shock; floridity and ruddiness suggest hypertension or polycythemia; flushing of the skin and erythema may be present in fever; icterus indicates hepatic or gall bladder disease or blood dyscrasia; cyanosis is found in cardiac disease, pneumonia, electric shock, and certain toxic states such as that following exposure to cyanide; a cherry-red color of the skin appears in carbon monoxide poisoning, and vasomotor dilation in alcoholic intoxication. Increased perspiration is evident in fever and in hypoglycemic shock. Petechiae are seen in blood dyscrasias, subacute bacterial endocarditis, and meningococcemia. Edema of the ankles suggests cardiac or renal disease. The odor of the breath should always be noted. An odor of acetone is characteristic of diabetic acidosis; an odor of household gas is sometimes found in carbon monoxide poisoning, and one of alcohol in acute intoxication. The odor of uremia is also characteristic, as is fetor hepaticus.

The patient should always be examined carefully for signs of injury, especially about the head. Bruises and hematomas, scalp wounds and lacerations, and bleeding from the orifices are all important, as are wounds, lacerations, and fractures of other parts of the body. **Battle's sign** is discoloration along the course of the posterior auricular artery with ecchymosis appearing near the tip of the mastoid process. This sign appears following a fracture of the base of the skull. It is always essential to remember that two conditions may occur together, such as trauma and alcoholic intoxication.

Special attention should be directed toward the blood pressure, temperature, pulse, and respiratory rate and rhythm. The blood pressure may be markedly increased in hypertensive states and in renal disease; it may be decreased in shock, and either increased or decreased when increased intracranial pressure is present. The temperature is elevated in pneumonia, meningitis, encephalitis, and other infections, and is sometimes moderately increased in cerebrovascular disease and subarachnoid hemorrhage; it may be decreased in carbon monoxide poisoning, diabetic coma, and many toxic states. The pulse may show variations; it may be rapid in infections, and slow, feeble, and irregular in toxic states and shock. It is full and bounding in hypertension, and irregular in cardiac disease. Bradycardia is often associated with increased intracranial pressure and also with heart block and Stokes-Adams disease.

Abnormalities of respiration are important in patients with depressed consciousness. The respirations may be depressed, stertorous, irregular, or of the Cheyne – Stokes type with severe neurogenic disturbances affecting central respiratory mechanisms, and of the Kussmaul variety, with evidence of air hunger, in diabetic coma. **Posthyperventilation apnea** may be present in patients with brain damage: a brief period of hyperventilation is followed by apnea that may persist for 15 – 30 sec or longer. In **respiratory ataxia** the pattern of breathing is irregular, and both shallow and deep respiratory movements occur; this may be present with medullary lesions. It may signify impending apnea. **Central neurogenic hyperventilation** refers to sustained, rapid, and regular hyperpnea. It occurs in patients with disease affecting the perimedian reticular formation in the low midbrain and upper pons regions. These respiratory alterations are associated with variations in pulmonary function and abnormalities in blood gas concentrations. Neurogenic disturbances of respiration may also accompany other disorders, such as metabolic or respiratory alkalosis, anoxia, and hypoglycemia. Cheyne-Stokes respirations may also be due to bilateral hemisphere lesions, as well as to increased intracranial pressure and cardiopulmonary dysfunction. Slow, regular respirations are noted with severe myxedema and a variety of substance or drug intoxications. Regular, even respirations occur after epileptiform seizures. When more than one cause of decreased alertness is present, respiratory patterns may be variable and confusing.

The association of disorders of consciousness with cardiac and pulmonary disease of various types is always important to remember. A detailed examination of the heart and lungs should be carried out on every comatose patient. The gastrointestinal and genitourinary systems are difficult to evaluate in states of coma, but vomiting, especially if projectile, and hematemesis should be noted, as well as retention or incontinence of urine or feces, and abdominal distention and rigidity. The examination of the eyes will be stressed under the neurologic appraisal, but it is important to remember that the pupillary and corneal reactions should always be tested and that a fundus examination has utmost importance in the diagnosis of states of disordered consciousness. Decreased intraocular tension may be present in diabetic coma. The ears, nose, mouth, and throat should also be investigated. An otoscopic examination may on occasion be indicated.

The Neurologic Examination

The details of the neurologic examination in the various states of disordered consciousness must vary with the degree of impairment and depth of coma. In stupor, for instance, the patient may respond to certain stimuli with muscular movements and even carry out some commands. The reflexes may be normal, swallowing and vegetative functions unimpaired, and some degree of speech present. In deeper coma, however, the patient may show little or no response to any type of stimulation, and even painful stimuli may evoke no muscular movements; the reflexes may be diminished to absent. Impairment of swallowing, alterations in the pulse and respirations, and failure of the pupils to react may be evident. Because the palatal muscles are relaxed, respirations may be stertorous.

The mental examination is, of course, carried out with difficulty. In confusional states and delirium, however, it may be possible to elicit evidence of failure of attention, loss of perception, illusions, hallucinations, and delusions, and in the amnesias the circumscribed memory defect may be apparent.

The Sensory Examination. Sensory perception varies with the degree of impairment of consciousness. The profoundly comatose patient does not perceive even the most painful stimulus, whereas the stuporous individual may respond to painful irritation by wincing, withdrawing the part of the body stimulated, or speaking. If the patient is unable to give relevant responses, however, it is impossible to evaluate the superficial and proprioceptive sensations and cortical sensory functions. Often the examination must be limited to observations of the response to painful stimulation and a comparison of the responses on each side of the body. The investigation is carried out by pinching the skin, pricking with a sharp object, pressing over the supraorbital notches, pressing on the knuckles, and squeezing muscle masses and tendons. If the depth of coma is not profound, the patient will respond to such testing by wincing, showing an expression of pain on the face, and attempting to withdraw the portion of the body that has been stimulated. The responses on each side of the body are compared. The examiner is able to determine whether painful stimuli are felt equally well. If there is paralysis, of course, the patient will not be able to withdraw the arm or leg when the skin is pinched, but general reactions, such as wincing or attempting to withdraw the entire body may indicate that sensation is present on the paretic side. With cerebral lesions there is often hemihypesthesia as well as hemiplegia, but the sensory defects are rarely complete and the patient may show an expression of pain on stimulation of the paretic extremity although no attempts are made to withdraw it.

The Examination of the Cranial Nerves. This cannot be performed in detail when consciousness is decreased to any significant degree, and often must be limited to an appraisal of those nerves that are essentially motor in function. It may be possible, however, to test pain sensation on the skin of the face, the cornea, and the conjunctiva, and to elicit certain of the cranial nerve reflexes. The olfactory nerve cannot be examined in stuporous and comatose persons. The functions of the optic, oculomotor, trochlear, and abducens nerves are discussed with the examination of the eyes and pupils below. The sensory functions of the trigeminal nerve can be examined, on both the face and the mucous membranes (especially the cornea and conjunctiva), if coma is not too profound, but motor functions are difficult to test. Certain trigeminal nerve reflexes, however, such as the jaw jerk and the head retraction, corneal, and supraorbital reflexes, should be investigated.

The mouth may be either open or closed in stupor, and there may be resistance to passive opening and closing of the mouth in hysterical states or psychoses. There may be trismus in tetanus and allied conditions. Foaming at the mouth, holding of saliva, and drooling of saliva, especially if unilateral, are all significant. The patient may be unable to protrude his tongue, but the position in which it lies in the mouth may be important. The motor supply of the facial nerve to the muscles of facial expression may be evaluated in the examination of motor status (discussed subsequently); Chvostek's sign is significant in tetany, and a risus sardonicus in tetanus. The sensory functions of the facial nerve are insignificant in comatose states, but the presence of tears and an intact lacrimal reflex may be important.

In testing the acoustic nerve one notes the response to loud noises and the presence of the auditory-palpebral, auditory-oculogyric, and general acoustic muscle reflexes and caloric responses. It may be impossible to examine the functions of the palatal and pharyngeal muscles directly, but the examiner should note the patient's ability to swallow, and should test the palatal and pharyngeal reflexes on each side. Relaxation of the palatal muscles may cause the respirations to have a stertorous character, and impairment of the laryngeal functions may alter the tone of the voice and interfere with breathing and coughing.

Examination of the Eyes and Pupils and of the Functions of the Optic, Oculomotor, Trochlear, and Abducens Nerves. This is the most important part of the cranial nerve evaluation in coma. One should note whether the eyes are open or closed and also compare the width of the palpebral fissures on the two sides. When the eyelids are closed in a comatose patient, the lower pons is still functioning. In a facial paresis the palpebral fissure may be increased in width, and in a third nerve paresis it is decreased. However, when peripheral facial paralysis develops, the associated paralysis and sagging of the orbicularis oculi and frontalis muscles may result in pseudoptosis. Full elevation of the eyelid is usually accompanied by contraction of the frontalis muscle. If the eyes are partially or completely closed, the examiner may try to open them by gently raising the upper lids, and then note the speed with which the eyes close again. If weakness of one orbicularis is present, there will be less rapid closing on that side. Forceful closing of the eyes may follow painful pressure over the exit of the supraorbital nerve or over the eyeball. In deep coma the eyes may be open and a glassy stare evident. Often in profound illness the patient lies with the eyes only partially closed, even in sleep, so that a narrow portion of the cornea is visible between the upper and lower lids. In malingerers the eyes may be kept tightly closed and the patient may resist attempts to open them, yet, however, may open the eyes and make furtive glances when unaware that someone is observing the action.

The examiner should also note whether blinking, flickering, or tremor of the eyelids is present when the patient rests, when light shines in the eyes, and when sudden movements are made toward the eyes, and whether there is blinking or closing of the eyes in response to a loud noise (auditory-palpebral reflex). The corneal reflex should be tested, and both direct and consensual responses noted; in deep coma the reflex is absent. In lesions of either the fifth or seventh nerve the reflex may be absent on the involved side. In a seventh nerve lesion there is a retained consensual reflex, but not in a fifth nerve lesion. (It is obvious that the presence of contact, or corneal, lenses should be detected before the corneal reflexes are tested.) Inability to close an eye, so that it is open for a period of time, may cause decreased corneal sensitivity, corneal drying, and even scarring of the cornea.

The position of the eyes and function of the extraocular movements should always be noted. Conjugate deviation of the eyes or paralysis of conjugate gaze toward one side may follow either cerebral or brain stem lesions. Paralysis of individual ocular movements may be apparent from the position of the eyes at rest, and occasionally nystagmus may be seen in the resting state. In meningitis and terminal illness there may be either loss of coordination or dissociation of ocular movements. In both coma and sleep the eyeballs may turn upward.

Attempts should always be made to elicit some movement of the eyes. If the stupor is not profound, the patient may attempt voluntary eye movements in response to verbal commands or may follow movements of the examiner or of moving objects within his field of vision. In deep stupor there may be only a fixed, staring gaze, although it may be possible to elicit reflex movements. Rapid turning of the head to one side should be followed by contralateral ocular deviation (the normal oculocephalic or vestibular

oculogyric reflex, also known as the doll's head maneuver). Absence of movement to one side indicates that there is paralysis of conjugate gaze to that side. Dissociation of responses or their total absence indicates that there is interruption of descending oculogyric pathways in the brain stem. Ice water calorics to check the oculovestibular response are used if the oculocephalic reflex is abnormal, to confirm dysfunction of the brain stem. Absence of response to ice water calorics has grave prognostic significance unless there is evidence of a vestibular disorder or the exposure to vestibular-suppressant drugs. If the patient is not fully comatose, testing for caloric and optokinetic nystagmus may also give important diagnostic information. Caloric nystagmus is absent if there is interruption of the descending oculogyric pathways, and is dissociated with other lesions of the brain stem. Absence or abnormalities of optokinetic nystagmus may indicate the presence of either cerebral or brain stem lesions. In hysteria and malingering there may be furtive glances and evasion of the use of the eyes.

The size, shape, position, equality, and reaction of the pupils are all important. In the various degrees of stupor and coma the pupils may be dilated or contracted. In certain toxic states, especially after the ingestion of opiates, they are often pinpoint in size. With either thrombosis or hemorrhage of the basilar artery and other lesions of the pons the pupils are also pinpoint in size. Unilateral lesions of the brain stem, especially of the medulla, may involve the descending pupillodilator fibers on that side and cause the miosis of the Horner's syndrome. In other varieties of stupor, such as those associated with head trauma, alcoholism, diabetes, uremia, and carbon monoxide poisoning, the pupils may be unequal. The pupillary reflexes may vary, regardless of the degree of depressed consciousness, but in deeper stages there is usually loss of the light reflex and also loss of the reflex response to painful stimulation applied to the eyeball (oculosensory reflex) or to the skin of the neck (ciliospinal reflex). The accommodation-convergence reflex cannot be tested in coma.

In increased intracranial pressure associated with a unilateral expanding supratentorial lesion, such as a brain tumor or abscess, subdural hematoma, cerebral hemorrhage, or skull fracture with an associated middle meningeal artery hemorrhage and subsequent epidural hematoma, the pupil may become dilated and unresponsive on the side of the lesion. With a unilateral increase in intracranial pressure the uncus and hippocampal gyrus may herniate through the tentorium cerebelli and press the third nerve against the sphenoid bone. The pupilloconstrictor fibers are the most accessible to such pressure, so that they are first affected and mydriasis results. Patients who have suffered head trauma or who show signs of increasing intracranial pressure should be observed closely for the development of anisocoria. It is said that occasionally, but rarely, the midbrain is pushed to the opposite side and it is the contralateral pupil that dilates first.

No neurologic evaluation of coma, stupor, or disordered consciousness is complete without an ophthalmoscopic examination. The presence of either early or fully developed papilledema is, of course, indicative of some process causing increased intracranial pressure. The ophthalmoscopic examination is also important, however, in the diagnosis of various systemic diseases responsible for disorders of consciousness, namely, diabetes, uremia, hypertension, atherosclerosis, and blood dyscrasias. It is not possible to test either visual acuity or the visual fields reliably if significant impairment of consciousness is present. If there is only partial impairment, however, the examiner should note whether the patient has a fixed gaze, follows objects, makes furtive glances, or evades the use of his eyes. It may be possible to demonstrate a hemianopia in stuporous patients by the absence of defensive closing of the eyes when objects are brought into the field of vision or when a sudden threatening movement is made toward the eyes; the response on the two sides must be compared.

The Examination of the Motor Status. This is one of the essential parts of the neurologic examination in disorders of consciousness. Reference has already been made to the position assumed by the body as a whole and by its parts, the degree of activity, the presence of tension or relaxation, and the appearance of tremors, spasms, and convulsions. It is always important to examine the patient carefully in order to see whether paralysis is present. If a patient is comatose and shows no motor activity, no paralysis may be apparent, and it may require skilled observation to elicit the presence of motor dysfunction.

The paralysis that follows cerebral lesions is contralateral and may involve either the entire opposite half of the body, or the lower part of the face or upper and lower extremities, alone or in combination. The paralysis is usually a flaccid one at the outset, although it later becomes spastic, with hyperactive muscle stretch reflexes and corticospinal tract responses. If the face is affected, there will be a central type of facial paresis with the lower portion of the face involved and the upper portion spared. There will be increased width of the palpebral fissure, drooping of the angle of the mouth, and a shallow nasolabial fold on the affected side. There may be drooling of saliva out of the angle of the mouth, and a pronounced puffing out of the cheek on expiration and retraction of the cheek on inspiration. Respirations may be more difficult if the patient is placed on the nonparetic side. Firm pressure over the supraorbital notch or the eyeball is followed by retraction of the facial muscles on the normal side, but no movement on the paretic side. If the examiner attempts to open the firmly closed eyes, there may be resistance on the normal side but none on the paretic side; paresis of the orbicularis oculi causes the eye to close slowly.

The position of the arms and legs and the response to passive movement may show evidence of paralysis of the extremities. There is usually flaccidity with marked relaxation and loss of tone of recently paralyzed limbs. If the two arms are lifted and then released by the examiner, or if they are placed with the elbows resting on the bed and the forearms at right angles to the arms, the affected extremity falls in a flaillike manner, whereas the normal extremity drops slowly and may even remain upright for a brief period before falling. If the arms are passively rotated before they are released, the affected hand may strike the face in falling; the normal hand rarely, if ever, strikes the face. If the lower extremities are lifted from the bed and then released, the affected extremity falls rapidly, whereas the normal limb gradually drops to the bed. If the lower extremities are passively flexed with heels resting on the bed and then released, the paretic limb rapidly falls to an extended position with the hip in outward rotation, whereas the unaffected limb maintains the posture for a few moments and then gradually returns to its original position. If depression of consciousness is not deep, there may be some response to painful stimulation: pinching of the skin on the normal side is followed by a withdrawal, whereas a painful stimulation on the paretic side causes no local movement, although grimacing or movements of the opposite side of the body may show that sensation is retained. Other tests of motor function, such as evaluation of coordination and active movement, cannot be performed on patients in deeper states of stupor and not at all when coma is present. In the lighter stages of depressed consciousness movements may be irregular, suggesting a disturbance of cerebellar and vestibular function, but this is of no localizing or diagnostic significance when evident bilaterally. It is important, however, to appraise the tonus, or resistance to passive movement, and to observe carefully any hyperkinesias, or abnormal movements. Occasionally spasticity instead of flaccidity develops after acute cerebral lesions, and in brain stem lesions there is especially apt to be hypertonicity of a decerebrate type involving all four extremities. It is important to remember that a previous spastic hemiplegia or extrapyramidal syndrome may have caused an alteration in tone that persists even in coma, and that arthropathies and skeletal abnormalities may also interfere with movements of joints. In catatonia there may be a waxy resistance resembling that of extrapyramidal disease. All hyperkinetic phenomena such as twitches, tremors, muscle spasms, choreiform movements, and focal and generalized convulsive movements should be described in detail.

The Examination of the Reflexes. The most objective part of the neurologic appraisal, this can be performed without the cooperation of the patient. As a consequence it has special value in the examination of comatose and stuporous individuals. All important muscle stretch reflexes and superficial reflexes should be tested, and the major tests of corticospinal tract dysfunction should be performed. In comatose states that are not associated with focal cerebral lesions both muscle stretch and cutaneous reflexes may be abolished, but if there is focal disease, abnormalities of the muscle stretch reflexes and corticospinal tract responses may be detected. In acute cerebral hemiplegia with flaccid paralysis of the extremities the muscle stretch and superficial reflexes may be either normal or diminished, but an extensor plantar response is frequently present. Later the muscle stretch reflexes are hyperactive, the cutaneous reflexes are absent, and the corticospinal tract responses become more definite. In brain stem lesions either tonic neck reflexes or signs of decerebrate rigidity may be detected. In every comatose patient one should attempt to elicit signs of meningeal involvement. After cervical spine fracture has been ruled out, the neck should be flexed passively and rotated from side to side in order to determine whether there is nuchal rigidity, and Kernig's and Brudzinski's signs and related signs should always be investigated. In tetany a Chvostek's sign and related phenomena may be found.

The Laboratory Examinations

Under many circumstances auxiliary examinations including laboratory tests have inestimable value in the differential diagnosis of the cause of coma. A urinalysis should be carried out in every instance, and if the patient has retention or if he voids without control, catheterization may be necessary in order to obtain a urine specimen, which should be examined for the presence of glucose, acetone, acetoacetic acid, protein, leukocytes, erythrocytes, casts, and toxins or drugs. The blood count is important to aid in determining the presence of infections, anemia, and hemorrhagic states. Further blood studies include determinations of glucose, ammonia, electrolytes, and certain enzymes, and analysis of blood gases; blood cultures may also be indicated. Thyroid function tests may be necessary. In cases of possible poisoning it may be valuable to examine the blood for determination of the alcohol level and for the presence of toxins, drugs, and street drugs. In most cases of suspected poisoning it is advisable to do a gastric lavage and examine the gastric contents for the presence of pills, capsules, toxins, or other substances. An electrocardiogram should be obtained in most instances; cardiac and blood pressure monitoring may become necessary. Roentgenograms of the chest, neck, and skull are usually needed, to be followed, or in the case of skull roentgenograms, to be replaced by computed tomography or magnetic resonance imaging of the cranium and its contents. After these imaging studies, or if there is no contraindication to lumbar puncture (such as the presence of papilledema, infections about the head, or infections about the puncture site) and if indications for such an examination are present, it should be performed. The pressure should be determined and the cerebrospinal fluid examined (Ch. 57 and 58). Electroencephalography may aid in some instances; it aids in ruling out electrical or absence status epilepticus presenting as coma or stupor, and it can serve as a baseline in the longitudinal evaluation of states of altered consciousness.

DIFFERENTIAL DIAGNOSIS OF THE CAUSES OF LOWERED CONSCIOUSNESS

Coma, semicoma, stupor, and related conditions may be the result of any one of a multiplicity of processes, including trauma, cerebrovascular disease, intoxications, infections, and metabolic disturbances. Convulsions and coma may constitute the terminal states of serious systemic disease and may be preceded by other signs and symptoms of disordered function, or they may be the first manifestations in a serious illness and appear precipitously before other evidence of disease becomes manifest. The relative incidence of different causes of coma should be remembered since the frequency of their occurrence may assist in the diagnosis. Incidence figures vary, however, depending on the circumstances under which data are collected. In large city hospitals, alcoholism or substance abuse are probably the most common cause of coma, followed in frequency by trauma and then cerebrovascular accidents. Cardiac arrest and poisoning are also relatively frequent. Epilepsy, diabetes, meningitis, pneumonia, cardiac decompensation, and other less frequent causes of coma must also be considered. Statistics that were based on studies of autopsies showed trauma to be the most common cause of coma that ends fatally, and this, in turn, was succeeded in frequency by vascular disease, meningitis, pneumonia, uremia, and diabetes. However, such studies were conducted before the prompt resuscitation measures following cardiac arrest were developed; thus, cardiac arrest is now a more frequent cause of coma, which often terminates fatally. Among the cases seen by the general practitioner of medicine, vascular lesions are the most common; these are followed, in turn, by trauma, postconvulsion states, poisoning, diabetes, and meningitis. It is important in all cases to arrive at a correct diagnosis as rapidly as possible, because immediate treatment may save the life of the patient in conditions such as diabetes, hyperinsulinism, poisoning, overdoses, trauma, shock, cardiac arrest, exsanguination, subarachnoid hemorrhage, meningitis, and eclampsia.

Loss of consciousness may occur with either diffuse or focal cerebral lesions, as well as with various alterations in cerebral function associated with metabolic disorders, deficiency in blood or oxygen supply, exposure to toxins, infectious processes, and other disturbances of structure or function. The suggestion has been made, in the past, that there is a specific "center of consciousness," disease of which causes alterations in the state of awareness. It is probable that no such center exists, but the smallest focal lesions that are followed by loss of consciousness are those of the diencephalon and brain stem, and more specifically those of the posterior hypothalamic and midbrain regions. The reticular activating system in the cephalad portion of the brain stem is important in attention and awareness. Stimulation of this area or of the afferents to it causes awakening or arousal; disease of this area or impaired conduction of impulses to or from it causes loss of awareness and somnolence; destruction of this center or its isolation from other parts of the nervous system may result in complete loss of consciousness. A purely unilateral cerebral lesion rarely causes coma unless it is accompanied by increased intracranial pressure. Bilateral lesions, however, especially if extensive, may result in a significant impairment of consciousness. Extensive bilateral cerebral lesions, such as those occurring in anoxic encephalopathy, may result in a marked depression of consciousness, including coma.

The degree of impairment of consciousness in many conditions in which there is either stupor or coma may be compared with the stages of surgical and barbiturate anesthesia. In the first stage there is clouding of consciousness, with impairment of contact with the environment, loss of discrimination, and, often, some euphoria; these phenomena are caused by slight to moderate depression of cortical activity. In the next stage there is loss of consciousness due to complete suppression of cortical control, and motor and reflex functions are carried out by subcortical structures. In still deeper stages there is loss of reflex response and of many visceral functions owing to depression of midbrain structures. In the final stage, just preceding death, there is a gradual abolition of respiratory and circulatory control owing to depression of brain stem activity.

CAUSES OF COMA

Cerebrovascular Disease

Vascular lesions of the brain constitute one of the most important causes of disturbances of consciousness and are responsible for the symptoms in about 10% of patients in coma. The various syndromes of cerebrovascular disease are discussed in Chapters 51 and 53.

Acute lesions of the intracerebral arteries usually cause both disturbances of consciousness and hemiplegia. The patient may be either deeply comatose or stuporous with responses to painful stimuli; occasionally there is no disturbance of consciousness. There is paresis of one side of the face and body, with drooping of the angle of the mouth, bulging of the cheek, and flaccidity of the affected extremities. The upper portion of the face is rarely affected, although the corneal reflex is often absent on the side of the paresis. There may be turning of the head and conjugate deviation of the eyes toward the nonparalyzed side, with paralysis of conjugate gaze toward the affected side. The flaccid extremities drop heavily if raised and allowed to fall, whereas the arm and leg drop slowly on the normal side. There is often anisocoria; in the case of a large intracerebral lesion the ipsilateral pupil is dilated, owing to pressure on the third nerve by herniation of the uncus and hippocampal gyrus through the incisura of the tentorium cerebelli, although occasionally the ipsilateral pupil is constricted. Both pupils may dilate as coma deepens, the one on the side of the lesion doing so first. The light reflex disappears in profound coma.

With intraventricular hemorrhage there may be coma and shock without localizing signs, followed by increasing paralysis of all four extremities, decerebrate rigidity, and signs of meningeal irritation.

In intracerebral hemorrhage the onset is usually sudden, although there may be a gradual development of coma. The ictus is usually the result of a sudden increase in blood pressure in an individual whose blood pressure is already elevated, although occasionally it is caused by the rupture of an anomalous cerebral artery, or for other reasons, such as amyloid degeneration of the vessel. The patient often has the hypertensive or apoplectic habitus: he is moderately obese, with a short, thick neck, broad chest and shoulders, and ruddy, flushed cheeks. There may be a history of previously diagnosed hypertension or of former strokes. The onset of symptoms often takes place during violent exercise or emotional stress. Some 90% of patients are over 40 years of age. Impending symptoms of intracerebral hemorrhage include severe occipital or nuchal headache, vertigo, drowsiness, confusion, stupor, forgetfulness, epistaxis, and retinal hemorrhages. Preceding the hemorrhage there may have been transient focal manifestations consisting of brief attacks of paresis, paresthesia, diplopia, or dysarthria, or fleeting localized convulsive seizures. In intracerebral hemorrhage the coma may be profound, and often there is some evidence of shock. Convulsions are infrequent at the outset. The respirations may be stertorous or of the Cheyne–Stokes type, and the temperature may be below normal. There may be signs of increased intracranial pressure with a slowing of the pulse. The patient is often incontinent. The pupils may fail to react to light. Examination of the retinal arteries may show evidence of hypertensive hemorrhages or related changes. The lesion of intracerebral hemorrhage is readily demonstrated on computed tomography or magnetic imaging. There may be an increase in the cerebrospinal fluid pressure and in the protein and cell content of the spinal fluid; there may be frank blood in the fluid. Lumbar puncture is not routinely necessary if the hemorrhage is in a usual location and seen on imaging studies.

Cerebral thrombosis, with resulting infarction and encephalomalacia, may have either a precipitous or a gradual onset. The symptoms may appear while the patient is idle or during sleep. There may be a history of previous transient ischemic attacks, atherosclerosis, hypertension, diabetes, or syphilis, and there may have been premonitory symptoms similar to those occurring with cerebral hemorrhage. Coma is less profound; in fact the patient often fails to lose consciousness. The patient may be younger, and there is less apt to be hypertension. The blood pressure is frequently normal, although cerebral thrombosis as well as intracerebral hemorrhage may occur in hypertensive individuals. Computed tomography may not demonstrate the cerebral infarct for hours or days; with contrast enhancement it is shown within 3–7 days as a rule. Magnetic resonance imaging usually can demonstrate the infarct earlier. The cerebrospinal fluid is clear and the pressure is normal.

With cerebral embolism the onset is sudden; the loss of consciousness may be transitory. It is often possible to determine the source of the embolus, and there may be a history of cardiac or pulmonary disease. Cerebral fat and air embolisms occur but are rare. The appearance of cerebral infarcts due to occlusion of vessels from local thrombosis and from emboli is often similar on imaging studies. Magnetic imaging may at times outline the actual clot in the affected vessel, while arteriograms show occlusions or lack of perfusion or flow in vessels.

Loss of consciousness is uncommon with lesions of the cortical branches of the major cerebral arteries or of the branches of the vertebral or basilar arteries; either thrombosis or hemorrhage of the basilar artery, however, may cause coma, as may cerebellar hemorrhage or infarction. Cerebellar vascular lesions usually cause coma by compression of the brain stem or by its upward herniation. Coma is also uncommon with transient ischemic attacks secondary to insufficiency of the extracranial arteries unless such insufficiency in the vertebrobasilar system interferes with the blood supply to the reticular activating system. If this is the case, there may be transient "blackouts" or "drop attacks" that are occasionally brought on by extension of the neck, especially if there is extensive cervical arthritis as well as stenosis of the vertebral arteries.

When subarachnoid hemorrhage occurs there is usually the sudden onset of an intense headache in the occipital region or the back of the neck. The coma comes on gradually and convulsions may or may not occur. The pulse is often slowed (50 – 60/min) and there may be vertigo, vomiting, and lethargy. Characteristically there are marked signs of meningeal irritation, with photophobia, Kernig's and Brudzinski's signs, and nuchal rigidity developing within a few hours. The diagnosis is confirmed by imaging studies or lumbar puncture; the cerebrospinal fluid contains fresh blood that does not clot, and later there is xanthochromia with crenation of the red cells. Bloody fluid and xanthochromia may also be found in intraventricular hemorrhage and in intracerebral hemorrhage accompanied by subarachnoid bleeding. In the latter condition, however, there are signs of both localization and meningeal irritation, as well as evidence of focal accumulation of blood on imaging studies.

In hypertensive encephalopathy, or acute hypertensive crisis, there may be a sudden onset of coma with or without convulsions. There is usually a history of kidney disease, severe hypertension, or both, and often of severe headaches, irritability, fatigue drowsiness, vomiting and failing vision. Severe hypertensive retinopathy with papilledema may be present. The cerebrospinal fluid pressure is moderately elevated.

Thrombosis of the venous sinuses is an uncommon cause of coma. Hyperviscosity syndromes including polycythemia, cryoglobulinemia, sickle cell anemia, and macroglobulinemia may result in depressed consciousness as can widespread small vessel occlusion syndromes associated with disseminated intravascular coagulation, lupus erythematosus, thrombotic thrombocytopenic purpura and related conditions, and bacterial endocarditis.

Trauma

Trauma is responsible for the symptoms in some 13% of the comatose patients who are admitted to large general hospitals and for a much larger percentage of patients who die in coma. The Glasgow Coma Scale (see above) is a widely used grading system for the severity of cerebral injury; it has some relationship to the prognosis. It is usually possible to obtain a history of an accident, although the type of injury may not be known. Automobile accidents, gunshot wounds, or blast concussions are common causes. There is usually evidence of injury on physical examination. There may be bruises and hematomas of the face; lacerations or hemorrhages about the scalp; depressions or other injuries of the skull; bleeding from the ears, nose, or mouth; or cerebrospinal fluid rhinorrhea. In cerebral concussion there may be an immediate brief period of loss of consciousness with no permanent symptoms, prolonged coma, late development of coma, or delirium. On regaining consciousness the patient may be dazed and confused, with retrograde and anterograde amnesia. With more severe injuries there may be petechial hemorrhages and cerebral edema that lead to prolonged stupor. Cerebral contusions and lacerations show focal signs on examination, and evidence of damage on imaging studies. In middle meningeal hemorrhage there is coma immediately after the accident; this may be followed by a lucid interval and then, in turn, by gradually deepening coma resulting from expansion of an epidural hematoma. With subdural hematoma and hygroma the symptoms may become apparent days to weeks after an injury. There is first confusion with slight lowering of consciousness, followed by stupor, gradually increasing coma, and progressive hemiparesis. The pupil, if enlarged, is usually dilated on the side of the lesion. In all traumatic states the physician should be especially concerned about the blood pressure, pulse, respirations, and temperature, and should watch closely for signs of shock (drop in blood pressure) or increasing intracranial pressure (papilledema, bradycardia, vomiting). The patient should be moved as little as possible and roentgenologic studies should be deferred until definite information has been obtained regarding the general status of the patient. Then, roentgenograms of the cervical spine, computed tomography of the head (or neck), or magnetic resonance imaging of these structures is usually indicated.

Alcohol Ingestion

Acute alcohol intoxication is a common cause for loss of consciousness in patients admitted to general hospitals in large cities. The history of previous alcoholism or acute alcoholic intoxication may be obtained. On examination the patient shows a flushed face, injected throat and conjunctivae, and diminished to absent reflexes. The pulse may be full and respirations deep, and the patient can usually be aroused lightly. The pupils are dilated and react normally. There are often minor injuries over the body; vomiting is common, and occasionally there are convulsions. There is evidence of alcohol on the breath, in the gastric contents, and in the blood. One should remember that patients in states of alcoholic intoxication may become comatose for other reasons. They may have suffered from cerebral hemorrhage and trauma, and many instances of subdural hematoma have been reported in alcoholism.

Wernicke's syndrome is a nutritional disorder secondary to thiamine deficiency that usually develops in undernourished alcoholic patients. Various alterations develop in the state of consciousness, ranging from mild confusion to coma. In addition, other neurologic alterations develop, including extraocular muscle weakness, ataxia, and tremors. This disorder can often be acute in onset and if the diagnosis is even entertained, the patient should immediately receive thiamine and other B complex vitamins in order to avoid irreversible neurologic deficits. It is wise, and essentially harmless, to administer thiamine to anyone in coma of uncertain cause. Thiamine will prevent the development of alcohol-related complications such as Wernicke's syndrome, and, to a lesser degree, delirium tremens and other sequelae of alcohol abuse.

Postconvulsion Coma

Coma or stupor may be a sequel of a recent convulsion in an epileptic patient or in a patient who has convulsions of another etiology, al-
though it may not be possible to obtain a history of either a recent convulsion or previous attacks. The patient may show evidence of tongue-biting, with frothing at the mouth and bloody sputum, and there may be incontinence and lacerations or other injuries to the body. Old scars may be found on the tongue. The stupor is usually brief in duration, but may be followed by either profound sleep or confusion and irrational behavior. In the absence of a history of previous convulsions it may be difficult to differentiate between the postconvulsive state and cerebral trauma. In status epilepticus there are repeated convulsions and the patient fails to regain consciousness between them. In so-called absence status there is lowering and clouding of consciousness and the patient may appear to be in a trancelike stupor suggesting drug abuse or psychiatric disorders.

Diabetes

Diabetic coma is encountered less frequently than in past years, probably because of the earlier diagnosis and treatment of diabetes. Coma, however, occasionally is the first clinical manifestation of the disease. If no history can be obtained regarding the patient who is first observed in coma, diabetes must always be considered as a possible factor. Most diabetic patients are now advised to carry cards, necklaces, or bracelets stating that they are afflicted with the disease. The loss of consciousness may be profound. The muscle stretch reflexes are often decreased or absent; there may be Babinski responses. The temperature is subnormal, the blood pressure depressed, and the pulse increased in rate. The respirations are rapid and may be of the Kussmaul type, with air hunger. The eyeballs may be soft, owing to decreased intraocular tension, and the pupils may be constricted and fail to react to light. There may be evidence of dehydration, with dry skin and tongue, and the feet are often cold. The characteristic odor of acetone is often noticed on the breath. The presence of acetone, acetoacetic acid, and large amounts of glucose in the urine will confirm the diagnosis, as will determinations of blood glucose and CO_2 combining power. Nonketotic hyperglycemic coma with associated serum hyperosmolarity and dehydration may develop, often accompanied by focal seizures; diabetes mellitus may initially present in this way.

Poisoning

Various types of poisoning may be responsible for either coma or stupor. The poisons are frequently self-administered in street drug use or suicidal attempts, although they may have been ingested accidentally, been given with homicidal intent, or been associated with industrial intoxication.

Coma may follow ingestion of opium or its derivatives. The patient is pale and cyanotic; the skin is cold; the temperature is subnormal; the respirations are slow, feeble, and irregular; the pulse is slow and feeble. The face may be livid and the extremities clammy. The pupils are markedly constricted, but may still react to light. The reflexes are diminished; there may be Babinski signs. There may be a history of drug addiction; often needle marks are found on the arms and legs.

Intoxication with barbiturates and other sedatives, hypnotics, and minor tranquilizers (Ch. 53) is commonly encountered. Drug overdosage with street drugs, including heroin, cocaine, phencyclidine, and others, must always be considered in the etiology of coma. Large doses of these drugs may be taken either in a suicidal attempt or accidentally by a patient who is already confused from the use of them. Alcohol may have been ingested simultaneously. It may be possible to obtain a history of excessive use of barbiturates or similarly acting drugs, or of depression that might lead to suicide attempts. The patient may be deeply comatose. The face is pale; the skin is cold and clammy; the respirations are deep, slow, and irregular; the pulse is slow. The pupils are not constricted, but the extraocular movements are often dissociated and there may be nystagmus. The reflexes are abolished and there may be Babinski signs. In profound coma the reflexes may be hyperactive. There may be pills or capsules in the gastric contents. Blood screens help to identify the abused substances. It is not possible to differentiate readily between short-acting and long-acting barbiturates on the basis of blood examinations, but coma develops with a lesser concentration of the former.

Coma due to the inhalation of carbon monoxide may be the result of either suicidal attempts or accidental exposure. It may follow the inhalation of either household gas or exhaust gas from automobiles. The skin is often described as cherry-red in color, but it may be pale and cold. The lips and nail beds are also a cherry-red color.

The temperature is subnormal; the pulse and respirations may vary and may be irregular, rapid, or shallow. There may be an odor of household gas on the breath. A history of the circumstances under which the patient was found aids in the diagnosis, as do blood studies for carbon monoxide, methemoglobin, and carboxyhemoglobin. Headache, vertigo, nausea, vomiting, and convulsions may precede the loss of consciousness.

Many of the other poisons listed in Chapter 53 cause coma and/or convulsions only when ingested in excessive amounts; confusion and delirium more often follow ingestion of or exposure to them. Salicylate intoxication, especially in infants and children, may cause coma, with changes in the respiratory rate, temperature, and reflexes, and with moderate dilation of the pupils; vomiting frequently precedes loss of consciousness. In cocaine and strychnine intoxication there may be a history of excitement and delirium preceding the coma. Lead poisoning causes convulsions and coma in children more frequently than in adults. Disordered consciousness is an early and important symptom in the hemorrhagic encephalitis associated with the use of organic arsenicals. Methyl bromide and chloride, aniline dyes, benzene derivatives, carbon disulfide, carbon tetrachloride, and many other industrial poisons may also cause disturbances of consciousness. Organic toxins that may cause coma and convulsions include those of botulinus, tetanus, and the poisonous mushrooms, as well as the endogenous toxins associated with anemias, hepatic dysfunction, uremia, extensive burns, and infections such as pneumonia.

Meningitis

Meningitis, especially the acute variety, must always be kept in mind as one of the relatively common causes of coma. The symptoms may come on abruptly, with severe headache, and loss of consciousness may follow soon afterwards. This is especially apt to be true in meningococcal meningitis. In streptococcal, pneumococcal, and staphylococcal meningitis there may be a history of infectious processes of some type, especially in the middle ear, about the head, or in the paranasal sinuses. Examination of the patient with meningitis shows evidence of infection (fever, leukocytosis). A rash on the skin is particularly common in meningococcal meningitis. Actually, this develops during the bacteremia that precedes the meningitis. The eruption consists of petechial hemorrhages occurring in the skin and mucous membranes in any portion of the body. They may coalesce to cause purpuric patches that occasionally become necrotic. The most important diagnostic signs are those of meningeal irritation (nuchal rigidity, Kernig's and Brudzinski's signs); the patient often is in a position of opisthotonos. Sometimes, however, the signs of meningeal irritation are absent or minimal, especially early in the disease, and in neonates. Other important abnormalities are altered pupillary responses, dissociation of ocular movements, convulsive manifestations, and focal neurologic involvement. Signs of increased intracranial pressure may be present. The patient with focal neurologic deficits will need immediate cranial imaging studies before a lumbar puncture is performed. In the absence of a significant focal intracranial mass or focal deficits on examination, the diagnosis may be confirmed by lumbar puncture, which shows increased pressure, pleocytosis, increased protein, and marked decrease in glucose, and often the presence of the infectious organisms. Tuberculous meningitis is less rapid in onset; it may occur in any age group, and no history of previous tuberculous infection may be evident. Other forms of meningitis are mentioned in Chapter 53.

Brain Tumors and Brain Abscesses

Brain tumors and brain abscesses may cause coma with or without paralysis. The disturbance of consciousness may be related to the localization of the lesion within the nervous system or may be secondary to an increase in intracranial pressure. If a history can be obtained, there is usually a story of gradual onset of symptoms, with headaches, vomiting, focal signs, convulsions, apathy, stupor, failing vision, and personality changes; however, with certain rapidly growing neoplasms and with brain abscesses the symptoms and signs may come on precipitously. A sudden hemorrhage into a tumor or sudden obstruction of the ventricular system may cause an abrupt onset or increase in symptoms. With brain abscesses there may be a history of some coexisting infectious process. If there is coma, there often are signs of increased intracranial pressure: vomiting, stupor, papilledema, bradycardia, and changes in the blood pressure and respirations; and there may be evidence of localization of disturbed cerebral function. The symptoms and signs of subdural hematoma and hygroma may be similar to those just described, but there is usually a history of an antecedent injury followed after some time by decreasing levels of consciousness, then stupor and coma; progressive hemiparesis and hemisensory deficits also occur. These mass lesions are usually readily demonstrated by computed tomography or magnetic resonance imaging. These studies also give hints as to the nature of the lesion, whether it is solid, cystic, likely primary or metastatic, or even multiple.

Encephalitis

Encephalitis causes a lowering of consciousness on most occasions, although hypersomnia may be present rather than stupor or coma, and the patient frequently can be aroused for short periods. With the viral encephalitides there often are dissociated eye movements, other abnormalities of the cranial nerves, and hyperkinetic phenomena. Toxic or hemorrhagic encephalitis may follow exposure to various toxins. Demyelinating encephalitis may be associated with vaccinia, smallpox, measles, and similar conditions. Dementia paralytica, which is a syphilitic encephalitis, usually has a subacute onset with a history of intellectual deterioration and delusional manifestations; the symptoms may, however, come on precipitously with convulsive manifestations and apoplectic phenomena that suggest cerebral hemorrhage. Usually, however, the history and the characteristic signs, including pupillary abnormalities and hyperactive reflexes as well as the blood and spinal fluid serologic findings, lead to a correct diagnosis. Meningoencephalitic manifestations may accompany many types of infectious disease. The rarer causes of infectious disease are especially likely to produce meningoencephalitic pictures in persons with immunosuppressed states, including the acquired immune deficiency syndrome and iatrogenically produced such states.

Reye's syndrome is a postviral syndrome of children, possibly related to treatment of the preceding viral infection; it is characterized by vomiting, glucose and liver disturbances, and progressive coma beginning within a few days of the original viral illness. The pathogenesis is unclear. The altered consciousness reflects both increased intracranial pressure and metabolic derangements of this syndrome.

Hypoglycemia

Hyperglycemia, usually accompanied by acidosis, may cause coma in diabetes, but hypoglycemia may also be responsible for coma. The loss of consciousness is often preceded by convulsions. A hypoglycemic state may be the result of any of the following: hyperinsulinism associated with either pancreatic or liver disease, hyperinsulinism caused by the production of an excessive amount of insulin by an adenoma of the pancreas, or the administration of large doses of insulin in the treatment of either diabetes or psychotic states. The convulsions and loss of consciousness are usually preceded by symptoms that consist of nervousness, weakness, fatigue, hunger, tremulousness, irritability, pallor, increased sweating, and psychic manifestations. Examination of the comatose patient shows dilation of the pupils, hyperhidrosis, cold skin, and tremors. The tendon reflexes may be retained and are often exaggerated, even in deep coma, and there may be a Babinski response. The coma may be brief in duration. The convulsive manifestations and the bodily responses may call forth additional glucose from storage in the liver, so that by the time the patient is examined the blood glucose determinations may be within the normal range. Nevertheless, all persons in coma for which the cause is not apparent at once should, after a blood sample for glucose determination has been drawn, receive a bolus of intravenous glucose. This will reverse serious hypoglycemia and will not harm persons with other causes of coma, even diabetics in acidosis.

Pneumonia and Other Infections

Pneumonia has been reported to be responsible for some 2% of the cases of coma admitted to general hospitals. The coma may be caused by either the infectious process itself or endogenous toxic substances produced by the infection. Since pneumonia is diagnosed much earlier than it was formerly, and since specific therapeutic measures can be instituted earlier in the course of the disease, coma due to pneumonia is less common than it once was. Other infections such as malaria, typhoid fever, scarlet fever, osteomyelitis, and septicemia may also cause loss of consciousness, and coma may be the terminal stage of any infectious process, as, for instance, the Waterhouse–Friderichsen syndrome in meningitis.

Cardiac Decompensation and Heart Failure

Heart disease of various types, with resulting cardiac decompensation and heart failure, must always be considered in the diagnosis of coma. Cardiac arrest is a frequent cause of coma. In the Stokes-Adams syndrome there is profound loss of consciousness with or without convulsions; the manifestations are accompanied by bradycardia, and may be preceded by vertigo. This syndrome may be caused by heart block with cardiac standstill, ventricular tachycardia and fibrillation, carotid sinus stimulation, and atherosclerosis of the vertebral and basilar arteries. Either transient or prolonged loss of consciousness may also occur with other types of heart disease, including paroxysmal tachycardia, coronary insufficiency, and aortic stenosis and insufficiency, as well as with pulmonary hypertension.

Metabolic Disturbances

In addition to the comas of diabetes and hypoglycemia, which have been discussed separately, many other metabolic disturbances may cause disorders of consciousness. These are generally referred to as secondary metabolic encephalopathies.

Uremic coma may result from a variety of renal lesions. There are complex metabolic disturbances including the retention of nitrogenous waste products and disorders of acid–base balance, water, and electrolyte balance. The coma may be relatively slow in onset and is often preceded by headache, vomiting, dyspnea, muscular twitching, diarrhea, and lethargy. There may have been a period of confusion with gradual lowering of consciousness, followed by delirium and convulsions, and then by coma. Examination often shows peripheral edema; the breath is uriniferous, and there may be "uremic frost" about the nose and lips. Urinalysis shows excessive protein along with large numbers of erythrocytes and casts, although there may be anuria. Ophthalmoscopy may reveal the presence of albuminuric retinitis with hemorrhages and exudates. Chemical studies on the blood show a marked increase in urea nitrogen. The cerebrospinal fluid pressure is often increased.

Hepatic coma may be a complication of cirrhosis, acute and chronic hepatitis, and disturbances of the portal and hepatic circulation, including portacaval anastomoses. The clinical picture shows fluctuation, and the coma may be preceded by apathy, lethargy, irritability, confusion, delirium, and motor symptoms consisting of coarse postural to-and-fro movements (asterixis) of the outstretched extremities. Actual loss of consciousness may come on spontaneously or be precipitated by increased dietary protein, inadequate nutrition, alcohol, drugs, infection, or hemorrhage. Additional motor disturbances include rigidity, dysarthria, grimacing, hyperreflexia, Babinski signs, sucking and grasping reflexes, and convulsions. The presence of large amounts of toxic nitrogenous substances in the systemic circulation may be responsible, and in a majority of patients there are high blood ammonia levels, but other metabolic abnormalities doubtless contribute to the production of neurologic symptoms.

The coma of eclampsia may have features resembling both uremic and hepatic coma, along with manifestations of hypertensive encephalopathy.

Coma may occur with chronic pulmonary insufficiency and respiratory failure secondary to emphysema, pulmonary fibrosis, and marked obesity (pickwickian syndrome). Headache, confusion, somnolence, and stupor may precede the coma, and there may be papilledema and other signs of increased intracranial pressure. The symptoms are related to carbon dioxide retention and anoxia.

Disturbances in the concentration of the electrolytes, acid-base dysequilibrium, dehydration, and water intoxication can all cause an encephalopathy with lethargy, depression, confusion, delirium, the syndrome of inappropriate antidiuretic hormone secretion, and either convulsions or coma (Ch. 53). Such disturbances may also contribute to the symptoms in comas of other etiologies. Coma may follow acidosis and alkalosis, both metabolic and respiratory, hyperkalemia and hypokalemia, hypernatremia and hyponatremia, hypermagnesemia and hypomagnesemia, hypercalcemia and hypocalcemia.

Comas secondary to disturbances of the endocrine glands are occasionally encountered. Myxedema coma occurs with long-standing, greatly depressed thyroid function. It is often precipitated by cold and is accompanied by profound hypothermia. In Addisonian coma, from adrenocortical failure, there are associated hypotension, hypoglycemia, and electrolyte disturbances. Hypopituitary coma is most commonly seen in women who have suffered ischemic necrosis of the anterior lobe of the pituitary during or after childbirth (**Sheehan's syndrome**), but

also occurs with pituitary cachexia (**Simmond's disease**). Adrenocortical deficiency and hypoglycemia contribute to the symptoms.

Anemia, Anoxia, and Nutritional Deficiency

Profound anemia may cause coma but the modern and simple methods for the blood count render anemia rare as a cause of coma in patients who consult a physician routinely. Complaints of weakness, fatigue, and many other symptoms precede the onset of stupor and coma. Loss of consciousness associated with a deficiency of the blood supply to the brain is usually associated with either exsanguination or some vasomotor disturbance such as vasodepressor syncope or shock. Anoxia may also cause coma; in exposure to high altitudes the loss of consciousness is usually transient, but deficient oxygenation associated with surgical anesthesia, lack of oxygen in the surrounding air, obstruction of the airway, paralysis of the muscles of respiration, impaired transport of oxygen by the blood, smothering, drowning, electric shock, cardiac insufficiency, methemoglobinemia, or cyanide intoxication may constitute the pathologic mechanism underlying coma. In profound nutritional deficiencies such as starvation, beriberi, pellagra, and severe cachexia and dehydration in the aged, there may be coma, as well as in the terminal stages of Wernicke's syndrome and untreated pernicious anemia. Coma associated with ruptured ectopic pregnancy is caused by exsanguination and shock. Profound hypothermia and hyperthermia may also cause coma, as may decompression sickness.

Stupor, coma, delirium, and other disorders of consciousness may develop as the result of multiple underlying metabolic alterations and deficiencies (Ch. 53).

Sun Stroke, Heat Exhaustion, and Electric Shock

Sunstroke and heat exhaustion may cause either stupor or convulsions. The collapse is usually ushered in by pallor, headache, vertigo, lethargy, confusion, and muscle cramps. The patient is restless, often with a high fever; the skin is hot and dry; the pupils are dilated; respirations are shallow and the pulse is weak. Elderly people with parkinsonism who live in warm climates and receive cholinergic drugs may develop heat exhaustion with far less exposure than healthy young people. Malignant hyperthermia, an unexpected reaction to certain antipsychotics and, rarely, other drugs, may also cause coma.

In lightning and electric shock there may be coma and convulsions associated with either pathologic changes in the brain or anoxia resulting from paralysis of respiration and cardiac arrhythmias.

OTHER STATES OF DISORDERED CONSCIOUSNESS

Syncope

Syncope, or fainting, may be difficult to differentiate from episodic coma resulting from other causes, but the loss of consciousness is usually transient and may be incomplete. The most common type is so-called vasodepressor syncope, and it is this variety that is often referred to as simple fainting. It may occur at any age, and often affects young and otherwise healthy individuals. The attacks usually take place while the patient is in the upright position, and may be precipitated by pain, loss of blood, the sight of blood, excessive heat, fatigue, hunger, nausea, worry, fear, shock, prolonged standing, sudden change in position, or psychic or emotional upsets. Often there is no warning, although the patient may notice giddiness, vertigo, numbness and tingling of the hands and feet or paresthesias of other parts of the body, tremors, sweating, lightheadedness, palpitations, muscle weakness, yawning or belching, nausea, scotomas, or blurring of vision just before the loss of consciousness. The patient may fall before becoming unconscious. The attacks are very brief and usually there is a return of consciousness within 15 seconds, although occasionally the syncope may last longer. Recovery is accelerated by placing the patient in a supine position with the head lower than the body, or, when he is seated, by placing his head between his knees. The patient usually feels perfectly normal afterwards, and notices no headache or sleepiness. There need not be complete loss of consciousness ("near-syncope"); the patient may notice only a transient "blackout" or period of giddiness, and may be able to avoid falling.

During syncope the bodily musculature is flaccid, and tongue-biting, rigidity, muscular contractions, cyanosis, and incontinence are absent, although the patient may injure himself in falling. Occasionally there are brief muscular twitchings or clonic jerks during the attack or while regaining consciousness. There is usually pallor, with increased perspiration, and cold, clammy hands and feet. The temperature, pulse, respirations, and blood pressure may be normal, but often there is a rapid, feeble pulse with rapid respirations and an abrupt fall in blood pressure, all of which soon return to normal. The eyes may be fixed or deviated upwards, and the pupils dilated.

Various causes for syncope have been postulated, and it is believed that both pathophysiologic and psychologic factors may, through vasodepressor action, produce transient cerebral anemia or anoxia, perhaps with alterations in blood chemistry. There is a fall in mean arterial pressure and a decrease in cerebral blood flow. The manifestations are similar to those that occur with sudden deprivation of oxygen in high-altitude flying and with low oxygen tension in experimental studies. It has been stated that when primitive reflex preparations for flight or struggle are initiated, but for some reason appropriate action becomes impossible or must be inhibited, physiologic changes take place in the autonomic nervous system; insufficient blood is delivered to the brain, voluntary tone of muscles is inhibited, and fainting results. In hysterical fainting, without vasodepressor action, there is no preceding weakness or fatigue, and the symptoms are not relieved by change in position; there are usually no changes in autonomic nervous system function or in brain metabolism.

Syncope may also be a symptom of various circulatory, cardiac, cerebral, and other disturbances. Many of the causes of coma, if only transitory in action, may induce what might be interpreted as fainting. The following are among the more important etiologies.

In orthostatic syncope, associated with postural hypotension, there is transient loss of consciousness on assuming the upright position. This may occur in "idiopathic" postural hypotension; after prolonged illness with recumbency, especially in elderly individuals with flabby musculature; after sympathectomy, which abolishes vasodepressor reflexes; with adrenal insufficiency; in severe neuropathies and tabes dorsalis; after the ingestion of sympatholytic drugs, catecholamine-depleting agents, certain other antihypertensive substances, and certain tranquilizers; in some individuals with abnormal autonomic nervous system responses (possibly of psychogenic origin), leading to syncope without tachycardia, pallor, sweating, or nausea;

and in a specific neurologic syndrome in which there is postural hypotension, anhidrosis, fecal and urinary incontinence, impotence, and other evidence of nervous system involvement (*Shy – Drager syndrome*).

In carotid sinus syncope stimulation of either the carotid sinus or body, in certain susceptible individuals, causes vertigo, pallor, loss of consciousness, and occasionally convulsions; these phenomena are caused by slowing of the heart rate, decrease in cardiac output, fall in blood pressure, and peripheral vasodilation. Three types of pathologic carotid sinus syndrome responses have been described: the vagal type, in which the predominant response is slowing of the heart rate; the depressor type, in which fall in blood pressure is the principal manifestation; and the cerebral type, characterized by syncope and sometimes convulsions (Ch. 15). In individuals with atherosclerotic involvement of the carotid and/or the vertebrobasilar arterial system the syncope and occasional convulsions and contralateral hemiparesis that may follow pressure in the region of the carotid bifurcation are the result of cerebral ischemia rather than a reflex response.

In Stokes-Adams disease there is loss of consciousness, with or without convulsions, associated with heart block and ventricular standstill. Syncope may also occur as a symptom of coronary and myocardial insufficiency, cardiac decompensation, paroxysmal tachycardia, arrhythmias, valvular disease, or other conditions in which there is either reflex cardiac inhibition or decreased cardiac output; the loss of consciousness may be prolonged. With hypertension there may be transient fainting, especially on arising, induced by a sudden increase, not a drop, in blood pressure. Pulmonary hypertension syncope is usually precipitated by exertion.

Among the cerebral causes for syncope are conditions in which there is either impaired cerebral circulation or impaired cerebral metabolism. Decreased blood flow may be secondary to atherosclerosis, hypertension, vascular insufficiency, trauma, carotid sinus stimulation, or peripheral circulatory failure. Disturbed metabolism may be present in severe anemia, anoxemia secondary to cardiac or pulmonary disease, anoxia of high altitudes, hypoglycemia, acidosis, and drug intoxications. It is often difficult clinically to differentiate between syncope of cerebral or other origin and brief akinetic epileptic seizures. Also, some syncopal attacks are accompanied by brief clonic jerking movements that resemble those occurring in convulsions. Electroencephalographic monitoring may help differentiate syncope from seizures.

In the hyperventilation syndrome rapid breathing produces hypocapnia and respiratory alkalosis, with symptoms of numbness and tingling of the extremities, dizziness, palpitation, stiffness of the muscles, blurring of vision, light-headedness, confusion, and sometimes syncope, which may be accompanied by either convulsions or tetany. The syndrome occurs more frequently in women than in men, and is usually precipitated by anxiety, fear, or other psychic manifestations. It usually occurs in emotionally labile individuals, and many of the minor symptoms may be related to anxiety rather than to alkalosis. Hyperventilation is also used to activate the electroencephalogram in patients with epilepsy and occasionally brings on certain types of seizures in such patients.

There are varieties of syncope that are related in part to **Valsalva's maneuver** (increase of intrathoracic pressure by forcible exhalation against the closed glottis). Tussive, or cough syncope usually follows a paroxysm of coughing in a person with chronic pulmonary or bronchial disease, often with some tracheal or laryngeal obstruction. The fainting comes on suddenly and there is a rapid return of consciousness. This usually occurs in robust or obese men. The increased intrathoracic pressure may cause a decrease of venous return to the heart, a diminution of cardiac output, and temporary cerebral anoxia. A transient rise in cerebrospinal fluid pressure and extravascular pressure leading to relative cerebral anoxia may also contribute to the etiology. Similar fainting may occur with straining at stool, vomiting, sneezing, lifting, or excessive laughing. Micturition syncope occurs in men (usually healthy young adults) during or following forceful urination immediately after arising from a recumbent position. The mechanisms are similar to those of tussive syncope, but orthostatic hypotension and cardioinhibitory reflexes from the bladder causing cardiac standstill may also contribute to the syndrome. In older men bladder neck obstruction may be an aggravating factor. In the "fainting lark" or "mess trick," brief syncope is brought on by compression of the chest while the subject is forcibly expiring agaist a closed glottis. In breath-holding spells, which usually occur in infants and young children, there is loss of consciousness when the child holds his breath in expiration after a prolonged cry that has often been precipitated by fear, anger, or frustration. There may be associated flushing, cyanosis, upward deviation of the eyeballs, and either tonic muscular spasms or brief convulsive movements. The attack may be difficult to differentiate by observation alone from a convulsive seizure. Both hyperventilation and the factors that bring about cough syncope may be responsible for the loss of consciousness, but it is probable that anoxia is the principal cause. Among the more rare types of syncope are those occurring when a needle is introduced into the pleural space, after a distended bladder is drained, or following removal of ascitic fluid. The mechanisms of these are poorly understood.

Shock

Shock, or, as it is often termed, surgical shock, is closely related to vasodepressor syncope. The onset usually follows trauma, burns, severe pain, or surgical procedures. There is an acute peripheral circulatory failure that results in a sudden drop in the arterial blood pressure owing to loss of blood from the exterior of the body and vasodilation in the splanchnic areas. There is a reduction in the effective circulating volume of blood, and there may also be changes in the electrolytes. The loss of consciousness may be preceded by restlessness, and the coma may be gradual in onset. There is marked pallor, and the skin is cold and moist, with excessive perspiration; the pulse is feeble and rapid; respirations are decreased in amplitude and rapid in rate; the blood pressure is very low. The patient does not respond at once, as he does in syncope, and must be kept warm and given supportive treatment. The impairment of circulation may continue until there is a state of irreversible circulatory failure with resulting collapse. Transfusions, plasma replacement, fluids, change in body position (lowering the head), and analgesics may be necessary as emergency measures.

Confusion and Delirium

The same processes that cause lowering of consciousness (coma and stupor) may also be responsible for clouding of the consciousness (confusion and delirium). In addition to disturbances of memory, attention, perception, and orientation, there may be excitement with excessive motor activity, increased response to all types of stimuli, and mental symptoms in the nature of poverty of ideas, incoherence, emotional lability, illusions, hallucinatory manifestations, and delusional phenomena. **Confusion** is a state of lowered consciousness with disorientation, disturbed thinking, and defects in memory, attention, and perception. **Delirium** consists of confusion with inattention, excitement, agitation, motor and sensory irritability, increased motor activity, and abnormal mental phenomena. Confusion and delirium may precede the development of stupor and coma, and may have the same causes. Therefore, the emergency measures used for stabilizing and investigating comatose persons also must be available to confused and delirious patients.

Delirium may be considered a reversible psychotic episode that appears symptomatically in response to brain injury by trauma, after the ingestion of toxins, or during the course of some underlying disease. There are fluctuations in the patient's level of awareness, with loss of attention and memory, and impairment in the ability to think in the abstract. The memory loss may be caused by failure of registration, retention, or recall, especially the first. Lack of comprehension and insight, loss of personal identification, and flagging of attention are common symptoms. The disorientation for time is often more marked than that for either place or person. There often are disorders of mood, and marked fear and apprehension may be present. Owing to the release of cerebral inhibition and repression there is loss of normal emotional control, with excitement, stereotyped activity, and regression of behavior to a primitive level of integration. Overactivity of lower centers causes tremors, excessive motor activity, and increased responsiveness to all stimuli. There is restlessness, with overactivity and purposeless body movements. Carphology and jactitation are common; the patient may struggle to get out of bed and have to be restrained. Food may be refused.

Overactivity of the autonomic nervous system is shown by the presence of dilated pupils, tachycardia, and marked hyperhidrosis. There are nocturnal and diurnal variations, and the symptoms are often more marked at night ("sundowning"), when there is a physiologic lowering of consciousness. Misinterpretation of stimuli leads to illusions. The hallucinations are usually either visual or auditory and are often hypnagogic, becoming manifest in the drowsy state that just precedes sleep; they have a dream-like character, and the patient is often aware of their hallucinatory nature. The delusions are often brief and unsystematized.

Delirium may be psychogenic, but it is usually organic and occurs in toxic, infectious, deficiency, or traumatic states; impairment of the nutrition and circulation of the brain are important factors.

It may appear spontaneously in association with drug intoxication (prescription or street drugs), febrile or infectious states, or cardiac or renal disease in patients who have no preexisting structural cerebral abnormality, or it may follow specific head injuries or convulsions. It is precipitated more readily, however, in patients who already have some type of brain disease, such as presenile or senile dementia. It occurs most frequently as a toxic, exhaustive, or infectious state associated with somatic disease, and usually manifestations of systemic disease are apparent. One must bear in mind that individuals vary widely in their susceptibility to delirium; some persons react with symptoms of delirium to every illness, minor evidence of toxemia or infection, or only slight temperature elevations, whereas others show no signs of delirium in spite of marked evidence of infection or intoxication. Delirium may develop with lesser degrees of temperature elevation in the elderly than it does earlier in life when infection is present. Definite electroencephalographic changes are found in most cases of organic delirium.

Delirium occurs with intracranial infections such as meningitis and encephalitis, but febrile delirium may also appear in association with any severe systemic infection, including such diseases as septicemia, pneumonia, typhoid fever, malaria, scarlet fever, and erysipelas. Motor manifestations such as carphology and jactitation may be more apparent than illusions and hallucinations. The diagnosis of the underlying somatic disease can usually be made by physical examination and laboratory procedures.

Toxic delirium may be caused by ingestion of exogenous toxins or dissemination of endogenous poisons. Symptoms of delirium are found more frequently in chronic than in acute alcoholic intoxication, although acute alcoholic confusion may be considered a delirious state. Alcoholic hallucinosis and delirium tremens are usually regarded as withdrawal phenomena, and Korsakoff's syndrome as a deficiency state. The latter consists of polyneuritis accompanied by confusion and confabulation. The patient often resorts to evasions and generalities and fills in memory gaps by the use of inappropriate answers based on distorted time relations. A toxic etiology must always be suspected if delirium is sudden in onset, especially in younger people, and extensive screening tests may be necessary to determine the causative drug or toxin. Delirium may follow the sudden withdrawal not only of alcohol but also of sedative and other drugs.

Exhaustion, or deficiency, delirium occurs in pellagra, beriberi, inanition, primary or secondary anemia, and in any prolonged illness that may lead to the development of nutritional deficiencies. The delirium of hypoglycemia is secondary to a deficiency of glucose; that of cardiac insufficiency and heart failure is associated with impairment of the blood supply to the brain. Delirium due to dehydration, water intoxication, or disturbances of the electrolytes or of the acid–base equilibrium (Ch. 53) may be precipitated or aggravated by trauma, surgery, vomiting, diarrhea, diuretics or other drugs, or inadequately balanced intravenous fluids. Delirium may develop in hyperthyroidism, Addison's disease, and other endocrine disturbances. In many instances of delirium there are multiple underlying factors, including metabolic alterations, deficiencies in electrolytes or glucose, impairment of cerebral circulation and oxygenation, toxic and infectious processes, and inhibition of enzyme activity. This is especially apt to be the case in postoperative or posttraumatic syndromes in elderly or debilitated persons.

Organic brain diseases of various types, in addition to meningitis and encephalitis, may be accompanied by delirium. Cerebral edema associated with brain tumors or abscesses, and subdural hematomas, may be responsible. Specific cerebrovascular lesions may cause delirium; either the focal process, secondary cerebral edema, temporary cessation of function of the parts of the brain left intact, or the influence of preexisting vascular disease may be responsible. Visual hallucinations may occur in patients with severe visual loss as a result of disease of the eyes or with lesions of any part of the visual pathway, and auditory hallucinations with disease of any part of the auditory pathway. In the syndrome of peduncular hallucinosis there may be either visual or auditory hallucinations secondary to disease of the level of the midbrain. "Cataract delirium" comes on following surgical therapy for cataracts in some elderly persons, and is characterized by disorientation, hallucinations, and delusions. The sudden complete loss of vision owing to the presence of dressings, and the effects of drugs, deficiency factors, and underlying organic cerebral disease are all important. The so-called postepileptic confusion is actually a transient delirium. Following cerebral trauma there may be delirium alternating with fluctuations in the level of awareness; there is confusion, disorientation, lowering of the consciousness, and amnesia (especially retrograde), together with headaches and focal neurologic changes. After a subarachnoid hemorrhage there may be symptoms of confusion and confabulation that are similar to those seen in Korsakoff's psychosis.

Psychogenic delirium is often difficult to diagnose. It may be a symptom of one of the major psychoses (manic-depressive or schizophrenic), but it is more commonly encountered in hysteria. The nonorganic features can usually be identified. In hysterical delirium there may be evidence of Ganser's syndrome, in which the patient gives approximate but incorrect answers to all questions. So-called Bell's mania, or acute delirious mania, may come on precipitously with either the manic or the agitated depressive phase of manic-depressive psychosis. The motor overactivity and inadequate dietary and fluid intake lead to metabolic disturbances and electrolyte imbalance, increased temperature, and accentuation of the symptoms. Delirium may also follow sensory and sleep deprivation.

Epilepsy, or Convulsive Disorders

Although it is usually possible to perform the various diagnostic procedures and auxiliary examinations that are necessary to determine the etiology of a convulsive disorder during the interval between attacks, under certain circumstances it may be necessary to arrive at the correct diagnosis while observing a seizure, or during electroencephalographic and simultaneous video monitoring of such an attack. In either case it is essential to determine 1) whether the symptoms are those of so-called idiopathic (cryptogenic) epilepsy, or 2) whether the convulsions are caused by focal or generalized cerebral disease, systemic affections, exposure to or ingestion of toxic substances, metabolic disturbances, withdrawal of drugs, or other etiologic factors, or are precipitated by visual, auditory, or other stimuli. It is also important to differentiate between organic convulsions and psychogenic attacks, and to remember that organic attacks may be precipitated by emotional stimuli. Furthermore, organic and nonorganic attacks may occur in the same person.

The history is of prime importance in the diagnosis of convulsive disorder (Ch. 2). This should be obtained not only from the patient but also from relatives and observers. The history should contain not only the details of the present attack, including precipitating factors, development of the attack, the exact sequence of events leading to the seizure, the nature of any aura and of tonic and clonic phases, and postconvulsion manifestations, but also a detailed chronologic account of the entire history of the disease. Both the aura and the distribution of motor phenomena may be of localizing significance. The examination should include a thorough physical survey, in an attempt to demonstrate the presence of underlying somatic disease, as well as a detailed neurologic appraisal; special concerns must include signs of increased intracranial pressure and evidence of localized disturbance of cerebral function.

In most convulsions the loss of consciousness persists for only a short period, although it may vary from a few seconds to hours or even longer. In jacksonian attacks there may be no loss of consciousness, while in status epilepticus there are recurring convulsions with no restoration of consciousness between attacks. The patient may be either flaccid or rigid during the period of epileptic coma, but there is usually a tonic phase followed by a clonic phase. The distribution of the motor phenomena should be observed closely; in jacksonian, or focal, attacks the movements may be limited to one arm or leg, one side of the face, or one half of the body. The spread of the movements — *e.g.*, from the thumb to the fingers, wrist, forearm, arm, and then to the forehead and face — indicates the site of the epileptogenic focus. Generalized attacks may be focal in onset. Turning of the eyes and/or head, either at the outset or during the attack, may have localizing significance. The presence of an epileptic cry, cyanosis, stertorous breathing, tongue-biting, foaming at the mouth, bleeding from the mouth, incontinence of urine and feces, or evidence of physical injury during attacks are valuable diagnostic criteria, not only in determining the depth of the loss of consciousness, but also in differentiating between organic and hysterical convulsions. These, however, are not always reliable: many epileptics never bite their tongues, injure themselves, or become incontinent, and in hysteria there occasionally is evidence of injury, tongue-biting, or incontinence. During the postconvulsive state the presence of headache, drowsiness, and a tendency to sleep should be noted. Manifestations of focal disturbances of function such as residual paralysis, anesthesia, or aphasia, as well as psychic symptoms such as confusion, irritability, and amnesia give localizing information. It must be remembered that trauma and vascular accidents may result in convulsions, but also that an intracranial hemorrhage, or a severe head injury, even a skull fracture, may occur during an epileptic attack. A patient with a convulsive disorder may develop a subdural hematoma or a subarachnoid hemorrhage as a result of injury during a seizure. Furthermore, ingestion or withdrawal from the use of alcohol, barbiturates, and other drugs may precipitate epileptic attacks. Post-convulsion stupor and alcoholic stupor may occur simultaneously.

Epilepsy or the convulsive disorder is not a disease but a symptom complex characterized by transient episodes of alteration in the state of consciousness that may be associated with convulsive movements and/or disturbances of feeling or behavior. Epilepsy may be classified variously: clinically, by the seizure type; anatomically, by the site of the responsible lesion; physiologically, by the electrical or biochemical alterations underlying or accompanying the seizure; etiologically, by the primary causal agent; pathologically, by the structural alterations in the brain; therapeutically, by the response to drug therapy. Many classifications take into consideration more than one of these; that is, a clinical description may be given, along with a mention of the probable anatomic lesion and a description of the electroencephalographic changes. The latter are characteristic in certain varieties of epilepsy, which often may be differentiated on the basis of wave form, amplitude, frequency, temporal sequence of the wave pattern, and the localization of the abnormality (Figs. 54-1, 54-2, and 54-3). The electrical alterations, especially when recorded during an interseizure period, are not specific for all of the clinical types, but when analyzed along with an adequate history and a detailed neurologic examination constitute an important diagnostic aid. Prolonged electroencephalographic monitoring is often helpful in differentiating seizure types. Imaging studies, either computed tomography or magnetic resonance types, blood chemistries and blood counts, electrocardiography, and at times lumbar puncture are valuable in the initial assessment of a patient with seizures.

In the clinical classification of the epilepsies the generalized tonic–clonic or **grand mal** attack is the most frequent variety. In this form, generalized convulsive movements, tonic and clonic motor phenomena, loss of consciousness, and often tongue-biting or bodily injury during attacks are characteristic. The electroencephalo-

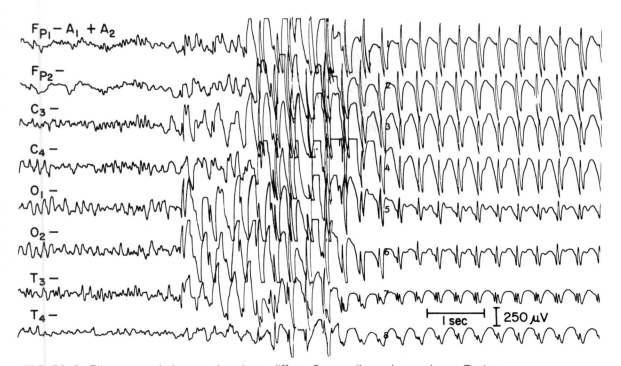

FIG. 54–1. Electroencephalogram showing a diffuse, 3 cps spike and wave burst. During this burst the patient was unresponsive and had eyelid fluttering. Electrode placement is according to the International System. (Courtesy of Dr. Richard P. Tucker)

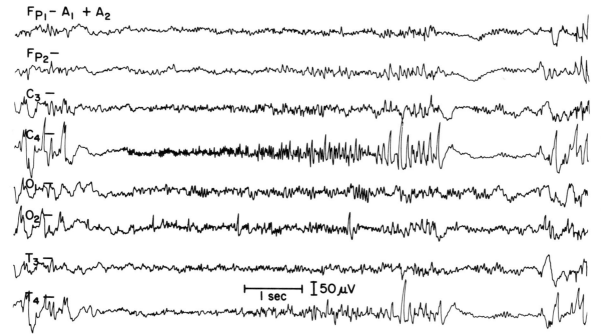

FIG. 54–2. Electroencephalogram showing a progressive ictal discharge originating in the right central area (C4). The patient had frequent focal seizures consisting of jerking of the left arm and, to a lesser extent, also of the left leg. Electrode placement is according to the International System. (Courtesy of Dr. Richard P. Tucker)

gram may show evidence of a diffuse dysrhythmia between attacks and high-voltage spike-like waves, usually of high frequency, but occasionally slow, during attacks. In **absence** seizures (formerly called petit mal), another form of generalized epilepsy, there is an extremely brief lapse of consciousness, usually without falling. The patient may stop talking for a moment, stare, and drop objects from the hands; brief slow movements of the eyes or eyelids, a droop of the head, or, rarely, movements of the extremities may be noted. The electroencephalogram shows an alternation of fast and slow cortical electrical activity, with a 2 – 3/sec high-voltage spike and wave pattern that is bilaterally synchronous and specific for this relatively rare disorder, usually occurring in young girls.

In **complex partial** (also known as temporal lobe or psychomotor) seizures there is a period of automatic or abnormal behavior during which the patient appears to be confused and may perform some unreasonable, unmotivated, purposeless or seemingly purposeful act. Although complete loss of consciousness is usually not present, patients may not be aware of what they are doing and may have complete amnesia for

what transpires during the attack. There usually are no convulsive movements. Accompanying or preceding the automatisms, or in place of them, there may be abnormalities of memory (*déjà vu*, *déjà pensé*, etc.), auditory or visual hallucinations or misinterpretations, olfactory or gustatory symptoms that may be accompanied by smacking or tasting movements of the lips and tongue, gastric or autonomic nervous system manifestations, or alterations of thinking or affect. These various phenomena, along with the usual electroencephalographic localization, indicate in most instances a disturbance of function in or near one or both temporal regions. In **focal motor** or **jacksonian** seizures (partial motor seizures) there are tonic and clonic movements that are confined to one extremity or one side of the body; they may begin in one extremity and spread to involve other parts. Often there is no loss of consciousness. The electroencephalogram is similar to that in generalized tonic-clonic attacks, but the abnormal waves originate locally in a specific area of the cortex and then spread; in the seizure-free period there may be a focus of slow waves.

It is not always possible to classify epileptic attacks into one of these four types. There may be

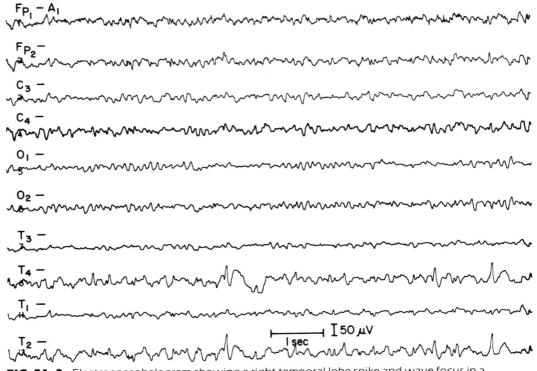

FIG. 54–3. Electroencephalogram showing a right temporal lobe spike and wave focus in a patient with both generalized tonic–clonic and complex partial seizures. Some theta–delta slowing is noted in the same area. Electrode placement is according to the International System. (Courtesy of Dr. Richard P. Tucker)

a variability of manifestations from time to time and no clearcut distinction between one type of attack and another; there may be *formes frustes* that cannot be classified. Many patients have more than one type of seizure. A seizure that starts as focal, or jacksonian, may become secondarily generalized.

There are other, less common, forms of epilepsy. In akinetic attacks there is sudden loss of postural control with nodding of the head or, if generalized, a sudden fall. In myoclonic epilepsy there are single, quick contractions of the muscles, especially those of the flexor groups, but occasionally of the trunk as well. Myoclonic jerkings may precede or accompany generalized tonic-clonic seizures or occur independently, usually without alteration of consciousness. The terms infantile spasm and massive epileptic myoclonus are used to describe seizure types that occur in infants and young children and are characterized by frequent, brief, bilaterally symmetric, jerky flexion movements of the neck, body, and extremities; mental deterioration and a diffuse electroencephalographic abnormality

(hypsarrhythmia) are usually associated. In cursive epilepsy there are running and other gross bodily movements that persist until the patient falls down and loses consciousness. A variety of reflex epilepsies have been described. Seizures may be triggered by laughing (gelastic epilepsy), bright lights, startles, reading, music, or other stimuli. In autonomic, or diencephalic, epilepsy, the attack consists of flushing of the head and neck, tachycardia, cutis anserina, hyperhidrosis, and other manifestations of autonomic nervous system activity. Epilepsia partialis continua is characterized by continuous clonic movements of a limited part of the body. In so-called brain stem and cerebellar fits there is rigidity of all four extremities, often with opisthotonos. A classification of the epilepsies formulated by the International League Against Epilepsy is given in Table 54-1; new versions are published every few years.

The diagnosis of epilepsy is established on the basis of observation of attacks, adequate history and description, and electroencephalographic criteria. It is valuable but often impossible to

TABLE 54-1. INTERNATIONAL CLASSIFICATION OF EPILEPTIC SEIZURES

1. Partial seizures (seizures beginning locally)
   (a) Partial seizures with elementary symptoms (generally without impairment of consciousness)
       (1) With motor symptoms (includes jacksonian seizures)
       (2) With special sensory or somatosensory symptoms
       (3) With autonomic symptoms
       (4) Compound forms
   (b) Partial seizures with complex symptoms (generally with impairment of consciousness) (Temporal lobe or psychomotor seizures)
       (1) With impairment of consciousness only
       (2) With cognitive symptoms
       (3) With affective symptoms
       (4) With psychosensory symptoms
       (5) With psychomotor symptoms (automatisms)
       (6) Compound forms
   (c) Partial seizures secondarily generalized
2. Generalized seizures (bilaterally symmetric and without local onset)
   (a) Absences (petit mal)
   (b) Bilateral massive epileptic myoclonus
   (c) Infantile spasms
   (d) Clonic seizures
   (e) Tonic seizures
   (f) Tonic–clonic seizures (grand mal)
   (g) Atonic seizures
   (h) Akinetic seizures
3. Unilateral seizures (or predominantly unilateral)
4. Unclassified epileptic seizures (data incomplete)

(Abstracted from Gastaut H: Epilepsia 11: 102–113, 1970)

have an opportunity to observe a convulsive seizure in order to appraise the patient's complaints, differentiate malingered or hysterical attacks from organic ones, and note the character of an organic seizure. Electroencephalography aids in the diagnosis, especially when it is difficult to obtain an adequate description of the seizure, and it may be of value in demonstrating the presence of either focal or generalized cerebral disease that may be responsible for the attacks. On occasion, if abnormality is suspected but not evident on routine recordings, diagnostic changes may be brought out by activating procedures such as hyperventilation, sleep, administration of stimulants, visual (photic) or auditory (sonic) stimulation or combinations of these. Electrical abnormalities, if the investigation is thorough enough, are found in 80%–90% of epileptics, between as well as during attacks. It is important to bear in mind, however, that occasional epileptics have normal recordings interictally, and their electroencephalogram may be abnormal only during attacks. Prolonged monitoring may help in their diagnosis. Also, some persons without evidence of central nervous system disease show electroencephalographic changes suggestive of epilepsy. Consequently, the diagnosis must not be based on electrical changes alone.

It must always be remembered that convulsions may be symptoms not only of epilepsy but also of some somatic disease, and careful physical, neurologic, and laboratory examinations should always be performed in order to determine their etiology. Convulsions in infancy may be caused by congenital abnormalities of the brain (cerebral dysplasia, hereditary defects, lipidoses, etc.), anoxia, trauma at the time of birth, antenatal or postnatal infections, hemorrhagic disease of the newborn (erythroblastosis fetalis), or infantile tetany; the last is diagnosed by the presence of Chvostek's and related signs, together with alterations in the blood calcium and phosphorus content. Convulsions in childhood may be caused by tetany, fevers, and acute infections (even in the absence of actual cerebral involvement by the inflammatory process), the ingestion of toxic substances (especially lead), trauma, brain tumors and abscesses, meningitis, encephalitis, vascular disease, tuberous sclerosis, and various metabolic disorders and diffuse degenerative diseases. Breath-holding spells in children are usually not related to convulsive diathesis. Convulsions in adolescents and adults may be caused by brain tumors or abscesses, trauma, meningitis or encephalitis, vascular disease, intoxications, hypoglycemia, uremia, eclampsia, tetany, tetanus, rabies, cardiac disease, hyperactive carotid sinus syndrome, cerebral degenerations, and other disease processes, as well as by the withdrawal of drugs or alcohol. Disturbances of consciousness and motor activity that resemble true convulsions may be symptoms of hysteria; the movements, however, are bizarre, and there may be no complete loss of consciousness. The differentiation between epilepsy (especially if the disturbance of consciousness is more outstanding than the convulsive manifestations), vasodepressor syncope, and hysteria is often difficult, and emotional stimuli may precipitate organic convulsions as well as true syncope or hysterical attacks.

Hypersomnia and Sleep Disorders

In hypersomnia and lethargy, which are states of pathologic sleepiness or continued or prolonged sleep, the symptoms closely resemble the manifestations of normal sleep. The patient can usually be aroused to consciousness by shaking, shouting, or other stimuli, and then appears to be in complete possession of his senses, but he may fall back into sleep as soon as the stimulus is removed. In normal sleep, however, unless it is the result of overpowering fatigue, the patient usually remains awake once he has been aroused, but in states of pathologic sleep the lethargy is continuous or prolonged. Hypersomnia is found in acute encephalitis, posttraumatic states, increased intracranial pressure, Wernicke's syndrome, intoxication by barbiturates and other sedatives and hypnotics, and brain tumors, especially those in the region of the third ventricle with pressure on or involvement of the posterior portion of the hypothalamus or the upper portion of the midbrain. The abnormal sleep may be the result or interruption of connections between the hypothalamus and portions of the reticular activating system, or between these structures and other parts of the brain (Ch. 50). Hypnotic trance and hysteria may simulate hypersomnia. In states of pathologic sleep, however, the electroencephalogram resembles that found in sleep, whereas in hysteria and malingering the electroencephalogram is no different from that obtained in the normal waking state.

Narcolepsy is a disorder, usually genetically determined, in which there are brief attacks of uncontrollable sleep that appear precipitously. There may or may not be warning drowsiness, and the patient may fall asleep while walking, talking, or eating; the symptoms leave rapidly or after a short nap. Occasionally there is sustained drowsiness between episodes of sleep. The narcoleptic attacks may be associated with periods of cataplexy, in which there is sudden loss of muscular power and tone, especially in the lower extremities, in association with laughter, anger, or other emotional feelings overt or suppressed; the knees may give way and the patient collapses. Less frequent, but occasionally part of the narcolepsy syndrome, are attacks of paralysis on relaxation or on going to sleep or awakening (sleep paralysis) and hypnagogic hallucinations. The electroencephalogram or polysomnogram is helpful in differentiating narcolepsy from other conditions characterized by excessive daytime sleep. Abrupt and early onset of rapid eye movement patterns (see below) on going to sleep are characteristic of this entity.

In the **Kleine–Levin syndrome** there are periodic attacks of hypersomnia with associated bulimia, irritability, behavioral changes, and uninhibited sexuality, usually occurring in young males. The **pickwickian syndrome** is a complex of obesity, somnolence, hypoventilation, and carbon dioxide retention.

Sleep apnea consists of temporary cessation of respiration during sleep. The resulting hypoxia may rouse the patient, who soon falls asleep again. It occurs in insomnia, narcolepsy, the pickwickian syndrome, and as central or obstructive sleep apnea. It occurs in virtually all infants between the ages of 1 and 3 months. In children and adults sleep apnea may be caused by hypoventilation secondary to intrinsic disease of the brain stem (infarction, poliomyelitis, degenerative disorders, syringobulbia) or may be an idiopathic disorder. It may develop as obstructive sleep apnea from conditions interfering with the upper airway or hypotonia of the muscles of the floor of the mouth (myotonic muscular dystrophy, tonsillar enlargement, obesity, myxedema, and other causes). Excessive daytime sleepiness may be a symptom of narcolepsy, but also occurs in patients with sleep apnea, the pickwickian syndrome, or drug dependency. It has been described in association with a variety of nocturnal disorders, including the restless legs syndrome, nocturnal myoclonus, paroxysmal nocturnal dystonia, and others.

Phases of Sleep. Studies on sleep have shown that it has two phases that differ physiologically. So-called initial, or forebrain, sleep is characterized electroencephalographically by slow waves and spindles. During a normal night's sleep, however, most individuals have four or five periods of paradoxic or activated (hindbrain) sleep that constitute 20%–25% of the total sleeping time. This latter variety is accompanied by rapid eye movements (REM) and shows a low-voltage, fast pattern on the electroencephalogram. REM sleep is accompanied by motor inhibition and dreaming. Explanations for the normal cycling of sleep are still incomplete; they include the action of the pontine reticular formation (as well as other sites) and various excitatory and inhibitory neurotransmitters.

Amnesia

In amnesia there is no loss of consciousness, but there is a memory defect that usually affects only a circumscribed period of time or certain experiences. Except for the period of time or the experience involved, registration, retention, and recall are normal. There usually is no loss of orientation for the immediate environment. Amnesia may be organic, psychogenic, feigned, or mixed in origin.

Amnesia of organic origin may be secondary to trauma, epilepsy, toxic states, cerebrovascular disease, fever, hypoglycemia, drug administration, brain tumors, or other causes. It is believed that involvement of the hippocampal-fornical-hypothalamic system is usually responsible, although amnesia may be caused by lesions of the amygdala and the temporal cortex. It has been stated that memory is dependent upon the intramolecular composition of neuronal proteins, including the continuous replenishment of ribonucleic acid.

Following trauma there may be both retrograde and anterograde (posttraumatic) amnesia. With improvement there is gradual lessening of the span of the former, but often a short period of retrograde amnesia remains. The posttraumatic amnesia is somewhat longer and covers the period of disordered consciousness that follows the injury. In epilepsy there is often amnesia for the convulsions and attacks, and the patient may fail to recall the aura of the seizures because of retrograde amnesia. In complex partial epilepsy there is amnesia for the period during which the patient exhibits automatisms and abnormal behavior. Amnesia may be a symptom of acute alcoholic intoxication and of Korsakoff's syndrome; in the latter the patient attempts to compensate for the amnesia by confabulation. Transient attacks of amnesia sometimes occur in older persons. In

these there is an abrupt onset of disorientation due to loss of recent memory and immediate recall, but there is retention of alertness and responsiveness. The term transient global amnesia has been given to this syndrome. It is felt to be a cerebrovascular event akin to transient ischemic attacks. A memory loss similar to amnesia has followed unilateral or bilateral temporal lobectomy. Either amnesia or more prolonged loss of memory may follow electroshock therapy. Senescent forgetfulness is usually a memory loss rather than an amnesia.

Psychogenic amnesia may occur as a symptom in hysteria; it is usually brought on by specific emotional trauma. The amnesia may persist from hours to days and during it the patient may carry out purposeful activities. Such dissociative reactions are referred to as **fugue states.** Feigned amnesia occurs in malingering.

Akinetic Mutism and Related Conditions

Akinetic mutism is a variety of altered consciousness in which the patient lies speechless and motionless in bed and appears to be asleep but can be aroused. Cycles of sleeping and wakefulness seem to be present. He makes little response to stimuli and no signs suggest that he is aware of what is happening in his environment. His eyes, however, may follow moving objects and deviate in response to loud noises. No voluntary or reflex movements of the extremities take place, but there is reflex withdrawal to painful stimuli. The patient has to be fed and cannot chew, but is able to swallow. There is incontinence of urine and feces. This syndrome has also been referred to as **coma vigil.** It occurs with basilar artery thrombosis, encephalitis, Wernicke's syndrome, and traumatic and neoplastic lesions of the upper brain stem, with pathologic changes affecting the corticospinal and corticobulbar pathways and the reticular activating formation in the posterior diencephalon, midbrain, and upper pons.

The term **locked-in syndrome** has been used to describe a state of similar etiology in which there is complete paralysis of all four extremities and the lower cranial nerves but no associated impairment of consciousness. If the supranuclear ocular pathways, which pass rostrally to the other corticobulbar and corticospinal pathways, are spared, the patient may retain the ability to move the eyes in the vertical plane and to blink. He may be able to reveal his awareness by eye movements and blinking, to indicate "yes" and "no," and even to communicate ideas by such movements.

The term **apallic state** has been used to describe the syndrome that develops with diffuse bilateral cerebral cortical degeneration that sometimes follows anoxia, trauma, and encephalitis. The patients may be rigid or spastic, but are immobile. The condition is closely allied to akinetic mutism.

Persistent, or **chronic, vegetative state** denotes the condition of patients who survive for prolonged periods (sometimes years) after severe brain injury without recovering any manifestations of higher mental activity. These patients are no longer actually comatose, but are in a state of markedly lowered consciousness; not all of them are akinetic. The term vegetative state is not an anatomic one but stresses the severe behavioral limitations of the patient; it is useful for physicians in providing information about the patient to others.

Hysteria

In hysteria the loss of consciousness is not deep and is rarely complete. The patient often responds to painful stimuli, unless there is associated hysterical anesthesia, and the reflexes are normal, with no pathologic responses. The corneal and pupillary reflexes and the temperature, pulse, respirations, and blood pressure are normal. The eyes may be closed tightly, and the patient may resist attempts to open them; vigorous contraction of the orbiculares oculorum often interferes with testing both the corneal and pupillary reflexes. Other diagnostic procedures may be resisted, and the patient may be seen to make furtive glances when not aware that he is being watched. If the latter is the case, care must be taken to differentiate between hysteria and malingering (Ch. 55). Complete loss of consciousness, however, is difficult to simulate and, therefore, is rare in malingering.

Hysterical impairment of consciousness is usually precipitated by emotional stress, and the onset is often dramatic. The patient may appear to be in a trance, or coma may alternate with weeping and thrashing movements. The performance is appropriately staged, and occurs when observers are in the vicinity. Movements, if present, are not stereotyped, but appear to be coordinated and purposive. The patient may struggle, clutch at objects or parts of the body, or attempt to tear off clothes. The tongue is only rarely bitten. Injuries when falling are uncom-

mon, the patient sagging slowly to the floor. There is no sleepiness or headache after the attack. Although the patient appears to be unconscious, some response to external stimuli may be evident. If there is hypertonicity of the muscles, it is usually of a rigid type, and there may be opisthotonos with the *arc de cercle*. If the patient can be stimulated to talk, his responses may be the type seen in Ganser's syndrome: he evades answers to questions and makes approximate but consistently inaccurate replies. The electrical activity of the brain is normal, and the electroencephalogram can be differentiated from that of normal and pathologic sleep, vasodepressor syncope, and organic brain disease. Insight into the condition and return of consciousness can often be obtained by the intravenous administration of drugs such as sodium amobarbital.

It is important to bear in mind that vasodepressor syncope and epileptic attacks may also be precipitated by emotional stimuli. Hyperventilation, brought about by either fear or anxiety, may cause loss of consciousness or hasten the onset of convulsions. The electroencephalogram, at times with prolonged monitoring, has distinct value in aiding one to differentiate between hysteria, vasodepressor syncope, and epilepsy, but it must not be considered the final criterion in diagnosis.

Psychotic States

There is rarely complete loss of consciousness in psychotic states. In severe depression, schizophrenia, and organic psychoses there may be mutism in which the patient is either completely withdrawn from the environment or refuses to speak. Negativism, either passive or active, may be a symptom of various psychoses, but especially of schizophrenia. In severe depression the patient may show both physical and psychomotor retardation that may simulate lowering of consciousness because of organic disease. In catatonic stupor there is apathy, mutism, and negativism; there often is a waxy rigidity of the musculature of the extremities, and the patient may hold his limbs or entire body in bizarre and seemingly uncomfortable positions for long periods of time. Food may be held in the mouth.

BRAIN DEATH

Traditionally death has been defined as the cessation of vital functions (specifically, heartbeat and respiration). Brain function usually ceases at approximately the same time. Legal definitions of death (and of brain death) vary from place to place. Using the criterion of cessation of blood circulation and breathing, it is relatively simple, under most circumstances, to determine the exact time of death. The developments of modern methods of resuscitation have made it possible to restore heartbeat and respirations, and to provide "life-support" measures. As a result, the formerly accepted criteria for death are not always valid. Accurate determination of the exact time of death has become increasingly important to physicians and the general public since organ transplantation has become refined and often life-saving. If the classic concept of cessation of heartbeat and respiration continues to be used as the sole criterion for death, delay in the removal of organs to be transplanted may cause them to be irreparably damaged, and the success of the transplant operations severely jeopardized.

Along with the development of transplant surgery, information about normal and abnormal cerebral function has been significantly increased. The concept of **brain death** has evolved. The term is used to include both **cerebral death** (irreversible loss of function resulting from bilateral destruction of the supratentorial structures, including the cerebral cortex, white matter, thalamus, and basal ganglia) and also loss of function of the infratentorial structures, namely, the brain stem and cerebellum. Numerous investigations have been made to determine exactly when the brain ceases to function. Most physicians believe that the brain, the organ of the mind, regulates all bodily functions and is essential to life. When irreversible generalized brain damage has occurred, the patient is, in effect, dead, regardless of whether respiration and heart beat can be sustained by mechanical and chemical procedures. Severe, widespread pathologic alterations develop rapidly in the brain after brain death. Neuropathologists have used the term **respirator brain** for the brains of patients who have been kept alive by artificial means after death has actually taken place.

This alteration in the definition of the time of death has resulted in much study and discussion, and, not infrequently, disagreement, not only among physicians but also among lawyers, theologians, and the general public. The determination of brain death has also resulted in a great impact on the practice of medicine, and many hospitals now require that more than one person, preferably a committee, make the decision about the time of brain death in a possible transplant donor.

Most neurologists accept the conclusions of the 1973 resolution adopted by the American Neurological Association, which states:

> The essential element in meaningful human existence is the viability of the brain. Without brain function, the activity of the rest of the body has no significance. Whereas in the past the destruction of the brain by injury or disease inevitably led to prompt cessation of respiration and early destruction of all vital organs, this situation has been altered by modern scientific resuscitation techniques. Medical science now has the ability to maintain respiration and circulation for a period of time after the brain is dead.
>
> As a result, cessation of respiration and heart action can no longer be relied upon as the sole valid indicators that life has ceased. When respiration and heart action have ceased, one can, indeed, be assured that the brain is dead, but with artificial respiration and circulatory support, the brain may be dead while the heart and other organs continue their vital functions.
>
> It is of practical and humanitarian concern that this situation be clarified, for effects to maintain life after the individual is dead pose unnecessary distress and expense on the family and a burden on our medical facilities.
>
> In view of these considerations, the American Neurological Association recommends that it be generally recognized that when satisfactory scientific evaluation has established that the brain is dead, the person is in fact dead, whether the heart and other vital organs continue to function or not.

More recently (1981) the President's Commission for the Study of Ethical Problems in Medicine and Biomedical and Behavioral Research established guidelines for brain death including cessation of brain function and its irreversibility. The American Academy of Neurology agrees with these criteria.

Characteristics of Brain Death

The criteria listed below follow, in general, the report of the Ad Hoc Committee of the Harvard Medical School to Examine the Definition of Brain Death.

> The patient should be totally unaware of external stimuli and completely unresponsive to them. Even intensely painful stimuli should evoke no vocal response, movement of the body, or alteration of respiration.
>
> The patient should be observed for at least one hour to note that there are no spontaneous muscular or respiratory movements.

When the patient is receiving mechanical respiratory assistance, it should be discontinued for at least 15 min to determine whether spontaneous respiration develops. To satisfy the criteria for brain death, no respiratory response of any type should occur. Alternative methods for apnea testing are advocated by some but are not uniformly adhered to (*e.g.*, preventilation with pure oxygen, then disconnection of the respirator along with delivery of 6 L of oxygen per min by endotracheal tube, for up to 10 min).

The pupils are nonreactive. They are usually dilated but occasionally fixed in midposition. An intense light source must be used before deciding that the pupils are nonreactive. Observing the pupils through a magnifying glass also ensures that no response is present.

There should be no eye movement in response to brisk head turning or irrigation of the external auditory canals with ice water. Blinking in response to these and other stimuli must be absent.

Swallowing, yawning, and, as mentioned, any type of vocalization, however feeble, should not occur.

Corneal, pharyngeal, and all other reflexes related to cranial nerve function must be absent.

Muscle stretch reflexes are usually absent and plantar stimulation should result in no response. There is no evidence of postural activity, decerebrate or otherwise.

The President's Commission suggests observation of the persistence of cessation of brain function for 6 hours when confirmatory tests such as electroencephalography are used, and for 12–24 hours without the use of such tests.

For children, a task force recommended certain modifications of the criteria. Two electroencephalograms separated by at least 48 hours are advocated for children aged 7 days to 2 months, and two electroencephalograms 12 hours apart (or one such study followed by another confirmatory test 12 hours later) apply to children aged 2 to 12 months. For those 1–4 years old, a 12 hour observation period is adequate. Neonates up to 6 days of age have special requirements. It has been suggested by some authors that clinical criteria alone may be more precise than neurodiagnostic studies in preterm and newborn infants.

While the electroencephalogram has been used in the determination of brain death, the neurologist, by utilizing the criteria just listed, can usually make the determination of brain death. However, it is desirable to obtain an electroencephalogram in many instances and particularly when the patient's organs are being considered for transplantation. The electroencephalogram should be isoelectric (flat, or showing no variation in potential). It is assumed, of course, that the electrodes are properly applied, that the apparatus is functioning normally, and that personnel in charge are competent.

A description of the detailed factors entering into the determination of an isoelectric encephalogram is beyond the scope of this work; they have been outlined by the Ad Hoc Committee of the American Electroencephalographic Society on EEG Criteria for Determination of Cerebral Death.

Other tests useful in the determination of brain death include several that establish the cessation of cerebral perfusion, such as transcranial Doppler, intravenous isotope angiography, contrast bolus computed tomography, and angiography. Auditory and somatosensory evoked potential studies have also been advocated.

There must be absence of hypothermia and absence of prior ingestion of drugs that can depress the nervous system before a definitive decision is reached concerning brain death. There have been rare instances in which patients who are hypothermic or who have ingested large amounts of barbiturates or other depressant drugs enter a state fulfilling the requirements for brain death (including an isoelectric electroencephalogram) but have recovered. The presence of hypothermia (temperature below 90° F) is simple to detect. However, a patient admitted to the hospital with unexplained coma should not be considered to be in a state of irreversible brain death until it can clearly be established by appropriate blood tests that depressants have not been ingested.

Further refinements in the definition of brain death are likely to occur, especially for young infants.

BIBLIOGRAPHY

Adams RD, Victor M. Principles of Neurology, 4th ed. New York, McGraw–Hill, 1989

Ajmone–Marson C, Ralston BL. The Epileptic Seizure. Springfield, IL, Charles C Thomas, 1957

Arnold H, Kühne D, Rohr W, Heller M. Contrast bolus technique with rapid CT scanning. A reliable diagnostic tool for the determination of brain death. Neuroradiology 1981;22:129

Ashwal SE, Schneider S. Brain death in the newborn. Pediatrics 1989;84:429

Beecher HK, Adams RD, Barger AC et al. A definition of irreversible coma: Report of the ad hoc committee of the

Harvard Medical School to examine the definition of brain death. JAMA 1968;205:85

Besser R, Dillmann U, Henn M. Somatosensory evoked potentials aiding the diagnosis of brain death. Neurosurg Rev 1988;11:171

Brain WR. The cerebral basis of consciousness. Brain 1950;73:465

Cairns S. Disturbances of consciousness with lesions of the brain-stem and diencephalon. Brain 1952;75:109

Cravioto H, Silberman J, Feigin I. A clinical and pathologic study of akinetic mutism. Neurology 1960;10:10

DeJong RN. "Psychomotor" or "temporal lobe" epilepsy: A review of the development of our present concepts. Neurology 1957;7:1

DeJong RN. The hippocampus and its role in memory: clinical manifestations and theoretical considerations. J Neurol Sci 1973;19:73

Dement W, Kleitman N. Cyclic variations of EEG during sleep and their relation to eye movements, body motility, and dreaming. Electroencephalog Clin Neurophysiol 1957;9:673

Dermksian G, Lamb LE. Syncope in a population of healthy young adults. JAMA 1958;168:1200

Earnest MP, Beresford HR, McIntyre HB. Testing for apnea in suspected brain death: Methods used by 129 clinicians. Neurology 1986;36:542

Edwards RH, Simon RP. Coma. In Joynt RJ (ed). Clinical Neurology. Philadelphia, JB Lippincott, 1989

Engel GL. Fainting, 2nd ed. Springfield, IL, Charles C Thomas, 1962

Fazekas JF, Alman RW. Coma: Biochemistry, Physiology and Therapeutic Principles. Springfield, IL, Charles C Thomas, 1962

Fisher CM. The neurological examination of the comatose patient. Acta Neurol Scand (suppl) 1969;45:5

Fisher CM, Adams RD. Transient global amnesia. Acta Neurol Scand (suppl) 1964;40:7

French JD. Brain lesions associated with prolonged unconsciousness. Arch Neurol Psychiatry 1952;68:727

Garland H, Summer D, Forman RP. The Kleine–Levin syndrome. Neurology 1965;15:1161

Gastaut H. The Epilepsies: Electro-clinical Correlations. Springfield, IL, Charles C Thomas, 1954

Gastaut H. Clinical and electroencephalographical classification of epileptic seizures. Epilepsia 1970;11:102

Gastaut H, Tassinari CA, Duron B. Polygraphic study of the episodic diurnal and nocturnal (hypnic and respiratory) manifestations of the Pickwick syndrome. Brain Res 1966;2:167

Gibbs FA, Gibbs EL, Lennox WG. Electroencephalographic classification of epileptic patients and control subjects. Arch Neurol Psychiatry 1943;50:111

Goldie WD, Chiappa KH, Young RR, Brooks EB. Brainstem auditory and short-latency evoked responses in brain death. Neurology 1981;31:248

Goodman JM, Heck LL, Moore BD. Confirmation of brain death with portable isotope angiography: a review of 204 consecutive cases. Neurosurgery 1985;16:492

Guilleminault C, Dement WC. Two hundred thirty-five cases of excessive daytime sleepiness: Diagnosis and tentative classification. J Chron Dis 1976;29:733

Halmos PB, Nelson JK, Lowry RC. Hyperosmolar non-ketoacidotic coma in diabetes. Lancet 1966;1:675

Ivan LP. Spinal reflexes in cerebral death. Neurology 1973;23:650

Kales A, Kales JD. Sleep disorders: recent findings in the diagnosis and treatment of disturbed sleep. N Engl J Med 1974;290:487

Kershman J. Syncope and seizures. J Neurol Neurosurg Psychiat 1949;12:25

Kiersch TA. Amnesia: A clinical study of 98 cases. Am J Psychiatry 1962;119:57

Korein J, Braunstein P, George A et al. Brain death. I. Angiographic correlation with the radiosotopic bolus technique for evaluation of critical deficit of cerebral blood flow. Ann Neurol 1977;2:195

Lennox WG. Amnesia, real and feigned. Am J Psychiatry 1943;99:732

Lennox WG, Lennox MA. Epilepsy and Related Convulsive Disorders. Boston, Little, Brown & Co, 1960

Leon–Sotomayor L, Bowers CY. Myxedema Coma. Springfield, IL, Charles C Thomas, 1964

Maccario M, Lustman LI. Paroxysmal nocturnal dystonia presenting as excessive daytime somnolence. Arch Neurol 1990;47:291

Maclagan NF. The biochemistry of coma. In Cumings JN, Kremer M (eds). Biochemical Aspects of Neurological Disorders. Springfield,IL, Charles C Thomas, 1964

Manolis AS, Linzer M, Salem D, Estes NA III. Syncope: Current diagnostic evaluation and management. Ann Intern Med 1990;112:850

Martin JP. Consciousness and its disturbances. Lancet 1949;1:1, 48

Merlis JK. Proposal for an international classification of the epilepsies. Epilepsia 1970;11:114

Mount LA. The differential diagnosis of coma. Med Clin North Am 1948;32:795

Noble RJ. The patient with syncope. JAMA 1977;237:1372

Parkes JD. Sleep and Its Disorders. London, WB Saunders, 1985

Penfield W, Jasper H. Epilepsy and the Functional Anatomy of the Human Brain. Boston, Little, Brown & Co, 1954

Plum F, Posner JB. The Diagnosis of Stupor and Coma, 3rd ed. Philadelphia, FA Davis, 1980

Plum F, Swanson AG. Abnormalities in the central regulation of respiration in acute and chronic poliomyelitis. Arch Neurol Psychiatry 1959;81:535

Powers AD, Graeber MC, Smith RR. Transcranial doppler ultrasonography in the determination of brain death. Neurosurgery 1989;24:884

Sabin TD. The differential diagnosis of coma. N Engl J Med 1974;290:1062

Saper JR, Lossing JH. Prolonged trance-like stupor in epilepsy: Petit mal status, spike-wave stupor, spaced-out status. Arch Intern Med 1974;134:1079

Sherlock S. Hepatic coma. Practitioner 1963;191:18

Shewmon DA. Commentary on guidelines for the determination of brain death in children. Ann Neurol 1988; 24:789

Shuttleworth EC Jr, Morris CE. The transient global amnesia syndrome. Arch Neurol 1966;15:515

Shy GM, Drager GA. A neurological syndrome associated

with orthostatic hypotension: a clinicopathologic study. Arch Neurol 1960;2:511

Silverman D, Saunders MG, Schwab RS et al. Cerebral death in the electroencephalogram: Report of the ad hoc committee of the American Electroencephalographic Society on EEG criteria for determination of cerebral death. JAMA 1969;209:1505

Silverman D, Masland RL, Saunders MG et al. Irreversible coma associated with electrocerebral silences. Neurology 1970;20:525

Solomon P, Aring CD. The causes of coma in patients entering a general hospital. Am J Med Sci 1934;188:805

Steinmetz EF, Vroom FQ. Transient global amnesia. Neurology 1972; 22:1193

Task Force for the Determination of Brain Death in Children. Guidelines for the determination of brain death in children. Neurology 1987;37:1077

Teasdale G, Jennett B. Assessment of coma and impaired consciousness. A practical scale. Lancet 1974;2:81

Vatne K, Nakstad P, Lundar T. Digital subtraction angiography in the evaluation of brain death. Neuroradiology 1985;27:155

Victor M. The amnesic syndrome and its anatomical basis. Can Med Ass J 1969;100:1115

Walker AE. Post-traumatic Epilepsy. Springfield, IL, Charles C Thomas, 1948

Walker AE. Cerebral Death. Dallas, TX, Professional Information Library, 1977

Walker AE. Cerebral death. In Tower DB, Chase TN (eds). The Nervous System. Vol 2, Clinical Neurosciences. New York, Raven Press, 1975

Walker AE. The neurosurgeon's responsibility for organ procurement. J Neurosurg 1976;44:1

Walker AE, Bickford R, Aung M et al. An appraisal of the criteria of cerebral death: A summary statement. A collaborative study. JAMA 1977;237:982

Walker AE, Diamond EL, Moseley JI. The neuropathological findings in irreversible coma: A critique of the respirator brain. J Neuropathol Exp Neurol 1975;34:295

Whitty CMW, Zangwill Ol (eds). Amnesia. London, Butterworths, 1967

Wolff HG, Curran D. Nature of delirium and allied states. Arch Neurol Psychiat 1935;33:1175

Chapter 55
EXAMINATION IN CASES OF SUSPECTED HYSTERIA AND MALINGERING

In the evaluation of every patient who has symptoms of nervous system dysfunction it is essential to differentiate between those manifestations that are organic in origin (*i.e.*, caused by pathoanatomic and pathophysiologic changes) and those that are psychogenic in origin. Furthermore, if nonorganic changes are present, it is essential to distinguish between those that are consciously induced, or feigned (malingered), and those that are unconsciously motivated (hysterical).

Psychogenic manifestations may closely resemble organic ones, and the differentiation between the two may present difficulties. It must be borne in mind, in the appraisal of every patient, that the presenting symptoms as well as the signs of disease may not be of organic origin. This is especially apt to be true if the manifestations are bizarre and do not seem to fit readily into any specific category. Furthermore, organic and nonorganic disease may exist simultaneously; the latter may precipitate manifestations of the former, or organic disease may be accompanied by psychogenic variations and accentuations. An individual with a convulsive disorder, for instance, may on occasion have attacks that are psychogenically precipitated and may, in addition, have occasional pseudoconvulsions (either consciously or unconsciously motivated) that may closely resemble the true organic seizures. If the patient is seen only during the malingered or hysterical attacks, his entire illness may appear to have a psychogenic origin, and the organic features may be overlooked.

The distinction between hysteria and malingering (or between unconscious and conscious motivation) is even more difficult than the differentiation between organic and psychogenic disease, and requires greater diagnostic acumen. Furthermore, hysteria and malingering may occur simultaneously, especially in instances where there is exaggeration of symptoms. By definition, hysteria and malingering are extreme opposites, and for diagnostic purposes one should always attempt to distinguish between them. This differentiation, however, is not always possible, especially in the presence of so-called neurotic malingering.

Hysteria is, by definition, a neurosis, or a disease of psychic origin. There is no known underlying organic basis for the patient's complaints, and the manifestations are produced by conversion mechanisms; *i.e.*, emotions are transformed into physical symptoms. The patient has no control over his acts and emotions; he is unconscious of the genesis of the symptoms, and is not aware of the absence of an organic basis for them. The emotional conflict that is responsible has been completely repressed, and the patient believes his symptoms to be the result of organic disease. The manifestations may be either brought on or altered by suggestion.

Malingering is defined as a willful, deliberate, and fraudulent imitation or exaggeration of illness, usually intended to deceive others, and, under most circumstances, conceived for the purpose of gaining a consciously desired end, such as financial compensation or obtaining drugs to sustain an addiction. **Simulation (positive malingering)** is the feigning or pretense of nonexisting symptoms by word, gesture, action, or behavior; **dissimulation (negative malinger-**

ing) is the concealment of existing symptoms by similar means. Three varieties of malingering have been described: (1) **Pure malingering** is the deliberate and designed feigning of disease or disability, or, if disease exists, its intentional concealment. This may be done by false allegation (untrue attestation that symptoms exist, or spurious denial of existing or previously acquired disease), imitation (feigning or simulation of symptoms of disease), or provocation (intentional production of lesions or symptoms by artificial means). (2) **Partial malingering,** or **exaggeration,** is the magnification or intensification of symptoms that already exist. It is usually conscious and voluntary, and the patient may exaggerate symptoms of real disease and cause an illness that is already present to assume greater severity, superimpose factitious symptoms on a substratum of real disease, or aggravate and protract the course and duration of a disease or injury. Unconscious and involuntary exaggeration may take place through ignorance, fear, or deficient powers of subjective analysis; such exaggeration closely resembles hysteria. (3) **False imputation** is the ascribing of morbid phenomena or symptoms to a definite cause although this cause may be recognized or ascertained to have no relationship to the symptoms. The patient may attempt to blame an innocent episode for manifestations that were present previously or that appeared from some other cause. False imputation may take place through design or through ignorance.

According to the above definitions, hysteria and malingering are widely divergent in both motivation and origin. In hysteria the symptoms are unconsciously determined, and the patient is not aware of their lack of an organic basis; they develop without apparent design; they are real to him and he deceives himself and often others. The manifestations of hysteria are often influenced by suggestion, and therefore signs and symptoms vary from time to time. There may be contradiction of responses, vagueness of history, and disproportion between the symptoms and the patient's general state of well-being, as well as disproportion between the subjective complaints and the objective manifestations. The symptoms are bizarre and do not fit into any organic pattern that may be explained by a specific anatomic lesion. The patient's attitude varies from complete indifference toward the illness and the examination to which he is subjected, to a state of marked apprehension and anxiety. He may appear to be unconcerned in spite of what seem to be incapacitating symptoms, or may appear to be in great discomfort with emotional display. Although the symptoms may fluctuate in severity, there is some involvement at all times; paralyzed extremities cannot be used for either work or play.

Hysteria is a disease of the personality. It represents the unconscious transfer, by the patient, of a psychic difficulty to a somatic one. The hysterical patient often welcomes examinations, and may be eager for repeated examinations, although occasionally he resents and avoids such studies. He is often pleased and reassured at the absence of organic disease. He is usually anxious to follow all recommended treatment procedures, takes whatever medications are prescribed, and is willing to submit to surgical operations. He may accept employment and attempt to work. He is honest and reliable in his contacts with physicians and usually has a good employment record. He frequently shows anxiety concerning his hospitalization and the episode that brought him to the hospital. Because hysteria is a disease, posttraumatic and other neuroses are considered compensable by most workmen's compensation laws and insurance contracts.

In malingering, on the other hand, the patient is conscious of the unreality of the symptoms, and manufactures them with definite intent. There is usually but slight variability in symptoms from time to time, and they are not influenced by suggestion; the responses are consistent, and the history is specific, especially in regard to the onset of disability following an accident or injury. Usually, however, the disability appears to be much greater than one would assume from the injury described; the pain is out of proportion to the injury sustained or the disability claimed, and the recovery period has been prolonged beyond clinical expectancy. Malingered symptoms also fail to fit an organic pattern that may be explained by a specific anatomic lesion and often assume bizarre characteristics. The malingerer plans to deceive, and his symptoms are fraudulently and deliberately produced. As a result, the patient is usually defensive, hostile, and suspicious of examinations, fearing, resenting, and attempting to avoid them. Repeated examinations may be resisted or refused because each new procedure may impose an ordeal requiring much concentration. The patient is aware of the need for consistency in symptoms and in disability, so that he will not give himself away. To avoid being enmeshed, he chooses his words carefully. Consequently, answers are evasive, and it frequently is impossible to obtain an exact description of symptoms. The patient is often sullen, ill at ease, suspicious, uncooperative, resentful, and tense during the examination. He often declines to cooperate in recommended therapeutic procedures and refuses surgical operations. He may claim that the investigative tests have aggravated the symptoms. He may refuse employment, claiming inability to work, even though he can use an allegedly paralyzed limb for other purposes. In personality the malingerer is apt to be greedy and dishonest, unpleasant and demanding, and may have a poor employment record and a history of previously incapacitating injuries, for which he may have received compensation. Because the malingerer is essentially a deceiver and the symptoms claimed are fraudulent, simulated diseases are not compensable by law. In the medicolegal setting, however, it is very difficult to substantiate the diagnosis of malingering, particularly when the complaint is headache, back pain, or some other subjective complaint not capable of being objectively disproved. It is true that autonomic responses are often associated with pain but tests are not sufficiently reliable to constitute legal evidence. A simple example is the law's refusal to allow the admission as evidence in court of information obtained in polygraph tests that may be used to detect deception.

Too often, especially among the laity and the legal profession, malingering and hysteria are regarded as more or less synonymous terms. In both conditions the symptoms have no organic basis, there is an incongruity of manifestations, many of which may be bizarre in character, and there may be a disproportion between the patient's disability and his general physical status. As a consequence, the symptoms of each are frequently referred to as "imagined." In hysteria, however, the manifestations are unconsciously determined and real to the patient. The arm is paralyzed because he believes it to be, and the patient has no voluntary power over it. In malingering, on the other hand, the patient alleges, falsifies, and feigns the paralysis, knowing that the arm is not paralyzed, but failing to move it and resisting attempts to move it passively. The difficulties are simulated for the patient's own gain. He consciously attempts to reproduce symptoms that have been seen or heard of in others and exaggerates or prolongs a disability.

Either hysterical or simulated symptoms may follow injuries and industrial accidents, but malingering is most apt to follow such accidents if the symptoms are associated with attempts to secure compensation. One must be especially concerned with the possibility of malingering in the following types of individuals: those who have had an injury, especially an industrial accident allegedly suffered in employment, the disability resulting from which is compensable by benefits payable under workmen's compensation laws or by damages based on alleged negligence (the accident and the injury may both be feigned, or the accident real but the injury feigned); those who have suffered either accidents that are payable by insurance benefits or injuries from which monetary gains may be expected; those who wish to obtain insurance benefits for illness or disability; civilians who wish to evade military service during times of conscription, or members of the armed forces who wish to obtain discharge from such service; those who develop symptoms in order to avoid disagreeable duties, evade legal and other responsibilities, gain sympathy or attention, or force others to bow to their will; addicts who feign symptoms to obtain drugs.

Although hysteria and malingering are essentially different, in many instances the distinction between them cannot be made with the ease that these definitions imply. The same tests to distinguish organic from nonorganic or psychogenic disease are used in both hysteria and malingering, and the results are usually the same in both. The procedures that rule out organic disease do not differentiate between hysteria and malingering. In the tests used to differentiate between true blindness or deafness and either hysterical or malingered loss of vision or hearing, for instance, it may be possible to determine that the patient has no organic defect, but may not be possible to state with certainty whether the difficulty is a conscious or an involuntary one. One must remember, that although hysteria and malingering are diametric opposites, the two may occur together in the same patient and they may blend into each other with a gradual transition from one to the other. In the midposition between the two extremes are the neurotic patient who exaggerates symptoms and the malingerer who has neurotic traits. The two are especially apt to occur together in post-traumatic syndromes where compensation or other medicolegal elements are involved (the so-called compensation or traumatic neurosis). The similarity between the two may be so great that it is not possible to distinguish between them and evaluate conscious and unconscious exaggeration of symptoms, and thus appraise the patient's difficulties. Furthermore, it must be borne in mind that either hysteria or malingering or both may occur in association with organic disease, especially if there is an exaggeration of symptoms. Under such circumstances the organic and nonorganic features must be appraised individually. Even experts in the fields of neurology and psychiatry disagree as to what may be nonorganic symptoms; for example, hysterical regional pain is considered rare by some and common by others.

The actual differentiation between hysteria and malingering depends upon the goal sought by the patient. If the goal is an intangible one, such as an escape from the responsibility of life, one should suspect hysteria; if it is tangible, such as an attempt to secure monetary gain or drugs, the evidence favors malingering. Perhaps the most important criteria in the distinction between hysteria and malingering are the past history and the personality inventory. Knowledge of the patient's past performances under similar circumstances aids in evaluation. Patterns of behavior and reactions to emotional situations and trauma in early life are important. In the hysterical patient there may have been similar episodes associated with emotional stress and strain, fears, anxieties, shocks, and disappointments, and there may be a past history of psychophysiologic symptoms starting at an early age that were not specifically related to the nervous system. These include anxiety attacks, tachycardia, respiratory difficulties, cardiospasm, anorexia nervosa, psychogenic vomiting, aerophagia, spastic constipation or emotional diarrhea, urinary disturbances, difficulties in sexual function, pseudocyesis, dementia factitia, neurotic excoriations, or other symptoms that may be referred to any of the organs or systems of the body. There is a striking tendency for the manifestations to return from time to time throughout life; they may be brought on by suggestion, and the form they take may be determined by suggestion. Furthermore, in hysterical patients there may be both past history and present evidence of autonomic nervous system imbalance, with tachycardia, hyperhidrosis, vasomotor instability, pupillary dilation, and labile blood pressure. In malingerers, on the other hand, if there have been previous episodes, they have all been related to minor traumas and industrial situations; oftentimes there is a history of previous conflict with the law, aggressive and antisocial behavior, prior litigation, and a poor employment record. There may be evidence that the patient has a sociopathic or antisocial personality disturbance or harbors paranoid ideas.

There is some controversy about whether or not to continue use of the term hysteria (a mental mechanism operating unconsciously, by which intrapsychic conflicts that would otherwise give rise to anxiety are instead given symbolic external expression). In some psychiatric classifications of disease, the term hysteria is dropped and the following categories are described: conversion reaction in which localized sensory and/or motor complaints develop; dissociated reactions in which alterations of consciousness or identity predominate; general anxiety states and psychophysiologic disorders in which symptoms are associated with complaints referable to the autonomic nervous system. One form of the last-named has been called **Briquet's syndrome,** a polysymptomatic disorder usually beginning in adolescence, affecting chiefly women, and characterized by multiple recurrent complaints that are often described dramatically. Patients with multiple psychogenic complaints of this type often come in with a paper or notebook describing in detail myriads of complaints, dates of onset, tests that have been performed, and other doctors' comments. Charcot used the colorful term *"la malade avec un petit papier"* for such situations.

Despite the controversy over the term hysteria, most physicians feel that it does exist and can be diagnosed if there are no signs of physical or morphologic disease, if there are signs that contraindicate the diagnosis of organic disease, and if the patterns of dysfunction suggest a psychogenic origin. Hysterical (or psychogenic) symptoms, or those of a conversion reaction, from a neurologic point of view, include such manifestations as loss of function (paralysis, anesthesia, blindness, deafness), disorders of consciousness (varying from syncope to coma and including convulsive phenomena), simulation of organic disease (hyperkinesias, dizziness, dysphonia), syndromes in which pain is the predominant symptom, and combinations with both organic and either conversion or psychophysiologic features such as abdominal or respiratory dysfunction.

THE EXAMINATION

There is no special routine for the neurologic examination in the attempt to detect hysteria and malingering. The complete procedures for the neurologic appraisal must be carried out in detail in every case. There is scarcely a symptom or sign of organic disease that cannot be assumed in either hysteria or malingering. The examiner must be alert for signs of dysfunction not fitting into an organic pattern, and if such appear, certain special tests and modifications of the routine procedure have to be performed. This is often apt to be the case in patients whose symptoms have a post-traumatic origin (especially if associated with industrial accidents), have medicolegal complications, or are related to military service. In all these circumstances psychogenic, predominantly malingered, symptoms are common. A common cause is the feigning of symptoms, usually pain, in order to receive prescriptions for narcotics, barbiturates, minor tranquilizers, or other drugs to which the patient is addicted.

In taking the history one should attempt to differentiate between organic and nonorganic factors; this applies not only to the symptoms that are directly referable to the nervous system, but also to somatic symptoms in general. The history of previous fainting attacks, cardiac or gastrointestinal symptoms of psychic origin, multiple illnesses or complaints, and vague manifestations of disease may help to explain the presence of bizarre neurologic complaints. The history of previous adjustment to the environment, the home situation, employment, and emotional stresses and strains has great significance. Such information should be obtained not only from the patient but also from relatives and friends. In the history of the present episode, the details of the precipitating experience (trauma, emotional strain, or mental shock) and of the evolution of the symptoms following their first appearance should be included. If there was an accident, details should be obtained. It is important to know how the injury occurred, whether witnesses were present, and whether the accident was reported. One should inquire whether the patient suffered loss of consciousness, whether he was able to move parts of his body or to walk after the injury, and whether he was given immediate medical treatment. It may help to have the patient reenact the injury and compare his present muscle power with that before the accident. A naive malingerer may move the allegedly paralyzed limbs freely to demonstrate his former strength or show the position of his body before or during the accident.

In carrying out the neurologic examination it must be remembered that findings that do not fit into an organic pattern may have a psychic origin. The patient should be examined in great detail with attempts to distract his attention from the symptoms and break down his guard. It may

be important to employ ruses to trick him into making false responses and to carry out repeated examinations to determine whether he is consistent. Apparatus may be employed to confuse and bewilder him. He should be watched carefully but discreetly while he dresses and undresses himself, walks into and out of the examining room, and turns his head to hear or eyes to see. He may be noted to carry out movements and use parts of his body whose functions, during the examination, seem to be impaired. He may, for instance, be unable to stand on one foot without falling while being examined, or even to stand on both feet in the Romberg test, yet be able to perform these acts without difficulty when putting on his trousers or lacing his shoes. The examiner should never allow the patient to gain the impression that either malingering or hysteria is suspected. He should approach the patient in a manner that gives utmost confidence. He should be sympathetic and never use harsh or inquisitional methods, threats, or intimidations, and should not attempt to force admission. He should avoid asking leading questions or making suggestions, and should never give away his feelings about the patient. Friends and relatives should usually be excluded from the examining room. Continued observation, often indirect, and repeated examinations may be necessary.

The patient's facies and general reactions often aid the examiner in his evaluation. Real pain, for instance, often affects the eyes, facies, pulse, blood pressure, respirations, and pupillary reactions; there may be grimacing, weeping, tachycardia, pupillary dilation, vasomotor changes, withdrawal of the part, and defense attitudes and postures to relieve or prevent pain. In both hysteria and malingering these are usually absent. Hysterical patients may show either excessive reactions to painful stimulation, but without physiologic accompaniments, or, conversely, decreased response to pain. They may appear indifferent and unconcerned while describing excruciating pain. The mode of speech, physiognomy, demeanor, and deportment may also aid in appraisal. In hysteria there may be either bland indifference with no signs of alarm and a cheerful smile in spite of what appears to be severe incapacity, or an excessive emotional reaction. In malingering the patient may betray deceit by blushing confusion or cast-down eyes; there is no open-eyed candor, and there may be either surly reserve or frank ill temper.

In general, hysteria may be diagnosed if there is absence of objective physical signs to substantiate the patient's subjective symptoms, evidence that the complaints had their onset in association with either emotional stress or suggestion, the presence of positive findings of hysteria in the neurologic examination (glove-and-stocking anesthesias, tubular vision), and a therapeutic response to suggestion. Malingering may be diagnosed if there is absence of objective physical signs to substantiate the patient's complaints, together with the absence of the above criteria of hysteria; the personality pattern and apparent purpose of the illness, however, are essential. Neither should ever be diagnosed merely by the absence of organic features or on the basis of one or two tests. It is necessary to substantiate the impression by the presence of positive features of either hysteria or malingering, and a conclusive diagnosis can be made only after a thorough analysis of the history, the patient's reactions toward his illness, and the findings elicited during a complete neurologic examination. It is important to remember that bizarre symptoms and signs may also occur in organic disease, and that in many somatic disorders there are no objective physical criteria of dysfunction.

Special diagnostic procedures occasionally are useful in the differentiation between organic and psychogenic disease, and in the distinction between hysteria and malingering. Tests of autonomic nervous system function, such as determinations of skin resistance (as used in the polygraph) or of reflex erythema, may provide some information. The electroencephalogram and prolonged recording of the electrical activity of the brain along with video monitoring may also aid, but their value is limited because many individuals without neurologic disease show some abnormality on electroencephalography. To aid in the exclusion of organic disease, computed tomography or magnetic resonance imaging may be useful when symptoms and signs suggesting a brain disease are present, and the electromyogram, nerve conduction studies, and sensory evoked potential studies when peripheral nerves and nerve root lesions must be excluded. Visual and auditory evoked potential studies, as well as noninvasive appraisals of cerebral blood flow or studies of cerebral metabolism may also be helpful at times. It must be stressed, however, that the normality of these procedures does not invariably exclude the presence of organic disease and that the history and physical examination are usually much more important in making a definitive decision as to the hysterical nature of the patient's complaints.

Psychologic tests may also provide useful information. Hypnosis or interviews using sodium amobarbital may also be useful but only when performed by a physician well experienced in their evaluation and limitations.

NERVOUS SYSTEM SYMPTOMS IN HYSTERIA AND MALINGERING

Either hysteria or malingering may appear to affect any part of the nervous system, and the symptoms may resemble those of any organic neurologic disturbance. By careful examination, however, together with diagnostic acumen, the examiner is able in most instances to make a differentiation and a diagnosis.

The Sensory System

Either pain, perversion of sensation, or decrease in sensation may be present on a nonorganic basis. Psychogenic pain is more difficult to evaluate than a nonorganic decrease in sensation. Pain is subjective, and the examiner must rely to a great extent upon the patient's account of his symptom. In analyzing the complaint one should obtain an accurate description of its exact location and distribution, areas of radiation, mode of onset, severity, type, character, duration, and periodicity, as well as factors that accentuate and decrease it. If paresthesias, dysesthesias, and phantom sensations are present, these should be analyzed in the same manner.

The differentiation between genuine, feigned, and exaggerated pain is usually difficult. Psychogenic pain may affect any portion of the body and may closely simulate organic pain, although it is more apt to be vague, inconstant, and poorly localized, and fails to correspond to any true nerve or nerve root distribution. In general, psychogenic pain is not accompanied by alterations in function and attitude, such as defense movements, withdrawal of the part, spasm of the muscles, and suppression of motion; it is not attended by changes in pulse rate, blood pressure, respiratory depth and rate, pupillary diameter, vasomotor and trophic function, or sweat secretion; it is not reflected in the facial expression; it is not intensified by pressure over the painful area; it is not associated with such phenomena as swelling, redness, and heat. There is often a lack of consistency between the severity of the pain that the patient describes and the intensity of the discomfort that he seems to be experiencing. There may be either a decreased response or an excessive reaction to the painful stimulus. The patient may complain of intense, unbearable pain, yet he may, at the same time, either smile or exhibit a bland, unconcerned facial expression. On the other hand, there may be such manifestations as dramatizations, theatrical gestures, and facial expressions that are out of proportion to the severity of the symptoms described. In spite of what is claimed to be great discomfort, the patient may be able to eat and sleep without difficulty, and is often able to pursue pleasurable activities. Psychogenic pain of long duration may be accompanied by no disturbance in general nutrition or loss of weight. The pain often is influenced by suggestion; it may be diminished by slight physical measures that should not be of therapeutic value, or it may, by the physician's suggestion, travel from one spot to another and change in type during the examination. Psychogenic pain is often relieved by placebos, but on the other hand most individuals are influenced to a certain extent by suggestion, and organic pain may also be diminished by the use of placebos. Furthermore, on occasion psychogenic pain is characterized by the fact that it is relieved by no medication, even the most powerful narcotic.

The determination of the sensory threshold and the patient's reaction to painful stimulation may aid in the evaluation of the severity of pain. The hysterical individual often overreacts to all painful stimuli, sometimes with an exaggerated motor response. There is no significant difference between neurotic and normal individuals in the pain *perception* threshold, but there may be a definite lowering of the pain *reaction* threshold in neurotics. This overreaction may be demonstrated by means of the test described by Libman (Ch. 5). The lowered pain reaction threshold in neurosis is not necessarily a manifestation of the conversion process, as such lowering may also occur in anxiety states, neurasthenia, and hypochondriasis. It is important to recall that there is a marked variability of the pain reaction threshold in normal individuals in states of fatigue and anxiety. The threshold varies, furthermore, with age, sex, and state of health.

The term **psychogenic headache,** which is often misunderstood, should be used for headaches in which the clinical disorder results from delusional or conversion reactions and when there is no evidence that peripheral pain mechanisms are affected. The term must be used with caution, for in the past it has been confused with muscle contraction headaches that, although often resulting from psychic stress and therefore psychogenic, have a demonstrable mechanism in that muscle contraction can produce severe and very real pain. In true psychogenic headache the pain is often bandlike in distribution, and it may be the so-called clavus type, which is specifically localized and characterized by a sensation of a nail being driven into the skull. The patient may have pain for which there is no organic basis, or he may exaggerate a minimal discomfort.

Hyperesthesia and tenderness are found in both malingering and hysteria. In the former they are usually localized to the involved area, and may be inconstant. The patient may wince and complain of intense tenderness when the affected portion of the body is barely touched, yet if attention is distracted deep pressure on the same area may cause no flinching or other objective change. If the patient is examined while his eyes are closed or his attention distracted, he may be found to contradict himself. **Mannkopf's sign** may be used in differentiating between organic and malingered pain. Pressure over a painful area usually causes a temporary acceleration of the pulse rate of from $10-30$ beats/min; in the presence of malingered pain there is no change. The hysterical patient often reacts like the normal individual in this test.

The most significant changes in sensation in both hysteria and malingering are those in which there is a decrease in sensibility. Areas of hypesthesia, hypalgesia, anesthesia, and analgesia are commonly encountered and may have diagnostic significance; these may be complete, partial, or dissociated, and may affect all modalities or may be selective. Anesthesias of various types are encountered somewhat more frequently in hysteria than in malingering. Even a normal individual, however, is suggestible, and the examiner must avoid suggesting such sensory changes. Occasionally one may be able to confuse the patient who complains of nonorganic changes in sensation by instructing him to say "yes" every time he feels the stimulus and "no" when he does not. The malingerer, and less commonly the hysterical patient, will say "no" every time the so-called anesthetic region is stimulated.

In both consciously and unconsciously motivated anesthesia the distribution of the sensory loss fails to correspond to any organic distribution, either peripheral nerve, nerve root, or segmental. In the extremities the changes frequently have the so-called glove-and-stocking distribution, with complete loss of all modalities below either the wrist or elbow in the arm and below either the ankle or knee in the leg. There may be loss of tactile, superficial pain, temperature, vibratory, and position sensations, without dissociation, and usually with an abrupt, well-demarcated border, which may, however, vary from examination to examination. This change must be differentiated from the peripheral blunting of sensation in the peripheral neuritides, where there is a suggestive glove-and-stocking change, but with a gradual transition rather than an abrupt border. In hysteria, furthermore, there is often an inconsistency in responses that cannot be explained by an organic lesion; in spite of complete loss of cutaneous sensibility, the patient may have intact stereognostic sensation and graphesthesia, or in spite of complete loss of position sense, he may be able to use the digits or the distal portions of the extremity without difficulty in the performance of skilled movements and fine acts. In carrying out the finger-to-nose test the hand may wander widely, but the patient is always able to find his nose eventually. The Romberg sign may be negative in spite of claimed absence of position sense. It may be possible to bewilder the patient and confirm the absence of organic changes by examining him while his hands are crossed behind his back. Comparison of sensation on the palmar and dorsal surfaces of the hands also may show an inconsistency in replies. In a test for hysterical hemianalgesia described by Bowlus and Currier the hands are first rotated so that the little fingers are up and the palms are outward. Then the arms are crossed, the palms are placed together, and the fingers interlocked. The hands are then rotated downward, inward, and upward, so that the interlocked fingers are against the chest. At the conclusion of this maneuver the fingertips are on the same side as the respective arm, but the thumbs are not interlocked and are on the side opposite the fingers (Fig. 55-1). When the fingertips and thumb are stimulated alternately and irregularly, the patient with nonorganic hemianalgesia may make errors, while the one with organic loss will not. Furthermore, the patient with nonorganic loss may respond slowly, delay his answers, or show sweating or other signs of tension. It must be remembered, however, that with practice the patient may learn to identify the stimulus correctly, so the test gives most conclusive results the first time it is done.

Over the face and body the sensory change is usually in the so-called midline distribution:

there is complete loss of sensation of one half of the body, and the change takes place either at the midline or beyond it (when stimulating from the anesthetic to the normal area), whereas with organic lesions sensation begins to return slightly before the midline is reached. In psychogenic disorders the midline change may include the penis, vagina, and rectum, a finding that is rare in organic hemianesthesia. Again, there often is loss of all types of sensation, with a midline change over the skull and sternum even for vibratory sensation; this latter phenomenon cannot be explained on an organic basis, because vibratory sensation is in part conducted through bone, and as a consequence a midline change is not possible. If midline sensory changes are found, one should compare the cutaneous reflexes on the two sides; if these reflexes are retained, there can be no anesthesia. In the evaluation of what appear to be psychogenic changes in sensation, it is always essential to recall that there is some variation in the nerve supply in normal individuals. Furthermore, hysterical and malingered changes may be superimposed on organic anesthesia in peripheral nerve lesions and other neurologic disorders. Hysterical or malingered hemianesthesia, which almost invariably occurs on the left side, may occasionally be accompanied by an ipsilateral decrease or loss of the senses of vision, hearing, smell, and taste.

Auxiliary diagnostic measures are sometimes used to differentiate between organic and psychogenic changes in sensation. If a peripheral nerve, nerve root, or segmental lesion is suspected, sweating tests, the dermometer (electrical skin resistance), the cutaneous histamine reaction, and the psychogalvanic reflex may be used for confirmation (Ch. 41). One may also note the galvanic skin response elicited by pinprick and light touch: currents are obtained from a normal portion of the body and recorded on an oscillograph, and the biochemical changes that accompany sweat gland and vasomotor activities of a normally functioning autonomic nervous system are recorded. In organic anesthesia no galvanic skin reflex is obtained when the anesthetic zone is stimulated, whereas in hysterical and malingered anesthesia the reflex is normal. The histamine flare reaction is normal in both hysteria and malingering. In hysteria, however, the reaction is painless, and in malingering it usually is painful. Electrical testing may also aid in the differentiating between genuine and malingered hyperesthesia. Even a mild faradic current over a painful area increases the pain in it;

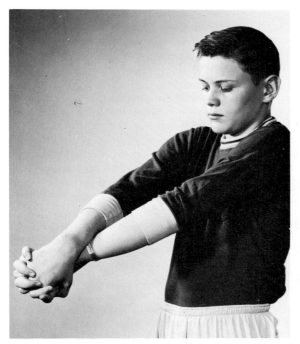
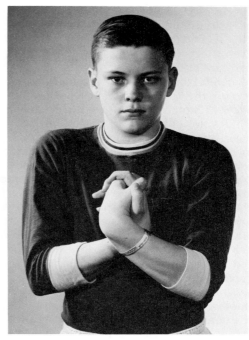

FIG. 55–1. Maneuver used in testing for hysterical hemianesthesia.

an insufficient current from an apparatus in action may produce a response in malingered hyperesthesia. Somatosensory evoked potential studies may also aid in differentiating organic from nonorganic sensory loss.

The Motor System

Abnormalities of the motor system that may be manifestations of both hysteria and malingering include disturbances of muscle strength and power, disorders of tone, dyskinesias, and abnormalities of coordination, station, and gait. There are rarely changes in volume or contour, except for wasting from disuse, and no organic abnormalities on electromyography or nerve conduction tests. However, with nonorganic weakness there may be a lack of recruitment of normal appearing motor units on the electromyogram, attesting to a lack of "effort" to contract the supposedly weak muscle. Electrical stimulation of a muscle during "maximum" contraction effort may also be used to assess the presence of functional weakness. Motor changes of psychic etiology may resemble almost any type of motor disturbance that is brought about by organic disease of the nervous system (see Table 21-1).

Psychogenic disturbances of muscle strength and power may cause various types of paresis and paralysis, and may even result in contractures and deformities. They may affect any portion of the body that is subject to voluntary control. Although the changes may be limited to certain movements or to part of a limb, an entire limb may be paralyzed or there may be a hemiparesis or hemiplegia affecting one half of the body. Paraplegia with involvement of both lower extremities is less common. The paresis or paralysis may be hypotonic or flaccid and resemble that occurring with a lower motor neuron lesion, there may be apparent hypertonicity, or there may be no or variable disturbances in tone. Contractures may develop following longstanding hysterical paresis. The distribution of the paresis is often anomalous, failing to correspond to any organic nerve supply or muscle arrangement. In a psychogenic hemiplegia, for instance, the face, tongue, and platysma and sternocleidomastoid muscles are spared (instead there may be weakness in turning the face toward the hemiparetic side), and in psychogenic paraplegia there is no sphincter paralysis, although psychogenic urinary retention can result in a distended bladder and occasionally causes difficulty in evaluation until cystometrography is performed. There may be muscular wasting due to disuse in psychogenic paralysis, together with secondary contractures. The paralysis never affects isolated muscles; movements, instead, are impaired.

A careful and complete examination is necessary for the diagnosis of psychogenic disturbances of motor function. Such an examination includes not only tests of muscle strength and power, but also observation of muscle tone, volume, coordination, and evaluation of abnormal movements. Careful testing of the reflexes, including the associated movements, is an important part of the evaluation of the motor defect.

Detailed testing of muscle power must always be performed. In both hysterical and malingered paralyses the patient makes little effort to contract the muscles necessary to execute the desired movement. He may be calm and indifferent while demonstrating his lack of strength; he may show little sign of alarm at the presence of complete paralysis, and smile cheerfully during the examination. Reliable evidence that the patient is not exerting all his power in an attempt to carry out a voluntary movement can be elicited by watching and palpating the contraction of the antagonists as well as the agonists. The patient may, for instance, be contracting the antagonists in order to simulate weakness of the agonists (*e.g.*, he may be observed to be contracting the triceps muscle, the antagonist to flexion of the elbow, when asked to tense the biceps and thus flex the elbow). On passive movement there may be evidence of contraction of the apparently paretic agonists when the antagonists are moved. Various muscles, muscle groups, and movements should be tested individually. In nonorganic weakness the muscular contractions are poorly sustained and may give way abruptly, rather than gradually, as the patient resists the force applied by the examiner; there may be absence of follow-through when the examiner withdraws his pressure. The paretic extremities should be raised and then dropped by the examiner. If the paralysis is organic, the extremity drops rapidly (especially if the paralysis is a flaccid one or is the result of a recent cerebral lesion), whereas in psychogenic paralysis the limb may drop slowly to avoid hurting it. Furthermore, if the arm is raised in such a way that it would strike the face if it dropped flaccidly, it may actually be seen to be moved to one side in order to avoid inflicting discomfort on the face. The examiner may suddenly, while distracting the patient's attention, apply a painful stimulus to the paretic limb; if the patient withdraws it,

the paresis cannot be organic. On occasion "functional" testing may corroborate an absence of weakness that was suspected during the routine test. For example, there may be apparent paresis of either dorsiflexion or plantar flexion of the foot when the patient is examined in the seated or recumbent position, but when upright, he may stand on either the heel or the toes of that foot, and support the entire body while doing so. Valuable information is obtained while watching the patient's performance while dressing and undressing; movements may be carried out that cannot be performed during the motor examination. Repeated examinations may be used to exhaust and bewilder the patient.

Certain tests have special value in differentiating organic from nonorganic paresis. In psychogenic paralysis of the arm the latissimus dorsi may be found to be paretic when tested by having the patient exert downward pressure of the arm, but to contract normally on coughing. In simulated hemiplegia the patient may be unable to adduct either the affected arm or leg against resistance, yet if he is asked to keep both arms against the body or both legs close together, the adductors may be felt to contract strongly on both sides, since it is difficult to adduct one extremity without adducting its apparently paralyzed fellow. In testing paralysis of the finger muscles the patient may be asked to pronate the forearms and interlock the fingers in such a way that the left fingers are on the right and *vice versa* (see Fig. 55-1); the examiner then points to the individual fingers and tells the patient to move them. It is difficult for one to determine immediately whether the indicated finger is on the right side or on the left, and if the patient attempts to respond promptly, he makes many mistakes. Similar tests may be carried out by asking the patient to perform individual movements while his hands are behind his back. The dynamometer may be used to test strength of grip; in organic weakness there is progressive fatigue, whereas in simulated paresis the patient may show instead an increase of strength with repeated testing.

The differentiation between hysterical and malingered paralyses may impose a difficult problem. Hysterical paralyses are usually more extensive and more profound; they are rarely limited to isolated muscles or muscle groups, and are usually accompanied by hysterical sensory changes. Simulated paralysis cannot be continuously maintained for any long period of time, but there is usually more resistance to passive movement than in hysterical defects. Hysterical paralysis may disappear with suggestion, psychotherapy, or hypnosis. If, however, contractures have developed, physical therapy may be necessary, as in the treatment of contractures related to organic disease.

The examination of muscle tone gives information in the evaluation of psychogenic motor changes. Tonus may be normal, decreased, or variable, but is often increased, with pseudorigidity or pseudospasticity. Rigidity, if present, resembles voluntary resistance, and voluntary and hysterical rigidity may be difficult to differentiate. The part may be held firmly in a bizarre position. Abnormalities in tone usually vary from time to time, especially under the influence of suggestion.

Muscle volume and contour rarely show significant change in psychogenic disorders; there is no true atrophy, although in longstanding defects there may be wasting because of disuse. Occasionally, with prolonged psychogenic paralyses, there are contractures caused by fibrous alterations and periarticular adhesions about the joints, with secondary wasting of the musculature, and even trophic changes of the skin (cyanosis and edema) and bones (osteoporosis) that closely resemble those of organic dysfunction.

Tests for coordination aid in the differentiation between psychogenic and organic motor defects. The patient may exhibit bizarre muscular responses that change from time to time, especially under the influence of suggestion. There may be a "wild" ataxia when he attempts to carry out tests for synergy, but no difficulty in carrying out acts such as buttoning clothes and lacing shoes. The incoordination may be out of proportion with the motor dysfunction. Adiadochokinesis, dysmetria, and dyssynergia may be simulated, but are usually not accompanied by the changes in tone, position, or reflexes that are found in either cerebellar or spinal ataxias.

Dyskinesias and hyperkinesias of various types are found in both hysteria and malingering. Their characteristics tend to change from time to time in the same individual. They may take the form of tremors, spasms, tics (habit spasms), convulsions, or very bizarre motor anomalies. In hysteria one may find medium-sized arrhythmic tremors, usually accentuated by voluntary movement, or bizarre habit spasms that consist of grimaces, blepharospasms, shrugging movements of the shoulders, twisting movements of the neck, and spasms of the larynx or diaphragm. These latter movements may be in the nature of compulsions, and may closely resemble those seen in organic torticollis, Hunt-

ington's chorea, Tourette's syndrome, and dystonia musculorum deformans. True fasciculations are considered to be pathognomonic of organic disease, but benign fasciculations, myokymic movements, and muscle tremors resulting from excitement, fright, fatigue, or cold may have to be differentiated from them. It is important to bear in mind that tremors, especially of the hands and fingers, may be symptoms of either tension or fatigue in any normal individual, and that psychogenic tremors may disappear with involuntary movement and increase with attention.

Observation of the station and gait may also furnish useful information in the detection of hysteria and malingering. The patient should be asked to stand with his feet together, first with his eyes open and then with them closed, and then to stand on his heels, on his toes, and on one foot at a time. The patient should walk forward, backward, tandem, and around chairs, with the eyes both open and closed. In so-called hysterical astasia-abasia (or *stasibasiphobia*) the patient is unable either to stand or to walk. When tested in the Romberg position, however, he may be seen to sway from the hips instead of from the ankles, and to tremble and shake without showing signs of fear or pain. The truly ataxic patient makes every effort to maintain the erect posture and to avoid falling, whereas the simulator or hysteric usually reels from side to side or falls *en masse* without the slightest attempt to maintain his equilibrium. The patient with organic ataxia can usually maintain an upright position with very slight support from a wall or table, or by lightly touching the examiner's hand, by watching the floor, or by placing the feet a short distance apart; the patient with psychogenic ataxia is not aided by these measures.

If a patient with either hysteria or malingering is asked to carry out various commands, such as touching a finger to the nose or alternately pronating and supinating the hands, while standing with feet together, he may "forget" to sway and fall. Furthermore, in hysterical astasia-abasia, although the patient seems unable to stand or walk, he may be able to move his limbs for other purposes, and may skip, jump, run, and walk backwards without difficulty. Tests for power, tone, and coordination may be normal if carried out while the patient is lying down. As he attempts to walk, he may show a nondescript type of gait, with swaying far to the side, stumbling, and skipping. Locomotion is accompanied by superfluous movements of other parts of the body. The patient may appear to be about to fall to the floor, but either catches himself or, if he does fall, does so in a theatrical manner, without injury. In other types of hysterical gaits, and in simulated paresis, there may be various changes from the normal. The patient may be unable to stand or walk because of a psychogenic hemiplegia or paraplegia, apparent foot-drop, pain on movement of the limbs, stiffness of the joints, shortening or anomaly of one leg, or ataxia, and may show bizarre disturbances of both station and gait. Some persons with nonorganic weakness of one lower extremity may claim to require a cane or other device for support but use it on the wrong side.

Testing of reflexes is essential to the appraisal of motor function (see Table 33-1). Although the muscle stretch reflexes are not specifically altered in psychogenic pareses, they may be modified by the tension of the muscles and there may be changes that resemble those seen in organic disease. In hysteria and other nonorganic states there frequently is a peculiar hyperactivity of the muscle stretch reflexes characterized by an increase in the range of movement rather than in the speed of response. This change may be present to a marked degree, so that a minimal stimulation of the patellar tendon, for example, may be followed by an extensive kick of the leg at the knee that resolves slowly and that may be accompanied by jerking movements of the other limbs and sometimes of the entire body. On the other hand, owing to tension of the muscles, the reflexes may be diminished or appear to be absent; in such circumstances, however, they can usually be obtained with reinforcement. The responses on the two sides must always be compared. The cutaneous reflexes, too, are not characteristically affected in psychogenic paralyses, although the abdominal reflexes are occasionally increased in hysterical patients.

The corticospinal tract responses are exceptionally important in the diagnosis of psychogenic disorders. There is no Babinski sign or related dorsiflexor and fanning response in nonorganic disease. There may be pseudoclonus at the knee or ankle, but it is irregular and poorly sustained; it can usually be differentiated from organic clonus since it is not stopped by plantar flexion of the foot. Although a Hoffmann sign is usually present in corticospinal tract disease, it is also present with the generalized reflex hyperactivity of tension states and neurosis, and may be found (usually bilaterally and incomplete) in normal persons. As a consequence this sign does not have diagnostic value unless it is unilateral and associated with other signs of corticospinal tract involvement.

Changes in the associated, or synkinetic, movements are valuable signs in the differentiation between organic and psychogenic paralysis. Testing for Hoover's sign, the trunk-thigh sign of Babinski, combined flexion of the thigh and leg (Neri), the various pronation tests, Bechterew's sign, the arm and leg signs of Raimiste, and other procedures to demonstrate the presence or absence of normal or abnormal coordinated associated movements that accompany voluntary contraction of muscles may give diagnostic information (Ch. 38).

Organic and psychogenic paralysis may be differentiated by the presence of many of the changes that have been mentioned. In organic hemiparesis there is involvement of the entire half of the body, with sparing only of the upper portion of the face; in psychogenic paralysis there is sparing of the face, tongue, and platysma and sternocleidomastoid muscles. In organic hemiparesis the muscle stretch reflexes are exaggerated, the abdominal reflexes are diminished or absent, the Babinski and other corticospinal tract responses are present, and there may be clonus; in psychogenic paresis the muscle stretch reflexes are normal or increased in range but have normal speed, the abdominal reflexes are normal or increased, there are no corticospinal tract responses, and there is no true clonus. In organic hemiparesis spasticity is present and there are contractures and the limbs assume a characteristic position (flexion of the upper extremity and extension of the lower extremity); in psychogenic paresis there may be variable changes in tone, and contractures, if present, are irregular and atypical. In organic hemiparesis the gait is of the unilateral spastic variety with circumduction of the leg; in psychogenic paralysis the gait is bizarre and there may be dragging of the foot. In organic hemiparesis Hoover's sign and other associated movements show certain changes that are reversed in psychogenic paralysis. Anesthesia on the affected half of the body is rare in organic hemiparesis, and if present, the changes are those seen in cerebral lesions; in psychogenic hemiparesis there is frequently a hemianesthesia that extends to the midline, affects all modalities of sensation, and may occasionally be accompanied by an ipsilateral decrease or loss of vision, hearing, taste, and smell.

It has been mentioned that in psychogenic as well as in organic paralysis there may be secondary contractures and vasomotor changes. Prolonged disuse of either an organically or hysterically paralyzed limb may lead to wasting of muscles that may resemble true atrophy, and there may be associated joint changes in the digits, periarthritis of the shoulder, and periarticular adhesions elsewhere that may lead to deformities and contractures. There may be trophic changes in the skin and nails; vasomotor changes with cyanosis, edema, and abnormalities of sweating; and even osteoporosis. The late sequelae of long-standing psychogenic paralysis may be almost impossible to differentiate from those of organic paralysis. If the immobile extremity is painful such diagnoses as shoulder-hand syndrome, reflex sympathetic dystrophy, and Sudeck's atrophy may have been applied to it.

Articulation

Dysphonia and aphonia are among the more common paralytic phenomena of hysteria; the manifestations usually come on suddenly, in association with shock or fright, and may disappear abruptly. Articulation may be completely absent, the patient may be able to speak only by whispering, or speech may be lost while the patient retains his ability to sing, whistle, and cough. There may be hypesthesia of the pharynx and larynx, with a diminished or absent pharyngeal reflex. Laryngeal examination shows bilateral paresis or paralysis of adduction, and the vocal cords remain in abduction during attempts at phonation, although they meet in the midline on coughing; abduction is unimpaired, and inspiration is normal. There may be associated dysphagia, laryngospasm, and globus hystericus. In both hysteria and malingering there may be lalling (the perfect enunciation of so-called baby talk), mutism, or anarthria. True aphasia is always of organic origin, but may occasionally be confused with hysterical or simulated mutism. An aphasic, however, no matter how speechless, at least occasionally tries to speak; a hysterical mute may appear to make a great effort but be unable to produce a tone; in simulated mutism the patient makes no effort to speak. One must bear in mind, however, that mutism may also be encountered in catatonia and severe depression. Stuttering, stammering, and tremulousness of speech are commonly encountered in tense and nervous individuals; true stuttering can usually be differentiated from a simulated difficulty.

The Special Senses

Smell and Taste

Hysterical anosmia is not commonly encountered, and malingered anosmia is rare. Patients with either condition may retain their ability to distinguish the flavor of foods, which is an olfactory function, in spite of an alleged loss of smell. In hysterical anosmia the patient may be unable to identify acetic acid, formaldehyde, and ammonia (substances that stimulate the trigeminal rather than the olfactory nerve) as well as volatile oils, whereas the patient with organic anosmia retains the ability to identify irritating substances, but not volatile oils. The patient with simulated anosmia may make grimaces and involuntary withdrawal movements when a disagreeable substance is placed in front of his nose. Hysterical patients may also complain of hyperosmia and parosmia; malingerers rarely describe such phenomena.

Although ageusia is an infrequent complaint in both hysteria and malingering, complete absence of taste is usually psychogenic, since such a defect would imply bilateral involvement of the gustatory functions of the seventh, ninth, and tenth cranial nerves. The edges and dorsum of the anterior two-thirds of the tongue are the most sensitive areas; a unilateral facial nerve lesion can cause loss of taste in this distribution on one side of the tongue, but this produces subjective loss of taste in only the most discriminating individual.

Vision

Both hysterical and malingered defects in the visual apparatus are occasionally encountered. These include disturbances not only of vision itself, but also of the sensibility and motility of the eye and of secretion. Exaggeration of a pre-existing visual defect resulting from corneal opacity or refractive errors may be either consciously or unconsciously motivated. In hysteria there may be either blindness (amaurosis) or impairment of vision (amblyopia). Amaurosis, if present, is usually bilateral. Amblyopia, however, is more frequent, and is usually associated with tubular or spiral constriction of the visual fields. There may be other disturbances of vision such as blurring, photophobia, ocular fatigue, polyopia, or monocular diplopia. In malingering, many of these symptoms are also present, but amaurosis is more common than field constriction, and it is usually unilateral and of sudden onset. It may be intermittent or shifting and may be accompanied by discrepancies, bizarre exaggerations, and contradictions. Occasionally a self-inflicted or factitious conjunctivitis or keratitis is encountered.

In the detection of psychogenic blindness the eyes themselves should first be carefully inspected, and the routine neurologic procedures, including testing of acuity and fields, together with ophthalmoscopy, should be carried out. The testing of pupillary reflexes is an important part of the examination. The pupil of a blind eye is usually dilated and does not react to direct light; the maintenance of a moderate amount of vision, however, may be associated with a persistent light reflex, and the pupillary reflexes may be normal in blindness that is due to a cortical lesion. Loss of reflexes, especially of the light reflex, as a result of iritis, keratitis, or trauma must be remembered; the Argyll Robertson pupil is rarely unilateral. In tense and agitated individuals the pupils are often dilated, but react normally. Occasionally either miotics or mydriatics are used to alter the pupillary reaction by malingerers with access to these agents. A normal ophthalmoscopic examination does not eliminate the possibility of organic disease, since there is no change in either the optic disk or the retina in some cases of retrobulbar neuritis and in blindness due to cortical lesions. Visual evoked potentials are preserved in psychogenic blindness and are usually abnormal or even absent in cortical blindness. Blink responses to threat and the elicitation of optokinetic nystagmus are generally preserved with psychic visual loss.

If blindness is bilateral and complete, it is usually possible to differentiate that of psychogenic origin from that due to organic disease. If a blind person attempts to look at his hand when it is either in front of his face or placed to one side, he fixes his eyes in a position so that the vision would be directed toward his hand if he could see, since his proprioceptive sensations are intact; a simulator will make no attempt to fix the eyes on the hand and may gaze in any direction (**Schmidt – Rimpler test**). A blind person is able to touch his forefingers together without difficulty; a malingerer will cause them to wander idly. A simulator may betray himself by lowering his eyelids or wrinkling his forehead in response to a sudden strong light (emergency light reflex), and the presence of normal visual, menace, and fixation reflexes precludes organic blindness. An alleged inability to read anything but the large type of the Snellen chart may be unmasked by

the following device: The patient is asked to stand 20 feet from a mirror that is covered by a testing chart; after the patient reads the smallest line that he states can be seen, the chart is removed from in front of the mirror and the patient is asked to stand 10 feet nearer the mirror. Another Snellen chart with letters the same size as the first chart, but printed backward, is then placed in front of the patient's chest as he faces the mirror and he is asked to read the letters seen in the mirror. Being half the original distance from the mirror, the patient may be induced to read twice the number of lines read when 20 feet away, assuming that he is ignorant of the laws of reflection.

The detection of psychogenic unilateral amaurosis may be more difficult. It is important to remember, however, that the amaurotic eye usually deviates when the sound eye is fixed. Feigned unilateral blindness may be unmasked by placing a pencil vertically in front of a page of small type while the patient is reading; if bilateral vision is present, the patient will continue to read, since he can see around the pencil, but if one eye is blind, one or two words on each line will be hidden by the pencil. Testing of visual acuity with the use of a strong convex lens, a prism, or a colored lens may aid in the detection of unilateral simulated blindness. While the patient is reading test type with both eyes open and lenses in front of both, a strong convex lens is placed in front of the good eye, and either a plain lens or a weak minus lens in front of the defective eye; if the patient continues to read distant type, he must be using the allegedly blind eye. While the patient is looking at a light, a prism of 6° with the base outward is placed before the defective eye; if the eye deviates inward and returns to the midposition when the prism is removed, the eye cannot be completely blind. While the patient is reading aloud a prism with the base outward, upward, or downward is placed before the allegedly blind eye; if the vision in that eye is defective, there will be no change in the patient's ability to read, but if the vision is retained, the prism will produce double images and inability to continue to read, and at the same time the eye will be seen to deviate. The patient is asked to look at a chart with alternate red and black letters, and a red lens is placed in front of the good eye; the red letters should disappear, and if the patient can read all the letters, he is using the allegedly blind eye.

Harman's diaphragm test is another device for determining monocular blindness. It is based on the facts (1) that a person is unable to tell which eye is being used when both eyes are open, and (2) that when objects are viewed through a small aperture properly placed, the right eye sees only those on the left side and the left eye only those on the right. The test is performed as follows: A flat ruler 18 in. long is constructed so that at one end there is a wooden carrier, set at right angles, on which is placed a small card with letters or numbers on it; 5 in. from the carrier there is a small vertical screen, pierced by a hole ¾ in. in diameter. The end of the ruler opposite the carrier is placed on the patient's upper lip. and he is asked to read the letters and numbers on the card through the hole in the screen. If the card has the letters ABCDEFG on it, and the patient reads only DEFG, it is obvious that the patient does not see with his right eye, whereas if only ABCD are read it is equally clear that only his right eye is being used and that the left is defective. If all the letters are read, both eyes must be used. Testing near vision after dilating the pupil of the good eye and instilling saline in the affected eye may also reveal the presence of simulated blindness.

There are many other tests and devices whereby hysterical and simulated blindness may be detected, but most of them involve complicated ophthalmologic instruments and procedures, and the tests just described usually give adequate information. A criterion of complete bilateral amaurosis may rest upon the use of the electroencephalogram. Normal alpha waves are present only when the eyes are closed, and they disappear when the patient opens his eyes and looks around. If alpha waves disappear when he opens his eyes, the patient must have a certain amount of vision. If alpha waves persist when the patient attempts to look at objects, one may conclude that there is true organic blindness. The response to photic stimulation and evoked potentials also give information about vision.

Changes in visual fields are encountered more frequently in hysteria than in malingering. The so-called tubular fields are common in hysteria; spiral and star-shaped fields may also be found (Figs. 10-10 and 10-11). These defects, however, may also be obtained in fatigue states, and the examiner must always bear in mind that concentric contraction, suggestively tubular in type, may occur in organic defects, in states of fatigue or poor concentration, and when severe refractive errors are present. Hemianopia, either homonymous or heteronymous, is not found in psychogenic disorders.

Psychogenic diplopia may be difficult to differentiate from organic diplopia, but can usually be distinguished by the use of the Lancaster chart (Ch. 11). Monocular diplopia and polyopia are encountered more commonly than true diplopia in both hysteria and malingering; these symptoms often have no organic etiology, although they occasionally result from dislocation of the lens and other disorders related to the eye itself; only rarely are they due to cerebral lesions. Blurring of vision may be difficult to appraise. Micropsia, macropsia, scotomas, flashes of light, and hallucinations may be psychogenic or may occur in association with migraine or temporal or occipital lobe irritations. Myopia secondary to spasm of accommodation is said to occur on a psychogenic basis, but is probably infrequent. Color blindness may be simulated, but such change is rarely significant.

Disturbances of sensibility, such as anesthesia or hyperesthesia of the skin and conjunctiva, or pain, burning, or itching of the eyes, can be diagnosed only by a complete history and examination. Photophobia may be either hysterical or simulated in origin. The patient with psychogenic photophobia may be able to keep his eyes open in the presence of intense illumination and may show no blinking, blepharospasm, or lacrimation when a strong light is flashed into the eyes. Disturbances of secretion (excessive or decreased lacrimation) are usually diagnosed without too much difficulty.

Spasm of the extraocular and associated muscles is common in psychogenic disorders, but paralytic phenomena are rare, and their presence throws doubt upon the diagnosis. Blepharospasm is at times a compulsive manifestation, although it may be a reflex response to photophobia and irritation of the eyes or cornea, or it may be part of an organic movement disorder. Real ptosis of psychogenic origin is rare, and impairment of raising the eyelids is usually a pseudoptosis brought about by spasm of the orbiculares oculorum; it is most commonly bilateral. When the patient who has a psychogenic ptosis attempts to raise the eyelids, there is no compensatory overactivity of the frontalis (an invariable accompaniment of true ptosis). When the patient who has a psychogenic pseudoptosis attempts to look upward, he may contract the levators and raise his eyelids as he raises his head. In unilateral simulated and hysterical ptosis the affected eyebrow is lower than the unaffected one; in true ptosis it is higher. Spasm of the individual ocular muscles may occur in psychogenic disorders. Spasm of convergence is most frequently encountered; this is usually bilateral and disappears when the patient looks quickly to one side or in an upward direction. Spasmodic conjugate deviation of psychogenic origin is rare. Spasm of accommodation occasionally causes myopia. Both voluntary and hysterical varieties of nystagmus have been described, but such instances are rare, and their existence is doubtful.

Hearing

Both hysterical and malingered deafness may be either partial or total and either unilateral or bilateral; there may be an exaggeration of a previously existing defect. Hysterical deafness is usually bilateral and total; the patient makes no attempt to hear what is said or to read the speaker's lips. In most instances it is a transitory symptom that appears suddenly after mental excitement or emotional stress. It may be associated with hysterical mutism and blindness. If hysterical deafness is unilateral, it is usually incomplete and is on the same side as hysterical motor and sensory disturbances. Simulated deafness is usually unilateral and has its onset following trauma where secondary gain, financial or otherwise, is sought. It is rare, however, to have unilateral deafness of posttraumatic origin without impairment of vestibular function. As a consequence, marked depression of the vestibular responses, especially the caloric, supports the assumption that the cochlear division of the acoustic nerve is also impaired. Conversely, normal labyrinthine responses suggest that the claimed loss of hearing is either simulated or exaggerated.

In cases of suspected hysterical and malingered deafness it is very important to obtain a detailed past history; this should include reference to any type of deafness, otitis, ear pain, vertigo, tinnitus, past infections such as measles, scarlet fever, meningitis, or syphilis, and occupation, as well as a history of the mode of onset of the deafness. The external auditory canals and tympanic membranes should be carefully examined, and all hearing tests, for both air and bone conduction, should be carried out while the patient is blindfolded. The Rinne, Schwabach, and Weber tests should be carefully performed. Inconsistent responses suggest that the deafness may not be organic. Repeated audiometric examinations are important; discrepancies and inconsistencies in the tests are common with hysterical and simulated deafness, and it may be difficult to obtain two or three successive audiograms that are comparable. The preservation of auditory brain stem evoked responses indicates that at least some hearing is present.

Simulated bilateral deafness, if the person under examination persistently refuses to give evidence of any hearing power, is usually easy to detect. Individuals who have been deaf for long periods of time usually raise their voices during conversation and keep their eyes fixed on the speaker's face and lips, watching for every gesture of the speaker that may aid in their interpretation of what he is saying. A deaf man who is eager to hear will automatically turn his best ear toward the speaker. A clearly enunciated whisper is sometimes more audible than a loud, indistinct shout. Even an experienced lip reader has difficulty with certain letters, especially the consonants, and may not be able to differentiate "mutton" from "button," "no" from "toe," "die" from "tie," and "most" from "post." A person who is simulating partial deafness may be able to differentiate these words by appearing to read lips. Sometimes the patient with bilateral simulated deafness can be caught off guard, and the making of disparaging remarks about him may cause changes in his facial expression.

Many tests have been devised for the detection of unilateral simulated deafness. The normal ear may be partially occluded with cotton or a perforated plug. Words and numbers are then repeated, starting with a low voice and progressively raising it. The voice should be heard by the sound ear, and if the patient states that he cannot hear he is probably malingering. The normal ear may then be completely occluded with a closed speculum, and the test repeated; if the patient hears, the so-called affected ear cannot be completely deaf. The stethoscope test is sometimes employed in detecting unilateral feigned deafness. An ordinary stethoscope, one earpiece of which is occluded, is used. First the occluded earpiece is put into the "deaf" ear, and the examiner says a few words into the funnel; the patient should be able to repeat these words because the sounds are coming into the normal ear. The stethoscope is then removed and placed with the occluded earpiece in the sound ear, and the process is repeated. If the patient is able to hear as well as before, it means that hearing is present in the so-called deaf ear. It may be of value to reverse the procedure and first put the closed earpiece into the normal ear and the open earpiece into the affected ear. If the patient comprehends what is said, he must have hearing in the "deaf" ear. The reliability of the stethoscope test, however, is doubtful.

Lombard's test is carried out by first asking the patient to read a selected passage aloud. As long as he hears his own voice, there is no change in pitch. Then a Bárány noise apparatus is inserted into the normal ear, and he is asked to read again; if he is actually deaf, the pitch and intensity of his voice will be raised while reading, and the voice will return to normal when the noise stops. If he continues to read in a normal voice, the allegedly deaf ear is probably hearing.

Teal's test is performed in the following manner: If the patient cannot hear by either air conduction or bone conduction, a blindfold is applied and a nonvibrating tuning fork is placed over the mastoid area on the affected side. Then a vibrating tuning fork is placed a short distance from the same ear. If the patient is truly deaf, he will not hear, and if he is able to hear, some air conduction must persist. In the **Doerfler – Stewart test** speech is introduced from a soundproof control room to the patient, wearing binaural headphones, in an adjacent soundproof room. The patient is asked to repeat what he hears, and auditory thresholds for speech and for static noise are determined. Then speech is introduced at a constant intensity level of 5 decibels louder than the established threshold and the patient is asked to continue to repeat what is heard while noise at increasing intensity is superimposed as a background. The normal person continues to perceive speech until the noise is 10 – 25 decibels more intense than the speech. In either hysteria or malingering the patient loses perception of speech before the noise reaches the intensity level of speech.

The auditory – palpebral, or cochleoorbicularis, reflex may also be used as a criterion in unilateral deafness. The normal ear is closed tightly and a loud noise is made near the supposedly deaf ear. A slight winking movement or contraction of the lid on the corresponding side means that the sound was heard. The cochleopupillary reflex, in which there is dilation, or constriction followed by dilation, of the pupils in response to a loud noise, has the same significance. Other more detailed tests for psychogenic deafness may require more complex equipment.

Vestibular Function

It may be difficult to differentiate between simulated and true vertigo. True vertigo, however, is usually rotatory in type and is accompanied by nausea, vomiting, pallor, hyperhidrosis, difficulty with equilibrium, and nystagmus. The absence of these manifestations, however, does not rule out true vertigo. The various examinations of vestibular function, which include the rotating chair, caloric tests, and electronystagmography, are evaluated entirely by objective criteria, and it is not possible to alter the responses to these tests in either hysteria or malingering. A history of ataxia, staggering, or syncope with change of position is helpful in evaluation of vestibular function. Tests for coordination are also important.

Disorders of Consciousness

States of disordered consciousness, with or without convulsive motor manifestations, may occur in either hysteria or malingering. In hysteria the loss of consciousness is not deep and is rarely complete. Unless there is an associated hysterical anesthesia, the patient usually responds to painful and unpleasant stimulation. The reflexes are normal, and there are no pathologic reflex responses. The temperature, pulse, respiration, and blood pressure are normal. The eyes may be tightly closed, and the patient often resists attempts on the part of the examiner to open them. There may be vigorous contraction of the orbiculares oculorum, rendering it difficult to test the corneal and pupillary reflexes. Careful observation may show the patient to be aware of what is happening in his environment despite apparent complete loss of consciousness. In malingering there is rarely complete loss of consciousness, and the patient may be seen to be making furtive glances when he is not aware that he is being watched.

Hysterical loss of consciousness is usually precipitated by emotional stress, and the onset is frequently dramatic. The patient may appear to be in a trance, or coma may alternate with weeping and laughing. The performance is appropriately staged and occurs when observers are present. The movements are coordinated and purposive. The patient may struggle, clutch at objects or parts of the body, or attempt to tear off clothes. Insight into the condition and return of consciousness may frequently be brought about by the intravenous injection of a barbiturate. Simulated loss of consciousness may often be terminated by painful stimulation, cold, water, or apparent neglect. It is important to bear in mind that vasodepressor syncope may also follow emotional shock. This syndrome, however, is usually preceded by a transient period of giddiness, weakness, fatigue, nausea, or vomiting. The attack is usually brief, with return to consciousness in a very few minutes. Recovery may be accelerated by placing the head lower than the body.

Hysterical and malingered convulsions may resemble organic convulsions. They are usually, however, more bizarre, and are unpredictable in their course. There is no manifestation of epilepsy that cannot be duplicated in either hysteria or malingering, but in both the attacks more closely resemble grand mal than absence or jacksonian seizures. The attack is not preceded by an aura, and may follow immediately after emotional stress or mental shock. As with psychogenic loss of consciousness, the performance is appropriately staged, and the onset is usually dramatic. A significant time and place are chosen for the attack, usually when spectators are present. The patient may fall to the floor, but he is usually careful to avoid injury. Biting the tongue and loss of sphincter control are rare. There is no cyanosis or frothing at the mouth. There are no pupillary changes or loss of reflexes, and no Babinski signs. Loss of consciousness is rarely complete. There may be generalized muscular rigidity, sometimes with retraction of the head and true opisthotonos, and the patient may be in the position of the *arc de cercle*; in the past this was called major hysteria (hysteroepilepsy). The patient may laugh or weep throughout the attack, or laughter and crying may alternate. Muscular movements are much more purposive than in true epilepsy. Sleepiness, headache, and confusion are absent after the attack and there are no other postconvulsion manifestations. Complex partial seizures are sometimes difficult to differentiate from psychogenic ones with a similar clinical picture or from similar syndromes precipitated by rage or frustration. Often the automatisms and bizarre movements of complex partial seizures are thought to be of psychogenic rather than organic origin.

Repeated observations, a detailed history, including inquiry into the presence of epilepsy in relatives and friends, and a thorough neurologic examination may, on occasion, be necessary in order to differentiate psychogenic from organic seizures, and, if psychogenic, those of hysterical from those of malingered origin. It is important to bear in mind that emotional stimuli may also precipitate organic attacks and, in addition, that epilepsy and hysteria may coexist. Response to medication may give helpful but not conclusive information, since anticonvulsants, which may also be sedatives, can favorably influence psychogenic as well as organic seizures, or may have a placebo effect, and furthermore not all epilepsies respond satisfactorily to the usual anticonvulsants. The objective information obtained from the electroencephalogram may be essential in the differential diagnosis, as may videotape and prolonged electroencephalographic monitoring. Certain serum enzymes may rise with organic but not psychogenic seizures.

Abnormal Mental States

The mental symptoms of hysteria vary widely, but usually follow a fairly definite pattern. Both mental and somatic symptoms may be associated with anxiety, conversion manifestations, and depression. The somatic symptoms may be referable to any organ or system of organs of the body. The mental symptoms may vary from moderate anxiety to severe depression and suggestive schizoid manifestations. In addition to disturbances of consciousness and convulsions, there may be amnesia, fugues, trance states, emotional instability, insomnia, and fatigue states. The diagnosis can usually be made by a review of the past history, assessment of the total personality, and the positive findings of hysteria in the neurologic examination.

Simulation of mental disease is less common than the presence of abnormal mental states in hysteria, but it may occur. It may be practiced in order to void or nullify civil contracts, escape conviction for crime, evade military duty, or obtain addictive drugs. Dissimulation, or concealment, of mental disease is occasionally practiced by alcoholics and paranoiacs in order to obtain release from mental hospitals or to remove previously adjudicated incompetence. Insanity is a legal term, and in most instances the diagnosis of either simulated or dissimulated insanity must be made by a competent medicolegal expert and psychiatrist. Psychologic tests and the use of intravenous barbiturates may aid in diagnosis. Simulation, however, is usually found only in individuals with personality disturbances, and malingering in general, as well as simulation of mental disease, implies the need for psychiatric management. Only rarely, however, will the malingerer admit to his disability and submit to psychotherapy.

BIBLIOGRAPHY

Adams RD, Victor M. Principles of Neurology, 4th ed. New York, McGraw – Hill, 1989

Baker JH, Silver JR. Hysterical paraplegia. J Neurol Neurosurg Psychiat 1987;50:375

Bowlus WE, Currier RD. A test for hysterical hemianalgesia. N Engl J Med 1963;269:1253

Briquet P. Traite Clinique et Therapeutique à l'Hysterie. Paris, JB Ballière et Fils, 1859

Carter AB. The functional overlay. Lancet 1967;2:1196

Chodoff P. The diagnosis of hysteria: An overview. Am J Psychiatry 1974;131:1073

Ewalt JR, Strecker EA, Ebaugh FG. Practical Clinical Psychiatry, 8th ed. New York, Blakiston Division, McGraw–Hill, 1957

Farley J, Woodruff RA, Guze SB. The prevalence of hysteria and conversion symptoms. Br J Psychiatry 1968;114:1121

Gorman WF. Defining malingering. J Forensic Sci 1982; 27:401

Gould R, Miller BL, Goldberg MA, Benson DF. The validity of hysterical signs and symptoms. J Nerv Ment Dis 1986;174:593

Guze SG. The diagnosis of hysteria: What are we trying to do? Am J Psychiatry 1967;114:491

Howard JE, Dorfman LJ. Evoked potentials in hysteria and malingering. J Clin Neurophysiol 1986;3:39

Keane JR. Hysterical gait disorders: 60 cases. Neurology 1989;39:586

Keschner M. Simulation (malingering) in relation to injuries of the brain and spinal cord and their coverings. In Brock S (ed). Injuries of the Brain and Spinal Cord and Their Coverings, 4th ed. New York, Springer, 1960

Koller W, Lang A, Vetere–Overfield B et al. Psychogenic tremors. Neurology 1989;39:1094

Krumholz A, Niedermeyer E. Psychogenic seizures: A clinical study with follow-up data. Neurology 1983;33:498

Leavitt F, Sweet JJ. Characteristics and frequency of malingering among patients with low back pain. Pain 1986; 25:357

Magee KR. Hysterical hemiplegia and hemianesthesia. Postgrad Med 1962;31:339

Marsden CD. Hysteria–a neurologist's view. Psychol Med 1986;16:277

McComas AJ, Kereshi S, Quinlan J. A method for detecting functional weakness. J Neurol Neurosurg Psychiatry 1983; 46:280

Merskey H. Regional pain is rarely hysterical. Arch Neurol 1988;45:915

Miller H, Cartlidge N. Stimulation and malingering after injuries to the brain and spinal cord. Lancet 1972;1:580

Naish JM. Problems of deception in medical practice. Lancet 1979;2:139

Perley MJ, Guze SB. Hysteria: The stability and usefulness of clinical criteria. A quantitative study based on a follow-up period of six to eight years in 39 patients. N Engl J Med 1962;266:421

Raskin M, Talbott JA, Myerson AT. Diagnosis of conversion reactions: predictive value of psychiatric criteria. JAMA 1966;197:102

Robins E, Purtell JJ, Cohen ME. "Hysteria" in men: A study of 38 patients so diagnosed and 194 control subjects. N Engl J Med 1952;246:677

Rolak LA. Psychogenic sensory loss. J Nerv Ment Dis 1988;176:686

Stephens JH, Kamp M. On some aspects of hysteria: A clincial study. J Nerv Ment Dis 1962;134:305

Walshe FMR. Diagnosis of hysteria. Br Med J 1965;2:1451

Woolsey RM. Hysteria: 1875–1975. Dis Nerv Sys 1976; 37:379

Woodruff RA Jr, Clayton PJ, Guze SB. Hysteria: Studies of diagnosis, outcome, and prevalence. JAMA 1971;215:425

Woodruff RA, Goodwin DW, Guze SB. Psychiatric Diagnosis. New York, Oxford University Press, 1974

Ziegler FJ, Imboden JB, Meyer E. Contemporary conversion reactions. Am J Psychiatry 1960;116:901

PART J

Lumbar Puncture and the Examination of the Cerebrospinal Fluid

Chapter 56

THE CEREBROSPINAL FLUID

The existence of the cerebrospinal fluid has been known since antiquity, but recognition of the functions and clinical significance of the fluid is of fairly recent date. It is common knowledge that craniotomies and trephines were performed by the ancients, probably in cases of trauma, hydrocephalus, and undiagnosed intracranial disease. Herophilus (280 B.C.) was aware of the presence of the cerebral ventricles and the choroid plexus. Galen (150 A.D.) considered the cerebrospinal fluid a watery excretion going from the brain to the nasal cavity. Vesalius (1552) recognized that the content of the ventricles was a watery humor.

Cotugno (1764) described the cerebrospinal fluid and subarachnoid spaces. Haller (1776) first postulated the circulation of the fluid. Magendie (1825 – 1842) expressed the modern concept of the protective nature of the fluid and brought its existence and functions to the attention of the medical profession. Faivre (1853 – 1854) and Luschka (1855) studied the formation and circulation of the fluid. In 1875 and 1876 Key and Retzius published their researches on the physiology of the formation, circulation, and absorption of the fluid. The first monograph on the subject was that of Mestrezat (1912), who described the chemical composition of the fluid in health and disease; his quantitative determinations allowed certain syndromes to be described. Further knowledge on the physiology of the fluid was contributed by the researches of Weed and his associates (1914 – 1927) and Dandy (1919).

Corning, in 1885, was the first to puncture the subarachnoid space of a living person; this was done for the purpose of introducing cocaine. Wynter and Morton, in 1891, drained the spinal fluid in the treatment of cases of tuberculous meningitis; this was done with a trocar and cannula, through an incision in the skin. Quincke, also in 1891, simplified the procedure, using a plain needle that he introduced through the skin and into the subarachnoid space. He was the first to remove spinal fluid for diagnostic purposes. Since that time modifications have been made in the examination and technic, namely, the Wassermann reaction (1908), since followed by numerous improved methods for the detection of syphilis; the Lange colloidal gold test (1912), since shown to relate to the IgG content of the cerebrospinal fluid; the Queckenstedt procedure (1916); and puncture of the cisterna magna (Ayer, 1920). Pneumoencephalography was introduced by Dandy (1919); and myelography by Sicard and Forstier (1921). More recently, computed tomography and magnetic resonance imaging of the head and spine have largely supplanted pneumoencephalography and myelography in the study of the ventricular and subarachnoid spaces. The need for lumbar puncture to study cerebrospinal fluid dynamics has also lessened with the arrival of modern imaging procedures. However, examination of the cerebrospinal fluid continues to be an important and often necessary test.

FORMATION, CIRCULATION, ABSORPTION, AND FUNCTIONS OF THE CEREBROSPINAL FLUID

The concepts of the formation, circulation, and absorption of the spinal fluid have varied. It has been generally believed, however, that under normal circumstances the major portion of the fluid originates in the choroid plexus of the ventricles of the brain, although there is also some production of cerebrospinal fluid through the ependymal lining of the ventricles and in the subarachnoid and perivascular spaces. It is discharged into and fills the ventricles, basal cisterns, and subarachnoid spaces (Fig. 56-1). The most important source is the choroid plexus of the lateral ventricles, although the plexuses in the roof of the third and fourth ventricles (that in the latter extending into the lateral recesses and protruding slightly through the foramina of Luschka into the subarachnoid space) also contribute to the formation. There is movement of the fluid from the lateral ventricles through the foramina of Monro and into the third ventricle, and then through the aqueduct of Sylvius into the fourth ventricle. The last-named structure communicates with the subarachnoid space through the two foramina of Luschka, one of which is situated in each of its lateral recesses, and through the midline foramen of Magendie. From the fourth ventricle the fluid may also go into the central canal of the spinal cord.

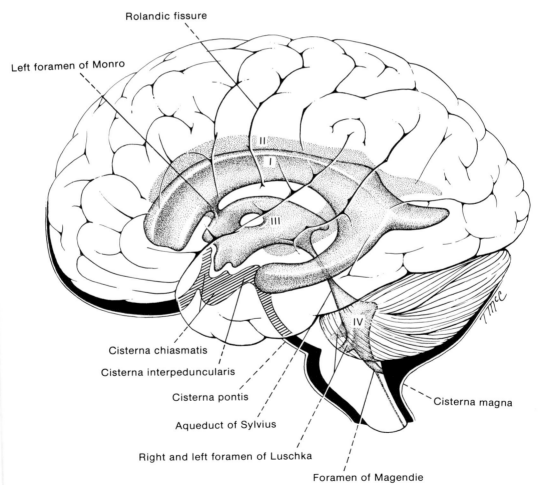

FIG. 56–1. Diagram of the cerebrospinal fluid spaces, showing lateral, third, and fourth ventricles, foraminal connections with the subarachnoid space, and some of the major subarachnoid cisterns. **I** and **II.** Lateral ventricles. **III.** Third ventricle. **IV.** Fourth ventricle. (Modified from Dandy WE. Bull Johns Hopkins Hosp 1921; 32:67–123)

In the subarachnoid space the fluid lies between the arachnoid and the pia mater. Within the space weblike strands of arachnoid extend between the arachnoid and pia. The pia closely invests the surface of the brain and spinal cord, dipping into the fissures and sulci. The arachnoid, however, bridges the fissures and sulci. As a consequence, the subarachnoid space varies greatly in depth, especially between the gyri and convolutions. At the base of the brain the pia and the arachnoid are widely separated to form enlargements or cisterns. The largest of these are the following: cisterna pontis, situated ventral to the pons; cisterna interpeduncularis (basalis), cephalad to the cisterna pontis and between the cerebral peduncles and the tips of the temporal lobes; cisterna chiasmatis, between the optic chiasm and the rostrum of the corpus callosum, and above the pituitary body; and cisterna magna (cerebellomedullaris), situated in the angle between the cerebellum and the posterior surface of the medulla.

The blood vessels that penetrate the nervous tissue go through the subarachnoid space and become invested with two layers of arachnoid; these subarachnoid cuffs, which accompany the vessels for varying distances into the nervous tissue, are known as the perivascular spaces of Virchow – Robin (Fig. 56-2). The spinal fluid flows into these, and thus it is carried for a certain distance into the substance of the brain and spinal cord. It is also carried outward from the subarachnoid cavity for varying distances in the periradicular, perineural, and perivascular spaces. In the spinal canal there is a large subarachnoid sac that extends from the termination of the spinal cord at the lower limits of the first lumbar vertebra to about the second sacral vertebra. This sac, which contains the cauda equina, is the usual site for performing the spinal puncture. The ventricles and central canal have been spoken of as the internal cerebrospinal fluid system, and the subarachnoid spaces including the cisterns and the perivascular and perineural spaces, as the external system. They communicate by means of the foramina of Luschka and Magendie.

The choroid plexus is a rich network of pial vessels within the ventricles of the brain. It is, in reality, a vascular invagination of the pia into the

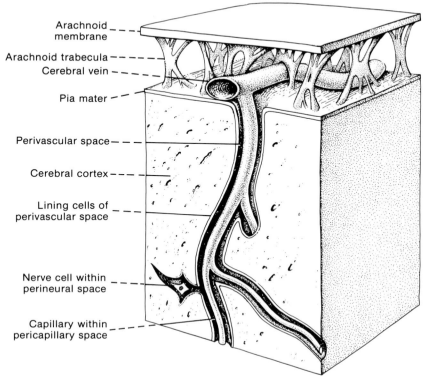

FIG. 56–2. Schematic diagram of the leptomeninges and nervous tissue, showing the relationship of the subarachnoid space, perivascular channels, and nerve cells. (Modified from Weed LH. Am J Anat 1923; 31:191–207)

Arachnoid membrane

Arachnoid trabecula

Cerebral vein

Pia mater

Perivascular space

Cerebral cortex

Lining cells of perivascular space

Nerve cell within perineural space

Capillary within pericapillary space

ventricles, and is covered by a layer of ependymal cells continuous with the lining of the ventricles. The choroid plexus of the lateral ventricles is present only in the body and inferior horn and not in the anterior and posterior horns. The arterial supply of the choroid plexus is provided by the anterior choroidal artery, a branch of the internal carotid artery, and by the posterior choroidal branches of the posterior cerebral artery. The innervation of the choroid plexus is largely from the superior cervical ganglion and the network around the internal carotid artery. Stimulation of the cervical portion of the sympathetic division of the autonomic nervous system causes constriction of the vessels of the choroid plexus, whereas stimulation of the vagus is said to cause a dilation of these vessels.

The mechanism of the formation of the cerebrospinal fluid has been a matter of controversy. Faivre and Luschka both believed it to be secreted by the cells of the choroid plexus, but Mestrezat, on the basis of chemical studies, suggested that it is a dialysate (or filtrate) in equilibrium with the blood plasma, and stated that the ependyma of the choroid plexus acts as the dialyzing membrane. In fact, both diffusion and secretion are involved. Evidence in favor of diffusion includes the fact that the cerebrospinal fluid is isotonic with the blood plasma and tends to remain in osmotic equilibrium with the blood when the latter is changed either experimentally or in disease. The pressure and volume of the cerebrospinal fluid can be changed by varying the osmotic or hydrostatic pressure of the blood; there is increased flow when the blood is made hypotonic, and a reversal of the direction of flow when the blood is made hypertonic. Serum proteins enter the cerebrospinal fluid by diffusion, and the exchange of carbon dioxide also seems to be dependent upon this process. However, there is considerable evidence to show that ionic exchange between the plasma and the cerebrospinal fluid is dependent upon secretory processes, or so-called active transport. Studies of the transport of constituents from the blood into the spinal fluid have been increasingly more accurate since the development of radioisotopic technics.

Although the cerebrospinal fluid does not circulate in the manner that the blood does, with an organ such as the heart to provide energy for motion of the fluid, there is a definite movement of the fluid from the lateral ventricles downward and into the subarachnoid spaces. It is constantly circulating in the sense that it is being constantly secreted and absorbed, and is in continuous movement in a definite direction

through a highly specialized pathway. There is a flow from the lateral ventricles through the foramina of Monro into the third ventricle, and then through the aqueduct of Sylvius into the fourth ventricle. The fluid goes through the foramina of Luschka and Magendie into the subarachnoid space about the medulla. Some of it then flows into the spinal subarachnoid space. The major portion, however, passes forward between the incisura tentorii and along the base of the brain through the pontine, interpeduncular, and chiasmatic cisterns to reach the sylvian fissure, and then ascends in the subarachnoid spaces over the convexity of the brain to spread over the hemispheres. It has been demonstrated, for instance, that obstruction of one foramen of Monro will cause a unilateral hydrocephalus, and that occlusion of the aqueduct of Sylvius will cause a bilateral hydrocephalus involving the third as well as both lateral ventricles. This so-called circulation of the spinal fluid and its rate of flow are influenced or brought about by arterial pulsations within the choroid plexuses, respiration, increase in the venous pressure by thoracic and abdominal movements, changes in position and other movements of the head and body, filtration and secretion pressures, and other factors. Pulsatile flow of cerebrospinal fluid can be demonstrated by magnetic resonance imaging.

The spinal fluid is absorbed into the venous system. It was originally stated that the major portion was absorbed through the arachnoid villi or pacchionian granulations and discharged into the dural sinuses and thence into the peripheral venous circulation. The arachnoid villi are small convolutions that penetrate the venous lacunae in the dura mater adjoining the sinuses. They lie directly beneath the vascular endothelium of the dural sinuses. No subdural space is present, and the cerebrospinal fluid in the villi is separated from the venous blood by only a layer of mesothelial arachnoid cells and a layer of vascular endothelium (Fig. 56-3). When enlarged, these villi are known as **pacchionian granulations.** They are most numerous in the superior sagittal sinus but are also found in the other sinuses and along the spinal cord. It has been suggested that they act as valves for the unidirectional flow of cerebrospinal fluid into venous blood. Evidence suggests that there is a passive transport of certain constituents of the cerebrospinal fluid through these granulations, while others are moved by active transport across the endothelial cells of the arachnoid villi, using micropinocytosis and vacuolization processes. It

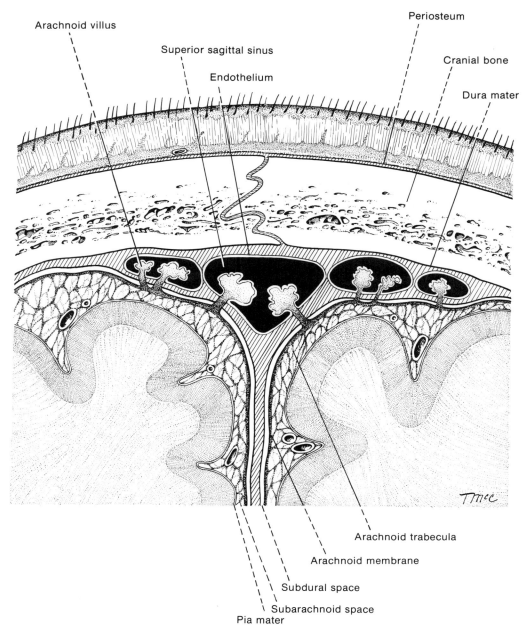

Arachnoid villus

Superior sagittal sinus

Endothelium

Periosteum

Cranial bone

Dura mater

Arachnoid trabecula

Arachnoid membrane

Subdural space

Subarachnoid space

Pia mater

FIG. 56–3. Schematic diagram of a coronal section of the meninges and cerebral cortex, showing the relationship of the arachnoid villus to the subarachnoid space and superior sagittal sinus. (Modified from Weed LH. Am J Anat 1923; 31:191–207)

is probable that a part of the spinal fluid is absorbed into the venous system from the periradicular and perineural spaces along the spinal roots and cranial nerves, and from the perivenous spaces. Studies suggest that there is also some absorption through the ventricular ependyma and in a reverse direction through the cho-

roid plexus. Ventriculocisternal perfusion studies suggest that some organic acids and bases, including penicillin, are removed from the cerebrospinal fluid through the choroid plexus. Some fluid may be absorbed by osmosis directly into the pial veins on the surface of the brain and by capillaries of the pia-arachnoid.

The concept of the **blood – brain, or hemato-encephalic, barrier** (including also the blood – cerebrospinal fluid and cerebrospinal fluid – brain barriers) has been developed to explain the mechanism that regulates the passage of various substances from the blood into the fluid or into the brain. The permeability of the barrier to substances that are normally in the blood or are introduced experimentally or therapeutically may be altered by various disease states. The site of this so-called barrier is at the level of the pial-glial membranes and the cerebral capillaries, which are distinguished by having tight cellular junctions, unlike those of capillaries in other parts of the body. These tight junctions, also a feature of the epithelial cells of the choroid plexus, restrict passive movement of macromolecular substances across the cellular barrier. The increase or decrease in permeability of this barrier found in certain disease states may be caused by chemical or physical alterations in the blood, changes in the meninges or nervous tissues, or variations in the permeability of the vascular structures. Knowledge about this barrier and the effect of disease upon it is important to the understanding of the action of drugs and other substances on the meninges and central nervous system.

Investigations on the secretion, flow, and absorption of the spinal fluid, using multiple simultaneous radioisotopic tracers, have materially altered earlier concepts. These studies show that water, electrolytes, and protein all enter and leave the cerebrospinal fluid in both the ventricles and the subarachnoid space at rates that vary with the site of formation or absorption and with the nature of the substance concerned. The rate of exchange varies inversely with the molecular size, the rate for water being most rapid, then electrolytes, and finally protein. Water exchange is more rapid in the region of the cisterna magna than through the walls of the ventricles, suggesting that water molecules are more retarded in their motion by the ependyma and choroidal epithelium than by the pia and pial – glial membranes. The electrolytes enter the fluid more rapidly in the ventricles than in the cortical, cisternal, or lumbar subarachnoid spaces, suggesting specific secretory activity of the choroidal epithelium. Protein appears to enter into the ventricles more rapidly than into the subarachnoid space, and leaves the cisternal region more rapidly than it leaves the ventricles. Minor injuries in the region of the ventricles cause a more rapid and erratic entry and departure of substances. These studies also suggest that the cerebrospinal fluid is both a secretion and an ultrafiltrate. It has been shown that certain substances enter the cerebrospinal fluid (or the brain) by passive transport or diffusion, others by active transport or by carrier-mediated transport (glucose) or secretion. Movement of substances from the cerebrospinal fluid to brain and back appears to occur mainly by passive mechanisms.

The functions of the cerebrospinal fluid are many but are chiefly mechanical. It serves as a water-jacket for the brain and spinal cord, bathing and protecting them. It helps to support the weight of the brain and acts as a cushion for it. It serves as a lubricant between the brain and the spinal cord on the one side and the skull and spinal column on the other. It acts as a buffer to distribute the force of a blow on the head. It serves as a space-compensating mechanism in regulating the contents of the cranium and aids in keeping the intracranial pressure relatively constant: if there is an increase in arterial pulsations, blood content, or brain volume, there is a decrease in the amount of cerebrospinal fluid, and if there is degeneration or atrophy of brain tissue, there is an increase in the amount of fluid. It is a medium for the transfer of substances from within the brain and spinal cord to the blood stream; it receives metabolic waste products and aids in eliminating them, and is important for the removal of pathologic products in disease and for the circulation of drugs in therapy. It does not, however, contain sufficient nutritive material to have much value in the metabolism of nervous tissue, and it does not actually penetrate the brain tissue. The work of Davson and others indicates that the spinal fluid has a "drainpipe" or "sink" action for the extracellular fluid of the brain. According to this concept, solutes and products of metabolism diffuse from the extracellular fluid to the cerebrospinal fluid, from which they may be removed by the bulk-flow reabsorption of the cerebrospinal fluid into the venous system as well as by active transport via the choroid plexus into the blood.

The amount of cerebrospinal fluid is about 90 – 150 ml in the normal adult, and 40 – 60 ml in the newborn. The rate of formation is related to factors such as the osmotic and hydrostatic pressures of the blood and variations in venous pressure. The volume of fluid is increased by either excessive formation or deficient absorption. Excessive formation can be caused by various factors. There may be a decrease in the osmotic pressure of the serum; this may be brought about by intravenous injections of hypotonic solutions. There may also be increased formation in meningitis and other infections, and also in association with increase of the venous pressure within the skull. Decreased absorption may be brought about by a blockage in the flow of the spinal fluid from (1) obstruction caused by processes such as tumors or stenosis of the aqueduct, resulting in a noncommunicating hydrocephalus, or from (2) obstruction of the arachnoid villi and perivenous spaces by the presence of blood, serum or inflammatory processes, resulting in a communicating hydrocephalus. Increased formation and decreased absorption may occur simultaneously. The technic of ventriculocisternal perfusion has shown that the normal rate of formation of cerebrospinal fluid seems to be about 0.35 ml/min or 500 ml/day. Thus, considering that the total volume is approximately 150 ml, the total volume of fluid is reformed frequently.

Katzman and his associates have developed a constant-infusion manometric test for the measurement of cerebrospinal fluid absorption based upon application of the ventriculocisternal perfusion studies of Pappenheimer and associates. The test is of value in the study of communicating hydrocephalus. The presence of hydrocephalus or other changes in the configuration of the ventricles is, however, nicely shown on cerebral imaging studies.

BIBLIOGRAPHY

Bakay L. The Blood – Brain Barrier With Special Regard to the Use of Radioactive Isotopes. Springfield, IL, Charles C Thomas, 1956

Bering EA Jr. Circulation of the cerebrospinal fluid: Demonstration of the choroid plexus as the generator of the force for flow of fluid and ventricular enlargement. J Neurosurg 1962;19:405

Bering EA Jr. Hydrocephalus: Changes in formation and absorption of cerebrospinal fluid within the cerebral ventricles. J Neurosurg 1963;20:1050

Bowsher D. Cerebrospinal Fluid Dynamics in Health and Disease. Springfield, IL, Charles C Thomas, 1960

Corning JL. Spinal anesthesia and local medication of the cord. NY Med J 1885;42:483

Cutler RWP, Page I, Galicich J et al. Formation and absorption of cerebrospinal fluid in man. Brain 1969;91:707

Dandy WE. The cause of so-called idiopathic hydrocephalus. Bull Johns Hopkins Hosp 1921;32:67

Davson H, Welck K, Segal MB. Physiology and Pathophysiology of the Cerebrospinal Fluid. Edinburgh, Churchill Livingstone, 1987

Faivre E. Recherches sur la structure de conarim et des plexus choroides chez l'homme et des animaux. CR Acad Sci 1854;39:424

Fishman RA. Cerebrospinal Fluid in Diseases of the Nervous System. Philadelphia, WB Saunders, 1980

Grant R, Condon B, Patterson J, Wyper DJ et al. Changes in cranial CSF volume during hypercapnia and hypocapnia. J Neurol Neurosurg Psychiatry 1989;52:218

Hochwald GM. Cerebrospinal fluid. In Joynt RJ (ed). Clinical Neurology. Philadelphia, JB Lippincott, 1989

Hussey F, Schanzer B, Katzman R. A simple constant-infusion manometric test for measurement of CSF absorption. II. Clinical studies. Neurology 1970;20:665

Katzman R, Hussey F. A simple constant-infusion manometric test for measurement of CSF absorption. I. Rationale and method. Neurology 1970;20:534

Key EAH, Retzius G. Studien in der Anatomie des Nervensystems und des Bindegewebes. Stockholm, Samson och Wallin, 1875 – 1876

Levinson A. Cerebrospinal Fluid in Health and in Disease, 3rd ed. St Louis, CV Mosby, 1929

Lups S, Haan AMFH. The Cerebrospinal Fluid. Amsterdam, Elsevier, 1956

Luschka H. Die Adergeflechte des Menschlichen Gehirns. Berlin, 1853.

Magendie F. Recherches Physiologiques sur le Liquide Céphalorachidien ou Cérébrospinal. Paris, Mequignon – Marvis, 1842

Merritt HH, Fremont – Smith F. The Cerebrospinal Fluid. Philadelphia, WB Saunders, 1937

Mestrezat W. Le Liquide Céphalorachidien Normal e Pathologique: Valeur Clinique de l'Examen Chimique; Syndromes Huroraux dans les Diverses Affections. Paris, A Maloine, 1912

Millen JW, Wollam DMH. The Anatomy of the Cerebrospinal Fluid. London, Oxford University Press, 1962

Morton CA. The pathology of tuberculous meningitis, with reference to its treatment by tapping the subarachnoid space of the spinal cord. Br Med J 1891;2:840

Oldendorf WH, Davson H. Brain extracellular space and the sink action of cerebrospinal fluid. Arch Neurol 1967;17:196

Pappenheimer JR, Heisey SR, Jordan EF et al. Perfusion of the cerebral ventricular system in unanesthetized goats. Am J Physiol 1962;203:763

Plum F, Siesjo BK. Recent advances in CSF physiology. Anesthesiology 1975;42:708

Quincke H. Die Lumbalpunction des Hydrocephalus. Berl Klin Wochenschr 1891;28:929, 965

Ridgway JP, Turnbull LW, Smith MA. Demonstration of pulsatile cerebrospinal-fluid flow using magnetic resonance phase imaging. Br J Radiol 1987;60:423

Russell DS. Observations on the Pathology of Hydrocephalus. London, His Majesty's Stationery Office, 1949

Schaltenbrand G. Normal and pathological physiology of cerebrospinal fluid circulation. Lancet 1953;1:805

Tourtellotte WW, Shorr RJ. Cerebrospinal fluid. In Youmans JR (ed). Neurological Surgery, 3rd ed. Philadelphia, WB Saunders, 1990

Weed LH. The cerebrospinal fluid. Physiol Rev 1922;2:171

Wolstenholme GEW, O'Connor CM. Ciba Foundation Symposium of the Cerebrospinal Fluid: Production, Circulation and Absorption. Boston, Little, Brown & Co, 1958

Woolam DHM. The historical significance of the cerebrospinal fluid. Med Hist 1957;1:91

Wynter WE. Four cases of tubercular meningitis in which paracentesis of the theca vertebralis was performed for the relief of fluid pressure. Lancet 1891;1:981

Yamashima T. Functional ultrastructure of cerebrospinal fluid drainage channels in human arachnoid villi. Neurosurgery 1988;22:633

Chapter 57
LUMBAR PUNCTURE

INDICATIONS AND CONTRAINDICATIONS

The term *lumbar puncture* has become the name routinely used for puncture of the lumbar subarachnoid space (lumbar subarachnoid puncture), although *spinal puncture, spinal tap,* and *Quincke's puncture* are also used as synonyms.

Although the technic of lumbar puncture is relatively simple, and the procedure has come to be almost routine in neurologic diagnosis, it must be remembered that withdrawal of the cerebrospinal fluid is not without danger under certain circumstances, and should not be done unless necessary for either diagnosis or treatment.

Indications. The indications for lumbar puncture are either diagnostic or therapeutic, but principally the former. Diagnostic punctures are performed for the purpose of examining either the fluid itself or the hydrodynamics of the fluid. Under most circumstances the test is performed to withdraw cerebrospinal fluid for examination, in order to observe the physical, chemical, cytologic, serologic, or bacterial composition of the fluid in the diagnosis of nervous system or somatic disease. It is an indispensable part of the neurologic investigation of diseases of the meninges and of many organic diseases of the nervous system. Changes in the composition of the fluid may aid in establishing a diagnosis, confirm a suspected diagnosis, assist in estimating the prognosis, and provide information essential to deciding on the most correct method of treatment. Alterations in the cerebrospinal fluid may also assist in the diagnosis of obscure nervous system diseases and of conditions in which the diagnosis is not apparent on clinical grounds alone. The usefulness of cerebral computed tomography and magnetic resonance imaging of the head and spine have reduced the need for lumbar puncture in disorders characterized by structural distortions or mass lesions. Lumbar puncture is also performed to determine the cerebrospinal fluid pressure, to investigate abnormalities in pressure in such conditions as spinal subarachnoid block, and as a part of special procedures and methods of investigation such as myelography and radioisotope cisternography.

Therapeutic lumbar punctures have been done for various reasons, although they are rarely performed at the present time. In the past, removal of fluid was occasionally done to relieve increased intracranial pressure. Under nearly all circumstances, however, it is best to relieve increased intracranial pressure by means other than spinal puncture, for example, by the administration of hypertonic solutions such as mannitol, or steroids for more chronic therapy.

Lumbar puncture is also used to introduce substances into the subarachnoid space for diagnosis, as in myelography and radioisotope cisternography, and for spinal anesthesia. Alcohol and phenol have been injected into the spinal subarachnoid space in attempts to relieve intractable pain and spasticity. The intrathecal administration of drugs and serums for therapy is now considered inadvisable in most instances. An exception is the intrathecal use of drugs for the treatment of certain leukemic and other forms of meningitis. Intrathecal medication may produce an aseptic meningitis and may be followed by arachnoiditis with spinal subarachnoid block and significant neurologic complications. Furthermore, most drugs are just as effective, or more so, when administered by intravenous and other routes.

Contraindications. The contraindications to lumbar puncture are even more important to bear in mind than the indications. They include infections in the skin or subcutaneous tissues, such as erysipelas, boils, carbuncles, or infected decubiti in the region of the puncture site. Under most circumstances spinal puncture is contraindicated in cases of septicemia or general systemic infection, and in persons with severe blood clotting deficiencies. Introduction of a needle into the subarachnoid space or a change in the pressure relationships of the spinal fluid may cause transmission or spread of a focal infection to the meninges and subarachnoid space. Spinal puncture is also contraindicated, or should be done with extreme caution, in all instances where there is an increase in intracranial pressure. This is especially true if the increase in pressure is caused by an expanding lesion of the posterior cranial fossa, such as a cerebellar tumor, or if there is a possibility that the increase in pressure is caused by a brain abscess. A sudden change of pressure in posterior fossa lesions may force the tonsils of the cerebellum and the medulla into the foramen magnum, with pressure on the respiratory and circulatory centers, causing respiratory failure, stupor, and sudden death. A sudden decrease in the subtentorial pressure in supratentorial lesions may cause herniation of the hippocampal gyrus through the incisura of the tentorium cerebelli, producing pressure on the midbrain, also with fatal results. Pressure changes in brain abscess may cause rupture of the abscess and dissemination of the infection. Computed tomography or magnetic resonance imaging should precede any decision about lumbar puncture if an intracranial mass is suspected. It is obvious but not always remembered that spinal puncture is contraindicated whenever the diagnosis is evident from the history and examination, and no additional information can be obtained from the procedure, but frequently the procedure is still used as a routine approach to diagnosis.

Under all circumstances the indications and contraindications must be weighed and evaluated before the procedure is carried out. It may be necessary, in certain cases, to perform punctures in spite of contraindications. The procedure may be essential in the presence of septicemia,

especially if the diagnosis of meningitis is suspected. The puncture under such circumstances should be done, however, only if absolutely necessary. A spinal puncture should never be performed before the patient has had a complete examination, especially a neurologic appraisal. An ophthalmoscopic examination of the optic disks for the evidence of papilledema is a prerequisite in every case, and under most circumstances, except in acute meningitis or subarachnoid hemorrhage, head imaging studies should precede lumbar puncture.

TECHNIC

Lumbar puncture is performed by introducing a needle into the subarachnoid space, usually below the level of the termination of the spinal cord. In the adult the spinal cord ends at the lower level of the first lumbar vertebral body, or between the first and second bodies (although in women it may extend to the second lumbar body), but the subarachnoid and subdural spaces extend to about the second sacral body. Within the lumbosacral sac are the roots of the cauda equina, but no spinal cord. It must be remembered, however, that in infants and children the spinal cord may extend to about the third lumbar vertebral body. The puncture is usually done in the interspace between the second and third, third and fourth, or fourth and fifth lumbar spinous processes. The site of preference is usually between the third and fourth vertebrae (Fig. 57-1), or, alternatively, at the level where the separation between the spinous processes is the widest. In infants and children the interspace between the fourth and fifth lumbar spinous processes is the one of choice. The procedure may be carried out with the patient either seated or in the lateral recumbent position, but if accurate pressure studies are to be made, the latter position is essential. The patient lies in this position on a relatively hard and firm table or stretcher, or, if in bed, is brought to its edge. The patient should be comfortable, warm, and relaxed, and reassured of the simplicity and relative painlessness of the test. If the patient is tense or nervous, some sedation by mouth may be administered before the puncture is to be done. It is desirable that the bowels and bladder be empty.

The position of the patient is very important. The back should be parallel with the edge of the bed. If the neck and trunk are acutely flexed and the hips and knees are flexed, the spinous pro-

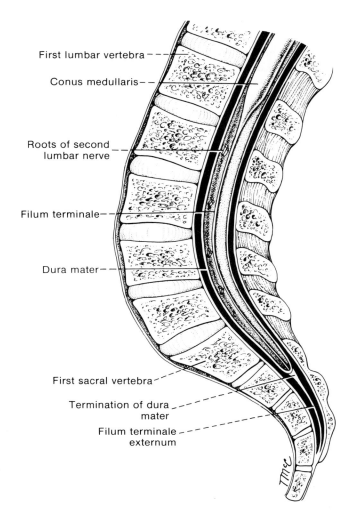

First lumbar vertebra

Conus medullaris

Roots of second
lumbar nerve

Filum terminale

Dura mater

First sacral vertebra

Termination of dura
mater

Filum terminale
externum

FIG. 57–1. Sagittal section of the vertebral canal, showing the lower end of the spinal cord, filum terminale, and subarachnoid space. (Modified from Larsell O. Anatomy of the Nervous System. New York, D Appleton–Century, 1939)

cesses are separated as widely as possible. It is often desirable to have the neck flexed so that the chin is on the chest, and the knees drawn up to the abdomen and clasped by the hands, which are in the popliteal fossae. The head may approximate the knees. The shoulders and pelvis should be vertical. A small pillow should be placed under the head so that the entire spine is horizontal. Most difficulties in performing spinal punctures are due to inadequate positioning of the body.

Lumbar puncture should always be carried out with aseptic precautions. The skin in the region of the puncture site and for some distance beyond should be washed with soap and water, and if necessary shaved. This same area should then be covered with an antiseptic preparation. Sterile towels or surgical drapes are placed around the puncture site; sterile instruments are used and the examiner should wear sterile surgical gloves. In most instances it is valuable to use local anesthesia, such as 1% lidocaine or some similar preparation. A small amount is infiltrated into the skin and subcutaneous tissues with a very small hypodermic needle, and then a slightly larger amount may be injected with a somewhat larger needle into the deeper structures, namely the muscles and fasciae, the interspinal ligament in the interspinous space, and the vicinity of the periosteum and the outer meninges. Many physicians do not use local anesthetics, especially if a small gauge needle (22 or smaller) is used for the puncture. If the patient is very tense or nervous, it may be necessary to have an assistant hold him firmly. Occasionally, if he is excited or delirious, it may be necessary to use general anesthesia or intravenous sedation for the test; since inhalation anesthesia increases the venous congestion of the brain, intravenous barbiturates are usually preferable. Such measures are rarely necessary, however, and under most circumstances the puncture can be performed without difficulty by first reassuring the patient, using oral sedation if necessary, employing a trained aide, and carrying out the test rapidly and skillfully.

The lumbar puncture needle should be well sharpened, and have a short bevel with a well-fitting stylet. The needle used should be as small as possible. If the determination of the hydrodynamics is an important part of the procedure, an 18- or 20-gauge needle should be used, but if the Queckenstedt test is not necessary, and especially if increased intracranial pressure is suspected, a 21- or 22-gauge or even smaller needle may be employed. In the adult a needle 3 – 4 in or 8 – 12 cm in length is preferable unless the patient is obese; in infants and children the needle may be much smaller and shorter.

The site for the puncture is determined by drawing a line between the iliac crests or placing the fingers between them. This line crosses the vertebral column at the level of the interspace between the third and fourth lumbar vertebrae, or at that of the fourth lumbar spinous process. By palpating the spinous processes, the correct site may be determined. Careful positioning and time taken to select the correct interspace are important. After a wait of a few minutes for the local anesthesia to take effect (if it is used), the needle is inserted in the midline and directed at right angles to the plane of the back and parallel to the plane of the floor; on some occasions it is tilted slightly cephalad. Some neurologists insert the needle 1 cm or 2 cm lateral to the midline and advance it at a slight angle. The needle should be grasped firmly by the hilt with one hand, and the point guided by holding the shaft with the other. After the skin has been punctured the needle should be realigned and pushed deeper slowly and carefully by pressure with both hands. The bevel of the needle is kept parallel to the dural fibers (which are parallel to the long axis of the body), in order to separate the fibers and avoid cutting through them. The needle penetrates the skin, subcutaneous tissues, supraspinal ligament, ligamentum flavum, epidural fat, dura, and arachnoid, and enters the subarachnoid space. In adults it usually must be introduced 5 – 6 cm in order to reach the subarachnoid space, the depth depending on the thickness of the lumbar muscles and the amount of subcutaneous tissue. One should not change the course of the needle during the puncture, and if obstruction is met or bone is encountered, the needle should be withdrawn to the subcutaneous tissues and reintroduced at another, slightly different angle.

Usually the examiner can feel a slight "give" or a sharp "click" when the resistance of the deep tissues is suddenly released as the needle goes through the ligamentum flavum. The stylet is then withdrawn to see whether the needle is in the subarachnoid space. If no fluid is obtained, the stylet is reintroduced and the needle is inserted for a few more millimeters. Usually another "give" is felt as the needle penetrates the dura. The stylet is then withdrawn again, and if no fluid is obtained the position of the needle is readjusted slightly, or it is rotated about 90°, since its point may be obstructed by a nerve root or a film of arachnoid tissue. If fluid is still not obtained, the point of the needle is withdrawn almost to the skin and redirected. A change in the direction of the needle cannot be made by shifting the hilt while the point is deep in the tissue.

The needle should not be introduced too far, since it may damage the intervertebral disks or traumatize the extradural venous plexuses. If blood is obtained before the arachnoid has been penetrated, it is well to used a clean needle and introduce it at a slightly different site.

Once fluid is obtained, the stylet is reintroduced, or the stopcock is turned to a neutral position. The patient is now reassured, and to assist him in relaxing may be told that the puncture has been successful and that no more discomfort will be felt. If necessary, the patient is asked to slowly partially straighten his legs and neck and to breathe easily so as to avoid a Valsalva effect, raising the pressure of the fluid. The manometer is next attached rapidly to the needle to avoid losing fluid; it is placed in a vertical position and the pressure is determined. Air bubbles should be removed from the manometer since they alter the pressure readings and the determination of the hydrodynamics. If the patient is tense, the examiner should wait a few moments before determining the pressure. It is sometimes necessary to wait several minutes to secure adequate relaxation. Not infrequently a pressure of over 200 mm of water will fall to a normal range with adequate relaxation. It is important to be certain that the needle is in the subarachnoid space and that there is free communication between this space and the manometer; this is ascertained by the presence of normal oscillations and a normal pressure rise in response to coughing and straining. Then, if necessary, the hydrodynamics are determined, as will be described and, following this, the fluid, usually not more than 16 ml, is removed for examination. The fluid is collected in three or more clean, dry, sterile test tubes to be used for cell count, study of cell content and structure, quantitative tests for protein and protein fractions, determination of glucose, serologic tests, culture, and other determinations as indicated in individual cases. Pressure readings are again taken, the stylet is reintroduced, and the needle is withdrawn slowly. The puncture site is then resterilized with an appropriate antiseptic; pressure is applied for a minute or two to prevent oozing, the wound may be covered with a bit of liquid collodion that is allowed to dry and adhere, and a sterile dressing is applied. A record should be made of the initial and final pressures and the amount of fluid removed, as well as of the color and turbidity of the fluid and any unusual circumstances encountered during the puncture.

The patient usually experiences pain only when the skin and the dura are penetrated. If local anesthesia is used, this pain may be eliminated. If the periosteum of the spinous processes or the vertebral bodies is traumatized there may be pain, and in certain instances where there is arthritis of the spinal column, the puncture may be quite painful. Occasionally there is a brief lancinating pain shooting down one leg; this indicates that one of the roots of the cauda equina was traumatized. This pain usually disappears immediately.

It is best not to change the position of the needle during puncture. If the puncture is performed with difficulty, or if blood is encountered, the puncture should be attempted at another level, preferably a higher one. If the fluid is slightly blood-tinged, a few ml should be allowed to escape before the fluid for examination is collected; under such circumstances, or if red blood cells are seen on microscopic examination, red blood cell counts should be made on specimens from three successive tubes to see whether there is a decline in the number of cells. If the fluid is grossly bloody, unless this is because of subarachnoid hemorrhage, the examination of the fluid is unreliable, and the puncture should be repeated in 1 – 5 days. If there is a rapid fall of pressure or a deterioration of the patient's condition during drainage of the fluid, the procedure should be stopped immediately. Some authorities advise the injection of 10 ml of

normal saline if there is a change in respiration during the test.

Theoretically, it should be possible to perform a spinal puncture and to obtain spinal fluid in every patient, but occasionally the procedure is difficult or even impossible to perform. If the subarachnoid space cannot be entered, one of the following may be the cause. The needle may be incorrectly placed: it may be lateral to the canal or introduced obliquely and not directed straight toward the canal. The needle may have been introduced too far or not far enough, or may be at the wrong level. The needle may be too blunt, and the dural sac pushed forward or to one side. A root of the cauda equina or a fold of arachnoid may be obstructing the point. (Under most of the above circumstances, a slight adjustment in the position of the needle will lead to a free flow of spinal fluid.) The needle may be plugged with foreign material such as pus or coagulated spinal fluid that will not flow freely. An anomaly of the lumbar spine (scoliosis) or severe spondylitis may be present. An obstructing tumor in the region of the conus medullaris or cauda equina may be present. A complete block of the subarachnoid space above the puncture site may be present. The intracranial pressure may be too low to allow free flow of fluid. If the latter is the case, the use of gentle suction with a syringe may be folllowed by some flow of fluid.

PRESSURE DETERMINATIONS AND THE HYDRODYNAMICS OF THE SPINAL FLUID

No lumbar puncture is complete without a determination of the spinal fluid pressure. Various glass or disposable plastic manometers are acceptable. The normal spinal fluid pressure with the patient in the lateral recumbent position is from 50 – 180 mm of cerebrospinal fluid, and it is identical, or nearly so, in the lumbar sac, cisterna magna, and ventricles. If the head and body are raised, however, the ventricular and cisternal pressures drop and the lumbar pressure rises. Pressures of 180 – 200 mm are considered borderline or at the upper limits of normal, and those over 200 mm as definitely elevated if the patient is relaxed. The pressure is lower in children than in adults. In the normal newborn, it varies from 0 – 76 mm. If the needle is in the subarachnoid space, minor oscillations of the spinal fluid pressure are seen on the manometer. There are relatively small oscillations (4 – 10 mm) that are synchronous with the respiratory rate (Fig. 57-2), and even finer oscillations (2 – 5 mm), synchronous with the pulse. In addition to these, it is not unusual to observe spontaneous fluctuations of 5 – 15 mm with slight movement of the body and alterations of neuromuscular tension, and even more marked and irregular fluctuations in some patients with increased intracranial pressure, especially after trauma or cerebral hemorrhage. If the needle is properly positioned in the subarachnoid space, the pressure increases with coughing and decreases with deep inspiration.

Manometry is not reliable if the patient is tense or excited, and it is important to wait for adequate relaxation. Instructing the patient to take a few deep breaths or engaging him in conversation may be helpful. One should not attempt to estimate the cerebrospinal fluid pressure by noting the rate or force of flow, size of drops, or number of drops per minute; these are dependent not only upon the size of the needle, but also upon the position and relaxation of the patient, surface tension of the fluid, and pulse and respiratory fluctuations. There is no accurate method of pressure determination without the use of a manometer. It has been stated that if the pressure is obtained with the patient seated, the reading is equal to the pressure in the lateral recumbent position together with the pressure of the column of fluid above the level of the puncture site. Experimental investigations have shown, however, that there is no precise mathematical relationship between the lumbar spinal fluid pressures in the erect and recumbent positions; neither can be computed from the other, even though the pressure in the erect or seated position has been found to be approximately equivalent to that in the lumbar recumbent position plus the millimeters in the vertical distance from the needle to the cisterna magna.

FACTORS AFFECTING THE SPINAL FLUID PRESSURE

The spinal fluid pressure is influenced by many factors. It is said to reflect the intracranial venous pressure and to be about equal to the venous pressure in the confluence of sinuses (torcular Herophili). It is not definitely related to either the diastolic or systolic arterial pressures, although a rapid rise in arterial pressure causes a transitory elevation of spinal fluid pressure. Arterial hypertension, on the other hand, sometimes occurs with increased intracranial pressure if the cerebrospinal fluid pressure is elevated to a level approaching that of the diastolic blood

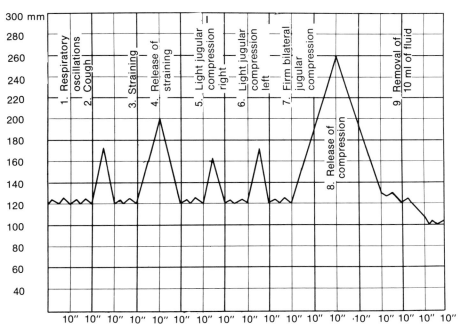

FIG. 57–2. Manometric chart showing respiratory oscillations and the normal response of the cerebrospinal fluid pressure to coughing, straining, light and firm jugular compression, and removal of fluid.

pressure. The rate of production, rate of absorption, osmotic pressure, hydrostatic pressure, rate of diffusion and secretion, elasticity of the vertebral and cerebral dura, size of the subarachnoid reservoir, osmotic equilibrium with the blood, blocking of the circulation of the fluid, disease states, and drugs also affect spinal fluid pressure. The cranial cavity is relatively fixed in volume. It is completely filled by the brain, cerebrospinal fluid, and blood vessels and blood. An increase in the volume or pressure of one of these is carried out at the expense of the volume or pressure of the others. An increase in intracranial pressure may result from an increase in the volume or pressure of either the blood and blood vessels, the brain or its coverings, or the cerebrospinal fluid. The spinal fluid pressure, consequently, is increased under a variety of circumstances.

The Blood and Blood Vessels

The venous pressure and the volume of blood within the skull are among the most important factors in determining the spinal fluid pressure. Changes in the intracranial venous pressure are transmitted through the entire ventriculosubarachnoid space and are quickly followed by changes in spinal fluid pressure, although the latter may not be maintained. The systemic venous pressure is influenced by the position of the heart, the volume of blood in the great veins, the weight of the viscera, and the tension of the abdominal and thoracic muscles. It may be increased with cardiac decompensation, obstruction of the venous trunks in the thorax and neck by tumors and anomalies, emphysema and other pulmonary disorders, or elevation of the intrathoracic and abdominal pressures by coughing, straining, or compression. The elevation of systemic venous pressure is accompanied by an increase in intracranial venous pressure and then of spinal fluid pressure. Manual compression of the jugular veins (**Queckenstedt maneuver**) interferes with the venous drainage from the head and causes an increase in intracranial pressure. Venous pressure within the skull may be increased by interference with venous drainage by neoplasms or other expanding masses or by obstruction of venous circulation by thrombosis of major channels or dural sinuses, especially the lateral or superior sagittal sinuses. So-called otitic hydrocephalus, one of the causes of benign intracranial hypertension, may follow thrombosis of one of the lateral sinuses. Alterations in the relationship between lumbar and ventricular pressures secondary to changes in posture may be due to changes in the intracranial venous pressure.

Variations in the cerebral blood supply also influence the intracranial pressure, which may be raised with increased blood flow and blood volume within the skull. Drugs and other substances that dilate the cerebral blood vessels (amyl nitrite, histamine, carbon dioxide), as well as those that cause a sudden elevation of the arterial and sometimes the venous pressure (epinephrine) increase the volume of the intracranial contents and thus the intracranial pressure. Inhalation of 5% carbon dioxide increases cerebral blood flow and causes a prompt rise in intracranial pressure. The pressure is decreased by caffeine and other substances that constrict cerebral blood vessels, increase the cerebrovascular resistance, and lessen the blood flow. Intracranial pressure is also elevated by the presence of free or clotted blood within the skull, as in intracerebral, subarachnoid, or extradural hemorrhage or subdural hematoma. With polycythemia there may be both increased blood volume and venous thromboses. Hyperventilation decreases cerebral blood flow and thus reduces intracranial pressure.

The Brain and its Coverings

An increase in the volume of the brain or its coverings also increases the intracranial pressure. The presence of a foreign body or an expanding lesion such as a neoplasm, abscess, granuloma, cyst, or hematoma may increase the pressure by an increase in bulk alone as well as by obstructing the circulation of the blood and the cerebrospinal fluid. A slow increase in brain volume, however, is compensated for by a decrease in the amount of cerebrospinal fluid, and it is often possible for the intracranial pressure to be normal with slowly growing brain tumors. Normal pressure, however, is rare with tumors in the posterior fossa, especially those of the cerebellum, although with pontine gliomas a rise in pressure is often a late manifestation. Contributing to or associated with cerebral edema there may be increased permeability of the capillaries, venous congestion, and petechial hemorrhages. Fishman categorizes cerebral edema into vasogenic, cytotoxic (cellular), and interstitial (hydrocephalic) types, each with its own location, pathogenesis, and other features. Cerebral edema occurs in the immediate posttraumatic state, with strokes, acute alcoholic intoxication, other drug intoxications, lead encephalopathy, meningitis, uremia, eclampsia, respiratory acidosis, anoxia, severe anemia and deficiency states, vitamin A intoxication, certain allergic and metabolic disorders, water intoxication, and alterations in electrolyte balance, to name some. The edema causes tissue hydration, an increase in brain volume, and elevation of intracranial pressure. Some cases of benign intracranial hypertension, or pseudotumor cerebri, may be the result of such alterations, others have no known mechanisms of pathogenesis. Suppuration of the meninges and the presence of inflammatory exudate also increase the intracranial pressure.

The Cerebrospinal Fluid

Pressure is elevated when the amount of cerebrospinal fluid is increased or its absorption is impaired. There are increases in the amount of fluid under the following circumstances: decrease in osmotic pressure of the blood serum by the intravenous injection of hypotonic solutions; decrease in osmotic pressure of the serum at the onset of febrile illnesses, especially in children, leading to the syndrome of meningismus; alterations of the vascular endothelium in encephalitis, meningitis, and other infections; increase in venous pressure within the skull causing greater filtration; obstruction of the arachnoid villi and perivenous spaces by an inflammatory reaction or by blood serum causes decreased absorption and a subsequent rise in pressure. A similar decrease in absorption and rise in pressure may occur with a significant elevation of the protein content of the cerebrospinal fluid; this has been observed in the Guillain – Barré syndrome, in late poliomyelitis, and with some brain and spinal cord tumors. There is also increased pressure if circulation is interfered with by neoplasms or adhesions, narrowing of the foramina of Luschka, Magendie, or Monro, or stenosis of the aqueduct. Internal, or noncommunicating hydrocephalus results from obstruction of the foramina or aqueduct, and external, or communicating hydrocephalus from impaired absorption by the arachnoid villi or within the perivenous spaces. The presence of pus or blood in the spinal fluid may also increase the pressure of the fluid. Increased pressure of the fluid and decreased absorption may occur simultaneously, as they do in meningitis and encephalitis; the increase in the volume of the cerebrospinal fluid may be accompanied, furthermore, by edema of the brain and venous congestion, all of which lead to great elevation of spinal fluid pressure.

Spinal fluid pressure is decreased in shock, fainting, dehydration, degenerative processes of the brain, wasting and cachectic diseases, asthenia, depression, and decrease in the systemic arterial and venous pressures. The pressure may be low owing to decreased formation or withdrawal of fluid following spinal puncture, trauma, or intracranial surgery, and occasionally in the presence of a subdural hematoma. Schaltenbrand has described the **syndrome of spontaneous aliquorrhea,** characterized by decreased fluid formation and very low pressure; the etiology of this is not known. The pressure may be decreased, either because of diminished formation of fluid, under circumstances in which there is increased viscosity of the blood. The pressure may also be low with complete subarachnoid block and with continued leakage of fluid following a spinal puncture, or from a spontaneous or traumatic fistula; it may appear to be low if there is inadequate communication between the lumen of the needle and the subarachnoid space. Under most circumstances, however, low spinal fluid pressure has little significance.

Drugs and other substances that raise the osmotic pressure of the blood serum also lower the intracranial pressure by decreasing the formation and pressure of the cerebrospinal fluid as well as by counteracting cerebral edema. Hypertonic solutions of dextrose, sucrose, or sodium chloride, administered intravenously, have been used, but their efficacy is hampered by the rebound of pressure that may occur after a few hours. The intravenous administration of a 25% solution of mannitol brings about a more prolonged decrease in pressure, with a less abrupt secondary rise. The glucocorticoids, in large doses, have also been shown to be of value in decreasing cerebral edema, and acetazolamide slows the secretion of cerebrospinal fluid in some types of hydrocephalus and pseudotumor cerebri through inhibition of the carbonic anhydrase in the choroid plexus. Oral glycerol has also been used in the treatment of pseudotumor cerebri.

Once the spinal fluid pressure has assumed a constant level, it is important under some circumstances to examine the hydrodynamics further in order to determine whether there is any interference with the flow of the fluid. The patient is first asked to cough; the pressure is normally seen to increase 40 – 50 mm (depending upon the normal pressure and the intensity of the cough) and it descends about as rapidly as it ascended (see Fig. 57-2). The patient is then asked to strain, as in moving his bowels; the pressure goes up 50 – 100 mm, and again descends after straining ceases. Both coughing and straining cause compression of the thorax and abdomen, and by retarding the venous return to the thorax, they produce an increase in intracranial pressure that is transmitted to the fluid in the ventricles and the subarachnoid space. The increase of the intraabdominal and intrathoracic pressures also interferes with the return of blood through the spinal veins and thus elevates the intraspinal venous pressure. If there is no rise on abdominal pressure, coughing, and straining, it is probable that the lumen of the needle is obstructed or that there is lack of free communication between the subarachnoid space and the manometer, and further adjustment of the needle is necessary.

THE QUECKENSTEDT TEST

If the presence of an obstructive lesion of the spinal cord is suspected, the jugular veins can be constricted by an assistant (Queckenstedt maneuver); this increases the intracranial venous pressure by obstructing the venous return from the head, causing a rise in intracranial pressure. The veins may be compressed either manually or with an inflatable cuff, such as that used in a sphygmomanometer. In performing manual compression, the veins on each side are first constricted lightly, one at a time, then firmly, one at a time, and then the two are constricted simultaneously, first lightly, then firmly. There should be a prompt rise in the spinal fluid pressure followed by a fall to about the original pressure. With firm jugular compression for about 10 sec there is a rise of 100 – 300 mm, depending on the degree of constriction, and within 10 sec after release the pressure falls to its original level, or to within a few mm of it.

In the Queckenstedt test the neck is constricted near the trachea (to include the internal jugular veins) with sufficient pressure to collapse the veins, but not sufficient to compress the carotid arteries, interfere with respirations, cause pain, or stimulate the carotid sinus reflex. If pressure is applied to the larynx, the patient may cough and there may be elevation of the spinal fluid pressure, even when a complete block is present. If the jugular veins are constricted by a sphygmomanometer cuff, the ex-

aminer first inflates the cuff 20 mm Hg, notes the height of the cerebrospinal fluid pressure at 10 sec, and then releases the pressure and takes readings at 10 and 20 sec. After an interval of 10 – 15 sec, the test can be repeated with the cuff inflated to 40 mm, and again with the cuff inflated to 60 mm (Fig. 57-3).

It is important to stress that the Queckenstedt test should never be carried out if the cerebrospinal fluid pressure is abnormally elevated (over 200 mm), if a brain tumor or other expanding intracranial mass is suspected, or if there is grave intracranial disease such as a subarachnoid hemorrhage. It is a useful diagnostic test, but one that should be performed only when indicated and not routinely with every spinal puncture. The Queckenstedt test has been largely replaced by magnetic resonance imaging of the spine in the assessment of patency of the subarachnoid space.

DETERMINATION OF SPINAL SUBARACHNOID BLOCK

Spinal subarachnoid block may be either partial or complete. It is caused by some interruption in the continuity of the spinal fluid along the spinal subarachnoid space. This may be the result of compression of the spinal subarachnoid space by a neoplasm, granuloma, or abscess of the spinal cord; by a spinal epidural abscess or a centrally herniated nucleus pulposus; by deformity of the vertebrae by fracture, dislocation, Paget's disease, Pott's disease, or nontuberculous kyphoscoliosis; by meningeal arachnoiditis with adhesions; or by other rare causes.

If there is a complete spinal subarachnoid block, the pulse and respiratory oscillations of the cerebrospinal fluid pressure are usually somewhat decreased, and the pressure is often low. There will, under most circumstances, be a normal rise in pressure on coughing and straining, since the intraspinal pressure is still increased by these maneuvers. Occasionally there is an exaggerated response on coughing and straining in a high block, at least exaggerated in comparison to the response to jugular compression, although if the block is in the lower thoracic or upper lumbar region there may be little change in pressure on coughing and straining, or a slow rise and a delayed fall. With a complete block, however, there is no change in the spinal manometric pressure following jugular compression (Fig. 57-4 and 57-5). With a partial spi-

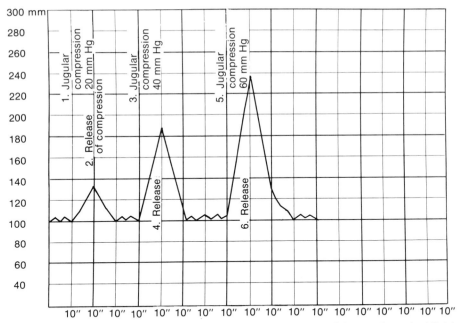

FIG. 57–3. Manometric chart showing the normal response of the cerebrospinal fluid pressure to jugular compression by means of a sphygmomanometer cuff.

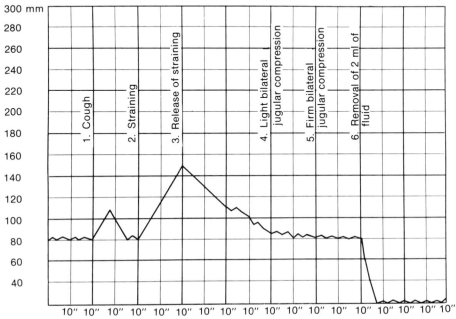

FIG. 57–4. Manometric chart in a case of complete spinal subarachnoid block.

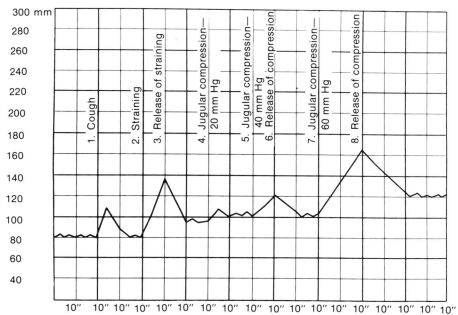

FIG. 57–5. Manometric chart showing complete spinal subarachnoid block as determined by means of a sphygmomanometer cuff.

nal subarachnoid block the response to coughing and straining will be normal or show very slight modifications, depending upon the level of the partial obstruction. In partial block, however, while there is a definite rise and fall on firm jugular compression, there is very little rise or a delayed rise followed by a slow, delayed fall on light jugular compression (Fig. 57-6). The pressure may fail to fall to its original level, and a new, higher level may be maintained. Occasionally, especially in a partial block, the response to jugular compression may falsely appear normal if the patient strains, coughs, or holds his breath during the test. In cervical lesions the response to the Queckenstedt test may be modified by either flexion or extension of the neck during the study of the pressure relationships. Under certain circumstances the dynamics may be normal if they are tested with the head in the neutral position, but either a partial or a complete block may be apparent when they are tested with the neck in either full flexion or full extension. Such maneuvers are especially helpful in the diagnosis of lesions in the cervical region.

With both partial and complete block there is a rapid fall in pressure on removal of spinal fluid. If a complete, or even a partially complete, block is found, very little fluid should be re-

moved, usually not more than 1 or 2 ml, and it is usually advisable in such cases to inject a contrast medium for myelography at once. When spinal cord tumors and similar obstructions of the spinal subarachnoid space are present, the removal of fluid from the lumbar region may increase the relative pressure above the tumor and force it downward in the spinal canal. This may be followed by an increase in symptoms and signs and even the sudden development of total paralysis below the level of the lesion. Therefore, if available, magnetic resonance or computed tomography imaging of the spinal subarachnoid space should precede lumbar puncture and/or be used in place of the Queckenstedt test when a mass lesion of this space is suspected.

COMPLICATIONS OF LUMBAR PUNCTURE

Complications of lumbar puncture are infrequent and rarely have serious prognostic import if clinical judgment is used in the performance of the procedure and if the various contraindications mentioned earlier in this chapter are not present. The development of a purulent meningitis or herniation of the medulla and/or cere-

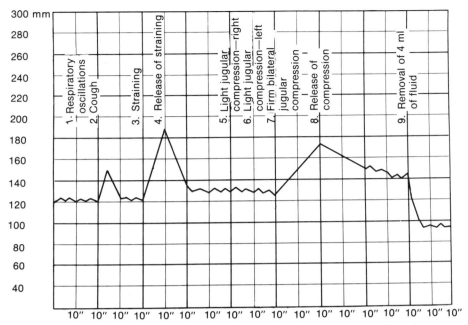

FIG. 57–6. Manometric chart in a case of partial spinal subarachnoid block.

bellar tonsils into the foramen magnum or the hippocampal gyrus through the incisura, with respiratory and circulatory distress, usually indicates that the puncture was ill-advised or was performed without the usual precautions. It is usually possible, however, to carry out a spinal puncture without dire effects even in the presence of papilledema and other signs of increased intracranial pressure unless a focal mass is present intracranially.

Pain in the nerve roots, which may occur during the puncture, is usually brief in duration and rarely causes persisting symptoms. The same is true of back pain that follows a puncture performed with difficulty in the presence of arthritis or skeletal anomalies. Patients in whom back or leg pain persists are often suggestible or hypochondriacal. Rare cases of injury to the intervertebral disks, vertebrae, interarticular facets, or venous sinusoids of the vertebrae have been reported with lumbar puncture. It has been postulated that in the exaggerated flexion of the torso the pressure is increased within the intervertebral disks and puncture of a disk with a needle may cause rupture of the nucleus pulposus into the canal. Osteomyelitis of the vertebrae has been reported on a few occasions following spinal puncture, as have extradural hemorrhage and extradural abscess.

Temporary meningitic signs are occasionally encountered following spinal puncture. Either a slight pleocytosis or a moderate increase in cerebrospinal fluid pressure may develop, usually with fever but no organisms; this may be taken to indicate either a slight inflammatory reaction (aseptic meningitis) or toxic sequelae due to the presence of foreign matter in the needle from disinfectants or detergents (chemical meningitis). Either temporary or permanent paralysis of the oculomotor, abducens, or other cranial nerves has been reported following spinal puncture or spinal anesthesia. The removal of spinal fluid in the presence of a complete or a partially complete subarachnoid block may force the obstructing lesion downward in the spinal canal, change a partial to a complete block, or cause the development of a complete paralysis below the level of the lesion. The dangers of puncture in the presence of brain tumor and other causes of increased intracranial pressures have been mentioned. It has often been stated that spinal puncture may cause an increase in the symptoms of multiple sclerosis and some myelopathies, but there is no scientific evidence for this. Breaking of the spinal puncture needle is rare if equipment is good and technic adequate. Intraspinal injection of drugs and foreign substances sometimes leads to the development of an aseptic meningitis, sensory and paralytic phenomena, and arachnoid adhesions with a consequent complete subarachnoid block.

The most frequent and most annoying sequel of lumbar puncture, distressing both the patient and physician, is the postpuncture headache that occurs in some form in a certain percentage of patients. Statistics vary widely regarding the frequency; it has been stated that a residual headache occurs in 10% – 50% of patients on whom spinal punctures are performed. Possibly it occurs in a very mild form in a fairly large number of patients, but it appears as a definite complication in 15%—— 30% of patients. The headache is usually occipital in site and may be accompanied by pain and stiffness in the back of the neck and in the back. It is usually present when the patient is upright and is relieved by recumbency. It may throb with the pulse and be increased by coughing, shaking of the head, sudden movement, and jugular compression. If severe, it may be accompanied by vertigo, nausea, vomiting, blurred vision, tinnitus, and transient deafness. If the complication is transitory, it lasts for only 1 – 2 hours; if moderate, it generally lasts but 1 or 2 days; in severe cases the patient may be incapacitated for 1 week, 10 days, or even 2 weeks. Sometimes there is a latent period of 1 – 3 days before the development of the headache.

Continued escape of fluid at the puncture site, mainly into the subdural space and subcutaneous tissues, is generally said to be the cause of postpuncture headache, along with traction on structures about the base of the brain displaced by the lowered pressure. Some patients who have had several punctures have developed headaches on some occasions and not on others. The headache does not seem to be dependent upon the amount of fluid withdrawn, unless more than 30 ml are removed. The symptom has been known to occur in patients in whom the dura was punctured but no fluid removed. It is rare after puncture of the cisterna magna. The reported increased frequency of postpuncture headache in patients with certain neurologic disorders such as multiple sclerosis has never been statistically proved. Some patients with postpuncture headaches have been found to have a slight pleocytosis, others not; some have a decrease in cerebrospinal fluid pressure, some an increase, and others normal pressure.

Studies have shown that the complication occurs much more frequently if the puncture is done with a large, 16- gauge needle than with a 22- gauge or smaller needle, so that physiologic factors such as leakage are probably more important than psychologic ones.

The best mode of treatment for postpuncture headaches is complete bed rest with the head as low as or lower than the rest of the body, together with the use of analgesics and sedatives if necessary. A generous fluid intake is probably advisable. Rarely, for severe, persistent postpuncture headaches, epidural injections of some of the patient's own blood ("blood patch") will be necessary to stop the cerebrospinal fluid leak.

BIBLIOGRAPHY

Adams RD, Victor M. Principles of Neurology, 4th ed. New York, McGraw – Hill, 1989

Ayala G. Ueber den diagnostischen Wert des Liquordruckes und einen Apparat zu seiner Messung. Z Gesamte Neurol Psychiatrie 1923;84:42

Baker CC. Headache due to spontaneous low spinal fluid pressure. Minnesota Med 1983;66:325

Cantore GP, Guidetti B, Virno M. Oral glycerol for the reduction of intracranial pressure. J Neurosurg 1965;21:278

Dunbar HS, Guthrie TC, Kardell PA. A study of the cerebrospinal fluid pulse wave. Arch Neurol 1966;14:224

Ecker A. Irregular fluctuation of elevated cerebrospinal fluid pressure. Arch Neurol Psychiatry 1955;74:641

Fisher RG, Copenhaver JH. The metabolic activity of the choroid plexus. J Neurosurg 1959;16:167

Fishman RA. Cerebrospinal Fluid in Diseases of the Nervous System. Philadelphia, WB Saunders, 1980

Foley J. Benign forms of intracranial hypertension — "toxic" and "otitic" hydrocephalus. Brain 1955;78:1

Gilland O. Cerebrospinal fluid dynamics in spinal subarachnoid block. Acta Neurol Scand 1962;38:285

Gilland O. Cerebrospinal fluid dynamic diagnosis of spinal block. V. Uniform lumbar electromanometrics. Neurology 1966;16:1110

Gilland O, Nelson JR. Lumbar cerebrospinal fluid manometrics with a minitransducer. Neurology 1970;20:103

Grant WT, Cone WV. Graduated jugular compression in the lumbar manometric test for spinal subarachnoid block. Arch Neurol Psychiatry 1934;32:1194

Kaiser AM, Whitelaw AG. Normal cerebrospinal fluid pressure in the newborn. Neuropediatrics 1986;17:100

Kaplan L, Kennedy F. The effect of head posture on the manometrics of the cerebrospinal fluid in cervical lesions: A new diagnostic test. Brain 1950;73:337

La Fia DJ. Abuse of the Queckenstedt test. N Engl J Med 1956;251:348

Luse SA, Harris B. Brain ultrastructure in hydration and dehydration. Arch Neurol 1961;4:139

Lysak WR, Svien HJ. Long-term follow-up on patients with diagnosis of pseudotumor cerebri. J Neurosurg 1966;25:284

Maren TH, Robinson B. The pharmacology of acetazolamide as related to cerebrospinal fluid and the treatment of hydrocephalus. Bull Johns Hopkins Hosp 1960;106:1

Myerson A, Loman J. Internal jugular venous pressure in

man: Its relationship to cerebrospinal fluid and carotid artery pressure. Arch Neurol Psychiatry 1932;27:836

O'Connell JEA. The vascular factor in intracranial pressure and the maintenance of the cerebrospinal fluid circulation. Brain 1943;66:204

O'Connell JEA. The cerebrospinal fluid pressure as an aetiological factor in the development of lesions affecting the central nervous system. Brain 1953;76:279

Queckenstedt ME. Zur Diagnose der Rückenmarks-kompression. Dtsch Z Nervenheilk 1916;55:325

Rubin RC, Henderson ES, Ommaya AK et al. The production of cerebrospinal fluid in man and its modification by acetazolamide. J Neurosurg 1966;25:430

Ryder SW, Espey FF, Kimbell FD et al. Effect of changes in systemic venous pressure on cerebrospinal fluid pressure. Arch Neurol Psychiatry 1952;68:175

Ryder SW, Espey FF, Kimbell FD et al. Influence of changes in cerebral blood flow on the cerebrospinal fluid pressure. Arch Neurol Psychiatry 1952;68:169

Sahs AL, Joynt RJ. Brain swelling of unknown cause. Neurology 1956;6:791

Schaltenbrand G. Die akute Aliquorrhoe. Verh Dtsch Ges Inn Med 1940;52:473

Shenkin HA, Finneson BE. Clinical significance of low cerebrospinal fluid pressure. Neurology 1958;8:157

Symonds C. Otitic hydrocephalus. Neurology 1956;6:681

Tourtellotte WW, Haerer AF, Heller GL, Somers JE. Post-lumbar Puncture Headaches. Springfield, IL, Charles C Thomas, 1964

Von Storch TJC, Carmichael EA, Banks TE. Factors producing lumbar cerebrospinal fluid pressure in man in the erect posture. Arch Neurol Psychiatry 1937;38:1158

Wise BL, Chater N. Effect of mannitol on cerebrospinal fluid pressure. Arch Neurol 1961;4:200

Chapter 58

EXAMINATION OF THE CEREBROSPINAL FLUID

Under most circumstances lumbar puncture is carried out for the purpose of examining the cerebrospinal fluid: the physical, cytologic, chemical, serologic, and bacteriologic compositions of the fluid are examined as part of the diagnosis of nervous system and somatic disease.

Normal spinal fluid is clear and colorless. Its specific gravity is low, ranging from 1.006 – 1.009, and that of ventricular fluid is even lower (1.002 – 1.004); the specific gravity is increased with elevation of the protein content and presence of abnormal constituents. It is slightly alkaline in reaction, with a pH of 7.3 – 7.4 (about the same as that of blood). Its total solids constitute about 1%, and the water content is about 99%. The freezing point is from 0.53 – 0.58°C, with an average of 0.57°C. There are about 3 – 5 mononuclear cells/cu mm. The various chemical constituents are listed subsequently. The serologic tests for syphilis give normal results, and no organisms are present.

APPEARANCE OF THE CEREBROSPINAL FLUID

The appearance of the fluid is noted with the naked eye. This is done most satisfactorily if the fluid is held up to the light against a dark background, although slight discoloration is sometimes more apparent against a white background. Moderate changes in color and turbidity may often be evaluated by comparing the spinal fluid with a like amount of clear water in a similar tube, or by observing the fluid by looking through the depth of the tube. The presence of foam on shaking may indicate the presence of pathologic constituents.

As was stated, the normal cerebrospinal fluid is clear and colorless. Physical alterations may be present in the form of either color change or turbidity. The most common physical change is a pinkish to red discoloration. This usually indicates the presence of blood or blood pigments in the fluid, and in every case in which such discoloration is found it is essential to determine whether the blood was present before the puncture was carried out (because of subarachnoid or intracerebral hemorrhage) or whether the blood entered the fluid at the time of the puncture (because of "traumatic tap" or venipuncture). Even the most skilled technician, performing a puncture under the most favorable circumstances, may occasionally traumatize some of the small vertebral, meningeal, or other veins and obtain fluid that is contaminated by the presence of blood. The following criteria may be used to differentiate between a "bloody tap" and subarachnoid and related bleeding: (1) three to four specimens of fluid are obtained. If the blood is present as a result of trauma during the puncture, each consecutive tube will be progressively clearer than the preceding one, and the last one may be colorless; also, there will be a progressive fall in the erythrocyte and hemoglobin content of the serial tubes. (Spinal fluid appears colorless to the naked eye if it contains fewer than 360 erythrocytes/cu mm.) On the other hand, if there has been a subarachnoid hemorrhage, each tube will be equally discolored. (2) The fluid is centrifuged. If the blood is fresh and due to trauma, it will not be mixed with the fluid; the supernatant fluid will be clear and colorless (unless the amount of blood is excessive). If there has been subarachnoid bleeding, the supernatant fluid will be xanthochromic (see next paragraph). (3) The fluid is allowed to stand. Blood present as a result of trauma may clot (if the erythrocyte count exceeds 200,000), whereas that from a subarachnoid hemorrhage will not. (4) The erythrocytes are examined under a microscope. The cells present as a result of recent trauma will appear as normal, biconcave disks (if examined immediately); the cells present from subarachnoid hemorrhage will be seen as crenated. (5) If it is felt that the blood is present as a result of trauma at the time of the puncture, the procedure may be repeated on the following day. The fluid should then be clear if the blood was present only as a contaminant. It is important to remember the following: Traumatic and subarachnoid bleeding may both be present; the lumbar fluid may be clear for a period of up to 2 or 3 hours after a spontaneous subarachnoid hemorrhage, but will be uniformly bloody thereafter; if normal fluid in the subarachnoid space is grossly contaminated by a traumatic venipuncture, some blood may be apparent for as long as 2 – 5 days after the original puncture.

The next most common type of discoloration of the spinal fluid is xanthochromia, or the appearance of a yellow color. This occurs with subarachnoid hemorrhage, and is seen in the supernatant fluid both soon after such a hemorrhage and also during convalescence, long ofter the gross and microscopic blood have both disappeared. It is not present immediately, but develops within 3 or 4 hours; it assumes its greatest intensity in about 1 week (the erythrocytes begin to disappear within 2 or 3 days), and may last for 3 – 4 weeks. Xanthochromia is also seen in association with the excessive protein content of fluid removed below a spinal subarachnoid block. In **Froin's syndrome** there is xanthochromia with increased protein, often to such a degree that the fluid clots spontaneously; there may or may not be a pleocytosis. This is usually found in complete spinal subarachnoid block that is due to the presence of spinal cord tumor, arachnoiditis with adhesions, severe cervical spondylosis, or traumatic compression of the spinal cord. Xanthochromia is also present, on occasion, in polyradiculoneuritis, acute and chronic meningitis, subdural hematoma, brain tumor, recent infarcts, progressive brain and spinal cord lesions, and other conditions in which there is excessive protein without block. It has been stated that the fluid always has a faint yellowish discoloration when compared with water if the protein content is more than 100 – 150 mg/100 ml of cerebrospinal fluid.

A slight xanthochromia has been reported in the spinal fluids of a large percentage of newborn infants, especially premature ones; this gradually disappears within 1 month. In jaundice, whether associated with liver disease of various types, biliary obstruction, or hemolytic anemia, the spinal fluid is discolored along with other body fluids; a yellow color is usually seen in cerebrospinal fluid with bilirubin values in the serum of 5 or greater. Other conditions in which the color of the body fluids is altered, such as hypercarotenemia, may produce similar discoloration in the cerebrospinal fluid. With meningeal melanosarcomatosis the fluid may be deeply colored. The supernatant fluid following a traumatic puncture will be xanthochromic if the fluid contained more than 150,000 – 200,000 erythrocytes/cu mm. The fluid will also be xanthochromic if the protein content was excessive prior to contamination, or if the tube had been washed with a markedly hemolytic substance such as a detergent. Xanthochromia and traumatic bleeding may be present simultaneously.

Spectrophotometric examination of xanthochromic spinal fluid is not usually necessary for diagnosis. It has been shown that the discoloration is due to the presence of both protein and products of red blood cell disintegration, namely, oxyhemoglobin, bilirubin, and, more rarely, methemoglobin. Oxyhemoglobin, which is red but with dilution varies from orange to orange-yellow, is the first pigment to appear after a subarachnoid hemorrhage; it is a product of hemolysis and may be found within 2 hours of onset. It increases rapidly, becoming maximal in the first few days, and gradually diminishes over a week or 10 days if no further bleeding occurs. Its presence may be ascertained by a positive benzidine test. Bilirubin, the iron-free derivative of hemoglobin, is yellow in color. It also appears in hemorrhagic fluids following hemolysis of erythrocytes; it is first apparent in 2 or 3 days and increases as the amount of oxyhemoglobin decreases. It may persist for 2 or 3 weeks. Bilirubin is also the predominant pigment present in the spinal fluid in cases of subarachnoid (and ventricular) block, as the result of transudation from the blood plasma, and it is the only pigment detected in the fluid in jaundice and liver disease. With subarachnoid block, however, it is accompanied by excessive protein, whereas with jaundice the protein content is normal. Methemoglobin, which is brown but becomes yellow with dilution, is found most commonly in fluids from subdural and intracerebral hematomas and in fluid near the encapsulated blood; its presence can be confirmed by a potassium cyanide test. Although the supernatant fluid is usually clear in traumatic punctures, it has been shown that oxyhemoglobin may be found by spectrophotometry if there are more than 12,000 erythrocytes/cu mm.

The cerebrospinal fluid may vary from opalescent to turbid in appearance owing to the presence of foreign or pathologic matter; this is usually the result of either an increase in cellular content (more than 500 cells/cu mm), the presence of organisms or fibrin, an increase in globulin or other protein, or contamination by blood. Degenerated cells are especially apt to cause the fluid to be turbid in appearance. A slightly bloody fluid may be turbid as well as discolored, and a grossly bloody fluid is opaque. In tuberculous meningitis with a moderate increase in cells (mainly lymphocytes), the fluid may vary from a ground-glass appearance to opalescence. In suppurative meningitis, with a marked increase in cells along with organisms and protein, the fluid may be cloudy or purulent, and may have a yellow or green discoloration. If the fluid is opalescent or cloudy, meningitis should be suspected and additional specimens should always be obtained for direct examination for bacteria and other microorganisms, including fungi, for cultures and quantitative glucose and protein tests, and some should be set aside for observation of a pellicle formation (see below). Fat globules have been demonstrated in the cerebrospinal fluid in cases of traumatic fat embolism and with ruptured cysts from a craniopharyngioma.

In certain conditions, such as tuberculous meningitis and other diseases in which there is an increase in protein, a pellicle or fibrin web appears if the fluid is allowed to stand. The fluid should be set aside for this purpose immediately after it has been drawn; it may be either left at room temperature or placed in a refrigerator. The formation of a pellicle or web indicates the presence of fibrinogen or fibrin ferment. A fine cobweb-like pellicle appears in tuberculous and other subacute meningitides, and occasionally in poliomyelitis and brain tumor; a coarse fibrin clot is seen in the acute meningitides. Cells and organisms, if present, may be studied more advantageously by examination of this web.

If the protein content is sufficiently increased, the entire specimen may solidify. This occurs in xanthochromic fluid, the Guillain – Barré syndrome, Froin's syndrome, and meningitis. The clot may be jellylike in appearance. It may be possible to precipitate the clotting by adding a single drop of blood to the spinal fluid.

CYTOLOGIC EXAMINATION OF THE CEREBROSPINAL FLUID

The fluid normally contains no erythrocytes and fewer than 5 cells of the leukocyte group (mononuclear cells or possibly lymphocytes) per cubic millimeter. The count is slightly lower in cisternal and ventricular fluid. The determination of the presence, number, and kind of cells is an essential part of every spinal fluid examination. The cell count should be done at once, or within 1 hour after the fluid has been drawn, since with longer standing the cells may adhere to the walls of the specimen tube or become disintegrated, making the estimation inaccurate. The cell count is usually carried out in the improved Neubauer or Thoma – Zeiss blood counting chamber; if available, a Fuchs – Rosenthal chamber may be used. If the fluid appears clear, it is not diluted and the number of cells in the entire chamber is noted. Since the ruled surface of the Neubauer or Thoma – Zeiss chamber (the 9 large squares) has an area of 9 cu mm and a depth of $1/10$ mm, to obtain the number of cells in 1 cu mm of fluid, the number of cells counted is multiplied by $10/9$. If the number of cells is too great to count satisfactorily without dilution, the fluid is diluted with the usual acetic acid solution used for leukocyte counts on the blood, and the cell content determined proportionately. If red blood cells are present, one should also note their number, diluting the fluid if necessary. Then the erythrocytes are eliminated by rinsing the pipette in glacial acetic acid several times before drawing spinal fluid into it. This dissolves the erythrocytes, and a cell count repeated after this should show only white blood cells. The fluid is allowed to stand in the pipette for 2 or 3 minutes, the first few drops are discarded, and the count is made on the next drop. The fluid is undiluted (except for the volatile acetic acid) and the red cells are either hemolyzed or badly crenated. This procedure should also be carried out whenever a count of more than 6 cells is made.

Many alternative methods of performing the cell count on the spinal fluid are in use. Many clinicians add a drop of some stain such as thionin, methylene blue, gentian violet, or Unna's polychrome methylene blue to the fluid. These aid in the differentiation between leukocytes and erythrocytes since they stain the nuclei of the former but do not affect the latter; they also aid in the differentiation between mononuclear and polymorphonuclear cells. If stain is used in making the routine cell count, it may be possible to do an approximate differential estimation in the counting chamber. Others use both acetic acid, to dissolve the red cells, and stain. The dilute acetic acid solution used for white blood counts usually contains a small amount of stain. An ordinary pipette, such as is employed for blood leukocyte counts, is filled to the 1.0 mark with acetic acid, and then to the 11 mark with spinal fluid. The fluid and the diluent are shaken in the pipette for 1 min, they are allowed to stand for 2 min, the first few drops are discarded, and then a drop is applied to the counting chamber. At least 2 counts are made, and an average is taken. The total is multiplied by 10/9, since $^9/_{10}$ cu mm were counted, and again by 11/10 to compensate for the dilution. If the Fuchs-Rosenthal chamber is used, the total count of cells from undiluted fluid is divided by 3.2 to obtain the number of cells per cubic millimeter.

Currently most determinations are made with automated and other sophisticated equipment; this includes the cytologic study of blood and other body fluids. The physician rarely performs the cell count on cerebrospinal fluid at present, and if he does, it is only in emergency situations when laboratory technology is not immediately available.

In most clinical laboratories the cells in the cerebrospinal fluid are counted in an automated cell-counting machine. If it is suspected that the cell count is considerably elevated, an isotonic diluent can be added to the fluid before the cells are counted. The count is first made with the setting at the red cell level. Then a fluid can be added to lyse the red cells, and a second count is made. The difference between the first and second readings gives a simple determination of the red and white cells. The cytocentrifuge is also available to allow concentration of cells when few are present. The concentrate can be stained with Wright's stain to allow the differential cell count.

The sedimentation and filtration methods for the study of cerebrospinal fluid cytomorphology are felt by those familiar with them to be improvements over the counting chamber, direct smear, and centrifugation technics. The filtration procedure is adequate for identification of most neoplastic cells, but for wider range and more precise studies the sedimentation procedure has been shown to be superior. Another innovation in the cytologic study of the cerebrospinal fluid has been the processing of the fluid immediately after the lumbar puncture. This delays the lysis and distortion of the cells, and they may be studied up to 2 weeks after collection without loss of morphologic detail.

The few cells normally found in the spinal fluid are mononuclear in type. Some of these may be lymphocytes, but the majority are probably mesothelial cells derived from the meninges, the ependymal lining of the ventricles, and the perivascular spaces of Virchow – Robin. In disease states other cells are present, including lymphocytes, neutrophils, eosinophils, plasma cells, and fibroblasts. They may be hematogenous in origin, or may be derived from the meninges or perivascular spaces. A count of 5 – 10 cells/cu mm is considered borderline, and one of over 10, definitely elevated. Many authors feel that the presence of even a single polymorphonuclear leukocyte is abnormal. An increased number of cells in the cerebrospinal fluid is known as a **pleocytosis;** this may be lymphocytic, polymorphonuclear, or mixed. The presence of 5 – 10 cells is known as a slight pleocytosis; 11 – 50 cells indicate a moderate pleocytosis; 50 – 250, a severe pleocytosis; more than 250, an extreme pleocytosis.

If an increase in the number of cells is present, a smear should be made and stained with gentian violet, methylene blue, Wright's, or some related stain, and a differential count made. If the fluid is purulent or the pleocytosis is marked, the smear is made directly from the fluid; if a pellicle is present, it is stained. If there is no opalescence and the cell count is not excessive, the fluid should be centrifuged and the supernatant decanted; then some sediment is placed on a slide and allowed to dry. The preparation may be fixed by drying, but better fixation is obtained by adding egg, bovine, or commercial albumin. If meningitis is suspected, a Gram or Ziehl – Nelson stain may be made at the same time. A careful study of the stained smear may be essential to the diagnosis of the disease process. It is possible to differentiate lymphocytes, neutrophils, eosinophils, monocytes, and phagocytes. In addition it is sometimes possible to identify tumor cells, cryptococci, actinomycotic granules, and fragments of echinococci and cysticerci. In estimating the number of cells present, the physician should always remember that tumor or yeast cells may resemble leukocytes under the low-power objective of the microscope. Special technics, such as staining with India ink, may aid in identifying cryptococci. If the presence of tumor cells is suspected, the fluid should be centrifuged and the sediment fixed and stained. In all patients with suspected meningitis the fluid should be cultured.

Red blood cells may be present in the cerebrospinal fluid as a result either of disease or of trauma to the vertebral or meningeal vessels at the time the puncture was performed. With the latter the cells may appear normal if examined immediately, but crenation occurs promptly. In general, if the cerebrospinal fluid is contaminated by large amounts of blood as a result of trauma at the time of the puncture, it is best to centrifuge the fluid, and to decant the supernatant fluid and use only that for the various diagnostic tests. Blood may be present in substantial amounts in the case of subarachnoid and intraventricular hemorrhages, as well as in a large percentage of intracerebral hemorrhages, and occasionally in association with subdural hematomas and extradural hemorrhages. Blood is also found in the spinal fluid in posttraumatic states (cerebral contusions and lacerations), brain tumor (especially vascular or degenerating neoplasm), subarachnoid or meningeal angiomatosis, meningeal inflammations with congestion of the meningeal vessels and diapedesis of cells through their walls, congestion of the meningeal vessels in association with spinal cord tumor or subarachnoid block, blood dyscrasias, and hemorrhagic encephalopathy or myelopathy.

A leukocyte count can never be considered accurate if the fluid is contaminated by the presence of blood. On occasion, however, an approximate correction for the blood cells may be made by this formula:

$$\frac{\text{Leukocytes (blood)} \times \text{erythrocytes (fluid)}}{\text{Erythrocytes (blood)}} = \text{Leukocytes (fluid)}$$

About 1 white cell/cu mm is added to the fluid by enough blood to add 600–700 red cells/cu mm.

A pleocytosis in the cerebrospinal fluid usually indicates the presence of meningeal irritation, but not necessarily meningeal infection. Whether these cells are polymorphonuclear, lymphocytic, or mixed depends upon the type of irritation, the nature and site of the pathologic process, and the nature of the infecting organism. The presence of polymorphonuclear cells is indicative of an acute process or an exacerbation of a chronic inflammation caused by a pyogenic organism. The process is usually close to or involves the meninges and ependyma, but polymorphonuclear cells may be present in association with a pyogenic infection in the neighborhood of the meninges (in the mastoid cells, or within the brain tissue), with no actual contamination of the meninges. The presence of lymphocytes usually indicates either a chronic or low-grade inflammatory process of the meninges or ependyma (not necessarily due to infection), a more extensive process at some distance from the meninges and ependyma, or an inflammation caused by a neurotropic virus. A mixed pleocytosis suggests that the process is a subacute one. The presence of eosinophils indicates an infection by parasites, yeasts, or fungi, or an allergic or foreign body reaction.

A slight to moderate lymphocytic pleocytosis (5–50 cells) is found in a variety of diseases, some of the more important of which are as follows: viral infections of the central nervous system and/or meninges (viral encephalitis and meningitis, poliomyelitis, rabies, herpes zoster, human immunodeficiency virus); multiple sclerosis; brain or spinal cord tumors near the meninges or ependyma; sterile or toxic meningitis following the intraspinal injection of serum, air, anesthetics, iodized oil, penicillin, streptomycin, or other substances, or in association with the presence of blood in the subarachnoid spaces; aseptic meningitis associated with some focus of infection within the cranium, such as sinus thrombosis, mastoid disease, brain abscess, subdural and epidural abscesses, or osteomyelitis; trauma to the central nervous system; cerebrovascular disease (cerebral infarction secondary to thrombosis or embolism); subdural hematoma; toxic processes or degenerative diseases of obscure etiology; tetanus; some varieties of polyneuritis; central nervous system complications of systemic diseases (syphilis, malaria, mumps, measles, whooping cough, vaccinia, varicella, lymphogranuloma venereum, infectious mononucleosis, Weil's disease, Lyme disease, undulant fever, sarcoidosis, collagen disorders), reactions to yeasts, fungi, and parasites; meningeal carcinomatosis; leukemic infiltrations and other hematologic disorders. There is often a slight pleocytosis in premature and newborn infants that disappears by 3 months. A mild pleocytosis is sometimes seen after a major motor seizure.

A severe to extreme lymphocytic pleocytosis (50–500 or more cells) is observed in chronic or subacute inflammations of the meninges. The more important conditions in which such a cell change occurs include tuberculous and cryptococcal meningitis, lymphocytic choriomeningitis, trypanosomiasis, and central nervous system involvement by acquired immune deficiency syndrome or its secondary infections. Occasionally, with brain tumors that are near the meninges or ependyma, or with aseptic meningitis, viral encephalitis, herpes zoster, carcinomatous meningitis, infections by fungi or parasites, and the meningoencephalitides and encephalomyelitides associated with the systemic diseases listed previously, the pleocytosis may be severe rather than moderate. In almost none of these conditions with a moderate or severe pleocytosis is the increase in cells entirely an elevation in the number of lymphocytes, and the percentage of polymorphonuclear cells may give some clue in regard to the activity or the chronicity of the process.

A polymorphonuclear pleocytosis of mild degree is rarely seen; it occurs in the preparalytic stage of poliomyelitis, where there may be 50 – 100 or even more polymorphonuclear cells, and occasionally along with a parameningeal inflammatory process, or a neoplasm near or in the subarachnoid space. Occasionally there is a slight increase in neutrophils in cases of vascular disease, hypercoagulable states, and trauma without bloody spinal fluid. In status epilepticus, the earliest stages of purulent meningitis, and in meningitis that has been suppressed by prior inadequate antibiotic or steroid treatment there may be a slight increase in either neutrophils or lymphocytes. If there is an increase in polymorphonuclear cells, however, it is usually to a significant degree, varying from 300 – 5,000 or more. This is indicative of a suppurative meningitis, usually of a coccal origin, namely the meningococcal, streptococcal, pneumococcal, or staphylococcal varieties, but it is occasionally seen in influenzal meningitis. If a large number of cells is found, with a high percentage of neutrophils, a tentative diagnosis of acute meningitis must be made. In such cases additional tests such as stained smears, cultures, and both blood and cerebrospinal fluid glucose determinations are essential. If organisms are found or the sugar is low, the patient must be treated for purulent meningitis. Counterimmunoelectrophoretic studies or other antigen studies for specific organisms may help if no organisms are seen in the cerebrospinal fluid. If no organisms are found and the glucose is normal, it is probable that the patient has an aseptic meningitis in association with some process such as brain abscess or sinus thrombosis. However,

the decision cannot await the results of culture, and when other aspects of the clinical features and cerebrospinal fluid examination suggest that a purulent meningitis is present, prompt antibiotic treatment is indicated.

A mixed pleocytosis, with an increase in both lymphocytes and polymorphonuclear cells, usually indicates a subacute meningeal inflammation, and is found in influenzal meningitis, in the more malignant varieties of tuberculous meningitis, and in aseptic meningitis associated with brain abscess or some other intracranial infection. The relative percentage of polymorphonuclear cells and lymphocytes is indicative of the activity of the infection. In later stages of tuberculous meningitis the proportion of neutrophils may be increased to one-third or more.

Carcinomatous meningitis may be difficult to differentiate from infectious meningitis; the cellular response may be similar in the two conditions, and the glucose content is often low in both. If carcinomatous meningitis is suspected, special stains of the concentrated sediment (Wright, Leishman, Papanicolaou, or others) and occasionally paraffin fixation with tissue-staining technics are indicated. Some of the cells first thought to have been lymphocytes or monocytes may be found to be neoplastic instead, but more characteristic are larger cells with multiple nuclei and mitotic figures (Fig. 58-1). Such cells are occasionally found with primary tumors of the nervous system, but occur more commonly with metastatic involvement.

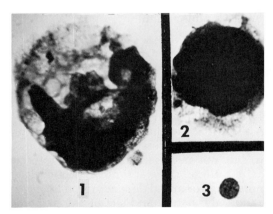

FIG. 58–1. Cells found in the cerebrospinal fluid of a patient with metastatic malignant melanoma. **1.** and **2.** Neoplastic cells. **3.** Normal mononuclear cell. Wright's stain. (Courtesy of Dr. W. W. Tourtellotte)

CHEMICAL EXAMINATION OF THE CEREBROSPINAL FLUID

The chemical examination of the cerebrospinal fluid may include many different determinations, but the most important from a clinical point of view are the estimation of the protein and glucose contents and analysis of the protein constituents.

The Protein Content

The total protein content of the spinal fluid normally ranges from 15 – 40 mg/100 ml (in contrast to the blood serum protein of 6.3 – 8 g/100 ml). This varies, however, with the site from which the fluid is obtained, and the above figure applies to the lumbar fluid; that obtained from the cisterna magna has from 15 – 25 mg/100 ml of protein, that from the ventricles, 5 – 15 mg/100 ml. The protein content of the fluid is normally lower in children and slightly higher in elderly persons. It is said to be slightly higher in males than in females. Some clinicians consider a protein content of up to 35 mg/100 ml as normal, 35 – 50 mg/100 ml as borderline, and over 50 mg/100 ml as abnormal. The cerebrospinal fluid protein consists mainly of albumin and globulin, with the former normally somewhat in excess. These can be partitioned into fractions, such as the prealbumin, alpha-, beta-, and gamma-globulins, and further into subfractions. A significant change in the ratio of these constituents can occur without an increase in the total protein content, as will be described.

The older qualitative tests for protein are no longer in general use in the analysis of cerebrospinal fluid. Quantitative protein tests are usually carried out in clinical laboratories. The physician does not perform them but should be able to interpret them. Their reliability depends upon the laboratory. The normal range may vary. The physician should know the technic used in the laboratory, recognize its advantages and possible shortcomings, and be able to rely upon the results.

It is important to determine not only the total protein content of the spinal fluid, but also the quantitative albumin and globulin (usually IgG) fractions, the albumin – globulin ratio, and the individual globulin components. These have been differentiated and analyzed by various technics. The protein content of the cerebrospinal fluid is increased in many diseases of the meninges and nervous system. In fact, an elevation of the proteins under most circumstances indicates the presence of an organic disease of the central nervous system or its membranes. Many factors are responsible. There is always an elevation of the protein content of the fluid in association with an increase in the cellular constituents, and especially with cellular disintegration and the presence of organisms. Except when it is associated with blood, cells, or organisms, increased protein comes mainly from the blood vessels and perineural spaces. With either gross or microscopic blood in the spinal fluid there is direct invasion of the subarachnoid channels by blood proteins. With inflammatory processes and associated congestion of the meningeal and other vessels there is an increased permeability of the blood – cerebrospinal fluid barrier, allowing transudation of blood proteins into the spinal fluid. With edema of the nervous tissues and meninges there may be transudation of serum from the perineural spaces. With damage to or destruction of nervous tissue in encephalomalacia, trauma, or degenerative or neoplastic processes there may be either actual formation of protein or release of it to the spinal fluid pathways, although edema, congestion, and hemorrhage may instead be responsible mechanisms. With stagnation or blockage of the spinal fluid there may be both increased permeability and decreased absorption of proteins. With a marked elevation of protein there may be spontaneous clotting and xanthochromia (Froin's syndrome).

Among those conditions (mainly neurologic and meningeal, but including some systemic disorders) in which an elevation of the cerebrospinal fluid protein is a significant and more or less consistent finding are the following: acute and chronic meningeal inflammations (carcinomatous meningitis, reactive and aseptic meningitides), arachnoiditis, acute and chronic encephalitides and meningitides, poliomyelitis (especially in the postparalytic phase), central nervous system syphilis (tabes dorsalis, dementia paralytica, meningovascular syphilis, and symptomatic central nervous system syphilis), brain neoplasms and abscesses (especially if near the meninges or ventricles, or if they obstruct the flow of blood or cerebrospinal fluid), vascular malformations and neoplasms (angiomas, arteriovenous malformations, ruptured aneurysms), subarachnoid and cerebral hemorrhage, posttraumatic states, subdural hematoma, multiple sclerosis, certain of the leukodystrophies and degenerative diseases of the brain and/or spinal cord, leprosy, diphtheritic and diabetic polyneuropathies (and occasionally diabetes without overt neurologic involvement), some chronic progressive neuropathies, myxedema, hyperparathyroidism, multiple myeloma, spondylitis, and rheumatoid arthritis.

There is a marked increase in the protein content in the lumbar fluid below a spinal cord tumor or other causes of spinal subarachnoid block, probably due to congestion of the meninges. This same factor may be responsible for the increase in protein in the spinal fluid in many cases of herniation of an intervertebral disk in the lumbosacral region, even though the fluid is obtained from above the level of the herniation. In certain types of polyneuritis or polyradiculoneuritis, especially in the Guillain-Barré syndrome, there may be a marked elevation in protein without a parallel pleocytosis (**albuminocytologic dissociation,** perhaps more precisely designated by the more accurate but less common term **protein-cytologic dissociation**). Similar dissociations, however, may also be observed with spinal cord tumors, some brain tumors, postparalytic poliomyelitis, and, rarely, other conditions. A moderate elevation of the protein occurs with nonhemorrhagic vascular disease, certain slowly progressive cerebral degenerations (such as presenile dementia), and many toxic and metabolic encephalopathies, as well as after convulsive seizures. The protein is also moderately elevated in premature and newborn infants, but assumes normal values at the age of 2 or 3 months. Occasionally no cause is found for elevated protein. The spinal fluid protein is diminished in children in the early stages of acute infections, in meningismus, in some types of communicating hydrocephalus, in some cases of pseudotumor cerebri, and at times with water intoxication. If a large amount of fluid is removed, the protein content of the last specimen is lower than that of the first (*i.e.*, the fluid is obtained from higher levels, and probably from the ventricles).

If gross blood is present in the fluid as a result of actual trauma to the venous plexus during the puncture, a rough correction can be made for the protein content contributed from the blood by subtracting 1 mg of protein/ 100 ml for every 750 erythrocytes/cu mm of fluid.

The differential quantitative determination of the albumin and globulin fractions of the spinal fluid and of the specific globulin components is important in the study of certain diseases of the nervous system. Of particular importance are the gamma-globulins, a variable group of proteins with similar electrophoretic properties. Various technics measure these as well as IgG, IgM, and IgA. IgG is of the most importance for neurologic diagnosis, particularly in the evaluation of multiple sclerosis. Measurements have been expressed in terms of the ratio of IgG to total protein in the cerebrospinal fluid, amounts of IgG produced in the central nervous system per day, and as the IgG/albumin index. In disorders such as multiple sclerosis, electrophoresis of cerebrospinal fluid may show the presence of oligoclonal bands of IgG. The oligoclonal pattern, representing discrete populations of IgG, has been shown to have a high sensitivity and specificity for confirmation of the diagnosis of multiple sclerosis. The oligoclonal pattern may be present in the cerebrospinal fluid of patients with multiple sclerosis even if the total IgG is not elevated. Oligoclonal bands, however, may also be present at times with any diseases that include proliferation of the plasma cell clones in the cerebrospinal fluid with *in situ* production of immunoglobulins. These include tertiary syphilis, subacute panencephalitis, fungal, viral (including human immunodeficiency virus), and chemical encephalitides, the Guillain-Barré syndrome, optic neuritis, and others.

The relative and absolute values for the various protein constituents, other than albumin and IgG, are of lesser diagnostic significance. Their ranges are listed by Fishman and others in texts devoted to cerebrospinal fluid. Amino acids normally present in blood are also found in small quantities in the cerebrospinal fluid but have little diagnostic significance.

The presence of excessive amounts of myelin basic protein in cerebrospinal fluid is a nonspecific indicator of active demyelination, whatever the etiology.

The Glucose Content

The glucose content of the cerebrospinal fluid is approximately one half to two thirds of the glucose content (80 – 120 mg/100 ml) of the blood plasma. The normal values are usually considered to be from 50 – 65 mg/100 ml, although some authorities believe values as high as 80 mg/100 ml to be within the normal range. The glucose content is higher in ventricular fluid, although not as high as in the blood. Cerebrospinal fluid glucose levels lag in their changes behind those of serum glucose levels for 30 – 60 minutes. A normal value for the spinal fluid glucose in association with an elevated blood glucose may indicate a pathologic decrease in the glucose content of the spinal fluid.

The glucose content of the spinal fluid is most important, from a diagnostic point of view, if it is decreased. It is decreased to a major degree principally with inflammation and infiltration of the meninges. Hypoglycorrhachia is an early and important diagnostic sign of meningitis. In tuberculous meningitis the spinal fluid sugar is often between 20 and 40 mg/100 ml, and in the acute pyogenic meningitides it is often below 20 mg/100 ml. The spinal fluid glucose is also often decreased in cryptococcal meningitis, but is usually normal in viral, aseptic, and reactive meningitides. It is markedly decreased in carcinomatous meningitis and in the meningitides associated with sarcomatosis and leukemia. There is probably an interference with glucose transport across the infiltrated meningeal membranes and a decreased entry into the cerebrospinal fluid. Possibly lack of transport and glycolysis both play a part in lowering cerebrospinal fluid glucose in infections. The glucose content of the cerebrospinal fluid is also low in insulin shock, hyperinsulinism, and often in subarachnoid hemorrhage.

An elevation of the glucose content of the spinal fluid, or hyperglycorrhachia, usually occurs in association with elevation of the blood glucose. Consequently the spinal fluid glucose is increased in diabetes. It may also be moderately elevated in certain of the acute encephalitides, namely Japanese type B encephalitis and the eastern and western equine varieties of encephalomyelitis.

Alimentary hyperglycemia causes only a small to moderate rise in the spinal fluid glucose, probably through a selective action of the choroid plexus in regulating the glucose content of the fluid, although a more pronounced elevation of the spinal fluid glucose accompanies the hyperglycemia produced by an injection of epinephrine. Simultaneous examinations of the glucose levels in the spinal fluid and blood are necessary, and these are best performed when the patient is in the fasting state, when the cerebrospinal fluid glucose will be in equilibrium with the blood glucose, unless emergency lumbar puncture is called for.

Other Chemical Constituents

The protein and glucose are the major chemical constituents of the cerebrospinal fluid that are examined routinely, but there are other substances that may be investigated experimentally or in individual cases.

The chloride content of normal cerebrospinal fluid varies between 118 and 130 mEq/ liter, whereas that of blood serum is from 96 – 103 mEq/ liter. The spinal fluid chloride is dependent on the plasma concentration. A low spinal fluid chloride is commonly noted in meningitis, especially in tuberculous meningitis, but also accompanies the decrease in the blood chloride that occurs in all acute and chronic infections. It is also decreased secondarily in the presence of increased spinal fluid protein. Routine examination of spinal fluid chloride has been abandoned because it contributes little to diagnosis.

The calcium content of spinal fluid varies from 2.2 – 3.4 mEq/liter, with an average of 2.4 mEq/ liter. This is approximately one-half of the blood serum content of 4.5 – 6.0 mEq/ liter. The calcium of the spinal fluid is decreased in conditions such as tetany in which the blood calcium is low, and is also decreased on occasion in tetanus and tumors of the diencephalon. It is increased with elevation of the blood calcium (as in hyperparathyroidism), and is sometimes slightly increased in meningitis and other conditions in which there is an elevation of the spinal fluid protein.

The inorganic phosphorus content of the spinal fluid is also about one half of the blood serum content, varying from 1.25 – 2.1 mg/100 ml with an average of 1.53 mg. (The blood serum inorganic phosphorus varies between 2.5 – 4.5 mg/100 ml.) It is increased with an increase of the blood phosphorus (tetany), in encephalitis, poliomyelitis, and other viral diseases of the nervous system, and in meningitis and other conditions in which there is an elevation of the protein content of the spinal fluid.

The sodium content of the cerebrospinal fluid varies from 130 – 152 mEq/ liter, with an average of 143 mEq/ liter. This is slightly in excess of the normal serum sodium content, which averages about 138 mEq/ liter.

The potassium content of the cerebrospinal fluid varies from 2.5 – 3.5 mEq/ liter, with an average of 2.8 mEq/ liter. This is slightly lower than the blood serum potassium, which averages from 4.0 – 5.5 mEq/ liter.

The magnesium content of the spinal fluid is 2.7 mEq/ liter, or slightly higher than the blood plasma content, which averages 1.3 mEq/ liter. The magnesium content of the spinal fluid is said to be slightly elevated in purulent meningitis and slightly decreased in tuberculous meningitis.

The bicarbonate content of the cerebrospinal fluid averages 23 mEq/ liter, about equal to the blood plasma content. The total base of the spinal fluid averages 157 mEq/ liter, again about equal to the blood plasma content of 155 mEq/ liter; it is increased in tuberculous meningitis and uremia. On occasion the acid – base balance, oxygen tension, carbon dioxide tension, osmolarity (normally the same as in serum), and hydrogen ion concentration are also determined.

The nonprotein nitrogen of the cerebrospinal fluid varies from 10 – 25 mg/100 ml, with an average of 19 mg/100 ml, or about two-thirds that of the blood plasma (25 – 35 mg/100 ml). The urea nitrogen ranges from 8 – 17 mg/100 ml, or about the same as that of the blood plasma. The creatinine of the spinal fluid ranges from 0.5 – 2.0 mg/100 ml with an average of 1.1 mg/100 ml, or again about the same as that of the blood plasma. The uric acid content of the spinal fluid ranges from 0.3 – 1.3 with an average of 0.7 mg/100 ml, in contrast to the blood serum uric acid of 3 – 5, with an average of 4.0 mg/100 ml. The ammonia content of the spinal fluid averages 30 µg/100 ml, whereas the blood ammonia is from 40 – 70 µg/100 ml. All of these spinal fluid contents increase, but not always proportionately, in uremia and other conditions in which the blood levels are elevated. The parallel between the blood and the spinal fluid urea content, however, is not as great as that of the others. In addition, the ammonia content is increased in hepatic disease, and the uric acid content has been said to be elevated in association with cerebral atrophy.

Many other chemical determinations may be performed under special circumstances. Studies of the content and distribution of the various lipid constituents of the cerebrospinal fluid have been done in certain of the demyelinating diseases as well as the lipidoses. Among the substances investigated are the total lipids, fatty acids, neutral fat, free and esterified cholesterol, phospholipids (cephalin, lecithin, and sphingomyelin), nonphosphorus sphingolipids (cerebrosides, sulfatides, and gangliosides), and the lipoproteins. By means of ultramicrochemical technics it is possible to differentiate and quantitate each of these. Certain carbohydrate constituents may also be assayed, including pyruvate, lactate, and α-ketoglutarate. Their changes are usually nondiagnostic.

Investigation of enzymes and enzyme activity in the cerebrospinal fluid has been the subject of many reports. Creatine phosphokinase, glutamic oxaloacetic transaminase, and lactic dehy-

drogenase and its isoenzymes have received much attention. Normally, the levels of such enzymes are significantly lower in the cerebrospinal fluid than in the blood. Elevation of the levels of these enzymes in the spinal fluid following cerebral infarction, subarachnoid hemorrhage, infections, multiple sclerosis, cerebral atrophy, and, at times, seizures has been reported.

Studies of the isoenzymes of lactic dehydrogenase are of interest. In normal spinal fluid, serum fractions 1 and 2 predominate. In bacterial meningitis isoenzymes 4 and 5, derived from leukocytes, have been elevated. Thus, an increase in isoenzymes 4 and 5 indicates pleocytosis of the polymorphonuclear type. Other enzymes have also been studied. For example, an elevated glucose isomerase in cerebrospinal fluid is said to be a marker for leptomeningeal metastases. In general, however, changes in the levels of the enzymes in the cerebrospinal fluid have yet to be determined to have precise, specific diagnostic or prognostic significance.

Assays of catecholamines and certain other substances related to neurotransmitters in the cerebrospinal fluid have mainly research applications.

BACTERIOLOGIC EXAMINATION OF THE CEREBROSPINAL FLUID

In every case in which a smear of the spinal fluid is made and stained for the study of the cellular constituents, a careful search should be made for the presence of organisms. Under many circumstances an ordinary gentian violet or methylene blue stain will suffice, but if the spinal fluid picture is even slightly suggestive of purulent meningitis, a Gram's stain should always be made to differentiate meningococci (gram-negative, intracellular organisms) from streptococci, staphylococci, and pneumococci. If pleocytosis is predominantly lymphocytic, a Ziehl – Nelson stain should be made to search for tubercle bacilli. In suspected cryptococcal meningitis the fluid is stained with India ink or fluorescein. Sometimes the examination for organisms is carried out more successfully if the fluid is first centrifuged, and the sediment examined, or, in the case of tuberculous meningitis, if a pellicle appears and can be examined, although the diagnosis can usually be entertained or established before this occurs. Tubercle bacilli are very difficult to demonstrate in many patients with tuberculous meningitis. Not only should the examiner search the smear closely for evidence of bacteria, especially cocci and bacilli, but also for evidence of yeasts, other fungi, and parasites.

If no organisms are found on the examination of the direct smear, cultures and other studies are indicated in all cases that show evidence of meningeal infection. An ordinary pyogenic culture is sufficient in most cases of purulent meningitis, but special culture media are necessary in suspected tuberculous and other less common varieties of meningitis. Sabouraud's medium is used if cryptococcosis is suspected. After the growth in the culture is observed, further smears and studies may be made to determine the identity of the infecting organism and its sensitivity to antibiotics. In brucellosis meningoencephalitis, especially if caused by *Brucella abortus*, the culture may have to be grown under anaerobic conditions. In every case of suspected tuberculous meningitis in which the diagnosis is not established on the basis of the direct smear, guinea pig inoculations should be made. Cultures should be started before the administration of antibiotics has been instituted. Further bacteriologic examinations include agglutination, precipitation, complement fixation, neutralization, and flocculation tests for special organisms, as well as counterimmunoelectrophoretic and other antigen studies of the serum; cryptococcal serum antigen tests may help establish a diagnosis of infection by that organism. In suspected invasion by neurotropic viruses, such as those of the St. Louis and Japanese B types of encephalitis, lymphocytic choriomeningitis, and the eastern and western varieties of equine encephalomyelitis, titers should be obtained on the blood during the acute and convalescent stages of the disease. In these, as well as in poliomyelitis and other viral infections, the virus can on occasion be isolated from the cerebrospinal fluid by special cultures and inoculation of experimental animals.

SEROLOGIC TESTS FOR SYPHILIS IN CEREBROSPINAL FLUID

The VDRL (Venereal Disease Research Laboratory) test has been the test of choice for syphilis on the cerebrospinal fluid in most laboratories. This is a rapidly performed slide-technic flocculation test employing cardiolipin antigen, and is highly sensitive and specific. A positive spinal fluid reaction may be considered diagnostic of certain types of central nervous system syphilis, especially if there are also abnormalities in the cell count and protein.

If there is a large amount of blood in the spinal fluid, from cerebral or subarachnoid hemorrhage or a traumatic spinal puncture, a falsely positive reaction may be obtained. In such cases it is necessary to repeat the test when the blood has disappeared from the fluid. Falsely positive reactions are also sometimes found in the spinal fluid, as well as in the blood, in cases of infectious mononucleosis, yaws, trypanosomiasis, cerebral malaria, lymphosarcoma, the collagen disorders, and some other systemic disorders. It must be remembered that a negative serologic test for syphilis does not rule out the possibility of some type of central nervous system syphilis, since in a certain percentage of cases of tabes dorsalis and meningovascular syphilis, especially those who have undergone some treatment, the serologic reactions may be normal; serologic studies are only rarely normal, however, in dementia paralytica. A confirmatory test in the presence of a positive VDRL test in the cerebrospinal fluid is the FTAabs test in the blood (a fluorescent treponemal antibody absorption test). The colloidal tests (colloidal gold curve and others) of cerebrospinal fluid, once helpful in the diagnosis of syphilis, multiple sclerosis, and other entities, are no longer in use.

BIBLIOGRAPHY

Adams RD, Victor M. Principles of Neurology, 4th ed. New York, McGraw – Hill, 1989

Barrows LJ, Hunter FT, Banker BQ. The nature and clinical significance of pigments in the cerebrospinal fluid. Brain 1955;78:59

Bauer CH, New MI, Miller JM. Cerebrospinal fluid protein values of premature infants. J Pediatr 1965;66:1017

Bulger RJ, Schrier RW, Arend WP et al. Spinal fluid acidosis and the diagnosis of pulmonary encephalopathy. N Engl J Med 1966;274:433

Chow G, Schmidley JW. Lysis of erythrocytes and leukocytes in traumatic lumbar puncture. Arch Neurol 1984;41:1084

Crosby RMN, Weiland GL. Xanthochromia of the cerebrospinal fluid. II. Preliminary description of several new colored substances. Arch Neurol Psychiatry 1953;69:732

Davis LE, Sperry S. The CSF-FTA test and the significance of blood contamination. Ann Neurol 1979;6:68

Devinski O, Madi S, Theodore WH, Porter RJ. Cerebrospinal fluid pleocytosis following simple, complex partial, and generalized tonic-clonic seizures. Ann Neurol 1988;23:402

Dyken PR. Cerebrospinal fluid cytology: Practical clinical usefulness. Neurology 1975;25:210

El-Batata M. Cytology of cerebrospinal fluid in the diagnosis of malignancy. J Neurosurg 1968;228:317

Evans JH, Quick DT. Polyacrylamide gel electrophoresis of spinal fluid proteins. Arch Neurol 1966;14:64

Fishman RA. Cerebrospinal Fluid in Diseases of the Nervous System. Philadelphia, WB Saunders, 1980

Greenawald KA, Speicher CE, Evers W et al. Glucose content in cerebrospinal fluid. Am J Clin Pathol 1973;59:518

Haerer AF. Citrate and alphaketoglutarate in CSF and blood. Neurology 1971;21:1059

Hochwald GM. Cerebrospinal fluid. In Joynt RJ (ed). Clinical Neurology. Philadelphia, JB Lippincott, 1989

Johnson KP, Arrigo SC, Nelson BJ et al. Agarose electrophoresis of cerebrospinal fluid in multiple sclerosis. Neurology 1977;27:273

Johnson KP, Nelson BJ. Multiple sclerosis: Diagnostic usefulness of cerebrospinal fluid. Ann Neurol 1977;2:425

Kabat EA, Glusman M, Knaub V. Quantitative estimation of the albumin and gamma globulin in normal and pathologic cerebrospinal fluid by immunochemical methods. Am J Med 1948;4:653

Kalin EM, Tweed WA, Lee J et al. Cerebrospinal fluid acid – base and electrolyte changes resulting from cerebral anoxia in man. N Engl J Med 1975;293:1013

Katzman R, Fishman RA, Goldensohn ES. Glutamic oxaloacetic transaminase activity in spinal fluid. Neurology 1957;7:853

Kolar O, Zeman W. Spinal fluid cytomorphology: description of apparatus, technique and findings. Arch Neurol 1968;18:44

Krentz MJ, Dyken PR. Cerebrospinal fluid cytomorphology: Sedimentation vs. filtration. Arch Neurol 1972;26:253

Lange C. Ueber die Ausflockung von Goldsol durch Liquor cerebrospinalis. Berl Klin Wochenschr 1912;49:897

Link H. Immunoglobulin G and low molecular weight proteins in human cerebrospinal fluid: Chemical and immunologic characterization with special reference to multiple sclerosis. Acta Neurol Scand (suppl) 1967;43:1

Lowenthal A. Agar Gel Electrophoresis in Neurology. Amsterdam, Elsevier, 1964

Marks V, Marrack D. Tumour cells in the cerebrospinal fluid. J Neurol Neurosurg Psychiatry 1960;23:194

Pesce MA, Strange CS. A new micromethod for the determination of protein in cerebrospinal fluid and urine. Clin Chem 1973;19:1265

Petito F, Plum F. The lumbar puncture. N Engl J Med 1974;290:295

Posner JB, Plum F. Spinal fluid pH and neurologic symptoms in systemic acidosis. N Engl J Med 1967;277:605

Posner JB, Plum F. Independence of blood and cerebrospinal fluid lactate. Arch Neurol 1967;16:492

Posner JB, Swanson AG, Plum F. Acid – base balance and cerebrospinal fluid. Arch Neurol 1965;12:479

Riddoch D, Thompson RA. Immunoglobulin levels in cerebrospinal fluid. Br Med J 1970;1:396

Schmidley JW, Simon RP. Postictal pleocytosis. Ann Neurol 1981;9:81

Sornas RA. A new method for the cytological examination of the cerebrospinal fluid. J Neurol Neurosurg Psychiatry 1967;30:368

Stokes HB, O'Hara CM, Buchanan RD et al. An improved method for examination of cerebrospinal fluid cells. Neurology 1975;25:901

Svennilson E, Dencker SJ, Swahn B. Immunoelectrophoretic studies of cerebrospinal fluid. Neurology 1961;11:989

Thompson EJ. Laboratory diagnosis of multiple sclerosis. Br Med Bull 1977;33:28

Thompson WO, Thompson PK, Silveus E et al. The cerebrospinal fluid in myxedema. Arch Intern Med 1929;44:368

Tourtellotte WW, Shorr RJ. Cerebrospinal fluid. In Youmans JR, (ed). Neurological Surgery, 3rd ed. Philadelphia, WB Saunders, 1990

Tourtellotte WW. Study of lipids in the cerebrospinal fluid. VI. The normal lipid profile. Neurology 1959;9:375

Tourtellotte WW, Quan K-C, Haerer AF et al. Neoplastic cells in the cerebrospinal fluid. Neurology 1963;13:866

Chapter 59
RELATED EXAMINATIONS AND PROCEDURES

PUNCTURE OF THE CISTERNA MAGNA

In 1919 Wegeforth, Ayer, and Essick first described the approach to the cisterna magna for the removal of cerebrospinal fluid based on preliminary studies on the cadaver, and in 1920 Ayer described the puncture of the cisterna magna as a clinical diagnostic procedure. The cisterna magna (cerebellomedullaris) is the largest of the subarachnoid cisterns. It is situated at the base of the brain and is below the inferior surface of the cerebellum, behind the posterior surface of the medulla and upper cervical spinal cord, and above and in front of the dura covering the posterior atlantooccipital membrane. A needle can be introduced into this space without contact with the nervous tissues.

For a cisternal puncture the patient is placed on an examining table in the lateral recumbent position with his shoulders perpendicular to the table and his neck slightly flexed. A firm pillow or small sandbag is placed under his head to make certain that the plane of the cervical spine is horizontal. The position of the patient is very important. The skin is prepared by shaving the hair over the area from the occipital protuberance to the midcervical level. As for a spinal puncture, sterile rubber gloves are worn, aseptic technics and sterile instruments are used, and the skin around the area of the puncture is sterilized and infiltrated with a local anesthetic preparation. An 18- to 20- gauge needle is most often used for the puncture. Many technicians prefer to use a needle that is marked in centimeters, or

to have a guard on the needle to indicate when a depth of 6.5 or 7 cm has been reached.

The needle is inserted in the suboccipital depression, at a point just below the external occipital protuberance and just above the spine of the axis, or second cervical vertebra (the highest palpable spinous process), exactly in the midline. It is then directed inward and slightly upward in a plane that passes through the external auditory meatus and continues to the glabella. It penetrates the skin, subcutaneous tissues, superficial muscles of the neck, ligamentum nuchae, posterior atlantooccipital membrane, dura mater (to which this ligament is intimately adherent), and arachnoid, and enters the subarachnoid cistern between the medulla and the cerebellum. After the needle has been introduced about 3 cm, the stylet is withdrawn to note whether fluid has been obtained. If not, the stylet is replaced, the needle is introduced another ½ cm, and the stylet is again withdrawn. This procedure is repeated every ½ cm until fluid is obtained. Usually a "give" is felt when the needle goes through the atlantooccipital membrane and dura. If the base of the occiput is encountered, the needle should be withdrawn slightly and then depressed enough to pass through the dura at the upper limits and posterior margin of the foramen magnum. If blood is encountered, the needle should be withdrawn and a clean one used or the procedure should be discontinued. The distance from the skin to the cisterna magna averages between 4 and 6 cm, although occasionally in extremely muscular individuals the needle may have to be introduced as far as 7.5

789

cm. Under most circumstances it is unwise to insert the needle more than 7.5 cm. The testing of the dynamics, removal of the fluid, withdrawal of the needle, and care of the puncture site are the same as with a puncture in the lumbar region.

A cisternal puncture can be done with ease and with a minimum of discomfort to the patient in most cases. It is less likely to be followed by a headache than is lumbar puncture, and there is less danger of continued leakage of cerebrospinal fluid or herniation of the medulla into the foramen magnum. It is more hazardous than spinal puncture, however, because of the proximity of the needle to the medulla and the possibility of hemorrhage resulting from trauma to abnormally placed blood vessels. It should always be performed by an experienced technician; authorities recommend practicing on a cadaver before performing the examination on a patient.

Cisternal puncture may be performed under the following circumstances: 1) for routine examination of the spinal fluid in those cases in which puncture at the lumbar area is either inadvisable or contraindicated by local conditions such as infections, and in cases where lumbar puncture is unsuccessful because of deformities or anomalies of the spine or spinal subarachnoid block; and 2) for the introduction of contrast medium in myelography when it is necessary to determine the upper level of a tumor or obstruction. Cisternal puncture is contraindicated if there is either subcutaneous infection at the puncture site or septicemia, if there is increased intracranial pressure (especially if caused by a posterior fossa tumor), or if the presence of a brain abscess is suspected.

AIR CONTRAST PROCEDURES

Pneumoencephalography. The withdrawal of the cerebrospinal fluid and its replacement with air or gases via a lumbar puncture was first described by Dandy in 1919 as an ancillary diagnostic procedure in neurologic evaluation. Pneumoencephalography has been largely abandoned in favor of computed tomography and magnetic resonance imaging.

Ventriculography. This procedure (described by Dandy in 1918) is the withdrawal of cerebrospinal fluid and injection of air or contrast material directly into the ventricles. It is a neurosurgical procedure, rarely needed when computed tomography or magnetic resonance imaging are available to study the intracranial contents.

MYELOGRAPHY

Myelography is performed by introducing a radiopaque contrast medium into the spinal canal for the purpose of roentgenologically evaluating the cause of a spinal subarachnoid block and for the diagnosis of other space-occupying lesions within the spinal canal, including ruptured intervertebral disks. It may also provide pertinent information in the interpretation of cervical spondylosis and lesions at or above the foramen magnum. Iophendylate or water-soluble contrast materials may be used.

The contrast medium is injected into the spinal canal at the usual site for lumbar puncture, and the patient is placed on a tilting table under a fluoroscope. If the lower portion of the canal is to be examined, as in cases of suspected lumbosacral herniation of the nucleus pulposus, the table is tilted so that the lower portions of the body are downward, the course of the radiopaque substance is followed, and roentgenograms are taken. If an obstruction is suspected above the level of the puncture site, the table is tilted so that the upper portions of the body are downward, and the same procedure is carried out. Sometimes, if lumbar myelography is impossible or unsuccessful, or if it is important to determine the upper limits of the lesion, the contrast medium is introduced into the cisterna magna, and the body is tilted so that the lower portions are downward. Myelography is indicated in cases of either partial or complete subarachnoid block in which the exact extent or location of the lesion is not apparent; in the diagnosis of conditions affecting the cauda equina, conus medullaris, and nerve roots; in lesions affecting the spinal cord or nerve roots at cervical (or, rarely, thoracic) levels; and occasionally in the study of lesions at or above the foramen magnum that are affecting the lower brain stem (cisternography or posterior fossa myelography). It is contraindicated if there is evidence of infection of the nervous tissues or meninges. Complications and sequelae of myelography occur infrequently, but include meningeal irritation, headache, and rarely meningitis or arachnoiditis. Myelography is less often necessary now that magnetic imaging and computed tomography frequently outline spinal lesions adequately.

RADIOISOTOPE CISTERNOGRAPHY

Studies of the intracranial distribution of radio-activity by scintillation scanning of the head after either ventricular or intrathecal injection of radioiodinated serum albumin or similar substances are referred to as radioisotope ventriculography and radioisotope cisternography, respectively. The former has had very little clinical application, but the latter has proved to be helpful in the diagnosis of occult or normal pressure hydrocephalus. External scans of the cranial vault are made at 4, 18, and 24 h after the injection of 85 – 100 μc of radioiodinated serum albumin into the lumbar subarachnoid space following lumbar puncture. In the normal person the material flows upward into the subarachnoid spaces and basal cisterns, with little concentration in the ventricles. In normal-pressure hydrocephalus, on the other hand, the radioisotope is concentrated in the ventricles, with little or no radioactivity over the cerebral hemispheres. In patients with cerebral atrophy, the radioisotope concentration in the ventricles is normal but the band of cortical radioactivity may be heavier than usual, presumably being related to a widening of the subarachnoid space secondary to the loss of cerebral substance.

BIBLIOGRAPHY

Ayer JB. Puncture of the cisterna magna. Arch Neurol Psychiat 1920;4:529

Benson F, Le May M, Patten DH et al. Diagnosis of normal pressure hydrocephalus. N Engl J Med 1970; 283:609

Bull JWD. Positive contrast ventriculography. Acta Radiol 1950;34:253

Dandy WE. Ventriculography following the injection of air into the cerebral ventricles. Ann Surg 1918;68:5

Dandy WE. Roentgenography of the brain after the injection of air into the spinal canal. Ann Surg 1919;70:397

Di Chiro G, Reames PM, Matthews WB Jr. RISA-ventriculography and RISA-cisternography. Neurology 1964;14:185

Jacobeus HC. On insufflation of air into the spinal canal for diagnostic purposes in cases of tumors of the spinal cord. Acta Med Scand 1921;21:555

Orrison WW. Introduction to Neuroimaging. Boston, Little, Brown & Co 1989

Schnitzlein HN, Murtagh FR. Imaging Anatomy of the Head and Spine. Baltimore, Urban & Schwarzenberg, 1985

Shapiro R. Myelography, 2nd ed. Chicago, Year Book Medical Pub, 1968

Sicard JA, Forestier J. Méthode radiographique d'exploration de la cavité épidural par le lipiodol. Rev Neurol 1921; 27:1264

Taveras JM, Wood EH. Diagnostic Neuroradiology, 2nd ed. Baltimore, Williams & Wilkins, 1976

Chapter 60

CEREBROSPINAL FLUID SYNDROMES

In the lumbar puncture of the normal individual, as has been stated previously, the pressure may vary from 50 – 180 mm of water, and its response to coughing, straining, and jugular compression is normal. The normal cerebrospinal fluid is clear and colorless, with no clot or web. There are fewer than 5 mononuclear cells/cu mm. The protein varies from 15 – 40 mg/100 ml, and the glucose from 50 – 65 mg/100 ml, assuming a normal blood sugar. No bacteria or other organisms are present. The serologic tests for syphilis are negative, and the IgG contents are within normal limits. The cell count and protein content are slightly less in cisternal and ventricular fluid, whereas the glucose content is slightly higher in ventricular fluid.

If blood is present in the normal fluid because of trauma to the spinal venous plexus or the meningeal or vertebral veins, the pressure relationships will be normal but the fluid will be blood-tinged, varying from a pink to a deep red color; the presence of blood may also give a turbid appearance to the fluid. If successive specimens of fluid are taken, the later ones will be more clear than the first ones. If much blood is present, a clot will form spontaneously. When the fluid is centrifuged, the supernatant fluid is clear and colorless, unless the amount of blood is excessive. The erythrocytes appear normal microscopically. No organisms are present. Contamination of the spinal fluid by blood will influence the leukocyte count and protein determination, but not the glucose content to any appreciable degree (see Ch. 58).

Specific cerebrospinal fluid syndromes have been described in association with certain disease processes. The more important of these are listed.

MENINGITIS

Acute Purulent, or Suppurative, Meningitis.
In acute meningitis there is a marked elevation of spinal fluid pressure, which may reach as high as 500 or even 1,000 mm. There is no block early in the course of the disease, but block may develop later due to the formation of arachnoid adhesions. (These may also form as a result of intrathecal administration of serums and drugs.) The fluid may vary in appearance from faintly cloudy to turbid, purulent, or opaque, owing to the presence of leukocytes and organisms. It may be slightly xanthochromic owing to elevated protein, or even greenish due to the presence of pus; it sometimes is blood-tinged. The fluid may be viscid and may clot on standing. There is a marked pleocytosis, sometimes reaching from 1,000 – 5,000 or even 50,000 cells/cu mm; nearly 100% of the cells are polymorphonuclears. As a reaction to the presence of debris in the fluid, the cell count may remain elevated even after the fluid is sterile. There is a distinct increase in the total protein, which may reach 1,000 mg/100 ml; both albumin and globulin may be increased. The glucose is diminished, often below 20 or even 10 mg/100 ml; Organisms are usually found on the direct smear; these may be either meningococci (gram-negative, intracellular cocci), pneumococci, streptococci, or influenzal bacilli; occasional instances of purulent meningitis may be

caused by other agents, including *S. typhosa* and *E. coli.* Occasionally multiple organisms are found. The organisms may be isolated from cultures even if not found on direct smear. If, however, antibiotics had been given to the patient prior to the examination of the cerebrospinal fluid, no organisms may be found in the fluid and it may be impossible to obtain any by culture. In such cases, cerebrospinal fluid antigen tests or counterimmunoelectrophoresis may help establish the etiology.

Tuberculous Meningitis. In tuberculous meningitis the pressure is also elevated, although rarely beyond 300 – 500 mm. There may be a spinal subarachnoid block late in the course of the disease. The fluid may be clear and colorless early in the course of the disease, but it is often opalescent or ground-glass in appearance. Occasionally it is blood-tinged or faintly xanthochromic. A fine, cobweblike fibrin web or pellicle appears after the fluid has stood for 24 hours. There is a pleocytosis, often ranging between 100 and 500 cells/cu mm, but sometimes going as high as 1,000/cu mm. The cells are predominantly lymphocytes (usually 85% – 95%, with the other 15%–5% polymorphonuclears). In terminal stages the percentage of polymorphonuclears increases; neutrophils also appear early in infants. The protein content is increased, often to 500 mg/100 ml or higher, and is both albumin and globulin. The glucose is decreased, and is usually between 20 and 40 mg/100 ml, although in terminal stages it may go lower. Acid-fast organisms may be found, especially if the pellicle is examined; they frequently are difficult to demonstrate on the direct smear, but cultures and guinea pig inoculations are positive.

Cryptococcus (Torula) Meningitis. In the meningitis caused by *Cryptococcus neoformans (Torula histolytica)* the spinal fluid picture closely resembles that of tuberculous meningitis, with moderately elevated pressure, no block, faintly cloudy fluid, a pleocytosis that is predominantly lymphocytic, and a moderate increase in protein. The glucose is significantly decreased in about 60% of patients. Tubercle bacilli are not found, however, and in most cases budding forms of the yeasts may be seen on direct smear or obtained by cultures, using either ordinary culture media or Sabouraud's medium (Fig. 60-1). They may also be demonstrated by mouse inoculation. Occasionally the yeast cells are mistaken for lymphocytes when seen in the counting chamber, but when stained with India ink their refractive

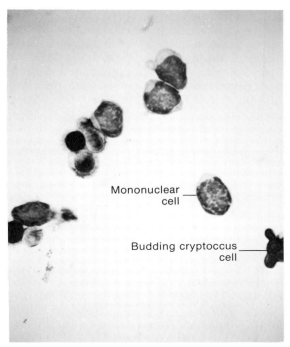

Mononuclear cell

Budding cryptoccus cell

FIG. 60–1. *Cells found in the cerebrospinal fluid of a patient with cryptococcal meningitis; the budding form of Cryptococcus as well as a mononuclear cell may be seen. Wright's stain. (Courtesy of Dr. W. W. Tourtellotte)*

capsules may be observed. They may also be identified by fluorescent technics. Eosinophils are sometimes demonstrated in the differential count. A similar spinal fluid picture may be found in meningitides caused by other fungi. Cryptococcal antigen studies of the cerebrospinal fluid and serum help in making the diagnosis.

Acute Syphilitic Meningitis. Rarely seen at the present time, acute syphilitic meningitis most characteristically develops during the secondary stage of syphilis. There is a moderate to severe lymphocytic pleocytosis, and moderate elevation of the pressure and protein. The glucose is normal or slightly decreased. The serologic tests for syphilis are positive in over 95% of the cases, and there is an increase in the amount of IgG.

Lymphocytic Meningitides. There are many meningitides in which the cerebrospinal fluid response is predominantly a lymphocytic one, with 25 – 200 cells or sometimes more. There are few other changes in the fluid, and the course is usually benign. These are often called instances of aseptic meningitis because no organism is found in the fluid on direct examination or by the usual culture methods. Many of them, however, are of viral origin, and in some of them the virus has been isolated from the fluid by special technics; in others it has been found in the feces or in the nasal and pharyngeal washings, or the diagnosis has been confirmed by neutralization or complement fixation tests done on blood serum. Among the most common viral etiologies are lymphocytic choriomeningitis, the Coxsackie and ECHO viruses, and those of mumps, herpes zoster, and herpes simplex. Poliomyelitis virus and the arboviruses may cause a similar meningeal response. A benign recurrent meningitis for which no etiology has been found is known as **Mollaret's meningitis;** its existence as a disease is controversial. Cerebrospinal fluid pleocytosis, however, is not invariably present in all of these conditions; occasionally, normal counts are present, notably in herpes simplex infections.

Human Immunodeficiency Virus Infections. The causative virus may attack any and all portions of the central and peripheral nervous systems primarily, or cause secondary infections by a host of opportunistic agents. In the primary infection, a lymphocytic or mixed pleocytosis is seen in the cerebrospinal fluid. In many cases elevated protein and IgG as well as the presence of oligoclonal bands of IgG are noted. The virus can sometimes be isolated from the cerebrospinal fluid, but this is not a routine procedure.

Aseptic Meningitis. An aseptic meningeal reaction occurs when there is a pyogenic infection near the meninges that has not yet invaded them, namely, in mastoid suppuration, paranasal sinus infections, cavernous or lateral sinus thrombosis, osteomyelitis of the skull, brain abscess, and subdural or extradural abscesses. A similar process (chemical or irritative meningitis) may occur as a meningeal reaction to the intraspinal injection of air, drugs, serums, or other foreign substances. Aseptic meningitis has also been reported on rare occasions as an idiosyncratic reaction to orally ingested medications. Recurrent episodes have been the result of the use of ibuprofen, trimethoprim with sulfamethoxasole, and other drugs. There is an increase in the spinal fluid pressure and often a marked pleocytosis (lymphocytic, mixed, or polymorphonuclear). The protein content of the fluid is usually elevated to a significant degree, but the glucose content is not reduced, the smears show no organisms, and cultures are sterile.

Carcinomatous Meningitis. With diffuse involvement of the meninges by carcinoma, sarcoma, leukemia, and related neoplasms, there may be a pleocytosis that is predominantly lymphocytic. In addition there may be a definite elevation of the pressure and the spinal fluid protein, and a significant reduction of the glucose content, so that the illness may at times be mistaken for a subacute infectious meningitis. Special staining of the cells and histologic studies of the stained sediment may demonstrate the presence of neoplastic cells, and certain of those cells first interpreted as being lymphocytes and monocytes may in reality be cancer cells. Beta glucuronidase and carcinoembryonic antigen are usually elevated in cerebrospinal fluid when the meninges are infiltrated with malignant cells.

ENCEPHALITIS AND MYELITIS

Viral Encephalitis. With the various arthropod-borne encephalitides such as the St. Louis, Eastern and Western equine, and Japanese B varieties, the spinal fluid changes are minimal to moderate. There is variable pleocytosis ranging from 25–600 or more cells, especially during the first few days of the illness and in the more serious cases. At the outset the cells are predominantly polymorphonuclear, but during the second week they are largely lymphocytes. The pressure is usually normal. There may be a moderate elevation of the protein, the extent depending upon the activity of the disease process. There is often a relative and sometimes a definite increase in the glucose content. Serologic tests for syphilis are normal. The fluid is sterile and no organisms are found. Occasionally the virus can be isolated from either the blood or spinal fluid by intracerebral inoculation of mice or other experimental animals, but usually the etiology is determined only retrospectively by means of titers done on blood serum obtained during the acute illness and during convalescence.

In subacute sclerosing panencephalitis there may be fairly typical changes in the spinal fluid. A slight pleocytosis and elevation of the protein may be present. However, there is usually a marked elevation of IgG, to as much as 60% of the total protein. Oligoclonal IgG bands may be present as well. Serum globulins, pressure, and glucose are normal. High measles antibody titers have been found in the serum and cerebrospinal fluid.

Encephalomyelitis or Meningoencephalitis Associated With Systemic Disease.

In encephalomyelitis or meningoencephalitis associated with various systemic diseases there may be characteristic changes in the cerebrospinal fluid. In the meningoencephalitis associated with mumps there may be a pronounced pleocytosis, often 500 – 1,000 cells, with 80% – 100% lymphocytes. In meningoencephalitis associated with infectious mononucleosis there may be a lymphocytic pleocytosis with an increase in protein; the blood picture and the heterophile antibody test may aid in making the diagnosis. In meningoencephalitis associated with undulant fever (brucellosis) there may be a pleocytosis with an increase in protein. A precise diagnosis is made by finding positive agglutination reactions and blood cultures. The organism is occasionally isolated from the spinal fluid. In meningoencephalitides associated with lymphogranuloma venereum and listeriosis there may be a pleocytosis of 50 – 1,000 cells, 90% of which are lymphocytes.

In sarcoidosis and Behçet's disease there is often a subacute meningeal reaction, with a slight increase in cells and protein. Angiotensin-converting enzyme levels may be elevated in the cerebrospinal fluid of patients with sarcoidosis. In trypanosomiasis there is a pleocytosis of varying degree, with 10 – 500 cells, mainly lymphocytes, along with an increase in protein; the organism may be isolated from the spinal fluid. In the cerebral complications of subacute bacterial endocarditis there may be neutrophils as well as lymphocytes, because of the presence of multiple infected emboli, and both pressure and protein may be elevated. In toxoplasmosis there may be a fairly marked pleocytosis (50 – 1,000 cells), principally lymphocytic, with occasional erythrocytes; there is a moderate increase in protein, the glucose is normal, and the organism may be isolated from the spinal fluid. In spirochetal jaundice (Weil's disease) there is a moderate lymphocytic pleocytosis with a slight increase in protein; the spinal fluid may be icteric. In Lyme neuroborreliosis the cerebrospinal fluid findings are variable, but intrathecal synthesis of antibodies against the organism can often be demonstrated; oligoclonal bands are usually present as well. In the meningoencephalitides associated with cysticercosis, echinococcosis, and schistosomiasis there may be mild meningeal changes, with a moderate increase in pressure and protein and a moderate pleocytosis (up to 300 cells). The presence of eosinophils in the spinal fluid is often suggestive of a parasitic infection. Fragments of the parasites or cysts may be found in the fluid. In the meningoencephalitides associated with measles, rubella, malaria, whooping cough, typhus, scarlet fever, typhoid fever, varicella, variola, vaccinia, Rocky mountain spotted fever, psittacosis, trichinosis, and other systemic infections there are slight or nonspecific changes in the spinal fluid, characterized usually by a slight to moderate increase in cells and total protein.

Acute Anterior Poliomyelitis.

The examination of the spinal fluid once had paramount importance in the diagnosis of poliomyelitis and may again in the future. The pressure is normal or slightly increased; there is no evidence of block. The fluid is clear and colorless, except in rare instances when the cell count is markedly elevated. Pellicle formation is rare. There is a mild to moderate pleocytosis. The cell count is highest in the preparalytic stage of the disease, when it may rise to from 50 – 100 or even 300 – 500 cells/cu mm. Over 50% and sometimes as many as 80% of these may be polymorphonuclears. This is thought to be an expression of the mesodermal reaction to the virus, and does not necessarily parallel the severity of the infection or the amount of paralysis to be expected. After the onset of paralysis the cell count drops rapidly (it is often only 10 – 50 in the early paralytic stage), and at this time the cells are predominantly lymphocytes. The cell count may be normal after the first week or 10 days, although it often remains elevated until the third or fourth week in severe cases.

As the cell count falls, the protein, which is normal or only slightly elevated during the first week of the illness, rises, usually reaching its maximum by the end of the second week of illness. It rarely exceeds 50 – 100 mg/100 ml during the paralytic period, but occasionally it continues to rise during the convalescent period and may remain elevated for a month and reach levels as high as 200 – 300 mg/100 ml. At this time there is an albuminocytologic dissociation resembling that of the Guillain – Barré syndrome. The glucose content of the cerebrospinal fluid is usually normal. The serologic tests for syphilis are normal. It is important to bear in mind that there may be significant cerebrospinal fluid changes in the nonparalytic and subclinical varieties of poliomyelitis, and also increased protein during convalescence from these varieties, but it is also possible to have entirely normal spinal fluid in acute poliomyelitis. Some of the infections mentioned previously (Coxsackie and ECHO) may cause clinical and spinal fluid pictures that closely simulate those seen in poliomyelitis.

Myelitis. If an acute inflammatory transverse myelitis is suppurative in type and is secondary to meningitis, adjacent infections, or infections elsewhere in the body, there may be a marked increase in cells and protein in the cerebrospinal fluid. Transverse myelitis, however, may come on acutely without evidence of coexisting infection. In such cases the spinal fluid may be normal or there may be only a slight to moderate increase in cells (lymphocytes) and protein, with normal pressure and no block. This last criterion is important in differentiating inflammatory myelitis, spinal cord tumor, and other conditions in which there is a sudden development of paraplegia due to spinal cord compression. The cerebrospinal fluid in tropical chronic myelitis (HTLV-I) is nondiagnostic.

INTRACRANIAL LESIONS

While spinal puncture and examination of the fluid may occasionally be of some aid in the diagnosis of brain tumor, it should be stressed that often the spinal fluid shows little or no abnormality and the puncture gives no information that may not be obtained by other means. Furthermore, if there is an increase in intracranial pressure, the procedure may be harmful. A lumbar puncture should never be carried out in a patient suspected of having an intracranial tumor unless the procedure is necessary to establish the diagnosis. Imaging studies should precede (or take the place of) the puncture.

Brain Tumor. The most characteristic finding with brain tumors is an increase in the spinal fluid pressure, which varies, of course, with the amount of elevation of the intracranial pressure. This is most marked in association with neoplasms of the posterior fossa, principally of the cerebellum, or with rapidly expanding neoplasms such as glioblastoma multiforme. Paradoxically, posterior fossa neoplasms such as gliomas involving the medulla, pons, and midbrain frequently cause no elevation of intracranial pressure. The spinal fluid pressure need not be proportional to the amount of papilledema: the pressure at spinal puncture may be markedly elevated in cases with no papilledema, or, on the other hand, nearly normal in cases with advanced papilledema. The fluid is usually normal in appearance, although occasionally it is slightly yellow or blood-tinged. There may be a pleocytosis, sometimes relatively high, if the tumor is near to or encroaches on either the meninges or the ventricles; the cells are predominantly lymphocytes. Occasionally tumor cells may be found in the centrifuged sediment (see Fig. 58-1). There may be erythrocytes in the fluid in association with vascular tumors (angiomas and hemangioblastomas) or degenerating neoplasms. The protein is often moderately elevated, especially with neoplasms near the meninges or ventricles, with those that obstruct the flow of blood or cerebrospinal fluid, and with vascular tumors. It is characteristically high with cerebellopontine angle tumors, and often with those of the parasellar region. Occasionally the glucose content of the spinal fluid is elevated. The bacteriologic and serologic examinations are normal. The spinal fluid findings in meningeal carcinomatosis (carcinomatous meningitis) have been discussed.

Benign Intracranial Hypertension. In the syndrome known variously as benign intracranial hypertension, pseudotumor cerebri, and brain swelling of unknown etiology there is increased intracranial pressure with headache and papilledema. There may be blurring or loss of vision, but usually no other significant neurologic abnormalities. Spinal puncture shows increased pressure but usually normal (or low) protein and cells and no other definite changes. There are probably multiple etiologies for this syndrome, which must be differentiated from some of the more malignant causes of increased intracranial pressure.

Brain Abscess. Cerebrospinal fluid study is also no longer done routinely when brain abscess is suspected or present. Computed tomography and magnetic resonance imaging are very sensitive diagnostic tools for abscesses. If lumbar puncture is contemplated, imaging should precede it, and the same precautions taken as with brain tumors. The spinal fluid findings are those of an expanding intracranial lesion together with those of an aseptic meningeal reaction. The pressure is usually elevated, especially with posterior fossa abscesses. In addition, there is often evidence of meningeal irritation, with a pleocytosis. There may be 100 – 200 cells/cu mm and occasionally as many as 1,000 cells/cu mm. The differential count varies, depending on the location of the abscess and the meningeal reaction to it. If the lesion is near the meninges or the ventricles, the cells may be predominantly polymorphonuclears, whereas if it is deeper in the brain tissue, they are mainly lymphocytes. The cell count and the percentage of neutrophils are both higher in acute than in chronic abscesses. The number and nature of the cells may indicate the progress of encapsulation; the percentage of polymorphonuclear cells is high in acute abscesses that are not yet walled off, and it decreases after encapsulation has taken place. The persistence of neutrophils may indicate failure of encapsulation. If the pleocytosis is marked, the fluid may be cloudy or turbid. The protein is increased, sometimes markedly, but the glucose is usually normal. If the abscess ruptures into the ventricles or subarachnoid space, the spinal fluid picture is that of a pyogenic meningitis.

The spinal fluid picture in an epidural, subdural, or extradural abscess is identical with that of an intracerebral abscess, and they cannot be differentiated by spinal fluid study. These types of abscesses are also well delineated with imaging studies.

Lateral Sinus and Cavernous Sinus Thrombosis. The cerebrospinal fluid findings in the now rare instances of lateral sinus and cavernous sinus thrombosis may be either those of an aseptic meningitis, if there is a pronounced meningeal reaction to the disease, or those of benign intracranial hypertension. They often closely resemble the changes seen in brain abscess, with a mixed pleocytosis, increased protein, and normal glucose, but the pressure is usually not elevated to the same degree. Occasionally with thrombosis of the lateral sinus, and more often with that of the cavernous sinus, there is an associated meningitis with its characteristic spinal fluid picture.

Cerebral Trauma. The cerebrospinal fluid findings in cerebral trauma are dependent upon the amount of damage to the cerebral tissues, meninges, and meningeal vessels. In cases of concussion there may be a significant elevation of the cerebrospinal fluid pressure, secondary to cerebral edema, a marked lymphocytic pleocytosis, and a slight increase in protein. If there have been contusions or lacerations of the brain or of one or more of the meningeal vessels, there may be a more marked elevation of spinal fluid pressure, and the fluid may contain erythrocytes or be xanthochromic; there is also a more marked increase in cells (mainly lymphocytes)

and protein. More significant changes in the spinal fluid are noted if there is an associated subarachnoid hemorrhage or subdural hematoma. Lumbar puncture is not needed in the evaluation of head trauma unless infection is suspected.

Subdural Hematoma. The cerebral imaging studies, and at times angiography are superior to cerebrospinal fluid examination in the demonstration of intracranial hematomas. In subdural hematoma the spinal fluid picture varies with the age of the hematoma. Early in the development of the clot the fluid often contains gross blood and increased protein, owing to associated subarachnoid bleeding and concomitant cerebral contusion; there is usually increased pressure as well. Later, after the disappearance of the blood cells, there is xanthochromia with increased protein, and a continued elevation of pressure. Still later the fluid is normal in appearance, without blood cells or xanthochromia, but there is evidence of gradually increasing intracranial pressure; there may be increased protein and a moderate pleocytosis, owing to transudation of serum and an associated meningeal reaction. The bacteriologic examination and the serologic tests are normal. Slightly xanthochromic fluid under increased pressure but with only moderately increased protein is very suggestive of a developing subdural hematoma.

In extradural hemorrhage there may be an increase in spinal fluid pressure; if there is associated damage to the brain or the meninges, there may be erythrocytes, leukocytes, and increased protein in the spinal fluid.

Lead Encephalopathy. Lead encephalopathy is encountered primarily in children. The pressure is usually elevated, sometimes to 1,000 mm of water, and there is often a pleocytosis, predominantly lymphocytic. The protein and glucose are normal or slightly elevated. Lead may be detected in the cerebrospinal fluid.

Epilepsy. In so-called idiopathic, or cryptogenic, epilepsy interictally the spinal fluid is normal in all respects. Occasionally there is a slight increase in pressure and protein during and immediately after convulsions, and a mild pleocytosis, usually of mononuclear cells may be noted at times. Some cerebrospinal fluid enzymes may be elevated transiently immediately after organic seizures. If a patient with a convulsive disorder is found to have definite abnormalities interictally in the nature of increased pressure, pleocytosis, and elevated protein, the probability that the attacks are symptomatic, or secondary to some intracranial abnormality such as brain tumor, abscess, or encephalitis, should be seriously considered. The diagnosis of idiopathic epilepsy should be made with caution if there are abnormalities in the cerebrospinal fluid between attacks.

Miscellaneous Conditions. The conditions characterized by low spinal fluid pressure and the syndrome of spontaneous aliquorrhea are discussed in Chapter 57. Usually there are no changes in the fluid itself, but occasionally slight xanthochromia with a moderate elevation in protein is present. In the syndrome of symptomatic occult hydrocephalus with "normal" pressure in the cerebrospinal fluid, or "normal pressure hydrocephalus," usually no alterations are detected in the fluid. In cerebrospinal fluid rhinorrhea and otorrhea, which are usually posttraumatic, the escaping fluid is normal except for an occasional slight increase in lymphocytes, unless infection supervenes. Spontaneous spinal fluid rhinorrhea has been reported with neoplasms in the vicinity of the sella turcica.

LESIONS OF THE SPINAL CORD

Spinal Cord Tumor. Imaging studies should precede cerebrospinal fluid investigations if masses are suspected of encroaching on the spinal subarachnoid space. Cerebrospinal fluid is obtained when and if myelography is done, or if infection is suspected. When a spinal cord tumor develops the fluid pressure may be normal or decreased. If the tumor encroaches on the spinal subarachnoid space, interfering with the flow of the fluid, there may be either a partial or a complete block, which appears earlier and is more marked with extradural and extramedullary intradural tumors than with intramedullary ones. The characteristics of the fluid depend upon the presence, location, and degree of block. Its appearance may be normal, or it may be markedly xanthochromic and may clot spontaneously (Froin's syndrome). The cell count may be normal or moderately elevated; the protein varies from normal to markedly increased. The glucose and the bacteriologic and serologic examinations are normal. Malignant cells may sometimes be present in the fluid. If the block is found and had not been expected, myelography should be performed. There may also be pleocytosis and increased protein with spinal cord and cauda equina tumors that are below the site of the

puncture, but block, of course, cannot be demonstrated. It is important to remember that a partial block may be changed to a complete block by removal of spinal fluid, and that complete paralysis sometimes follows spinal puncture in patients with spinal cord tumors. The reservoir is small, and if the pressure drops rapidly, the needle should be withdrawn.

Pott's Disease, Vertebral Compression, and Adhesive Arachnoiditis. In Pott's disease, vertebral compression from trauma, neoplasm or spondylosis, adhesive arachnoiditis, and hypertrophic cervical pachymeningitis, any of which may cause spinal subarachnoid block, the spinal fluid findings are identical with those in spinal cord tumor and depend on the degree and location of the block.

Spinal Epidural Abscess. If a spinal puncture is performed below the level of the abscess in a patient with a spinal epidural abscess, the findings will be similar to those in spinal cord tumor, depending upon the degree of block. There may, however, be a pleocytosis, largely polymorphonuclear. If the examiner accidentally punctures the abscess, he may encounter pus when the epidural space is reached. It is important to use care to avoid puncturing the dura.

Syringomyelia. The spinal fluid findings are essentially normal in syringomyelia unless swelling of the cord causes a partial spinal subarachnoid block. In some patients there is a slight increase in protein and cells. The syrinx can be demonstrated by magnetic resonance imaging.

Herniated Nucleus Pulposus. With rupture of an intervertebral disk and herniation of the nucleus pulposus, the spinal fluid picture varies. If the herniation is in the cervical region (or, as is much less frequent, in the thoracic spine) the findings depend upon the degree of protrusion and the extent to which the flow of spinal fluid is interrupted. There may be no change in the fluid, or a moderate increase in the protein content, or there may be a partial to complete block, with an increase in protein (and occasionally of cells), sometimes with xanthochromia. The picture under such circumstances is similar to that found in spinal cord tumors and vertebral compression.

If the herniation is in the lower lumbar or lumbosacral area, where it most frequently occurs, the findings at spinal puncture and on examination of the fluid may be normal, since the lesion is below the site of the puncture. In a fairly large percentage of cases (at least 50%), however, there is a slight increase in protein. If the elevation of protein is marked, some diagnosis other than herniated nucleus pulposus must be considered.

LESIONS OF THE NERVE ROOTS AND PERIPHERAL NERVES

Polyneuritis and Polyradiculoneuritis. In most cases of toxic polyneuritis (*i.e.*, those due to lead, mercury, arsenic, thallium, etc.) spinal fluid abnormalities may not be present. In so-called alcoholic polyneuritis and the other vitamin-deficiency neuritides there is a pleocytosis (5 – 25 cells/cu mm) in 10% and a slight increase in protein (to 75 or 100 mg/100 ml) in 15%. In diphtheritic polyneuritis, however, there is often an increase in the protein content of the fluid, sometimes to 250 mg/100 ml, without an associated pleocytosis. In diabetic polyneuritis, also, there may be a marked elevation of the protein content. Other peripheral nerve disorders in which the spinal fluid protein may be increased are leprosy, some of the chronic progressive neuropathies, hereditary sensory neuropathy, hereditary ataxic polyneuropathy (Refsum's syndrome), the neuropathy associated with primary familial amyloidosis, and neurofibromatosis.

In the form of polyradiculoneuritis called the Guillain – Barré syndrome there is a significant elevation of the total protein, sometimes delayed for a few days after the onset of symptoms, which in most cases is over 100 – 150 mg/100 ml, and may reach as high as 1,000 mg/100 ml. Sometimes the protein content continues to rise during the course of the disease, often for 4 – 8 weeks, and even after convalescence has started. It may rise to a plateau and then gradually decline. In rare cases the clinical syndrome is characteristic of the disorder but no elevation of the spinal fluid protein is detected. Nerve conduction studies are helpful in such cases, demonstrating multifocal asymmetric axonal blocks and slowing. Of importance in the diagnosis is the fact that the increase in protein is not accompanied by a proportionate increase in cells, and in most cases, even though the protein is elevated to a marked degree, the cell count is normal. This so-called albuminocytologic dissociation (although the globulin may also be elevated) is characteristic of the Guillain – Barré syndrome, and is important in differentiating it from poliomyelitis, which it may resemble closely from a clinical point of view. There may also be an albuminocytologic dissociation in the convalescent stage of poliomyelitis, but elevation of the protein does not last long (usually 2 – 4 weeks) and is not as high. Albuminocytologic dissociation is also encountered in spinal cord tumors and brain tumors. Consequently, the diagnosis of Guillain – Barré syndrome should not be made on the basis of the spinal fluid findings alone—the clinical manifestations of the illness are exceedingly important, as are electromyographic findings. The cerebrospinal fluid in chronic intermittent demyelinating neuropathy, clinically somewhat similar to Guillain – Barré syndrome, shows abnormalities of the same type.

VASCULAR DISEASES

Subarachnoid and Intraventricular Hemorrhage. In subarachnoid and intraventricular hemorrhage the spinal fluid examination may be needed for diagnosis if cerebral imaging procedures are unavailable or do not clearly demonstrate the hemorrhage. There is often a marked increase in pressure. The fluid is grossly bloody (within about 2 hours after the onset of the hemorrhage), and it is uniformly bloody throughout; *i. e.*, there is no clearing of the fluid as additional samples are obtained. There may be 1,000 – 3,500,000 erythrocytes/cu mm. The blood does not clot. On microscopic examination the cells are crenated. The erythrocytes begin to hemolyze within 12 – 24 hours, and have usually completely disappeared by 7 – 9 days. Within a few hours after the hemorrhage slight xanthochromia may be noted in the supernatant fluid on centrifuging (oxyhemoglobin may be detected by spectrophotometry within 2 hours), and the color change is grossly visible by 12 – 24 hours. The color deepens during the first few days, as bilirubin appears in the fluid, and assumes its greatest intensity at the end of a week. The xanthochromia may leave by the sixteenth day but may last 28 days or longer. There may be an increase in both mononuclear and polymorphonuclear cells, out of proportion to those contained in the blood, as a result of the reaction of the meninges to the presence of blood. The protein is markedly elevated. Occasionally the glucose is slightly decreased. There are no organisms; the serologic tests are usually negative. During the period of recovery from an acute subarachnoid hemorrhage there is a progressive decrease in the number of erythrocytes (which may be absorbed directly into the blood stream, phagocytized by mesothelial cells lining the subarachnoid space, or enmeshed and fixed in the arachnoid), and also a progressive disappearance of pigments and lowering of the protein level. Occult hydrocephalus may develop up to months or years after a subarachnoid hemorrhage.

Intracerebral Hemorrhage. The spinal fluid is grossly bloody in some cases of intracerebral hemorrhage, when the bleeding does not remain localized or confined, and it may be turbid or xanthochromic in others. Occasionally red cells may be observed microscopically in certain of the remaining cases. The spinal fluid pressure is often elevated. A moderate to significant increase in the protein content is common, and is usually proportional to the amount of blood present. As with subarachnoid hemorrhage, there may be an irritative meningitis, with a leukocyte elevation out of proportion to the amount of blood.

Cerebral Infarction. With cerebral infarction secondary to either thrombosis or embolism there are no characteristic changes in the cerebrospinal fluid, and lumbar puncture is not routinely needed. Occasionally, however, one finds microscopic blood, slight xanthochromia, or a moderate elevation in the cell count and/or protein. This occurs more frequently with embolism (in which case the infarct may be hemorrhagic) than with thrombosis, and there may even be gross blood in the fluid with cerebral embolism. With septic embolism the fluid may be turbid, with pleocytosis and elevated protein, and occasionally organisms are found.

Extracranial Vascular Disease, Cerebral Atherosclerosis, and Arterial Hypertension. With transient cerebral ischemic attacks secondary to extracranial vascular insufficiency and atherosclerosis, and arterial hypertension, there are no characteristic changes in the spinal fluid unless these conditions are complicated by cerebral hemorrhage or infarction, congestive heart failure, or uremia. The pressure is usually normal, even with extremes of hypertension. With cardiac decompensation and elevation of the systemic venous pressure, however, the cerebrospinal fluid pressure is also elevated, and there may be a high intracranial pressure with papilledema. In hypertensive encephalopathy, also, papilledema may be found; the spinal fluid pressure is increased, and there may be a moderate pleocytosis and a protein elevation. These conditions must be differentiated from brain tumor.

SYPHILIS

Primary Syphilis. There may be occasional changes in the spinal fluid in the primary stage of syphilis. In 15% – 35% of patients there is a slight lymphocytic pleocytosis (5 – 10 cells/cu mm) or a slight increase in the protein content. These changes usually disappear either spontaneously or as a result of treatment. Serologic reactions are usually negative.

Secondary Syphilis. Spinal fluid changes are somewhat more common in secondary syphilis. In 35% – 45% of patients there is a moderate pleocytosis (10 – 50 cells/cu mm), with increased protein and a positive serologic reaction. With the exception of the serologic reaction, spinal fluid abnormalities usually clear with treatment.

Dementia Paralytica. The spinal fluid changes in dementia paralytica are important. The pressure is normal or very slightly increased, without block, and the fluid is normal in appearance. There usually is a meningeal reaction with a mononuclear pleocytosis of 10 – 50 cells/cu mm, sometimes as high as 150 – 200 cells/cu mm. The protein is definitely elevated, and may range from 50 – 150 mg/100 ml. It occasionally is elevated as high as 300 – 400 mg/100 ml. The IgG is increased more than the albumin. The glucose content is normal or slightly decreased. The serologic tests for syphilis are strongly positive in 95% – 100% of cases, and the blood serologic reactions are positive in 85% – 95%. There is an increase in the IgG-albumin and IgG-total protein ratios. The diagnosis of dementia paralytica, however, must always be made on the basis of clinical findings, not laboratory results.

Tabes Dorsalis. The spinal fluid findings in tabes dorsalis depend upon the activity of the process. In early cases they are very similar to those in dementia paralytica. In late cases the abnormalities are less marked. The serologic tests are not positive as frequently.

Acute Syphilitic Meningitis. This has been discussed earlier in the chapter (see under "Meningitis").

Meningovascular Syphilis. The spinal fluid findings vary in meningovascular syphilis. If the meningeal reaction is pronounced, there may be increased pressure, pleocytosis, and elevated protein. On occasion the fluid is turbid and the cell count reaches 500 lymphocytes/cu mm. The serologic reactions on the spinal fluid are positive in about 90% of cases. In predominantly vascular involvement the pressure and cytology are more apt to be normal, but there may be an increase in protein. The various types of central nervous system syphilis are now rarely encountered.

OTHER DISEASES OF THE NERVOUS SYSTEM

Multiple Sclerosis. There is a wide variation in the spinal fluid findings in multiple sclerosis. In about 25% of the cases the routine constituents of the fluid are normal or nearly so. In 50% there are nonspecific changes characterized by a slight increase in lymphocytes (10 – 15, rarely as high as 50/cu mm), a moderate increase in protein (from 50 – 75 mg/100 ml), and in another 25% there are more marked changes, with a pleocytosis (25 – 100 lymphocytes/cu mm) and an increase in protein (up to 100 mg/100 ml). In no case, however, is there characteristically any change in pressure, block, abnormality in appearance of the fluid, alteration in the glucose content, or positive serologic reaction for syphilis. It is often important, in the diagnosis of multiple sclerosis, to observe each of the individual constituents of the spinal fluid as well as the spinal fluid picture as a whole. The IgG-albumin ratio, the IgG index, and the IgG synthesis rate in the central nervous system as reflected in the cerebrospinal fluid are abnormal in over 90% of cases. Oligoclonal bands of IgG are present in a high percentage. Abnormalities of the kappa-lambda ratios of the immunoglobulins are frequently present, with elevated kappa fragments, as are reversals of the percentages of subtypes of lymphocytes in the cerebrospinal fluid. Myelin basic protein may be elevated in spinal fluid during exacerbations, reflecting active demyelination in the vicinity of the subarachnoid spaces, and antibodies against this protein have been found in cerebrospinal fluid cells. There may also be significant alterations in the lipid constituents of the spinal fluid in demyelinating disorders.

Occasionally there is some degree of correlation between the severity of the clinical picture in multiple sclerosis and the presence of abnormal cerebrospinal fluid findings, and an elevated cell count may be present with an exacerbation. Most often, however, there is no definite relationship between the abnormalities in the fluid and the clinical course, duration, or severity of the disease.

Neuromyelitis Optica. In neuromyelitis optica (**Devic's disease**) and acute encephalomyelitis the spinal fluid changes may resemble those of multiple sclerosis, but often they are more marked. A pleocytosis of 25 – 50 mononuclear cells/cu mm, and even up to 200 cells/cu mm, is almost characteristic. The protein is elevated in 60% of the cases. The other cerebrospinal fluid abnormalities are similar to those of multiple sclerosis. In fact, some authorities believe that neuromyelitis optica is not a clinical entity but represents an acute form of multiple sclerosis.

Amyotrophic Lateral Sclerosis and Related Disorders. Characteristically there are no spinal fluid changes in amyotrophic lateral sclerosis, primary lateral sclerosis, progressive bulbar palsy, or progressive spinal muscular atrophy, although on occasion there may be a slight increase in the protein and/or cells. The protein may be increased in one third of the cases, but it usually is not over 75 mg/100 ml. The presence of pronounced alterations in the cerebrospinal fluid should lead to the consideration of other diagnoses.

Posterolateral Sclerosis. There are no significant or characteristic changes in the cerebrospinal fluid in posterolateral sclerosis, although there may be a slight pleocytosis (as many as 10 cells in 20% of patients) or a protein level varying from about 45 – 100 mg/100 ml.

Other Diseases. In some of the leukodystrophies and other progressive cerebral deteriorations of infancy and childhood, as well as in some of the toxic and metabolic encephalopathies, nonspecific changes in the spinal fluid may develop, with borderline to marked elevations of the pressure, protein, and cells. In the lipidoses there is often a change in the lipid profile of the cerebrospinal fluid, as well as some increase in protein, and large, vacuolated foam cells have been observed in the fluid of patients with Tay-Sachs disease (Fig. 60-2). In the de-

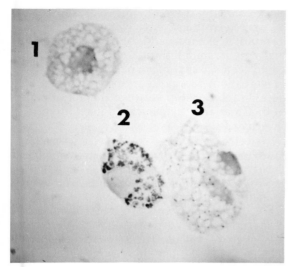

FIG. 60–2. *Vacuolated foam cells in the cerebrospinal fluid of a patient with Tay–Sachs disease. Wright's stain. (Courtesy of Dr. W. W. Tourtellotte)*

mentias such as Alzheimer's and Pick's diseases, on the other hand, the spinal fluid is essentially normal, although in advanced cases an increase in protein may develop. There are no characteristic changes in the spinal fluid in Huntington's chorea, Parkinson's disease, Friedreich's ataxia, myasthenia gravis, migraine, narcolepsy, or the myopathies.

MISCELLANEOUS DISORDERS

Diabetes. The most characteristic alteration of the cerebrospinal fluid in diabetes mellitus is an increase in the glucose content, which usually parallels the hyperglycemia. With ketosis, acetone bodies may be found in the fluid. In diabetic neuropathy, as well as in association with the cerebrovascular complications of diabetes, there is often an increase in the spinal fluid protein, which is sometimes present in significant amounts; the same change is sometimes found in diabetes without neurologic or vascular involvement.

Myeloma. Multiple myeloma may cause spinal cord compression, with the spinal fluid changes of spinal subarachnoid block. In addition, however, the paraproteins associated with the disorder may also be found in the spinal fluid and may cause elevated globulins. Spinal fluid abnormalities may also be found with

some of the other serum protein disturbances such as macroglobulinemia, cryoglobulinemia, and other gammopathies.

Leukemia. Leukemic infiltrations may affect the meninges and the nervous tissues, and in the various types of leukemia, as well as in lymphosarcoma and Hodgkin's disease, there may be an increase in leukocytes in the spinal fluid, sometimes with an associated rise in the protein content and the pressure. The type of cell found (lymphocytic, neutrophilic, etc.) depends upon the variety of leukemia.

Polycythemia. Changes in the cerebrospinal fluid appear in polycythemia only if there have been intracranial complications. With cerebral and meningeal hemorrhage blood and xanthochromia may be found in the fluid; with cerebral thrombosis there may be slight elevations in the cell count and protein content.

Thyroid Disorders. In myxedema the spinal fluid pressure is normal or slightly elevated. The protein content of the fluid is often increased, sometimes to 200 mg/100 ml or more. The increased protein has been suggested to result from an increase in the permeability of the blood-brain barrier, but in some patients the spinal fluid IgG is elevated, suggesting increased synthesis of IgG in the central nervous system. The spinal fluid abnormalities return to normal when the patient becomes euthyroid.

The spinal fluid in hyperthyroidism is usually normal except that the protein has been reported to be lower than normal in some patients.

Hypoparathyroidism. Hypoparathyroidism may be associated with pseudotumor cerebri, and in such instances the cerebrospinal fluid pressure may be markedly elevated. The protein may also be increased. The amount of calcium in the spinal fluid may be somewhat depressed.

Collagen Disorders. Central nervous system manifestations may occur with the various collagen disorders, especially with systemic lupus erythematosus and polyarteritis nodosa. With such involvement there may be spinal fluid changes consisting of protein elevation (especially IgG) and a lymphocytic pleocytosis. The serologic tests for syphilis done on the blood serum may be falsely positive. The spinal fluid protein may also be elevated with rheumatoid arthritis and spondylitis. The increased protein that has been reported with rheumatoid arthritis may be secondary to spondylitis and due to either interference with the circulation of the fluid or to increased permeability of the blood vessel walls or the meninges.

Alcoholic Intoxications. The spinal fluid pressure is often markedly increased in acute alcoholic intoxication with cerebral edema. There may also be some increase in the cells and protein, and there is often a positive test for alcohol in the fluid. It has been said that in about 20% of chronic alcoholism there is an increase in the spinal fluid protein.

The Psychoses. Many studies have been made of the cerebrospinal fluid findings in the functional psychoses — schizophrenia, manic-depressive psychosis, and involutional melancholia. It has been stated that the protein may be increased in 3% – 5% of cases of schizophrenia, 3% – 5% of cases of manic-depressive psychosis, and 5% of cases of involutional melancholia. Other minor changes that have been reported are elevations in the pressure, cell count, glucose content (especially in senile psychoses), and potassium, calcium, lactic acid, and cholesterol content. In general it may be said that the spinal fluid should be normal in the functional psychoses, and that the presence of any significant deviation from the normal casts serious doubt on the validity of the diagnosis.

BIBLIOGRAPHY

Antonen J, Syrjälä P, Oikarinen R, Frey H et al. Acute multiple sclerosis exacerbations are characterized by low cerebrospinal fluid suppressor/cytotoxic T-cells. Acta Neurol Scand 1987;75:156

Bell WE, Joynt RJ, Sahs AL. Low spinal fluid pressure syndromes. Neurology 1960;10:512

Bronsky D, Kaplitz SE, Ade RD, Dubin A. Spinal fluid proteins in cerebrovascular disease. Am J Med Sci 1962;244:54

Bruetsch WL, Bahr MA, Dieter WJ, Skobba JS. The cerebrospinal fluid protein in the psychoses. Dis Nerv Syst 1941;2:319

Campbell WG. Diagnosis of poliomyelitis. Ariz Med 1951;8:25

Chofflon M, Weiner HL, Morimoro C, Hafler SA. Decrease of suppressor inducer (CD4+2H4+) T cells in multiple sclerosis cerebrospinal fluid. Ann Neurol 1989;25:494

Dattner B. Significance of the spinal fluid findings in neurosyphilis. Am J Med Sci 1948;5:709

Dencker SJ (ed). Vessel-plaque and cerebrospinal fluid and brain tissue changes in multiple sclerosis. Acta Neurol Scand (suppl) 1964;40:9

Fishman RA. Cerebrospinal Fluid in Diseases of the Nervous System. Philadelphia, WB Saunders, 1980

Ford GD, Eldridge FL, Grulee CG Jr. Spinal fluid in acute poliomyelitis. Am J Dis Child 1950;79:633

Fredrikson S, Ernerudh J, Olsson T, Forsberg P et al. Mononuclear cell types in cerebrospinal fluid and blood of patients with multiple sclerosis. Quantitation by immunoenzyme microassay with panel of monoclonal antibodies. Arch Neurol 1989;46:372

Freedman DA, Merritt HH. The cerebrospinal fluid in multiple sclerosis. Assoc Res Nerv Dis Proc 1950;28:428

Fremont – Smith F. Cerebrospinal fluid in differential diagnosis of brain tumor. Arch Neurol Psychiat 1932;27:691

Greenfield JG, Carmichael EA. The Cerebrospinal Fluid in Clinical Diagnosis. London, Macmillan, 1925

Greenlee JE, Brashear HR, Jaeckle KA, Stroop WG. Anticerebellar antibodies in sera of patients with paraneoplastic cerebellar degeneration: studies of antibody specificity and response to plasmapheresis. Ann Neurol 1986;20:139

Hafler DA, Duby AD, Lee SJ, Benjamin D et al. Oligoclonal T lymphocytes in the cerebrospinal fluid of patients with multiple sclerosis. J Experiment Med 1988;167:1313

Halperin JJ, Luft BJ, Anand AK et al. Lyme neuroborreliosis: central nervous system manifestations. Neurology 1989;39:753

Hochwald GM. Cerebrospinal fluid. In Joynt RJ (ed). Clinical Neurology. Philadelphia, JB Lippincott, 1989

Ivers RR, McKenzie BF, McGuckin WF, Goldstein NP. Spinal-fluid gamma globulin in multiple sclerosis and other neurologic diseases. JAMA 1961;176:515

Jacobi C, Reiber H, Felgenhauer K. The clinical relevance of locally produced carcinoembryonic antigen in cerebrospinal fluid. J Neurol 1986;233:358

Johnson KP, Nelson BJ. Multiple sclerosis: Diagnostic usefulness of cerebrospinal fluid. Ann Neurol 1977;2:425

Kilham L, Levens J, Enders JF. Nonparalytic poliomyelitis and mumps meningoencephalitis: Differential diagnosis. JAMA 1949;140:934

Kutt H, Hurwitz LJ, Ginsburg SM, McDowell F. Cerebrospinal fluid protein in diabetes mellitus. Arch Neurol 1961;4:31

Locoge M, Cumings JN. Cerebrospinal fluid in various diseases. Br Med J 1958;1:618

McFarland HR, Heller GL. Guillain – Barré disease complex. Arch Neurol 1966;14:196

McMenemy WH, Cumings JN. The value of the examination of the cerebrospinal fluid in the diagnosis of intracranial tumors. J Clin Pathol 1959;12:400

Oksanen V, Fyrquist F, Somer H, Grönhagen – Riska C. Angiotensin converting enzyme in cerebrospinal fluid: a new assay. Neurology 1985;35:1220

Olsson T, Baig S, Höjeberg B, Link H. Antimyelin basic protein and antimyelin antibody-producing cells in multiple sclerosis. Ann Neurol 1990;27:132

Rosenblum ML, Levy RM, Bredesen DE. AIDS and the Nervous System. New York, Raven Press, 1988

Rudick RA, French CA, Breton D, Williams GW. Relative value of cerebrospinal fluid kappa chains in MS: Comparison with other immunologic tests. Neurology 1989;39:964

Salonen R, Ilonen J, Jägerroos H, Syrjälä H et al. Lymphocyte subsets in the cerebrospinal fluid of active multiple sclerosis. Ann Neurol 1989;25:500

Stark E, Haas J, Malin JP, Brunkhorst U. Immunocytochemical demonstration of human immunodeficiency virus infected cells in the cerebrospinal fluid. J Neurol Neurosurg Psychiatry 1988;51:977

Tallman RD, Kimbrough SM, O'Brien JF, Goellner JR et al. Assay for beta-glucuronidase in cerebrospinal fluid: Usefulness for the detection of neoplastic meningitis. Mayo Clin Proc 1985;60:293

Tourtellotte WW. A selected review of reactions of the cerebrospinal fluid to disease. In Fields WS (ed). Neurological Diagnostic Techniques. Springfield, IL, Charles C Thomas, 1966

Tourtellotte WW. Cerebrospinal fluid in multiple sclerosis. In Vinken PJ, Bruyn GW (eds). Handbook of Clinical Neurology, vol 9. Amsterdam, North Holland, 1970

Tourtellotte WW, Metz LN, Bryan ER, DeJong RN. Spontaneous subarachnoid hemorrhage: Factors affecting rate of clearing of the cerebrospinal fluid. Neurology 1964; 14:301

Tourtellotte WW, Shorr RJ. Cerebrospinal fluid. In Youmans JR (ed). Neurological Surgery, 3rd ed. Philadelphia, WB Saunders, 1990

Townsend SR, Craig RL, Braunstein AL. Neutrophilic leucocytes in spinal fluid associated with cerebral vascular accidents. Arch Intern Med 1939;63:848

Walton JN. Subarachnoid Hemorrhage. Edinburgh, E & S Livingstone, 1956

Watkins AL. The cerebrospinal fluid in optic neuritis, "toxic amblyopia" and tumors producing central scotomas. N Engl J Med 1939;220:227

Whitaker JN. Myelin encephalitogenic protein fragments in cerebrospinal fluid of persons with multiple sclerosis. Neurology 1977;27:911

Whitaker JN, Herman PK. Human myelin basic protein peptide 69–89: Immunochemical features and use in immunoassays of cerebrospinal fluid. J Neuroimmunol 1988; 19:47

Wiederholt WC, Mulder DW. Cerebrospinal fluid findings in the Landry–Guillain–Barré–Strohl syndrome. Neurology 1965;15:184

Index